CURRENT
ISSUES in
NURSING

CURRENT ISSUES in NURSING

Seventh Edition

Perle Slavik Cowen, PhD
Associate Professor
College of Nursing 472 NB
The University of Iowa
Iowa City, Iowa

Sue Moorhead, PhD, RN
Associate Professor and Director of Center for Nursing Classification
  and Clinical Effectiveness
Colonel US Army Retired 458 NB
College of Nursing
The University of Iowa
Iowa City, Iowa

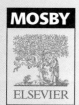

MOSBY

ELSEVIER

MOSBY
ELSEVIER

11830 Westline Industrial Drive
St. Louis, Missouri 63146

Notice

Neither the Publisher nor the Authors assume any responsibility for any loss or injury and/or damage to persons or property arising out of or related to any use of the material contained in this book. It is the responsibility of the treating practitioner, relying on independent expertise and knowledge of the patient, to determine the best treatment and method of application for the patient.

The Publisher

Previous editions copyrighted 2001, 1997, 1994, 1990, 1985, 1981

ISBN-13: 978-0-323-03652-8
ISBN-10: 0-323-03652-X

Acquisitions Editor: *Yvonne Alexopoulos*
Senior Developmental Editor: *Lisa P. Newton*
Publishing Services Manager: *John Rogers*
Senior Project Manager: *Beth Hayes*
Design Direction: *Teresa McBryan*

Printed in the United States of America

Last digit is the print number: 9   8   7   6   5   4   3   2   1

Contributors

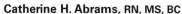

Catherine H. Abrams, RN, MS, BC
Vice President of Nursing
Mercy Hospital
Iowa City, Iowa

Janet D. Allan, PhD, RN, CS, FAAN
Dean and Professor
University of Maryland
School of Nursing
Baltimore, Maryland

Mary Ann Anderson, PhD, RN
Associate Professor
University of Illinois at Chicago
College of Nursing
Chicago, Illinois

Ida M. Androwich, PhD, RNC, FAAN
Professor and Director, Health Systems Management
  Marcella Niehoff School of Nursing
Loyola University Chicago
Maywood, Illinois

Jo Ann Appleyard, PhD, RN
Clinical Assistant Professor
College of Nursing
University of Wisconsin–Milwaukee
Milwaukee, Wisconsin

Suzanne Bakken, RN, DNSc, FAAN
Alumni Professor of Nursing
Professor of Biomedical Informatics
Columbia University
New York, New York

Marjorie Beyers, PhD, RN, FAAN
Patient Care Consultant
Barrington, Illinois

Sandra C. Garmon Bibb, DNSc, RN
Acting Chair
Department of Health Systems Risk and Contingency
  Management
Associate Professor
Uniformed Services University of the Health Sciences
Graduate School of Nursing
Bethesda, Maryland

Kathy A. Boyle, RN, MSN
Senior Director, Patient Services
University of Colorado Hospital Anschutz Inpatient Pavilion
Aurora, Colorado

Cheryl L. Brandi, DNSc, RN
Student, Adult NP Post-Masters Certificate Program
University of South Florida
Former Professor of Undergraduate and Graduate Nursing
Aichi Medical University College of Nursing
Aichi-ken, Japan

Rosalind Bryant MN, APRN, BC, PNP
Pediatric Nurse Practitioner
Texas Children's Hospital
Instructor
Baylor College of Medicine
Houston, Texas

Vern L. Bullough, PhD, D Sci, RN
Distinguished Emeritus Professor
State University of New York–Buffalo
Buffalo, New York
Emeritus Professor
California State University, Northridge
Northridge, California

Howard Karl Butcher, RN, PhD, APRN, BC
Associate Professor
The University of Iowa
College of Nursing
Iowa City, Iowa

Patricia T. Castiglia, RN, PhD, PNP, FAAN
Private Consultant in Issues in Higher Education
Professor Emeritus
University of Texas at El Paso
El Paso, Texas
Associate Professor Emeritus
The State University of New York
Buffalo, New York

Helen Castillo, PhD, RN, FAAN
Dean, College of Health and Human Development
California State University–Northridge
Northridge, California

Mary W. Chaffee, ScD(h), MS, RN, CNAA, FAAN
Captain, Nurse Corps, U.S. Navy
Doctoral Student, PhD Program, Uniformed Services
  University of the Health Sciences,
Bethesda, Maryland

Mary T. Champagne RN, PhD, FAAN
Dean Emerita
Duke University School of Nursing
Durham North Carolina

Peggy L. Chinn, RN, PhD, FAAN
Professor Emerita
University of Connecticut
Storrs, Connecticut

Kristine J. Chirlin, RN, BA, MSN
Adventist HealthCare
Rockville, Maryland

Thomas R. Clancy, MA, MBA, RN
Vice-President, Professional Services
Mercy Hospital
Iowa City, Iowa

June Clark DBE, PhD, RN, RHV, FRCN
Professor Emeritus
University of Wales–Swansea
Swansea, England

Mara M. Clarke MS, RN, FNP
Clinical Instructor
University of Illinois at Chicago–College of Nursing
Quad Cities Regional Program
Family Nurse Practitioner
Valley View Family Practice
Moline, Illinois

Patricia Clinton, PhD, RN, CPNP, FAANP
Clinical Associate Professor
College of Nursing
The University of Iowa
Iowa City, Iowa

Perle Slavik Cowen, PhD, RN
Associate Professor
The University of Iowa
College of Nursing
Iowa City, Iowa

Kennith Culp, PhD, RN
Associate Professor
The University of Iowa
College of Nursing
Iowa City, Iowa

Leanne M. Currie, RN, DNSc
Assistant Professor
Columbia University School of Nursing
Nurse Researcher
New York Presbyterian Hospital
New York, New York

Connie Davis, MN, ARNP
Geriatric Program Development Specialist
Fraser Health
Abbotsford, British Columbia
Canada

Betty Pierce Dennis, Dr P.H.
Professor and Dean
School of Nursing
Dillard University
New Orleans, Louisiana

Catherine J. Dodd, MS, RN, FAAN
District Director
U.S. House of Representatives Democratic Leader
  Nancy Pelosi
San Francisco, California

Kathryn J. Dolter, PhD RN, LTC USA (Retired)
Chair, Nursing Department
University of Dubuque,
Dubuque, Iowa

Marie E. Dusio, C, MS, RN
Assistant Professor of Nursing
Black Hawk College
Moline, Illinois

Joellen B. Edwards, PhD, RN
Professor
East Tennessee State University
Director, Organization Development
Mountain States Health Alliance
Johnson City, Tennessee

Nancy Edwards, RN, PhD
Associate Professor
Purdue University
West Lafayette, Indiana

Jo Eland PhD RN FNAP FAAN
Associate Professor of Nursing
The University of Iowa
College of Nursing
Iowa City, Iowa

Karen L. Elberson, PhD, RN
Associate Dean
Associate Professor
Doctoral Program Director
Uniformed Services University of the Health Sciences
Graduate School of Nursing
Bethesda, Maryland

Charlotte Eliopoulos RN, MPH, ND, PhD
Author and Speaker
President, Health Education Network
Glen Arm, Maryland

Anne M. Fiedler, Ph.D.
Professor of Management
Andrea School of Business
Barry University
Miami Shores, Florida

Terry Fulmer, PhD, RN, FAAN
The Erline Perkins McGriff Professor and Dean
College of Nursing
New York University
New York, New York

Richard Garfield RN DrPH
Henrik H. Bendixen Professor of Clinical International
    Nursing
Deputy Director for Public Health, Operation Assist
Center for Emergency Preparedness
Columbia University
New York, New York

Mary M. Gibson, MPH, MBA
Health Policy Analyst
University of Illinois at Chicago Medical Center
Chicago, Illinois

Nancy Girard, RN, PhD, FAAN
Associate Professor and Chair
Department of Acute Nursing Care
University of Texas Health Science Center–San Antonio
San Antonio, Texas

Colleen J. Goode, RN, PhD, FAAN
Vice President Patient Services and Chief Nursing Officer
University of Colorado Hospital
Denver, Colorado

Victoria T. Grando, PhD, RN
Associate Professor
Department of Nursing Science
University of Arkansas for Medical Science
Little Rock, Arkansas

Cecelia Gatson Grindel, PhD, CMSRN, FAAN
Associate Director for Graduate Programs
Professor
Byrdine F. Lewis School of Nursing
Georgia State University
Atlanta, Georgia

Susan M. Grover, PhD, RN
Professor and Chair
Family/Community Nursing
College of Nursing
East Tennessee State University
Johnson City, Tennessee

Sara Groves DrPH, APRN, BC
Assistant Professor
Johns Hopkins University School of Nursing
Baltimore, Maryland

Sheila A. Haas, PhD, RN, FAAN
Dean and Professor
Niehoff School of Nursing,
Loyola University Chicago
Chicago, Illinois

Mary Fran Hazinski, RN, MSN, FAAN
Clinical Nurse Specialist
Monroe Carroll Children's Hospital at Vanderbilt
Vanderbilt University Medical Center
Nashville, Tennessee

Ann Henrick, PhD, RN, FAAN
Lecturer
Degree Program
School of Nursing
Galway-Mayo Institute of Technology
Castlebar County
Mayo, Ireland

Ada Sue Hinshaw, PhD, RN, FAAN
Dean and Professor
University of Michigan
School of Nursing
Ann Arbor, Michigan

Marilyn J. Hockenberry, RN-CS, PhD, PNP, FAAN
Professor of Pediatrics
Baylor College of Medicine
Nurse Scientist/Director of Nursing Research
Texas Children's Hospital
Houston, Texas

Rufus Howe, RN, MN
Vice President, Clinical Programs
Healthways, Inc.
Nashville, Tennessee

Jillian Inouye, PhD, APRN-BC
Professor and Director of the Office of Faculty Research
Director of the PhD Program
University of Hawaii at Manoa
School of Nursing and Dental Hygiene
Honolulu, Hawaii

Lucille A. Joel, RN, EdD, APN, C, FAAN
Professor
Rutgers–The State University of New Jersey
College of Nursing
Newark, New Jersey

Tess Judge-Ellis, MSN, ARNP, FNP
Assistant Professor (Clinical)
University of Iowa
College of Nursing
Iowa City, Iowa

Gail Keenan, PhD, RN
Associate Professor
Director
Nursing Informatics Initiative
University of Illinois–Chicago
Chicago, Illinois

Bette Keltner, PhD, FAAN
Dean, Georgetown University
School of Nursing and Health Studies
Washington, DC

Noel Kerr, MN, RN, CMSRN
Clinical Nurse Specialist, Medical-Surgical Nursing
Director–Academy of Medical-Surgical Nurses
Washoe Medical Center
Reno, Nevada

Diane K. Kjervik, JD, MSN, RN, FAAN
Professor (Nursing) and Director, Carolina Women's Center
The University of North Carolina at Chapel Hill
Chapel Hill, North Carolina

Rose P. Knapp, MSN, RN, ACNP-C
Clinical Faculty
New York University
College of Nursing
New York, New York

Phyllis Beck Kritek, PhD, RN, FAAN
Consultant, Trainer, Facilitator, and Coach in Conflict
    Transformation
Proprietor
Courage: Conflict Transformation Services
Richmond, Virginia

Chris L. Latham, Professor
Nursing Department
Director of Extramural Funding
California State University, Fullerton
Fullerton, California

Roberta P. Lavin, MSN, APRN, BC
Captain, Nurse Corps
U.S. Public Health Service
Chief Policy Officer, Office of Public Health Emergency
    Preparedness
U.S. Department of Health and Human Services
    Washington, DC
Doctoral Student, PhD Program
Graduate School of Nursing
Uniformed Services University of the Health Sciences
Bethesda, Maryland

Judy Lee, RM, CPM
MBA Management Group, Vice President
San Miguel, New Mexico

Kristin Lemko, RN, BSN, MSNc
New York University
Division of Nursing
New York, New York

Karen Dunn Lopez, RN, MPH, PhD(c)
Doctoral Candidate
The University of Iowa
College of Nursing
Iowa City, Iowa

June R. Lunney, PhD RN
Associate Dean for Research
West Virginia University School of Nursing
Morgantown, West Virginia

Virginia A. Lynch, MSN, RN, FAAN
International Consultant in Forensic Nursing Science
Faculty,
Beth El College of Nursing and Health Sciences
University of Colorado
Colorado Springs, Colorado

Meridean L. Maas, PhD, RN, FAAN
Professor Emerita
Sally Mathis Hartwig
Professor of Gerontological Nursing Research
College of Nursing,
The University of Iowa
Iowa City, Iowa

P. J. Maddox. RN, MSN, EdD
Professor and Director, Office of Research
Center for Health Policy, Research, and Ethics
College of Nursing and Health Science
George Mason University
Fairfax, Virginia

Karen Markus, AS, BA, JD, RN
Law Faculty
Santa Clara University School of Law
Santa Clara, California

Jeanne M. Martinez RN, MPH, CHPN
Quality and Education Specialist
Northwestern Memorial Home Health Care
Chicago, Illinois

María Mercedes Durán De Villalobos, MSN
Titular and Emeritus Professor
Facultad de Enfermería
Universidad Nacional de Colombia,
Bogotá, Colombia

Paula R. Mobily, PhD, RN
Associate Professor
University of Iowa
College of Nursing
Iowa City, Iowa

Mary Margaret Mooney, PBVM, DNSc, RN,CS, FAAN
Professor and Chair
North Dakota State University
Fargo, North Dakota

V. Jane Muhl, PhD, RN
President and Chief Executive Officer
Bellin College of Nursing
Green Bay, Wisconsin

Audrey Nelson, PhD, RN, FAAN
Director of the Veterans Health Administration
    Patient Safety Center of Inquiry
Tampa, Florida

Adele W. Pike, RN, EdD
Director, Center for Excellence in Home Care Education
    and Practice
Visiting Nurse Association of Boston
William F. Connell School of Nursing at Boston College
Chestnut Hill, Massachusetts

SueEllen Pinkerton, PhD, RN, FAAN
Independent Consultant
Star 7 Strategies
Indialantic, Florida

Ian Portelli, PhDc, MScCRA, PCNS, BSc, SRN
Project Director, Organization Based Incident
    Management (OBIM) and Large Scale
    Emergency Readiness Project (LaSER)
New York University
David B. Kriser College of Dentistry and Nursing
New York, New York

G. Jeanne Potter, RN, MS, BSN
Senior Director of Clinical Operations/Nurse Executive
Adventist Home Health
Silver Spring, Maryland

Gail Powell-Cope, PhD, RN, FAAN
Assistant Director of Clinical Nursing
The University of South Florida
College of Nursing
Tampa, Florida

Anne Marie Rafferty, RN, PhD
Professor
Florence Nightingale School of Nursing and Midwifery
King's College
London, England

Marilyn J. Rantz, PhD, RN, NHA, FAAN
Professor, School of Nursing
University Hospital and Clinics Professor of Nursing
University of Missouri–Columbia
Sinclair School of Nursing
Columbia, Missouri

Terri Rebmann, PhDc, RN, CIC
Associate Director for Curricular Affairs Institute
    for Biosecurity
Saint Louis University
School of Public Health
St. Louis, Missouri

Ann M. Rhodes, RN, MA, JD
Assistant to the Provost and HIPAA Privacy Officer
The University of Iowa
Iowa City, Iowa

Rose Rivers, PhD, RN, CNAA
Vice President and Chief Nursing Officer
Shands at the University of Florida
Gainesville, Florida

Kathleen Rice Simpson, PhD, RNC, FAAN
Perinatal Clinical Nurse Specialist
St. John's Mercy Medical Center
Clinical Professor
Saint Louis University School of Nursing
St. Louis, Missouri

Cheryl Rodgers, MSN, RN, CPNP, CPON
Clinical Instructor
Baylor College of Medicine
Pediatric Nurse Practitioner
Texas Children's Cancer and Hematology Service
Houston, Texas

Janet C. Ross-Kerr, BScN, MS, PhD
Professor Emeritus
Faculty of Nursing
The University of Alberta
Edmonton, Alberta, Canada

Pam Scheibel, RN, MSN
Clinical Professor
University of Wisconsin
School of Nursing
Madison, Wisconsin

Esther Salang Seloilwe, RN, RM, PhD
Head, Department of Nursing Education
University of Botswana
Gabarone Botswana

Mary Cipriano Silva, PhD, MS, RN, BS
Professor Emerita
School of Nursing
College of Health and Human Services
George Mason University
Fairfax, Virginia

Diane J. Skiba, PhD, FAAN, FACMI
Professor and Project Director
The I-Collaboratory, Partnerships in Learning
University of Colorado at Denver and
    Health Sciences Center
Denver, Colorado

Capt Lynn A. Slepski, RN, MSN, CCNS
United States Public Health Service
PhD Student, Uniformed Services University of the
    Health Sciences
Washington, DC

Mechem Slim, RN
(Navajo)
Critical Care Staff Nurse
Albuquerque, New Mexico

Debra Smith
(Shoshone)
Evaluation and Development Coordinator
    Human Services Division
Fond du Lac Reservation, Minnesota

Linda S. Smith, MS, DSN, RN, CLNC
Associate Professor/Director
Idaho State University
Pocatello, Idaho

P. Ann Solari-Twadell, RN, PhD, MPA, FAAN
Assistant Professor of Nursing
Director of the Center for Spiritual Leadership
    in Health Care
Marcella Niehoff School of Nursing
Loyola University Chicago
Chicago, Illinois

Bernard Sorofman, PhD, RPh
Professor and Head
Clinical and Administrative Pharmacy
College of Pharmacy
The University of Iowa
Iowa City, Iowa

Janet P. Specht, PhD, RN, FAAN
Associate Professor
College of Nursing
The University of Iowa
Iowa City, Iowa

Sharon Staib, MS, RN
Associate Professor
Ohio University–Zanesville
Zanesville, Ohio

Anita M. Stineman, PhD, RN
Assistant Professor (Clinical)
The University of Iowa
College of Nursing
Iowa City, Iowa

Nancy A. Stotts, RN, EdD, FAAN
Professor
School of Nursing
University of California–San Francisco
San Francisco, California

Gail W. Stuart, PhD, APRN, BC, FAAN
Dean and Professor
College of Nursing
Medical University of South Carolina
Charleston, South Carolina

Teruko Takahashi, PhD, RN
Dean and Professor
Aichi Medical University
College of Nursing
Aichi-ken, Japan

Janette Y. Taylor, PhD, RN, ARNP, WHCNP
Assistant Professor
The University of Iowa
College of Nursing
Iowa City, Iowa

Rebecca A. Terranova, MA, RN.BC.
Nursing Arts Laboratory Manager
New York University
College of Nursing
New York, New York

Sheila Dinotshe Tlou, PhD
Minister of Health of Botswana
HIV/AIDS Coordinator
University of Botswana
Garborone Botswana

Sara Torres, PhD, RN, FAAN
Dean
University of Medicine of Dentistry of New Jersey School
of Nursing
Newark, New Jersey

Dana Tschannen, PhD, MS, BSN
Lecturer and Research Associate
University of Michigan
School of Nursing
Ann Arbor, Michigan

Michele J. Upvall, PhD, CRNP
Associate Dean and Director
School of Nursing
Carlow University
Pittsburgh, Pennsylvania

Joy E. Wachs, PhD, APRN, BC, FAAOHN
Professor
East Tennessee State University
Johnson City, Tennessee

Patricia Hinton Walker, PhD, RN, FAAN
Dean
Graduate School of Nursing
Uniformed Services University of
Health Sciences
Bethesda, Maryland

Maria R. Warda, RN, PhD
Dean and Professor
School of Nursing
Georgia Southwestern State University
Americus, Georgia

Kathleen O. Williams, RN, PhD
Associate Professor
Jefferson College of Health Science
Roanoke, Virginia

Deidre Wipke-Tevis, RN, PhD
Associate Professor
MU Sinclair School of Nursing
University of Missouri, Columbia
Columbia, Missouri

Joseph W. York, PhD
Associate Dean for Graduate Medical Education
University of Washington
School of Medicine
Seattle, Washington

Donna Zazworsky, MS, RN, CCM, FAAN
Manager
Diabetes Care Centers and Parish Nursing Program
Carondelet Health Network
Tucson, Arizona

Polly Gerber Zimmermann, RN MS MBA CEN
Assistant Professor
Harry S. Truman College
Chicago, Illinois
Associate Editor, Journal of Emergency Nursing
Bedford Park, Illnois

Margo R. Zink, RN, BSN, MS, EdD
Home Health Care Consultant
Self-Employed
Arlington, Virginia

Laurie Zoloth, PhD, RN, MA
Professor, Medical Humanities and Bioethics and Religion
Director, Center for Bioethics, Science and Society
Northwestern University
Chicago, Illinois

Mary Zwygart-Stauffacher, PhD, RN, BC-APRN, FAAN
Professor and Chair-Department of Nursing Systems
Interim Associate Dean-College of Nursing and Health
Sciences
University of Wisconsin-Eau Claire
Eau Claire, Wisconsin
Gerontological Nurse Practitioner
Red Cedar Clinic/Mayo Health System
Menomonie, Wisconsin

Preface

Welcome to the seventh edition of *Current Issues in Nursing*. Previous editions of this book were published in 1981, 1985, 1990, 1994, 1997, and 2001 by Joanne McCloskey Dochterman and Helen Grace. Current Issues has provided a means to discuss the important issues faced by nurses over this period of time. Reflecting back over these issues provides a synopsis of the challenges nurses have faced over a 20-year period when change was the norm in health care. Some issues presented in the past are still unresolved over this time period, and new issues have certainly been identified. What is clear is that nursing is a profession that accepts these challenges and welcomes discussion of the issues. The purpose of this edition, as with past editions, is to provide a forum for knowledgeable debate on the important issues that nurses face today so that intelligent decision-making can occur. We are excited to be the "new editors" of *Current Issues in Nursing* and have enjoyed working with the many authors of the chapters in this edition and our editors.

We believe that, given the rapidity of changes in the health care environment, a book like this that attempts to describe and discuss all the current issues in nursing is important. In periods of rapid change, decisions must often be made quickly. With many issues confronting such a large and diverse profession, there is danger that decisions will be made without full knowledge or without sufficient opportunity for discussion and debate. Or, worse yet, issues may be ignored and decisions not made. The chapters in this book provide excellent information and thoughtful comment on the important issues currently facing the nursing profession. We hope these chapters help foster debate in practice and educational settings and help set an insightful path to the future of nursing.

As in the previous editions, the issues are identified and addressed in sections. The seventh edition includes 12 sections: Definitions of Nursing; Changing Education; Changing Practice; Quality Improvement; Governance; Health Care Systems; Health Care Costs; Role Challenges, Collaboration and Conflict; Cultural Diversity; Ethics, Legal and Social Issues; Violence Prevention and Care: Nursing's role; and International Nursing. As a new feature of this edition, we have added a section on victims of violence. We believe this section addresses issues faced by nurses in practice today in all settings within health care. Most sections include an overview of the section, a debate chapter, and several viewpoint chapters. Past editions have had from 75 to 103 chapters. This edition continues that trend with 91 chapters. The 12 sections begin with an overview in which we briefly introduce the section. These overviews highlight some of the important points in each chapter, raise some related issues, and assist readers to select chapters for in-depth reading.

Following the overview for all but two sections (the international section and victims of violence) there is a debate chapter, featuring the pros and cons of one of the problematic issues in nursing. A listing of the titles of debate chapters in the seventh edition gives some idea of the scope of the issues:

- What is nursing and why do we ask?
- The future direction for nursing education: Educational models for future care.
- Moving the care: From hospital to home.
- Institute of Medicine recommendations: Can we meet the challenges?
- Who should provide nursing care?
- From a medical system for a few to a comprehensive health care system for all
- Controlling health care costs: Is there an answer?
- Collaboration issues between nurses and physicians.
- Why isn't nursing more diversified?
- Ethics of health care reform: Should health care be rationed?

The bulk of the book is composed of viewpoint chapters. In these, each author provides her or his own view and critical analysis of one particular aspect of the section's general topic. Viewpoints are those of the individual authors and provide an opportunity for posing a controversial stand on the issue, presenting a case study or results of some research, reviewing the past and current status of a topic, or outlining problems and future directions. The viewpoint chapters differ from the debate chapters as the words *viewpoint* and *debate* differ: the viewpoint chapters, for the most part, offer only one side or a piece of an issue. It is hoped that the viewpoint chapters provide material and ideas for other debates that readers will agree with or take issue with, so that after reading a viewpoint they will be stimulated to think and seek out more information. It is impossible to list all the many viewpoints here but a sample list of titles will, we hope, make you eager to read these and more.

- ◆ Nursing faculty: Opportunties and challenges.
- ◆ Web-based education.
- ◆ Moving the care: From hospital to home.
- ◆ Alternative and complementary therapies: Recent changes and current issues.
- ◆ Nursing care priority area: Patient safety.
- ◆ Are drugs are too cheap?
- ◆ Nursing employment issues: Unions, mandatory overtime, and patient staff ratios.

- ◆ Nurse practioners: Issues within a managed care environment.
- ◆ Impact of Health Insurance Portability and Accountability Act (HIPAA).
- ◆ Nursing at the crossroads: Men in nursing.
- ◆ Health care for the poor and underserved.
- ◆ Nursing care during terrorist events.
- ◆ Nursing in wars.

This edition of *Current Issues in Nursing,* as others in the past, offers a fairly complete analysis of all of today's important nursing issues. Careful reading, thought, and debate today can result in good decisions, actions, and achievements tomorrow. We hope readers will enjoy the work of the many talented contributors who collectively represent the diversity and wisdom of nursing. We thank them for their contributions to this edition. We also want to thank Sharon Sweeney for helping us with the many details of editing a book with 91 chapters.

Perle Slavik Cowen and **Sue Moorhead**

Who Is Current Issues For?

urrent Issues in Nursing is appropriate for several audiences. First, it is an ideal book to use in a senior level undergraduate or graduate level issues course. Faculty who are teaching courses designed to help associate degree and diploma RNs make the transition to university will also find this particularly useful. A teacher using this book could easily have students orally present the debates written here or could structure a whole new set of debates using the readings as source material. The book is also useful for international students who are trying to compare the issues in their country with those faced by nurses in the United States. In addition, the international section provides further comparisons of nursing across the globe.

Second, it is a good book to use as a core text for a graduate curriculum. There is something here that will fit with most graduate nursing courses. For example, the section on education for education course; the sections on practice, quality improvement, and health care systems for advanced practice and nursing administration courses; the section on governance and role transition for leadership classes; and so on. By picking and choosing from the numerous viewpoints, every class in the graduate curriculum can benefit from the use of this book. By using one text throughout the curriculum, there is financial savings for the individual student and consistency in expectations from the faculty.

Third, the book is an excellent source of information about nursing and about the issues confronting the profession. The chapters are written by experts in the area and include many well-known nursing leaders. The book is stimulating and invigorating, and the challenges within will revitalize and energize the reader. It would make a good gift for a new RN or for a nurse going back to graduate school.

Acknowledgments

We have many people to thank for helping us with the seventh edition:

- We want to thank Joanne Dochterman and Helen Grace for entrusting this edition to our care. We appreciate the opportunity to continue the traditions and unique perspectives this book provides to nurses.
- A special thank you to Sharon Sweeney, who assisted us every step of the way. Without her assistance and dedication to this book we would have been unable to meet the many challenges in editing a book with over 90 chapters. She helped identify authors, communicate with the authors and our publishers, and proofread and edit the final chapters.
- Yvonne Alexopoulos, Lisa Newton, and Michael Ledbetter, Editors at Elsevier, who helped us plan this edition and work our way through the process.
- Our authors for taking the time from busy schedules to think and write about their topics in an interesting and helpful manner. This book is only as good as their contributions.
- Our readers in the United States and other countries for their continued support and enthusiasm for this book. We hope that this edition continues to meet your needs.
- Our immediate families, who continue to be our main supporters. Thank you Jessie, Leah, Don, Brian, Sara, and Scott.

Perle Slavik Cowen and **Sue Moorhead**

Contents

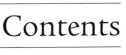

CURRENT
ISSUES in
NURSING

DEFINITIONS OF NURSING

The Richness of Nursing

PERLE SLAVIK COWEN ◆ SUE MOORHEAD

Nursing is a profession with rich career opportunities that change and reflect the society in which nurses live. Over the years the role of the nurse has changed to meet the needs of patients. Much of nursing history is focused on the role of the nurse as a direct patient care provider, mainly in hospitals. As the health field changes, so do the roles of nurses and the places in which they work. Today, nurses are experiencing a rapid shift to care in the community rather than the hospital. As care shifts into community settings, patients return to their homes after brief hospital stays and need assistance to make this transition to care outside the walls of the hospital. Because of this, the family is more involved with providing care to loved ones in the home environment. Families are faced with complex care issues that challenge their ability to provide appropriate care to family members. Services such as hospice care, home care with intensive treatment protocols, assisted-living facilities, and new models for nursing home care for the elderly are examples of how the health care system has changed to meet these needs. To their credit nurses have been key in making these changes happen. In addition to nurses in direct practice roles, the opportunities for nurses as faculty members, researchers, and administrators in a variety of systems are expanding, and critical shortages in every area of nursing are presenting new challenges.

Not only is the organizational context of practice changing, but also the forms of practice are shifting as the health care system changes to address current challenges. Increasingly, nurses, especially nurse practitioners, are developing their own group practices and are working in new forms of collaboration with physicians and other health care providers. Physicians are incorporating nurse practitioners into their practice structures and care delivery models; for example, obstetricians/gynecologists now integrate nurse-midwives as practice partners, cardiologists add nurse practitioners to their staffs, and critical care practitioners are found in

hospitals alongside physicians and physician assistants. Whereas in the past, nurses' roles have been defined primarily in relationship to practice and practice settings, the "business" world of health care has opened up new opportunities for nursing in the management of health care. Nursing educational programs have entered into partnership relationships with schools of business for nurses who want to build careers in the "business" side of nursing. This business model also is affecting the types of courses offered in undergraduate programs. The world of information technology is opening up other vistas as nurses influence and help design an electronic health record. Monitoring of patient care through use of computer technology is another example of a potential career track for nurses merging nursing knowledge with that of information-communication expertise. The impact of technology is present in any role of nursing one explores. Technology is no longer an issue but a reality of the practice environment.

Traditionally, nurses in the past tended to develop career paths opportunistically. Today's students enter nursing with a clearer sense of what they want to do. One commonly hears a newly admitted student to an undergraduate program state that she (or increasingly he) would like to be a pediatric nurse practitioner in the future. Hopefully, this trend will continue, and persons entering the nursing field will be knowledgeable about the opportunities for career development in the field and have more clearly delineated career paths to a variety of opportunities within nursing that are matched by a commensurate reward system. What is evident is that the roles open to future nurses will continue to evolve to meet the care needs of patients. This first section serves as an introduction to some of the potential career fields in nursing. This section certainly is not an exhaustive list by any means. Subsequent sections introduce many other possibilities in terms of the organizational context and practice patterns. Nurses have the responsibility to make these opportunities known to future generations of potential nurses.

Perhaps no other profession has been so obsessive and diligent in attempting to define its field. Historically, the first chapter of this book has focused on defining nursing, and in the past Donna Diers has differentiated dictionary definitions that record common usage from legal definitions that serve to regulate and establish the boundaries for the field. Because medicine was first to develop a regulatory framework that is so broad that "practically anyone's work including a mother's may be captured within it," all other professions have had to contend with this "first mover" effect and build their definitions in ways that are not duplicative. Thus defining the field of nursing is a political process, according to Diers, rather than an intellectual and logical exercise. In this edition, Meridean Maas offers a new perspective on defining nursing for today and adds a second question to the discussion. Historically, the question has been, "What is nursing?" Maas also discusses the question, "Why do we ask?" This chapter discusses nursing from the viewpoint of the public view of nursing, the legal view of nursing, the nursing discipline view of nursing, and other definitional challenges. In conclusion, Maas advocates for abandoning the preoccupation with defining nursing and suggests that building the science of nursing and translating the science to nursing practice is a better use of nurses' efforts. If these practices show a benefit, society will define nursing and resist challenges to legitimacy for the nursing profession.

In the first viewpoint chapter, Grando traces the history of nursing in hospitals focused specifically on hospital nursing. The hospital of today presents formidable challenges to nursing related to the greater intensity of care required, the sophisticated technology in the care setting, and the creation of new roles for nurses to fill. The declining proportion of nurses practicing in hospital settings, the aging of the nursing population, and the lag in diversifying the nursing profession to match that of the general population are some of the challenges. Increased specialization and cross-training of nurses, delegation of tasks to assistive personnel, and the need to accelerate nursing work such as patient teaching create increased pressure on nurses in hospital settings. In addition to traditional roles, nurses are assuming greater responsibility for management of patient care as case managers and discharge planners. Within this context, nurses in hospital settings live with the constant fear of health risks in the workplace, such as the danger of being infected with human immunodeficiency virus or hepatitis C by needle prick, and the relatively new phenomenon of violence in the workplace. Hospital nursing is responding favorably to these challenges while dealing with a shortage of nurses at the bedside.

Some form of nurse specialization has been in place in the nursing profession throughout its history. In the next viewpoint chapter, Appleyard and Henrick describe and trace the origins of the clinical nurse specialist. This specialty role developed primarily in hospital settings related to areas of specialty medical practice and care of severe conditions. Clinical nurse specialty areas developed around intensive care, for example, and in medical, surgical, and obstetrical specialty areas. The clinical nurse specialist has become one of four advanced practice registered nurse roles described in *Nursing's Social Policy Statement* (American Nurses Association, 2003). Clinical nurse specialist roles traditionally have focused on direct patient care, patient and staff education, and to a lesser extent, research and health care administration. This chapter provides excellent examples of the clinical nurse role in practice. The chapter summarizes the current challenges faced by nurses choosing this role.

The next viewpoint chapter focuses on the role of the nurse practitioner. Clinton describes the 40-year history of this role in nursing. The chapter summarizes the struggles nurse practitioners have faced in the legislative arena, on medical turf, and within the corridors of nursing and its historical development. The role of nurses in this specialty is influenced greatly by Nurse Practice Acts in each state. The chapter includes a description of the current practice environment in which these nurses work, the educational requirements for this role, and current challenges such as reimbursement, future educational models, and access to clients. Clinton believes the future for nurse practitioners is optimistic but that nurses must be diligent in establishing and protecting their practice alongside medicine.

Just as the care environment is changing, the roles of nurses in management positions also are changing. Traditionally, nurse managers were limited to the management of nursing services, but today the responsibilities of nurse executives have broadened in scope, and many times their responsibilities include all patient care services. Pinkerton and Rivers focus this chapter on nurse executives in acute care settings. Challenges faced by nurse executives include the recent resurgence of the importance of Magnet status and the current nursing shortage. These authors define the nurse executive role as maximizing the quality of patient care, maximizing the professional satisfaction of the nursing staff, meeting the cost-effectiveness goals of the organization, and participating in long-range strategic planning, including nursing. Nurse executives are clinical and business leaders in the organization and are experts in coordinating care and the cost of such care. At a time when the opportunities for nurse executives are increasing, programs to prepare nurses in the field of administration are declining. The current nursing shortage presents a formidable challenge for nurse executives, who are pushed by hospital executives who tend to see the solution to the problem as bringing additional assistive personnel into the care setting—the "slice and dice" approach. Pinkerton and Rogers advocate that nurse executives have a clear set of standards and a line they will not cross in compromising patient care. The chapter ends with a case study that clearly illustrates the dilemmas facing nurse executives.

In another viewpoint chapter, Mobily and Stineman discuss some of the major issues affecting nursing education as nurse educators prepare nurses for the twenty-first century. One of the most pressing problems facing the profession is the shortage of nursing faculty that will only intensify in the years ahead. Two major factors—the aging of current faculty, often referred to as the "graying of the professoriate," and declining interest in an academic career—provide a framework for the discussion of this shortage. The chapter outlines the challenges nurse faculty members face and discusses external and internal challenges in this current shortage of faculty. This chapter illustrates the complex issues facing nurses in this role. This is an important chapter for understanding the issues today in educating nurses for the future.

Ending this section, Stotts and Wipke-Tevis address the role of nurse researchers. Nurse researchers focus on understanding the science of care through systematic investigation. Nurse researchers design studies, participate in the conduct of research, and disseminate findings at professional meetings and in peer-reviewed journals. This chapter outlines pathways to research careers. Successful researchers are adept at problem definition, and their expertise in research methods permits them to gather data to address the problem. Ability to attract funding for research, grant-writing skills, publishing of research results, and participation in scientific discourse are talents integral to the role of a researcher. Particular challenges are the tendency for nurses to be overly critical of others whose substantive content or research methodologies differ from their own, their dependence on others for generating a caseload of research subjects, and the limited funding available to support nursing research. The work of nurse researchers to generate new knowledge is vital to the nursing profession.

The introductory section of this book illustrates the richness of nursing as a career choice. Few professions offer the expanse of roles that nurses can pursue. In this changing health care environment, nursing faces the challenge of keeping grounded in the positive traditions of the past—concern for the well-being of patients and participation and leadership in the here-and-now complex problems of providing cost-effective quality care—while embracing technology and shaping health policy for a future that will fully actualize the potential of nursing. All nurses have an obligation to assist the profession to keep this richness alive in the profession while building the science of nursing.

What Is Nursing, and Why Do We Ask?

MERIDEAN L. MAAS

The question "What is nursing?" has perplexed nurses and nursing students for some time. I was asked to answer the question for a class assignment in one of my first nursing classes in the early 1950s. I thought it a strange question then because I had come to school to be taught what nursing is and how to do it. It was my introduction to the identity crisis in nursing.

Why do we ask? Why is it important to define nursing? In previous editions of this book, Donna Diers (1994; 2001) suggested that definition is necessary if we are to teach nursing, study nursing, and make policy decisions about nursing. Diers also maintained that nursing is not defined by what nurses do. More accurately, nursing cannot be defined solely by what nurses do, even though the definition is the major concern of most nurses and training in tasks is historically the predominant reason for schools of nursing. For what do nurses do what they do, why do they do what they do, and what is achieved by what they do also must be addressed in a definition of nursing. Definitions also vary by purpose and perspective, but the definitions tend to become more concordant as professions mature. In this chapter, common usage definitions of nursing, legal definitions, and definitions by the discipline are explored. The purpose of the definition from each perspective and the implications for nursing are discussed. Finally, a recommendation to replace the preoccupation of nursing with definition is proposed.

THE PUBLIC VIEW OF NURSING

Common usage definitions are contained in dictionaries and reflect the customary meaning among members of the public at the time they are written. For example, in the Merriam-Webster Online dictionary (2005), meanings of *nurse* are "to promote the development or progress of," "to manage with care or economy," "to take charge of and watch over," "to care for and wait on," and

"to attempt to cure by care and treatment." Synonyms found in the *Merriam-Webster's Collegiate Thesaurus* (1994) for the term are likewise for the verb form: "to cherish, cultivate, foster, nourish, nursle, nurture, advance, forward, further, promote; humor, indulge, pamper." The word *nursing* yields similar action meanings, such as "treatment," "nurture," "tending," and "attention." In the Britannica Concise Encyclopedia Online (2005), the word *nurse* is reported to mean a health care professional who is skilled or trained and provides physical and emotional care to the sick and disabled and promotes health in all individuals through activities including research, health education, and patient consultation.

Although the progress in defining what a nurse is is an encouraging note, nurses still should understand that common usage lags behind definitions in the discipline and often behind legal definition. Common usage reflects the public view of nursing, a view that often does not distinguish nurses from others who care and nurture or nursing as a profession with a body of scientific knowledge. The common usage meanings of nurse and nursing affect who is recruited into the discipline, their socialization into and within the discipline, their contributions to nursing science and practice, legal and policy constraints on nursing, relationships with other providers, and the resources that are available to support the development of nursing science and translation for practice.

THE LEGAL VIEW OF NURSING

The public and nurses seek legal definitions for protection. The public legal definition describes the individuals who can advertise themselves as nurses (use the title of registered nurse, licensed practical nurse, or advanced practice nurse) and the scope within which the nurse with a specific title can practice legally. Legal definitions exist in all state codes for the registered nurse, licensed practical (or vocational) nurse, and for advanced

practice registered nurse. The public seeks these definitions purportedly to protect members of the public
from practitioners who might provide services for
which they are not qualified. Nurses seek legal definitions to protect their practice from others who might
offer the same services and to enable their own practice
according to definitions and standards established by
the discipline (profession). In truth, legal definitions
are highly political, fairly ambiguous, and do not enable
nurses to practice the full scope that is defined by the
profession.

Licensing laws vary from state to state, so it is important that nurses are familiar with the Nurse Practice Act
in the state in which they are practicing. Because licensing laws are relatively vague, they are subject to interpretation by boards of nurse examiners, staff of boards
of nurse examiners, and by attorneys general in state
jurisdictions. Thus refinement of licensing laws is a
political process. This is important for nurses to recognize because interpretations will depend on how well
decision makers understand current nursing practice and
how effective the collective of nurses is in influencing
their decisions.

A problem for nursing and most other health
care disciplines is that the medical profession obtained
licensing laws first and defined the practice of medicine
so broadly that it encompasses almost everything that
could be done to assist another person with health and
well-being. In carving out its legal prerogatives, nursing
usually is required to show how the practice of nursing
does not encroach on medical practice. This is not only
an arduous political process, but combined with vague
nurse practice acts, it also heightens the potential for
nurses to be accused of practicing medicine without a
license.

In 1903, North Carolina passed the first licensing
law for nursing. The law was intended mostly to protect
the title. Under this law, most anyone could perform
nursing functions as long as that person did not use
the title "registered nurse" (Hadley, 1989). In was not
until 1938 that New York passed a licensing law that
included a definition of nursing (Driscoll, 1976). With
this law, nursing sought to protect the positions and
compensation of registered nurses (RNs) from unlicensed
and unqualified persons who were using the title registered nurse. Like other professions, including medicine
with its broad definition, nursing seeks to use licensure
to protect its own interests.

The word *diagnosis* was especially provocative when
considered for inclusion in nursing licensing laws.
Medicine successfully protected the term to refer only

to medical practice until New York redefined nursing in
the state Nurse Practice Act in the late 1970s.

> The practice of the profession of nursing ... is defined as
> diagnosing and treating human responses to actual or
> potential health problems through such services as casefind-
> ing, health teaching, health counseling and provision of
> care supportive to and restorative of life and well-being
> (Driscoll, 1976, p. 59).

The New York law broadened the definition of
nursing and served to differentiate nursing from medicine. The law also heightened awareness of the need to
define and classify the human responses to actual or
potential health problems that nurses could treat.
Coincidentally, in 1973 Kristine Gebbie and Mary Ann
Lavin organized an invitational conference of nurses
at St. Louis University to identify, define, and classify
nursing diagnoses. Subsequently, the North American
Nursing Diagnosis Association (NANDA) was formed.
The definition of nursing diagnosis that was adopted
by NANDA in 1990 was "Nursing diagnosis is a clinical
judgment about individual, family, or community
responses to actual and potential health problems/
life processes. Nursing diagnoses provide the basis for
selection of nursing interventions to achieve outcomes
for which the nurse is accountable" (North American
Nursing Diagnosis Association, 1992, p. 5). In 1980
the American Nurses Association published the monograph *Nursing—A Social Policy Statement* containing a
definition of nursing based on the New York State
Nurses Association definition. Although nursing had
legitimized diagnosis as a function and drawn a seman-
tic line between the focus of nursing and that of medicine, it also was controversial within nursing and
constrained the evolution of the scope of nursing practice. This constraint was most apparent for advanced
practice nurses (APNs) and some nurses working with
acutely ill patients in hospitals.

Some nurses argue that defining nursing as the diagnosis of actual or potential responses to illness places
nursing in a practice cul-de-sac, closing off expansion
of the scope of practice and limiting economic gain.
Others argue that the definition describes nursing practice that is independent and autonomous. At the ninth
conference of NANDA a nursing diagnosis was defined
as "a clinical judgment about individual, family, or
community responses to actual or potential health
problems/life processes which provides the basis for
definitive therapy toward achievement of outcomes for
which the nurse is accountable" (Carpenito, 1991, p. 65).
This definition expanded the phenomena that nurses are

accountable to treat to include family and community units and health states other than illnesses.

In reality, nurses have not assumed the autonomy and accountability for their practice that is prescribed by Nurse Practice Acts, largely because of the policies and politics in employing organizations and because the diagnosis and treatment of human responses mostly are not reimbursed by third-party payers. However, APNs are not supported by the definition of nursing as the diagnosis and treatment of human responses. To accommodate advanced practice nursing, Nurse Practice Acts were split with separate definitions of nursing for RNs and APNs. Although RNs and APNs continue to press for expanded definitions of the scope of their practice, they are divided by definition. Both groups often hesitate to open practice acts because they fear that the political power of the medical profession will be stronger than their own and thus APNs might lose rather than gain prerogatives.

Advanced practice nurses have made gains in most states in expanding the scope of their practice into the domain of medicine to enable the diagnosis and treatment of disease. Yet a number of states still require APNs to have a formal "collaborating" relationship with a physician, a euphemism for a dependent, supervised relationship with a medical professional. Advanced practice nurses in some states have gained prescriptive authority and the authority to admit patients to hospitals, but these privileges are by no means the case in all 50 states. Advanced practice nursing, however, has increased the overlapping prerogatives of nursing and medicine.

Although advanced practice nursing has gained and is continuing to gain prerogatives that expand the scope of nursing into what heretofore has been the sole domain of medicine, there is no consensus within nursing that this is the way that all of nursing should go. Many nurses fear that gains in medical prerogatives will distract nursing from its calling to advocate and care for the health and well-being needs of individuals, families, and communities holistically. A closer look at definitions of nursing within the discipline will account for the lack of consensus. Historical efforts and differing conceptions used to define nursing by members of the discipline influence how nurses are socialized and their subsequent individual and collective behaviors.

THE VIEW OF THE DISCIPLINE

Many definitions of nursing exist within the discipline, beginning with Nightingale (1859/1946), who claimed, "a nurse is any person in charge of the personal health

of another," nursing is "the act of using the environment of the patient to assist him in his recovery," and "what nursing has to do … is put the patient in the best condition for nature to act upon him" (p. 75). Nightingale must be understood in the context of the time and circumstances when she wrote. The view of nursing she advanced greatly influenced subsequent definitions. Virginia Henderson's much-used definition, which she calls her personal concept and not a definition of nursing, reveals Nightingale's influence (Henderson, 1961):

> Assisting the individual sick or well in the performance of those activities contributing to health, its recovery or peaceful death that he would perform unaided if he had the necessary strength, will, or knowledge and to do this in such a way as to help him gain independence as rapidly as possible (p. 2).

Years later, Henderson revised her personal concept to include primary care as a function of nursing and that nurses "diagnose and treat as well as 'care'" (Henderson, 1961, p. 98). Nightingale and Henderson emphasize what nurses do rather than what nursing is. Whether nursing should be defined by what nurses do is a question to consider as further attempts within the discipline to define nursing are explored.

In the latter half of the 1950s and throughout the 1960s, during the time that nursing programs were moving rapidly into universities, a number of nurse grand theorists emerged, prompted by the need to describe and justify nursing as an academic discipline. Nursing grand theories—such as the "science of unitary man" (Rogers, 1970), Roy's "adaptation theory" (1970), Orem's theory of "self-care deficits" (1971), and King's "human interaction" theory (1971)—were mostly conceptual models or frameworks, each containing four major constructs: person, environment, health, and nursing (Fawcett, 1980). Although nursing was struggling for definition, these grand theories offered none but did provide broad concepts that were intended to form the basis of the development of the science of the discipline. The grand theorists proposed conceptual frameworks from which propositions were expected to be derived deductively and tested to generate the science/ knowledge of nursing.

Other nurse theorists, mainly Orlando (1961, 1972), Wiedenbach (1964), and Travelbee (1966), developed practice theories. These theories began with the assumptions that nursing is an independent profession and what nursing is, is known. The purpose of the practice theories was to guide practice and practice research, underscoring that the most pressing need was to describe the outcomes of nursing. In this same vein, Hildegard Peplau (1987) described nursing diagnoses as the problems that nurses fix.

Nursing was the object of study in the 1960s and 1970s by sociologists who mostly were concerned with describing the efforts of nursing to be recognized as a profession and its relationships with medicine and other health disciplines. Despite the efforts of nursing to describe its uniqueness, in academia and in hospitals that at the time employed 80% or more of active nurses, sociologists offered little in the way of definition. An exception was Hans Mauksch, a medical sociologist who advanced a humorous definition of nursing largely influenced by hospital nursing. Paraphrasing Mauksch (1963), he observed that nursing is the cookie dough that is left over after all other health care disciplines have cut out their cookies. This definition illustrates the difficulty nursing was having defining its identify but also may foretell the holism, coordination, case management, and advocacy concepts of nursing that became prominent in the last decade.

Another approach to defining nursing and to building nursing theory began with the NANDA work to define and classify nursing diagnoses (Gebbie & Lavin, 1975). Nursing diagnoses are concepts that describe the phenomena (human responses) that nurses treat. A decade later, the Nursing Interventions Classification (NIC) research team began work at the University of Iowa, funded by the National Institutes of Health, National Institute of Nursing Research, to identify, define, and classify nursing interventions (Iowa Interventions Project, 1992). NIC interventions describe the actions and strategies that nurses use to treat nursing diagnoses. In 1989 the Nursing Outcomes Classification (NOC) research team also funded by the National Institute of Nursing Research, developed and defined patient outcomes that are sensitive to nursing interventions and constructed and evaluated measurement scales for nurses to use in their practice (Johnson & Maas, 1996). NOC outcomes describe variable patient, family, or community states, perceptions, or behaviors that are measured on a continuum in response to nursing interventions (Moorhead, Johnson, & Maas, 2004). The NIC and NOC research continues through the Center for Nursing Classification and Clinical Effectiveness in the College of Nursing, the University of Iowa. As the NANDA, NIC, and NOC are implemented in electronic clinical nursing information systems, opportunities for the development of nursing clinical data repositories that can be used to evaluate the effectiveness and

cost-effectiveness of nursing interventions will result. Evaluating the effectiveness and cost-effectiveness of nursing interventions to produce desired patient outcomes is the accountability expected of a profession and is consistent with the view of practice theorists. Rather than being concerned about the definition of nursing, it is more important to diagnose, treat, and evaluate the outcome effects of interventions with patients.

The development and classification of concepts that describe the phenomena that nurses treat (nursing diagnoses), the nursing treatments that are used (nursing interventions), and the effects of the interventions (patient outcomes) is an inductive theory–building strategy. These descriptive concepts, labeled with standardized terms, are the building blocks of nursing practice theory. Recent activities of the NANDA, NIC, and NOC Alliance produced an initial, unifying taxonomy to advance the development of propositions linking nursing diagnosis, intervention, and outcome concepts to build middle-range theories and encourage research to test the theories (Dochterman & Jones, 2003). Blegen and Tripp-Reimer (1997) argue that classifications of nursing diagnoses, interventions, and outcomes should be used to form middle-range nursing theories.

The knowledge or science of a discipline is the result of building and testing theories. No better definition of a practice discipline exists than the science upon which it bases its practice. Rather than debating the issues of definition, nursing will be better served by focusing those energies on its science and the translation of the science in nursing practice. Armed with science-based nursing practice, nursing will better resist other definitional challenges.

OTHER DEFINITIONAL CHALLENGES

Medicine and nursing challenge advanced practice definitions of nursing. The challenge from medicine is mostly political, whereas the challenge from nursing is mostly philosophical. Both challenges are over economic resources. Physicians resist the encroachment into what they view as their domain of practice and the corresponding economic loss. To reduce the threat of advanced practice nursing, the medical profession challenges a definition of nursing that includes the diagnosis and treatment of disease and illness. Advanced practice nurses challenge the definition of nursing as the diagnosis and treatment of human responses to actual or potential health problems. As primary health care providers, APNs expand the definition of nursing to include the diagnosis and treatment of illnesses and expect greater remuneration because of their expanded practice. Advanced practice nurses claim that the primary care they deliver is comparable in quality to that delivered by physicians, but more cost-effective. Some nurses question whether advanced practice nursing is within the scope of nursing practice or is delegated medical functions (Bates, 1974; Edmund & Ruth, 1991; Henrick & Appleyard, 1997). Others fear that as advanced practice expands into the domain of medicine, "nursing" functions will be neglected (Henrick & Appleyard, 1997). It seems reasonable that with the appropriate training, nurses' scope of practice should expand and that consumers should have a choice of providers of primary care. This definitional challenge, however, quickly becomes a political and economic challenge.

Other economic and political challenges come from nurse employer and health policy sources. Employers use nurses however it best suits their economic and political interests. Much of what nurses do when there is an ample supply of RNs and wages are lower is determined to be done as well by lesser-trained personnel when RNs are in short supply and wages are higher. Breaking nursing into activities that can be delegated to lesser-trained persons results in fragmented nursing care. The most recent illustration of the dangers of a view of nursing as tasks occurred with the reengineering in hospitals that followed the advent of managed care. Responding to consultants and seeking to advantage their bottom line, hospital administrators split up the work of nurses and assigned the tasks to ancillary and assisting personnel while downsizing the number of RN positions. Soon enrollments in schools of nursing dropped sharply, job dissatisfaction escalated among RNs who remained, the "bottom line did not improve," and the quality of patient care was greatly eroded (Kovner & Gergen, 1998; Shindul-Rothchild, Berry, & Long-Middleton, 1996). These results focused attention on the quality of care, the relationship of RN staffing to quality outcomes, and patient safety (Institute of Medicine, 1996).

Clearly, what nursing is or becomes depends on the influence it is demonstrated to have on its clients' outcomes, whether the clients are individuals, families, or communities. Building the science of nursing and translating the science to nursing practice that is shown to benefit the society will define nursing and resist challenges to legitimacy. Broad conceptions of nursing that encompass the client, health, environment, and nurse will guide the development of the science. Forming and testing propositions that link the concepts that describe the phenomena that nurses diagnose, the interventions that nurses use, and the outcomes achieved will build the science of nursing. The science of nursing is what will move definitions from different viewpoints ever closer together.

Advanced practice nursing likely will continue to expand practice into areas previously claimed by medicine as APN programs and graduates consume and master the enabling medical science. Without continued development of the science of nursing, the diagnosis and treatment of responses to actual or potential illness or injury and the translation of research evidence for nursing practice and policy decisions, nursing will continue to be defined by tasks rather than the outcomes that are achieved. The knowledge that is needed to achieve the outcomes, including making the correct nursing diagnoses and prescribing the most effective nursing treatments, will not be defined regardless of who performs specific tasks. Rather than being overly preoccupied with defining nursing, consumers of nursing and the profession would be better served by an obsession with building the science of nursing. A better question to ask and answer is, What nursing interventions for specific nursing diagnoses are effective in achieving desired outcomes? When this question is answered, public, legal, and discipline perspectives will be less disparate and "What is nursing?" will be of less concern.

REFERENCES

American Nurses Association. (1980). *Nursing: A social policy statement.* Kansas City, MO: Author.

Bates, B. (1974). Doctors and nurses: Changing roles and relations. *New England Journal of Medicine, 283*(3), 129-134.

Blegen, M A., & Tripp-Reimer, T. (1997). Implications of nursing taxonomies for middle-range theory development. *Advances in Nursing Science, 19*(3), 37-49.

Britannica Concise Encyclopedia Online. (2005). *Nurse.* Retrieved June 1, 2005, from http://www.britannica.com/ebc/article?tocId=9373777

Carpenito, L. J. (1991). The NANDA definition of nursing diagnosis. In R. M. Carroll-Johnson (Ed.), *Classifications of nursing diagnosis: Proceedings of the ninth conference* (pp. 65-71). Philadelphia: Lippincott.

Diers, D. (1994). What is nursing? In J. C. McCloskey & H. K. Grace, *Current issues in nursing* (4th ed., pp. 5-14). St. Louis, MO: Mosby.

Diers, D. (2001). What is nursing? In J. C. McCloskey & H. K. Grace, *Current issues in nursing* (6th ed., pp. 5-13). St. Louis, MO: Mosby.

Dochterman, J., & Jones, D. (Eds.). (2003). *Unifying nursing languages: The harmonization of NANDA, NIC, and NOC*. Washington, DC: American Nurses Association.

Driscoll, V. M. (1976). *Legitimizing the profession of nursing: The distinct mission of the New York State Nurses Association*. Albany, NY: Foundation of the New York State Nurses Association.

Edmund, M. W., & Ruth, M. V. (1991). NPs who replace physicians: Role expansion or exploitation? *Nurse Practitioner, 16*(9), 46, 49.

Fawcett, J. (1980). A framework for analysis and evaluation of conceptual models of nursing. *Nurse Educator, 5,* 10-14.

Gebbie, K., & Lavin, M. A. (Eds.). (1975). *Classification of nursing diagnosis: Proceedings of the first national conference*. St. Louis, MO: Mosby.

Hadley, E. H. (1989). Nurses and prescriptive authority: A legal and economic analysis. *American Journal of Nursing, 15,* 245-300.

Henderson, V. (1961). *Basic principles of nursing care*. Geneva, Switzerland: International Council of Nurses.

Henrich, A., & Appleyard, J. (1997). Clinical nurse specialists and nurse practitioners. In J. McCloskey & H. Grace (Eds.), *Current issues in nursing* (5th ed., pp. 18-24). St. Louis, MO: Mosby.

Institute of Medicine. (1996). *Nursing staff in hospitals and nursing homes: Is it adequate?* Washington, DC: National Academy Press.

Iowa Intervention Project. (1992). *Nursing interventions classification (NIC)*. St. Louis, MO: Mosby.

Johnson, M., & Maas, M. (1996). *Nursing outcomes classification (NOC)*. St. Louis, MO: Mosby.

King, I. M. (1971). *Toward a theory for nursing: General concepts of human behavior*. New York: John Wiley & Sons.

Kovner, C., & Gergen, P. J. (1998). Nursing staffing levels and adverse events following surgery in US hospitals. *Image, 30*(4), 315-321.

Mauksch, H. O. (1963). Becoming a nurse: A selective view. In J. Skipper & R. Leonard. (Eds.), *Social interaction and patient care*. Philadelphia: J.B. Lippincott.

Merriam-Webster's collegiate thesaurus. (1994). Springfield, MA: Merriam-Webster.

Merriam-Webster Online. (2005). *Nurse* Retrieved June 1, 2005, from http://www.m-w.com/cgi-bin/dictionary

Moorhead, S., Johnson, M., & Maas, M. (2004). *Nursing outcomes classification (NOC)* (3rd ed.). St. Louis, MO: Mosby.

Nightingale, F. (1946). *Notes on nursing—What it is and what it is not*. Philadelphia: Lippincott. (Original work published 1859.)

North American Nursing Diagnosis Association. (1992). *NANDA nursing diagnoses: Definitions and classification 1992*. St. Louis, MO: Mosby.

Orem, D. E. (1971). *Nursing: Concepts of practice*. New York: McGraw-Hill.

Orlando, I. J. (1961). *The dynamic nurse-patient relationship*. New York: G.P. Putnam's Sons.

Orlando, I. J. (1972). *The discipline and teaching of nursing process: An evaluative study*. New York: G. P. Putnam.

Peplau, H. (1987). ANA Social Policy Statement Part I. *Archives of Psychiatric Nursing, 1*(5), 301-307.

Rogers, M. (1970). *An introduction to the theoretical basis of nursing*. Philadelphia: Lippincott.

Roy, C. (1970). Adaptation: A conceptual framework in nursing. *Nursing Outlook, 18*(3), 42-45.

Shindul-Rothchild, J., Berry, D., & Long-Middleton, E. (1996). Where have all the nurses gone? Final results of our patient care survey. *American Journal of Nursing, 96*(11), 52-57.

Travelbee, J. (1966). *Interpersonal aspects of nursing*. Philadelphia: Lippincott.

Wiedenbach, E. (1964). *Clinical nursing: A helping art*. New York: Springer.

Staff Nurses Working in Hospitals

Who They Are, What They Do, and
What Are Their Challenges?

VICTORIA T. GRANDO

Hospital nursing in the United States has a long and diverse history. It began in the late 1700s, when hospitals were mostly charitable institutions that served the sick-poor. By the 1800s many hospitals were dirty, vermin-infested places that frequently spread disease. Nurses working in these marginal institutions had no formal training and were typically from the "bottom of female society." This grim picture changed quickly with the establishment of hospital-based schools of nursing in 1873 (Kalisch & Kalisch, 1995; Melosh, 1982; Reverby, 1987).

Acting on the belief that the upper class was entrusted to provide for the sick, poor, and working class, wealthy female reformers sought to improve hospital care in the late 1800s. To this end, they established nurses' training schools for women of good moral character that incorporated bedside training and strict discipline. These reforms were effective. Soon hospitals, staffed by student nurses, were clean and orderly environments in which patients received good care and became well. As a result of the improved care by student nurses and the developing sophistication of medicine, the number of hospitals grew drastically, increasing from 200 hospitals in 1870 to more than 4000 in 1910 (Ashley, 1976; Flood, 1981; Melosh, 1982; Reverby, 1987).

Hospitals continued to be staffed largely by student nurses until the late 1920s.* By the early 1930s, about a third of graduate nurses worked for hospitals as directors, supervisors, head nurses, and instructors. Private duty nurses also worked in hospitals during this period. By 1928, some estimate that perhaps as high as 60% of private duty nursing occurred in hospitals. Private duty nurses working in hospitals held a variety of roles.

Some worked for surgeons, some cared for the difficult patients, and others did general duty nursing for individual patients. As the 1930s progressed, hospital administrators began hiring graduate nurses to staff hospitals. This shift resulted from two societal events. One was the growth of hospital beds at a time when the availability of student labor was decreasing because of nursing leaders' pressure to close inadequate schools of nursing and decreased enrollments in nursing schools. The other was the depression, which rapidly brought about the collapse of home nursing because of the weakened economy. This led graduate nurses, unable to obtain private duty work in patient homes, to work as staff nurses for low wages, sometimes just for room and board. Thus hospitals found it economically feasible to hire graduate nurses to meet their increasing staff needs. In fact, paying staff nurses under these arrangements was often less expensive than educating students (Flood, 1981).

Hospital staff nursing as we know it today took shape after World War II. Although many hospitals still relied heavily on student labor from their schools of nursing, the number of paid staff nurses was increasing.* By 1945, hospitals employed 49% of all registered nurses (RNs) as administrators, supervisors, head nurses, and staff nurses. Nurses worked in a variety of inpatient clinical areas including communicable diseases, tuberculosis, operating rooms, orthopedics, pediatrics, medicine, surgery, psychiatry, obstetrics, and gynecology as well as in outpatient departments (American Nurses Association [ANA], 1946). Advances in surgery and medical technology lead to increasingly complex nursing roles. By the 1950s and 1960s, nurses were

---

*During this period, graduate nurses worked as private duty nurses in patients' homes and as public health nurses. Some served as administrators in hospitals.

*In 1945 most schools of nursing were hospital-based diploma schools of nursing.

providing care for patients recovering from open heart surgery, receiving hemodialysis, and on respirators. They also worked in newly emerging specialty units such as "preemi" centers that care for premature infants or special cardiac recovery units that took care of patients after cardiac surgery. Moreover, as physicians' roles expanded, nurses assumed many roles formerly done only by doctors. Nurses took over intravenous care, participated in cardiac resuscitation, and conducted psychotherapy (Grando, 1994; Kalisch & Kalisch, 1995).

As these clinical advances were occurring, nurses faced numerous challenges. The end of World War II began a long period of nursing shortages resulting from expanding job opportunities for women, a reemphasis on women's role in the family, poor working conditions in hospitals, and low wages (Grando, 2000). The nursing shortages in turn added to the stress of staff nurses who were working 44 to 48 hours per week, split shifts, and overtime without extra pay or comparable time off. Indeed, some questioned why nurses continued to work at all (Brown, 1948). Gradually, however, through the efforts of the ANA and local nurses across the country, wages and working conditions steadily improved (Grando, 1994, 1997, 2000).

TODAY'S PROFILE

Today, hospitals employ most working RNs, and this likely will be the case in the near future. The number of nurses working in hospitals has increased gradually to about 65% of all nurses by the 1960s and has remained constant until recently (Grando, 1994; ANA, 1985). In 2000, just under 60% of the almost 2.3 million employed RNs worked in hospitals* (U.S. Department of Labor, 2004). The profile of RNs working in hospitals is changing. In 2000, RNs in hospitals were younger than other employed RNs. Nearly 75% of all RNs 30 years old or younger worked in hospitals. The majority worked full time (71.8%) for an average of 42.2 hours a week, just slightly more than 39.3 hours per week they were scheduled to work. Many RNs worked in general/specialty units (31%), but most worked in critical care units such as intensive care (17%), step-down units (6%), operating rooms (9%), recovery rooms (3%), and emergency rooms (8%). Almost 75% worked in direct patient care

(U.S. Department of Health and Human Services, n.d.; ANA, 2000b).

To get a better understanding about staff nurses, we need to compare them to all other RNs in the United States.* In 2000 the estimated number of RNs licensed to practice was 2,696,540. The majority of these (81.7%) worked as RNs. Although nursing continues to be a predominately female profession, the number of male nurses is increasing steadily. The estimated number of male RNs in 2000 was 5.4%, a substantial increase from the 2.7% in 1980. The percent of RNs from racial/ethnic minorities also has increased. About 12% of RNs in 2000 were from racial/ethnic minorities, which is almost double the 7% of nurses from ethic and racial minorities in 1980s. But this is less than the 30% of ethic and racial minorities in the general population. In 2000 the distribution of RNs by ethnic and racially diverse backgrounds was as follows: 0.5% were two or more races, 1.2% were Native American/Alaskan Native, 2.0% were Hispanic, 3.7% were Asian/Pacific Islander, 4.9% were Black (non-Hispanic), and 86.6% were White (non-Hispanic). Registered nurses vary greatly regarding their educational preparation. In 2000 the majority of RNs (40%) were prepared at the associate degree level, whereas 30% entered nursing with a baccalaureate degree and 30% entered with a diploma in nursing. Nine percent of RNs had a master's as their highest degree, whereas 0.6% had a doctoral degree. The average salary of a full-time RN in 2000 was $46,782, which was an 11.2% increase over RN salaries in 1996 (U.S. Department of Health and Human Services, n.d.)

The aging American RN workforce is another important issue that is receiving increased attention. The average age of RNs has increased steadily over the past 25 years because fewer young persons are entering nursing and increasing numbers of RNs are retiring (American Association of Colleges of Nursing, 2000). This trend of fewer young nurses, added to other recent statistics, gives cause for concern. In 2000, only 9.1% of RNs were under 30 years old, and 31.7% were under 40 compared with 1980 when 25.1% of RNs were under 30 and 52.9% were under 40 (U.S. Department of Health and Human Services, n.d.). The aging of the RN workforce is the result of three related social forces: increasing job opportunities for women, more individuals choosing nursing as a second career, and the declining

---

*The most current information we have on hospital nurses comes from the March 2000 National Sample Survey of RNs (U.S. Department of Health and Human Services, n.d.).

*The most current information we have on RNs is from the March 2000 National Sample Survey of RNs (U.S. Department of Health and Human Services, n.d.).

attractiveness of nursing as a career.* These factors work together to keep young persons from choosing nursing as a career and bring older individuals into the profession. These nursing trends, added to the aging of the current nursing workforce, are driving nursing shortages today and are certain to influence hospital supply needs in the future.

TODAY'S ROLES

An important trend in hospital care that is shaping nurses' roles is the increased complexity of care rendered in hospitals. Although hospital staff nurses continue to provide the essential 24-hour care and management of patients, they do this within environments transformed by technological and communication advances, and economic restraints. Furthermore, many sophisticated hospital services once offered as inpatient care now are provided on an outpatient basis. These trends have resulted in increased patient acuity and shorter hospital stays. They also have led to several shifts in nurses' roles within hospitals, including subspecialty roles within traditional nursing specialties, increased delegation of traditional nursing duties to unlicensed assistive personal, and increased cross-training of nurses. How these changes affect nurses depends largely on where they work. For nurses working in large hospital centers, increased specialization is common, but at the same time, they also are expected to become cross-trained in related areas. In small rural hospitals, however, nurses often are called upon to be generalists, to be competent in caring for an older person with a cardiac condition and in the emergency room treatment of an injured child.

Within hospitals today, nurses are caring for sicker, often older patients, with complex care needs during shorter hospital stays with ever more sophisticated technology (Benefield et al., 2000; Brown, 2004; Clark, 2004; Hudak, Gallo, & Morton, 2003; Porter-O'Grady, 2001a, 2001b). To meet this challenge, hospital staff nurses require expert clinical and communication skills to do the following:

1. Provide evidenced-based care.
2. Use information systems to manage patient care.
3. Provide culturally sensitive care within a holistic framework.
4. Maintain the "human caring" component of patient care.

5. Counsel patients' families.
6. Focus on the system level while providing direct care.
7. Interface and collaborate with other health care providers.
8. Keep up with rapid technological advances while adapting to change and chaos.
9. Participate in clinical research.

Nurses in this new era are assuming greater responsibility in the management of acutely ill patients in hospitals. Today hospital staff nurses run cardiac resuscitation, monitor patients on complex ventilation and intravenous systems, and provide crisis counseling to patients and their families. To manage these complex care needs, staff nurses need to (1) critically evaluate all pertinent patient information from varied sources; (2) understand the perspective of all key persons including the patient, the patient's family, and other health care professionals; (3) make rapid and precise clinical judgments; (4) have impeccable clinical skills; (5) set and evaluate outcomes; and (6) work independently and in collaboration with other health care professionals (Comer, 2005; Hudak et al., 2003). These greater responsibilities have also led to increased subspecialization. Many hospital RNs are becoming certified as oncology nurse specialists; diabetes educators; wound, ostomy, and continence nurse specialists; lactation nurse specialists; trauma nurse specialists, and psychiatric nurse liaison specialists. Some nurses are taking the next educational step by becoming advanced practice nurses such as geriatric clinical nurse specialists and acute care nurse practitioners.

Effective discharge planning and patient education also have evolved and become increasingly complex as hospitals shift to shorter stays and outpatient surgery. No longer do nurses have the luxury of longer hospital stays in which to develop patient relationships fundamental to patient teaching or the time necessary to teach patents how to care for themselves, take medications, and cope with complex health conditions (Clark, 2004; Maramba, Richards, Myers, & Larrabee, 2003). For example, it is common to discharge patients receiving outpatient surgery within hours of awaking from anesthesia. This makes it difficult for nurses to instruct patients how to care for themselves postoperatively. Short and often unplanned hospitalizations cause patients and their families stress, making it difficult for them to assimilate patient education. Before surgery, patients may be too stressed, and afterward they may not be alert enough to remember the information taught. Furthermore, patients discharged early from hospitals require complex, high-tech home care. As a

---

*This is related to increased publicity of the many work-related problems such as forced overtime, understaffing, and increased workloads connected to hospital downsizing.

result, hospital RNs have to provide not only discharge education but also comprehensive discharge planning. To do this effectively, they need to be knowledgeable about available community resources and Internet-based health care information.

The supervision of unlicensed assistive personnel continues to be a major part of the nurse's role within hospitals. Hospitals began employing unlicensed assistive personnel in the 1930s, but the practice did not become routine until the severe nursing shortages of the late 1940s and early 1950s (Grando, 1998, 2000). Today's hospitals employ a mix of nursing staff, and given today's complex hospital environment, RNs need to consider the following issues to use unlicensed assistive personnel safely (Cohen, 2004; Fisher, 1999; King, 1995):

1. Are duties delegated to unlicensed assistive personnel allowed under state scope of practice acts?
2. Are protocols developed to guide the delegation of nursing acts to unlicensed assistive personnel?
3. Do RNs train unlicensed assistive personnel to perform delegated nursing tasks or to monitor patients?
4. Do RNs supervise unlicensed assistive personnel?
5. Do RNs know exactly what unlicensed assistive personnel are trained to do?
6. Do RNs understand how to delegate effectively?

These are important questions for all staff nurses to consider when delegating tasks to unlicensed personnel.

Nursing case management is a more recent role for hospital nurses that emerged in the late 1980s in response to unpredictable patient outcomes, poor-quality care, high health care costs, and the advent of prospective payment systems. Hospital-based nurse case management has proved to be an effective way to improve patient outcomes, reduce fragmented hospital services, and prevent unnecessary hospital days. Currently four models of nurse case management are being practiced. Use of nurse case managers blends traditional utilization review with a focus on reimbursement and discharge planning. Insurance-based nurse case managers act as liaisons between the hospital administrators and the insurance providers. They deal with a wide range of health plan benefits to ensure continuity of care and cost containment by focusing on use of resources, benefits management, and discharge planning. Another nurse case management model is a primary nurse case manager. The primary nurse case manager assumes 24-hour accountability for patients, collaborates with the patient's health care team, and provides direct care. The newest nurse case management model is the advanced practice nurse case manager. In this role the nurse case manager identifies populations at risk and develops an interdisciplinary coordinated plan of care (Wayman, 1999).

Hospital nursing of the future will be influenced by the sweeping changes that are expected to reshape hospitals. Hospital inpatient services will shrink while outpatient services soar, and hospitals will focus increasingly on critically ill and surgery patients (Hupfeld, 2000). Computer technology also will transform the hospital environment in numerous ways. Pervasive computing, computer devices connected across the hospital, will allow nurses to be interconnected to all aspects of the hospital information system from virtually any place in the hospital. Software analytic systems that gather, organize, and analyze patient data also will assist nurses planning patient care (Simpson, 2004).

TODAY'S CHALLENGES

Staff RNs face many challenges, some of which have been revisited from the past. Hospital staff nursing shortages that result in overwork, work-related stress, and mandatory overtime are one challenge that nurses have faced before. Nursing has experienced numerous periods of short staffing, and often the forces causing the shortages are similar. The underlying causes of today's hospital staff shortage have been seen before, such as drops in student enrollment, cost cutting by hospitals, and increased job opportunities for women (Trossman, 2000). However, some aspects to the current nursing shortage are different. The present aging of the nursing labor force is one. Not only are fewer persons coming into nursing, but also more nurses are being lost to retirement. Another aspect of the current nursing shortage is the failure of nursing to increase the diversity among nurses. Ninety percent of nurses are Euro-American compared with roughly 72% of the general population. Not only does it appear that we do not have enough nurses to meet government projections for 2008, but also we are likely not to have increased the percentage of nurses who share the heritage with the many minority groups in our nation (Trossman, 1998; U.S. Department of Labor, 2004).

Health risks at the workplace are also a major challenge for today's hospital nurses and have new aspects. Nurses are being assaulted from many different fronts. The risks from needle sticks are especially troublesome. Although nurses have faced the threat of infections transmitted from patients before, the threats nurses face today are different. The danger from being infected with a deadly disease such as human immunodeficiency virus and hepatitis C is shockingly real. Health care workers are estimated to receive from 600,000 to 1 million injuries from needles and sharps every year, and at least 1000 nurses contract a serious illness (ANA, 2000a). This is not the same as a time-limited situation such as the influenza outbreak in 1918 to 1919: this is the stress of working day in and day out with the knowledge that an accidental slip of a needle can be life changing and ultimately deadly. Another health-related threat that is causing nurses increased stress is the sensitivity many nurses are developing to latex, a material found in many more areas of a hospital than just in latex gloves (Trossman, 1999).

The last major challenge facing hospital staff nurses is workplace violence. Workplace violence is increasing across the nation, and the health care industry is no exception. Hospitals and nursing homes account for 64% of workplace violence, and health care workers have a 16 times greater risk of sustaining a fatal injury on the job (ANA, 2000c; Smith-Pittman & McKoy, 1999). The ANA (2000c) reports that it is getting increasing reports submitted by members who have sustained workplace violence. Workplace violence is becoming a concern for all hospital nurses, not just those who work in emergency rooms or psychiatric units. Sexual harassment in the workplace also is an ongoing problem (Valente & Bullough, 2004). Studies have shown that this is a widespread problem troubling many RNs that often goes unreported.

Hospital staff nurses are facing today's challenges with courage, professional competence, and commitment. They are striving in the face of numerous obstacles to improve the quality of patient care at the same time that they are responding to changes of new technology, increased responsibility, hospital downsizing, and managed care. Hospital staff nursing today is still one of the major practice areas in nursing that continues to move the profession forward as it did in the past.

REFERENCES

American Association of Colleges of Nursing. (2000). *Nursing school enrollments decline as demand for RNs continues to climb.* Retrieved February 28, 2005, from http://www.aacn.nche. edu/Media/NewsReleases/Archives/2000/2000feb17.htm

American Nurses Association (Ed.). (1946). *Facts about nursing: A statistical, 1946.* New York: Author.

American Nurses Association (Ed.). (1985). *Facts about nursing: 84-85.* Kansas City, MO: Author.

American Nurses Association. (2000a). *Nursing facts: Needlestick injury.* Retrieved February 28, 2005, from http://www. nursingworld.org/readroom/fsneedle.htm

American Nurses Association. (2000b). *Nursing facts: Today's registered nurse—Numbers and demographics.* Retrieved February 28, 2005, from http://www.nursingworld.org/ readroom/fsdemogr.htm

American Nurses Association. (2000c). *Real news: Art imitates life: TV show, "ER," highlights threat of workplace violence.* Retrieved February 28, 2005, from http://www.nursingworld.org/ pressrel/2000/pr0209.htm

Ashley, J. A. (1976). *Hospitals, paternalism, and the role of the nurse.* New York: Teachers College Press.

Benefield, L. E., Clifford, J., Cox, S., Hagenow, N. R., Hastings, C., Kobs, A. E. J., et al. (2000). Nursing leaders predict top trends for 2000. *Nursing Management, 31*(1), 21-23.

Brown, B. J. (2004). From the editor: Restoring caring back into nursing. *Nursing Administration Quarterly, 28,* 237-238.

Brown, E. L. (1948). *Nursing for the future: A report prepared for the National Nursing Council.* New York: Russell Sage Foundation.

Clark, J. S. (2004). An aging population with chronic disease compels new delivery systems focused on new structures and practice. *Nursing Administration Quarterly, 28,* 105-115.

Cohen, S. (2004). Delegating vs. dumping: Teach the difference. *Nursing Management, 35*(10), 14, 18.

Comer, S. (2005). *Delmar's critical care: Nursing care plans* (2nd ed.). Clifton Park, NY: Thomson, Delmar Learning.

Fisher, M. (1999). Do your nurses delegate effectively? *Nursing Management, 30*(5), 23-26.

Flood, M. E. (1981). *The troubling expedient: General staff nursing in United States hospitals in the 1930s, a means to institutional, educational, and personal ends.* Ann Arbor, MI: University Microfilms International, No. 8211927.

Grando, V. T. (1994). *Nurses' struggle for economic equity: 1945 to 1965. Dissertation Abstracts International, 55*(09B), 3815. (University Microfilms International, No. 9504017).

Grando, V. T. (1997). ANA's economic security program: The first 20 years. *Nursing Research, 46,* 111-115.

Grando, V. T. (1998). Making do with fewer nurses in the United States, 1945-1965. *Image, 30,* 147-149.

Grando, V. T. (2000). Hard day's work: Institutional nursing between 1945-1950. *Nursing History Review, 8,* 169-184.

Hudak, C. M., Gallo, B. M., Morton, P. G. (2003). *Critical care nursing: A holistic approach* (8th ed.). Philadelphia: Lippincott.

Hupfeld, S. (2000). Through the looking glass: Tomorrow's hospital. *RN, 63*(6), 52-59.

Kalisch, P. A., & Kalisch, B. J. (1995). *The advancement of American nursing* (3rd ed.). Philadelphia: J. B. Lippincott.

King, B. A. (1995). Working with the new staff mix. *RN, 58*(6), 38-41.

Maramba, P. J., Richards, S., Myers, A. L., & Larrabee, J. H. (2003). Discharge planning process: Applying a model for evidence-based practice. *Journal of Nursing Care Quarterly, 19,* 123-129.

Melosh, B. (1982). *The physician's hand: Work culture and conflict in American nursing.* Philadelphia: Temple University.

Porter-O'Grady, T. (2001a). Into the new age: The call for a new construct for nursing. *Geriatric Nursing, 22*(1), 12-15.

Porter-O'Grady, T. (2001b). Profound change: 21st century nursing. *Nursing Outlook, 49,* 182-189

Reverby, S. (1987). *Ordered to care: The dilemma of American nursing.* Cambridge: Cambridge University Press.

Simpson, R. (2004). Information technology: Where will we be in 2015? *Nursing Management, 35*(12), 38-44.

Smith-Pittman, M. H., & McKoy, Y. D. (1999). Workplace violence in healthcare environments. *Nursing Forum, 34*(3), 5-13.

Trossman, S. (1998). Diversity: A continuing challenge. *The American Nurse, 30*(1), 24-25.

Trossman, S. (1999). When workplace threats become reality. *The American Nurse, 31*(3), 1, 12.

Trossman, S. (2000, January/February). Nurses fight short staffing on several major fronts. *The American Nurse, 32*(1), 1-2.

U.S. Department of Health and Human Services, Health Resources and Service Administration, Bureau of Health Professions, Division of Nursing. (n.d.). *The registered nurse population, March 2000.* Retrieved February 1, 2005, from http://www.bhpr.hrsa.gov/healthworkforce/reports/rnsurvey/rnss1.htm

U.S. Department of Labor, Bureau of Labor Statistics. (2004). *Occupational employment and wages, May 2004 29-1111 registered nurses.* Retrieved February 1, 2005, from http://www.bls.gov/oes/current/oes291111.htm#(1)

Valente, S. M., & Bullough, V. (2004). Sexual harassment of nurses in the workplace. *Journal of Nursing Care Quality 19*(3), 234-241.

Wayman, C. (1999). Hospital based case management: Role clarification. *Nursing Case Management, 4,* 236-241.

Clinical Nurse Specialist

*Who They Are, What They Do, and
What Are Their Challenges?*

JO ANN APPLEYARD ◆ ANN HENRICK

The clinical nurse specialist (CNS) is one of four advanced practice registered nurse (APRN) roles described in *Nursing's Social Policy Statement* (American Nurses Association, 2003). The other APRN roles include nurse practitioners, certified nurse-midwives, and certified registered nurse anesthetists. The CNS role was developed as the nursing profession sought to advance nursing practice after World War II in response to a need for nurses who focused on a specific segment of nursing and who developed expert knowledge and skills in a particular area of practice.

The criteria for specialists in nursing practice were identified first by the American Nurses Association (1980) in the first edition of *Nursing: A Social Policy Statement* as "a nurse, who through study and supervised practice at the graduate level (master's or doctorate), has become expert in a defined area of knowledge and practice in a selected clinical area of nursing" (p. 23). The recently published second edition of *Nursing's Social Policy Statement* (2003) states that APRNs possess expanded and specialized knowledge and skills, defining the term *expanded* as new knowledge and skills that may overlap with medical practice roles and defining the term *specialized* as concentrating on one specific part of the whole domain of nursing. Clinical nurse specialists originally were prepared for specialty nursing roles; however, in recent years there has been some movement toward blending the CNS role with the nurse practitioner (NP) role, resulting in CNSs who can perform medical diagnoses and prescribe medicines. In addition, a new master's-level nursing program preparing clinical nurse leaders has emerged, and there is some overlap between the CNS and clinical nurse leader roles.

The concept of role blending is one of the challenges that face CNSs in today's health care environment. Other challenges include the regulatory process that legitimizes CNS practice, chronic pressures regarding job loss related to health care financing issues, and a new movement toward requiring doctoral preparation for APRNs.

HISTORICAL ORIGINS OF THE CLINICAL NURSE SPECIALIST

Nursing has always had "specialists" who acquired specialized knowledge and skill through practice and on-the-job instruction. During the 1930s and 1940s, many nurses attended short-term postgraduate educational programs sponsored by hospitals and became the specialists in their particular fields (Donahue, 1985; Hamrick, 1989). The modern CNS emerged, however, in response to the recognized need to improve the quality of patient care and the clinical practice of professional nursing, primarily in the acute care setting (Berlinger, 1973; Georgopulous & Christman, 1970; Koetters, 1989; Padilla, 1973; Reiter, 1973; Vaughn, 1968).

Nursing care had deteriorated seriously during and immediately after World War II, in large part because of the dramatic decrease in the numbers of registered nurses practicing in hospitals (Sample, 1987). Many nurses returning from the war used the GI Bill to go back to school and become teachers and administrators, and a number of nurses were no longer content to work in the paternalistic environment of the hospital, where low salaries and substandard working conditions were the norm (Donahue, 1985).

The quick fix (replacing registered nurses with less-qualified health care providers) to the acute nursing shortage and substandard patient care failed to address the nurses' concerns. Despite emerging technology and increased complexity of care, hospitals continued to use wartime measures to fill the gap; volunteers became paid nurses' aides and vocational (practical) nurses were introduced to provide the major portion of the direct care for patients (Berlinger, 1973; Donahue, 1985; McClure, 1990; Reiter, 1966; Stafford, 1988). Team nursing was introduced, but it further fragmented patient care and frustrated the registered nurses, who continued to leave the hospital (Donahue, 1985). The registered nurse felt devalued because others with less education and professionalism took over the nursing care of patients while the professional nurse "nursed" the desk. In addition, the development of shortened programs in hospital diploma schools and associate degree programs in community colleges contributed little to the recognized need for increased knowledge and skill at the bedside.

In 1947 a National Nursing Council (representing the American Nurses Association and other health care organizations) obtained a grant from the Carnegie Foundations and commissioned Esther Lucille Brown to study and determine how professional nursing schools could meet the demand for nursing services. One result of the study was Brown's publication *Nursing for the Future* (1948), in which she strongly proposed that basic schools of nursing be part of universities and colleges. She stated, in addition, that

> provision for the development of some specialists within clinical nursing has been viewed in this report as necessary, if the base on which nursing service rests is to be strengthened, and if the profession is to look forward to a sound healthy development (p. 95).

Following this report, nurse educators met at the historic Williamsburg Conference and strengthened the resolve to initiate clinical nursing specialty education at the master's level (National League for Nursing, 1958). Hildegard E. Peplau established the first specialty graduate program in psychiatric nursing at Rutgers University in 1954 (Donahue, 1985). In 1961, Frances Reiter (1973) presented a paper enunciating her concept of the nurse clinician, which is virtually synonymous with the CNS of today: "one ... who consistently demonstrates a high degree of clinical judgment and an advanced level of competence in the performance of nursing care in a clinical area of specialization" (p. 9).

During the 1960s, publications expressing the need for clinical nursing to keep abreast of the knowledge explosion in technological and behavioral sciences flourished (Berlinger, 1973). Federal funding was obtained to support this level of learning, and in the early 1960s, programs to prepare CNSs in many areas of clinical practice were established (Hoeffer & Murphy, 1984). In 1966 a change in the structure of the American Nurses Association to include divisions of clinical practice gave

further impetus to the development of master's-prepared clinicians (Donahue, 1985; Hoeffer & Murphy, 1984). Since the 1960s, CNS roles have continued to develop and, in some instances, flourish. Currently, in the first decade of the twenty-first century, there are more than 300 graduate programs in the United States to educate CNSs (Walker et al., 2003).

CLINICAL NURSE SPECIALISTS TODAY

Estimates indicate that approximately 69,000 registered nurses are educated and credentialed to practice as CNSs in the United States (National Association of Clinical Nurse Specialists, 2005b). Although most CNSs practice in acute care hospitals, an increasing number of them are found in a wide variety of other settings, including community and public health agencies, outpatient clinics, long-term care agencies, and organized medical group practices. According to the National Association of Clinical Specialists, the specialty practice of the CNS may be identified in terms of a particular population, a setting, a disease, a particular type of care, or type of problem. Populations are defined according to client groups, such as pediatrics, geriatrics, or women's health. Settings include critical care and the emergency room, whereas type of care refers to areas such as psychiatry and rehabilitation. The disease frame of reference includes disease entities, such as diabetes, and medical subspecialty areas, such as oncology. Type of problem refers to broad health problems such as wounds, pain, and stress.

Clinical nurse specialist roles traditionally have focused on direct patient care, patient and staff education, and to a lesser extent on research and health care administration. Clinical nurse specialist "practice is consistently targeted toward achieving quality, cost-effective outcomes within 3 spheres of influence—patients, nurses and nursing personnel, and organizations/systems" (National Association of Clinical Nurse Specialists, 2003, p. 164). Clinical nurse specialist roles within these spheres of influence vary according to practice settings and specific job descriptions, but most CNSs have responsibilities in all three of these areas. This concept is exemplified by the following CNS practitioners with brief descriptions of their practice roles in hospital and outpatient settings. These examples, gleaned from personal contact and interaction, are not intended to be all-inclusive, but rather to illustrate the breadth and depth of the CNS role in current health care organizations.

◆ Angie Brechlin is a psychiatric CNS who practices in a community hospital with inpatient and outpatient behavioral health programs. At this point, her direct patient care activities are limited to leading groups for medication and cognitive behavioral training; however, she has a collaborative practice agreement with a psychiatrist and is in the process of establishing hospital credentialing. She will soon be doing psychotherapy and medication management in the behavioral health day program of the hospital. Angie does a great deal of staff education among all disciplines within the hospital. She regularly participates in the employee orientation program, training staff in restraint use and verbal intervention, and she oversees the orientation program for all staff in the behavioral health units of the hospital. She also provides in-service training to unit staff throughout the hospital on communication, team-building, professional boundaries, and suicide prevention. When patients with behavioral health problems are admitted to nonpsychiatric units, Angie consults with the nursing staff and assists them in developing appropriate care plans for the patients. She has administrative responsibilities in hospital committee leadership and quality improvement, chairing the restraint committee and reviewing all quality concerns from the behavioral health programs, including identifying trends and designing and implementing training to address practice issues. Angie currently is not participating in any research studies, but she stays current with the research literature in her specialty and works to encourage evidence-based practice within the behavioral health programs of the hospital. Angie's community outreach activities are an important part of her practice. She serves on a local suicide prevention committee and on a work group for the statewide suicide prevention task force, and she performs community-based workshops on suicide prevention. Angie also is a clinical instructor in behavioral health for two local nursing programs.

◆ Cathy Gentz is a CNS specializing in cardiovascular disease and is employed in a community hospital. Her focus is telemetry care and noninvasive cardiac testing, and she provides patient care support and staff education in the telemetry unit, as well as in the oncology and combined orthopedics/neurosurgery unit where there are also several telemetry beds. Her primary patient care role is assisting the nurses in those units in caring for patients with complex needs. Cathy is called to consult on patient care for unusually long lengths of stay or when patients have multiple comorbidities or are undergoing complex medical procedures. Her staff education responsibilities include unit-based training on new technologies and/or cardiovascular care practices. She also develops competency criteria for telemetry staff and performs quarterly and annual skills evaluations. Hospital-wide, Cathy delivers part of the core orientation and participates in regularly scheduled education on the care of patients with cardiac disease. In the area of administrative responsibilities, Cathy recently was in charge of a hospital-wide project to implement a new intravenous pump system, and she is currently the chair of a committee developing strategies for rewarding and retaining bedside nurses. She also actively participates in the planning activities for a new cardiovascular center being built on the hospital campus. Cathy's research activities focus on quality improvement and implementation of evidence-based practice within the hospital. She is active in interdisciplinary work, serving on the committees for conscious sedation, medication review, infectious disease, and diabetic education. In addition, Cathy teaches clinical cardiovascular nursing for a local nursing program.

◆ Nora Ladwig is a CNS in outpatient neurology and neurosurgery services in a tertiary medical center, which is part of a large multihospital system. Her work is multidisciplinary, involving support to nursing staff, physicians, and technicians in radiology and electroencephalography. She provides direct patient care on a consultation basis to patients and families who are struggling with managing their conditions and to acutely ill patients with neurological or neurosurgical needs who present in the outpatient clinics. In addition, she often coaches patients in how to discuss their conditions effectively with their physicians, and she leads support groups for patients with brain tumors and multiple sclerosis. Nora spends about half of her time in staff education activities focused on new technologies, new practice models, and new evidence-based practice interventions. She also does systemwide formal education presentations in neurology/neurosurgery and systems thinking. Nora has several administrative responsibilities, including participating in new staff interviews and in staff evaluations, chairing a hospital-wide committee on clinical policies and procedures, and participating on a regional system professional development council. She recently facilitated staff group discussions on diversity and age-specific interventions for the accreditation program of the hospital, and she works with a shared governance practice council to define practice competencies for outpatient staff in neurology and neurosurgery. Nora's employer has a robust nursing research program, and she is currently a data collector in a study examining nurse behaviors as they progress through novice to expert levels within the clinical practice model framework used at the medical center. In the quality improvement arena, Nora works closely with the staff in her units to identify quality concerns and to evaluate the outcomes of corrective actions implemented to resolve quality issues.

◆ Jeanne Stadler is a CNS specializing in wound and enterostomal care in a community hospital. She spends at least 50% of her time in direct patient care, doing assessments, care plans, and treatments for patients with significant skin, wound, or ostomy problems. She works collaboratively with other nursing staff and interdisciplinary team members to plan patient discharges and provide teaching to patients and family members regarding postdischarge wound and ostomy care. On a consultation basis, she also assesses and treats ambulatory patients referred to her by local physicians. Another function Jeanne provides is ongoing staff education to nurses and other team members regarding skin, wound, and ostomy care. She is responsible for identifying nursing competencies in this area and for developing self-study modules and other forms of learning for the staff. In addition, Jeanne functions as the academic liaison with 10 schools of nursing in the area, with the responsibility for arranging for student clinical practicum experiences at her hospital each semester. She is the lead in quality improvement monitoring for prevalence of incidents related to pressure ulcers, and she participates in unit-based research activities. Finally, Jeanne has several community-based responsibilities, including serving on advisory boards to two local nursing programs, sitting on the clinical board for the local home health and hospice agency, and representing her hospital on a community-based nursing research consortium. She also participates actively in her local specialty organization and supports her state nurses' association.

CURRENT CHALLENGES OF CLINICAL NURSE SPECIALIST PRACTICE

The health care system continues to be challenged by severe financial constraints, and mergers, reorganization, reengineering, and staff reductions often are used in response to this pressure. Some organizations have reduced or eliminated CNS positions in their quest to remain financially viable (Cohen et al., 2002; Dabbs,

Curran, & Lenz, 2000; Morrison, 2000). Increasingly, health care providers are being pressured to demonstrate the actual outcomes of their practice in order to justify their roles.

In part, because of the 50-year history of CNS practice, there is consistent evidence that CNS practice does improve health care outcomes, particularly in terms of quality, safety, and cost-effectiveness. In 2004, Fulton and Baldwin (2004) published their article "An Annotated Bibliography Reflecting CNS Practice and Outcomes" in the journal *Clinical Nurse Specialist*. This bibliography contains 70 research articles reflecting CNS practice outcomes, 7 of which were described as randomized clinical trials, the gold standard of clinical research. In addition, the bibliography contains 31 articles describing CNS program development and evaluation and 55 articles with anecdotal descriptions of CNS practice. Another recent article reviews studies regarding the outcomes of NP and CNS practice in acute and critical care settings (Kleinpell, 2002).

Fulton and Baldwin (2004) argue that "building an evidence base for practice is of the utmost importance" (p. 21). Certainly many CNSs would agree with this assertion. One significant barrier in this area is the lack of a standardized way to describe CNS practice. A pilot study in this area was published in 2000 (Dabbs, Curran, Lenz, 2000), but the work in developing a standardized database for CNS practice is in its beginning stages. Such a database would facilitate a standardized way of describing CNS practice, which could assist in the pursuit of receiving independent third-party reimbursement for CNS services. Currently, most third-party reimbursement for advanced practice nursing is limited to those APRNs who for the most part are carrying out diagnostic and treatment interventions for which physicians also are reimbursed (National Heritage Insurance Company, 2004). Unfortunately, the health care reimbursement system remains firmly geared toward physician practice, and in most instances, nurses are able to be reimbursed as independent practitioners only when they are performing in substitute roles for physicians. The issue here is that traditional nursing services, whether or not such services are specialized or expert, usually are not reimbursed independently by insurance carriers.

The lack of third-party reimbursement for CNS practice is one of the reasons there has been recent pressure to combine the CNS and NP roles (Lincoln, 2000; Scharer et al., 2003). During the past 20 years, the focus has been increasingly on developing innovative, sophisticated health care systems in ambulatory and community settings. Historically and currently, most persons receive the vast majority of their health care services outside of acute care hospitals. However, advanced practice nursing roles in ambulatory and community settings still are being established, and third-party reimbursement for such services is key to increasing nursing roles in this arena because most community-based settings cannot pay APRNs without some level of direct reimbursement for their practice. Literature describing CNS practice in ambulatory and community settings increasingly refers to clinical specialists with NP credentials (Girard, 2001; Hardin & Hussey, 2003; Scharer et al., 2003). In addition, many current studies regarding the outcomes of nursing practice roles do not distinguish between CNSs and NPs; the research models examine both roles under the concept of advanced practice nurse specialists (Brooten et al., 2002; Kleinpell, 2002).

More than a decade ago, Williams and Valdivieso (1994) published a descriptive study demonstrating significant differences in how CNSs and NPs carried out their practice roles. More recently, this study was replicated, and again CNS and NP practice roles were substantially different (Lincoln, 2000). Although CNSs and NPs perform essentially the same practice activities, the percentage of time spent in 22 out of 25 of those activities varies significantly between the two advanced practice specialties. Nurse practitioner practice focuses substantially on direct patient care (physical examinations/prescribing medications), whereas the CNS role includes a greater emphasis on patient care consultation, staff education, and research. Both roles include a great deal of patient teaching, but CNSs conduct more support groups. This leads to the conclusion that CNSs and NPs have overlapping roles, but the roles are distinct enough that both are needed in today's vast and complex health care system. "Instead of debating whether CNS and NP roles should be separated or merged, all APNs should be acknowledged for their contributions encouraging the continued variety, diversity, and evolution of APN roles" (p. 271).

Licensure at the advanced practice level is another challenge for CNS practice. For many years, the CNS practiced under his or her basic registered nurse license, which "authorizes the nurse to diagnose (nursing diagnoses) and to treat (nursing therapeutics) health related problems, as well as to execute prescribed medical regimens" (National Association of Clinical Nurse Specialists, 2003, p. 163). During the past three decades, advanced registered nurse practice has grown substantially, especially with the advent of the NP role. Although master's

degree preparation is rapidly becoming the current standard, it is not universally required for NP practice, and State Boards of Nursing became concerned about ensuring public safety with this new role. States began amending their Nurse Practice Acts by adding a new category of licensure and/or recognition for APRNs, for the most part including all four categories of advanced practice nurses. Currently all 50 states and the District of Columbia recognize APRNs in their practice acts, and 39 states and the District of Columbia include CNSs in their definitions of the APRN (Phillips, 2005).

One of the problems with current licensure laws is that many of the states require that APRNs be certified in their specialty, but for many CNSs, there are no certification examinations for their areas of practice. The other significant problem is that the APRN regulations tend to homogenize the distinct practice roles of advanced practice nurses, particularly blurring the distinctions between the NP and CNS roles. In some states, these two roles are combined into one, and CNSs have had to return to school to get NP training in order to continue to practice as APRNs (Lyon, 2004). This of course is a hardship and is inappropriate for those CNSs whose roles focus on specialty nursing practice rather than the more medically oriented NP practice. Another confusing area related to APRN regulation is prescriptive authority. Although it is a clear advantage for some CNSs to obtain prescriptive privileges as defined by their state Nurse Practice Acts, many CNSs can continue to practice successfully using standardized procedures, practice guidelines and protocols, and standing physician orders to provide care to their patients on drug regimens (O'Malley & Mains, 2003).

The National Association of Clinical Nurse Specialists is working proactively with the American Nurses Association, credentialing boards, other specialty organizations, and the National Council of State Boards of Nursing to clarify regulatory requirements and ensure that specialty certifications are available for all CNSs (National Association of Clinical Nurse Specialists, 2004a, 2004b). The National Association of Clinical Nurse Specialists has model state Nurse Practice Act language, as does the National Council of State Boards of Nursing, and there are substantial differences between the two (National Association of Clinical Nurse Specialists, 2005a; National Council of State Boards of Nursing, 2000). The issues are difficult, but given time, they probably will be resolved as the nursing profession continues to define and clarify the multiple roles and practice scopes that characterize this large, diverse profession.

Finally, the issue of appropriate educational preparation for CNS practice is a current challenge as the American Association of Colleges of Nursing continues to explore ways to prepare nurses appropriately in today's complex and knowledge-dependent health care system. The American Association of Colleges of Nursing (2005) recently proposed a master's-level program for a new role titled clinical nurse leader. In addition, this organization is recommending that master's programs preparing APRNs enrich and upgrade their programs to provide a doctor of nursing practice degree by 2015 (American Association of Colleges of Nursing, 2004a).

Compared with the CNS specialty practice role, the clinical nurse leader role has been characterized as an innovative leadership role practicing in all types of care settings. Educated at the master's level, clinical nurse leaders will have a solid theoretical foundation in health promotion, disease prevention, and risk reduction, as well as advanced concepts in illness and disease management, information technology, and diversity and global health perspectives (American Association of Colleges of Nursing, 2005). A recent publication from the American Association of Colleges of Nursing (2004b) developed by a group of CNS educators and American Association of Colleges of Nursing representatives compared the CNS and clinical nurse leader roles, concluding that despite some overlapping functions, both roles have different and complementary functions. The publication emphasized that CNSs function as expert clinicians, assisting nurses and patients while using specialized, advanced nursing practice competencies, whereas clinical nurse leaders function as generalists who manage and coordinate comprehensive care for populations and patient cohorts. At this time it is too early to predict the impact this new master's-prepared nursing role will have on CNS education or practice, but there is always the possibility that scarce resources may be directed away from CNS positions and educational programs to fund the implementation of this new role.

Likewise, the American Association of Colleges of Nursing position statement on substituting practice-focused doctoral degree programs for master's programs preparing advanced practice nurses will have a significant impact on nurses currently in those roles and on nurses who plan to become APRNs in the near future. Given the rapid evolvement of practice doctorates for many health care practitioners, including pharmacists, physical therapists, and occupational therapists, it is not unreasonable that the nursing profession move toward the practice doctorate as the preferred level of preparation for all nurses in advanced practice roles.

This level of preparation of course will be controversial within our large, diverse profession, but clinical specialists have a long tradition of "being ahead of the curve" in terms of graduate-level preparation, and after some dialogue with the multiple stakeholders in the ongoing debate over the DNP proposal, one can anticipate that they will support this latest effort to enhance and improve their educational preparation.

Despite many challenges facing CNSs, as expert clinician role models, teachers, and researchers, these APRNs have a profound impact on health care today. Their contributions to bringing about evidence-based practice changes are well-documented, and CNSs will continue to design and participate in studies that identify nursing outcomes and will serve as leaders in disseminating the findings of nursing research. In addition, they will continue to serve as direct care specialty practitioners, teachers, mentors, and researchers in our increasingly complex health care delivery system.

REFERENCES

American Association of Colleges of Nursing. (2004a). *AACN position statement on the practice doctorate in nursing: October 2004.* Retrieved April 25, 2005, from http://www.aacn.nche.edu/DNP/pdf/DNP.pdf

American Association of Colleges of Nursing. (2004b). *Working statement comparing the clinical nurse leader and clinical nurse specialist roles: Similarities, differences and complementarities.* Retrieved April 25, 2005, from http://www.aacn.nche.edu/CNL/pdf/CNLCNSComparisonTable.pdf

American Association of Colleges of Nursing. (2005). *Working paper on the role of the clinical nurse leader.* Retrieved October 30, 2005, from http://www.aacn.nche.edu/Publications/Whitepapers/ClinicalNurseLeader.htm

American Nurses Association. (1980). *Nursing: A social policy statement.* Kansas City, MO: Author.

American Nurses Association. (2003). *Nursing's social policy statement* (2nd ed.). Washington, DC: Author.

Berlinger, M. R. (1973). The preparation and roles of the clinical nurse specialist. In J. P. Riehl & J. W. McVay (Eds.), *The clinical nurse specialist: Interpretations* (pp. 100-107). New York: Appleton-Century-Crofts.

Brooten, D., Naylor, M. A., York, R., Brown, L. P., Munro, B. H., Hollingsworth, A. O., et al. (2002). Lessons learned from testing the quality cost model of advanced practice nursing (APN) transitional care. *Journal of Nursing Scholarship* 34(4), 369-375.

Brown, E. L. (1948). *Nursing for the future.* New York: Russell Sage Foundation.

Cohen, S. S., Crego, N., Cuming, R. G., & Smyth, M. (2002). The synergy model and the role of clinical nurse specialists in a multihospital system. *American Journal of Critical Care, 11*(5), 436-446.

Dabbs, A. D. V., Curran, C. R., & Lenz, E. R. (2000). A database to describe the practice component of the CNS role. *Clinical Nurse Specialist, 14*(4), 174-183.

Donahue, M. P. (1985). *Nursing: The finest art.* St. Louis, MO: Mosby.

Fulton, J. S., & Baldwin, K. (2004). An annotated bibliography reflecting CNS practice and outcomes. *Clinical Nurse Specialist, 18*(1), 21-39.

Georgopulous, B., & Christman, L. (1970). The clinical nurse specialist: A role model. *American Journal of Nursing, 70*(5), 1030-1039.

Girard, N. (2001). An overview of advanced practice nurses. *Seminars in Perioperative Nursing, 10*(4), 156-158.

Hamrick, A. B. (1989). History and overview of the CNS role. In A. B. Hamrick & J. A. Spross (Eds.), *The clinical nurse specialist in theory and practice* (2nd ed., pp. 3-18). Philadelphia: Saunders.

Hardin, S., & Hussey, L. (2003). AACN synergy model for patient care: Case study of a CHF patient. *Critical Care Nurse, 23*(1), 73-76.

Hoeffer, B., & Murphy, S. (1984). Specialization in nursing practice. In American Nurses Association (Ed.), *Issues in professional nursing practice,* part 2 (pp. 1-5). Kansas City, MO: American Nurses Association.

Kleinpell, R. M. (2002). What advanced practice nursing outcomes research is out there? *Critical Care Nursing Clinics of North America, 14*(3), 269-274.

Koetters, L. (1989). Clinical practice and direct patient care. In A. B. Hamrick & J. A. Spross (Eds.), *The clinical nurse specialist in theory and practice* (2nd ed., pp. 107-123). Philadelphia: Saunders.

Lincoln, P. E. (2000). Comparing CNS and NP role activities: A replication. *Clinical Nurse Specialist, 14*(6), 269-277.

Lyon, B. L. (2004). The CNS regulatory quagmire: We need clarity about advanced nursing practice. *Clinical Nurse Specialist, 18*(1), 9-13.

McClure, M. L. (1990, October 14-15). *Differentiating nursing practice into the 21st century.* Paper presented at the American Academy of Nursing 18th Annual Meeting, Charleston, SC.

Morrison, J. D. (2000). Evolution of the perioperative clinical nurse specialist role. *AORN Journal, 72*(2), 227-232.

National Association of Clinical Nurse Specialists. (2003). Regulatory credentialing of clinical nurse specialists. *Clinical Nurse Specialist, 17*(3), 163-169.

National Association of Clinical Nurse Specialists. (2004a). Executive summary of clinical nurse specialist regulatory summit. *Clinical Nurse Specialist, 18*(3), 116-117.

National Association of Clinical Nurse Specialists. (2004b). Proceedings: Clinical nurse specialist regulatory summit, July 16, 2004, Indianapolis, IN. *Clinical Nurse Specialist, 18*(6), 275-278.

National Association of Clinical Nurse Specialists. (2005a). *Model rules and regulations for CNS title protection and scope of practice.* Retrieved October 30, 2005, from http://www.nacns.org/updates/model_language.pdf

National Association of Clinical Nurse Specialists. (2005b). *What is a clinical nurse specialist? FAQs.* Retrieved January 4, 2005, from http://www.nacns.org/faqs.shtml/

National Council of State Boards of Nursing. (2000). *Proposed uniform advanced practice registered nurse licensure/authority to practice requirements: A supporting paper.* Retrieved April 22, 2005, from http://www.ncsbn.org/resources/complimentary_nocost_ncsbn.asp

National Heritage Insurance Company. (2004). *Physician assistant, nurses practitioner & clinical nurse specialist billing guide* (pp. 1-25). Los Angeles: Author.

National League for Nursing. (1958). *The education of the clinical specialist in psychiatric nursing.* New York: Author.

O'Malley, P., & Mains, J. (2003). Update on prescriptive authority for the clinical nurse specialist. *Clinical Nurse Specialist, 17*(4), 191-193.

Padilla, G. (1973). Clinical specialist research: Evaluation and recommendations, conclusions and implications. In J. P. Riehl & J. W. McVay (Eds.), *The clinical nurse specialist: Interpretations* (pp. 283-334). New York: Appleton-Century-Crofts.

Phillips, S. J. (2005). Seventeenth annual legislative update: A comprehensive look at the legislative issues affecting advanced nursing practice. *The Nurse Practitioner, 30*(1), 14-47.

Reiter, F. (1966). The clinical nursing approach. *Nursing Forum, 5*(1), 39-44.

Reiter, F. (1973). Improvement of nursing practice. In J. P. Riehl & J. W. McVay (Eds.), *The clinical nurse specialist: Interpretations* (pp. 9-18). New York: Appleton-Century-Crofts.

Sample, S. A. (1987). Justifying and structuring the CNS role within a nursing organization. In A. B. Hamrick & J. A. Spross (Eds.), *The clinical nurse specialist in theory and practice* (2nd ed., pp. 251-260). Philadelphia: Saunders.

Scharer, K., Boyd, M., Williams, C. A., & Head, K. (2003). Blending specialist and practitioner roles in psychiatric nursing: Experiences of graduates. *Journal of the American Psychiatric Nurses Association, 9*(4), 136-144.

Stafford, M. J. (1988). Margaret Stafford. In T. M. Schorr & A. Zimmerman (Eds.), *Making choices, taking chances: Nurse leaders tell their stories* (pp. 330). St. Louis, MO: Mosby.

Vaughn, M. (1968). Difficult task: Defining role of the clinical specialist. *Hospital Topics, 5*(18), 93-94.

Walker, J., Gerard, P. S., Bayley, E. W., Coeling, H., Clark, A. P., Dayhoff, N., et al. (2003). A description of clinical nurse specialist programs in the United States. *Clinical Nurse Specialist, 17*(1), 50-57.

Williams, C. A., & Valdivieso, G. C. (1994). Advanced practice models: A comparison of clinical nurse specialist and nurse practitioner activities. *Clinical Nurse Specialist, 8,* 311-318.

Nurse Practitioners

*Who They Are, What They Do, and
What Are Their Challenges?*

PATRICIA CLINTON

Nurse practitioners have provided health care for 40 years. For most, if not all, of that time, such care has been at considerable cost. Nurse practitioners have had to fight for every inch of their respective scopes of practice. These struggles have occurred in the legislative arena, on medical turf, and within the corridors of nursing. Yet they have persisted. The nurse practitioner role has expanded from primary care to include acute, chronic, and specialty care (Table 4-1).

Nurse practitioners were able to broaden their practice in many states through their legislative efforts and by educating health care institutions, providers, and the public about the value nurse practitioners bring to health care. At the national level, nurse practitioners have well-established professional organizations that employ professional lobbyists to move their legislative agendas forward. But the hard work still remains at the grass-roots level. In every state nurse practitioners need to be vigilant and prepared to protect their practice acts and to seek opportunities to expand their practice. In the words of Dr. Loretta Ford (Pearson, 2004, p. 9), "NPs are well prepared, politically savvy, committed to professional nursing values, and ready and willing to be counted on as patient advocates, case managers, and leaders in health care."

Despite Dr. Ford's words, nurse practitioners still find themselves all too frequently having to define who they are and what they do. Who they are is more often than not a function of which agency or organization is supplying the definition. State Boards of Nursing define nurse practitioners, state and national professional organizations define nurse practitioners, certification agencies define nurse practitioners, and federal law defines nurse practitioners. Although there are common threads in the definitions across these agencies, varying definitions do create problems. In general,

most definitions refer to a nurse practitioner as a registered nurse with additional knowledge and skills that permit the nurse practitioner to diagnose, treat, manage, and provide health services to a specific population. A nurse practitioner practices first under the registered nurse license and, depending on which state the nurse practices in, gains additional practice privileges and scope of practice by authority of the state. This differs from physician assistants who are not autonomous but practice under their supervising physician's license.

The nurse practitioner's scope of practice describes what nurse practitioners may do within a prescribed jurisdiction. Similar to the variety of definitions that describe nurse practitioners, scope of practice is defined by professional organizations (their own and others) and by state statutes and regulations. Definitions may be vague and general or specific and detailed about functions the nurse practitioner may perform, such as diagnosing, prescribing, and hospital admission privileges. Although the nurse practitioner practices independently of a physician's license, state statute or regulation may require some degree of physician involvement such as practice agreements, collaboratory agreements, or protocols.

Nurse practitioners must be absolutely clear about the scope of practice under which they provide services. In the event nurse practitioners deliver care outside of their scope of practice, they jeopardize their individual license to practice but also may threaten other nurse practitioners in the state by opening them up to scrutiny by competitors who would benefit by restricting nurse practitioner practice. For example, a pediatric nurse practitioner who prescribes drugs for the grandmother of a child seen in the nurse practitioner's practice is violating the scope of practice that is defined by the age of patients the nurse practitioner is permitted to attend.

TABLE 4-1

Nurse Practitioner Specializations

Primary Care	Acute Care	Specialty
Adult	Adult	Neonatal
Family	Pediatric	Psychiatric–
Gerontological		Mental Health
Pediatric		
Women's Health		

WHO THEY ARE

The role of the nurse practitioner emerged in the mid-1960s not solely as a response to physician shortage, but rather as an evolution of public health nursing. Two forces, the Western Interstate Commission on Higher Education for Nursing in which Dr. Loretta Ford played a prominent role and an encounter by Dr. Henry Silver at a Child Health Nursing Conference, resulted in a model of graduate nursing education that would focus on clinical specialization (Komnenich, 2005).

Primary Care Nurse Practitioners

In 1965 the first nurse practitioner program was opened in Colorado. The program was a pediatric nurse practitioner program that educated public health nurses in a model of well-child care, health promotion, and disease prevention. The paradigm of primary health care was used to prepare an advanced practice nurse who would specialize in pediatrics. These early practitioners would be known as pediatric associates or pediatric nurse practitioners. Other primary care clinical specializations soon followed and now include the adult nurse practitioner, the family nurse practitioner, the gerontological nurse practitioner, and women's health nurse practitioner.

A component of the scope of practice for each of the primary care nurse practitioner roles is defined by the population to whom the nurses provide care. Adult nurse practitioners care for adolescents and young, middle, and older adults. Family nurse practitioners provide care to persons from newborns to older adults including pregnant and postpartum women. The gerontological nurse practitioner directs care to elderly clients in classifications such as young-old, old, frail, and old-old clients. Pediatric nurse practitioners tend to children from birth to young adulthood according to developmental stages: newborns, infants, toddlers,

preschoolers, school-age children, adolescents, and young adults. The population on which women's health nurse practitioners focus includes women from menarche through the remainder of the life cycle. All of the primary care specialties share a common practice role: assessment of health status, diagnosis of health status, and treatment and management of health problems with the goal to return the client's health to a stable state and to optimize the client's health status (National Organization of Nurse Practitioner Faculties & American Association of Colleges of Nursing, 2002).

Primary care nurse practitioners practice in a variety of settings including community and public health clinics, private practice (both nurse practitioner and physician owned), school-based clinics, college health services, industrial sites, hospital clinics, and state and federal prisons. Additionally, nurse practitioners are an integral part of health care in the uniform services, providing health care services to personnel in the Army, Navy, Air Force, Public Health Service, and the Coast Guard.

Acute Care Nurse Practitioners

The additional knowledge and clinical skills used in assessing, diagnosing, and managing acute and chronic problems has enabled nurse practitioners to expand beyond the primary care model and now includes adult and pediatric acute care nurse practitioners, neonatal nurse practitioners, and psychiatric mental health nurse practitioners.

Acute care nurse practitioners are prepared in educational programs that focus on patients with complex acute, critical, and chronic health conditions that may include the delivery of acute care services (National Panel for Acute Care Nurse Practitioner Competencies, 2004). Programs for the acute care nurse practitioner may be oriented to adult or pediatric populations.

Most often, acute care nurse practitioners practice in critical care units and emergency departments, but they also may bridge care in specialty clinics. For example, a nurse practitioner with expertise in cardiac care may supervise a panel of patients and attend to them should they require hospitalization or critical care.

The neonatal nurse practitioner is an advanced practice nurse with extensive neonatal experience who manages the health care needs of newborns and infants and their families (National Association of Neonatal Nurses, 2001). "The NNP works within the context of the neonatal care unit in collaboration with neonatologists and pediatricians and makes independent and interdependent decisions in the assessment, diagnosis,

VIEWPOINTS

management, and evaluation of the health care needs of neonates and infants" (p. 1). Neonatal nurse practitioners function in all levels of newborn care, from normal newborn nurseries to level III neonatal units found in tertiary health care settings.

Blended Role

The psychiatric–mental health nurse practitioner represents the blended role of clinical nurse specialist and nurse practitioner. With the advent of the American Nurses Credentialing Center certification examination for adult and family psychiatric nurse practitioners, the clinical nurse specialist and nurse practitioner role and scope of practice have been more clearly differentiated. Bjorklund (2003) argues that the creation of a certification examination by American Nurses Credentialing Center was a positive step for self-realization by psychiatric nurses of the roles they perform. Because primary care adult and family nurse practitioners also screen and treat clients with mental health problems, it was important for psychiatric nurses to take ownership of the role and define their practice according to the scope and standards of practice of their specialty. Overlap remains between the clinical nurse specialist and nurse practitioner role in psychiatric nursing, and controversy related to which title is more appropriate for the individual practitioner undoubtedly will continue.

The psychiatric–mental health nurse practitioner's scope of practice is more restrictive than the primary care nurse practitioner's scope of practice. Primary care nurse practitioners screen clients for physiological pathological and mental health problems or illness within their specific population as defined by their scope of practice. Some primary care nurse practitioners also may manage clients with mental health illness. Psychiatric–mental health nurse practitioners are limited to the provision of psychiatric/mental health services only and not more general primary health care. The issue that arises is related to the link between education and practice. Adult and family nurse practitioners who were educated in programs that were focused only on primary care and did not receive additional psychiatric mental health content (such as group or individual counseling therapies) technically may be practicing outside of their scope of practice if their panel of patients is composed largely of clients with mental health diagnoses. These nurse practitioners could do postgraduate work in the psychiatric program to gain the additional knowledge and skills necessary. They may have to obtain certification and maintain dual certification in both specialties (Bjorklund, 2003).

CURRENT PRACTICE ENVIRONMENT

Nurse practitioners belong to the category of advanced practice nurses that includes clinical nurse specialists, certified registered nurse anesthetists, and certified nurse-midwives. Currently there are approximately 115,091 nurse practitioners in the United States (Phillips, 2005). Practice privileges vary widely across the country. Each state has an advanced practice nursing act that specifies who may be designated a nurse practitioner or advanced practice nurse and the practice privileges to which the nurse practitioner or advanced practice nurse is entitled. The ability to diagnose, treat, and prescribe drugs is specified in the state practice act. State Boards of Nursing, however, do not always have the final say in how the rules and regulations are applied to the nurse practitioner's practice. For example, boards of medicine and boards of pharmacy may be involved in determining and regulating prescriptive practice for nurse practitioners.

In 22 states the board of medicine has some control over the ability of the nurse practitioner to practice (Pearson, 2005). The extent of this control varies from some type of agreement or protocol between the nurse practitioner and the physician to direct supervision. In some states the agreements vary as to the degree of formality under which they exist. Some states require these agreements to be written, filed with the state, and regularly updated. In other states the requirement may be nothing more than a verbal agreement between the nurse practitioner and the physician.

Collaboratory agreements are common. Collaboration, as many nurse practitioners have discovered, is not always perceived by physicians as a reciprocal relationship between professionals, but rather, for some physicians, it is simply a euphemism for supervision. The ability of the medical profession to exercise power, influence, or authority over nursing practice, and especially advanced nursing practice, has been and is a source of frustration for nurse practitioners. Influence by the American Medical Association and the authority granted to the board of medicine in some states has affected the variation in nurse practitioner practice from state to state. For example, in Iowa, nurse practitioners practice with complete autonomy. They may diagnose, treat, and prescribe all types of devices and drugs, including schedule II through V controlled substances. Louisiana requires physician supervision over nurse practitioners who prescribe, although the supervision is not necessarily on site but clearly must be within a reasonable distance (Pearson, 2005).

Physician involvement in nurse practitioner practice most often involves the areas of diagnosis, treatment, and prescriptive privileges. Thirty states mandate some degree of physician involvement in these activities. A common method of involvement by physicians is the practice agreement discussed previously. Another type of physician involvement is chart review. Sixteen states require that a physician review charts. This may involve only an annual review of protocols or it may entail monthly review of charts and cosigning of certain orders to monthly review of a designated percentage of charts (Pearson, 2005).

EDUCATION

The education of nurse practitioners has changed since the early programs in the late 1960s and early 1970s. From the onset the educational programs always were intended to be at the master's level (Komnenich, 2005). However, as the need for advanced practice nurses became more acute, alternative programs emerged that, in some cases, granted a certificate verifying educational and clinical content. Programs for neonatal nurse practitioners and women's health practitioners are examples of advanced practice specialties for which the master's degree was not necessary when those roles first emerged.

Today virtually all nurse practitioner programs are at the graduate level or will be within the next few years. Some programs now grant a clinical doctorate as the entry into advanced practice. An interesting note is that only 32 states require the master of science in nursing (MSN) for nurse practitioner practice, and in a few states the degree is required only if the nurse practitioner seeks prescriptive authority. States may defer to certification agencies and educational institutions to set criteria for professional practice. Although eligibility requirements vary from certification agency to agency, most require the MSN as the educational base for advanced practice. Forty-two states require that a nurse practitioner hold certification as a prerequisite to practice (Pearson, 2005).

Many, if not most, nurse practitioner educational programs comply with educational standards and competencies developed by nursing and other institutions. Nurse practitioner programs most often frame their curriculum using the *Essentials of Master's Education for Advanced Practice Nursing* (American Association of Colleges of Nursing, 1996) and the *Criteria for Evaluation of Nurse Practitioner Programs* (National Task Force on Quality Nurse Practitioner Education, 2002) as guides. These documents identify core content and clinical skills that must be incorporated into master's-level education and advanced practice curriculum.

Professional organizations and certification agencies also may exert influence over nurse practitioner programs by requiring certain educational content pertinent to the specialty. Clinical practice hours and skills also may be specified by these institutions. The American Association of Nurse Anesthetists, the American College of Nurse-Midwives, and the Pediatric Nursing Certification Board are examples of organizations that directly or through certification councils stipulate educational and clinical requirements.

Continuing education for nurse practitioners varies. Maintenance of specialty certification may include requirements such as pharmacology content, advances in clinical knowledge, and clinical practice. State Boards of Nursing may require continuing education for license renewal and also may stipulate a specific number of content hours in pharmacology, for example, to retain prescriptive privileges.

CHALLENGES

Nurse practitioners represent the largest number of advanced practice nurses. Nurse practitioners vary by subspecialty and scope of practice, but they share similar challenges in the practice world. These challenges include reimbursement, education, and access to clients, and from the consumer's perspective, access to a nurse practitioner. Because of these challenges, nurse practitioners have found common ground in legislative and lobbying efforts to overcome issues of reimbursement, education, and access to care.

Reimbursement

Compensation for the provision of services is fundamental to professional viability. Education and certification are the primary criteria by which eligibility for nurse practitioner reimbursement is determined. For example, as of January 2003, nurse practitioners were required to obtain a provider number known as the unique physician identifier number (UPIN) for direct reimbursement from Medicare. To obtain the UPIN, the nurse practitioner was obliged to hold the MSN degree and to be certified by a recognized certification agency. Nurse practitioners without the degree or certification were able to obtain a Medicare provider number during a phase-in period before the January 2003 deadline. Those who failed to do so are now unable to receive direct reimbursement. The inability to receive Medicare reimbursement is a considerable impediment to practice for nurse practitioners. The circumstances just described illustrate a valuable lesson in responsibility and accountability that nurse practitioners should take to heart. Notification of this requirement was provided through professional organizations, professional newsletters, and other means of communication. Nurse practitioners continually must examine their practice, stay on top of rules and regulations (despite the burden that that task may occasion), and react accordingly. Accountability for the failure to respond and obtain the "credentials matched to their professional duties" (Buppert, 2004, p. 9) lies at the feet of the individual nurse practitioner, not with a State Board of Nursing, professional organization, or educational program.

Since 1997, nurse practitioners have been able to receive direct reimbursement from Medicare provided they have their UPIN and have complied with the requirements to obtain that number as discussed previously. Changes to this arrangement, however, are imminent. The Health Insurance Portability and Accountability Act passed in 1996 will require providers to use a new provider number for filing health care claims and transactions. The National Provider Identifier will replace all other numbers, including the UPIN. Phase-in for this program will occur from May 2005 to May 2008.

The greatest challenge to reimbursement for nurse practitioners, however, may come from physicians and their professional organizations. Health maintenance organizations and other providers are well aware of the cost savings and benefits of employing nurse practitioners. Yet it is not uncommon for nurse practitioners to bill under the physician title, in part because of the higher fees generated for billing under the physician provider number. Nurse practitioners in these situations are invisible to accounting. Aside from the revenue issue, billing under the physician title continues the myth of physician supervision. This is precisely why organized medicine fights so ferociously in many states at any attempt by nurse practitioners to broaden their scope of practice. The incentive for managed care is to control costs, keep premiums reasonable, and obtain satisfactory patient encounter outcomes (Kremer & Faut-Callahan, 2005). The bottom line of profits and losses in the end may prove more beneficial than legislative efforts to ensure reimbursement.

From a business standpoint, the strategy is to find the right provider mix of physicians, nurse practitioners, and physician assistants or other health care providers. Curiously, the Council on Graduate Medical Education that had long held the position that there was a physician surplus now contends that a significant shortage exists (Croasdale, 2003). Explanations of the change in predictions include younger physicians wanting to work fewer hours, aging population, increased demand for specialists, and liability issues (Croasdale, 2003; Elliott, 2004). The solution for the physician shortage according to the council is to increase medical school graduates by 15%. Increasing numbers of graduates does not address the issue of demographics (where physicians end up practicing) or how to distribute *health* services better and not *physician* services. Physicians tend to practice in metropolitan areas and shy away from underserved and lower socioeconomic populations (Elliott, 2004). Nurse practitioners traditionally have been the providers to step into this gap and provide health care, and there is no reason to believe that they will not continue to do so. Therefore nurse practitioners will need to continue to organize and invigorate their legislative efforts to secure recognition by third-party payers, to promote themselves as health care providers, and to resist efforts by physicians to limit nurse practitioner reimbursement or access to patients.

Nurse practitioners also may use interventions outside of traditional protocols such as complementary and alternative medicine to provide more integrative care. However, reimbursement for these therapies has been difficult to obtain. An alternative coding system known as the ABC code remedies this deficiency by providing a systematic process of applying appropriate codes and identification to alternative and complementary medicine and nursing interventions not otherwise covered. The ABC codes are under review by U.S. Department of Health and Human Services for inclusion under the Health Insurance Portability and Accountability Act. An extensive manual is available to assist nurses in using these codes (Alternative Link, 2005).

Education

The education of advanced practice nurses currently is part of a national debate revolving around entry into practice. The American Association of Colleges of Nursing (2004) has stipulated that by the year 2015 the educational preparation for advanced practice nurses (clinical nurse specialists, nurse anesthetists, nurse-midwives, and nurse practitioners) should be the doctor of nursing practice. This has raised a number of issues and concerns for academicians and clinicians alike. Task forces have been appointed to determine educational standards, clinical competencies, and how best to transition current MSN programs to the doctoral level.

Although change is generally uncomfortable, it is also a stimulus for growth. Raising the educational bar and requiring a practice doctorate for advanced practice nurses is a bold and (to some) controversial step. The development of core and specialty competencies through the National Organization of Nurse Practitioner Faculties has been a significant accomplishment that reaffirms the need for quality education but it also obliges programs to reevaluate their curricula and make the necessary curricular adjustments.

Many nurse practitioner programs today far exceed the academic credits for a master's degree required in other fields. Continuing to add courses to existing programs to bridge the knowledge gap only serves to increase the burden and undervalue the degree. The practice doctorate is envisioned as the terminal program for clinicians that will recognize the level to which practitioners must be educated to practice competently in today's health care environment.

If the practice doctorate is to be realized, it is imperative that deliberate and thoughtful conversations occur across professional organizations and academic institutions. These conversations must take a hard look at how practice would be affected and how educational programs would adapt. Healthy debate on the pros and cons of the standards and competencies that will emerge is the best way to guarantee excellence in programs. The concerns of nurse practitioners who are currently in practice are valid, and it is important to address these concerns. For example, how would nurse practitioners currently holding the MSN degree be able to obtain the doctor of nursing practice in an efficient manner? Will it be worth their while? Will State Boards of Nursing adopt the doctor of nursing practice as the entry for practice, and how will they deal with nurse practitioners who are not educated at that level? There is much to be gained in this endeavor, but the potential for failure is also possible. What the outcome will be remains to be seen, and it will be closely monitored by nurse practitioners, educators, and nursing leaders.

Access Issues for Nurse Practitioners and Clients

Safriet (2004) asserts that quality, cost-effective health care is in the public interest and that the issue of access plays an important role in serving the needs of the public. Nurse practitioners frequently cite access to clients as a significant barrier in their ability to practice. In part this may be attributable to a lack of knowledge of the nurse practitioner role by consumers, insurance carriers, legislators, or other health care providers. Despite the

40 years nurse practitioners have been providing care, they still must define themselves to patients, business managers, legislators, and sadly even other nurses.

Nurse practitioners experience a number of practice or role impediments that restrict access to clients. Among these are exclusion from provider panels, restrictive practice acts, opposition to independent nurse practitioner practice, and competition by other providers. To overcome these obstacles will require legislative action, education for the stakeholders, and aggressive grassroots activism. Access and reimbursement are intimately linked. If the desired outcome is to protect one's own economic well-being, then one strategy to accomplish that is to reduce competition from others. The previous discussion about physician shortage vis-à-vis financial motivation is pertinent in this case as well. If the problem truly is inaccessibility to health care services (and not physician services), then the solution must be to use the most qualified and effective health care provider, not necessarily increase the number of medical graduates (Pearson, 2004).

Legislators are lobbied heavily by the American Medical Association and other medical organizations to continue to restrict nurse practitioner practice by rules and regulations that require physician involvement through supervision, collaboration, or strategies such as chart review and practice agreements (Towers, 2004). No data exist that support the position that medical supervision is necessary for safe care. Physicians frequently state that their education and experience is necessary to diagnose the rare (zebras) and the common (horses) medical conditions. Aside from questioning how often physicians miss the zebras, it is important to remember that knowledge is not the exclusive domain of any one group (Safriet, 2004). Nurse practitioners through their education, experience, and clinical practice have ownership of that knowledge also; the science belongs to everyone.

The consumer also may encounter barriers that limit access to the nurse practitioner. For example, the ability to pay is crucial. If the consumer is uninsured or has limited health care coverage, access to care is not so much a barrier as it is a determination of whether health care is a right or a privilege. Ignoring the principles of preventative care and health promotion that are the cornerstone of primary care only delays the inevitable costly and chronic health problems that will occur. Other consumer barriers are related to urban planning issues such as lack of adequate transportation to health clinics, especially in rural areas but also in metropolitan areas with inadequate public transportation.

Communities without adequate (or any) health care providers should reexamine their request for a physician to provide care. Although the National Health Service Corps links providers to underserved communities, nurse practitioners are less likely to be marketed to these communities (Towers, 2004). Nurse practitioners must educate community leaders about the services they can provide and back up the education with the evidence available in the literature of quality, cost-effective care. The bottom line speaks to everyone. If nurse practitioners demonstrate to the consumer that they provide the same level of care as a physician and can provide care that embraces the nursing core values of holistic family-centered care, then half the battle will be won.

OPPORTUNITIES

The challenges that have been discussed are of course opportunities as well. Reimbursement may be problematic now, but if the barriers can be removed with continued pressure from nurse practitioners, consumers, and managed care, opportunities may arise for entrepreneurship and independent practice. Marketing to and educating consumers, legislators, and managed health care systems can affect accessibility issues by putting nurse practitioners where they can do the most good. Nurse practitioners must be able to participate at every level of policy making. Holding credentials that validate one's knowledge and expertise is fundamental to invitations to sit at the policy decision-making table. Raising the entry level into advanced practice from the master's degree to the practice doctorate is essential to realizing these goals.

The nurse practitioner of the twenty-first century must be able to participate fully in the delivery of quality and cost effective health care. The Institute of Medicine (2003) report *Health Professions Education: A Bridge for Quality* outlines five competencies that all health care professionals and clinicians should possess to deliver the type of care that will be needed in the twenty-first century:

◆ Provision of patient-centered care
◆ Interdisciplinary teams
◆ Evidence-based practice
◆ Quality improvement
◆ Informatics

Advanced practice nursing is well-positioned to incorporate and develop these competencies. Issues of patient safety, quality of care, and management of chronic conditions through skillful case management are fundamental to the core values of nursing. Informatics is an integral part of master's education, and evidenced-based practice is at the center of core competencies for advanced practice. More can be done to enhance and enlarge the depth and breadth of these competencies, but the foundation is there.

What appears to be the most prominent area of deficiency is the concept of interdisciplinary teams. Although lauded for years as the gold standard, interdisciplinary initiatives are relatively short-lived and depend on the vagaries of funding. An obstacle to realization of true interdisciplinary practice and education is that so much of one's professional identity is engaged in protecting an image and maintaining a prescribed role rather than reflecting on how the unique knowledge and skills one possesses could contribute to the best practice of health services for the consumer. Embracing the interdisciplinary model requires that one let go of outdated job descriptions and move in a different direction. The competencies proposed by the Institute of Medicine of patient centered care, evidenced-based practice, quality improvement and informatics are value neutral. No single profession can claim exclusive ownership of any of the competencies. However, everyone's best interest is to share the work that each profession has done in relation to each of the competencies and contribute that knowledge in an environment of interdisciplinary cooperation.

SUMMARY

Forty years ago the concept for the nurse practitioner was that of a nurse with additional skills that would alleviate provider shortages and deliver primary health care: screening, health promotion, and diagnosis and treatment of minor illness. Walk into hospitals across the country today and you will find nurse practitioners on virtually every service. Adult and pediatric acute care nurse practitioners practice in critical care units, neonatal nurse practitioners provide round-the-clock care to the sickest of newborns, and specialty services routinely have advanced practice nurses as part of the interdisciplinary team. Recent changes in resident medical training and a shortage of physician residencies has increased the demand for nurse practitioners (Cheek & Harshaw-Ellis, 2005). But the real benefits are the cost savings and improved patient outcomes when nurse practitioners care for patients (Brooten et al., 2002). Not surprisingly then, administrators are turning to nurse practitioners to assume more responsibilities and provide essential care in clinical settings strained by lack of health care providers.

Outside of the hospital, nurse practitioners are moving beyond a traditional physician practice and are setting up independent practices. Gaps in the health care system fueled by consumer demands for easy access to a health care provider for minor problems have resulted in drop-in, no-appointment, cash-only clinics in retail stores such as Target or Wal-Mart. These clinics provide consumers with health services such as screening, immunizations, and treatment for minor illnesses (Wojcik, 2004). They are not designed to be a medical home for the client. The advantage for the retail store is a customer base for their own on-site pharmacies. For the consumer, the advantage is no waiting and one-stop shopping for treatment of minor illnesses.

Expanding the role and services of nurse practitioners is an exciting opportunity, and the outlook for nurse practitioners in the next decade is optimistic. But nurse practitioners also must attend to the political and social ramifications that innovation generates. Once again, Dr. Lorretta Ford advises consensus among nurse practitioners and across professional nurse practitioner organizations:

> Change strategies will not lead to constructive action plans unless there is unity of philosophy and purpose in the nursing profession. Policy makers must sense our unity in our voices, our demands, and, if appropriate, our votes.
>
> If necessary, we should merge our organizations or form our own coalitions in order to prevent the erection of towers of Babel that will allow others to overpower and divide us (Pearson, 2004, p. 10).

Nurse practitioners have accomplished much in the past 40 years. But it is most important that nurse practitioners set aside disagreements among themselves and speak with one voice and one spirit. Nursing traditions and core values have positioned nurse practitioners in a place of trust and respect from the clients they serve. That trust and respect is what nurse practitioners must protect and nurture to ensure that they will be able to provide quality health care in an environment that supports independent and full scope of health care practice.

REFERENCES

Alternative Link. (2005). Retrieved October 13, 2005 from http://www.alternativelink.com/ali/home/

American Association of Colleges of Nursing. (1996). *Essentials of master's education for advanced practice nursing.* Washington, DC: Author.

American Association of Colleges of Nursing. (2004, October). *AACN adopts a new vision for the future of nursing education and practice.* Press release, retrieved January 22, 2005, from http://www.aacn.nche.edu/Media/NewsReleases/DNPRelease.htm

Bjorklund, P. (2003). The certified psychiatric nurse practitioner: Advanced practice psychiatric nursing reclaimed. *Archives of Psychiatric Nursing, 17*(2), 77-87.

Brooten, D., Naylor, M. D., York, R., Brown, L. P., Munro, B. H., Hollingsworth, A. O., et al. (2002). Lessons learned from testing the quality cost model of advanced practice nursing (APN) transitional care. *Journal of Nursing Scholarship, 34*(4), 369-375.

Buppert, C. (2004). Let's talk money: Match your activities with your credentials or get the credentials you need to do the job you want to do. *Nurse Practitioner World News, 9*(9), 1, 8.

Cheek, D. J., & Harshaw-Ellis, K. S. (2005). Advanced practice nurses in non-primary care roles: The evolution of specialty and acute care practices. In J. M. Stanley (Ed.), *Advanced practice nursing: Emphasizing common roles* (2nd ed., pp.146-157). Philadelphia: F.A. Davis.

Croasdale, M. (2003). *Federal advisory group predicts physician shortage looming.* Retrieved January 30, 2005, from http://www.ama-assn.org/amednews/2003/11/03/prsb1103.htm

Elliott, V. S. (2004). *Physician shortage predicted to spread.* Retrieved January 30, 2005, from http://www.ama-assn.org/amednews/2004/01/05/prl20105.htm

Institute of Medicine. (2003). *Health professions education: A bridge to quality.* Washington, DC: National Academies Press.

Komnenich, P. (2005). The evolution of advanced practice in nursing. In J. M. Stanley (Ed.), *Advanced practice nursing: Emphasizing common roles* (2nd ed., pp. 2-45). Philadelphia: F.A. Davis.

Kremer, M., & Faut-Callahan, M. (2005). Reimbursement for expanded professional nursing practice services. In J. M. Stanley (Ed.). *Advanced practice nursing: Emphasizing common roles* (2nd ed., pp. 187-225). Philadelphia: F.A. Davis.

National Association of Neonatal Nurses. (2001). *Position statement on advanced practice neonatal nurse role.* Petaluma, CA: Author.

National Organization of Nurse Practitioner Faculties & American Association of Colleges of Nursing. (2002). *Nurse practitioner primary care competencies in specialty areas.* Washington, DC: Department of Health and Human Services, Health Resources and Services Administration.

National Panel for Acute Care Nurse Practitioner Competencies. (2004). *Acute care nurse practitioner competencies.* Washington, DC: National Organization of Nurse Practitioner Faculties.

National Task Force on Quality Nurse Practitioner Education. (2002). *Criteria for evaluation of nurse practitioner programs.* Washington, DC: Author.

Pearson, L. J. (2004). Opinions, ideas, and convictions from NP's founding mother Dr. Loretta Ford. *Nurse Practitioner World News, 9*(12), 1, 9-10.

Pearson, L. J. (2005). The Pearson Report: A national overview of nurse practitioner legislation and healthcare issues. *American Journal for Nurse Practitioners, 9*(1), 9-136.

Phillips, S. J. (2005). Seventeenth annual legislative update. *The Nurse Practitioner, 30*(1), 14-47.

Safriet, B. (2004, June). *Regulatory issues for nurse practitioners.* Paper presented at the meeting of the Alliance for Nursing Certification Organizations, Washington, DC.

Towers, J. (2004, June) *Access 2010: Acting now for the future of healthcare.* Panel discussion at the American Academy of Nurse Practitioners, New Orleans, LA.

Wojcik, J. (2004). *Retail health clinics promise savings, convenience.* Retrieved June 2, 2005, from http://www.workforce.com/archive/article/23/82/35.php

Nurse Executives

Critical Thinking for Rapid Change

SUEEELLEN PINKERTON ◆ ROSE RIVERS

This chapter outlines several challenges that nurse executives face in rapidly changing health care environments. The purpose is to provide a basis for continued discussion, to stimulate readers to reflect on and think through the issues, and to motivate them to seek further information and dialogue.

The title of nurse executive is used for deans of colleges of nursing and vice presidents for nursing. However, in this chapter the focus is on nurses who fill the role of vice president for nursing or chief nursing officer (CNO) in acute care facilities or hospitals.

FACING RAPID CHANGE

Because the role of CNOs is broad, their preparation must be correspondingly broad. They are concerned with maximizing quality of patient care, meeting all regulatory requirements, maximizing competency and professional satisfaction of nursing staff, meeting the cost-effectiveness goals of the organization, maintaining relationships, and participating in short- and long-range strategic planning. As the lead professional nurse in the organization, the CNO is concerned with the governance and advancement of professional nursing practice. Additionally, the CNO serves as a liaison with the board of nursing to promote public safety; for example, systems in place to identify and manage impaired nurses.

Chief nursing officers are clinical and business leaders in the organization. They know how to coordinate care and the cost of such care. They can contribute to the growth of the organization and control patient outcomes. Nurses often have assumed responsibility for areas and departments other than nursing because of the breadth of their experience and talent. Also not unusual is to see nurses accept positions such as chief operating officer, chief executive officer, and human resource officer. Because of their knowledge and experience with coordinating care in the hospital 24 hours a day, 7 days a week, CNOs are prepared to step into many different operational roles in the organization. Given this shift in responsibilities, should nursing administration programs in schools of nursing offer courses or electives that help to prepare nurse executives for leadership in other departments? Is it limiting to the careers of CNOs to have the courses in the master's program focus exclusively on nursing?

Many different agencies seem to have an impact on restructuring and enhancing nursing and the CNO role. For example, some current job descriptions for CNO positions include as a candidate qualification a requirement that the nurse being recruited has had experience with a Magnet-designated facility. This is a result of the positive impact Magnet designation has had for health care facilities. The Forces of Magnetism, part of the criteria by which the Magnet-designated facilities are measured, also list requirements of the CNO in terms of education and impact within the organization. The CNO, for example, must possess a master's degree and by January 1, 2008, either the master's degree or baccalaureate degree must be in nursing (American Nurses Credentialing Center, 2004).

The Magnet application manual (American Nurses Credentialing Center, 2004) also lists the need for organizations to be in compliance with the practices recommended in the National Patient Safety Goals, which include things such as improving the effectiveness of communication among caregivers, the safety of using medications and infusion pumps, and reducing the risk of surgical fires and patient harm resulting from fires.

As part of their business role, nurse executives expect to be included in planning, development, and decision making of the governing body of the organization. Participation at the highest organizational level provides the CNO with an opportunity to influence organizational outcomes. However, for nurse executives to be excluded from business activities such as planning for new services still is not unusual, despite the fact that they are expected to support the services by providing competent nursing staff and in some instances leading the implementation. Nurse executives who are consistently excluded from such decision making yet are held accountable for nursing and patient-related outcomes eventually must confront the chief executive officer (CEO) or president with a rationale for inclusion. If a satisfactory resolution is not reached, the CNO must decide whether to leave or stay in the position. To stay is to support a system that may not value nursing contributions or to support a system that uses these tactics as a subtle devaluation of nursing participation and contributions. A CNO who stays also may miss an opportunity to develop business skills, which may mean restricting job mobility. In "Force 2: Organizational Structure," the Magnet application manual (American Nurses Credentialing Center, 2004, p. 38) states that "The CNO serves as an influential member of the organization's highest decision-making body for strategic planning and operations" and that supporting evidence must be supplied that demonstrates this involvement at the highest level of the organization.

This is an example of how an organization (American Nurses Credentialing Center) is helping to set the standards for the CNO and the responsibilities inherent in this role. This seems supportive to role development, especially in the aforementioned case, but is it where this influence should reside? What if there are standards and criteria that do not make sense for mainstream CNOs? How do CNOs influence the Magnet Commission if they are not a part of the Magnet application process? Does this situation limit the impact that a CNO can have on the standards being developed for her or his job, should they wish to comply or influence these standards without seeking Magnet designation? These are questions that need to be answered by CNOs as they refine their roles.

Another area of rapid change in nursing administration is related to the nursing shortage. The current shortage is predicted to have long-lasting effects because there are so many forces that are increasing the demand for nurses as the supply diminishes. Forces that repeatedly have been mentioned in the literature include (1) population growth, especially of the over-100 age group who need more care as they age because of the increased onset of illnesses and diseases, (2) an increase in chronic illness that requires more caregivers, and (3) advances in technology that require more skilled caregivers (nurses) to operate the technology and provide the complex care required as a result of the implementation of such technology (transplants). The decreasing supply of nurses is due to (1) a preference by women, traditionally the majority of nurses, for careers such as law, pharmacy, and medicine; (2) a decrease of nursing faculty resulting in limitations on nursing school enrollments; (3) a decline in growth of wages for nurses; and (4) the aging of the registered nurse workforce.

How should CNOs address the nursing shortage? Should they look for more roles to carve out of nursing? Should they try to take the issue to the policy level? The Robert Wood Johnson Executive Nurse Fellows Program brochure (Robert Wood Johnson Foundation, 2005, p. 2) states that the purpose of the program is to be "an advanced leadership program for nurses in senior executive roles in health services, public health and nursing education who aspire to help lead and shape the U.S. health care system." This is one way CNOs can learn how to influence policy and try to affect funding for research, training, and recruitment. Should CNOs contribute to the political action committee of the American Hospital Association to support candidates for public office or the political action committee of the American Nurses Association, which often supports opposing candidates? What is the impact of CNOs choosing not to be a member of the American Nurses Association since the association supports collective bargaining groups that are often at opposite sides of the table from the CNO at negotiations?

Should CNOs rely on national media campaigns, such as the Johnson & Johnson media campaign, to eventually change the image of nursing, especially negative images related to long working hours, hard work (mental and physical), and shift work? Will younger generations be driven by altruism to enter nursing, or will they remain true to their generation, seeking jobs that give them more freedom to pursue personal interests, with loyalty to self being more important than loyalty to the organization, a hallmark of the generation of nurses who are retiring?

Can the American Organization of Nurse Executives rally support for the nursing profession? Where is nursing leadership making an impact on factors that can address the nursing shortage? How should such efforts be organized? Which professional organization should nurse executives support? Are the nursing profession and its leadership still functioning as an oppressed group? Susan Roberts (1983) in her classic article "Oppressed Group Behavior: Implications for Nursing" purports that dominant groups, which in hospitals are hospital administrators (CEOs) and physicians, control and influence outcomes for subordinate groups such as nurses. The way to move groups out of the oppressed status is through deliberate and active nursing leadership, which brings us back to the question of current and future leadership of nurse executives. Are leaders supported? Is leadership united? Are we educating nurses as future leaders and future nurse executives? What is the CNO's role in succession planning?

CRITICAL THINKING

Embedded within the challenge of the nursing shortage, besides the challenge of leadership, are the challenges of relationships with hospital CEOs and physicians. Just how much can a nurse executive learn during her or his interview for a position? What critical thinking skills are needed to assess a position and the relationships that support the position? Can the nurse executive applicant get a sense of the support for nursing that the CEO demonstrates to the hospital board of directors? Does this really say anything about the CEO's support of nursing in daily operations of the organization? Is there a balance of discussions about financial and quality issues at the board of directors meetings? Does quality, when discussed, mean only medical care or does it include nursing care? Should the CNO be a voting member of the board of directors? Should this be negotiated before hire? What issues should a CNO consider in her or his decision to leave?

As the nurse leader in the organization, each nurse executive must have a "line" that she or he will not cross. If that line is crossed, the nurse executive seemingly has no choice but to resign. But what if leaving creates a worse situation for nursing staff and patients than remaining does for the nurse executive? Is the "line of no return" related to variance in staffing? Will the nursing shortage create situations intolerable for CNOs? Will "compassion fatigue" (Figley, 2003) be a factor for the CNO from her or his caring for the caregivers? Or can the CNO use the nursing shortage for some leverage? Is the line related to a continual devaluation of nursing? Is it related to sexual harassment? Is it related to substance abuse by the CEO? Where does the nurse executive find colleagues with whom to discuss such situations?

The other embedded relationships in the organization that are important to nursing are the relationships with physicians. What does it mean when a CNO addresses a group of physicians who will not return eye contact? Do physicians really want collaborative relationships with nurses? What are the generational differences among physicians that affect relationships with nursing? How much support should the CNO expect from the CEO in creating productive nurse/physician relationships? How strong should the relationship between the CNO and the physician chief of staff be to feel that there is a collaborative relationship between nursing and the physician staff?

SUMMARY

In all of the issues put forward, nursing leadership by the CNO is key, especially when the outlined situations occur in hospitals. The structures of hospitals and the nursing profession, however, are complex. Where does the CNO begin? Does it matter if a CNO focuses only on the hospital organization to promote change? Will CNO leadership in her or his hospital somehow affect another hospital? Should a CNO focus on creating excellence in her or his own hospital to attract and retain nurses and not worry about other hospitals? Are CNOs willing and able to "manage" other CNOs? Should the CNO abandon worrying about the direction and future of the nursing profession, essentially becoming isolated in her or his own environment? If not, how will nurses connect as a profession to ensure the continued development of nurse leaders and CNOs? Is there an organizational disadvantage to the CNO who has the responsibility of personal professional development that other leaders in operations do not have?

Will the spirit that nurses have always had be a central rallying point? Will the government through policy development help promote the continued growth of nursing? How should CNOs be involved? There is plenty to do. How will CNOs organize to do it? How will CNOs get it all done?

CASE STUDY

Ann Mason has been a vice president for 14 years. This is her second position as CNO, having been successful in her first position, which she left to take up the challenge of being a CNO in an academic health center with a college of nursing.

In her role as CNO, she is seen as a team player and has had responsibility for departments other than nursing. The nursing staff is unionized, but the union has not been active until recently. Ann is loyal to nursing. Actually, she is passionate about nursing. She has a PhD in nursing and is anxious to work in partnership with the college of nursing on research and knowledge generation. In her daily operations, Dr. Mason holds individuals accountable for their actions. She has been successful in putting a shared governance model in place and recently extended the model from nursing to include all departments.

Dr. Mason has a productive relationship with the medical staff. She is respected for her knowledge and actions. The quality of care is considered by physicians to be excellent. Ann is responsible to physicians, including them in decision making and working with them in collaborative partnerships. As part of the shared governance model, she established physician-nurse committees.

One week ago, Dr. Mason was told to make some budget cuts that would affect nursing practice at the bedside. She feels the cuts into her budget are too deep. Nonclinical vice presidents take a linear or oversimplified approach to address budget cut implications for nursing. They challenge Ann to divide the work among lesser-paid employees to achieve cost savings. Ann feels their suggestions do not take into account the complexities involved in delivering quality patient care.

Staff nurse reactions are starting to reach Dr. Mason. She thinks the staff feels she might be selling them out to a form of work redesign. How can Ann address staff nurse concerns? How can she communicate the principles driving her decision making? Her communication through the nurse managers is strained at this point because of their fear and what seems to be immobility and paralysis on their part. How can she gain the support and leadership of the nurse managers?

What should Ann lose sleep over? What evaluation criteria should she use to determine her effectiveness as the CNO? Ann wonders if she has a colleague with whom she can discuss these issues. Because she does not have a colleague in the institution, should she discuss her situation with a colleague at the local or national level? As Ann ponders the situation, she suddenly remembers the whimsical idea CNOs often entertain in tough situations: Is it time for me to leave and open my own boutique?

Should Ann leave or stay? Why? If she stays, what should her plan be for convincing her counterparts in administration? What elements can she use to make her points in a counterproposal (Kritek, 2002)? If her request for reconsideration is denied, should she rally the staff nurses and physicians?

How will she deal with the gap between staff nurses and the CNO? How can she convince the staff nurses she is not the enemy? What are the short- and long-term implications of involving other persons in the response to the request for budget cuts? Will it be seen as the CNO and her allies against the CEO and administration?

If she gets a positive response to her request, how will Ann work with administration to keep them updated about the needs of nursing at the bedside? Does she risk stepping over the hospital "loyalty" line in favor of the nursing profession? How as a CNO does she keep a balance?

Ann is all too aware of the potential human and business effects of a senior leader leaving an organization. If Ann decides to leave, what are some likely scenarios for the future of the staff nurses and for patient care? How will the change in nursing leadership affect nursing options? Will it make any difference if she leaves? Is a decision to leave from self-interest? How will she know if she is staying because she is afraid to leave? How can Ann ensure that she is playing to win instead of playing not to lose? Has she had all the crucial conversations necessary to make a decision? How can Dr. Mason get a good estimate of her own power in the organization?

Ann's situation is typical of the challenges many CNOs face in rapidly changing health care environments fraught with reimbursement issues, staffing shortages, increasing external regulations, and expanding scope of CNOs. Chief nursing officerss must possess highly developed critical thinking and negotiation skills to thrive in rapidly changing, volatile health care environments. Are CNOs adequately prepared to practice in such environments? Where do CNOs learn the necessary critical thinking skills to manage in rapidly changing environments?

REFERENCES

American Nurses Credentialing Center, Magnet Recognition Program. (2004). *Recognizing excellence in nursing services: Application manual 2005.* Silver Spring, MD: Author.

Figley, C. R. (2003). *Treating compassion fatigue.* New York: Brunner-Routledge.

Kritek, P. B. (2002). *Negotiating at an uneven table: Developing moral courage in resolving our conflicts* (2nd ed). San Francisco: Jossey-Bass.

Robert Wood Johnson Foundation. (2005). *Robert Wood Johnson executive nurse fellows program 2005 brochure.* Princeton, NJ: Author.

Roberts, S. J. (1983). Oppressed group behavior: Implications for nursing. *Advances in Nursing Science, 5*(4), 21-32.

Nursing Faculty

Opportunities and Challenges

PAULA R. MOBILY ◆ ANITA M. STINEMAN

T he nursing shortage has heightened the visibility of the nursing profession and has placed nursing education in the spotlight. Changes in the delivery of health care and the demographics of the population are requiring that nurses develop a different skill set to be effective leaders and patient care providers. This chapter discusses some of the major issues affecting nursing education as nurses prepare for the twenty-first century.

SHORTAGE OF FACULTY

In the past few years, considerable concern and attention have been devoted to the shortage of nurses, but somewhat less attention has been devoted to the current and impending shortage of nursing faculty. The shortage of nursing faculty, however, presents one of the most pressing problems facing the profession. A shortage of faculty is clearly interwoven with the current and projected national shortage of nurses. Educational programs are necessary to supply more nurses, but the shortage of available faculty will limit student enrollments and numbers of graduates. The shortage of nurses will offer additional career opportunities and job choices within the profession, thereby decreasing the number of nurses selecting graduate education and an academic career (Hinshaw, 2001; Lewallen, Crane, Letvak, Jones, & Hu, 2003). Because nursing faculty often are the primary source of nursing research, a decrease in the number of nursing faculty will decrease concomitantly the number of individuals conducting research and the development of the knowledge base required for excellence in nursing practice. These factors ultimately limit the number of professional leaders to shape health policy in the state, national, and international arenas (Hinshaw, 2001).

According to the American Association of Colleges of Nursing (2003, p. 1), "the deficit of faculty has reached critical proportions." In 2005, the American Association of Colleges of Nursing (AACN) released data noting a nurse faculty vacancy rate of 8.6%. This is an increase in the vacancy rate of 7.4% the AACN reported in 2000. Although this vacancy rate may seem insignificant, vacant positions can seriously affect the numbers of students admitted to existing programs and subsequently affect the workload of the remaining faculty. Further, despite accelerating interest in baccalaureate and graduate nursing education programs, not all applicants are being accepted at 4-year colleges and universities. The AACN (2005) reports that 32,797 qualified applicants were not accepted into schools of nursing in 2004 primarily because of a shortage of faculty and resource constraints. Of those who were denied admission, 29,425 had applied to entry-level baccalaureate programs; 422 to registered nurse–bachelor of science programs; 2748 to master's programs; and 202 to doctoral programs. Insufficient faculty was cited as the primary reason for not accepting all qualified students.

Multiple factors are creating this shortage of nursing faculty. Two major categories appear to encompass these factors and will be used as a framework for discussion: the aging of current faculty often referred to as the "graying of the professoriat" and declining interest in an academic career.

Graying of the Professoriat

The AACN conducts a survey of faculty in baccalaureate and higher-degree nursing programs each fall, and faculty age continues to climb. According to the most recent AACN report (2004a), the median age of full-time faculty in baccalaureate and graduate programs in nursing is 51.5 years; the average age of doctorally prepared nurse faculty holding the ranks of professor, associate professor, or assistant professor was 56.8, 54.6, and 50.8 years, respectively; and the average age for all faculty ranks prepared at the master's degree level was 49.0 years. Similarly, the proportion of faculty older than 50 years has increased from 50.7% in 1993 to 70.3% in 2001. This is a strong indicator of the problem that deans in nursing education face in the United States.

Given the average age of nursing faculty, it is not surprising that a wave of faculty retirements is expected over the next decade. On average, nursing faculty retire at the age of 62.5 years, and faculty 65 years and older account for only 3% or less of faculty (AACN, 2004a; AACN, 2003). The American Association of Colleges of Nursing projects that from the years 2003 to 2012, between 200 and 300 doctorally prepared nurse faculty will be eligible for retirement annually and that from 2012 to 2018, between 220 and 280 master's-prepared nurse faculty will be eligible for retirement. As many educational institutions face growing economic issues, early retirement incentives may increase faculty attrition further.

The problem of the nursing faculty shortage is compounded by the lack of individuals to replace the older generation of faculty. Not only has there been a concomitant decrease of 17.3% in the age groups of faculty 36 to 45 years (AACN, 2003), but other trends have surfaced that narrow the pipeline for replacing the current generation of nursing faculty. Master's and doctoral programs in nursing are not producing a pool of applicants sufficient to meet the future demand for nurse educators. Fewer graduate nurses are selecting academic or teaching careers in nursing, and those that choose nursing education tend to enter academia later in their careers and have fewer years of productivity (AACN, 2004a; Brendtro & Hegge, 2000; Hinshaw, 2001).

Declining Interest in an Academic Career

The reasons that fewer nurses with graduate degrees are selecting academic careers include increasing opportunities outside academia, noncompetitive salaries in academia, and faculty workload and expectation issues. A recent AACN (2003) White Paper on "Faculty Shortages in Baccalaureate and Graduate Nursing Programs" noted that "egression from academic life is the major reason for the loss of younger faculty members" (p. 2). An AACN survey of 280 nursing programs reporting faculty resignation data in 2002 revealed that 188 full-time doctorally prepared faculty and 202 master's-prepared faculty resigned from schools of nursing. Of these, 56.2% of those with doctoral degrees left to take other faculty or administrative positions in academia, but 43.8% left academia to assume nonacademic positions such as nursing service, private sector, or private practice positions; and 43% of those with master's preparation resigned to take nonacademic jobs.

Similarly, of the 457 doctoral graduates in 2001-2002, 28.6% reported employment commitments in nonacademic settings (Berlin, Stennett, & Bednash, 2003). Data from the *Survey of Earned Doctorates* (National Opinion Research Center, 2001) revealed that the percent of nursing doctoral recipients planning to be employed in nonacademic settings increased steadily from 15.5% for 1980 to 1984 to 26.9% for 1995 to 1999. Teaching as a primary employment activity decreased from 70.8% to 59.5% during the same two periods.

Why are the nonacademic positions becoming more appealing? Corporate organizations often use the leadership and research skills of doctorally prepared nurses in positions that reinforce and use competencies in research and administration most highly valued by doctorally prepared nurses (Hinshaw, 2001). Conversely, most graduate programs do not provide the opportunity for developing knowledge and expertise in teaching, and graduates may not be as comfortable with the teaching role inherent in academia.

In a recent editorial in *Nursing Outlook*, Marion Broome (2003) posits that one of the primary characteristics of nursing academia that makes it less than attractive to many potential doctoral students contemplating a career in nursing education is the lack of an intellectually stimulating and growth-enhancing environment. She argues that the majority of faculty has become "bored and tired" and the result is a lack of intellectual debate and creative dialogue that previously challenged those in an academic environment, sharpened critical thinking skills, and infused the environment with a sense of excitement. She believes these changes in the academic environment are recognized by doctoral students and diminishes their interest in an academic career.

Salary differentials between academic and other positions often are cited as an influential factor contributing to the nursing faculty shortage. When comparing the responsibilities and salaries associated with various employment opportunities open to nurses with graduate degrees, faculty positions are often less appealing. Given the economic constraints faced by most colleges and universities, average salaries for clinical positions have risen more than those for faculty positions (AACN, 2004a). Also, graduate study has become more expensive as the fees for tuition and expenses have increased, and many potential students weigh more carefully whether it profits them to seek graduate study and enter academia when they often earn better salaries in nonacademic clinical positions.

Anderson (2002) poses an intriguing and important question in terms of nursing faculty salaries. She concurs that nurses with advanced education can earn more in clinical or administrative positions, but she also notes that a discrepancy exists between academic and practice salaries in many disciplines such as the other health professions, law, and engineering. In these other professions, salaries of faculty typically are well above the campus mean because of the market. She questions why the economic concept of supply and demand does not work in terms of the nursing faculty shortage. Is this related to the fact that academic nursing is a female-dominated profession and therefore not as highly valued by the institution, or might it be related to the fact that many nurse educators lack the doctoral degree, thereby marginalizing nursing faculty?

Issues related to faculty workload and role expectations are connected closely to the faculty shortage. Those who select academic careers and are on the tenure track have high expectations related to teaching, research, and service; and balancing these is critical but often difficult. For many, the high expectations associated with these roles compromise the ability to do all of them well, thus contributing to role stress and job dissatisfaction. As many institutions strive to increase their national standing, expectations for promotion and tenure increase concomitantly. New faculty working toward tenure may be expected to do more than their senior colleagues, causing anxieties for the individual and additional tensions between the two groups. Many faculty perceive that expectations are unclear or evolving, further contributing to their sense of stress and overload.

Because of the shortage of faculty, many institutions now offer nontenured clinical-track positions. Faculty in these positions typically carry heavier teaching loads and provide the majority of the clinical teaching but also are expected to be "productive" in terms of service and professional scholarship or practice. As this new role evolves in academic settings, stress and job dissatisfaction for these faculty is common.

As noted by Longin (2002), the life of the college professor has changed considerably since the late 1980s. Now more than ever, faculty have varied responsibilities and stressors. In addition to the traditional teaching role, they also are expected to obtain extramural funding, conduct research, produce scholarship, and provide community and university service. In addition, most faculty spend a significant amount of time advising and mentoring students outside the classroom, updating curricula, developing new courses, maintaining their knowledge base and clinical expertise in an ever-expanding field, and mastering new advances in technology. As noted by Berberet and McMillin (2002),

73% of faculty express frustration at "never having time to complete a piece of work" (p. 9).

Diversity in Educational Preparation

Remember the era when there was much discussion about obtaining the correct patient care mix? How many registered nurses, licensed practical nurses, and unlicensed assistive personnel were needed to provide quality care? Now a similar discussion can be heard in the halls of academia—only it pertains to the educational preparation of faculty needed to maintain a quality nursing education program. What is the right mix of tenure-track and nontenure clinical-track faculty?

To maintain the mission of research-intensive institutions, there is no question that the faculty on the tenure track need to be doctorally prepared. These are the faculty who will be responsible for teaching courses in the doctoral programs. But what about the time-intensive clinical courses in the undergraduate programs and the nurse practitioner programs that require faculty certification in the specialty area? Tenure-track faculty cannot afford to be responsible for undergraduate clinical courses without sacrificing their program of research. Nursing programs are hiring faculty to fill these roles that do not meet criteria for tenure-track (i.e., not doctorally prepared) or are not interested in fulfilling the requirements of a program of research and grant writing to obtain external funding. These individuals often assume clinical-track positions that focus on excellence in clinical teaching and practice.

Ideally, the two groups would function in harmony, each respecting the contributions of the other, but as with anything new, pains occur with change. Equity issues abound related to workload, involvement in program governance, decision making related to curriculum matters, and criteria for promotion and retention.

Nurse practitioner faculty are essential for graduate programs preparing students to function as advanced practice nurses. However, to maintain their certification, they must verify completion of a specified number of practice hours. Institutions are working to establish faculty practice arrangements that would offer opportunities to implement best practices based on outcome research. This venue would enable clinical faculty to maintain and enhance their direct and/or indirect care skills—skills that are invaluable when mentoring nursing students during their learning process. However, financial sustainability remains one of the most formidable issues facing the establishment of these enterprises. Consequently, the issue of incorporating faculty practice time into the workload of clinical-track faculty remains unresolved for many nursing programs.

Scholarship is an expectation for tenure-track and clinical-track faculty. That tenure-track faculty are expected to have data-based publications in peer-reviewed journals is well established. What constitutes scholarship for clinical-track faculty? Publications that focus on clinical topics and use of research in clinical practice are appropriate. Are there other types of activities that also could constitute scholarship? Consider the contribution that could be made to the profession by development of a continuing education program related to a clinical topic, development of an innovative teaching method or materials, participation as a collaborator in a clinical study, or serving as an item writer for the National Council of State Boards.

Resolution of issues related to tenure-track and clinical-track equity must be resolved to prevent the development of a two-tier system in educational institutions. The contributions of each are significant to maintaining the quality of nursing education programs and to the advancement of the profession.

PREPARING NURSES FOR THE TWENTY-FIRST CENTURY

Significant and dynamic changes in society and the health care environment, coupled with the need to prepare nurses to practice in such an environment, have resulted in unprecedented challenges for nurse educators. These changes in turn create external and internal pressures on today's nursing faculty.

External Pressures

To prepare nurses with the knowledge and competencies needed to function effectively in the current and emerging health care delivery system, nursing education must respond to mandates and standards from nursing education organizations such as the AACN and National League of Nursing, among others, and mandates from health care and government bodies. Although it is essential that nursing education curricula reflect these mandates and standards, it becomes challenging and stressful for nurse educators to stay current with these and incorporate them into their courses and curricula. Although it is beyond the scope of this chapter to discuss all of the potential external mandates, a few are highlighted.

As major professional nursing organizations, the AACN and National League for Nursing provide direction for nursing education and the profession at large.

The AACN, the national voice for baccalaureate and graduate nursing programs, works to establish quality standards for bachelor's and graduate degree nursing education, assist deans and directors to implement those standards, influence the nursing profession to improve health care, and promote public support of baccalaureate and graduate education, research, and practice in nursing. In addition to identifying competencies for baccalaureate education (AACN, 1998), more recently the AACN (2004b) has developed position statements and recommendations related to the development of a master's-prepared clinical nurse leader, which builds on the identified baccalaureate competencies. In addition, the AACN has championed the establishment of accelerated bachelor of science in nursing and master of science in nursing programs, has accelerated bachelor of science in nursing to doctor of philosophy programs, and has endorsed the doctor of nursing practice.

The stated mission of the National League of Nursing is to advance quality nursing education to prepare the nursing workforce to meet the needs of diverse populations in an ever-changing health care environment. To this end the National League of Nursing sets standards to advance excellence and innovation in nursing education. Recent publications such as the position statement on "Innovation in Nursing Education: A Call for Reform" (2003) and the more recent position statement "Transforming Nursing Education" (2005) provide recommendations for changes in nursing education curricula.

In addition to professional nursing organizations, a number of external constituencies influence nursing education, including mandates from the government in the form of health objectives. Published by the U.S. Department of Health and Human Services, *Healthy People 2010* (2000) provides a comprehensive set of disease prevention and health promotion objectives for the United States to achieve over the first decade of the twenty-first century. The report identifies a wide range of public health priorities and specific, measurable objectives.

In 2001 the Institute of Medicine released a report, *Crossing the Quality Chasm: A New Health System for the 21st Century,* from the Committee on Quality of Health Care in America that makes an urgent call for fundamental changes in the American health care system by offering a set of performance expectations. This report provides overarching principles for specific direction for policy makers, health care leaders, clinicians, regulators, and health profession educators, among others. The report sets out a vision for all programs engaged in clinical education, recommending educational reform and the implementation of a core set of competencies.

More recently, the World Health Organization (2005) issued a publication titled *Preparing a Health Care Workforce for the 21st Century: the Challenge of Chronic Conditions.* This publication calls for the transformation of health care workforce training because of the rapid escalation in chronic health problems and presents a new and expanded training model based on a set of core competencies for all members of the health care workforce.

The need to address certain competencies in nursing education comes not only from organizations such as those noted but also from a myriad of professional or specialization groups within nursing. Nursing faculty increasingly are expected to capitalize on the most recent trends in knowledge and health care delivery by incorporating content and competencies related to evidence-based practice, informatics, and genetics, to name a few. Clearly, this need to make nursing education responsive to all of these differing but important groups can seriously challenge nursing faculty as they try to determine the principles and competencies that should or must be included and redesign courses and/or curricula to reflect these.

Internal Pressures

Notwithstanding the pressures and expectations from external constituencies, a number of internal factors create challenges for today's nurse educators. Change in academia is ever present: in the way higher education is conducted; in the traditional roles of teaching, research, and service; and in the characteristics of today's students. These changes challenge faculty and require time and preparation in order to be successful in the faculty role (AACN, 2004a).

A comprehensive discussion of all of the internal pressures facing faculty is not within the scope of this chapter; and, as such, those that are placing the greatest demands on today's nursing faculty are addressed briefly. These include fiscal challenges, maintaining or increasing enrollments, provision of quality experiences for today's diverse student populations, development and use of alternative teaching strategies, and recruitment and retention of students and faculty of diversity.

Despite the need to educate more nurses in response to the nursing shortage, most institutions of higher learning and nursing education programs are faced with economic and fiscal challenges. As more and more programs face the challenges of "doing more with less," faculty within these programs are affected significantly.

Times of resource constraint require nursing education programs to develop creative approaches to maximize faculty resources and to accommodate larger numbers of students. Resource constraint is forcing administrators to consolidate or eliminate courses, have faculty teach more courses, and often teach courses outside their area of expertise. To attract and reach a greater number of students, faculty are being asked to develop online courses—a task that can be time intensive and overwhelming. At the same time, efforts to secure research or extramural funding are intensifying. All of these situations create the need for additional faculty time and efforts when time is already a limited commodity.

Increasingly, nursing faculty are challenged to provide quality educational experiences for a more nontraditional population of students. According to the U.S. Department of Education (2002), almost 73% of undergraduate students are considered "nontraditional" by virtue of their older age, more independent financial status, delayed entry into higher education, and competing responsibilities such as jobs and families. These nontraditional students place new demands on faculty to provide a relevant, no-nonsense approach to education that is immediately applicable and complementary to their lives. The challenge for faculty is to plan more creative, practical, and interactive teaching-learning strategies. Though valued by the students, these strategies often are time intensive for faculty to develop and monitor.

Additionally, faculty are challenged by a broad range of student capabilities ranging from at-risk to exceptional. Those at-risk require additional academic help, advising, and monitoring, whereas those who are exceptional often are interested in advanced or enrichment opportunities. Faculty who provide clinical instruction are responsible for an increasing number of ill patients or are working to develop new partnerships with clinical agencies and clinical preceptors. No wonder then that many faculty may feel stressed with their teaching responsibilities; and, for those with research or scholarship expectations, this stress may contribute to job dissatisfaction, emotional exhaustion, burnout, and possibly resignation or retirement.

Reflective of the changing learning and work environments, faculty now increasingly are expected to develop proficiency in distance education/distance learning technologies. No longer is the lecture method of imparting information seen as ideal, but designing a course that replaces lectures with interactive and/or multimedia materials often requires more technical know-how than most faculty possess. The importance of distance technology and Web-based media to deliver educational course work is revolutionizing academia; however, developing well-designed and effective courses is daunting and time consuming.

Cultural competence throughout the health system will be strengthened with a health care workforce that is representative of the diversity in the population. The cultural challenges presented by patients with more diverse demographics can best be addressed by health professionals educated in a culturally dynamic environment (Sullivan Commission, 2004). To achieve this environment, academic institutions are incorporating student and faculty diversity into their strategic plans.

Increasing student diversity requires new and creative strategies for recruitment and retention of these students and new and creative nontraditional teaching strategies to meet their needs. New initiatives to improve the retention and graduation rates of students from different racial and ethnic backgrounds are essential to the success of this endeavor, but many faculty are challenged to relate to students from different cultures who having varying backgrounds, learning styles, and needs.

In 2002, more than 90% of the full-time faculty in nursing programs were white, and 95% or more were female. These figures have remained unchanged since 1996 (Rosenfeld, Kovner, & Valiga, 2002). This stagnation in the diversity of nursing faculty is occurring at a time when America's population is becoming increasingly diverse. A more diverse faculty will enhance the leadership and mentoring needed by minority students.

FACULTY DEVELOPMENT

The landscape for nursing education is changing. Some of the factors that have accelerated this change are the paradigm shift in educational methodology from teacher-centered learning to the focus on student-centered learning and an introduction of new types of technology that are not only altering the ways students can access courses but also challenging faculty to change the design, delivery, and evaluation of the courses they teach. To maintain quality in nursing graduates, nurse educators must maintain the skills needed by faculty to be able effectively to facilitate student learning. A comprehensive development program for "educators" at all levels of academic experience can contribute to maintaining quality outcomes in graduates, increasing satisfaction with the faculty role, and serving as a strong recruitment and retention strategy.

Public concern about the nursing shortage is driving nursing programs to increase enrollments in the midst of a faculty shortage. Nursing programs are increasing reliance on part-time clinical/adjunct faculty and are filling full-time positions with individuals who have limited, if any, teaching experience. When combined, these factors create a significant need for faculty development for new and experienced faculty. As the educational needs of faculty change throughout their careers, institutions need to take responsibility for meeting these ongoing developmental needs to increase the efficiency and effectiveness of faculty and to increase satisfaction with their careers in academia.

Nurse educators automatically envision some type of orientation for new faculty. But how well this is occurring is questionable. The norm for most institutions is that new faculty orientation, spanning a limited number of days, focuses on the policies and procedures for the nursing program and is a time to learn about the institution and the services offered to students and faculty. Although this information is needed, much more must be included to assist new faculty successfully to assume the role of a top-notch educator.

Orientation for new faculty should continue throughout their first year. New educators who have limited teaching experience and perhaps no background in educational principles will need additional support for the development of their courses, preparation for lecture/classroom activities, and construction of various tools to assess student learning. If their teaching assignments include any online instruction, additional support must be provided for the use of any course management system and its components, guidelines to facilitate successful online discussions, and innovative ways to engage students to create an active learning environment. Plans for this comprehensive orientation of new faculty must be individualized, requiring the faculty member to take an active role in identifying specific learning needs.

Teaching is only one part of the tripartite mission that must be addressed in the development of new faculty. Research/scholarship and service should not be overlooked. Without ongoing support, the new faculty member can become so overwhelmed with the new responsibilities of teaching that the development of a program of research suffers. Development of support groups can be effective. The benefits of a support group go beyond assisting new faculty to develop their research focus, it also is a mechanism for the socialization of individuals into the professional role of nursing educator and provides a network of individuals that the new faculty can feel comfortable turning to for advice.

Although a support group for new faculty can be effective, a mentoring program also should be established. This process involves a senior faculty member taking a personal interest in the success of the more junior individual and facilitating adjustment and success in the organization. The time commitment to mentor a new faculty member effectively may seem burdensome for the senior faculty member who is involved heavily in meeting her or his own tripartite responsibilities, but this type of sharing of skills and insights seems to be a critical component in successful faculty development programs and the retention of new faculty (Genrich & Pappas, 1997). The incorporation of innovative approaches to the mentoring of new faculty needs further investigation and development.

As enrollments in nursing programs increase, a growing number of individuals are being hired on a part-time basis to teach clinical courses. Many nursing programs are meeting the need for clinical instructors by moving to a preceptor model for student clinical experiences. To enable students to receive quality clinical experiences, nurse educators must properly prepare those who are facilitating that learning. Although use of the preceptor model is a key strategy for building capacity in nursing programs, the developmental needs of these individuals as "educators" must be addressed. Although they may be excellent clinicians who can expose students to innovative clinical practices, they often have no background in educational theory to guide their interactions with students.

Clinical instructors and preceptors must understand the outcomes to be accomplished by the students. With this as a basis, their developmental program can focus on how students learn in a clinical environment and effective methods to guide that process, ways to develop critical thinking, how to question students and provide feedback, and how to observe students to evaluate their performance and document achievement of course outcomes. If the time and energy is taken to prepare these individuals properly for their roles, they may become excited about the educator role and become future faculty. A quality experience does not happen by itself, the guidance of a prepared instructor is needed to plan and facilitate the learning.

This same philosophy also could be applied to teaching assistants, graduate students who are paid a stipend to assist faculty with their courses. The bottom line remains the same: greater satisfaction with their role as an educator can be gained by the teaching assistants if they participate in a developmental program to assist them in understanding how students learn and approaches they can use to be more effective in achieving their responsibilities. If nurse educators can excite teaching assistants about being nurse educators, they could include formal nursing education course work as a part of their graduate plan of study. When seeking their initial faculty position, they would be equipped with an entry-level educational skill set that would promote a beginning level of comfort with the educational component of their faculty role.

The developmental needs of individuals who have established careers as faculty in an academic setting should not be overlooked when it comes to the design of a comprehensive faculty development plan. Needs change over the course of a career. Many of these individuals may have developed expertise as a teacher, but with changes in the educational environment, new learning needs arise that must be addressed. Examples of some of these changes may include advancements in technology available for use in the classroom (simulators, handheld electronic devices) and the technology needed to offer online courses, how best to match outcomes and technology use, or knowledge about current student characteristics and learning needs. Finally, as faculty take on leadership positions, they may find that they need assistance in developing a new skill set to be effective in this new role.

SUMMARY

The expectations for a nursing educator are great. Nursing education is a demanding career that needs the brightest and most creative among its ranks. The dynamic challenges faced by educators should be seen as opportunities for leadership and professional growth. The bottom line is that nurse educators affect the lives of many students, patients, families, and populations. The rewards experienced are priceless to nurse educators and to society.

REFERENCES

American Association of Colleges of Nursing. (1998). *The essentials of baccalaureate education for professional nursing practice*. Washington, DC: Author.

American Association of Colleges of Nursing. (2000). *Special survey on vacant faculty positions (unpublished data)*. Washington, DC: Author.

American Association of Colleges of Nursing. (2002). *Faculty resignations and retirements (unpublished data)*. Washington, DC: Author.

American Association of Colleges of Nursing. (2003). *Faculty shortages in baccalaureate and graduate nursing programs: Scope of the problem and strategies for expanding the supply.* Retrieved May 19, 2005, from http://www.aacn.nche.edu/Publications/WhitePapers/FacultyShortages.htm

American Association of Colleges of Nursing. (2004a). *2004-2005 enrollment and graduations in baccalaureate and graduate programs in nursing.* Washington, DC: Author.

American Association of Colleges of Nursing. (2004b). *Working paper on the role of the clinical nurse leader.* Retrieved May 19, 2005, from www.aacn.nche.edu/Publications/docs/CNL6-04.DOC

American Association of Colleges of Nursing. (2005). *New data confirms shortage of nursing school faculty hinders efforts to address the nation's nursing shortage.* Retrieved May 29, 2005, from http://www.aacn.nche.edu/Media/NewReleases/2005/Enrollments05.htm

Berberet, J., & McMillin, L. (2002, Spring). The American professorate in transition. *AGB Priorities,* (18), 1-15. Washington, DC: Association of Governing Boards of Universities and Colleges.

Berlin, L. E., & Sechrist, K. R. (2002). The shortage of doctorally prepared nursing faculty: A dire situation. *Nursing Outlook, 50*(2), 50-56.

Berlin, L. E, Stennett, J., & Bednash, G. D. (2003). *2002-2003 enrollment and graduations in baccalaureate and graduate programs in nursing.* Washington, DC: American Association of Colleges of Nursing.

Brendtro, M., & Hegge, M. (2000). Nursing faculty: One generation away from extinction? *Journal of Professional Nursing, 16,* 97-103.

Broome, M. E. (2003). We are the future: Revisioning the faculty culture. *Nursing Outlook, 51*(3), 97-98.

Genrich, S., & Pappas, A. (1997). Retooling faculty orientation. *Journal of Professional Nursing, 13*(2), 84-89.

Hinshaw, A. S. (2001). A continuing challenge: The shortage of educationally prepared nursing faculty. *Online Journal of Issues in Nursing, 6*(1) Manuscript 3. Retrieved May 29, 2005, from http://www.nursingworld.org/ojin/topic14/tpc14_3.htm

Institute of Medicine (Committee on Quality of Health Care in America). (2001). *Crossing the quality chasm: A new health system for the 21st century.* Washington, DC: National Academic Press.

Lewallen, L., Crane, P., Levtak, S., Jones, E., & Hu, J. (2003). An innovative strategy to enhance new faculty success. *Nursing Outlook, 24*(5), 257-260.

Longin, T. C. (2002, Spring). Towards a 21st century academe. *AGB Priorities* (18), 16. Washington, DC: Association of Governing Boards of Universities and Colleges.

National League for Nursing. (2003). *Innovation in nursing education: A call to reform* [Position statement]. Retrieved May 25, 2005, from www.nln.org/aboutnln/PositionStatements/innovation.htm

National League for Nursing. (2005). *Transforming nursing education.* New York: Author.

National Opinion Research Center. (2001). *Survey of earned doctorates* [Unpublished special reports generated for the American Association of Colleges of Nursing]. Chicago: National Opinion Research Center.

Rosenfeld, P., Kovner, C., & Valiga, T. (Eds.). (2002). *Nurse educators 2002: Report of the faculty census survey of RN and graduate programs.* New York: National League for Nursing.

Sullivan Commission. (2004). *Missing persons: Minorities in the health professions.* Retrieved May 26, 2005, from http://www.aacn.nche.edu/Media/pdf/SullivanReport.pdf

U.S. Department of Education. National Center for Education Statistics. (2002). *Nontraditional undergraduates.* NCES 2002-012. Washington, DC: Susan Chong.

U.S. Department of Health and Human Services. (2000). *Healthy people 2010: Understanding and improving health* (2nd ed.). Washington, DC: U.S. Government Printing Office.

World Health Organization. (2005). *Preparing a health care workforce for the 21st century: The challenge of chronic conditions.* Retrieved May 29, 2005, from http://www.who.int/chronic_conditions/resources/en/workforce_report.pdf

Nurse Researchers

*Who They Are, What They Do, and
What Are Their Challenges?*

NANCY A. STOTTS ◆ DEIDRE WIPKE-TEVIS

Nurse researchers are scientists who seek to find answers to questions through methodical observation and experimentation. They design studies, conduct research, and disseminate findings at professional meetings and in peer-reviewed journals.

Nurse researchers seek to advance the science of care through systematic investigation. The work they do is diverse. The design of the studies spans the scope from qualitative to quantitative research. The research encompasses interviews, epidemiological surveys, large databases, controlled clinical trials, and basic science experiments. The topics addressed by their research are broad and divergent, reflecting the vast scope of practice of nursing and the rich heritage of nursing in the biological and social sciences. Nurse researchers study individuals, families, and communities and health care systems. Nurse researchers also are basic scientists whose laboratory work ranges from proteonomics to systems physiology. A great deal of variety exists in the cluster of persons who call themselves nurse researchers and in the nature of their work.

This chapter is designed to introduce you to the world of nurse researchers. It will answer the following questions: Who are nurse researchers? What do they do? What challenges do they face?

WHO ARE NURSE RESEARCHERS?

Nurse researchers are nurses who participate in systematic study of topics related to nursing. They seek to develop the science behind evidence-based practice and understand the fundamental cellular and humanistic laws that have implications for health and illness.

Historically, most nurse researchers began their career as staff nurses and progressed up the clinical ladder. Several pathways led to the role of the nurse researcher.

Some had always dreamed of being a faculty member in a school of nursing, and research is an integral part of that role in major research-intensive institutions. Others realized they did not want administrative responsibilities in the clinical arena, so they chose research as an alternative way to progress in nursing. Another group was overcome with a desire to understand "why" and "what is the mechanism," and they used research to find the answers. A fourth group just happened into a job and fell in love with the work of research. Today, a new breed of researchers is introduced to research early in nursing education, and they elect to prepare themselves as nurse researchers by moving rapidly into graduate programs, thus bypassing the many years of clinical practice that in the past have characterized nurse researchers.

As with most other disciplines, doctoral preparation is required to be a scientist and scholar in nursing. Although previously many nurses earned a doctor of philosophy (PhD) in another discipline (e.g., psychology, statistics, or physiology) or in an allied field such as education, this track has become less common in recent years. Usually the degree obtained is a PhD with a major in nursing, a doctor of nursing science (DNS, DSN, or DNSc), or a doctor of nursing. In the purest sense the PhD is designed to prepare a nurse researcher, and the DNS is conceptualized as preparing an advanced clinician, parallel to the doctor of medicine but with the substantive focus being nursing; however, in practice, there often has been little difference in the curriculum in the PhD program and the DNS program. Currently, there is interest in the development of a practice doctorate, with the nurse completing the program earning a doctor of nursing practice. This doctoral degree is designed to prepare nurses as advanced practice clinicians with expanded research and leadership skills (American Association of Colleges of Nursing, 2004).

Doctorally prepared nurses are equipped to carry out all aspects of the research process. They have been taught and actually have carried out the process of conceptualizing a problem, formulating a question and/or a hypothesis, designing the study, collecting the data, analyzing the data, and reporting the findings. This process is encompassed in their dissertation research, a requirement for graduation.

As nurses progress through the academic system, they begin to learn the research process by working initially as a research assistant. Classically, the research assistant is an undergraduate or graduate student who is working for a faculty member. The responsibilities of the research assistant include conducting a library search as the basis for the literature review, collecting data, or entering data into the computer for later analysis. In the most ideal world, the research assistant is an integral member of the research team, learning process and content through this paid or volunteer position.

The next level of researcher is a research nurse. This nurse usually is bachelor's or master's prepared and is hired to recruit subjects, collect and manage data, or to carry out specific aspects of the research that have been planned by the researcher(s) who wrote the grant. The term *project director* is used for the research nurse who assumes major responsibility for coordinating and implementing the research study.

Co-investigators are researchers who have expertise in a specific area and share the responsibilities of conceptualizing and conducting the study. They are asked to participate for a variety of reasons. They may have substantive expertise (e.g., wound healing or social support), exceptional knowledge in a research method (e.g., phenomenology or high-performance liquid chromatography), are recognized for understanding a statistical analysis technique (e.g., survival analysis or meta-analysis), or have access to a potential subject population (e.g., persons with diabetes). One or more co-investigators may be on a grant, depending on the nature of the project and the expertise of the various team members. Consultants also have expertise in a specific area, but their contribution is more circumscribed than that of a co-investigator.

The leader of the research team is the principal investigator, the person who is responsible not only for writing the grant but also ultimately for the scientific conduct of the research project. This means that this researcher needs to bring the team together, define the roles of the members, and see that the conceptual work is completed. Later, the prinicpal investigator will ensure that the study is conducted, the data are analyzed, and the results are presented and published. The prinicpal investigator sets the tone for how the team works together. The research team may be run with a democratic or autocratic style; one approach is not better than the other; the approaches just produce different dynamics, and each style has its own strengths and limitations. The prinicpal investigator also initiates discussions about authorship of articles and plans with team members the nature of publications and order of authorship. This proactive negotiation sets a tone for fairness and parity in the team. When students are part of the research team, their contribution and role needs to be addressed in the negotiations.

It is important to recognize that many research teams are interdisciplinary. The research team may consist of physicians, social workers, physical therapists, basic scientists, or other scholars with a PhD. The nurse may be the principal investigator or a co-investigator or may have any of the other roles described. To work on an interdisciplinary team is a rich experience, especially when all members of the team leave their titles behind and bring the full measure of their expertise to the research team and the research process. Ideally, a student experiences this as a member of the team.

Thus nurse researchers are nurses who do research. They usually are doctorally prepared. They may design and conduct the entire project or be responsible for only a portion of the research. They use a variety of research designs and methods, including surveys, interviews, clinical trials, evaluation research, and basic science techniques. They function with a variety of titles and roles. The work they accomplish is diverse and reflects the heterogeneity of nursing. The role a specific researcher occupies depends on the nature of the study, the various personalities of the team members, the expertise of the researcher, and timing or serendipity.

WHAT DO NURSE RESEARCHERS DO?

The research process outlines the type of thinking and activities in which nurse researchers engage. For a study to take place, the researcher must identify a problem and must have sufficient interest and expertise in the problem to address it. Seasoned researchers have an identified program of research and know the literature in that substantive area. Often they have a long list of questions that they would like to answer. They need only time and funding to address them. Newer researchers have an evolving set of research questions the foundation of which has come from their dissertation. This set of questions forms the basis for developing a program of research.

Knowledge of funding sources is an integral part of the role of the researcher, because without funding, research productivity is significantly limited. The major source of funding for health care research is the National Institutes of Health. Although the National Institute for Nursing Research (NINR) is an important source of funding for nursing research, other institutes such as the National Institute on Aging or National Heart, Lung, and Blood Institute may fund nurse researchers.

The researcher must understand the NINR and National Institutes of Health priorities for funding. The priorities are based on identification of needs for scientific knowledge for health care. The NINR Roadmap for the future indicates funding priorities in "changing lifestyle behaviors, managing effects of chronic illness to improve health and quality of life, identifying effective strategies to reduce health disparities, harnessing advanced technologies to serve human needs, enhancing the end-of-life experience for patients and their families" (Grady, 2004, p. 97). These topics have been identified as significant to the health and welfare of the American people, and so future NINR funding will focus on these topics.

Grants are also available from public and private foundations and professional organizations (Box 7-1). Each organization has its own funding priorities, budget limits, and application process. In the library are books that specifically address funding sources, and increasingly those data are available on the World Wide Web. The contracts and grants division in most research-intensive universities also provides assistance to faculty in understanding the multiple sources and processes for obtaining financial support for research. A specific funding source usually is targeted early in the proposal development process so the explicit criteria for a given funding source are incorporated into the proposal.

The first step to writing a grant proposal is the identification of an important research question. For the seasoned scientist, the next research study typically is formulated in the course of conducting and analyzing data from a previous study. For the novice researcher, generating a research idea usually involves analyzing the existing research literature to understand what has been done already in the field and identifying one or more "gaps" that need answering. Regardless of how the research idea is generated, the researcher critically analyzes the literature and puts the proposed study in the context of the published literature. The researcher makes a case for the significance of the problem to be studied. Reviewing the literature also helps in the development of the study procedures because using established approaches and instruments increases the validity and reliability of the data that are obtained in the study.

When a new area of study is embarked upon, often pilot work needs to be undertaken. The process for grant application for pilot work is the same as applying for a major grant; however, because pilot work usually can be done more inexpensively, the sources of funding may be different from those needed for a larger project.

A crucial aspect of grant writing is the development of a budget. This involves determining the costs for conducting the research. The researcher must step through the entire research process and estimate costs for a wide variety of expenditures including personnel, laboratory renovations, travel expenses, computers and specialty software, equipment and related supplies, laboratory fees, data collection tools, advertisements, photocopying and office supplies, subject and/or mileage reimbursement, data analysis, and publication costs. Although this sounds relatively easy to do, it is a sophisticated skill. For example, in calculating staff costs, one item to consider is recruitment of subjects. The researcher must know the number of subjects who must be screened, the proportion who will meet the study criteria, and some estimate of how many will consent to participate and in what time period. The researcher also must include in the calculation attrition rate from drop out or death. Part of the consideration is also how sick the potential subjects are, the amount of burden that the study imposes, and what the subject will gain by participating. All these factors need to be considered when calculating the amount of time it will take to recruit subjects, the level of personnel required to do the job, and the amount of subject reimbursement required to compensate participants fairly. Because a grant award is a fixed amount of money, the budget must be planned carefully, monitored closely, and adjusted throughout the study to account for unexpected expenses and inflation.

Thus far the general activities of the nurse researcher have been discussed. One must recognize that in part the researcher's employer determines what the nurse researcher does. Researchers are employed by colleges and universities or by industry, or they may be self-employed and work by contract or do consultation.

In the college or university community, researchers typically serve in the academic series or research series. The person in the academic series classically is in a tenure-track position in which research/creative work is one criterion for progression in rank. Research needs to be completed, but time also needs to be devoted to teaching, professional competence, and university and public service. Thus most nurse researchers in the academic series are not solely researchers. The nurse researchers in the academic series are usually on "hard money" (i.e., university or college funds), and grant funding is used to offset a part of their salary so release time is available to conduct the study. One also must realize that some colleges and universities allow their faculty little time to devote to research, and participation in research depends on the mission of the institution and how it is implemented.

In the research series the researcher is hired specifically to conduct his or her own studies or to be employed as a member of someone else's research team. Persons in the research series are funded entirely from grant money or "soft money." Successful nurses in this series are productive, flexible, and creative because their position lasts only as long as they are funded by grants. Individuals in the research series typically do not have a teaching assignment; however, some level of service to the institution may be a role expectation.

Nurse researchers employed by industry (e.g., pharmaceutical companies) often are hired because they bridge the gap between clinical practice and the basic sciences. They often are responsible for overseeing the clinical research testing of the company's products. This researcher often is responsible for locating sites to conduct the studies, identifying a principal investigator, setting up multisite studies, training the project coordinator at each site, performing site visits to ensure that the protocol is conducted consistently and that data are recorded in a manner that allows for analysis by site and for pooling of data across settings. Often the nurse researcher employed by industry must understand the requirements of the Food Drug Administration for the testing of new products, so that the protocol developed and data gathered will meet the scrutiny required for ultimate approval of the product.

Nurse researchers who are self-employed contract with others for specific services. The type of services offered and the cost vary widely. Some researchers do primarily data analysis, others assist with design of the study, and others combine their substantive nursing expertise (e.g., cardiovascular nursing of adults) with research skills. Their income depends on developing a set of clients with ongoing needs or being so well known that new clients are referred to them consistently.

Thus in summary, nurse researchers are prepared to actualize all aspects of the research process. They may be responsible for the entire study or a portion of it.

They may work in academia or industry or may be self-employed. Much heterogeneity exists in what nurse researchers do.

WHAT CHALLENGES DO NURSE RESEARCHERS FACE?

Nurse researchers face a myriad of challenges (Box 7-1). Among them are limited availability of start-up funding; defining why nursing research is important to nursing practice; developing intradiscipline respect for nurse researchers whose substantive focus or research methods differs from one's own; continuing to define the discipline of nursing through nursing research in a changing health care arena; limited availability of space for data collection; acquiring access to potential research subjects; obtaining national-level funding in a world of shrinking fiscal resources; and implementing the study.

In the basic science arena a newly hired researcher is given a start-up package. Depending on the type of research, the equipment necessary to perform the research, and whether the researcher is bringing any equipment from a previous job, the start-up package often consists of thousands of dollars. Historically, schools of nursing have not had the monies available to offer a start-up package to new faculty members. This can be particularly problematic in the case of biological research for which expensive instrumentation may be required. To obtain national-level funding, the gold standard in academia, preliminary data are necessary; however, the only grant funding with a sufficiently large budget to purchase much of the need equipment is a national-level grant. In many cases, nurse researchers become creative, however, and borrow equipment from a collaborator or rent equipment with funds from a small seed grant.

Within nursing and from outside the profession, there is limited appreciation of the need for nursing research. Research in nursing has been viewed as an activity of nursing students, one of the hoops to jump

BOX 7-1

Challenges Nurse Researchers Face

Limited start-up funding
Devaluation of nursing research
Disagreements about research methods
Limited availability of space for data collection
Limited access to population of interest
Limited availability of funding for ongoing research program

through to graduate rather than being important to the development of the discipline and practice of nursing. This conclusion does not seem overwhelmingly surprising, because in the past, few nurses conducted research. More recently, however, nurses are expected to use the best available evidence to make patient care decisions to improve health care outcomes and to decrease costs (Polit & Beck, 2004). Consequently, nursing research and the translation of nursing research to the bedside are becoming recognized as essential components of evidence-based nursing practice.

Only recently have researchers in nursing been recognized for their program of research. Drew and colleagues, whose research is in electrocardiography (Adams & Drew, 2002; Drew et al., 2002; Pelter, Adams, & Drew, 2003), are an example of important nursing research with significant clinical implications. Interdisciplinary work is illustrated by the work of Miaskowski et al. (2004) in behavioral strategies to modulate cancer pain. Multicenter studies also contribute significantly because large samples that would be unavailable at a single institution can be enrolled to answer clinically important questions (Puntillo et al., 2001).

Within the nurse researcher community there seems to be a lack of support for researchers whose substantive content or research methods differ from one's own. The battle is between quantitative and qualitative methods and between basic science laboratory research and applied clinical studies (Wipke-Tevis & Williams, 2002). Although some of the conflict is honest discussion and an effort to understand by comparing and contrasting, the lack of support has been divisive and detracts from nursing research. A kinder and more broad-minded approach that encourages understanding of differences and appreciation of the types of knowledge that can be produced with different approaches allows nurse researchers to focus their energies on generating science rather than defending their substantive content or research method. Ultimately, the research question being asked should drive the method(s) used, and a need exists for building a scientific basis for care, regardless of the research method selected.

Another challenge for nurse researchers is to continue to define the discipline of nursing through research in a changing health care arena. The nature of nursing is changing continually because of economic forces such as the costs of disease prevention and treatment rise. Less expensive care may not be better care. Nursing has not defined well its unique contribution to health care, and the discipline is in jeopardy of being marginalized in this period when interventions are being linked tightly to outcomes. Recently, nurse researchers whose research focus is health care systems and outcomes have begun to demonstrate the importance of quality nursing care in decreasing mortality in hospitalized patients (Aiken, Clarke, Sloane, Sochalski, & Silber, 2002; Aiken, Clarke, Cheung, Sloane, & Silber, 2003).

Because maintaining an active clinical practice typically is not required of faculty members within a school of nursing, nurse researchers seldom have their own caseload of patients. Thus when the time comes to recruit subjects for research, gaining access to potential subjects may be a challenge. If the sample needed is healthy subjects, physician approval may not be needed and advertising in newspapers or posting flyers in the community is sufficient. If the sample involves patients with a particular disease process, access to patients depends on the openness of the patient's primary care provider to having the subject studied and the collaborative relationship that the nurse researcher has established with health care providers. Other considerations that may affect access to patients are the numbers of studies being conducted at a given site, the direct potential financial benefit of the study to the health care team, and whether the researcher is seen as someone who might "steal" patients from the primary care provider's practice.

Another challenge is limited funding. Funding available from the NINR for nursing studies is limited, and nurse researchers compete directly with each other and with scientists in other National Institutes of Health institutes. The benefit of research to the consumer needs more emphasis to help leverage funding from the public and private sector. One approach to this is to focus for a period on translational research in which the emphasis is on research utilization and the effects research findings have on outcomes. However, there must be a fine balance between creating knowledge and finding ways to use it, and funding for the pipeline of knowledge must not be sacrificed for immediate use.

Implementing the research study brings its own unique challenges. A local committee called the institutional review board must review the proposal before initiation of the project. The institutional review board determines whether the risks associated with the study are reasonable with respect to the potential benefits and the knowledge to be gained. Potential risks include not only risk of physical harm (which may be negligible in many nursing research studies) but also emotional distress, breech of confidentiality, and legal risks. Furthermore, depending on the amount of risk involved with the project and type of data being collected (individually identifiable personal health information versus non–personally identifiable data), oral or written informed consent of the participants and a Health Insurance Portability and Accountability Act authorization may be required (Wipke-Tevis, 2001; Olsen, 2003).

Several categories of vulnerable populations for which the institutional review board requires special precautions include minors, cognitively impaired adults, pregnant women, fetuses, prisoners, and those who do not read, speak, or understand English. Depending on the type of vulnerability, the institutional review board will require special adaptations. For example, parents give approval for research with their children and when the child is of an age of understanding, the child must give assent. The same process is applicable when cognitively impaired adults are present; that is, the person with legal authority provides consent and the potential research subject provides assent, if able. Special guidelines are applicable for other categories of the vulnerable such as prisoners. The protections provided may increase the challenges of the researcher who must obtain informed consent. In fact, Geluda et al. (2005) suggest that third-party consent is a major obstacle to research in these populations and the researcher must accommodate the research plan to address the slow recruitment that often results.

Recruitment of subjects offers its own challenges, for example, developing the methods to screen and obtain consent from potential subjects. Perhaps your study examines pain in patients with long bone fracture and you want to follow them from the emergency department, through hospitalization, and into the community. How will you identify subjects? You could hire a research assistant to sit in the emergency department and identify cases as they enter the system. Or perhaps you might elect to pay the ward clerk a fee to page you when a person meeting the inclusion criteria arrives. Alternatively, you might invite the head nurse in the emergency department to work as a member of your research team and help you solve this critical issue. Depending on the characteristics of the desired sample, the researcher also may have to consider issues such as obtaining proxy or surrogate consent. Resourcefulness and creativity are important as you consider the issues related to recruitment of subjects.

Instrumentation also provides challenges. Some paper and pencil instruments are copyrighted, and you must obtain permission to use them. Other instruments require acknowledgment of the source. Still other instruments require copyright permission and a fee for use. Biological instruments provide other opportunities for growth. Training study staff in the proper use and routine maintenance and calibration of the instrument is critical to obtaining quality data. Where to place the sensor, how to get it to adhere to the site, and strategies to minimize subject burden with multiple biologic instruments are considerations that the researcher needs to address.

Adequate physical space in which to perform the research is a pivotal issue. In the ideal situation, the researcher has dedicated research space within the school of nursing. In the grant writing process, this allows the researcher to demonstrate to the potential funding agency that the researcher has institutional support for the research. During the implementation phase, dedicated space provides a controlled environment for data collection, entry, and management and space for study staff. Unfortunately, research space is often not readily available because most schools of nursing were designed with the mission of teaching in mind rather than research. Consequently, nurse researchers may have to negotiate research space in an affiliated health care facility or in a non–health care-related building on campus or in the community. If the actual data collection occurs in the clinical arena (e.g., nursing home or outpatient clinic), knowledge of the formal and informal lines of communication and refined diplomatic skills are needed to gain and maintain access to the site.

Hiring and maintenance of a research staff requires yet another skill set. The system may require advertising for a minimal period, and salaries may be dictated by standardized criteria. Knowledge of union standards and holiday/vacation time are hidden responsibilities of the researcher. Given the extensive, specialized training required to get research staff oriented to a project, it is important to select individuals who are compatible with the research team members and who are likely to stay throughout the duration of the project.

Thus nurse researchers face many challenges in their work. Anticipating the challenges assists the researcher in consciously devising approaches to mitigate them in order to focus their energies on generation of knowledge.

SUMMARY

Nurse researchers are a hearty group of nurses who seek to develop understanding of the basis for clinical care. For the most part, they are doctorally prepared persons who initiate or participate in all phases of the research process. They are engaged in diverse research methods, and their substantive content addresses the full life span and the health and illness spectrum and the health care system. They also work in a variety of settings. They face numerous challenges in their daily work. It is critical, however, to recognize that the work of the nurse researcher is pivotal to the profession and discipline because it directs the future path of nursing.

REFERENCES

Adams, M. G., & Drew, B. J. (2002). Efficacy of 2 strategies to detect body position ST-segment changes during continuous 12-lead electrocardiographic monitoring. *Journal of Electrocardiology, 35*(Suppl.), 193-200.

Aiken, L. H., Clarke, S. P., Cheung, R. B., Sloane, D. M., & Silber, J. H. (2003). Educational levels of hospital nurses and surgical patient mortality. *JAMA: The Journal of the American Medical Association, 290*(12), 1617-1623.

Aiken, L. H., Clarke, S. P., Sloane, D. M., Sochalski, J., & Silber, J. H. (2002). Hospital nurse staffing and patient mortality, nurse burnout, and job dissatisfaction. *JAMA: The Journal of the American Medical Association, 288*(16), 1987-1993.

American Association of Colleges of Nursing. (2004). *AACN position statement on the practice doctorate in nursing, October 2004.* Washington, DC: Author.

Drew, B. J., Pelter, M. M., Brodnick, D. E., Yadav, A. V., Dempel, D., & Adams, M. G. (2002). Comparison of a new reduced lead set ECG with the standard ECG for diagnosing cardiac arrhythmias and myocardial ischemia. *Journal of Electrocardiology, 35*(Suppl), 13-21.

Geluda, K., Bisaglia, J. B., Moreira, V., Maldonado, B. M., Cunha, A. J. L. A., Trajman, A. (2005). Third-party informed consent in research with adolescents: The good, the bad and the ugly. *Social Science & Medicine, 61,* 985-988.

Grady, P. A. (2004). Setting future directions at the National Institute of Nursing Research (NINR). *Policy, Politics, & Nursing Practice, 5*(2), 95-99.

Miaskowski, C., Dodd, M., West, C., Schumacher, K., Paul, S. M., Tripathy, D., et al. (2004). Randomized clinical trial of the effectiveness of a self-care intervention to improve cancer pain management. *Journal of Clinical Oncology, 22*(9), 1713-1720.

Olsen, D. P. (2003). HIPAA privacy regulations and nursing research. *Nursing Research, 52*(5), 344-348.

Pelter, M. M., Adams, M. G., Drew, B. J. (2003). Transient myocardial ischemia is an independent predictor of adverse in-hospital outcomes in patients with acute coronary syndromes treated in the telemetry unit. *Heart Lung, 32*(2), 71-78.

Polit, D. F., & Beck, C. T. (2004). *Nursing research: Principles and methods* (7th ed.). Philadelphia: Lippincott Williams & Wilkins.

Puntillo, K. A., White, C., Morris, A. B., Perdue, S. T., Stanik-Hutt, J., Thompson, C. L., et al. (2001). Patients' perceptions and responses to procedural pain: Results from Thunder Project II. *American Journal of Critical Care, 10*(4), 238-251.

Wipke-Tevis, D. D. (2001). Research column: What is research? *Journal of Vascular Nursing, 19*(2), 63-64.

Wipke-Tevis, D. D., & Williams, D. A. (2002). What is the difference between basic and applied research? *SVN … prn, 9*(5), 5.

CHANGING EDUCATION

Nursing Education in Transition

PERLE SLAVIK COWEN ◆ SUE MOORHEAD

It is, of course, a Chinese curse to say "may you live in interesting times" and who among us would deny that this is true for nursing education now. Although some of the current "interesting" educational challenges that nurses face have been with us for a long time (nursing shortages and entry into practice), others have appeared recently on the horizon (new educational paths and information technology). Our debate author, Mary Champagne, notes that our current nursing shortage is different and has resulted perhaps from a "perfect storm" of economic, social, technological, workplace, and demographic forces. Data from the U.S. Department of Health and Human Services indicates that by 2020, hospitals will be shy almost 800,000 nurses. Many complex problems underlie this shortage, and there are no easy solutions. A unique factor in today's shortage is the graying of nursing faculty and clinicians, with large numbers projected to retire in the next 20 years, paired with an insufficient pool of young replacements. The National League for Nursing reports that currently there are fewer than 20,000 nursing faculty, with a projected need for 40,000 to address the nursing shortage. This problem is the watershed of issues discussed throughout many of the chapters in this section.

Recent proposals for new educational paths in nursing, including the clinical nurse leader (CNL) and the doctor of nursing practice (DNP) have been met with mixed support and much discussion. Proponents view the CNL as a highly skilled generalist clinician who implements evidence-based, outcomes-focused, and quality improvement strategies. Others express concern that this new model threatens baccalaureate education and wonder how the new model will affect the work of master's-prepared clinical nurse specialists. Issues related to the DNP are debated openly in academic circles and professional journals. One camp believes this new degree will bring about parity with other health care disciplines and help address the complex issues of today's care system, whereas others express concerns for the negative, unintended consequences of this degree including a decrease in the number of PhD prepared nurses, erosion of nursing as a scientific discipline, and a further widening of the chasm between nurse scientists and clinicians. Several authors in this section delve into these issues.

Interwoven with these educational challenges is the informatics technology (IT) revolution. Nursing academia has been encouraged to use IT to increase access to nursing programs, remove geographic and time boundaries, increase interactive learning programs, develop simulation laboratories, facilitate course sharing across institutions, prepare students for use of IT in practice and to prepare nursing informatics specialists. For nursing to move forward as a scientific discipline we must generate data about patient encounters and the different systems of health care delivery. These data can then be organized in ways that yield information, and the information in turn can be organized, explored, and tested to confirm what nurses know or to reveal new knowledge. The links between practice, research, and theory are data links, and the science of nursing is only as good as the data and what nurses do with it. Several chapters address some of the new advances in this area of information management and education.

In the opening debate chapter, Champagne takes a historical look at nursing and nursing education and contrasts the conflicting perspectives of nursing as a craft versus nursing as a profession. She explores the current array of prelicensure and graduate nursing educational programs and contends that the need and timing of the proposed new models (CNL and DNP) can be decided best based on an understanding of the nurse and nurse faculty shortage and the issue of quality and safety. After exploring the many etiological factors related to the current shortages, Champagne deftly describes the genesis of the new models and details their potential and the concerns they have raised. She concludes her chapter by raising a series of questions, the answers for which lie in the future of nursing education.

In the first viewpoint chapter, Dolter questions whether there is a current crisis in nursing education. She approaches this through a quality assurance paradigm marching through indicators and outcome measurements that include production of adequate numbers of pre-licensure and graduate students, NCLEX pass rates, and employers' and graduate nurses' satisfaction with nurses' educational preparation. Dolter skillfully examines issues related to quality of care, particularly recent Institute of Medicine (IOM) findings, with implications for nursing and nursing education. She concludes her chapter with a solid health care cost and access discussion and a final outcome analysis of the answers she uncovered to her original question.

Expanding the scope to an international perspective, Upvall provides an interesting overview of varying approaches to international education and describes the vast differences in the maturity of international graduate education programs. She offers an insightful review of global nursing shortage issues and identifies internal and international migration as a critical challenge. Upvall notes, "The intense, active recruitment of nurses in developing countries in particular is a new phenomenon affecting the global shortage and negatively impacting health care in the home country." Although ICN supports the right of nurses to migrate, they recognize that this may negatively affect health care in the home country and condemn active recruiting by countries that have not addressed human resources and planned appropriately. Upvall concludes, "This issue will continue to be a matter of debate between the nursing leadership in Western and developing countries until the nursing shortage in Western countries eases."

At all levels of nursing education the future requires increased attention to critical thinking. Staib clarifies the concept, its critical elements, and the implications of critical thinking to altering approaches to curriculum design and process. Based on seven skills integral to critical thinking, as defined by an international panel of nursing experts, the author suggests ways in which learning experiences can be designed to hone these skills. Use of critical thinking skills as an organizing framework would allow students to acquire knowledge in a manner different from the traditional approach of teaching content. Staib notes, "If a change in students' critical thinking abilities is to take place, education practices must be interactive and participatory." The future requires nurses to be able to draw on an ever-increasing body of knowledge and to use their critical thinking abilities to seek the best ways of applying this knowledge and their thinking abilities to the care of patients.

Continuing the theme of lifelong learning, Muhl and Scheibel describe a statewide approach developed in Wisconsin, in which all baccalaureate nursing programs contribute to making nursing education readily available to nurses in their home settings. Their description of the way in which the curriculum has been developed and the way in which collaboration has been built among institutions provides a positive example of nursing education adjusting to the changing world in which we live. Their discussion of the faculty perspective in offering a nursing program through the collaborative efforts of five institutions provides for an interesting read.

Latham's chapter describes a related concept in the development of a partnership between an established academic nursing program and two separate, service-based clinical programs housed within a neighboring university and a large health care service provider organization in California. This collaboration resulted in three new programs: a statewide distance baccalaureate RN completion program and two master of science in nursing advanced practice specialties, including nursing anesthetist and family nurse practitioner concentrations. The American Association of Colleges of Nursing has supported the development of strategic partnerships to expand nursing programs in light of the current faculty shortage, insufficient clinical sites to support nursing student education, and academic fiscal constraints. This chapter provides an interesting operationalization of this concept.

The next chapter moves in a new direction in which Butcher provides a thought-provoking debate about the relationships among nursing theory, nursing research, and nursing practice. Butcher notes, "Increasingly, articles in nursing education encourage faculty to ground nursing knowledge in evidence-based practice, outcomes, research, and theory." After defining the terms, Butcher identifies three vantage points: knowledge based in nursing theory, knowledge based in practice, and knowledge based in research. Although a fully integrated discipline-specific nursing theory-research-practice model is the "ideal," he reviews three subtypes that approach his benchmark. This chapter should provide for much lively debate and discussion among all those interested in knowledge generation and use.

The link between knowledge development and the computer is explored in the next chapter. Bakken and Currie provide a thorough overview of the challenges related to transforming nursing data into knowledge. The authors begin by addressing the question of why traditional automated nursing systems have not fostered the development of nursing knowledge. They review the development of standardized nursing terminologies and the evolution of standards for data exchange in information systems. The role of informatics in fostering knowledge development in nursing is reviewed through the system design framework of the National Commission on Nursing Implementation Project. The framework's four types of information system processes (data acquisition, storage, transformation, and presentation) are reviewed. They give several examples that illustrate the interaction among information and information processes. These include data mining and knowledge discovery techniques for analysis of data repositories. The authors conclude that technological building blocks such as standardized terminologies and integrated systems are necessary but not sufficient for the development of nursing knowledge. Computer competencies related to the acquisition, organization, and analysis of large repositories of clinical data are required. The chapter ends with the formulation of three questions that demonstrate the evolution of nursing knowledge through the documentation of nursing care. Overall, the chapter illustrates the central role of the computer in building nursing science.

In the next chapter, Eland identifies some of the challenges and opportunities facing those involved in nursing education in the area of using online learning to provide quality education. This chapter is a good companion to the previous one. Eland details the technical support components that faculty and students require to make this a successful learning experience, provides a pragmatic do's and don'ts list for an effective virtual classroom, and details important operational considerations in an understandable and straight forward manner. This is an enjoyable chapter.

In the final chapter, Skiba supports the growth of online learning and summarizes the best practices in Web-based education. She also provides students with criteria to assess the quality of Web-based educational programs before selecting an online course or degree program. She reviews principles of quality for electronically offered degree or certificate programs under the areas of curriculum and instruction, institutional context and commitment, and evaluation and assessment. An overview of the *Evaluating Educational Uses of the Web in Nursing* (EEUWIN) Benchmarking Project is provided and includes interesting research findings related to differences in perceptions of undergraduate and graduate students' experiences in Web-based courses.

This section provides an interesting window on the far-reaching shifts and interesting times in contemporary nursing. The themes are amazingly consistent in detailing the threshold of change that nursing education has crossed.

The Future of Nursing Education

Educational Models for Future Care

MARY T. CHAMPAGNE

Recent developments in health care have led to proposals for new educational paths in nursing, including the clinical nurse leader (CNL) and the doctor of nursing practice (DNP). Support for these new pathways, however, is mixed. Debate about educational preparation in nursing is not new: it has been particularly fierce regarding entry into practice. The debate stems from the fact that varied educational paths lead to eligibility to sit for the NCLEX-RN, the examination for licensure as a registered nurse. Camilleri (2001) has explained the development of the confusing array of prelicensure educational programs through analysis of the social, economic, and political forces of the times. She notes that the growth of educational programs in nursing in the United States was a struggle between two traditions in nursing: between the "craft culture" that valued the daily work of nurses and the "professional culture," advocates of which dreamed of improving nursing care and the education of nurses. In the United States, as in Britain, nursing education began in hospitals based on an apprenticeship model, and students were awarded a diploma. Throughout the twentieth century, nurse leaders in the United States fought for better education for nursing students. They lobbied for classroom lecture time (dismissed as too theoretical by most physicians) and aimed to bring nursing into the system of higher education.

Over time, these leaders were successful in upgrading educational offerings, and nurse education transitioned from hospital programs to academic settings. The number of hospital-based diploma programs decreased (today fewer than 70 exist), and baccalaureate nurse education programs were established (today there are more than 560 entry-level baccalaureate programs). Then in response to a national nurse shortage following World War II, a "technical nurse" program in community colleges was implemented as an experimental model, and today there are more than 800 associate's degree programs (Berlin, Stennett, & Bednash, 2004;

Greene, Allan, & Henderson, 2003). As a result of this history, multiple educational paths (diploma, associate's degree, and bachelor's degree) lead to undifferentiated licensure as a registered nurse. And in recent years the accelerated bachelor of science in nursing (ABSN) program has been added for individuals who hold a college degree in another field and complete prerequisite courses. The ABSN programs have grown rapidly. In 2002, 105 such programs existed; the number increased to 151 programs in 2004; and 46 new ABSN programs are under development (American Association of Colleges of Nursing [AACN], 2005e). Other, less widely adopted prelicensure models include the doctor of nursing degree and the generic or accelerated master's. In addition, programs such as the registered nurse (RN) to bachelor of science in nursing (BSN) program, the accelerated RN to BSN program, and the RN to BSN external degree program serve to provide educational mobility to RNs with a diploma or associate's degree in nursing (Berlin et al., 2004) (Box 8-1).

In addition to programs designed for preparation for licensure, nursing education includes master's and doctoral preparation. Master's programs generally prepare graduates in a specialized area of nursing and admit individuals with a bachelor's degree in nursing.* Currently, 400 institutions offer master's programs in nursing in the United States and its territories. Specialties offered vary by institution and include

---

*Note that there are accelerated or generic master's programs in nursing for students who have bachelor's or higher degree in other fields. Most often these programs include an intensive period of nursing education that makes the student eligible to sit for the NCLEX-RN. Once the student passes the NCLEX-RN, the student continues with the master's portion of the program and completes a chosen specialty in nursing. Registered nurse to master's programs also admit RNs without bachelor's degrees in nursing and award a master's degree in nursing.

BOX 8-1

Pre–Registered Nurse Licensure Educational Nursing Programs (to Prepare Graduates Eligible for the NCLEX-RN)®

Diploma: A program that requires at least 2 to 3 years of full-time course work, usually within a hospital setting, and awards a diploma or certificate.

Associate's degree in nursing: A program that requires 2 to 3 years of full-time academic work, usually within a junior or community college setting, and awards an associate's degree in nursing.

Generic or entry-level bachelor's degree in nursing: A program that requires 4 to 5 years of full-time academic work for students who have no previous nursing education and awards a baccalaureate degree.

Accelerated bachelor's degree in nursing: A program that requires 12 to 18 months of full-time academic work for students who have a bachelor's or higher degree in another field and who have completed prerequisite course work. A bachelor's degree in nursing is awarded.

Generic master's degree: A program that usually requires 3 years of academic work for students who

have bachelor's or higher degree in other fields. Most often, these programs include an intensive period of nursing education that makes the student eligible to sit for the NCLEX-RN. Once the student passes the NCLEX-RN, the student continues with the master's portion of the program and completes a chosen specialty in nursing. A master's degree in nursing is awarded.

Doctor of nursing (ND): A program that usually requires 3 years of academic work, primarily for nonnursing baccalaureate-prepared college graduates. The doctor of nursing program is a generic doctoral program with a clinical focus. For non-nurses the program usually begins with an accelerated prelicensure component that qualifies the student to sit for the NCLEX-RN. Once the student passes the NCLEX-RN, the student then undertakes study the remainder of the curriculum. The doctor of nursing degree is awarded.

Adapted from Berlin, L. E., Stennett, J., Bednash, G. D. (2004). *2003-2004 enrollment and graduations in baccalaureate and graduate programs in nursing.* Washington, DC: American Association of Colleges of Nursing.

nonclinical practice areas such as administration, informatics, and education, as well as specialization in one of four major clinical advanced practice groups: nurse practitioners, nurse-midwives, clinical nurse specialists, and nurse anesthetists. Clinical nurse specialists and nurse practitioners further specialize, generally by age group (e.g., pediatric nurse practitioner) or by disease (e.g., oncology clinical nurse specialist). Most master's graduates take a certification examination in their specialty following graduation, and in the clinical advanced practice groups such certification generally is required for advanced practice (Table 8-1). Eighty-seven doctoral programs in nursing award the doctor of philosophy and the doctor of nursing science (DNSc or DNS) degree and prepare graduates for research careers.* In the fall of 2003, 3198 students were enrolled in doctoral study; around 400 students graduate each year with a research doctoral degree in nursing (Berlin et al., 2004).

---

*Eight doctoral programs have a clinical or practice focus, and these programs offer the doctor of nursing degree or the doctor of nursing practice degree, and one offers the doctor of nursing science (DNSc) degree.

ARE CURRENT EDUCATIONAL MODELS SUFFICIENT TO MEET CONTEMPORARY AND FUTURE HEALTH CARE NEEDS?

Although there are multiple nursing educational paths, in general, prelicensure programs prepare graduates for licensure as a RN and general nursing practice, master's degree programs prepare graduates in a specialized area of practice, and doctoral programs prepare graduates for a research career. Two new models of education, the CNL and the DNP, currently are being developed. The CNL will be prepared at the master's level as a generalist clinician, and the DNP is a terminal practice doctorate for those who provide care for individuals, groups, and populations and for those who influence care through administration or policy. Whether these two new models are needed and whether the timing of their introduction is optimal can be decided best based on an understanding of the nurse and nurse faculty shortage and the issue of quality and safety.

THE NURSE SHORTAGE

Since the late 1990s, education in nursing has been dominated by a focus on the existing and future shortage of nurses and to a lesser extent the shortage of nurse

TABLE 8-1

Master Degree Programs, Fall 2003

Major Area of Study	Number of Schools Offering the Major	Number of Students
Administration	198	4,995
Case management	17	215
Clinical nurse specialist	199	3,506
Combined clinical nurse specialist/nurse practitioner	52	982
Community health/public health	25	213
Education	148	2,873
Health policy/systems	16	112
Informatics	26	318
Nurse anesthetist*	45	2,424
Nurse-midwifery*	41	657
Nurse practitioner	301	18,163
School nursing	12	183
Other clinical majors	24	381

From Berlin, L. E., Stennett, J., Bednash, G. D. (2004). *2003-2004 AACN enrollments and graduations in baccalaureate and graduate programs in nursing.* Washington, DC: American Association of Colleges of Nursing.
*Some additional nurse anesthetist and nurse-midwifery programs are not within schools of nursing.

faculty. In the past, nurse shortages were cyclical and were tied closely to market demands; the current shortage, however, is different and has resulted perhaps from a "perfect storm" of economic, social, technological, workplace, and demographic forces. A recent story in *US News & World Report* (Marek, 2005), "More Nurses Needed," called today's shortage "the shortage that won't quit" and cited data from the U.S. Department of Health and Human Services indicating that by 2020, hospitals will be shy almost 800,000 nurses. This shortage involves supply and demand issues and represents a complex system problem with no easy solutions. One clearly unique factor in today's shortage is that large numbers of nurses are projected to retire in the next 20 years, without a sufficient influx of young nurses to replace them (Buerhaus, Staiger, & Auerbach, 2000). The faculty shortage is related most directly to the aging of the professoriat, lack of competitive salaries, and an inadequate educational pipeline for new faculty (AACN, 2005e).

Numerous public and private groups have addressed the nurse and nurse faculty shortage and have recommended interventions at multiple levels, including improving media coverage, instituting state and federal government programs to support students and faculty, increasing capacity at educational institutions, and improving the work environment in health care settings.

Progress is being made. Media coverage, including the national Johnson & Johnson Campaign for Nursing's Future, has increased public awareness of the value of nurses and the work they do in caring for patients. Hospitals and other health care organizations have developed hiring and retention strategies, have engaged in partnerships with educational programs to fund faculty and students, and have made efforts to improve the work environment. In 2002, hospital nurse wages, which had been flat for years, showed a real increase of about 5% (Buerhaus et al., 2003). Federal dollars have been allocated for student loans and scholarships and for loans for faculty education, as well as special workforce improvements; and even in tight budget times, some states are working to improve the workplace environment, expand the number of faculty, and support students (AACN, 2002a; Greene et al., 2003; H.R. No. 3457, Nurse Reinvestment Act, 2002). Educational programs have increased enrollments significantly; in the academic year 2003-2004, prelicensure programs were up 50.3% from the academic year 2002-2003 (National League for Nursing, 2004). And the number of candidates for the RN examination (NCLEX-RN), which had decreased 27% between 1996 and 2001, is showing an upturn. However, in 2004 the number of students who passed the NCLEX-RN as "first time exam takers" was lower than that in 1995 (Table 8-2).

Master's and doctoral degree enrollments also have increased over the last 5 years; in 2004, master's degree enrollments increased 13.7% to 42,751, and doctoral enrollments increased 7.3% to 3439. The numbers of graduates from these programs also have begun to increase slightly: 6.9% for master's graduates (669 additional

TABLE 8-2

Number of Candidates Taking the NCLEX-RN: First-Time, U.S. Educated Candidates Only									
Program	1995	1996	1997	1998	1999	2000	2001	2002	2003	2004
Diploma	7,335	6,346	5,240	3,978	3,161	2,679	2,310	2,424	2,565	3,162
Baccalaureate	31,195	32,278	31,828	30,142	28,107	26,048	24,832	25,806	26,630	30,648
Associates	57,908	55,554	52,396	49,045	45,255	42,665	41,567	42,310	47,423	53,648
Total	96,438	94,178	89,464	83,165	76,523	71,392	68,709	70,540	76,618	87,458

From National Council of State Boards of Nursing. (1995-2004). Quarterly examination statistics: Volume, pass rates & first-time internationally educated candidates' countries. Retrieved January 25, 2005, from http://www.ncsbn.org/pdfs/NCLEX_fact_sheet.pdf.

graduates) and 2% for doctoral programs (8 additional graduates). The diversity in nursing students also is increasing: the proportion of racial and ethnic minorities enrolled in baccalaureate, master's, and doctoral programs has increased steadily over the last 10 years (Berlin et al., 2004).

Yet the shortage remains problematic. Demand for nurses continues to be strong. A human resources report from the U.S. Department of Labor ("BLS Releases," 2004) projects that more than a million new and replacement nurses will be needed by 2012, and the U.S. Department of Labor ("High-Paying," 2004) has identified registered nursing as the top occupation in terms of job growth through the year 2012. A survey of 138 hospitals by the Hodes Group (2004) from July to November 2004 noted that despite an overall increase of 8% in total nurses employed in these hospitals, the RN turnover rate was 13.9%, and RNs were the health care group with the highest vacancy rate (16.1%). Buerhaus et al. (2003) have reported employment of RNs in hospitals increased 9% between 2001 and 2002, an increase that represented 100,000 nurses. However, the increase reflected employment of older nurses (those 50 years of age and older) who perhaps were returning to work or moving from part-time to full-time employment and increased hiring of foreign-born nurses. Indeed, in recent years the greatest increase in those passing the NCLEX-RN has been in "foreign educated nurses," an increase from 7506 in 2000 to 18,285 in 2004 (National Council of State Boards of Nursing, 2000, 2004).

More students are interested in entering the nursing profession; however, academic institutions are unable to accommodate all qualified applicants. The AACN (2005e) reported that in the fall 2004, more than 29,000 qualified baccalaureate applicants were turned away because of insufficient numbers of faculty and resources. A report from the National League for Nursing (2004) gave an even higher number of rejected qualified applicants: 125,037 from all prelicensure nursing programs,

including 36,615 from baccalaureate programs. The faculty shortage continues to be the most commonly cited reason for turning away qualified applicants, and it is obvious that the small increase in doctoral students will be insufficient to fill current and future faculty vacancies. Clearly, nurse educators need to bring more RNs into the workforce and prepare more nurse faculty. Nurse educators have responded positively to the nurse shortage through increasing enrollments. However, more support for academic institutions in faculty development and resource development (such as space and clinical sites) is necessary for further enrollment growth to occur.

Is the Focus on Numbers Sufficient?

In general, efforts to address the nurse shortage have paid little attention to the knowledge, skills, and educational qualifications needed for nurses; the focus has been on numbers. However, this issue was raised in a recent article (Aiken, Clarke, Cheung, Sloane, & Silber, 2003) that reported that after controlling for other variables, hospitals with larger proportions of nurses educated at the baccalaureate level or higher had lower mortality and failure-to-rescue rates for surgical patients. This raises the question of whether nursing should look not only at the numbers of nurses needed to provide care but also at the level of education they receive. This is not a new issue; it is at the heart of the "entry into practice debate" that has been waged between associate's degree and bachelor's degree education for decades. In 1996 the National Advisory Council on Nurse Education and Practice, a policy advisory group to Congress and the U.S. secretary for Health and Human Services on issues relating to nursing, recommended that at least two thirds of the nurse workforce hold baccalaureate degrees by 2010. Other reports also have supported the baccalaureate degree as the desired degree for professional nursing practice. And a survey of employers indicated that they had a clear preference for hiring experienced BSN graduates for management and specialty positions (National Council of State Boards of Nursing, 2002). Chief nurse officers in university hospitals prefer to hire nurses with baccalaureate degrees, and federal entities such as the U.S. Army, U.S. Navy, U.S. Air Force, U.S. Public Health Service, and the U.S. Department of Veterans' Affairs have recognized the baccalaureate degree as the desired educational level for nursing (AACN, 2003b; Goode et al., 2001). Nevertheless, with an undifferentiated license, the debate on "entry into practice" is unlikely to come to resolution. In 2003 the AACN, a strong proponent of baccalaureate education, noted, "In general, we have not succeeded in differentiating practice of RNs with different educational preparation" (AACN, 2003a).

Given the nurse shortage, clearly we need graduates of all programs that prepare students for the RN examination, and nurse educators perhaps should focus not only on enrollment in baccalaureate nursing programs but also on promoting baccalaureate education for those initially educated at the associate's degree level. Over the years, community colleges and universities have worked together to make a seamless transition from an associate degree in nursing to a baccalaureate nursing program (RN to BSN); however, enrollments in RN to BSN programs declined after 1999 and showed only a modest increase of 6.2% in the academic year 2003-2004 (Berlin et al., 2004). Overall, only 17.4% of nurses educated in associate degree programs go on to complete a 4-year nursing degree program. Nurse educators need to increase this percentage. Although this is reasonable, the question remains, What is the needed education for nurses in today's and tomorrow's health care systems? In a time of shortage, should resources be focused only on enhancing existing models of education, or should nursing education move to new models such as the CNL or DNP to serve as even greater magnets for highly qualified students who would better meet the health care needs of the public and increase the numbers of clinical nurse faculty.

QUALITY AND SAFETY

Questions about the knowledge, skill, and education needed in nursing are related to issues of quality and safety of care. Patients are older and frailer with more chronic illnesses, care is more complex and costly, consumers are more aware and demanding, and there is widespread concern regarding the quality of health care. Thus in the last decade, questions have been raised about the quality of education of nurses and indeed all health care professionals (Joint Commission on Accreditation of Healthcare Organizations, 2002; Kimball & O'Neil, 2002).

In 1996 the Institute of Medicine began a quality initiative with the aim of improving health care and meeting the health care needs of contemporary society. The first report, *To Err Is Human: Building a Safer Health System* (Kohn, Corrigan, & Donaldson, 2000), documented that the fragmented health care system results in serious medical errors that lead to more deaths per year than motor vehicle accidents or AIDS, whereas other, less serious medical errors unnecessarily increase the cost of health care. The report concluded that the burden of harm and the collective impact of health care quality problems are staggering. This study was followed by *Crossing the Quality Chasm: A New Health System for the 21st Century* (Institute of Medicine, 2001). This report emphasized that reform around the "margins" will not suffice; the current health care system is not structured to promote quality and safety or to make the best use of its resources. The report called for all health care professional groups and systems to adopt health care practices that promote care that is "safe, effective, client-centered, timely, efficient, and equitable" (p. 6). Reasoning that our health system cannot be transformed without changing the education of health professionals, the Institute of Medicine issued a call for an interdisciplinary summit to develop the next step: reform of health professional education in order to enhance patient care quality and safety. Thus the third report in the quality trilogy was *Health Professions Education: A Bridge to Quality* (Greiner & Knebel, 2003). This report focused on the knowledge that health care professionals need to provide optimal care in the twenty-first century. Specifically, the report stated that students in the health professions are not prepared to address the shifts in the country's demographics (in particular the aging of the society), nor are they educated to work in interdisciplinary teams, access evidence for use in practice, analyze root causes of errors and markers of quality, use informatics to access the latest literature, or use systems to enhance teamwork and minimize errors. The report noted that in order to improve quality and safety of care, education needs to change and concluded that "All health professionals should be educated to deliver patient-centered care as members of an interdisciplinary team, emphasizing evidence-based practice, quality improvement approaches and informatics" (p. 3).

The report identified five core competencies that all clinicians should possess, regardless of their discipline (Box 8-2). Challenges in implementing these

BOX 8-2

Core Competencies for All Health Professionals

Provide patient centered care: Identify, respect, and care about patients' differences, values, preferences, and expressed needs; relieve pain and suffering; coordinate continuous care; listen to, clearly inform, communicate with, and educate patients; share decision making and management; and continuously advocate disease prevention, wellness, and promotion of healthy lifestyles, including a focus on population health.

Work in interdisciplinary teams: Cooperate, collaborate, communicate, and integrate care in teams to ensure that care is continuous and reliable.

Use evidence-based practice: Integrate best research with clinical expertise and patient values for optimum care, and participate in learning and research activities to the extent feasible.

Apply quality improvement: Identify errors and hazards in care; understand and implement basic safety design principles, such as standardization and simplification; continually understand and measure quality of care in terms of structure, process, and outcomes in relation to patient and community needs; and design and test interventions to change processes and systems of care, with the objective of improving quality.

Utilize informatics: Communicate, manage knowledge, mitigate error, and support decision making using information technology.

From Greiner, A. C., & Knebel, E. (2003). *Health professions education: A bridge to quality* (p. 4). Washington DC: National Academies Press.

competencies and the role of licensure, accreditation, and certification are discussed in the report, with recommendations and strategies for the reform of clinical education.

The report raises questions about the adequacy of current education in nursing at all levels, but particularly at the prelicensure and master's degree levels. The core competencies reflect advances in scientific and health care knowledge, the complexity of the health care delivery system, and the responsibility of all health care professionals to provide safe, high-quality care. The core competencies are certainly reasonable, but it is difficult to imagine how a 2-year associate's degree program can address all of these competencies, and even baccalaureate program faculty may find it difficult to include the additional content and learning experiences required. At the master's level, programs might find it a struggle

to supplement specialty knowledge and clinical experiences with all of the core competencies. New models of nurse education, including the CNL and the DNP, are being developed in part to address the need for these competencies. The new models will add to the complexity of nurse education and thus may further confuse students, professionals, and the public regarding nurse education. The question is whether these new models are needed to meet contemporary needs for care, or whether it would be better to focus resources on modifying existing programs.

TWO NEW MODELS

Clinical Nurse Leader

In 1999 the AACN convened a Task Force on Education and Regulation for Professional Nursing (TFER 1) to develop a response to declining enrollments in baccalaureate educational programs, concerns about the quality of patient care, and the increasing complexity of care. This task force consulted with leaders from service and regulatory agencies, elicited input from focus groups and membership surveys, and determined that a new nursing role was needed to best meet health care needs and differentiate scope of nursing practice (AACN, 2002b, 2003a). In 2002, TFER 2 was convened to continue this work and more specifically to identify the competencies needed to improve patient care and envision the role of a new CNL (AACN, 2004f). The CNL, which has been accepted by the AACN (2005c), is a clinical leader who is a provider and manager of care to individuals and populations. The CNL oversees the coordination of care for a group of patients, assesses cohort risk, provides direct patient care in complex situations, and functions as part of an interdisciplinary team to communicate, plan, and implement comprehensive care. The CNL will be prepared at the master's level as a generalist clinician and leader in health care delivery and will work across settings and assume accountability for health care outcomes for a clinical population or specified group of patients (AACN, 2004c, 2004g).

The CNL role addresses the recommendations of the Institute of Medicine report: the CNL will be a highly skilled generalist clinician who implements evidence-based, outcomes-focused quality improvement strategies. Most notably, the CNL is not an administrator but a clinical leader who will enhance interdisciplinary care across settings and bring the latest in evidenced-based practice to patients. The preparation of a generalist at the master's level is a new model in nursing education, but this new model already has been recognized by the

American Association of Nurse Executives, which will join the AACN in planning and overseeing implementation of the new role (AACN, 2005b).

Some are concerned that this new model threatens baccalaureate education; others wonder how the new model will affect the work of master's-prepared clinical nurse specialists (AACN, 2004h). However, proponents of the CNL note that the role already has emerged in practice but is being developed there on an ad hoc basis without the needed formal education. Thus educational preparation for the role is essential. Nevertheless, the AACN is taking a careful approach to implementing this educational innovation and is recruiting education/practice partners to pilot CNL programs. Links between service and education in piloting this new educational program are critical to ensure that the CNL is prepared for practice and has a well-defined scope of practice. At this writing, more than 70 educational programs and 140 service organizations have signed on with the AACN to conduct pilot studies that will experiment with the CNL role (AACN, 2005a). A draft curriculum has been developed (AACN, 2004d), as have potential pathways to education as a CNL (these include pathways for those with a BSN and for those entering college). Although initially a new license for those educated as CNLs was considered, it now appears that this will not be the case; rather the CNL program graduate will be eligible to sit for a certification examination developed under the auspices of the AACN. The hope is that this new model of nurse education will result in better use of the full scope of knowledge and skill of nurses and in better patient outcomes, as well as in recruitment of highly qualified candidates to nursing and retention of nurses in the profession.

Doctor of Nursing Practice

The idea of a practice doctoral degree in nursing is not new. In 1979, Case Western Reserve University began offering the doctor of nursing degree as an entry-level educational program for nursing (AACN, 2004b). Since that time, several other practice doctoral degrees have been established. However, none of these degrees resulted in fundamental change in nursing education, and to some extent they have been seen as confusing to students, professionals, and the public. In 2002 the AACN established a Task Force on the Practice Doctorate to examine the current status of clinical or practice doctoral programs and to make recommendations on the development of future practice doctorates. The establishment of the task force grew out of the Institute of Medicine reports, the movement in other health care professions to the practice

doctorate (for example, the doctor of pharmacy, the doctor of physical therapy, the doctor of public health, and the doctor of psychology), and from analysis of current curricular requirements for the master of science in nursing degree. The task force noted that many master's degree programs in nursing require far more credits and didactic and clinical hours than master's programs in other disciplines. In particular, the task force noted that in nurse practitioner programs that the credit hours had remained stable over the last several years, but didactic and supervised clinical hours had increased. After meeting with a variety of constituents and stakeholders, including the National Organization of Nurse Practitioner Faculties, practicing advanced practice nurses, and organizations affiliated with the Alliance for Nursing, the task force concluded that it was time for nursing education to focus on a terminal practice degree that encompassed any form of nursing intervention that influences health care outcomes for individuals or populations, including the direct care of individual patients, management of care for individuals and populations, administration of nursing and health care organizations, and the development and implementation of health policy (AACN, 2004b). Thus those obtaining a practice doctorate will include not only traditional advanced practice nursing students (nurse practitioners, clinical nurse specialists, nurse anesthetists, and nurse-midwives) but also those whose study focuses on management, administration, or health policy (indirect care). The task force was clear that the practice doctorate is an alternative to the research doctorate, and graduates will be prepared to blend clinical, economic, organizational, and leadership skills and to use science in improving the direct care of patients, care of patient populations, and practice that supports patient care (management, administration, and health policy). The task force made 13 specific recommendations (Box 8-3).

The recommendations of the Task Force were endorsed by the AACN membership on October 25, 2004, which voted to move the educational preparation of advanced practice nurses, broadly defined, from the master's level to the practice doctorate level (DNP) by 2015 (AACN, 2004a). Two additional AACN task forces have been established to facilitate the transition. The Task Force on the Roadmap to the DNP will study the full array of issues that this new educational direction brings to nursing education. The Task Force on the Essentials of Nursing Education for the DNP will address a set of core competencies that graduates must possess. The Commission on Collegiate Nursing Education has

BOX 8-3

Summary of Recommendations From the AACN Task Force: Position Statement on the Practice Doctorate in Nursing

1. The term *practice doctorate* be used instead of clinical doctorate.
2. The practice-focused doctoral program be a distinct model of doctoral education that provides an additional option for attaining a terminal degree in the discipline.
3. Practice-focused doctoral programs prepare graduates for the highest level of nursing practice beyond the initial preparation in the discipline.
4. Practice-focused doctoral nursing programs include seven essential areas of content. The seven essential areas of content include:
   - Scientific underpinnings for practice;
   - Advanced nursing practice;
   - Organization and system leadership/management, quality improvement, and system thinking;
   - Analytic methodologies related to the evaluation of practice and the application of evidence for practice;
   - Utilization of technology information for the improvement and transformation of healthcare;
   - Health policy development, implementation and evaluation; and
   - Interdisciplinary collaboration for improving patient and population healthcare outcomes.
5. Practice doctoral nursing programs should include development and or validation of expertise in at least one area of specialized advanced nursing practice.
6. Practice-focused doctoral nursing programs prepare leaders for nursing practice. The practice doctorate prepares individuals at the highest level of practice and is the terminal practice degree.
7. One degree title should be chosen to represent practice-focused doctoral programs that prepare graduates for the highest level of nursing practice.
8. The Doctor of Nursing Practice (DNP) be the degree associated with practice-focused doctoral nursing education.
9. The Doctor of Nursing (ND) degree title be phased out.
10. The practice doctorate be the graduate degree for advanced nursing practice preparation, including but not limited to the four current APN roles: clinical nurse specialist, nurse anesthetist, nurse midwife, and nurse practitioner.
11. A transition period be planned to provide nurses with master's degrees, who wish to obtain the practice doctoral degree, a mechanism to earn a practice doctorate in a relatively streamlined fashion with credit given for previous graduate study and practice experience. The transition mechanism should provide multiple points of entry, standardized validation of competencies, and be time limited.
12. Practice doctorate programs, as in research-focused doctoral programs, are encouraged to offer additional coursework and practica that would prepare graduates to fill the role of nurse educator.
13. Practice-focused doctoral programs need to be accredited by a nursing accrediting agency recognized by the U.S. Secretary of Education (i.e., the Commission on Collegiate Nursing Education or the National League for Nursing Accrediting Commission).

From American Association of Colleges of Nursing. (2004). AACN position statement on the practice doctorate in nursing (pp. 14-15). Retrieved January, 10, 2005, from http://www.aacn.nche.edu/DNP/DNPPositionStatement.htm.

agreed to develop a process for the accreditation of programs that offer practice doctorates. The impact of the recommendations already is being felt: schools that earlier offered a practice or clinical doctorate under a different title (such as the doctor of nursing) are transitioning to the DNP, and as of spring 2005, more than 40 additional DNP programs are under development (AACN, 2005d). However, the AACN vote in favor of the DNP in 2004 was not unanimous (160 for and 106 against), and although the AACN collaborated with the National Organization of Nurse Practitioner Faculty, as of this writing that organization has not yet endorsed the proposal. Other advanced practice organizations,

including the National Association of Clinical Nurse Specialists, American Association of Nurse Anesthetists, and the American College of Nurse-Midwives also are considering whether to endorse the proposal. Deanne R. Williams, MS, CNM, executive director of the American College of Midwives, noted that her organization was surprised by the proposal and noted that there was no evidence that the DNP degree would improve care from the perspective of the client (Nelson, 2005).

The DNP raises a number of questions for educators, advanced practitioners, and potential students. As one might expect, practicing advanced practice nurses worry that their preparation and credentials might be devalued, school of nursing faculty are concerned that their master's degree programs will become obsolete and that they may not have the institutional support or ability to develop a DNP program, administrators and faculty question where additional faculty will be found to teach the additional courses required in the DNP program, and students wonder whether enrolling in a master's program at this time is wise. The AACN has said that it supports the education of master's-prepared nurses, that it will help educational programs transition from the master's to the DNP, and that students should continue with their current educational plans (AACN, 2004e). Other concerns are these: Will students be willing to pay for and complete a program that is longer than a master's program? Will certification agencies offer examinations to graduates of both master's programs and the new DNP programs? Will the graduates of DNP programs be accepted by interdisciplinary colleagues? And how will programs educating nurse anesthetists and nurse-midwives that are not located in a nursing school be affected? (AACN, 2004e; Marion et al., 2003; O'Sullivan, 2005). The fundamental question is whether the current education of advanced practice nurses is optimal, or whether the increased complexity of the care environment warrants education at the doctoral level. All of these issues call for further discussion among a broad constituency of stakeholders.

FINAL CONSIDERATIONS ON EDUCATIONAL MODELS FOR THE FUTURE

We live in a time of rising expectations for health care, declining resources, quality concerns, and in the case of nursing, a major and continuing shortage of personnel. Nursing education has (at best) used a patchwork approach to providing students with an education that prepares them to meet health care needs. Nurse educators have been unsuccessful in resolving the differences in prelicensure programs. Further, service organizations for the most part have given little support to efforts to differentiate among the graduates of bachelor's degree, associate's degree, and diploma programs. At the master's level, nurse educators have had remarkable success in educating advanced practice nurses in clinical areas (nurse practitioners, nurse anesthetists, clinical nurse specialists, and nurse-midwives). Many of these programs began as certificate programs (some in schools of medicine) and only in the last 3 or 4 decades have they moved to schools of nursing and master's preparation. Doctoral education, which focuses on preparing nurse researchers,

is a relatively new phenomenon, and such doctoral programs have grown considerably in the last 50 years. Thus the educational system currently is poorly defined at the prelicensure level but much better defined at the master's and doctoral levels.

Nevertheless, reports from national sources such as the Institute of Medicine indicate that nurse educators need to overhaul the educational preparation of health professionals and embrace a paradigm that focuses on patient-centered care, interdisciplinary teams, and use of evidence-based practice, quality improvement, and informatics. The CNL and the DNP are being designed in large part to address the issues raised by the Institute of Medicine. Both models are being developed carefully using a consensus approach among colleges and schools of nursing, professional organizations, and affiliated partners. Both programs will have a major impact on educational preparation at the master's level. The CNL will introduce a generalist practitioner, although master's programs traditionally have focused on the preparation of specialists. The DNP will move the specialist education of advanced practice nurses (broadly defined) from the master's level to the doctoral level. These innovations also could affect baccalaureate education, which in the college and university traditionally has prepared generalists, and perhaps the research doctorate, which has been the primary mechanism for doctoral education in nursing.

Nursing has a strong history of educational experimentation. The two new educational models, the CNL and the DNP, offer promise and raise concerns: Will the new models better prepare nurses to meet the health care needs of people? Will the new models be affordable for students and educational institutions? Will the new models recruit a larger, more diverse, and talented applicant pool? Will graduates of the new models be accepted and rewarded by colleagues and employers? What will be the effect of the new models on the current structure of baccalaureate and master's education in nursing? Clearly, these questions will be answered in the near future as the two new models of nurse education are implemented and evaluated. And the way that the profession addresses the answers to these questions may help ensure that nursing accrues more benefits with the new and fewer difficulties with the old educational models. In the spirit of evidence-based innovations, nurse educators should welcome the experimentation and evaluate the results regarding future education. The outcomes of such experimentation may cement the current educational system or issue a call for nurse educators to embrace "good transitions."

REFERENCES

Aiken, L. H., Clarke, S. P., Cheung, R. B., Sloane, D. M., & Silber, J. H. (2003). Educational levels of hospital nurses and surgical patient mortality. *JAMA: The Journal of the American Medical Association, 290*(12), 1617-1632.

American Association of Colleges of Nursing. (2002a). *Media relations: AACN applauds the swift passage of the Nurse Reinvestment Act in both the House and the Senate.* Retrieved January, 15, 2005 from http://www.aacn.nche.edu/Media/NewsReleases/NRApass.htm

American Association of Colleges of Nursing. (2002b). *Report of the Task Force on Education and Regulation for Professional Nursing Practice 1.* Retrieved December 30, 2004, from http://www.aacn.nche.edu/Education/edandreg02.htm

American Association of Colleges of Nursing. (2003a). *Clinical nurse leader: Remarks delivered by AACN president Kathleen Ann Long at the business meeting on Monday, October 27, 2003.* Retrieved January 10, 2005, from http://www.aacn.nche.edu/CNL/History.htm

American Association of Colleges of Nursing. (2003b). *The impact of education on nursing practice.* Retrieved January 10, 2005, from http://www.aacn.nche.edu/edimpact

American Association of Colleges of Nursing. (2004a). *AACN adopts a new vision for the future of nursing education and practice: Position on the practice doctorate approved by AACN member schools.* Retrieved January 10, 2004, from http://www.aacn.nche.edu/Media/NewsReleases/DNPRelease.htm

American Association of Colleges of Nursing. (2004b). *AACN position statement on the practice doctorate in nursing.* Retrieved January 10, 2005, from http://www.aacn.nche.edu/DNP/DNPPositionStatement.htm

American Association of Colleges of Nursing. (2004c). *The clinical nurse leader: Developing a new nursing role.* Retrieved January 15, 2005, from http://www.aacn.nche.edu/CNL/index/htm

American Association of Colleges of Nursing. (2004d). *Draft curriculum framework.* Retrieved January 10, 2005, from http://www.aacn.nche.edu/CNL/index.htm

American Association of Colleges of Nursing. (2004e). *Frequently asked questions: Position statement on the practice doctorate in nursing.* Retrieved January 2, 2005, from http://www.aacn.nche.edu/DNP/DNPFAQ.htm

American Association of Colleges of Nursing. (2004f). *Task Force on Education and Regulation for Professional Nursing Practice #2.* Retrieved on January 2, 2005, from http://www.aacn.nche.edu/ContactUs/tfer2.htm

American Association of Colleges of Nursing. (2004g). *Working paper on the role of the clinical nurse leader.* Retrieved on January 15, 2005, from http://www.aacn.nche.edu/Publications/WhitePapers/CNL.htm

American Association of Colleges of Nursing. (2004h). *Working statement comparing the clinical nurse leader and clinical nurse specialist roles: Similarities, differences and complementarities.* Retrieved January 15, 2005, from http://www.aacn.nche.edu/CNL/index/htm

American Association of Colleges of Nursing. (2005a). *Partnership resources/CNL partnerships.* Retrieved February 1, 2005, from http://www.aacn.nche.edu/CNL/ index.htm

American Association of Colleges of Nursing. (2005b). *Clinical nurse leader update.* Retrieved February 1, 2005, from http://www.aacn.nche.edu/CNL/updates.htm

American Association of Colleges of Nursing. (2005c). *CNL frequently asked questions.* Retrieved January 15, 2005, from http://www.aacn.nche.edu/cnl/FAQ.htm

American Association of Colleges of Nursing. (2005d). *Doctor of nursing practice (DNP) programs.* Retrieved January 30, 2005, from http://www.aacn.nche.edu/DNP/DNPProgramList.htm

American Association of Colleges of Nursing. (2005e). *New data confirms shortage of nursing school faculty hinders efforts to address the nation's nursing shortage.* Retrieved February 1, 2005, from http://www.aacn.nche.edu/Media/NewsReleases/205Enrollment05.htm

Berlin, L. E., Stennett J., Bednash, G. D. (2004). *2003-2004 AACN enrollments and graduations in baccalaureate and graduate programs in nursing.* Washington, DC: American Association of Colleges of Nursing.

Buerhaus, P., Staiger, D., & Auerbach, D. (2000). Implications of a rapidly aging registered nurse workforce. *JAMA: The Journal of the American Medical Association, 283*(22), 2948-2954.

Buerhaus, P., Staiger, D., & Auerbach, D. (2003). Is the current shortage of hospital nurses ending? *Health Affairs, 22*(6), 191-198.

Camilleri, D. C. (2001). The century ahead: Old traditions and new challenges for nursing education. In J. M. Dochterman & H. K. Grace (Eds.), *Current issues in nursing* (pp. 90-98). St. Louis, MO: Mosby.

Goode, C. J., Pinkerton, S., McCausland, M. P., Southard, P., Graham, R., & Krsek, C. (2001). Documenting chief nursing officers' preference for BSN-prepared nurses. *Journal of Nursing Administration, 31*(2), 55-99.

Greene, D. L., Allan, J. D., & Henderson, T. (2003). *The role of states in financing nursing education.* Denver, CO: Institute for Primary Care and Workforce Analysis, National Conference of State Legislatures.

Greiner, A. C., & Knebel, E. (2003). *Health professions education: A bridge to quality.* Washington, DC: National Academies Press.

Hodes Group. (2004). *Health care metrics study, 12.15.04. Bernard Hodes Health Care Division.* New York: Author.

H.R. No. 3487, Nurse Reinvestment Act. (2002).

Institute of Medicine. (2001). *Crossing the quality chasm: A new health system for the 21st century.* Washington, DC: National Academies Press.

Joint Commission on Accreditation of Healthcare Organizations. (2002). *Health care at the crossroads: Strategies for addressing the evolving nursing crisis.* Chicago: Author.

Kimball, B., & O'Neil, E. (2002). *Health care's human crisis: The American nursing shortage.* Princeton, NJ: Robert Wood Johnson Foundation.

Kohn, L. T., Corrigan, J. M., & Donaldson, M. S. (Eds.). (2000). *To err is human: Building a safer health system.* Washington, DC: National Academies Press.

Marek, A. C. (2005, January 31/February 7). More nurses needed. *US News & World Report,* pp. 68-69.

Marion, L., Viens, D., O'Sullivan, A. L., Crabtree, K., Fontana, S., & Price, M. M. (2003). The practice doctorate in nursing: Future or fringe? *Topics in Advanced Practice Nursing eJournal, 3*(2).

National Advisory Council on Nurse Education and Practice. (1996). *Report to the secretary of the Department of Health and Human Services on the basic registered nurse workforce.* Washington, DC: United States Department of Health and Human Services, Health Resources and Services Administration, Bureau of Health Professions, Division of Nursing.

National Council of State Boards of Nursing. (2000). *Quarterly examination statistics: Volume, pass rates & first-time internationally educated candidates' countries.* Retrieved January 25, 2005, from http://www.ncsbn.org/about/annual reports.asp

National Council of State Boards of Nursing. (2002). *2001 employer's survey.* Chicago: Author.

National Council of State Boards of Nursing. (2004). *Quarterly examination statistics: Volume, pass rates & first-time internationally educated candidates' countries.* Retrieved January 25, 2005, from http://www.ncsbn.org/about/annual reports.asp

National League for Nursing. (2004). *Startling data from the NLN's comprehensive survey of all nursing programs evokes wake-up call.* New York: Author. Retrieved December 30, 2004, from http://www.nln.org/newsreleases/datarelease05.pdf

Nelson, R. (2005). Is there a doctor nurse in the house? A new vision for advanced practice nursing. *American Journal of Nursing, 105*(5), 28-29.

O'Sullivan, A. L. (2005). President's point: The practice doctorate in nursing. *The Mentor: The NONPF Newsletter, 16*(1), 1-2, 11.

U.S. Department of Labor, Bureau of Labor Statistics. (2004). *BLS releases 2002-12 employment projections.* Retrieved January 15, 2005, from www.bls.gov/news.release/ecopro.nr0.htm

U.S. Department of Labor, Bureau of Labor Statistics. (2004, Spring). High-paying occupations with many openings, projected 2002-12. *Occupational Outlook Quarterly.* Washington, DC: Author. Retrieved February 10, 2005, from http://www.bls.gov/opub/ooq/2004/spring/ oochart.pdf

CHAPTER
9

Educational Challenges

The Crisis in Quality

KATHRYN J. DOLTER

The first thing to do in a crisis is to determine whether a crisis really exists: *Is* the sky falling? Once one establishes that a crisis exists—the sky *is* falling—one then would analyze the situation systematically to determine possible courses of action to prevent the sky from falling further, get the sky back up to its original position, and remediate the consequences of the sky falling. This viewpoint chapter proposes to identify whether there a crisis in prelicensure nursing education through an examination of the outcomes of prelicensure nursing education. The chapter then presents a systematic analysis of inputs and processes that might have led to such a crisis, if one exists.

IS THERE A CRISIS IN PRELICENSURE NURSING EDUCATION?

The first question in analyzing any purported crisis is to determine whether that purported crisis exists. Determination of the existence of a crisis in the quality of nursing education would lead one to examine the trends in the outcomes of nursing education. Intermediate and final outcomes of nursing education that exist would need to be assessed over time to determine the existence of a crisis.

The primary outcome of nursing education would be the production of an adequate number of competent nurses to meet health care demand. The number of competent nurses produced per year is therefore a major outcome indicator. So then, what is a "competent nurse"? The National Council of State Boards of Nursing (NCSBN, 1996) defined the characteristics of a competent nurse (Box 9-1) and identified stakeholder accountability for nurse competency (Figure 9-1). Nursing education outcome indicators of prelicensure graduate nurse competency include first-time U.S.-educated NCLEX-RN pass rate, employer assessment of prelicensure graduate nurse competencies/satisfaction with

graduate competency, and graduate self-assessment of competency/satisfaction with competency preparation. However, these are only intermediate outcome indicators of nurse competency. End or terminal outcome indicators of nursing education include quality of care measures such as iatrogenic morbidity and mortality rates, quality of care process measures, patient satisfaction, cost of care measures, and access to care measures. Box 9-2 lists intermediate and final indicators of the nursing education outcome of nurse competency.

The outcomes indicators of nursing education listed in Box 9-2 are themselves the result of many variables. One first would have to established that a statistically significant trend occurred in one or more of those variables to determine whether a crisis really existed. What is the current status/trend in these nursing education outcome variables?

Question: Is There a Trend in the Number of Competent Graduate Nurses Produced?

The number of professional nursing graduates declined precipitously from 1995 to 1999 (Figure 9-2). However, the number of professional nursing graduates has been increasing since 2000. The number of competent professional nursing graduates as demonstrated by the number of graduates passing the NCLEX-RN on the first attempt also declined in the 1990s but since 2001 has been increasing (Figure 9-3).

Question: Is There a Downward Trend in First-Time U.S.-Educated NCLEX-RN Pass Rate?

The NCLEX-RN measures the competencies needed to practice safely and effectively as a newly licensed entry-level registered nurse. This examination is used by boards of nursing throughout the United States and its territories to assist in making licensure decisions. The NCLEX-RN is based on an incumbent job analysis of

BOX 9-1

Characteristics of a Competent Nurse

In addition to the definition of competence, the National Council of State Boards of Nursing developed the following standards.

The nurse is expected to do the following:

1. Apply knowledge and skills at the level required for a particular situation

Indicators:
- Determines actions needed to achieve desired outcomes
- Performs nursing activities in a safe/effective manner
- Demonstrates current knowledge necessary to provide safe client care
- Delegates in accordance with established guidelines
- Collaborates with appropriate professionals to attain client health care outcomes

2. Demonstrate responsibility and accountability for practice and decisions

Indicators:
- Exhibits ethical behavior
- Ensures that client welfare prevails

- Establishes and maintains therapeutic boundaries
- Limits practice to current knowledge, skills, and abilities
- Clarifies expectations of the role
- Intervenes when unsafe nursing practice occurs
- Practices within the legal authority granted by the jurisdiction
- Implements professional development activities based on assessed needs

3. Restrict and/or accommodate practice if the nurse cannot safely perform essential functions of the nursing role because of mental or physical disabilities

Indicators:
- Identifies abilities necessary to perform the essential functions of the nursing practice role
- Implements accommodations when needed
- Safely performs essential functions of the nursing practice role
- Limits practice when accommodations are not sufficient to enable safe performance of essential functions of the nursing practice role

From National Council of State Boards of Nursing. (1996). *Assuring competence: A regulatory responsibility.* Retrieved August 1, 2005, from http://www.ncsbn.org/resources/complimentary_ncsbn_competence.asp.

The Regulatory Board
- Establishes standards for competence
- Communicates standards
- Engages in a collaborative model to ensure ongoing standards
- Identifies mechanisms to demonstrate competence
- Holds individual nurses accountable through disciplinary process

The Individual Nurse
- Conducts self-assessment
- Develops developmental criteria to facilitate professional growth
- Accepts legal and ethical obligations of the profession
- Limits nursing practice and/or implements accommodations
- Participates in peer review

The Employer
- Incorporates standards into institutional policies
- Assesses nurses' performance
- Evaluates nurses upon report of poor performance
- Performs evaluations based upon standards
- Reports nurses who fail to meet standards to Board of Nursing

The Educator
- Incorporates standards into curriculum
- Promotes integration of standards by student
- Evaluates student performance based upon standards
- Provides first role model for student as to the expectation of life-long learning, professional accountability

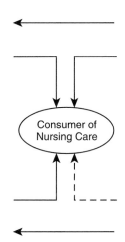

Consumer of Nursing Care

FIGURE 9-1 Stakeholder accountability for nursing competence. (From National Council of State Boards of Nursing. [1996]. *Assuring competence: A regulatory responsibility.* Retrieved August 1, 2005, from http://www.ncsbn.org/resources/complimentary_ncsbn_competence.asp.)

VIEWPOINTS

BOX 9-2

Outcome Indicators of Nursing Education

INTERMEDIATE OUTCOME INDICATORS: NATIONAL, STATE, AND PROGRAM LEVEL OUTCOMES
NCLEX pass rate
Employer satisfaction with graduate nurse educational preparation
Graduate nurse satisfaction with education preparation
Number of registered nurse graduates produced annually

END/TERMINAL OUTCOME INDICATORS: NATIONAL, STATE, AND HOSPITAL/PROVIDER LEVEL
Global Hospital Level
Iatrogenic morbidity and mortality rates
Adverse event rates
Patient satisfaction with care
Patient satisfaction
Cost of care
Supply cost
Access to care

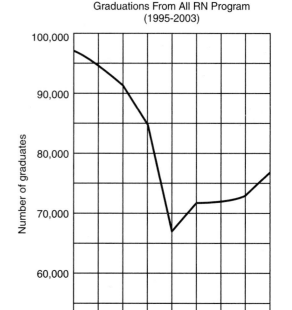

The number of nursing school graduates has begun to edge upward after a 31% decline (1995-1999), but many barriers to creating an adequate supply of nurses still exist.

FIGURE 9-2 Graduations from all registered nurse programs (1995-2003). (From Robert Woods Johnson Foundation. [2005]. Addressing the nursing shortage: Partnerships among governments, schools, and employers are getting results. *Charting Nursing's Future.* Retrieved August 1, 2005, from http://www.rwjf.org/files/publications/other/nursing_issue1_final2%20(2).pdf.)

newly licensed entry-level registered nurses. This analysis addresses critical nursing activities, the frequency of performance, and their impact on client safety. The job analysis is the foundation for development of a test plan that ensures that each unique NCLEX-RN reflects the knowledge, skills, and abilities essential for the registered nurse to meet the needs of clients requiring the promotion, maintenance, and restoration of health (NCSBN, 1999).

The NCLEX-RN has transitioned from a paper and pencil examination available intermittently throughout the year to a computer-adaptive testing examination available continuously.

Assessment of NCLEX-RN pass rates over time is important. Pass rates are cyclical when compared over the course of any given year (NCSBN, 2002) (Figure 9-4). The highest pass rates for any given year are in the April-to-June 30 time frame (NCSBN, 2005a). Figure 9-5 provides the trend of NCLEX-RN pass rates for first-time U.S.-educated candidates for the April-June time frame and the total for each year, obtained from review of NCLEX-RN statistics available on the NCSBN Web site:http://www.ncsbn.org/testing/psychometrics_nclexpassrates.asp (NCSBN, 2005a). A downward trend in NCLEX-RN pass rates appears for first-time U.S.-educated examination candidates from 1992 to 2000. This downward trend matched a previous trend in the years 1988 to 1990. The trend in pass rates of U.S.-educated first-time NCLEX-RN candidates has been upward from 2002 to 2005.

Answer

Currently, the trend in NCLEX-RN pass rates is not downward but rather upward. The NCSBN is revising and updating the NCLEX-RN constantly to ensure that the examination measures graduate nurse competence.

Question: Is There a Downward Trend in Employer and Graduate Nurse Satisfaction and With Graduate Nurse Preparation/Competency?

The NCSBN surveyed nurse employers in 2001 and 2003. Nurse employers were asked "if the various groups of newly licensed nurses were prepared to provide safe, effective care. Positive ratings were given to both ADN and BSN graduates by 41.9% of overall respondents,

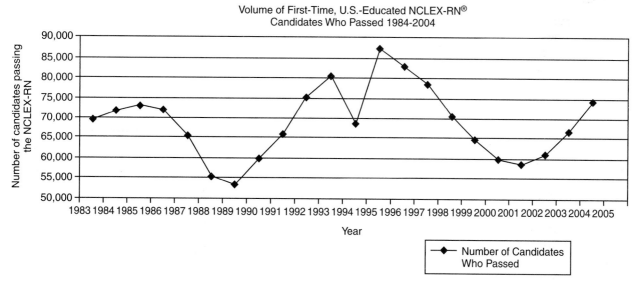

FIGURE 9-3 Number of U.S.-educated first-time candidates who passed the NCLEX-RN. (From National League for Nursing. [2005]. NLN board of governors takes faculty shortage to the Hill. *NLN Nursing Education Policy.* Retrieved August 1, 2005, from http://www. ctleaguefornursing.org/pdf/nursingeducationpolicy_june05.pdf.)

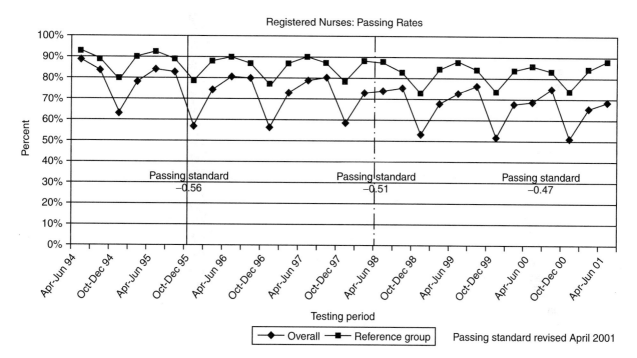

FIGURE 9-4 The cyclical nature of NCLEX-RN pass rates. (From National Council of State Boards of Nursing. [2002]. *NCLEX research report.* Retrieved August, 1, 2005, from http://www.ncsbn.org/pdfs/RecentNCLEXResearch_Web_Testing017B02.pdf.)

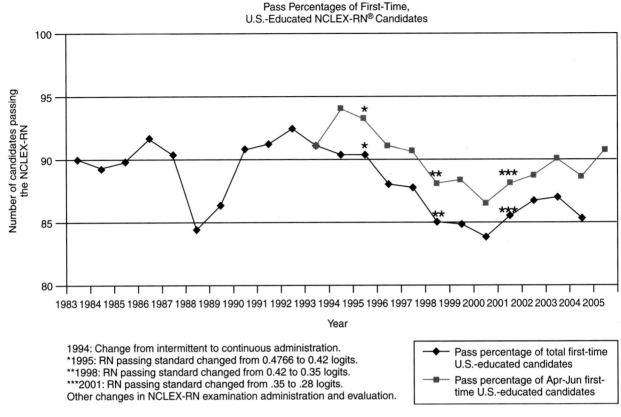

FIGURE 9-5 Pass percentages of U.S.-educated first-time NCLEX-RN candidates. (From National League for Nursing. [2005]. NLN board of governors takes faculty shortage to the Hill. *NLN Nursing Education Policy.* Retrieved August 1, 2005, from http://www.ctleaguefornursing.org/pdf/nursingeducationpolicy_june05.pdf.)

to diploma graduates by 48.8%, ..." (Smith & Crawford, 2004). Though 41.9% and 48.8% of employers gave positive ratings to nurses with bachelor of science in nursing (BSN) degrees or associate's degrees in nursing (ADN) and to nurses with diplomas (respectively) regarding whether they were competent ("prepared to provide safe, effective care"), 58.1% and 51.2% of employers must have given negative or neutral safe and effective care ratings to BSN/associate's degree in nursing and diploma graduates.

The Joint Commission on Accreditation of Healthcare Organizations (JCAHO, 2002) cites the NCSBN in its *Health Care at the Crossroads* report:

> In two recent studies from the National Council of State Boards of Nursing which asked entry-level nurses and employers of newly licensed nurses to rate the adequacy of nurses' preparation to perform a variety of patient care tasks, both groups ranked the adequacy of preparation low. Employers' rankings were much lower for every variable. Among these tasks, the ability of new nurses to respond to emergency situations, supervise the care provided by others, and perform psychomotor skills were rated at the lowest levels. (p. 3)

Answer

The NCSBN surveys were conducted at two points in time, 2001 and 2003. Employer satisfaction and graduate nurse satisfaction with graduate nurse competence/preparation was not positive. Data is available (to me) for only two points in time, 2 years apart. Therefore discernment of any trend in employer and graduate nurse satisfaction with graduate nurse competency is difficult. It would be interesting to assess and compare overall and task-specific employer and graduate satisfaction rates over time and their correlation with NCLEX-RN results.

Question: Is There a Trend in Terminal Nursing Education Outcome Indicators—Quality, Cost, and Access?

The 2.8 million nurses—with the 2.3 million nursing assistants that they supervise—compose 54% of the health care provider population in the United States (Greiner & Knebel, 2003). Though the health care outcomes of quality, cost, patient, and provider satisfaction are multi-factorial, nursing has a major impact on these outcomes.

Status of Quality Care in the United States. The Institute of Medicine has called into question the quality of health care in its two reports, *To Err Is Human* (1999) and *Crossing the Quality Chasm* (2001). These reports outlined the quality issues in the U.S. health care system and made recommendations for addressing identified problems. The *To Err Is Human* report (Kohn et al., 1999) cited estimates of hospital deaths caused by iatrogenic injuries ranging from 44,000 to 98,000 per year and indicated that the number of errors in hospitals exceeded that of the eighth leading cause of death in America. In the United States, iatrogenic hospital deaths exceeded deaths from breast cancer (45,297), motor vehicles (42,297), and acquired immunodeficiency syndrome (16,516). This iatrogenic mortality estimate is based on hospital errors alone and does not include iatrogenic deaths in outpatient clinics, same-day surgical settings, long-term care facilities, or other health care settings. Other safety statistics indicate that 7% of hospital patients experience a serious medication error and that 11% of hospital admissions are due to adverse drug events.

The *Crossing the Quality Chasm* report (Institute of Medicine, 2001) concluded that the American health care delivery system is lacking in each of the six dimensions of quality it defines within the report. Specifically, the report charges that U.S. health care is not the following:

◆ Safe: avoiding injuries to patients from the care that is intended to help
◆ Effective: providing services based on scientific knowledge
◆ Patient-centered: providing care that is respectful and responsive
◆ Timely: reducing waits and harmful delays
◆ Efficient: avoiding waste, including waste of supplies, ideas, and energy
◆ Equitable: providing care that does not vary in quality because of personal characteristics such as geographic location and socioeconomic status

Health care quality issues continue to exist following the publication of the *Crossing the Quality Chasm* report

(Institute of Medicine, 2001). In December 2003 the Agency for Healthcare Research and Quality (AHRQ) reported that "37 of 57 areas with trend data presented in the report have either shown no improvement or have deteriorated" (p. 2). Compared with similar countries—Australia, Canada, France, Germany, and the United Kingdom—the United States appears to offer lower quality of care. The United States has the highest infant mortality rate; the lowest length of life at birth for males and females; and the lowest disability-free life expectancy at birth (58.2 years) of any comparable Organization of Economic Cooperation and Development nation (Anderson, 1998). A second report indicated that although there have been improvements in some measures, "the gap between best possible care and actual care remains large" (AHRQ, 2004b)

Root causes of quality of care issues in hospitals identified by the Institute of Medicine in its *To Err Is Human* (1999), *Keeping Patients Safe: Transforming the Work Environment of Nurses* (Page, 2003), and *Health Professions Education: A Bridge to Quality* (Greiner & Knebel, 2003) reports included the following:

◆ Insufficient number of nurses
◆ Loss of the best nurses
◆ High nursing turnover
◆ Overworked nurses
◆ Unfocused nursing roles
◆ Too much wasteful work
◆ Process breakdowns
◆ Missed handoffs
◆ Interdisciplinary breakdowns
◆ Low compliance with best practices
◆ Insufficiently prepared nurse leaders
◆ Lack of reward systems
◆ Increased patient condition severity
◆ Shorter hospital stays
◆ Redesigned work
◆ Change in total nursing personnel in relationship to adjusted patient days
◆ High patient turnover
◆ Long work hours
◆ Rapid increases in new knowledge and technology
◆ Increased interruptions and demands on nurse's time
◆ Inadequate health professional preparation for the complexities of the environment of the twenty-first century health care system

Aiken, Clarke, Sloane, Sochalski, & Silber (2002) and others (AHRQ, 2004a) illustrated the importance of nursing on patient outcomes. Aiken et al. (2002) demonstrated the importance of the ratio of registered nurses to patients in patient outcomes, with higher morbidity and mortality noted on surgical units with lower BSN nurse-to-patient ratios. Aiken, Clarke, Cheung, Sloane, & Silber (2003) also found lower mortality and morbidity in hospitals with higher proportions of BSN nurses. "Higher rates of RN staffing were associated with a 3- to 12-percent reduction in adverse outcomes, depending on the outcome. Higher staffing at all levels of nursing was associated with a 2- to 25-percent reduction in adverse outcomes depending on the outcome" (AHRQ, 2004a). Nurse-to-patient ratios and proportion of BSN-prepared nurses affect health care. Population-specific nurse knowledge also has been associated with lower mortality rates. Dolter (1995) identified an association between greater knowledge of intensive care unit nurses regarding hemodynamic assessment techniques— the basis of cardiovascular therapy in the postoperative open heart surgery patients—and lower mortality in open heart surgical units.

Health care in the United States has quality issues, with studies demonstrating associations between quality of health care and the number, education level, and knowledge level of nurses.

Status of the Cost of Care in the United States.
The cost of health care in the United States exceeded $1.7 trillion in 2004 (Centers for Medicare and Medicaid Services, 2004). The approximately $4200 per capita health care spending in the United States exceeds the per capita health expenditures of comparable Organization of Economic Cooperation and Development (OECD) countries (Anderson, Petrosyn, & Hussey, 2002), with U.S. per capita health care expenditures being 2 to 3 times that of most OECD nations. Health care dollars in the United States are not spent on preventive services; 75% of health care dollars are spent on the care of chronic illness (U.S. Department of Health and Human Services, 2003). With 1% of people accounting for more than a quarter of all health spending (Centers for Medicare and Medicaid Services, 2004), the fairness of U.S. health care spending also is called into question. Research suggests that a sizable percentage of U.S. health care spending can be traced to the higher administrative costs required by the complexities of the U.S. system (Reinhardt, Hussey, & Anderson, 2004).

Cost of care issues in U.S. health care include the high costs related to morbidity (AHRQ, 2004a):

> While inadequate staffing levels place heavy burdens on the nursing staff and adverse events are painful for patients, there is also a considerable financial cost to be considered. An AHRQ-funded study found that all adverse events studied (pneumonia, pressure ulcer, UTI, wound infection, patient fall/injury, sepsis, and adverse drug event) were associated with increased costs. Treating pneumonia raised total treatment costs by $22,390-$28,505… Pressure ulcers are estimated to cost $8.5 billion per year.

The relationship between cost of health care and the number, education level, or knowledge level of nurses requires further study.

Status of Access to Health Care in the United States.
Even though the United States spends more on health care, health care is inaccessible to a greater percentage of its population relative to the other comparable OECD nations, with 16% of the U.S. population lacking health care coverage (National Center for Health Statistics, 2003). In the United States, approximately 43 million persons—including 8.5 million children—do not have health insurance (Institute of Medicine, 2004). Access to health care in the primarily employer-based health insurance system is decreasing because of the continued rise in health care costs leading to employer reduction of health benefits for full-time employees; increased use of part-time employees to avoid health care benefit provision; and reduction or elimination of retiree health benefits.

Health care in the United States has access issues. The relationship between access to health care and the number, education level, or knowledge level of nurses has not been studied.

Answer

Despite high health care expenditures in the United States, health care is inaccessible and poor quality. The Institute of Medicine (2001) in its *Crossing the Quality Chasm* series emphasizes that quality of care issues are primarily system issues, stating that "Health care has safety and quality problems because it relies on outmoded systems of work. Poor designs set the workforce up to fail, regardless of how hard they try. If we want safer, higher quality care, we will need to redesign systems of care" (p. 4). The Institute of Medicine concludes, "The current system cannot do the job. Trying harder will not work. Changing systems will" (p. 4).

The Institute of Medicine indicts the system of care rather than health care providers for the current crisis in health care quality. However, current health care providers, especially nurses—who make up 54% of the health care provider workforce—bear a major responsibility for the current and future status of quality, cost, and access of health care. Although advocating for changes in the system by current providers, the *Crossing the Quality Chasm* report (Institute of Medicine, 2001) also concluded that health professions education must ensure that future health professionals have the skills necessary to face these twenty-first century challenges in cost, quality, and access if the U.S. health care system is to improve. The report recommended that a multidisciplinary health care summit be convened to address "restructuring clinical education to be consistent with the principles of the 21st century health system throughout the continuum of undergraduate, graduate, and continuing education for medical, nursing, and other professional training programs" (p. 19). The Institute of Medicine convened this multidisciplinary summit, which culminated in the publication of *Healthcare Professions Education: A Bridge to Quality* (Greiner & Knebel, 2003). This report defined the changes in heath professions education that are needed to overcome the quality issues in U.S. health care system and other challenges of twenty-first century health care.

Within the *Healthcare Professions Education* report (Greiner & Knebel, 2003), the Institute of Medicine indicated that health professionals:

♦ "Are not adequately prepared to address shifts in the nation's patient population."

♦ "Are not educated or trained in team-based skills."

♦ "[Are not] schooled in how to search and evaluate the evidence base and apply it in practice."

♦ "Have few opportunities to avail themselves of coursework and other educational interventions that would aid them in analyzing the root causes of errors and other quality problems and designing system-wide fixes."

♦ "[Are] not provided a basic foundation in informatics."

The report ultimately recommended that "accreditation bodies should … revise their standards so that programs are required to demonstrate—through process and outcome measures—that they educate students to … deliver patient care using a core set of competencies". Box 9-3 lists other recommendations from the report. Currently, the NCSBN, the National League for Nursing, and the American Association of Colleges of Nursing do not incorporate the five competencies identified by the Institute of Medicine (Tables 9-1 and 9-2).

The NCSBN currently is studying post-entry practice to determine the impact of nursing education and other factors on the competence/safe practice of nurses and licensed practical nurses in response to calls since the *Crossing the Quality Chasm* report for health care regulatory bodies to ensure safe practices of those they regulate and calls by advocates for BSN-level of entry into the profession for a separate BSN licensure examination (NCSBN, 2005b). The NCSBN Post-Entry Competence Study initiated in August 2001 is a combined cross-sectional and longitudinal cohort study to answer the following questions:

1. What are the characteristics of post–entry-level practice?
2. How do the characteristics of practice change over time?
3. To what extent do factors specific to the individual nurse (e.g., age, gender, type of basic nursing educational program, and propensity for self-study) influence the evolution of practice?
4. To what extent do environmental factors (e.g., work setting, mentors or preceptors, continuing education, work experience, and knowledge resources) influence the evolution of practice?
5. What are the characteristics of safe versus unsafe practice?

Conclusion

Nursing outcomes indicators are mixed on whether there is a crisis in health care education. The number of graduates from registered nurse programs had been trending downward in the 1990s but has been increasing since 2000. Pass rates for the NCLEX-RN currently are trending upward after a downward trend from the early 1990s to 2002, and though employer and graduate nurse assessment of graduate nurse competency are low, data is insufficient to assess a trend. The quality, cost, and access issues in U.S. health care are the responsibility of nurses and other health care providers. Even though these global outcomes have multifactorial causes, the number of nurses, education level, and knowledge level have a demonstrated association with these outcomes. Nurse competency is a major issue. Nursing education must produce an adequate number of competent professional nurses to ensure the provision of quality health care.

PRELICENSURE NURSING EDUCATION INPUT ASSESSMENT

Inputs to nursing education include money, students, and faculty. An analysis of these inputs and discussion of input-specific issues, concerns, and recommendations follow.

Input: Funding for Prelicensure Nursing Education

The amount of federal funding for nursing education is far below that of medical education. In 2001, $78 million was appropriated to fund basic and advanced nursing

BOX 9-3

Institute of Medicine Recommendations

Recommendation 1: The Department of Health and Human Services and leading foundations should support an interdisciplinary effort focused on developing a common language, with the ultimate aim of achieving consensus across the health professions on a core set of competencies that includes patient-centered care, interdisciplinary teams, evidence-based practice, quality improvement, and informatics.

Recommendation 2: The Department of Health and Human Services should provide a forum and support for a series of meetings involving the spectrum of oversight organizations across and within the disciplines. Participants in these meetings would be charged with developing strategies for incorporating a core set of competencies into oversight activities based on definitions shared across the professions. These meetings actively would solicit the input of health professions associations and the education community.

Recommendation 3: Building upon previous efforts, accreditation bodies should move forward expeditiously to revise their standards so that programs are required to demonstrate—through process and outcome measures—that they educate students in academic and continuing education programs in how to deliver patient care using a core set of competencies. In so doing, these bodies should coordinate their efforts.

Recommendation 4: All health professions boards should move toward requiring licensed health professionals to demonstrate periodically their ability to deliver patient care as defined by the five competencies identified by the committee through direct measures of technical competence, patient assessment, evaluation of patient outcomes, and other evidence-based assessment methods. These boards simultaneously should evaluate the different assessment methods.

Recommendation 5: Certification bodies should require their certificate holders to maintain their competence throughout the course of their careers by periodically demonstrating their ability to deliver patient care that reflects the five competencies, among other requirements.

Recommendation 6: Foundations, with support from education and practice organizations, should take the lead in developing and funding regional demonstration learning centers representing partnerships between practice and education. These centers should leverage existing innovative organizations and be state-of-the art training settings focused on teaching and assessing the five core competencies.

Recommendation 7: Through Medicare demonstration projects, the Centers for Medicare and Medicaid Services should take the lead in funding experiments that will enable and create incentives for health professionals to integrate interdisciplinary approaches into educational or practice settings, with the goal of providing a training ground for students and clinicians that incorporates the five core competencies.

Recommendation 8: The Agency for Healthcare Research and Quality and private foundations should support ongoing research projects addressing the five core competencies and their association with individual and population health, as well as research related to the link between the competencies and evidence-based education. Such projects should involve researchers across two or more disciplines.

Recommendation 9: The Agency for Healthcare Research and Quality should work with a representative group of health care leaders to develop measures reflecting the core set of competencies, set national goals for improvement, and issue a report to the public evaluating progress toward these goals. The Agency for Healthcare Research and Quality should issue the first report, focused on clinical educational institutions, in 2005 and produce annual reports thereafter.

Recommendation 10: Beginning in 2004, a biennial interdisciplinary summit should be held involving health care leaders in education, oversight processes, practice, and other areas. This summit should focus on reviewing progress against explicit targets and setting goals for the next phase regarding the five competencies and other areas necessary to prepare professionals for the twenty-first century health system.

Reprinted with permission from *Health Professions Education: A Bride to Quality,* © 2003 by the National Academy of Sciences, courtesy of the National Academies Press, Washington, D.C.

education compared with $9 billion in federal funding of medical education. "During the last serious nursing shortage (1974), Congress appropriated $153 million for nurse education programs. In today's dollars that would be worth $592 million, approximately four times what the federal government is spending now" (National League for Nursing [NLN], 2005a).

Various stakeholders have recommended increased funding for nursing education, specifically nursing students and nursing faculty (JCAHO, 2002). The NLN

TABLE 9-1

Accrediting Organizations and Standards Addressing the Five Health Profession Competencies

Accrediting Organizations	Quality Improvement	Patient-Centered Care	Informatics	Interdisciplinary Teams	Evidence-Based Practice
MEDICINE					
Undergraduate					
Liaison Committee on Medical Education (2000) American Osteopathic Association (2002b)		X		X	X
Residency					
Accreditation Council for Graduate Medical Education (1999)	X	X	X	X	X
American Osteopathic Association (2002a)	X	X	X	X	X
PHARMACY					
Undergraduate					
American Council on Pharmaceutical Education (2002)	X	X	X	X	X
Residency					
American Society of Health-System Pharmacists (2001)	X	X	X	X	X
PHYSICIAN ASSISTANT					
Accreditation Review Commission on Education for the Physician Assistant (2001)	X	X		X	X
NURSING					
National League for Nursing Accrediting Commission (1999)		X		X	X
Commission on Collegiate Nursing Education (1998)				X	
OCCUPATIONAL THERAPY					
Accreditation Council for Occupational Therapy Education (1998)	X	X	X	X	X
CLINICAL LABORATORY					
National Accrediting Agency for Clinical Laboratory Sciences (2001)	X		X	X	X
RESPIRATORY THERAPY					
Committee on Accreditation for Respiratory Care (2000)		X	X		X

From Greiner, A. C., & Knebel, E. (Eds.). (2003). *Health professions education: A bridge to quality.* Washington, DC: National Academies Press.

(2005a) has advocated for increased expenditure on nursing education research to ensure evidence-based nursing education. Public-private partnerships are being advocated to assist in defraying costs related to faculty and equipment (Robert Woods Johnson Foundation, 2005). Lack of funding to support nursing education affects its other inputs, nursing students, and nursing faculty.

Input Assessment: Prelicensure Nursing Students

Before 2000, enrollment of students in U.S. nursing prelicensure programs was declining. Though enrollment has increased since 2000, the increase will be insufficient to meet the projected need for nurses in upcoming years with implications for the current and future quality of health care (Figures 9-6 and 9-7). The need for nurses in

TABLE 9-2

Licensure Examinations and Content Related to the Five Health Profession Competencies

Examination	Quality Improvement	Patient-Centered Care	Informatics	Interdisciplinary Teams	Evidence-Based Practice
MEDICINE					
USMLE (United States Medical Licensing Exam, 2002a)	X	X			X
COMLEX (National Board of Osteopathic Medical Examiners, 2002)		X			
PANCE (National Commission on Certification of Physician Assistants, 2002)		X			
PHARMACY					
NAPLEX (National Association of Boards of Pharmacy, 2002)		X			X
NURSING					
NCLEX-RN (National Council of State Boards of Nursing, 2000)	X	X		X	
ALLIED HEALTH					
NBCOT (National Board for Certification in Occupational Therapy, 2002a)	X	X			X
NBRC (National Board for Respiratory Care, 2001)					

From Greiner, A. C., & Knebel, E. (Eds.). (2003). *Health professions education: A bridge to quality.* Washington, DC: National Academies Press.

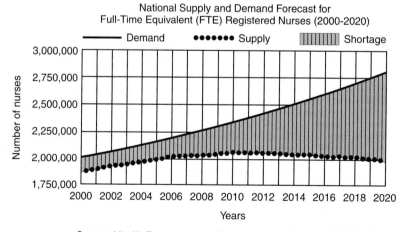

National Supply and Demand Forecast for Full-Time Equivalent (FTE) Registered Nurses (2000-2020)

Source: Health Resources and Services Administration (HRSA) 2002

FIGURE 9-6   Supply and demand forecast for registered nurses (2000-2020). (From Robert Woods Johnson Foundation. [2005]. Addressing the nursing shortage: Partnerships among governments, schools, and employers are getting results. *Charting Nursing's Future.* Retrieved August 1, 2005, from http://www.rwjf.org/files/publications/other/nursing_issue1_final2%20(2).pdf.)

The Growing Shortage of Full-Time Equivalent (FTE) Registered Nurses

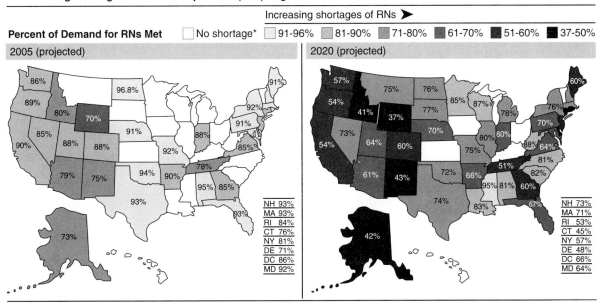

FIGURE 9-7   States affected by nursing shortage: 2005 and 2020.

the United States is projected to be 2.8 million by 2020 (Health Resources and Services Administration, 2002). Even with recent increases in young, U.S.-educated nurses and the recent increases in the recruitment of international nurses and older nurses returning to the workforce, the projected supply is only estimated to peak at 2.3 million, 500,000 short (Buerhaus, Staiger, & Auerbach, 2004).

Enrollments, though increasing from 2000, are still down from pre-1995 levels. A probable cause of decreased enrollments is the expanded employment opportunities that have developed for women. Flat salaries (Health Resources and Services Administration, 2000); a physically demanding and potentially dangerous work environment, which includes exposure to dangerous chemicals and biohazards; the constant high stress of performing in life-or-death situations; and scheduling demands affecting personal quality of life cause nursing to appear less desirable compared with the other more lucrative, less stressful employment opportunities that have opened up to women since the 1970s (American Association of Colleges of Nursing [AACN], 2005b). Other issues affecting enrollment in nursing programs include high

tuition rates, lack of scholarship or other funding opportunities, increasing attrition, and inadequate math and science preparation (Robert Woods Johnson Foundation, 2005). Enrolled students are older and include more nontraditional students (AACN, 2003a).

Even though nursing enrollments are increasing (NLN, 2003b), many "qualified" nurse applicants are being turned away from all levels of nursing education programs because of an inadequate number of spaces: "An estimated 125,000 applications were tuned away from nursing programs at all levels for the academic year 2003-2004" (NLN, 2004).

Currently, with not enough spaces for all of the qualified applicants to nursing programs, the primary strategy to increase the number of competent graduates from nursing programs would need to focus on increasing the capability to increase enrollments in those programs. An increase in enrollments could be achieved by (1) opening more nursing programs, which is constrained by lack of nursing faculty and clinical sites (nursing education inputs to be discussed later), and (2) redesign of current nursing programs to facilitate increased enrollments through more creative use of existing nursing faculty and more creative use of or development of alternatives to the limited clinical sites. Lack of faculty and clinical sites are major constraints to increasing enrollments. Creative solutions to increase enrollments by nursing education programs discussed by Oermann (2004) include "offering … nursing programs on site in clinical agencies … [where] advanced practice nurses and clinicians provide clinical teaching with academic faculty assuming responsibility for the class-room component and coordinating the course."

Secondary strategies that focus on increasing the enrollment of qualified students into nursing educa-tion programs include improved and earlier recruit-ment such as the Johnson and Johnson (http://www. discovernursing.com/) and Nurses for a Healthier Tomorrow (http://www.nursesource.org/mission.html) campaigns. Tertiary strategies to support those who become interested in a career in nursing would need to focus on (1) increasing the funding for nursing students through scholarships, grants, and service-cancelable loans (dollar input discussed previously) and (2) increasing the convenience of obtaining a nursing degree through implementation of accelerated nursing programs, time-saver programs embedded within the traditional setting to support those who must work to pay for their education, and Web-based nursing curricula. Primary, secondary, and tertiary enrollment strategies would need to be pursued simultaneously.

Another strategy not found in the literature but suggested by a colleague involves better matching of the supply of qualified applicants to nursing programs to the available nursing program "slots." This strategy would involve the development of a "match program" by which qualified applicants unable to gain entry at a local school because of local demand for nurse student spaces exceeds the supply for those spaces would be notified of approved/accredited nursing schools throughout the nation in which student spaces/slots were not filled (Rachel McDermott, RN, BSN, personal communication, spring 2005).

Input Assessment: Nursing Faculty

Currently, there are fewer than 20,000 nursing faculty, with a projected need for 40,000 to address the nursing shortage (NLN, 2005a). Reasons for the faculty short-age include the aging and retirement of current faculty; lack of competitiveness of nursing salaries in academia compared with industry; lack of funding for education of prospective nursing faculty; state budgets constrai-ning faculty hiring at public institutions; budgetary constraints in hiring at private institutions for what is perceived as a resource-intensive department; and faculty dissatisfaction. Faculty dissatisfaction relates to workload and role expectations, including the disparity between the "counting" of clinical hours versus didactic hours; the lack of value and incentives for the teaching role in the current tenure system; the need to accommodate the broad range of student capabilities (aging, nontraditional/ traditional, and multigenerational); and frustration with student study habits (AACN, 2003a; AACN, 2005c; JCAHO, 2002; Oermann, 2004; Robert Woods Johnson Foundation, 2005; Valiga, 2002).

Strategies to address the faculty shortage focus on improving (1) the use of faculty positions; (2) the recruitment of nurses into nursing education; (3) the retention of current faculty; and (4) the preparation of faculty for the educative role. Improved use of faculty positions includes the use of part-time faculty; joint appointments with industry; preceptorships; use of retired faculty; and use of interdisciplinary faculty (AACN, 2003a; JCAHO, 2002; Oermann, 2004; Robert Woods Johnson Foundation, 2005; Valiga, 2002). With the clinical component of nursing education the most labor-intensive faculty input, focused strategies that have been proposed or are already in use include decreasing faculty-to-student ratios in clinical rota-tions, expanding use of preceptorships throughout nursing curricula, and decreasing or eliminating the requirement for a clinical component to nursing educa-tion. Issues and concerns arise with the implementation of any of these strategies.

In light of studies by Aiken et al. (2002) and others (AHRQ, 2004a) relative to mandatory nurse-to-patient staffing ratios, the lowering of faculty-to-student ratios in the clinical arena would seem to be counterintuitive. Experienced nurses can safely provide care for a maxi-mum of five to six noncritically ill hospitalized patients. Therefore, how could a nurse educator be expected to safely supervise, teach, and evaluate more than eight students caring for eight similarly ill patients?

Examination of the expanded use of preceptorships has identified issues with that strategy. Within a precep-torship, staff nurses replace faculty in mentoring nurs-ing students, guiding students on a one-to-one basis in the clinical area, usually in the student's final semester. If the staff nurse preceptor is a volunteer appropriately qualified by education and extent of clinical experience, is appropriately educated in the preceptor role, is provided student learning objectives, is afforded lower patient load responsibilities during student precepting experi-ences, is afforded a break from the precepting role, and is compensated for the extra responsibility of education in addition to patient care, then preceptorship would appear to be an advantageous method of extending nurse faculty. Unfortunately, overuse of nurse preceptorships may lead to an abrogation of nurse faculty responsibility to overworked, underpaid, poorly prepared nonvolunteer staff nurse preceptors with resultant implications for the quality of nursing education and the quality of patient care.

The NLN is calling for innovation in nursing education (2003b) but is advocating that nursing education innovations be evidence-based and that nursing education research increase (2005b). No study of the preceptorship on nursing education outcomes was identified in a systematic review published by the NCSBN (2005c). Examination of the optimal ratio of nurse faculty to students also was not noted in the NCSBN systematic review.

Strategies to improve faculty recruitment and retention include increased funding for nurse faculty education and improved nurse faculty salaries in relation to industry, increased valuation of the teaching role of nurse faculty (as opposed to service and research roles in academia); and increased support of the administrative functions of nursing faculty (grading/paperwork). More controversial strategies to increase nurse faculty recruitment include elimination of the undergraduate degree as a prerequisite to graduate study and elimination of clinical experience requirements as a prerequisite to graduate study. Controversy in relation to these strategies relates to the ability of a faculty member of a practice profession who has never practiced a profession to teach that profession. With the majority of nurses working in hospitals or nonacademic, nonresearch positions (Health Resources and Services Administration, 2000), it is difficult to understand how faculty who have never had any clinical experience can teach or role-model effective nurse practice in those settings. The JCAHO white paper on nursing (2002, p. 30) comments about "the lack of awareness of nursing faculty about actual nursing practice today" and the "continental divide between nursing education and nursing practice." Improved preparation of nurse faculty has been suggested by others (Valiga, 2002) and includes expansion of graduate programs focused on nursing education. Nursing education–oriented service-cancelable loans also would increase the number of nurses choosing the faculty role rather than the industry role.

Input Assessment: Patient Care Experiences

A major limitation to the number of students a nursing program can matriculate is the availability of clinically relevant patient care experiences. With the decrease in patient admission and patient length of stay and closures of units and hospitals (American Hospital Association, 2002; U.S. Department of Health and Human Services, 2002), fewer clinical opportunities are available. Creative use of available clinical sites (weekends, evenings, nights, summer, winter) and less focus on hours spent in clinical settings and more focus on guided, reflective examination of clinical experiences are possible solutions, as are substituting the use of clinical simulation for clinical hours and decreasing or eliminating clinical experiences within nursing curricula. Elimination of clinical content in the curricula is controversial:

> AONE [American Organization of Nurse Executives] … believes that the education programs for the nurses of the future will require a balance of didactic content and supervised clinical instruction. Although innovative approaches may be developed, it is the position of AONE that all prelicensure nursing education programs must contain structured and supervised clinical instruction and that the clinical instruction must be provided by appropriately prepared registered nurses. (NCSBN, 2005c)

PRELICENSURE NURSING EDUCATIONAL PROCESSES

"Variation is the enemy of quality" is a pronouncement that has been attributed to Demming, the father of total quality management and the infamous plan-do-study-act quality cycle. Yet the hallmark of nursing and nursing education is variation. Variation is pervasive in the preparation of nursing graduates for registered nurse licensure and exists in types of programs, curricula within each type of program, mode of program delivery, and the amount and type of clinical/patient experience required. Nothing is standardized in nursing prelicensure programs.

Currently, various stakeholders are promoting changes in curricula such as the addition of end-of-life, gerontology, and bioterrorism content requirements. The Institute of Medicine (Greiner & Knebel, 2003) is advocating that nursing programs develop evidence-based medicine, informatics, quality improvement, patient-centered care, and teamwork competencies in its graduates, which requires further curricular change. Clinical simulation and Web-based education are being promoted, and the requirement for clinical experiences in prelicensure programs is being debated (NCSBN, 2005c). Employers advocate for those competencies they view as most important: critical thinking experiences and

TABLE 9-3

Joint Commission on Accrediation of Healthcare Organizations Recommendations for Bolstering Nursing Educational Infrastructure	
Tactics	**Accountability**
Fund nurse faculty positions and student scholarships for all levels of nursing education.	Federal and state governments Private industry Foundations
Increase federal funding for nursing education through the Nurse Education Act and Medicare monies appropriated for clinical education.	Federal government
Provide fast-track, low-cost opportunities for nurses to achieve higher levels of education.	Nursing schools Hospitals Private industry Foundations
Establish standardized postgraduate nurse residency programs,a nursing equivalent of the Accreditation Council for Graduate Medical Education, and funding to support this training.	Nursing schools in partnership with hospitals Federal government
Emphasize team training in undergraduate and postgraduate nurse education and training programs.	Nursing schools Medical schools Allied health schools Hospitals
Enhance hospital budgets for nursing orientation and in-service and continuing education.	Hospitals
Create nursing career ladders commensurate with educational level, training, and experience.	Hospitals Nursing schools

From Joint Commission on Accreditation of Healthcare Organizations. (2002). *Health care at the crossroads.* Retrieved August 1, 2005, from http://www.jcaho.org/about+us/public+policy+initiatives/nurse+staffing+crisis.htm.

therapeutic relationship skills (Smith & Crawford, 2004), whereas new graduates advocate for other competencies. Table 9-3 shows process recommendations by various stakeholders at a summit convened by the JCAHO (2002).

Meanwhile, change continues: baccalaureate programs may be offered at community colleges (AACN, 2005a); a clinical nurse leader program (AACN, 2003b) is being implemented at the master's level; others advocate for a postgraduation/licensure residency requirement before independent practice (JCAHO, 2002); and still others promote simulation as the answer to diminishing opportunities for clinical instruction within health care provider agencies. The NLN (2005b) currently is advocating for evidence-based nursing education innovation and centers of educational excellence, at the same time that non–evidence-based innovations are being implemented vigorously by others. Evidence is being gathered for some innovations: studies are ongoing relative to the effectiveness of the simulation (Jeffries & Rizzola, 2005) and postgraduation/licensure residencies (JCAHO, 2002).

PROCESS ASSESSMENT: PRELICENSURE REGULATION AND ACCREDITATION

Regulatory and accrediting agencies are facing ever greater challenges in the performance of their mission to protect the public. These agencies are charged with ensuring the competence of nurses and the adequacy of nursing education providers in the ever-changing, challenging health care environment of twenty-first century. Faced with competing demands of their various stakeholders, variation in the nursing education regulatory and accreditation process has become the norm. State Boards of Nursing have variable structure and process requirements for nursing education programs. Instead of one accrediting agency for all nursing education programs, there are two. Nursing education programs write self-assessments for accreditation and approval instead of being judged by standardized, evidence-based process and outcome measures. While variation is seen as the enemy of quality from a total quality management perspective, variation in regulation and accreditation requirements is also

BOX 9-4

Nursing Agenda for the Future: Education Strategies

- Establish congruence between the educational enterprise and societal needs (primary strategy).
- Enrich the high caliber of nursing faculty.
- Attain clarity in education about nursing roles and scopes of practice.
- Work for universal excellence in nursing education.
- Promote the value of nursing education to the profession and the public.

OBJECTIVES TO SUPPORT THE PRIMARY STRATEGY

- Redefine scopes of nursing practice and the educational preparation for each scope of practice to meet the general and specialized health care needs of society.
- Establish standards for the educational preparation of nurses for roles as nurse educators in academic and practice settings.
- Secure funding to establish Magnet models or centers of excellence in education. These centers will provide an environment for research and demonstration of new education models and partnerships.
- Pursue adequate funding for individuals who are seeking a nursing education to prepare for registered nurse licensure and for individuals seeking advanced education degrees for roles as nurse educators.

COCHAMPIONS

- American Association of Colleges of Nursing
- National League for Nursing

From American Nurses Association. (2002). *Nursing's agenda for the future.* Retrieved August 1, 2005, from http://nursingworld.org/naf/Nafa.pdf.

BOX 9-5

National Council on State Boards of Nursing Recommendations Regarding Prelicensure Clinical Instruction

The position of National Council on State Boards of Nursing is that

- Prelicensure nursing educational experiences should be across the life span.
- Prelicensure nursing education programs should include clinical experiences with actual patients; they might also include innovative teaching strategies that complement clinical experiences for entry into practice competency.
- Prelicensure clinical education should be supervised by qualified faculty who provide feedback and facilitate reflection.
- Faculty members retain the responsibility to demonstrate that programs have clinical experiences with actual patients that are sufficient to meet program outcomes.
- Additional research needs to be conducted on prelicensure nursing education and the development of clinical competency.

From National Council of State Boards of Nursing. (2005b). *Post-entry competence study research proposal August 2001.* Retrieved August 8, 2005, from http://www.ncsbn.org/regulation/researchregulation_research_post_entry_competencystudy.asp.

confusing to various stakeholders and may not serve the public well. Without standardized, evidence-based assessment of nursing programs, best practices cannot be identified. Just as there is need to increase the transparency of health care through publication of health care provider outcomes on the Web for easy access by the public by the Centers for Medicare and Medicaid (U.S. Department of Health and Human Services, 2005a, 2005b), there is a need for increasing transparency of nursing education provider outcomes via publication of NCLEX-RN pass rates on the Web for easy access by the public and nursing education stakeholders (Boxes 9-4 and 9-5).

SUMMARY

Assessment of the outcomes of nursing education produces mixed results as to whether there is a crisis in nursing education and its production of competent nurses. When nursing education is judged by NCLEX-RN outcomes alone, there is no crisis. However, when nursing education is judged by graduate nurse and employer assessment of graduate nurse competencies, there is a crisis. The crisis in health care quality and cost, for which nursing is accountable with other health care professionals, also forces nurses to question the adequacy of nursing education in developing competent nurses for twenty-first century health care systems.

Analyses of the inputs and processes of nursing education identified input problems and some strategies for input and process improvement. Controversies exist relative to some of the identified input and process strategies, especially relative to implementation of non–evidence-based nursing education process innovations. A major quality of nursing education and nursing education regulation and accreditation issue—process variation—was identified.

Nursing education, regulation, and accreditation process variation needs to be decreased for quality improvement to happen. Standardized, evidence-based outcome measures to supplement NCLEX-RN pass rates, such as employer and graduate nurse competence/ satisfaction surveys to be used by all programs of nursing need to be developed, implemented, and publicized. Nursing education outcome measurement should be a transparent process, with all data easily accessible to the public and other stakeholders.

Evidence-based nursing best practices then can be identified, based on these outcome measures, and process improvements can be implemented to achieve quality improvement in nursing education. The move to evidence-based nursing education outcomes measurement, identification of nursing education best practices/ processes, and dissemination of nursing education best practices/processes for quality improvement across all providers of nursing education is essential to ensuring the provision of quality health care in the twenty-first century.

REFERENCES

Agency for Healthcare Research and Quality. (2003). *National healthcare quality report, 2003*. Retrieved August 7, 2005, from http://www.qualitytools.ahrq.gov/qualityreport/ archive/2003/browse/browse.aspx

Agency for Healthcare Research and Quality. (2004a). Hospital nurse staffing and quality of care. *Research in Action*, (14). Retrieved August 7, 2005, from http:// www.ahrq.gov/research/nursestaffing/nursestaff.pdf

Agency for Healthcare Research and Quality. (2004b). *National healthcare quality report, 2004*. Retrieved August 7, 2005, from http://www.qualitytools.ahrq.gov/qualityreport/ browse/browse.aspx

Aiken, L. H., Clarke, S. P., Sloane, D. M., Sochalski, J., & Silber, J. H. (2002). Hospital nurse staffing and patient mortality, nurse burnout, and job dissatisfaction. *JAMA: The Journal of American Medical Association, 28*(16), 1987-1993.

Aiken, L. H., Clarke, S. P., Cheung, R. B., Sloane, D. M., & Silber, J. H. (2003). Educational levels of hospital nurses and surgical patient mortality. *JAMA: The Journal of American Medical Association, 290,* 1617-1623.

American Association of Colleges of Nursing. (2003a). *Faculty shortages in baccalaureate and graduate nursing programs: Scope of the problem and strategies for expanding the supply.* Retrieved August 7, 2005, from http://www.aacn.nche.edu/ Publications/pdf/TFFFWP.pdf

American Association of Colleges of Nursing. (2003b). *Working paper on the role of the clinical nurse leader.* Retrieved August 7, 2005, from http://www.aacn.nche.edu/ Publications/WhitePapers/ClinicalNurseLeader.htm

American Association of Colleges of Nursing. (2005a). *AACN's statement on baccalaureate nursing programs offered by community colleges.* Retrieved August 8, 2005, from http://www. aacn.nche.edu/Publications/positions/DRAFTCCBSNs Statement.htm

American Association of Colleges of Nursing. (2005b). *Nursing faculty shortage.* Retrieved August 1, 2005, from, http:// www.aacn.nche.edu/Media/FactSheets/facultyshortage.htm

American Hospital Association. (2002). *TrendWatch Chartbook 2002: Trends affecting hospitals and health systems, November 2002.* Retrieved, August 7, 2005, from http://www. hospitalconnect.com/ahapolicyforum/trendwatch/ chartbook2002.html

Anderson, G. F. (1998). *Multinational comparisons of health care: Expenditures, coverage, and outcomes.* Center for Hospital Finance and Management, John Hopkins University. Retrieved March 1, 2003, from http://www.cmwf.org/ usr_doc/Anderson_multinational.pdf

Anderson, G. F., Petrosyan, V., & Hussey, P. S. (2002). *Multinational comparisons of health systems data, 2002.* John Hopkins University. Retrieved August 1, 2005, from http://www.cmwf.org/usr_doc/Anderson_healthpop_ multi99_354.pdf

Buerhaus, P. I., Staiger, D. O., & Auerbach, D. I. (2004). New signs of a strengthening U.S. nurse labor market? *Health Affairs.* Retrieved August 1, 2005, from http://content. healthaffairs.org/cgi/content/full/hlthaff.w4.526/DC1

Centers for Medicare and Medicaid Services. (2004). *National health accounts: Definitions, sources, and methods used in the NHE 2003.* Retrieved November 12, 2004, from http:// www.cms.hhs.gov/statistics/nhe/definitions-sources- methods/

Dolter, K. J. (1995). *Identifying process variation via risk-adjusted outcome.* Unpublished doctoral dissertation, University of California, San Francisco.

Greiner, A. C., & Knebel, E. (Eds.). (2003). *Health professions education: A bridge to quality.* Washington, DC: National Academies Press.

Health Resources and Services Administration. (2000). *The registered nurse population: Findings from the National Sample Survey of Registered Nurses.* Retrieved April 13, 2005, from http://bhpr.hrsa.gov/healthworkforce/reports/rnsurvey/ default.htm

Health Resources and Services Administration, Bureau of Health Professions, & National Center for Workforce Analysis. (2002). *Projected supply, demand, and shortages of registered nurses: 2000-2020.* Retrieved August 14, 2005, from ftp://ftp.hrsa.gov/bhpr/nationalcenter/rnproject.pdf

Institute of Medicine. (2001). *Crossing the quality chasm.* Washington, DC: National Academies Press.

Institute of Medicine. (2004). *Insuring America's health: Principles and recommendations.* Washington, DC: National Academies Press.

Jeffries, P. R., & Rizzolo, M. A. (2005). *Progress report. Project title: Designing and implementing models for the innovative use of simulation to teach nursing care of ill adults and children: A national, multi-site, multi-method study.* Retrieved August 7, 2005, from http://www.nln.org/research/LaerdalReport05.pdf

Joint Commission on Healthcare Accreditation. (2002). *Health care at the crossroads.* Retrieved August 1, 2005, from http://www.jcaho.org/about+us/public+policy+initiatives/nurse+staffing+crisis.htm

Kohn, L. T., Corrigan, J. M., & Donaldson, M. S. (Eds.). (1999). *To err is human: Building a safer health system.* Washington, DC: National Academies Press.

National Center for Health Statistics. (2003). *Chartbook on trends in the health of Americans.* Retrieved November 12, 2004, from http://www.cdc.gov/nchs/data/hus/hus03cht.pdf

National Council of State Boards of Nursing. (1996). *Assuring competence: A regulatory responsibility.* Retrieved August 1, 2005, from http://www.ncsbn.org/resources/complimentary_ncsbn_competence.asp

National Council of State Boards of Nursing. (1999). *Uniform core licensure requirements.* Retrieved August 8, 2005, from http://www.ncsbn.org/resources/complimentary_ncsbn_uclr.asp

National Council of State Boards of Nursing. (2005a). *NCLEX® examination pass rates.* Retrieved August 1, 2005, from http://www.ncsbn.org/testing/psychometrics_nclexpassrates.asp

National Council of State Boards of Nursing. (2005b). *Post-entry competence study research proposal, August 2001.* Retrieved August 8, 2005, from http://www.ncsbn.org/regulation/researchregulation_research_post_entry_competencystudy.asp

National Council on State Boards of Nursing. (2005c). *Section II. 2005 NCSBN annual meeting.* Retrieved August 6, 2005, from http://www.ncsbn.org/pdfs/III_BB_2005_Section_II_Recommendation.pdf

National League for Nursing. (2003a). *Position statement: Innovation in nursing education: A call to reform.* Retrieved April 23, 2005, from http://www.nln.org/aboutnln/PositionStatements/innovation.htm

National League for Nursing. (2004). Alarming data from the NLN's comprehensive survey of all nursing programs evokes wake up call. *NLN News, 7*(25). Retrieved August 1, 2005 from http://www.nln.org/newsletter/dec202004.htm

National League for Nursing. (2005a). NLN board of governors takes faculty shortage to the Hill. *NLN Nursing Education Policy.* Retrieved August 1, 2005, from http://www.ctleaguefornursing.org/pdf/nursingeducationpolicy_june05.pdf

National League for Nursing. (2005b). *Transforming nursing education.* Retrieved May 10, 2005, from http://www.nln.org/aboutnln/PositionStatements/transforming052005.pdf

Oermann, M. H. (2004). Reflections on undergraduate nursing education: A look to the future. *International Journal of Nursing Education and Scholarship, 1*(1). Retrieved January 5, 2005, from http://www.bepress.com/ijnes/vol1/iss1/art5

Page, A. (Ed.). (2003). *Keeping patients safe: Transforming the work environment of nurses.* Washington, DC: National Academies Press.

Reinhardt, U. E., Hussey, P. S., & Anderson, G. F. (2004). U.S. health care spending in an international context. *Health Affairs, 23*(3), 10-25.

Robert Woods Johnson Foundation. (2005). Addressing the nursing shortage: Partnerships among governments, schools, and employers are getting results. *Charting Nursing's Future.* Retrieved August 1, 2005, from http://www.rwjf.org/files/publications/other/nursing_issue1_final2%20(2).pdf

Smith, J., & Crawford, L. (2004). *Executive summary: Report findings from the 2003 employers survey.* Retrieved August 1, 2005, from National Council of State Boards of Nursing Web site: http://www.ncsbn.org/pdfs/RB14_03Employers_Survey_ESforWeb.pdf

U.S. Department of Health and Human Services. (2002). *Health, United States, 2002.* Retrieved August 7, 2005, from http://www.cdc.gov/nchs/data/hus/hus02.pdf

U.S. Department of Health and Human Services. (2003). *Steps to a healthier US: A program and policy perspective.* Retrieved November 12, 2004, from http://www.healthierus.gov/steps/summit/prevportfolio/Power_Of_Prevention.pdf

U.S. Department of Health and Human Services. (2005a). *Hospital compare.* Retrieved August 15, 2005, from http://www.hospitalcompare.hhs.gov/

U.S. Department of Health and Human Services. (2005b). *Nursing home compare.* Retrieved August 15, 2005, from http://www.medicare.gov/NHCompare/Home.asp?version=alternate&browser=IE%7C6%7CWinXP&language=English&defaultstatus=0&pagelist=Home&CookiesEnabledStatus=True

Valiga, T. M. (2002). *The nursing faculty shortage: National League for Nursing perspective.* Retrieved August 7, 2005, from the National League for Nursing Web site: http://www.nln.org/Research/facultyshortage.htm

International Graduate Nursing Education

A Critical Examination

MICHELE J. UPVALL

Experienced, educated nurses are necessary throughout the world to ease and resolve complex health care needs of individuals and societies. The International Council of Nurses (ICN) and Sigma Theta Tau International (STTI) have documented global challenges affecting health care and the profession of nursing (Hegyvary, 2004; International Council of Nurses, 2004). Major challenges affecting global society include alleviation of poverty, care of refugees and migrant populations, violence, promotion of education and access to health care for women and children, and prevention of infectious diseases.

The internationally focused Arista conferences sponsored by STTI delineated issues and strategies for the nursing profession in creating healthy communities. One recommendation common to the participants from each of region of the world during the third Arista conference was development of "comprehensive, culturally sensitive, student-centered educational models" (Dickenson-Hazard, 2004, p. 8). This recommendation has implications for further evolution of existing graduate nursing programs while establishing the need for new programs. Clearly, graduate nursing education must become a priority from a global perspective, given the needs of society and nursing.

GRADUATE EDUCATION AROUND THE WORLD

Increasingly, countries are moving toward university-based models of nursing education (Jones & Coeling, 2000). This evolution from diploma to baccalaureate and graduate programs reflects expansion of nursing knowledge (Hinshaw, 2000) and awareness of the need for competent nurses to manage complex health care problems in society. The growth of international nursing (Gennaro, 2000) and the use of technology in education

have facilitated this educational evolution, although nurses remain one of the least educated among all types of health care professionals (Nelson, 2002). Countries are in the process of reversing this trend by developing graduate programs. Master's and doctoral programs can be found throughout Africa, Asia, Australia, Europe, and the Middle East. Many of these programs have been influenced by the development of nursing education in Canada and the United States, which presents its own set of issues. These issues are discussed later in the chapter.

Graduate programs are at various levels of development in Africa. Master's and Doctorate of Philosophy (PhD) programs extend from Egypt, Namibia, and the Republic of South Africa (Munodawafa, 2003). Other countries such as Zimbabwe have developed Master's programs only within the past 10 years and hope to expand to doctoral education in the near future. The University of Zimbabwe admits students from neighboring countries, including Zambia, Lesotho, and Swaziland. Students complete courses in a clinical major and research courses to support completion of a dissertation (Mapanga & Mapanga, 2000).

Complexity describes nursing education in Japan. Diploma programs are regulated by the Division of Nursing of the Ministry of Health and Welfare, whereas the Ministry of Education is responsible for baccalaureate and graduate programs. A proliferation of master's and doctoral programs has occurred since 1987. Thus far, there are more than 30 master's programs and 8 doctoral programs, with more being planned by the government (Primomo, 2000).

A similar phenomenon also can be found in Iran where at least 14 master's programs and 4 doctoral programs have been developed since 1986. Plans are to increase the number of doctoral programs by 1 every 2 years. Courses in the programs include those that support clinical practice and research (Nasarabadi, Lipson, & Emami, 2004).

Australian nurses can choose to pursue a graduate certificate in a 6-month program or a diploma in a 12-month program. Courses in both of these programs are divided further into practice and research. Students in research programs complete original studies contributing to nursing knowledge. This division between practice and research exists at the doctoral level as well. PhD degrees require original research, but the professional Doctor of Nursing and Doctor of Midwifery programs require research projects or series of projects with course work that is meant to be significant to nursing practice (Stein-Parbury, 2000).

DEVELOPMENT OF ADVANCED PRACTICE NURSING INTERNATIONALLY

Advanced practice nursing (APN)—encompassing the roles of nurse anesthetists, nurse-midwives, clinical nurse specialists, and nurse practitioners—is a natural development in graduate education in response to complex health care needs of society. Historically, APN began in the United States through the forces of the Civil War and the discovery of chloroform (Keeling & Bigbee, 2005). Sociopolitical forces and other factors also have shaped the development of APN from an international perspective.

Critical factors in the development of APN elsewhere in the world compared with the United States include the sociopolitical environment, health needs of society, supply and demand of nurses, government support, collaboration among nurses and between the health professions, nursing education specific to the advanced practice role, and documented effectiveness of the role (Styles, 1996). These factors provide a useful framework for tracing the evolution of advanced practice in other countries, as Ketefian, Redman, Hanucharurnkul, Masterson, and Neves (2001) illustrated in their study of Brazil, Thailand, and the United Kingdom. For example, health care reform and some government initiatives provide support of the advanced practice role in each of these countries. Also, pressing health care needs in each society, along with a maldistribution of health care professionals and active leadership in support of graduate education, were noted. A limited amount of research documents the effectiveness of the role, but this may be enhanced through graduate education.

A review of other countries also demonstrates the influence of these factors. In Botswana the number of nurses working in rural areas and the demand for quality health care by the people in these communities required the nursing profession and the government to establish the role of the nurse practitioner (Seitio, 2000). However, in other countries such as Japan and Taiwan, autonomy for nurses is limited by the influence of the medical community. The role of nurse practitioner does not exist, whereas clinical nurse specialists have more of a medical focus (Chen, n.d.; Primomo, 2000). Botswana and Japan support graduate education for APN, and this in turn will facilitate development of the advanced practice role.

Organizations such as the ICN will promote the further evolution of APN. The ICN International Nurse Practitioner/Advanced Practice Nursing Network (INP/APNN) is a subgroup of ICN providing a forum to discuss and deliberate advanced practice issues as they affect nurses globally. The network also supports member countries in process of developing APN programs and disseminates information related to APN issues. The INP/APNN also has developed a definition of APN along with scope and standards of practice. The ICN-approved definition is as follows (International Council of Nurses, 2003):

> The NP/APN is a registered nurse who has acquired the expert knowledge base, complex decision-making skills and clinical competencies for expanded practice, the characteristics of which are shaped by the context and/or country in which s/he is credentialed to practice. A Masters degree is recommended for entry level.

This definition is clear in its position of APN beginning with the credentials of a registered nurse with further clinical expertise. It allows for adaptation of the role depending on the societal and cultural context in which nursing is practiced.

The ICN scope and standards encompass APN in primary, secondary, and tertiary levels of care in rural or urban settings. Standards for regulation, education, and practice have been established and are retrieved easily from the ICN Web site (http://www.icn.ch). These standards have not yet been finalized but are expected to be completed and approved in the near future.

Another organization influencing standards and defining competencies for APN internationally is the National Organization of Nurse Practitioner Faculties. The competencies developed by the organization have served as a model for APN education in Canada and the United Kingdom (Crabtree & Hunter, 2005). Other countries such as Pakistan use the American Association of Colleges of Nursing (AACN) competencies (AACN, 1996; Upvall, Karmaliani, Pirani, Gul, & Khalid, 2004). In 2002 the National Organization of Nurse Practitioner

VIEWPOINTS

Faculties and AACN joined forces to develop further the core competencies for nurse practitioner specialties (Crabtree & Hunter, 2005). Regardless of the model used to guide APN education, all countries must adapt the standards and competencies to their unique setting.

ISSUES CONFRONTING INTERNATIONAL GRADUATE NURSING EDUCATION

A myriad of concerns are facing the development of graduate nursing education today. Some of the concerns are limited to a few countries, whereas others are more prevalent. For example, nursing faculty in the United States are becoming older, and replacing this faculty is becoming an issue in schools of nursing (AACN, "Faculty Shortages," 2003). Other countries may not have enough faculty educated even at a baccalaureate level, let alone those with graduate preparation. Selected issues and potential solutions are based on experience and are discussed in the literature.

Influence of Western Nursing

Nursing education has a long history of crossing national boundaries beginning with Florence Nightingale, who attended a 3-month nursing program in Kaiserwerth, Germany (Catalano, 2003). The number of nurse educators influencing nursing internationally continues to increase. However, documenting the number of nurses working outside of their home countries for short or extended periods is not possible.

Lash, Lusk, and Nelson (2000) studied the phenomenon of American nurses involved in international health. They surveyed nursing faculty in doctoral programs in the United States, focusing on scholarship and other professional activity from 1985 to 1995. Significant findings include a threefold increase of international activity during this time frame with a wide range of number of days abroad each year in 109 countries. Teaching was the most common faculty role, followed by consultation (curriculum development for undergraduate and graduate programs, implemention of the clinical specialist role, and research implementation), and conducting research. Assessing only doctoral programs in the United States and having a 50% rate of return of surveys limited this study. Faculty in U.S. programs offering master's degrees also may be involved in teaching, consultation, and research. In addition, nursing faculty in other countries such as Canada, the United Kingdom, and Australia also may be active internationally on a scale as large as or even greater than nursing faculty in the United States. Although the number of faculty from Western countries

working across their national boundaries is not known, those who do so may be assumed to exert at least some influence over nurses in host countries.

Davis (1999) documents the influence of American nursing in Japan. Important considerations discussed include the difference in values between the ways of life in the United States (individualism and self-reliance) as opposed to the value placed on group cohesion in Japan. Japanese nurses educated in the United States may experience much role confusion when they return home to teach after having experienced a vastly different ethical nursing system. This then raises the question, "Does nursing having universal values?" Nurses must examine their basic assumptions and be responsible for questioning the appropriateness of knowledge they bring to nursing in other cultures.

Migration

Movement of nurses from one country to another, especially that of nurses going from developing countries to Western countries, has increased with the worsening of the global nursing shortage (World Health Organization, 2000). A report from the ICN reviewing the global shortage identifies internal and international migration as a critical challenge (Buchan & Calman, 2004). Nurses not only are moving from country to country but also within their own country from rural to urban areas, from the public sector to private employment, and from nursing positions to nonnursing employment.

Intense, active recruitment of nurses in developing countries in particular is a new phenomenon affecting the global shortage and negatively affecting health care in the home country. Major shortages of nurses have been reported in sub-Saharan Africa, especially Malawi, where more than 50% of the nursing positions in a hospital are unfilled because of migration. Nurses migrate for financial reasons, poor working conditions, lack of opportunities for professional growth or promotion, and lack of autonomy. These nurses are often young and competent in nursing skills and may well have been future leaders in their home countries (Buchan & Calman, 2004).

Active recruitment of nurses also may occur when nurses are given opportunities for furthering their education in a Western country. Once they complete their degree, they may be offered a position as nursing faculty or clinical manager. Again, their potential for leadership in their home country is diminished.

The issue of nurse recruitment in developing countries has been debated by nursing organizations. The ICN does support the right of nurses to migrate but recognizes that this may affect health care in the home country negatively. Active recruiting by countries that have not addressed human resources and planned appropriately is condemned by the ICN (International Council of Nurses, 1999). This issue will continue to be a matter of debate between the nursing leadership in Western and developing countries until the nursing shortage in Western countries eases.

Developing Research Capacity

Nursing and health care research is still in its early phases of development in many countries. Lack of graduate programs and faculty with research skills are major obstacles for future development of nursing knowledge. The preconference on "Nursing and Midwifery Research for Development" before the International Conference on Health Research for Development deliberated the research challenges of developing countries (Vonderheid et al., 2000). Most of the participants were from Thailand, but the identified challenges would be familiar to anyone with international nursing experience.

Participants of the preconference recognized the need to develop a critical mass of nurse researchers and mentors for those with beginning research skills. A supportive research environment also was identified as a need at the institutional, community, national, regional, and international levels. National plans need to identify research priority areas and available funding to conduct research and to support a culture of research provided enough nurse researchers are available and have not migrated to more developed countries. Multidisciplinary research projects and teams could facilitate access to more funding sources as well (Vonderheid et al., 2000). Encouraging nurses who left the country for higher education to return and then providing the resources for them to conduct collaborative studies with their colleagues in hospitals and universities would begin to create the capacity for global nursing research.

Regulation of Advanced Practice Nursing

Issues of adapting nursing cultural values, migration, and research capacity are generic to international graduate nursing education. Regulating professional practice, including defining practice, licensure, and certification and developing standards of practice are more specific to APN. Regulation provides professional accountability to the public and facilitates safety and quality within nursing (Bednash, Honig, & Gibbs, 2005).

The INP/ANPP network of ICN has been in the process of surveying 120 ICN member countries to learn more about APN and how it has been implemented in these countries (International Council of Nurses, 2001). To date, 109 participants representing 40 countries have responded. Findings thus far indicate that 78% have accrediting or approval processes for APN programs, and 69% of the countries responding have formal APN education programs.

Despite progress made in regulating APN, many countries continue to struggle. Even before ANP is introduced into the country, the nursing hierarchy within the country must explore definitions, regulatory mechanisms, and ways to recognize the APN role (Pearson & Peels, 2002). This is may be difficult in countries such as Indonesia where registration and standardization of levels of practice do not even exist at the diploma level (Shields & Hartati, 2003).

PROMOTION OF QUALITY IN INTERNATIONAL GRADUATE NURSING EDUCATION

Factors influencing the quality of graduate education from an international perspective are similar to those for the successful development and implementation of undergraduate programs as well. Collaboration along with awareness of cultural values affecting the collaborative process is key to globalization in the nursing profession (Dougherty, Lin, McKenna, & Seers, 2004). Collaboration in nursing education occurs through international organizational networking, agreements between institutions across national boundaries, and expert nurses providing consultation on an individual basis.

The International Academic Nursing Alliance was created in 2001 with the support of Sigma Theta Tau International. Its purpose is to unite schools of nursing globally through an electronic alliance so that standards of nursing education can be improved throughout the world, thereby improving the health of all peoples. An international steering committee of at least 31 nurse leaders is attempting to provide mentoring, scholarship, and dissemination of knowledge through the alliance (Parker, 2001). Although not yet fully operationalized, the International Academic Nursing Alliance vision is to use partnerships among schools of nursing strategically to promote quality nursing education at all levels.

Formal partnerships between at least two schools of nursing can promote quality education in both institutions. Zheng, Hinshaw, Yu, Guo, and Oakley (2001) describe a 5-year partnership between the Peking University and the University of Michigan. Visits of the two deans and individual faculty members culminated in meeting the partnership objectives of providing academic learning in workshop, lecture, and consult formats; improving undergraduate and graduate education in both schools of nursing; and conducting cross-cultural nursing research. Two distinct outcomes as a result of the partnership include development of a community-based clinic at Peking University and demonstration and research projects with Chinese Americans living in Michigan. Each institution experienced growth and increased stature within their respective universities through the partnership.

An evaluative outcome of the Peking University and University of Michigan partnership was a study of communication modalities between the institutions. In-person visits of the deans and short-term visits by the faculty during the partnership were the most important elements contributing to the success of the partnership. Distance communication by e-mail, Web sites linking the institutions with chat room capability, fax machines, telephones, and the postal system were used during the project. Problems of computer access, slow servers, and even denial of access occurred because of government policy that affected use of these modes of communication (Oakley et al., 2004). Their experience of distance education has implications for future development of networks such as the International Academic Nursing Alliance that rely on distance communication for success.

Individual nurses also promote collaboration and quality nursing education. Schools of nursing in developing countries actively may seek nurses willing to make short- or long-term commitments to the institution as faculty members, administrators, or consultants. These nurses are hired by governments or the university and are provided individual contracts. This type of collaboration has a special significance and perhaps a greater impact when the nurse is of the same ethnic origin as the country seeking assistance. For example, Dr. Chien-Yun is a Chinese American who has reformed nursing education throughout China with the endorsement of the Chinese Ministry of Health and the Chinese Nursing Association (Xu, Xu, Sun, & Zhang, 2001).

Ongoing curriculum evaluation resulting in curriculum change also promotes quality graduate nursing education. Gagan, Berg, and Root (2002) present a model of evaluation and revision for nurse practitioner education that translates into a model for all graduate nursing curricula. Their model is based on the concept that curriculum goals are fluid and must be evaluated regularly according to feedback from students, faculty, alumni, the public, and government. A second concept

within the model evaluates health policy and state regulation that influence health care demands. Finally, the curriculum must respond to the needs and demands of the community.

The model can be adapted for use in developing countries, although it was conceptualized originally for use in the United States. The model emphasizes health policy and input from the public and government. Graduate nursing programs such as the first one developed in Pakistan (Upvall et al., 2004) could benefit from using concepts within the model for developing an evaluation plan. Curriculum changes have been made continually, but the model would promote inclusion of national nursing leadership as part of the process. This is crucial in a country where APN is not widely understood or recognized.

EMERGING GRADUATE NURSING EDUCATION MODELS

Graduate education is evolving in the United States and has the potential for influencing graduate nursing education internationally. Two of the most recent developments originated by the AACN ("Working paper," 2003; 2004) include the clinical nurse leader (CNL) and the doctor of nursing practice (DNP).

The CNL is a nurse generalist with leadership preparation and a master's degree in nursing. Various models for preparing the CNL are being tested now in partnerships between schools of nursing and clinical settings throughout the United States. The CNL is expected to provide and manage care of patients in a variety of clinical settings, not only hospitals. Clinical nurse specialists are not prepared as nurse administrators or managers, but are leaders through designing, implementing, and evaluating patient care. They also will delegate and supervise other health care providers while practicing from an evidence-based perspective.

The DNP will be considered the terminal degree for APNs. The DNP is based on the premise that current master's degree programs for APNs already require more credit hours than a typical 2-year master's program, and more educational demands are being placed on these programs. Doctor of nursing practice preparation will provide more education to allow APNs to remain current in practice. This exciting development allows nursing to meet the challenge of ever-increasing health care demands (Marion et al., 2003). The AACN (2004) recommends the DNP as the graduate degree for APNs and that a transition period be in place for those already prepared as APNs who wish to pursue a DNP. Seven areas of content have been identified for the DNP (p. 10):

1. Scientific underpinnings for practice
2. Advanced nursing practice
3. Organization and system leadership/management, quality improvement, and systems thinking
4. Analytic methodologies related to the evaluation of practice and the application of evidence for practice
5. Use of technology and information for the improvement and transformation of health care
6. Health policy development, implementation, and evaluation
7. Interdisciplinary collaboration for improving patient and population health care outcomes

Much work remains in realizing the vision for the CNL and DNP. Issues of licensing and credentialing must be addressed, and standards must be in place before more nursing schools develop these programs. At an international level, these new roles can transform graduate nursing education. To be successful, these programs would need to be implemented with the support of organizations such as the ICN and World Health Organization. Nursing councils worldwide and nursing associations should take an approach of "watchful waiting" as these new graduate roles evolve elsewhere. Lessons learned in the West then can be applied to other countries.

SUMMARY

Graduate nursing programs throughout the world are evolving in many ways. The need for APNs is being recognized, and development of new APN programs is occurring globally. New programs are being initiated in countries such as Botswana, Thailand, and Hong Kong while others are improving through international collaborative partnerships. Nurse educators and consultants from the West will need to take particular care to adapt their knowledge of graduate education for the cultural context in which they are working. Examples of successful partnerships should be scrutinized carefully for lessons learned before new partnerships are initiated. The problem of migration could interfere with partnerships if the nursing leaders in developing countries perceive they are having their human resources depleted by uncaring, wealthier countries also in need of well-educated nurses. Graduate nursing education will never be a finished product in any country. New roles are emerging in the United States, and new roles also may emerge from other countries. Creating and then accepting these new roles for graduate nursing will be a challenge in all countries, but the commitment to change is required if the nursing profession is to address today's health care needs adequately.

REFERENCES

American Association of Colleges of Nursing. (1996). *The essentials of master's education for advanced practice nursing.* Washington, DC: Author.

American Association of Colleges of Nursing. (2003). *Faculty shortages in baccalaureate and graduate programs: Scope of the problem and strategies for expanding the supply* [White paper]. Washington, DC: Author.

American Association of Colleges of Nursing. (2003, May). *Working paper on the role of the clinical nurse leader.* Retrieved March 25, 2004, from http://www.aacn.nche.edu/Publications/WhitePapers/ClinicalNurseLeader.htm

American Association of Colleges of Nursing. (2004, October). *AACN position statement on the practice doctorate in nursing.* Retrieved November 20, 2004, from http://www.aacn.nche.edu/DNP/pdf/DNP.pdf

Bednash, G., Honig, J., & Gibbs, L. (2005). For mutation and approval of credentialing and clinical privileges. In J. M. Stanley (Ed.), *Advanced practice nursing: Emphasizing common roles* (2nd ed., pp. 158-186). Philadelphia: F.A. Davis.

Buchan, J., & Calman, L. (2004). *The global shortage of registered nurses: An overview of issues and actions.* Geneva, Switzerland: International Council of Nurses.

Catalano, J. T. (2003). Historical perspectives. In J. T. Catalano (Ed.), *Nursing now* (3rd ed, pp. 25-36). Philadelphia: F.A. Davis.

Chen, C. H. (n.d.). *The current issues in advanced nursing practice in Taiwan.* Retrieved January 14, 2005, from http://www.aanp.org/NR/rdonlyres/ekuvhi5or3bq7tqiwakcw25u72nmwcmkfk3o3sstjhidqbvxi2jr2q2t7kvus7kwbs4sr55cyhsvnbmzxyfmoohvb2d/NPTaiwan.pdf

Crabtree, K. G., & Hunter, A. (2005). Advanced practice nursing and global health. In J. M. Stanley (Ed.), *Advanced practice nursing: Emphasizing common roles* (2nd ed., pp. 353-373). Philadelphia: F.A. Davis.

Davis, A. (1999). Global influence of American nursing: Some ethical issues. *Nursing Ethics, 6,* 118-125.

Dickenson-Hazard, N. (2004). Global health issues and challenges, *Journal of Nursing Scholarship, 36,* 6-10.

Dougherty, M. C., Lin, S. Y., McKenna, H. P., & Seers, K. (2004). International content of high-ranking nursing journals in the year 2000. *Journal of Nursing Scholarship, 36,* 173-181.

Gagan, M., Berg, J., & Root, S. (2002). Nurse practitioner curriculum for the 21st century: A model for evaluation and revision. *Journal of Nursing Education, 41,* 202-206.

Gennaro, S. (2000). International nursing: The past 25 years and beyond. *Maternal/Child Nursing, 25*(6), 296-299.

Hegyvary, S. T. (2004). Working paper on grand challenges in improving global health. *Journal of Nursing Scholarships, 36,* 96-101.

Hinshaw, A. S. (2000). Nursing knowledge for the 21st century: Opportunities and challenges. *Journal of Nursing Scholarship, 32,* 117-124.

International Council of Nurses. (1999). *Nurse retention, transfer and migration* [Position statement]. Retrieved January 19, 2005, from http://www.icn.ch/psretention.htm

International Council of Nurses. (2001, October). *Update: International survey of nurse practitioner/advanced practice nursing roles.* Retrieved January 20, 2005, from http://www.aanp.org/INP+APN+Network/Research/Survey+results/Internatio nal+Survey+October+2001.htm

International Council of Nurses. (2003). *Definition and characteristics of the role.* Retrieved January 14, 2005, from http://www. aanp.org/inp%20apn%20network/practice%20issues/role %20definitions.asp

International Council of Nurses. (2004). *Tackling the UN millennium development goals (2002-2003 Biennial Report).* Geneva, Switzerland: Author.

Jones, S. L., and Coeling, H. (2000). Nursing around the world: What are the commonalities and differences. *Online Journal of Nursing Issues.* Retrieved May 31, 2000, from http://www.nursingworld.org/ojin/topic12/tpc12ntr.htm

Keeling, A. W., and Bigbee, J. L. (2005). The history of advanced practice nursing the United States. In A. Hamric, J. Spross, & C. Hanson (Eds.), *Advanced practice nursing: An integrative approach* (3rd ed., pp. 4-45). St. Louis, MO: Elsevier Saunders.

Ketefian, S., Redman, R., Hanucharurnkul, S., Masterson, A., & Neves, E. (2001). The development of advanced practice roles: Implications in the international nursing community. *International Nursing Review, 48,* 132-163.

Lash, A., Lusk, B., & Nelson, M., (2000). American nursing scholars abroad, 1985-1995. *Journal of Nursing Scholarship, 32,* 415-420.

Mapanga, K. G., & Mapanga, M. B. (2000). A perspective of nursing in Zimbabwe. *Online Journal of Nursing Issues.* Retrieved May 31, 2000, from http://www.nursingworld. org/ojin/topic12/tpc12_2.htm

Marion, L., Viens, D., O'Sullivan, A., Crabtree, K., Fontana, S., & Price, M. (2003). The practice doctorate in nursing: Future or fringe. *Topics in Advanced Practice Nursing eJournal, 3.* Retrieved February 1, 2005, from http://www.medscape. com/viewarticle/453247

Munodawafa, A. C. (2003, October). *Developing global leaders through LMD Education.* Paper presented at the meeting of the International Network for Doctoral Education, Toronto, Canada.

Nasarabadi, A. N., Lipson, J. G., & Emami, A. (2004). Professional nursing in Iran: An overview of its historical and sociocultural framework. *Journal of Professional Nursing, 20,* 396-402.

Nelson, M. A. (2002). Education for professional nursing practice: Looking backward into the future. *Online Journal of Nursing Issues.* Retrieved May 31, 2002, from http:// www.nursingworld.org/ojin/topic18/tpc18_3.htm

Oakley, D., Yu, M.-Y., Lu, H., Shang, S., McIntosh, E., Pang, D., et al. (2004). Communication channels to help build an international community of education and practice. *Journal of Professional Nursing, 20,* 381-389.

Parker, J. (2001, June). *Nursing practice and scholarship: Approaches to effective international alliances.* Paper presented at the conference of the International Network for Doctoral Education, Copenhagen, Denmark.

Pearson, A., & Peels, S. (2002). Advanced practice in nursing: International perspective. *International Journal of Nursing Practice, 8,* 51-54.

Primomo, J. (2000). Nursing around the world: Japan— Preparing for the century of the elderly. *Online Journal of Nursing Issues.* Retrieved May 31, 2000, from http://www. nursingworld.org/ojin/topic12/tpc12_1.htm

Seitio, O. S. (2000, October). *The family nurse practitioner in Botswana: Issues and challenges.* Paper presented at the meeting of the 8th International Nurse Practitioner Conference, San Diego, CA.

Shields, S., & Hartati, K. (2003). Nursing and health care in Indonesia. *Journal of Advanced Practice Nursing Roles.* Retrieved January 20, 2005, from http://icn_opnetwork.org

Stein-Parbury, J. (2000). Nursing around the world: Australia. *Online Journal of Nursing Issues.* Retrieved May 31, 2000, from http://www.nursingworld.org/ojin/topic12/tpc12_3.htm

Styles, M. M. (1996). Conceptualizations of advanced nursing practice. In A. Hamric, J. Spross, & C. Hanson (Eds.), *Advanced nursing practice: An integrative approach* (2nd ed., pp. 25-41). Philadelphia: W.B. Saunders.

Upvall, M., Karmalian, R., Pirani, F., Gul, R., Khalid, F. (2004). Developing nursing leaders through graduate education in Pakistan. *International Journal of Nursing Education Scholarship, 1.* Retrieved from http://www.bepress.com/ijnes/vol1/iss1/art27/

Vonderheid, S., Persaud, V., Stein-Parburg, J., Ghebrehiwet, T., Hanuchararunkul, S., Boontong, T., et al. (2000, October). *Challenges, strategies, and priority areas for nursing and midwifery research: Report of the preconference on nursing and midwife research.* Retrieved January 5, 2005, http://www. nursingsociety.org/programs/building_global.html

World Health Organization. (2000, November). *Global advisory group on nursing and midwifery.* Retrieved January 1, 2005, from http://www.who.int/health-services-delivery/nursing/gagnm/who_eip_osd_2001.4en.htm

Xu, Z., Xu, Y., Sun, J., & Zhang, J. (2001). Globalization of tertiary nursing education in post-Mao China: A preliminary qualitative assessment. *Nursing and Health Sciences, 3,* 179-190.

Zheng, X. X., Hinshaw, A. S., Yu, M. Y., Guo, G. F., & Oakley, D. J. (2001). Building international partnerships. *International Nursing Review, 48,* 117-121.

Critical Thinking

What Is It and How Do We Teach It?

SHARON STAIB

Critical thinking, nursing process, problem solving, logical reasoning, or simply better decision making—are these terms synonymous? Critical thinking has been a buzz word in higher education for at least the last 20 years. Nurse educators have joined the crusade to make students better thinkers. Despite a growing body of literature on this topic, practical suggestions for improving these skills are limited. Throughout history, critical thinking has been expounded as an essential component of a well-educated person. The roots of critical thinking originate from Greek philosophers. Socrates extolled critical questioning, believing that thinking was driven by questions not answers. As early as 1605 in his book *Advancement of Learning,* Francis Bacon said knowledge is to be accepted with great limitation and caution (Wright, 1900). Since these early attempts to describe critical thinking and its importance in education, educators have tried to find ways to stimulate students to think. Nurse educators continue attempts to define critical thinking and to find ways to teach and evaluate the results. Nurse educators have developed models of critical thinking (Reising, 2004; Videbeck, 1997; Whiteside, 1997), have shared teaching methods, and have evaluated the results. Returning to the original question, yes, critical thinking is problem solving, logical reasoning, and good decision making; but as this chapter illustrates, these are only parts of a process that is more complex than the individual parts.

WHAT IS CRITICAL THINKING?

Toward a Definition of Critical Thinking

Whether teaching or measuring critical thinking, one of the first hurdles to overcome is establishing a consensus definition of critical thinking. One of the most frequently cited definitions of critical thinking comes from Richard Paul, widely known philosopher and founder of the Foundation for Critical Thinking. Paul (1993) describes critical thinking as the art of thinking about one's thinking while trying to make it better, clearer, more accurate, and defensible. This is a broad definition that has been used by many disciplines in an attempt to describe CT. Many other definitions of CT exist, no one definition is agreed upon by all disciplines, and most disciplines, including nursing, use various definitions depending on their purpose, to describe CT. The American Philosophical Association, under the direction of Facione (1990), conducted a survey among CT experts and through use of the Delphi technique, they arrived at a consensus statement of critical thinking. That statement reads, "We understand critical thinking to be purposeful, self-regulatory judgment which results in interpretation, analysis, evaluation, and inference as well as explanation of the evidential, conceptual, methodological, criteriological, or contextual considerations upon which judgment is based" (p. 2). This study came to be known as the Critical Thinking Delphi Report, and several critical thinking evaluation tools resulted from this study.

A Nursing Definition of Critical Thinking

Numerous definitions of critical thinking appear in nursing literature, many of them borrowed from other disciplines (Walthew, 2004). In the 1970s and 1980s, nursing process focused on problem solving, and for most nurse educators nursing process and CT were synonymous (Tanner, 2000). Apparently, not a great deal has changed since then. In her study surveying 201 baccalaureate nurse educators, Gordon (2000) reported that more than one half of those surveyed agreed with the statement that nursing process and CT are synonymous. According to Alfaro-LeFevre (2002), "critical thinking must be viewed as being more than a problem-solving method. If you have only a problem-solving mentality, you're not a critical thinker." One of the reasons CT may be confused with problem solving, is that problem solving implies the use of the scientific process to arrive at an answer. Follow a series of steps and the problem will be resolved. In CT, there are no assumptions and a clear answer may not be apparent. Facione (1990) describes CT as a cognitive engine that drives problem solving and decision making.

Despite interest in developing CT skills, a universally agreed upon definition of CT in nursing does not exist. In a landmark study, Scheffer and Rubenfeld (2000) used the Delphi technique to arrive at a consensus statement on CT in nursing. This study consisted of an international panel of experts from nine countries and 23 states. The panel arrived at a consensus definition that identified "ten habits of the mind and seven skills" (p. 352) used to advance understanding of the role of critical thinking in nursing. The habits of the mind include "confidence, contextual perspective, creativity, flexibility, inquisitiveness, intellectual integrity, intuition, open-mindedness, perseverance, and reflection. Skills included analyzing, applying standards, discriminating, information seeking, logical reasoning, predicting and transforming knowledge" (p. 352). This study also revealed different perceptions of CT between nurse educators and non-nurse educators. Furthermore, nurse educators were more likely to conceptualize critical thinking as a thinking process used to solve problems, whereas non-nurse CT experts were less likely to view decision making and problem solving as CT (Gordon, 2000). In a study by Walthew (2004) investigating nurse educators conceptions of CT, 12 nurse educators viewed rational, logical thinking as the main focus of CT.

Defining CT is fundamental to evaluating CT. Without a clear, concise definition of CT, one must question how tests of CT can evaluate accurately an increase in critical thinking or how any reliable statements can be made regarding increases in students' CT. A valid concern when choosing a definition of CT is the issue of whether each discipline has its own definition and views about the characteristics of CT, or is CT discipline specific? According to Gordon (2000), when nurse educators were asked if CT was conceptually different in nursing than in other disciplines, nurse educators indicated there was no difference. However, the results of a study by Gordon (2000) indicated that nurse educators differed significantly from the panel of experts in the Facione study on conceptualizing CT. Nurse educators were more likely to view affective characteristics of empathizing and sensing as skills that are part of CT (Gordon, 2000). This is consistent with the reports of Scheffer and Rubenfeld (2000) and of Zimmerman and Phillips (2000). Any definition of critical thinking, when applied to nursing situations, needs to be meaningful and useful to students and faculty. Therefore the definition of critical thinking for nursing may be different from that of other disciplines.

WHY SHOULD NURSE EDUCATORS ASSESS CRITICAL THINKING IN NURSING?

Critical thinking is considered vital to nursing practice. Nursing has changed from a task-oriented practice largely directed by others to a skilled profession with its own body of knowledge. Along with this change in practice comes a responsibility to be accountable for one's decisions and actions, decisions that often involve complex patient problems that can result in the life or death of the patient. Complex decision making is tied closely to CT. As patient status changes, the nurse immediately must recognize, interpret, and consider new information and make decisions based on knowledge and judgment. Members of a profession have their own body of knowledge. The members of a profession review and research that body of knowledge to find new and better ways of providing patient care. Critical thinking is part of the development of new knowledge. Nursing education has placed increased emphasis on CT in response to this change in the role of the nurse. Critical thinking is a criterion in the accreditation process for schools of nursing (American Association of Colleges of Nursing, 1998; National League for Nursing Accrediting Commission, 2002).

ASSESSMENT METHODS
Standardized Tests

A variety of standardized tests have been used to measure critical thinking. Standardized tests commonly are administered using a pre-post test design with the hope of showing increases in CT after an intervention is applied. None of the following standardized tests described were designed specifically for nursing. All were designed to be used across disciplines. The primary advantages to using a standardized test include the following: the test has been developed already, results may be compared with norms, and statistical data with reference to validity and reliability have been obtained.

In a literature review, one of the most frequently used standardized tests in nursing studies was the Watson-Glaser Critical Thinking Appraisal. This test consists of five subtests designed to measure different, though interdependent aspects of CT. The tasks of this test require consideration of a series of suggestions (inference, assumption, a conclusion, or an argument) relating to a statement. The task of the participant is to study each statement and to evaluate its appropriateness of validity in context to the suggestion. Each section consists of 16 questions for a total of 80 items (Watson & Glaser, 1991).

Another standardized CT assessment tool used in nursing is the California Critical Thinking Disposition Inventory. The inventory is a 74-item instrument that measures personality characteristics derived from the Dephi report of Facione. These characteristics include inquisitiveness, systematicity, analyticity, truth-seeking, and open-mindedness (Facione, 1990). According to Facione, these traits are consistent with CT. Another standardized measure of CT and a companion test to the California Critical Thinking Disposition Inventory, is the California Critical Thinking Skills Test. This test consists of 34 multiple-choice items designed to assess core CT skills of analysis, inference, and evaluation (Facione & Facione, 1992). Two forms of this test are available.

The Cornell Critical Thinking Tests also come in several forms. Levels X and Z are the most commonly used forms in higher education. These forms are in a multiple-choice format and test concepts such as induction, credibility, observation, prediction, fallacies, deduction, and assumption identification (Ennis, 2002). No nursing research studies were located in which this test has been used to evaluate CT (Staib, 2003).

Other standardized CT tests include the Ennis-Weir Critical Thinking Essay Test, this test uses written essays to evaluate skills such as "getting the point, seeing the reasons and assumptions, stating one's point, offering good reasons, seeing other possibilities and responding to and avoiding equivocation, irrelevance, circularity, reversal of an if-then relationship, overgeneralization, credibility problems and the use of emotive language to persuade" (Ennis, 2002, p. 2). This is the only CT test listed that uses an essay format.

Although other CT standardized tests exist, they are not as well known as these tests, and no research-based nursing studies were identified that reported using any of these tests. Also available are several subject-specific tests such as the Cornell Class Reasoning Test, Logical Reasoning, and Test on Appraising Observations; other tests that incorporate CT include the American College Test and Graduate Record Examination, but that is not the primary focus of these tests (Ennis, 2002). Many attractive and justifiable reasons exist for using commercially available tests of CT in nursing research, however, there remains the issue of whether this is the best way to measure an increase in CT. The literature is clearer about measures to facilitate development of critical thinking skills than about measures to evaluate the results of those efforts. Perhaps part of this problem is related to the use of objective, qualitative instruments when most of nursing research is quantitative. Rather than relying solely on standardized tests, nurse educators may need to focus on the development of measures that are more in tune with nursing curricula (Angel, Duffy, & Belyea, 2000). Although a body of evidence suggests that nursing education has little effect on CT abilities of students, this evidence is generally in the form of nonspecific changes on a standardized test with no insight given as to why this might be the case or how student nurses actually reason to arrive at professional judgment (Daley, 2001). According to Beckie, Lowry, and Barnett (2001), the use of standardized tests to measure CT in nursing is best supplemented with other evaluation methods.

Instructor-Made Tests

If a standardized test is not used to evaluate increases in CT, then a teacher-made test may be used. The obvious hurtle in this type of endeavor is the development of such an instrument. Besides development, the instrument will need to be tested for reliability and validity. This process can be time consuming and still may not yield the desired information. With the increased focus on CT and the drive to verify results, this may be an option researchers choose to pursue especially in light of the vast amount of qualitative research in nursing. According to Simpson and Courtney (2002), the challenge for nursing is the construction of CT instruments specific for measuring CT skills in nursing and instruments that measure teaching techniques for instructional effectiveness. Morrison and Free (2001) suggest that appropriately written multiple-choice test items can be a way to measure CT. Multiple-choice test items should focus on application of concepts, require a high level of discrimination, require multilogical thinking (student must know more than one concept to answer the question correctly), and must include a rationale for correct and incorrect answers.

Considerations When Choosing an Evaluation Instrument

Whether to use a standardized measure of CT or an instructor-made test is a decision only the research designer can make. One must take some factors into consideration when making this decision, however. One must begin by asking exactly what standardized tests measure. Is the test suitable for the purpose of the study? Is administration of the test feasible and cost-effective? Is there time to develop and pilot an instructor-made test? How will the validity and reliability of the instructor-made instrument be determined? There is no right or wrong answer to these questions, and there is no one way to assess changes in CT, but it is important to document the effectiveness of an intervention or strategy.

Without accurate measurement, nurse educators are just guessing as to the best approach for teaching CT.

TEACHING STRATEGIES

Although it generally is agreed that teaching students to think critically is an important part of nursing education, the best approach to achieve this objective is not always clear. Multiple strategies have been proposed in the literature as ways to improve student CT. Table 11-1 summarizes strategies, methods of evaluation, and results. The best approach seems to be to use a variety of techniques. In addition to evaluation, Morrison and Free (2001) state that students can learn CT from well-written multiple-choice test items. They believe that carefully written test item rationales can provide teaching and increase students' learning and thinking. Youngblood and Beitz (2001) suggest that CT skills can

TABLE 11-1

Strategies Used in Nursing Literature to Improve Critical Thinking			
Author	**Strategy**	**How Evaluated**	**Results**
Magnussen, Ishida, & Itano (2000)	Inquiry-based learning	Watson-Glaser Critical Thinking Appraisal	Posttest showed improvement in students with low pretest scores.
Su, Masoodi, & Kopp (2000)	Clinical laboratory activities	Faculty assessment of student thinking aloud through a clinical situation	Anecdotal assessment shows increase in critical thinking skills.
Saucier, Stevens, & Williams (2000)	Computer-assisted instruction	California Critical Thinking Skills Test	Did not demonstrate a significant increase in critical thinking.
Cioffi (2001)	Clinical simulations	Tested by a panel of experts for construct validity, determined to be unrealistic to test for reliability	Anecdotal feedback was positive.
Youngblood & Beitz (2001)	Active learning strategies	Student evaluations	Student anecdotal data revealed an increase in critical thinking.
Mattola & Murphy (2001)	Antidote dilemma	Reviewing responses	Participant verbal feedback showed an increase in critical thinking.
Van Eerden (2001)	Vignettes	Reliability study in progress	Faculty response was favorable.
Bell, Heye, Campion, & Hendricks (2002)	Process-focused learning strategy	None	Anecdotal observation appeared to strengthen theoretical and experiential knowledge.
Williams, Sewell, & Humphrey (2002)	Problem-based learning	Pre-post test of five areas established by the authors	Scores improved after the intervention.
Rutherman, Jackson, Cluskey, & Flannigan (2004)	Clinical journaling	Student and faculty	Results were inconclusive.
Morrison & Free (2001)	Multiple-choice test items	Faculty	The faculty prepare critical thinking test questions and evaluate the results.
Price (2004)	Reflection	No formal evaluation	Author suggests this technique may help learners develop collegial forms of learning.

be enhanced using different active learning strategies including case studies, group debates, concept analysis, reaction papers, clinical reports, and modeling of CT by faculty.

Many of the strategies are based on clinical experiences or are designed to enhance CT in the clinical setting. Several authors (Price, 2004; Ruthman, Jackson, Cluskey, & Flannigan, 2004) found journaling or postclinical reflection to be helpful in increasing CT. This strategy gives students a chance to reflect on clinical performance after the fact when there is less pressure to perform, thereby allowing the student a chance to review decisions and judgments in an effort to determine whether the patient received the highest level of care possible. Although it seems reasonable that journaling and postclinical reflection may increase CT, there is no evidence actually to support this assumption (Clarke & Holt, 2001).

Another way suggested to increase CT is through simulations in a laboratory setting (Cioffi, 2001; Su, Masodi, & Kopp, 2000; Van Eerden, 2001). Simulations bring real-life activity into a safe learning environment, thus facilitating CT. Many times students have a strong knowledge base in nursing but are unable to apply that knowledge in clinical situations. Students look for one answer to a problem; they do not always consider all mitigating circumstances. Nursing cannot be taught by memorization; at some point students must develop creative solutions to unpredictable problems. Clinical simulations and reflective thinking offer an opportunity to correct faulty thinking though discussion and education. The "safe" atmosphere of the clinical laboratory provides the perfect milieu for CT to take place. According to Cioffi (2001), clinical simulations can range from simple to complex, but to be effective, the simulation must have varying degrees of uncertainty present. In a complex simulation the degree of uncertainty is higher. Simpler simulations are constructed with a lower degree of uncertainty requiring simple decision making. Simulations help learners distinguish relevant from irrelevant information. The extent that the thinking process induced by simulations is a valid indicator of what happens in real practice, and the degree to which being distanced from the problem influences actual critical thinking is considered a limitation of clinical simulations.

Saucier, Stevens, and Williams (2000) compared the effect of computer-assisted instruction with written nursing process case studies and their effect on CT. Although the results of this study were inconclusive, and because many computer-assisted programs are available, it would

be beneficial to determine whether these programs actually improve students' CT abilities. A method that is similar to clinical simulations is an activity called antidote dilemma. In this activity, learners are given a scenario to which they are asked to respond. Additional information then is presented and discussion follows (Mattola & Murphy, 2001). A similar strategy is used in problem-based learning (Celia & Gordon, 2001; Williams, Sewell, & Humphrey, 2002) and closely related inquiry-based learning (Magnussen, Ishida, & Itano, 2000). In this approach, a series of realistic problems is presented. It is incumbent on learners to extract the relevant data, determine their existing knowledge, and conduct research to incorporate new knowledge into the problem (Celia & Gordon, 2001).

In a process-focused learning strategy, Bell, Heye, Campion, and Hendricks (2002) asked students to formulate a critical incident from their clinical experience. After students submitted the incidents, faculty selected one incident to which all students were to respond. This exercise was designed to clarify and focus student thought processes. CT was enhanced through experiential learning. Concept mapping, mind mapping, and concept analysis are related techniques that may be useful as strategies to increase CT, but according to Clarke & Holt (2001), these are advanced intellectual techniques that are most useful in postgraduate programs.

WHERE DO NURSE EDUCATORS GO FROM HERE

There seems to be little doubt that CT is vital to nursing. As nursing has progressed from a task-oriented occupation to a profession based on its own body of knowledge, it becomes imperative that nurses are able to make sound decisions that provide the highest level of patient care possible. Concern exists that there still remains a gap between CT skills in the classroom and CT skills exhibited in clinical practice (Seymour, Kinn, & Sutherland, 2003). Some (Seymour et al., 2003) believe that the successful development of CT skills for academic purposes does not necessarily mean the transfer of those skills to the clinical setting. Future research must focus on this issue and determine the best method of ensuring this transfer of CT from classroom to clinical practice.

Nurse educators must be willing to try new teaching approaches and provide sound research-based evidence to establish those teaching strategies that are most effective in promoting CT among students. Faculty need to be critical thinkers themselves. Nurse educators cannot assume that one strategy will work for all students.

They need to pursue those methods actively that provide the sought after results. Many of today's nursing faculties were educated in the old lecture regurgitation format. This teaching style does little to promote CT in students. Although some students prefer to be passive learners and like the lecture/memorization format, faculty who teach in this manner are not preparing students adequately for the rapidly changing profession of nursing. If a change in students' CT abilities is to take place, education practices must be interactive and participatory. CT is a skill that individuals can develop over a period of time. Nurse educators must help students develop that skill. Teaching critical thinking skills will require work, but the results will elevate the profession of nursing even further by educating practitioners who can actually think.

REFERENCES

Alfaro-LeFevre, R. (2002). Letter to the editor of AACN News. Retrieved January 17, 2006, from http://www.aacn.org/AACN/aacnnews.nsf/GetArticle/two199

American Association of Colleges of Nursing. (1998). *The essentials of baccalaureate education for professional nursing practice.* Washington, DC: Author.

Angel, B. F., Duffey, M., & Belyea, M. (2000). An evidence-based project for evaluating strategies to improve knowledge acquisition and critical-thinking performance in nursing students. *Journal of Nursing Education, 39*(5), 219-228.

Beckie, T. M., Lowry, L. W., & Barnett, S. (2001). Assessing critical thinking in baccalaureate nursing students: A longitudinal study. *Holistic Nursing Practice, 15*(3), 18-27. Retrieved December 3, 2004, from ProQuest database.

Bell, M. L., Heye, M. L., Campion, L., & Hendricks, P. B. (2002). Evaluation of a process-focused learning strategy to promote critical thinking. *Journal of Nursing Education, 41*(4), 175-181. Retrieved April 19, 2002, from ProQuest database.

Celia, L. M., & Gordon, P. R. (2001). Using problem-based learning to promote critical thinking in an orientation program for novice nurses. *Journal for Nurses in Staff Development, 17*(1), 12-19.

Cioffi, J. (2001). Clinical simulations: Development and validation. *Nurse Education Today, 21,* 477-486.

Clarke, D. J., & Holt, J. (2001). Philosophy: a key to open the door to critical thinking. *Nurse Education Today, 21,* 71-78.

Daley, W. M. (2001). The development of an alternative method in the assessment of critical thinking as an outcome of nursing education. *Journal of Advanced Nursing, 36*(1), 120-130.

Ennis, R. H. (2002). *An annotated list of critical thinking tests.* Retrieved January 17, 2006, from http://www.critical/thinking.net/CTTestList1199.html

Facione, P. A. (1990). *Critical thinking: A statement of expert consensus for purposes of educational assessment and instruction* (ERIC ED 315-423). Millbrae, CA: California Academic Press.

Facione, P. A., & Facione, N. C. (1992). *The California Critical Thinking Skills Test: Test manual.* Millbrae, CA: California Academic Press.

Gordon, J. M. (2000). Congruency in defining critical thinking by nurse educators and non-nurse scholars. *Journal of Nursing Education, 39*(8), 340-352. Retrieved November 14, 2001, from ProQuest database.

Magnussen, L., Ishida, D., & Itano, J. (2000). The impact of the use of inquiry-based learning as a teaching methodology on the development of critical thinking. *Journal of Nursing Education, 39*(8), 360-365. Retrieved December 3, 2004, from ProQuest database.

Mattola, C. A., & Murphy, P. (2001). Antidote dilemma: An activity to promote critical thinking. *The Journal of Continuing Education in Nursing, 32*(4), 161-164. Retrieved January 17, 2006, from ProQuest database.

Morrison, S., & Free, K. W. (2001). Writing multiple-choice test items that promote and measure critical thinking. *Journal of Nursing Education, 40*(1), 17-24. Retrieved October 19, 2001, from ProQuest database.

National League for Nursing Accrediting Commission. (2002). *The accreditation manual and interpretive guidelines by program type.* Retrieved January 17, 2006, from http://www. ntn. org/testprods/guideinterpretation.htm score report

Paul, R. (1993). *Critical thinking: How to prepare students for a rapidly changing world.* Santa Rosa, CA: Foundation for Critical Thinking.

Price, A. (2004). Encouraging reflection and critical thinking in practice. *Nursing Standard, 18*(47), 46-53. Retrieved December 3, 2004, from ProQuest database.

Reising, D. L. (2004). The outcome-present state-testing model applied to classroom settings. *Journal of Nursing Education, 43*(9), 431-432. Retrieved December 3, 2004, from ProQuest database.

Ruthman, J., Jackson, J., Cluskey, M., & Flannigan, P. (2004). Using clinical journaling to CAPTURE critical thinking across the curriculum. *Nursing Education Perspectives, 25*(3), 120-123. Retrieved December 3, 2004, from ProQuest database.

Saucier, B. L., Stevens, K. R., & Williams, G. B. (2000). Critical thinking outcomes of computer-assisted instruction versus written nursing process. *Nursing and Health Care Perspectives, 21*(5), 240-250. Retrieved July 11, 2002, from ProQuest database.

Scheffer, B. K., & Rubenfeld, M. G. (2000). A consensus statement on critical thinking in nursing. *Journal of Nursing Education, 39*(8), 352-360. Retrieved November 14, 2001, from ProQuest database.

Seymour, B., Kinn, S., & Sutherland, N. (2003). Valuing both critical and creative thinking in clinical practice: Narrowing the research-practice gap. *Journal of Advanced Nursing, 42*(3), 288-237. Retrieved December 9, 2004, from EBSCO.

Simpson, E., & Courtney, M. (2002). Critical thinking in nursing education: Literature review. *International Journal of Nursing Practice, 8,* 89-98.

Staib, S. A. (2003). Teaching and measuring critical thinking. *Journal of Nursing Education, 42*(11), 498-508.

Su, W. M., Masodi, J., & Kopp, M. (2000). Teaching critical thinking in the clinical laboratory. *Nursing Forum, 35*(4), 30-36. Retrieved December 3, 2004, from ProQuest database.

Tanner, C. A. (2000). Critical thinking: Beyond nursing process. *Journal of Nursing Education, 39*(8), 338-340. Retrieved December 3, 2004, from ProQuest database.

Van Eerden, K. (2001). Using critical thinking vignettes to evaluate student learning. *Nursing and Health Care Perspectives, 22*(5), 231-236. Retrieved October 19, 2001, from ProQuest database.

Videbeck, S. (1997). Critical thinking: A model. *Journal of Nursing Education, 36*(1), 23-28.

Walthew, P. J. (2004). Conceptions of critical thinking held by nurse educators. *Journal of Nursing Education, 43*(9) 408-412. Retrieved December 3, 2004, from ProQuest database.

Watson G., & Glaser, W. M. (1991). *Watson-Glaser Critical Thinking Appraisal manual.* New York: The Psychological Corporation, Harcourt Brace Jovanovich.

Whiteside, C. (1997). A model for teaching critical thinking in the clinical setting. *Dimensions of Critical Care Nursing, 16*(3), 152-162.

Williams, R. A., Sewell, D., & Humphrey, E. (2002). Implementing problem-based learning in ambulatory care. *Nursing Economics, 20*(3), 135-142. Retrieved December 3, 2004, from ProQuest database.

Wright, W. A. (Ed.). (1900). *Bacon: The advancement of knowledge.* Oxford, England: Clarendon Press.

Youngblood, N., & Beitz, J. M. (2001). Developing critical thinking with active learning strategies. *Nurse Educator, 26*(1), 39-42.

Zimmerman, B. J., & Phillips, C. Y. (2000). Affective learning: Stimulus to critical thinking and caring practice. *Journal of Nursing Education, 39*(2) 422-428. Retrieved November 14, 2001, from ProQuest database.

Collaborative Institutional Approches to Nursing Education

V. JANE MUHL ◆ PAM SCHEIBEL

This chapter discusses the process used for the development of the Collaborative Nursing Program. The chapter identifies the key collaborative participants, the elements of the facilitation process model used in the development of the program, a description of the characteristics of the Collaborative Nursing Program, the faculty perspective of offering a nursing program through the collaborative efforts of five institutions, and the positive aspects associated with the Collaborative Nursing Program.

BACKGROUND

Wisconsin is a large, rural, Midwestern state covering more than 54,000 square miles. In the Wisconsin system of higher education, of the 13 4-year institutions, only five offer baccalaureate nursing programs. These five institutions include an urban university, a land-grant research university, and three regional comprehensive universities. One of the regional comprehensive universities offers a baccalaureate completion program only, whereas each of the others offers basic nursing education through graduate education. Although part of a state system, each institution contributes to the vision of the state but maintains its own unique mission, including regional and nursing accreditation.

Faculty in the nursing programs recognized that because of the geographical location of the institutions, educational opportunities are limited for many of the registered nurses (RNs), especially those in the northern sector of the state. In addition, the deans of the nursing programs identified that resource limitations prioritized the focus of the programs on the needs of students who could come to campus. The demand for off-campus instruction, however, continued.

EDUCATIONAL NEEDS STUDY

To determine the extent of the need for baccalaureate education completion opportunities, a survey of RNs was conducted in 1993. At that time there were just more than 46,000 licensed RNs in the state. The total population was stratified geographically into four strata based on zip code. A sample of 1500 individuals was drawn and surveyed. The survey determined that more than 60% of the nurses in the state did not have a baccalaureate degree in nursing. Of the nurses who indicated that they were thinking of continuing their education in the next 5 years, 86% responded positively to the idea of obtaining the courses through distance education technology. Further, 67% stated that a degree-completion program delivered entirely by distance education technology would be very or somewhat attractive to them. From the stratified sampling process, it was extrapolated that nearly 9000 RNs were interested in baccalaureate education.

Conclusions of the study indicated that it was essential to make opportunities for degree completion available to RNs close to work or home and at a reasonable cost. This could be accomplished only through a collaborative effort of the five institutions using distance education technologies.

COLLABORATIVE PARTICIPANTS

The University of Wisconsin Board of Regents had a vision for the twenty-first century. They identified that bringing student-centered learning environments to the citizens of the state by removing time and place as barriers to learning and by using technologies that would expand the traditional walls of the campus should be a priority (The University of Wisconsin System Board of Regents, 1996). This set the educational climate for change and innovation.

The deans of the five nursing programs reported that, independently, they could not address the need of RNs across the state for baccalaureate completion. The University of Wisconsin Extension, a non–degree-granting entity of the University of Wisconsin system, offered to provide the leadership and personnel to facilitate the collaborative process among the five institutions.

The development of the Collaborative Nursing Program resulted from the combined energies of a university system interested in serving the educational needs of all of its citizens, without regard to time and place, to the dedication of the deans and faculty of the five institutions with nursing programs who were willing to risk entering into a collaborative approach to address the needs of RNs across the state, and to the insight of the personnel of the UW-Extension to provide an opportunity to facilitate a statewide collaborative effort.

FACILITATION PROCESS MODEL

The process used in the development of the Collaborative Nursing Program is described in the context of a facilitation model, which was developed and applied to this institutional collaborative effort by Offerman (1997), UW-Extension dean of continuing education. The process was facilitated by an external and objective team that was joined by a faculty "champion." For this situation, the facilitation team members were not nurses, had no vested interest in any of the existing nursing programs, and were not employed by any of the nursing schools. However, they were informed about collaboration, were knowledgeable about nursing education, and were able to engage with the planning group. The faculty "champion" was a known and highly regarded leader in the nursing education community. Even though she was from one of the University of Wisconsin schools of nursing, she was trusted and embraced by colleagues across the state as one of the nursing leaders in the state.

The process model consists of the following elements: (1) agreement to collaborate, (2) faculty control, (3) curriculum focus, (4) iterative planning, (5) attention to student needs, (6) structured curriculum planning, and (7) assertive conflict management. These elements are described, and the related actions are identified.

ELEMENTS OF THE FACILITATION MODEL

Agreement to Collaborate

The faculty champion and members of the facilitation team made visits to all five schools, asking the deans to enter into discussions for the purpose of determining whether a collaborative effort might assist in addressing the needs of RNs seeking a baccalaureate degree, using distance technology as the methodology for delivery. Schools were assured that their participation was voluntary, that they could withdraw from the discussions at any time, that faculty were to be involved actively, and

that decisions needed to be embraced by all. Each dean of the five nursing schools agreed to participate. In addition, the facilitators obtained the support of the vice-chancellor of each of the institutions and of the Wisconsin University system administration. This was done so that policies could be changed, if need be, to support the collaborative effort and address existing barriers.

Faculty Control

The initial joint meeting brought together one or two faculty members from each of the five nursing programs. The facilitators structured the meeting to allow faculty an opportunity to express concerns about a collaborative endeavor, to determine the operational ground rules, and to outline the expectations and responsibilities of the faculty. The facilitation team felt that by engaging faculty early in the process, faculty would be more willing to support an effort in which they had participated in its development stage.

Curriculum Focus

Although each of the institutions had its own baccalaureate completion curriculum, they agreed to engage in an exercise early in the process to develop an "ideal curriculum." Because the committee meetings were facilitated by persons without vested interests in any individual program and included one or two faculty from each of the participating institutions, each school could contribute to the evolving common nursing curriculum. In addition, by initially focusing on the curriculum, the potential logistical barriers did not surface or interfere with the development of the curriculum.

Iterative Planning

Committee members were asked to take information, ideas, and concerns back to their home institutions, where in turn they would receive support and input to share with the committee. Because one of the ground rules stated that decisions and issues could be revisited, all faculty had an opportunity for input at every juncture.

Attend to (Focus on) Student Needs

The vision of the curriculum was to attend to the needs of the adult employed learner, who had many roles and responsibilities and who was living at a distance from the campuses. During the curricular development process, the logistics of addressing the specific student needs were discussed.

VIEWPOINTS

Structured Curriculum Planning

Curricular planning considerations focused on the adult learner's needs, content needed to meet those needs, and the essential elements of an RN to baccalaureate nursing curriculum. With representatives from each of the five institutions, the essential elements of the curriculum were identified. The essential elements included five core courses in nursing, upper-level nursing electives, clinical experiences, and a capstone nursing course. This upper-division nursing curriculum would contain approximately 30 credits.

Further decisions about the curriculum included that nurses with an associate's degree in nursing (ADN) could transfer up to 60 credits of prior learning. The additional credits needed to obtain the baccalaureate degree would be institution-specific and would include the general education and nursing support courses unique to each institution (approximately 30 to 38 additional credits).

Once the curriculum was determined, the collaborative effort focused on developing common courses across the five institutions to offer the advanced nursing component content. Faculty groups with representatives from each institution developed the outlines and basic syllabi for the core courses. These five core courses included health assessment (including decision making based on data analysis), theoretical foundations of nursing practice, leadership/management (including change agent or multidisciplinary care issues), nursing research, and community health nursing (including health promotion, families and groups, and community-based practice).

Courses were approved on each campus through the approval process of the nursing program and institution. Each institution took responsibility for developing and delivering at least one of the core courses and one elective. Initially, each of the courses was developed to be delivered in a synchronous format to sites throughout the state. More than 30 sites were identified and contracted with for technology support. The distance education technologies identified for delivery of the courses included the following synchronous site-to-site modalities:

- Audio graphics: Combines audio teleconferencing with computer graphics. Students use a computer to view prepared graphics and a desktop microphone to communicate with the instructor.
- Interactive videoconferencing (compressed video): Students and instructors are linked through live audio and video.
- Telecourses: Broadcast on Wisconsin Public Television.

- Conference call service: Connects students and instructor through audio conference lines.

As the program has developed and with the assistance of grants, the courses also are being developed for online (Internet) delivery.

Transitioning to Online Courses

The vision of the program was to provide education to nurses who were bound by place and time. As the program progressed, it was evident that the goal of providing the courses synchronously met the place bound objective but not the time bound one. Because of the shortage of nurses in many areas, access to the course at the designated time and place was a hardship, limiting the number of students who could attend class. In some cases, RN students were still driving more than 1 hour to and from a delivery site (Muhl, 2002).

To address this problem, the faculty agreed to provide the courses in two formats, synchronous and online. The online option gave nurses access to the courses anytime, anyplace. The courses were structured as in a face-to-face class, with weekly or biweekly assignments, discussion groups, examinations and projects, and interaction with other students and with the instructor of the course. To facilitate study by those nurses who did not have access to a computer, laptops were made available for use during the students' tenure. An instructional technologist was sent to various sites to orient the students to online learning, software, and technical instruction. As the semesters continued, more and more students were opting for online learning versus synchronous. Eventually, all courses were placed in an online format and replaced the synchronous delivery course.

Assertive Conflict Management

The facilitation team was charged with managing the entire process, from objective facilitation of the agreement to collaborate, through the design and development of the curriculum, through the implementation of the program, including confronting conflict. This included making explicit the ground rules, which involved putting all the issues on the table and then addressing them. It focused on respect for all persons and ideas. It provided that all ideas would be heard and that all decisions could be revisited. It also identified that the outcome of the process needed to be a win-win situation for all. This last concept was especially vital to the one comprehensive institution that had as its only nursing program a baccalaureate completion program.

CHARACTERISTICS OF THE COLLABORATIVE NURSING PROGRAM

The Collaborative Nursing Program was implemented in spring 1996. The program is a multiple-institution collaborative effort to deliver a baccalaureate nursing degree by distance education technologies and the combined resources of the five nursing programs. The Collaborative Nursing Program began using synchronous technologies but now has expanded into the asynchronous, Web-based format, following the guidelines for use of technology as identified by the American Association of Colleges of Nursing (1999).

During the visioning and development process, the logistical considerations were deferred so that they would not emerge as barriers. However, before the program could be implemented, these considerations were addressed. The facilitation team worked with faculty, a steering committee that provided oversight to all components, an administrative committee that made decisions about cost of technology support and tuition issues, and the deans and administrators of each of the institutions. The following further describe how the program functions:

- ◆ Each institution maintains its own unique baccalaureate degree rather than offering a common degree.
- ◆ Each institution participates in developing and offering portions of a shared nursing curriculum.
- ◆ The home institution concept evolved to implement the program, so that students choose one of the five institutions to be their designated home institution, from which they receive their degree. The home institution provides the advising, financial aid, registration, and specified degree requirements. In most cases, students select the institution that is the closest to where they live or work. Students register and take courses through the home institution, although faculty from one of the other institutions might provide the instruction.
- ◆ A central coordinating body was identified to maintain a central database of class rosters and demographic information. It also coordinates the site assignments and rotation of courses.
- ◆ Tuition and fees are the same across the institutions to maintain a level playing field.

FACULTY PERSPECTIVE

The program has been widely accepted by students, who report many positive aspects: ease of use, availability of the courses, interaction with peers and faculty, access to library facilities, and accomplishment of personal educational goals. An important outcome of the program not often communicated is the beneficial affects this collaboration has had on the faculty between institutions and within institutions. The beneficial effect of this collaboration is best described globally as sharing ideas/online experience, sharing students, and sharing faculty.

Switching from synchronous to an online environment provided an important motivation for collaboration. Often faculty members new to software and online teaching relate only to technical support/instruction support persons who provide the basics necessary to teach online. The advantage of having multiple faculty placing courses online at once is the ability of the faculty to collaborate with one another and troubleshoot experiences, as well as personally to help each other. A meeting was held to convene all faculty who were part of the Collaborative Nursing Program. During this meeting, faculty members demonstrated their courses and described their challenges and ways they met these challenges. In addition, faculty shared ideas and experience that were helpful to the creation and teaching of the course. This sharing provided an excellent venue to make visible the teaching and learning that was being done in the course. Often most teaching is singular; that is, that between teacher and student. Rarely do faculty members have an opportunity to share their courses and their teaching with other faculty. This sharing provided a strong bond between the faculty members, who then could feel comfortable reaching out and discussing teaching and learning ideas and issues together.

A second benefit of the collaboration was the sharing of students. Because of the demographic difference in students from each of the campuses, the students shared different experiences, providing a rich learning environment to the class. Rural nurses worked in groups with urban nurses, for example, expanding each other's insight. Faculty also shared students, for example, by helping them find resources that might be needed for a class that a faculty member on a different campus was teaching. In addition, some faculty mentored a student whose interests were aligned with the faculty member's research or area of expertise.

The sharing of faculty provided an interesting collaboration within institutions. Once the course was designed and taught, a second faculty member was paired with the primary faculty member. This person was orientated to the course and often monitored the course for one semester. The point of this practice was to increase the faculty who knew how to teach online, to provide relief to the primary faculty member, and to expand the collaboration. This practice of pairing provided an easy way for faculty on other campuses to accept the new member. Ryan, Carlton, and Ali (2004) provide further insights on the role of faculty in distance learning education programs.

POSITIVE ASPECTS

Kuramoto (1999) identifies positive aspects of being involved in this multiinstitutional collaborative effort. These include a reduced sense of competition among the institutions because marketing, tuition costs, and the curriculum have been agreed upon previously. In addition, sharing of the teaching load by all five institutions reduces the duplication of efforts to deliver the program on a statewide basis. The central administrative office coordinates the selection of student information and scheduling of the courses. Further, instructional technology support for faculty and students has been positive. Increased communication among the five schools of nursing has resulted.

However, perhaps the most positive aspect of the collaborative effort is that RNs throughout the state now have access to a baccalaureate degree in nursing without having to relocate or travel great distances to a campus through the application of distance education. Nearly 400 students now have graduated from the Collaborative Nursing Program, and enrollment continues to be strong. The opportunities are expanding with the redesign of the synchronously delivered courses into delivery over the Internet. All of the core courses now are delivered over the Internet. Although the program has not changed significantly since its inception, the software platforms for delivery have changed to accommodate the changing technology requirements at the campuses. The program continues to provide educational opportunities for RNs that any one institution was unable to offer independently.

REFERENCES

American Association of Colleges of Nursing. (1999, July). *Distance technology in nursing education*. Washington, DC: Author.

Kuramoto, A. M. (1999). The challenges and rewards of institution collaboration in distance education. *Journal for Nurses in Staff Development, 15*(6), 236-240.

Muhl, V. J. (2002). RN to BSN online education: The University of Wisconsin's nation wide program. In M. Armstrong & S. Frueh (Eds.), *Telecommunications for nurses* (pp. 118-130). New York: Springer Publishing.

Offerman, M. J. (1997). Collaborative degree programs: A facilitation model. *Continuing Higher Education Review, 61,* 28-55.

Ryan, M., Carlton, K., & Ali, N. (2004). Reflections on the role of faculty in distance learning and changing pedagogies. *Nursing Education Perspectives, 25*(2), 73-80.

The University of Wisconsin System Board of Regents. (1996). *A study of the UW System in the 21st century*. Madison, WI: Author.

Using Academic-Service Collaborative Partnerships to Expand Professional Nursing Programs

CHRIS L. LATHAM

Many academic programs have embraced a closer link between nursing service and education to enhance professional nursing education (Sabatier, 2002). The American Association of Colleges of Nursing (2002) has supported the development of strategic partnerships to expand nursing programs in light of limited numbers of nursing faculty, insufficient clinical sites to support nursing student education, and academic fiscal constraints. The shortage of clinical sites, faculty, and academic funding for nursing education can be eased by partnerships between service and academic institutions. Faculty practice is not the norm in academic institutions with high teaching workloads; practice may not be valued or included in retention and promotion criteria. Increasing program capacity is difficult to accomplish without faculty who have current clinical expertise. Service-academic partnerships can enhance faculty practice expertise and add clinical sites that are essential for students to achieve clinical competency. Successful collaborative ventures between academic nursing programs and health care service entities have increased the capacity of academic institutions through resource-sharing endeavors (American Association of Colleges of Nursing, 2002; Kinnaman & Bleich, 2004; Stevens & Roper, 2004).

This chapter explores partnership development between an established academic nursing program and two separate, service-based clinical programs housed within a neighboring university and a large health care service provider organization. These partnerships used clinically competent specialty nursing faculty employed by service institutions to increase the nursing program capacity to meet regional health care needs while maintaining high student academic and clinical competency outcomes. Other resource-sharing components to the partnerships facilitated a high level of student achievement. The process to develop the partnerships was intensive and focused on meeting both partners' needs.

PARTNER BACKGROUNDS

The California State University system is one of the largest university systems in the United States. The system is a 24-campus, state-supported system with 17 campuses offering registered nurse entry-level and/or registered nurse completion bachelor of science in nursing and master of science in nursing programs. Increasing the academic institution capacity in state-supported higher-degree nursing programs is limited by a lack of faculty, shortage of university-based classroom space, competition for clinical sites, and insufficient funding (Russler, 2005). California has one of the lowest ratios of registered nurses to patients in the nation. Innovative models such as the ones discussed in this chapter are believed to help to increase the capacity of nursing academic institutions.

California State University, Fullerton (CSUF), is the third-largest California State University campus that serves a growing, diverse urban region of approximately 3 million people. For 25 years, CSUF had a registered nurse completion program. In 1996 the program was targeted for discontinuance because of low enrollment. As part of a necessary program expansion effort, three partnership programs were initiated. The three new programs included a statewide distance baccalaureate registered nurse completion program and two master of science in nursing advanced practice specialties, including nursing anesthetist and family nurse practitioner concentrations. The process and outcomes for the two advanced practice concentration partnerships are discussed in this chapter.

PARTNERING: DETERMINING THE NEED AND PROCESS

Based on a statewide registered nurse workforce assessment and increasing complexity of health care needs, there was a need for advanced practice nurses to care for patients of varying condition severity levels across hospital, outpatient, and community settings (California Strategic Planning Committee for Nursing, 1999). Partnering between academic and service to enhance an academic nursing program and meet community needs involved intensive interinstitutional collaboration that led to formal contracts to enhance both partners' ability to meet a common goal with mutually beneficial, long-term, positive outcomes. Many levels of collaboration are possible (Table 13-1). Each type of collaborative carries different levels of risk and commitment by partnering institutions, and the highest full partnership collaborative includes a legal contract. A high level of collaboration, or full partnership, was used to develop a new system of partner program delivery that enhanced

the capacity of both advanced nursing practice concentrations as part of a master of science in nursing program.

California State University, Fullerton, used four important collaboration principles to establish a working relationship for a partnership. The four collaboration principles are mutuality of goals and assumptions, intense involvement of participants, clarity of early and ongoing planning, and a reciprocity that includes discussion of the each partner's abilities, resources, and potential approaches to meet partnership goals (Meleis & Gray, 1998). As these principles were incorporated in partnership discussions, a better understanding of driving and restraining forces was developed. Driving forces for successful education partnerships include common goals and objectives, a high level of interest and ongoing motivation during the planning and initiation phases, previous experience with planning interinstitutional partnerships, and institutional support and resource commitment. *Restraining forces* for education partnering include turf issues; insufficient administrative or resource commitment; service/academic cultural differences; inability to

TABLE 13-1

Description and Examples of Various Levels of Collaborative Partnerships

Type of Collaborative Partnership	Characteristics of Collaborative Partnerships	Example of Academic-Service Partnership
Networking Partnership Definition: Informal partnering	Low risk to partnering organizations Low commitment Maintain separateness	Professional conference meetings with new or established partners
Coordinated Partnership Definition: Partnering to achieve a common purpose	Low risk to partnering organizations Low commitment May be joint or individual endeavor	Clinical rotations are altered to meet service demands, while achieving student educational needs
Cooperative Partnership Definition: Partnering to share resources and information and alter activities for mutual benefit	High risk to partnering organizations Higher commitment Joint work teams	Use of joint appointments from service in academic classes
Collaborative Partnership Definition: Partners share resources, alter activities to enhance capacity of other partners for mutual benefit and to achieve a common purpose	Very high risk to partnering organizations Phased-in relationship/closely work together Commit resources and seek joint funding, if necessary	Both partners need a valued commodity or product outcome and an enhanced capacity, such as agreeing to share expert lecturers
Full partnership Definition: Involves contracting and intensive collaboration to enhance bilateral partner capacity on relatively complex operations with mutually beneficial, long-term, positive outcome(s) for a common purpose	Very high risk to partnering organizations Legally determined Contractual in nature	Both partners are engaged in developing a new system of delivering a joint program that enhances capacity, such as jointly teaching a graduate specialty option

define common goals or reconcile logistics (scheduling, faculty workload/teamwork); lack of interest, motivation, or energy to sustain the planning phase; resistance to change; and inexperience or insecurity that hinders the collaborative partnership process (Kuehn, 1998). The pros and cons of partnering emerge as a relationship is initiated and the vision for a mutual goal is established. The partnership process evolves through relationship-building, formal need assessment, resource planning, and follow-through of each partnership phase with ongoing verbal and written agreements, such as minutes of meetings, memoranda of understanding, and formal contracts.

Preplanning the Partnerships/ Relationship Building

The preplanning phase to explore the possibility of partnerships included establishing a trusting relationship with ongoing communication, documenting the need to offer the program as a partnership, and deciding to commit resources to the ongoing partnership. The partnership-planning participants of both institutions previously had worked together in other forums and respected each others' talents and accomplishments. This assisted in the development of a trusting relationship. Communication started with individual meetings and was followed by formal presentations to administrators at both institutions.

Establishing the Need for the Program. The need for advanced practice nurses in these two specialties was established through state and local workforce planning studies. The California Strategic Planning Committee for Nursing conducted a study of the registered nurse workforce needs throughout the state of California, including the need for advanced practice nurses. The workforce analysis from the California Strategic Planning Committee for Nursing (1999) reported that family nurse practitioners, nurse anesthetists, clinical nurse specialists, and nurse-midwives were needed in California as calculated from the intention-to-employ data. National research revealed that almost 60% of patients needing procedures with anesthesia used nurse anesthetists, and there was a growing number of outpatient and pain clinics using procedures that required general or regional anesthesia administration. The proposed advanced practice nursing concentrations would become part of the first state-supported, campus-based master of science in nursing program in Orange County, the home base of the CSUF campus. The local need for advanced practitioners in nursing exceeded the national and state data, and health care service had to recruit from outside the region.

Resource Planning. The business plan for both advanced nursing practice programs was completed after the partnering relationship was established and goals were decided. The business plan explicated the outcomes, structure, governance, budget, and time period of the partnership. Later, the business plan was adapted to create a memorandum of understanding (MOU) to outline the shared governance, ongoing commitments, and financial aspects of the partnership. The MOU is a partnership agreement that details the processes used to meet goals that can be reviewed and changed annually. Identification of shared activities and the separate responsibilities of each institution ensures accountability. In addition to the MOU, a formal interinstitutional contract was completed. Formal contracts signed by administrators at each institution listed the major partnership goals, and after sustainability was ascertained, an evergreen contract (termination of the contract must be initiated by one of the institutions) was supported. Formal contracts often take longer to develop because they incorporate legalities of the relationship and need to be signed by high-level administrators from each partnering institution (e.g., university president and chief executive officer of the health care service entity). Both types of written agreements are discussed later in more detail.

The resource commitment was based on the fiscal requirements and in-kind contributions from each institution for the partnership. One of the programs was self-supporting and did not require CSUF to pay faculty salaries or other student resource and clinical needs. The other established program previously had used clinical nurse practitioner faculty to offer a post-master's certificate course of studies and required reimbursement of the portion of time that these clinicians taught in the advanced practice nurse courses, as well as reimbursement for performance testing and student equipment needs throughout the program. Both service-based programs had substantial in-kind resources that would support the partnership. For example, both institutions had experienced faculty with clinical expertise, off-campus training facilities, and established clinical affiliations for student practice, including contracts for clinical placement that used physicians and other advanced practice preceptors. Early in the preplanning phase, all institutions completed and shared formal budgets to determine the feasibility of the partnerships. After budget deliberations were completed, meetings were held to elicit both partners' perspectives about the infrastructure, instruction, and student and academic services aspects of the partnership.

Partnership Development Phases

Three phases of developing the partnership occurred once the participants and institutional administrators decided to embark on the endeavor. These phases were maintaining integrity of the relationship, establishing a project planning team that sought faculty acceptance and input into the partnership, and developing and executing the formal agreements.

Maintaining Integrity of the Relationship. Ongoing project planning team communication about the values, end goals, and accountability of each group was spelled out in written documents that helped to move the two groups forward. Visualizing the mutual gain from partnering and identifying potential pitfalls were important to maintain the momentum to formalize the partnership.

Project Planning Team and Faculty Participation. The project planning team from each institution met regularly to explore and develop the partnership. This team included administrators and faculty with previous advanced practice program experience. The participants included the department chair of the CSUF nursing program, an advance practice program consultant, and directors of each of the advanced practice programs. The advanced practice programs previously had been affiliated with a continuing education program or an academic setting. Both programs had a track record of successfully conducting an advanced practice program on a limited scale. The initial meetings dealt with sharing the vision for the partnership from both partners' perspectives. After the vision was agreed upon, the project planning team members consulted with executive level management at their institutions to discuss the need for the program and the philosophical (institutional mission compatibility and institutional motives), political, economic, legal, and operational feasibility of the partnership. Once the need and feasibility were established, faculty from all institutions met and formed specialty teams to determine the course work, student issues, and programmatic elements that needed to be merged within the academic and clinical frameworks of each institution.

As faculty worked together, differences in organizational cultures and difficulty with energy and time commitments to remain involved became evident. Organizational cultures varied in what is valued (e.g., amount of faculty practice), norms (e.g., degree of teaching/learning expertise), and expectations (e.g., explicit course syllabi and program outcome measures). The partnership accepted a "unified diversity" of cultures, based on a shared understanding and agreement about differences in the objectives, policies, procedures, and

skill level (academic versus clinical) in each organization (Rosenfeld, Richman, & May, 2004). A general meeting of academic and service faculty was held, followed by small team meetings combining academic and service faculty with similar specialty areas to share perspectives on course content.

These meetings highlighted the differences in clinical and academic viewpoints of culture in each institution. Both partners began to appreciate each other's educational perspectives and to view the partnership as strengthening student outcomes. For example, CSUF required prerequisite academic research and theory courses for advanced practice nurses, whereas multiple role courses were visualized as important to the partnering clinical faculty. Interinstitutional agreement emerged after both groups of faculty met together and formed small teams to consider the objectives, requirements, and teaching and assessment methodologies for each course. However, an intermediary advanced nursing practice program specialist, who worked as a consultant to write the final courses to meet curricular standards of the university, accomplished the final sculpting of courses within each program. The use of an outside consultant kept the program development moving forward, avoided turf issues, and resulted in a high-level, integrated program outcome.

Establishing Written Agreements. Two levels of agreements were used for partnering with off-campus advanced practice programs: the MOU and a formal contract.

MEMORANDUM OF UNDERSTANDING. The first type of agreement, the MOU, can be useful throughout the partnership discussion and implementation. During the planning phases, short MOUs can be used to document iterative agreements that are discussed. This is helpful if there is a long period devoted to planning the potential partnership because these iterative, signed agreements clarify the perspective of each institution on the partnership. Table 13-2 identifies some of the academic changes that must be considered when adding an off-campus program to the academic unit.

The MOU may be the outgrowth of the initial business plan. The business plan outlines the mission, structure, governance, partnership activities (joint and separate responsibilities), finances, and time line for partnership renewal and refinement. In this way the MOU can explicate shared responsibilities and conflict resolution strategies used during the partnering process. Partners should include a time line in the MOU to review and refine the partnership, usually every 1 to 2 years.

An important component of the MOU is to specify how often the partners will meet and how partners will

TABLE 13-2

Examples of Changes to Accommodate a Collaborative Partnership for an Academic Program	
Academic Department Partner	**Clinical Service Partner**
Increase the infrastructure for student services with additional student recruiters and admissions personnel	Formalize clinical contracts
Assist with student selection (shared interview committees)	Assist with student selection (shared interview committees)
Augment research input for students in the culminating outcomes requirements by adding a group seminar experience to add research faculty experience/input to students' work	Increased involvement of clinical faculty with student research
Institute student fee changes to support advanced practice costs of performance examinations and clinical laboratories	Increased faculty involvement with nonclinical curriculum
Share technology, for example, online software and access to training in technology	Attend on-campus committees and other student events
Share classroom space	Increased faculty involvement with technology
Change scheduling of classes to accommodate new cohort	Work collaboratively to schedule classes

be integrated into each other's institutional structure. For example, outside partners are required to attend the on-campus graduate program and evaluation committee meetings. Partners are voting members of each committee, and their input is solicited for program reviews, updates, and other student issues.

The MOU is a useful way to obtain a signed commitment for day-to-day decisions and expectations that may change over time, as the partners' operations (e.g., change in committee name/function) or program (e.g., culminating experience options are broadened) changes occur. The MOU can be revised every 1 to 2 years, and the existence of the MOU needs to be included in the formal interinstitutional contract. Box 13-1 contains some of the important components of an MOU.

LEGAL CONTRACT. The partnership contract is a legal document that outlines all aspects of the relationship, responsibilities, and expected outcomes. Each institution may need to decide on indemnity (institutional protection) clauses and other liability issues. The format for how decisions are made and dissolving the partnership are important parts of the legal contract.

ONGOING COMMUNICATION

Ongoing communication is a partnership imperative for sustainability and quality improvement. The partnership program, student, and fiscal outcomes are reviewed, as well as each partner's satisfaction with the agreement

and processes for decisions related to graduate programming. A collaborative partnership often needs many revisions as the partnership is operationalized. The aim is to eliminate boundaries by jointly working together to execute a program, including the assessment, ongoing planning, delivery, and evaluation.

PARTNERSHIP OUTCOMES

Both partnerships were based on solid relationships and focused discussions between faculty and administrators that resulted in a firm understanding of the contributions of each partner to a mutual goal of delivering competent advanced practice nurses to meet a community need. Since the partnerships were established, MOUs have been used to guide decisions when issues arise and are reviewed and updated after several years. Faculties continue to meet monthly to discuss student, course, and program issues. Students are given opportunities to work with clinically competent faculty in a wide array of clinical placements. Capacity of both service partners increased as a result of partnering; one increased from admitting 4 students to 20 students each year, and the other increased from an annual admission of 20 to 35 students each year. Although organizational cultures value different aspects of the student experience (clinical versus research emphasis), the structural integration of faculty and academic processes has resulted in a richer experience for faculty, students, and administrators.

BOX 13-1

Components of a Memorandum of Understanding: Fully Integrated Partnerships

I. Faculty Structure
   A. Approval and hiring of faculty
   B. Salaries: Who pays and at what level
   C. How will course review and faculty evaluation be conducted?
   D. How will faculty communicate? Is meeting attendance required?
   E. Process for clinical placement of students and affiliation agreements with clinical sites and preceptors
   F. Database of faculty qualifications and evaluations
II. Accreditation
   A. Who will participate in writing and preparing for accreditation?
   B. Funding of accreditation costs
   C. Quality improvement processes
III. Academic Processes
   A. Academic-service communication
   B. Coordination and review process for student evaluations
   C. Grading standards and course completion
   D. Program completion
   E. Use of technology in the program by students, faculty, and administrators
   F. Specific detail on which institution is responsible for course instruction or joint responsibility
   G. Program evaluation: Who is responsible?
   H. Course scheduling: Days, times, and responsibility for scheduling classroom space
IV. Students
   A. Numbers of students expected in each cohort
   B. Database responsibility
   C. Admission and advising policies: responsibility and process
   D. Student services: Library, e-mail, parking, financial aid
   E. Professional insurance requirements
   F. Student liability issues
   G. Student and faculty health requirements for clinical rotations
   H. Student registered nurse licensure requirements
   I. Worker's compensation issues
V. Finances
   A. Student fee structure
   B. Payments required between institutions: Faculty salaries, time line
   C. Other estimated costs
VI. Administrative Structure
   A. Director oversight: Each partner and jointly
   B. Staff required for administrative, student, and clerical services
   C. Technology oversight: staff and administrative
   D. Mechanism for conflict resolution
   E. Facilities and space considerations
   F. Integration of faculty between partnering institutions with administrative decisions and committee input

REFERENCES

American Association of Colleges of Nursing. (2002). Using strategic partnerships to expand nursing education programs. In *AACN Issue Bulletin*. Washington, DC: Author.

California Strategic Planning Committee for Nursing. (1999). *Nursing workforce projections for the state of California*. Irvine, CA: Author.

Kinnaman, M. L., & Bleich, M. R. (2004). Collaboration: Aligning resources to create and sustain partnerships. *Journal of Professional Nursing, 20*(5), 310-322.

Kuehn, A. E. (1998). Collaborative health professional education: An interdisciplinary mandate for the third millennium. In T. J. Sullivan (Ed.), *Collaboration: A health care imperative* (pp. 419-466). San Francisco: McGraw-Hill.

Meleis, A. I., & Gray, G. (1998). International collaboration: Principles and challenges. In T. J. Sullivan, *Collaboration: A health care imperative* (pp. 177-392). San Francisco: McGraw-Hill.

Rosenfeld, L. B., Richman, J. M., & May, S. M. (2004). Information adequacy, job satisfaction, and organizational culture in a dispersed network organization. *Journal of Applied Communication Research, 32*(1), 28-54.

Russler, M. (2005). Nursing shortage collides with CSU budget crisis. *California Faculty, 9*(1), 19, 22. Sacramento: California Faculty Association.

Sabatier, K. H. (2002). The Institute for Johns Hopkins Nursing: A collaborative model for nursing practice and education. *Nursing Education Perspectives, 23*(6), 178-182.

Stevens, R. H., & Roper, W. L. (2004). The North Carolina experiment: Academia-practice partnerships. *Journal of Public Health Management and Practice, 10*(4), 316-320.

Integrating Nursing Theory, Nursing Research, and Nursing Practice

HOWARD KARL BUTCHER

There should be little doubt that nursing has arrived as a scientific discipline. Significant emerging evidence supports the arrival of nursing as a scientific discipline. The National Institute of Nursing Research, initially created as a center at the National Institutes of Health in 1986, was established in 1993 and is now one of 25 centers in the National Institutes of Health. In 1986 the initial budget for the National Institute of Nursing Research was $16 million; for 2005 the appropriation has risen to $127,134,000 (National Institute of Nursing Research, 2005). More than 73% of the budget is used to fund extramural research project grants. Currently, more than 94 doctoral nursing programs in the United States are preparing future nursing researchers, scholars, and leaders (American Association of Colleges of Nursing, 2005a). In addition, more than 190 nursing journals are in continuous print with more than 15 journals having a clear research focus (University of Adelaide Library Guides, 2005).

Despite these impressive advances, much needs to be accomplished for the nursing discipline if it is to achieve full recognition as an academic, professional, and scientific practice discipline among peer health care disciplines. Although the National Institute of Nursing Research budget allocation has made significant gains since 1986, that budget represents only 0.045% of the total $28.8 billion National Institutes of Health budget (National Institutes of Health Office of Budget, 2005). Furthermore, year after year, the National Institute of Nursing Research budget increase is consistently smaller than most of the other 27 institutes and centers housed at the National Institutes of Health. Although university-based education is the hallmark of a professional discipline, currently only 43% of all nurses hold a baccalaureate degree or higher. More significantly, less than 1% of the 2.7 million nurses in the United States hold a doctor of philosophy, and less than 10% have a master's degree (American Association of Colleges of Nursing, 2005b).

Although establishment of doctoral education, a mass of published scholarly work, and recognition as an "institute" at the National Institutes of Health are hallmarks of the knowledge development and emergence of nursing as a science, nurse scholars have expressed concern about the divergent patterns of nursing knowledge development. Knowledge in nursing typically has developed along three separate areas: (1) theoretical knowledge, (2) practice knowledge, and (3) knowledge based in research or science. Early in the focus on knowledge development, many nurse scholars called for integrated knowledge (Conant, 1967; Fawcett, 1978; Fawcett & Downs, 1992; Jacobs & Huether, 1978; Kim, 2001), yet knowledge development processes have continued to develop separately. Concerns about the fragmentation of nursing knowledge and calls for "integrated knowledge" continue to be voiced (Chinn & Kramer, 2004; Fawcett, 2005; Fawcett & Bourbonniere, 2001; Kim, 2001; Meleis & Im, 2001). This concern about the lack of knowledge integration leads to the viewpoint addressed in this chapter: If nursing is to progress and receive recognition as a scientific practice discipline, nursing practice, theory, and research knowledge development need to be integrated into a seamless whole. The bringing together or nexus of nursing theory, practice, and research creates a true integration of knowledge designed to support the service to clients and the health of society.

KNOWLEDGE BASED IN NURSING THEORY

A major thrust in the ascent for recognition of nursing as a discipline and as a science has been the development of nursing theories. *Nursing theory* refers to extant grand theories, conceptual frameworks, and theories developed for the purpose of guiding nursing education, research, and practice. Nursing theories are designed to (1) provide a perspective for understanding the person the nurse is caring for, (2) direct the approach to be taken to deliver care, and (3) structure critical thinking, reasoning, and decision making in practice (Alligood, 2002). Nursing conceptual frameworks and theories therefore (1) guide all aspects of nursing research and (2) provide a general outline for organizing nursing knowledge (Fawcett, 2005).

An important note is that disciplines exist because of their unique body of knowledge. Although professional and occupational fields such as nursing also have roots or "linkages" in basic sciences, social science, humanities, and the arts (Stark & Lattuca, 1997), they also are characterized by a unique disciplinary perspective and knowledge structure. Donaldson and Crowley (1978) pointed out in their classic article that "a discipline is not global; it is characterized by a unique perspective, a distinct way of viewing all phenomena, which ultimately defines the limits and nature of its inquiry" (p. 113). Having a unique body of knowledge is the essence of a discipline. The academy is organized into colleges, schools, and departments according to disciplines or branches of knowledge. As early as the mid-1950s the National Science Foundation held that curricula should be formulated according to the structures of disciplines (Tanner & Tanner, 1975). If nurse educators do not take the structures of the disciplines into account in the curriculum, "there will be failure of learning or gross mislearning by our students" (Schwab, 1962, p. 197). According to the extensive studies by Phenix (1986) and Dressel and Marcus (1982) on the nature of disciplines, all disciplines have substantive structure, symbolic structure, syntactical structure, value structure, and organizational/conjunctive structure. Nursing theories are associated most closely with and are embedded within the substantive structure of the discipline because the substantive structure is concerned with assumptions and particular concepts of interest to the discipline. Nursing theories and classification systems such as the nursing diagnosis, nursing intervention, and Nursing Outcomes Classification contribute to delineating the syntactical structure of nursing.

Despite the presence of development of discipline-specific knowledge, nursing theories often are not used to guide research or practice. Many nursing theories emerged in the late 1960s to early 1980s as efforts to define the discipline and foster curricular reform. Although these models were historically essential in the articulation of nursing identity, they evolved parallel to, rather than interwoven with, research (Blegen & Tripp-Reimer, 1994). These models were statements of nursing philosophy and ideology but did not present knowledge that could be applied directly in practice. They were separate from the world of nursing practice and neither were developed from research nor were tested through research. A number of nursing scholars (Cody, 1994; Fawcett, 1999; Levine, 1995; Mitchell, 1997; Rawnsley, 1999; Reed, 1995) have noted the decreased emphasis on the application of unique nursing knowledge in nursing education and clinical practice. DeKeyser and Medoff-Copper (2002) commented that "over the decade of the 90s nursing theory seemed to take an increasingly smaller role in the content of schools of nursing" (p. 330) and "practicing nurses are continuing with their daily routines and are often unaware that the world of nursing theory is changing" (p. 329). The vast majority of published nursing research continues to be theory-isolated or conceptualized from theories borrowed from other disciplines. Fawcett (1999) reviewed all articles published in 1998 in *Research in Nursing and Health* and *Nursing Research* and noted that only 3% were guided by recognized nursing theories. When conducting research, there is nothing wrong with conceptualizing the research problem within a theory from another discipline.

Over the past 30 years, all the major nursing theories have evolved to the point they provide specific guidance for research and practice. The journal *Nursing Science Quarterly* consistently has published nursing theory testing research for the past 18 years. Fawcett (2005) references more than 200 refereed research-based articles testing Roy's adaptation model and lists more than 300 research-based articles testing Orem's self-care framework. The presence of just one example of the testing of nursing theory calls into question any claims that the models are untestable. The real question that should be asked is, Why do nurse educators, researchers, and practicing nurses opt for adopting primarily biomedical and psychological theories rather than embracing knowledge developed specific to the nursing discipline?

NURSING KNOWLEDGE AND PRACTICE

Nursing knowledge tends to be practical and is applied as soon as possible in a clinical setting. The ultimate purpose of knowledge development in nursing must be to serve as a foundation for guiding nursing practice. Practice refers to the professional health-related services nurses offer to individuals, families, communities, and populations. *Nursing practice* is the "protection, promotion, and optimization of health and abilities, prevention of illness, injury, alleviation of suffering through the diagnosis and treatment of human response, and advocacy in the care of individuals, families, communities,

VIEWPOINTS

and population" (American Nurses Association, 2003, p. 6). According to *Nursing's Social Policy Statement* (American Nursing Association, 2003), the social mandate of the nursing discipline includes the provision of the following health-related services: promoting health and safety; supporting self-care processes; providing physical, emotional, and spiritual comfort; facilitating adaptation to physiological and pathophysiological processes; assisting clients in dealing with the emotions related to the experiences of birth, growth and development, health, illness, disease, and death; helping clients find meaning in the health-illness experience; preventing disease; enabling client decision making; enhancing role performance and relationships; enacting social policies that promote human environment health and well-being; and facilitating clients' quality of life.

Nursing has a mandate from society to use its specialized knowledge and skills to promote the well-being and human betterment. The knowledge that nurses use while engaging in practice comes from many sources and is learned initially in the courses taken during undergraduate education. These courses are selected carefully from all disciplines: biophysical sciences, social sciences, humanities, and nursing science. The courses in nursing science present knowledge based in other disciplines and knowledge generated by nurses. When nurses are grounded in a clear and distinct philosophical and theoretical disciplinary perspective, knowledge borrowed from other disciplines can be reformulated and can take on new meaning as this knowledge is interpreted through the nursing disciplinary lens.

Practice knowledge, however, often is not informed or guided by nursing theory. Johnson (1987) pointed out that many nurses use "private" or "implicit" mental frameworks that are not informed by specific theories. These mental frameworks tend to be disconnected, diffuse, incomplete, and often are based on concepts and conceptual schema used by other disciplines such as medicine and psychology. Some critics of nursing theory believe that basing nursing practice on nursing theory is too narrow and that nursing is more than what is articulated in nursing theories. However, the use of non-nursing theory is what limits nursing, not the use of nursing theory. Practicing from a non-nursing theory base potentially limits the full extent of a nurse's contribution to promoting the health in persons needing nursing care. All nursing theories extend beyond any borrowed biomedical, psychological, sociological, or even critical theories. All nursing theories are inherently holistic, and therefore they provide a base for a practice more expansive than any particular sociological, psychological,

biological, biomedical, cultural, or spiritual theory. Most nursing theories are inclusive of all these components while at the same time organizing them all into a coherent, systematic, logical, and scientific whole. Conceptualizing and understanding nursing through the lens of a nursing theory opens up new possibilities. Nurses who base their practice on an explicit nursing conceptual framework are assured that they "follow in Nightingale's footsteps and articulate what nursing is and what it is not" (Fawcett & Bourbonniere, 2001, p. 312).

Nursing theory as a type of knowledge in that era often was considered by practitioners and researchers to be too abstract to be useful. As others have noted, nurses seemed to believe that in order to be theory, the knowledge needed to be obscure and lack immediate use and meaning (Levine, 1995). Therefore theory was relegated to a place separate from other types of nursing knowledge. Yet the "abstract" language embedded in their conceptual frameworks and theories characterizes all disciplines. Every discipline educates its future practitioners by immersing them in a knowledge and language base unique to that discipline. Nursing conceptual frameworks, theories, and classification systems provide the language of nursing. As Cody (1994) points out, "nurses who read in other disciplines take it upon themselves to learn the language ... shouldn't they be expected to do the same with regard to their own discipline" (p. 99). Watson (1995) has pointed out that if one does not have a language, one does not exist. "In a fundamental way, one is one's language" and "is a way of being" (Allen, 1995, p. 177). The nature of theory requires concepts and a specific language to provide clarity of meaning. The terminology in nursing conceptual frameworks and theories are abstract or difficult only to one who has not studied or learned the theory.

All theory by its nature is abstract. Practice by its nature is not abstract. DeKeyser and Medoff-Cooper (2002) point out that an inherent gap must exist between theory and practice and perhaps the problem is not that there is a gap between theory and practice but is in the expectations of what theory can do for practitioners. An important note is that nursing practice informs the development of nursing theory. Nursing theories are guides to practice and typically are not prescriptive. Nursing theory provides a way of thinking and being in nursing situations (Butcher, 2004). Each nursing conceptual framework provides a definition of nursing, identifies the major concepts of concern to nursing, and describes the purpose and goal of nursing care. More specifically, theories derived from conceptual framework are designed to *guide* all aspects of nursing care. A nursing theory gives direction to the focus of assessment by identifying the phenomenon of concern; providing a scientific basis for understanding the nature of patient problems; and providing the specifics for guiding all aspects of planning, implementing, and evaluating nursing care.

As a science matures, a more precise terminology is used to communicate abstract formulations in a clear and unambiguous way. For example, the language of psychoanalytic theory (i.e., ego, superego, transference, and counter transference) sounds equally meaningless and cumbersome when one first learns psychoanalytic theory. The terminology of nursing theory pales in comparison to the complex biomedical language of pathophysiology and pharmacology that all nurses must learn. Nurses first exposed to medical terminology often require a medical dictionary. Once familiar with the terminology, the meaning of these abstract concepts is so clear that most anyone understands their meaning. Clarity of meaning enhances communication and understanding of the theory.

Yet the reality is that few nurses are educated within a nursing theory perspective, so it is not surprising that few nurses come to use nursing theory in practice. Many practice settings continue to be dominated by physicians and their biomedical model. Throughout nursing history, nursing has adopted or adapted the language of other disciplines to explain nursing phenomena. Not surprisingly, when nursing adopts the language of medicine, nursing is seen as an extension of medicine rather than a separate and unique discipline. If the nurse uses only knowledge derived from other disciplines such as medicine or psychology, the nurse would have little to contribute to the care of the patient distinct from what physicians and psychologists contribute. If nurses use a particular nursing theory to guide assessment, the nurse would have information distinct from any other member of the team and therefore contribute to a new understanding of the patient's situation that likely is not otherwise addressed. Other nurses argue that nurse educators should abandon nursing theory because other health care professionals do not understand it and argue that all health care professionals should speak the same language. Such statements really translate into "we all need to speak the language of medicine." Why should the nurses relinquish their valued knowledge base? Other health care professionals, such as psychologists and social workers, do not abandon their theoretical heritage when working with the multidisciplinary team. Rather, other professionals translate abstract theoretical concepts in a manner that those unfamiliar with the theory can understand.

The lack of using nursing theory to conceptualize and guide nursing practice contributes to making nursing knowledge invisible in the eyes of the public, other disciplines, and most of all to nurses themselves. Fawcett and Bourbonniere (2001) call for nurses to end their intellectual and practice romance with the knowledge of other disciplines and to "fall in love with nursing knowledge and develop a passion for the destiny of the discipline of nursing" (p. 316).

KNOWLEDGE BASED IN NURSING RESEARCH

Nursing research is the "systematic, formal, rigorous, and precise processes employed to gain solutions to problems and/or to discover and interpret new facts and relationships" (Waltz & Bausell, 1981, p. 1). Research is primarily a means for theory development. Kerlinger (1986) pointed out that research is "guided by theory" (p. 10). Thus theory and research are intertwined because theory and research inform one another. Philosophers of science have advanced the idea that, whether identified or not, all research flows from an ontological, paradigmatic, and theoretical perspective (Bernstein, 1983; Guba & Lincoln, 1989; Hesse, 1980; Lauden, 1984; Morgan, 1983; Polkinghorne, 1983).

In a practice discipline, the role of research is to develop and test knowledge designed to guide practice. The fact that nursing research often is not informed explicitly by theory (theory-isolated) and is seldom applied in nursing practice has been lamented for some time. One view advanced by some nurse scholars is that research conceptualized using non-nursing theories or borrowed theories from other disciplines does not advance nursing science and does not advance the development of a unique body of disciplinary knowledge. Some of the inattention to theory-testing research comes from the researchers themselves. Researchers who continue to perpetuate the false notion that nursing theory is "untestable" (Acton, Irvin, & Hopkins, 1991) must not be familiar with the vast amount of evidence that clearly demonstrates not only the testability of nursing theories but also the ability of nursing theory to conceptualize nursing practice across populations, settings, and patient situations. Although optimistic about the increase in application of research findings, most authors point to significant barriers to research use (Baessler et al., 1994; Carroll et al., 1997; Coyle & Sokop, 1990; Pettengill, Gillies, & Clark, 1994; Titler, 1997).

The idea of applying knowledge from research to practice implies the crossing of a chasm. This chasm is created in part through difficulties in finding, reading, understanding, and preparing the research for application. Another part of the chasm between research and practice is the different orientations of nurses who conduct research and those who care for patients directly. The orientation of nurse researchers leads them to increase the validity of the general knowledge produced by their studies by removing or controlling the influence of unique individual characteristics of each patient or subject and the setting. Nurses oriented to practice must focus on those individual characteristics to provide care that truly meets each patient's needs. These different perspectives and tools continue to keep knowledge from research separate from knowledge used in practice until a nurse takes pieces of the knowledge from one arena and uses it in the other. Increasingly, articles in nursing education encourage faculty to ground nursing knowledge in evidence-based practice, outcomes, research, and theory. These exhortations often emphasize the existing separateness of research, theory, and practice.

MODELS FOR INTEGRATING NURSING THEORY, RESEARCH, AND PRACTICE

A unique body of knowledge is a foundation for attaining the respect, recognition, and power granted by society to a fully developed profession and scientific discipline. Furthermore, the autonomy of a profession rests most firmly on the uniqueness, recognition, and recognized validity of the theoretical knowledge of the discipline. Thus the profession and society are served best when the professional discipline of nursing has a body of knowledge that is unique, coherent, and as seamlessly as possible linking nursing theory, research, and practice. This unique body of knowledge consists of nursing philosophy, metaparadigm constructs, patterns of knowing, paradigms, conceptual frameworks, nursing theories, midrange theories derived from or linked to extant conceptual frameworks and theories, practice models derived from or guided by nursing theories, nursing classification systems, and finally empirical indicators linked to the nursing concepts composing the theoretical landscape of nursing (Butcher, 2004). This knowledge must have the following characteristics:

1. This knowledge must be organized by theoretically identified concepts, patterns, and relationships.
2. The statements of this knowledge must be generated from and tested by systematic research.
3. Knowledge needs must be identified in practice, and generated knowledge must be applied immediately to practice (Blegen & Tripp-Reimer, 2001).

Like practitioners in other disciplines, students are taught the philosophical and theoretical framework of the discipline. A host of nursing theories are integrated fully into all aspects of the curriculum, including clinical courses where nursing students learn how specific nursing theories guide practice and how nursing theories may be used to conceptualize and test knowledge derived from practice. Nursing theories and their corresponding practice models are standards of practice across clinical settings. Practice is grounded on research that is conceptualized within the discipline-specific knowledge of nursing. Anything less than full integration will continue the current pattern of separateness.

The ideal model brings together academic researchers, nurse theorists, and practicing nurses to identify knowledge needs, to carry out research projects, to create and refine theory, and to bring research findings systematically into nursing practice. Although few if any real-world examples exist of a fully integrated discipline-specific nursing theory–research–practice model, three subtypes can be identified. The first is the researcher-practitioner collaboration. Two examples of this model come from northern California and involve collaboration among several health care agencies and nurse research experts (Chenitz, Sater, Davies, & Friesen, 1990; Rizzuto & Mitchell, 1988). Another example comes from the Midwest and describes a collaborative research project that began as a utilization project, became a research conduction project because of the lack of adequate base for interventions, and concluded as the results of the research were used and evaluated in practice (Blegen & Goode, 1994). Yet another suggestion for increasing the connectedness of the production and use of research knowledge in practice is offered by Boyd (1993). The nursing practice research method features the relationship between the nurse researcher–as–clinician and the patient. The research process is collaboration between nurse and patient; it is therapeutic to the patient and leads to development of the nurse. One can question whether the knowledge produced by these efforts is generalizable beyond the setting and patients involved in the project. Even researchers from the "perceived" view call for the creation of knowledge that can be used by all nurses; that is, knowledge that is generalizable (Schumacher & Gortner, 1992). The greater the need for knowledge that is generally useful by all nurses, the less this approach will be satisfactory.

Another nurse researcher–practitioner model that is receiving increasing attention is the use of evidence-based practice. Titler (2001) explains that typically evidenced-based practice refers to the use of scientific information from randomized clinical trails as a guide for practice. In nursing, levels of evidence can range from randomized clinical trails to case reports and expert opinions. The development of research evidence used to create evidence-based protocols, practice guidelines, policies, procedures, or CareMaps requires researcher's close collaboration with expert clinicians and the evidenced-based nurse researcher.

The second type of collaboration is the theorist-practitioner model. Examples of this kind of collaboration are found in discussions of implementation of the conceptual models. Practitioners using nursing theories in practice have published a wide range of works describing how particular nursing theories are used to guide practice in specific patient populations (Alligood & Marriner-Tomey, 2002; Fawcett, 2005; Parker, 2006). A number of published examples, though not nearly enough, also focus on the implementation and integration of a conceptual model in the organization of a hospital or other patient care facility. Unfortunately, the success of these efforts is difficult to analyze. How can nurses determine whether implementing model A or model B in a hospital leads to better outcomes? Real-world problems are too complex to conclude unequivocally that the model implemented resulted in the changes specified and that the changes enhanced patient outcomes. Fawcett (1999) suggests that nursing needs two dominant provider types, which she labels nurse scholars. The first type, prepared in doctor of nursing programs, would integrate research and practice in caring for individual clients. The second type, prepared in doctor of philosophy programs, would integrate nursing theory and practice with groups of patients.

The third type of collaboration is the researcher-theorist group, which includes the research that is conceptualized within specific nursing theories. Fawcett's text (2005) includes a comprehensive listing of hundreds of nursing theory–based research studies organized by each of the major conceptual frameworks and theories. However, little of the nursing theory–based research is ever actually translated into practice, used by practitioners, or even included in educational programs.

No examples exist of models combining all three knowledge areas. Although needed—and this need often is discussed in published literature—no working models have been described. One recently suggested approach may be able to facilitate this. Theories can be tested using means other than traditional empirical research methods. Silva and Sorrell (1992) suggested that there are four approaches to testing theory: verification through correspondence with empirical research, testing to verify through critical reasoning, testing through verification

of personal experiences, and verification through assessment of problem-solving effectiveness. If a theory were tested with all these approaches, it clearly would increase the integration of practice, theory, and research. However, theory testing using any one of these four methods also involves advanced skills that many practicing nurses do not have or feel they have little time to use.

Although collaboration is generally to be recommended and is essential if nurse educators set out to develop one coherent, seamless body of knowledge, there are limitations to the extent of collaboration that actually can take place. Crossing the differing perspectives of the persons involved is difficult. Practitioners focus on individual and unique patients; researchers focus on systematically collecting knowledge that transcends the individual subjects from whom they collect data; and theorists focus on general and abstract concepts and relationships among them. A great deal of time and effort must be expended to enhance communication among collaborators.

This connected approach to nursing knowledge would put to rest the problem of separated areas of knowledge; however, working in teams that draw persons from multiple settings consumes a great deal of time and other resources. With a highly connected approach to nursing knowledge creation and use, the chasm-spanning activities encompassed by research use would no longer be needed. This would release some resources for use in the collaboration needed for the success of the connected approach.

Perhaps the most comprehensive and prominent model for integrating discipline-specific knowledge with research and practice is the conceptual-theoretical-empirical system–based nursing practice model described by Kenney (1995) and elaborated on by Fawcett (2005). The model includes not only how the nexus of metaparadigm concepts, philosophy, conceptual models and theories, and empirical indicators in nursing is translated into practice but also a 10-step process for implementing this discipline-specific knowledge into practice. In addition, Fawcett links the conceptual-theoretical-empirical model to research by describing how practitioner-researchers can use "single-case studies" to test outcomes based on interventions. The creation of a conceptual-theoretical-empirical system would include linking the empirical indicator to an appropriate discipline-specific conceptual frame of reference such as a grand theory, a conceptual model, or a middle-range theory. Fawcett notes that the "key to the integration of research and practice is the recognition and acceptance of the similarity between the process of research and the process of practice, and recognition that both the research and practice are guided by the same C-T-E [conceptual-theoretical-empirical] system" (p. 594).

STRENGTHENING THEORY-RESEARCH-PRACTICE INTERCONNECTIONS

Nursing knowledge is developed at different levels of abstraction. For example, philosophical inquiry is at a high abstract level of knowledge development, whereas the testing of a specific "micro-theory" that covers only a narrow range of phenomena may be tested in a highly controlled systematic study. Although the threads of knowledge development often develop separately along different levels of abstraction, what connects theory development at different levels of abstraction is the link of the inquiry to the conceptual-theoretical-empirical system of the discipline.

However, nurses need stronger integration, particularly connections that span the chasm separating nursing knowledge from practice. These connections should be structural and intrinsic to the knowledge itself rather than dependent on chasm spanner models. If the knowledge developed was closer to practice, amenable to research testing, and built around structures intrinsic to the discipline of nursing, nursing then would have stronger connectedness for application. One solution is to use middle-range theory as a connecting point between theory, research, and practice. Middle-range theory, when developed from research and thoughtful consideration of practice and tested by other research projects, does represent the most valid and useful type of knowledge available in nursing and other disciplines (Lenz, Suppe, Gift, Pugh, & Milligan, 1995).

Middle-range theory provides the means of articulating general knowledge, confirmed by the specific results of research projects, to nurses in clinical practice. When middle-range theory is used to guide research and knowledge development, the theorist and researcher are the same person or two persons focusing on the same carefully delineated topic. The scope of knowledge within the topic area is narrower than the grand theories and the metaparadigm concepts. The restriction of scope allows for far more precision and depth than the grand theories and conceptual models have allowed. This precise, in-depth, and focused knowledge then can be used to inform and guide practice in specific and useful ways. Each middle-range theory is more narrow and precise, and yet, as midrange theories develop, they eventually will produce a body of knowledge that covers a broad range of nursing activities.

Theories of the middle range were suggested first by the sociologist Robert K. Merton. The discipline of sociology also initially developed large theories attempting to differentiate sociology from other disciplines and to explain all of social phenomena with one effort. Merton (1967) responded by suggesting middle-range theories and differentiating them from the grand theories. Middle-range theory can be used to guide empirical inquiry because it lies between the minor working hypotheses that evolve in abundance during day-to-day practice and the all-inclusive systematic efforts to develop one unified theory that would explain all behavior. Middle-range theory is intermediate to the general theories, which are too remote from specific classes of behavior to account for what is observed and to those detailed orderly descriptions of particulars that are not generalized at all. Middle-range theory, according to Merton, involves abstractions, but these are close enough to observed data to be expressed in propositions that permit testing with systematic research.

Merton (1967) suggested that the search for the perfect grand theory led to a multiplicity of philosophical systems in sociology and further to the formation of schools, each with its own cluster of masters and disciples. Nursing perhaps has fallen to a similar fate. That is, nursing became differentiated from other disciplines but also became internally differentiated not in terms of specialization, as in other sciences, but in terms of schools of philosophy, held to be mutually exclusive and largely at odds. Although a diversity of paradigms and research traditions has value within a discipline, it is time to refocus from discussing these larger philosophical systems to producing knowledge that explains patient-related phenomena and helps in the evaluation of nursing care.

Merton (1967) further described the middle-range orientation as one that involves the specification of ignorance. Rather than pretend to have knowledge when it is in fact absent, the work on middle-range theories expressly recognizes what must yet be learned in order to lay the foundation for more knowledge. Middle-range theory does not begin with the task of providing theoretical solutions to all the urgent practical problems of the day but addresses itself to those problems that now might be clarified in the light of available knowledge and to the identification of problems about which nurses know very little.

The major task of nursing is to develop middle-range theory for the general advancement of nursing knowledge and to provide closer connections among theory, research, and practice. A large part of what now is described as theory consists of general orientations toward the discipline, suggesting types of variables that theories must take into account, rather than clearly formulated, verifiable statements of relationships between specified variables. Nursing has many concepts but few supported propositions relating them, many points of view but few confirmed theories. It is time to move on.

To make use of the knowledge provided by middle-range theories, practicing nurses would need some grasp of research methods, but they would not have to read and critique directly the often complex reports of research methods and findings. In addition, practicing nurses would not have to attempt to apply the global, highly abstract grand theories to everyday practice. Middle-range theories, developed and tested by research, would contain much more specific descriptions of human responses to health and illness and the nursing interventions applicable to these responses. Although understanding the theory and deriving specific nursing actions would be necessary, these activities would not be as daunting with theory developed in the middle range as they are with the grand theories. However, further fragmentation of knowledge will occur if middle-range theory development is detached from the extant conceptual systems of nursing.

Typically, middle range theory has developed around concepts that are relevant to nursing practice, such as pain, unpleasant symptoms, self-efficacy, empathy, chronic sorrow, comfort heath promotion, resilience, uncertainty, self-transcendence, informed caring, personal risk taking, illness trajectory, smoking relapse, family caregiving, and attentively embracing story (Chinn & Kramer, 2004; Peterson & Bredow, 2004; Smith & Liehr, 2003). Although the knowledge articulated with middle-range theories is much closer to practice, it still must be located and critiqued. Nurse educators and group leaders for evidence-based practice projects could provide this necessary assistance. Their job would be much easier with theory in the middle range that had been tested systematically by researchers. Knowledge built in this way is synthesized more easily: the accumulation of knowledge across individual studies occurs as part of the process of conducting research and testing a theory. Persons actively engaged in evidence-based practice could provide an additional service by formally feeding back to the researchers the evaluation of practice guidelines and protocols. This would provide a test of pragmatic usefulness for the knowledge.

Liehr and Smith (1999) list five approaches to developing middle-range theory: induction through research and practice; deduction from research and practice applications of grand theories; combination of existing

nursing and non-nursing middle-range theories; derivation from theories of other disciplines that relate to the disciplinary perspective of nursing; and derivation from practice guidelines rooted in research. However, to avoid further fragmentation of nursing knowledge, middle-range theory development should be connected to the theoretical, conceptual, and philosophical systems of nursing. One way that middle-range theory development has been connected to extant nursing knowledge is when midrange theories are derived from nursing theories. Middle-range theories have been derived from a number of nursing theories including the Roy adaptation model, King's systems theory, and Orem's self-care model (Butcher, 2004). Smith and Liehr (2003), in their book on middle-range theories, illustrate how particular midrange theories have been developed within one of the three extant paradigms of nursing.

Blegen and Tripp-Reimer (2001) suggest that recent developments in nursing knowledge structures provide another way to ground these theories within the discipline. Developments in the structure of nursing knowledge (the taxonomies for nursing diagnoses, interventions, and outcomes) hold great promise for capturing the middle-range theories within a thorough and extensive framework of nursing knowledge. The Iowa Intervention Project has advanced even beyond the taxonomy of interventions and has identified a three-dimensional structure underlying these interventions (Tripp-Reimer, Woodworth, McCloskey, & Bulechek, 1996). Classes of interventions were characterized along four factors that then were related to the dimensions. The dimensions indicated principal elements describing patient needs and setting characteristics that nurses use in selecting the interventions, and four factors characterized the interventions available. Combined, these produce three descriptive categories. The first dimension nurses might use in selecting interventions is the *intensity of care* dimension, and the groups of interventions range along two bipolar factors: healthy self-care to provider illness care and continuous routine care to sporadic emergency care. The second dimension describing intervention selection is *focus of care,* and the interventions range from individual independent to system collaborative. The third dimension is *complexity of care* and includes two groups of interventions: continuous routine to sporadic emergency and high-priority difficult to low-priority easy (Blegen & Tripp-Reimer, 1997, 2001). These three dimensions and the factors within them could serve as the framework for guiding development of middle-range theories describing nurses' decision making in the selection of interventions.

The taxonomies of nursing diagnoses, interventions, and outcomes provide a full skeletal framework for nursing knowledge. Although Blegen and Tripp-Reimer (2001) do not advocate that the midrange theories necessarily be connected to or derived from the philosophical, conceptual, and theoretical knowledge of the discipline, the viewpoint expressed in this paper is clear: midrange theory development linking nursing diagnoses, intervention, and outcomes should be informed by the unique body of discipline-specific knowledge in nursing. Nursing theories would suggest explanations and predictions of relationships between diagnoses of actual or potential health problems, nursing interventions chosen to deal with these problems, and the patients' eventual outcomes. Each theoretical linkage would need to be tested in systematic research studies. The theories and the framework itself would be modified as this research progressed.

To bring about the integration of theory, research, and practice using middle-range theories, nurses from each perspective must understand and appreciate the uniqueness of each perspective and the need to communicate across all perspectives. Researchers must accept the responsibility of truly testing the middle-range theories. That is, not only must their research be guided by the theory, but also their results must be used explicitly to develop and modify the theory (Blegen & Tripp-Reimer, 2001). In addition, the researchers must ensure that the theory is described comprehensively and is useful to practitioners. Nurse theorists must work to develop theories that are testable by researchers and that can be applied by practitioners. This knowledge, confirmed by research, could be incorporated into educational programs. Nurse educators would need to update continually their grasp of current research and the state of the knowledge pertaining to these middle-range theories (Blegen & Tripp-Reimer, 2001).

Blegen and Tripp-Reimer (2001) assert that even with well-grounded theories in the middle range, nurses still may need assistance in applying the knowledge in practice. As other disciplines have found, the time lapse from discovery of knowledge to full application is often long. This assistance could be less extensive and formal than the current research utilization process is. If research specifically tests middle-range theories and if the process of replication and extension is followed systematically, the knowledge would accumulate naturally and would be directly applicable in practice. Furthermore, if these middle-range theories are organized around knowledge structures as closely tied to practice as the taxonomies currently under construction, and if they are indexed using the standardized languages, they will be found readily and immediately pertinent.

Nurse educators and nurses formulating evidence-based practice guidelines are important to the goal of incorporating nursing knowledge produced by theory building and testing in practice. However, nurses in practice must accept the primary ongoing responsibility of seeking out the most current developments in a theory and applying it in practice or communicating to the researchers and theorists the reasons why it cannot be applied. Nurses in clinical practice provide the final test of the theories and the frameworks that organize these theories (Blegen & Tripp-Reimer, 2001). When discipline-specific theory, research, and practice knowledge coalesce into a seamless whole, then perhaps the recognition of nursing as an academic, professional, and scientific practice discipline among peer health care disciplines and the public will be fully realized.

REFERENCES

Acton, G. J., Irvin, B. L., & Hopkins, B. A. (1991). Theory-testing research: Building the science. *Advances in Nursing Science, 14*(1), 52-61.

Allen, D. G. (1995). Hermeneutics: Philosophical traditions and nursing practice research. *Nursing Science Quarterly, 8,* 174-182.

Alligood & A. Marriner-Tomey (Eds.)(2002), *Nursing theory: Utilization & application.* St. Louis, MO: Mosby.

Alligood, M. R. (2002). Philosophies, models, and theories: Critical thinking structures. In M. R. Alligood & A. Marriner-Tomey (Eds.), *Nursing theory: Utilization & application* (pp. 41-61). St. Louis, MO: Mosby.

American Association of Colleges of Nursing. (2005a). *Institutions offering doctoral programs and degrees conferred.* Washington, DC: American Association of Colleges of Nursing, Research and Data Center.

American Association of Colleges of Nursing. (2005b). *Testimony of Harriet R. Feldman, PhD, RN, FAAN, Dean and Professor, Lienhard School of Nursing, Pace University, on fiscal year 2006 appropriations for nursing education and research as recommended by the American Association of Colleges of Nursing on April 21, 2005, at 10 a.m. before the House Appropriations Subcommittee on Labor, Health and Human Services, Education and Related Agencies.* Retrieved on May 23, 2005, from http://www.aacn.nche.edu/Government/Testimony/Feldman.htm

American Nurses Association. (2003). *Nursing's social policy statement* (2nd ed.). Washington, DC: Author.

Baessler, C. A., Blumberg, M., Cunningham, J. S., Curran, J. A., Fennessey, A. G., Jacobs, J. M., et al. (1994). Medical surgical nurses' utilization of research methods and products. *Medical Surgical Nursing, 3*(2), 113-121.

Bernstein, R. J. (1983). *Beyond objectivism and relativism: Science, hermeneutics, and praxis.* Philadelphia: University of Pennsylvania Press.

Blegen, M. A., & Goode, C. (1994). Interactive process of conducting and utilizing research in nursing service administration. *Journal of Nursing Administration, 24*(9), 24-28.

Blegen, M. A., & Tripp-Reimer, T. (1994). The nursing theory-nursing research connection. In J. McCloskey & H. K. Grace (Eds.), *Current issues in nursing* (4th ed., pp. 87-91). St. Louis, MO: Mosby.

Blegen, M. A., & Tripp-Reimer, T. (1997). Implications of nursing taxonomies for middle-range theory development. *Advances in Nursing Science, 19*(3), 37-49.

Blegen, M. A., & Tripp-Reimer, T. (2001). Nursing theory, nursing research, and nursing practice: Connected or separated? In J. McCloskey Dochterman & H. K. Grace (Eds.), *Current issues in nursing* (6th ed., pp. 44-51). St. Louis, MO: Mosby.

Boyd, C. O. (1993). Toward a nursing practice research method. *Advances in Nursing Science, 16*(2), 9-25.

Butcher, H. K. (2004). Nursing's distinctive knowledge base. In L. Haynes, H. K. Butcher, & T. Boese (Eds), *Nursing in contemporary society: Issues, trends and transition into practice* (pp. 71-103). Upper Saddle, NJ: Prentice Hall.

Carroll, D. L., Greenwood, R., Lynch, K. E., Sullivan, J. K., Ready, C. H., & Fitzmaurice, J. B. (1997). Barriers and facilitators to the utilization of nursing research. *Clinical Nurse Specialist, 11*(5), 207-212.

Chenitz, W. C., Sater, B., Davies, H., & Friesen, L. (1990). Developing collaborative research between clinical agencies: A consortium approach. *Applied Nursing Research, 3*(3), 90-97.

Chinn, P. L., & Kramer, M. K. (2004). *Integrated knowledge development in nursing* (6th ed.). St. Louis, MO: Mosby.

Cody, W. K. (1994). The language of nursing science: If not now, when? *Nursing Science Quarterly, 7,* 98-99.

Conant, L. H. (1967). Closing the practice-theory gap. *Nursing Outlook, 15*(11), 37-39.

Coyle, L. A., & Sokop, A. G. (1990). Innovation adoption behavior among nurses. *Nursing Research, 39,* 176-180.

DeKeyser, F. G., & Medoff-Cooper, B. (2002). A non-theorist's perspective on nursing theory: Issues in the 1990s. *Scholarly Inquiry for Nursing Practice: An International Journal, 15,* 329-341.

Donaldson, S. K., & Crowley, D. (1978). The discipline of nursing. *Nursing Outlook, 26,* 113-120.

Dressel, P. L., & Marcus, D. (1982). *On teaching and learning in college.* San Francisco: Jossey-Bass.

Fawcett, J. (1978). The relationship between theory and research: A double helix. Advances in Nursing Science, 1(1), 49-62.

Fawcett, J. (1999). The state of nursing science: Hallmarks of the 20th and 21st centuries. *Nursing Science Quarterly, 12*(4), 311-318.

Fawcett, J. (2005). *Contemporary nursing knowledge: Analysis and evaluation of nursing models and theories.* Philadelphia: F.A. Davis.

Fawcett, J., & Bourbonniere, M. G. (2001). Utilization of nursing knowledge and the future of the discipline. In N. L. Chaska (Ed.), *The nursing profession: Tomorrow and beyond* (pp. 311-320). Thousand Oaks, CA: Sage.

Fawcett, J., & Downs, F. (1992). *The relationship of theory and research* (2nd ed.). Philadelphia: F.A. Davis.

Guba, E. G., & Lincoln, Y. S. (1989). *Fourth generation evaluation.* Newbury Park, CA: Sage.

Hesse, M. (1980). *Revolutions and reconstructions in philosophy of science.* Bloomington, IN: Indiana University Press.

Jacobs, M. K., & Huether, S. E. (1978). Nursing science: The theory practice linkage. *Advances in Nursing Science, 1*(1), 63-73.

Johnson, D. E. (1987). Guest editorial: Evaluating conceptual models for use in critical care nursing practice. *Dimensions of Critical Care Nursing, 6,* 196-197.

Kenney, J. W. (1995). Relevance of theory-based nursing practice. In P. J. Christensen & J. W. Kenney (Eds.), *Nursing process: Application of conceptual models* (4th ed., pp. 1-25). St. Louis, MO: Mosby.

Kerlinger, F. N. (1986). *Foundations of behavioral research* (3rd ed.). New York: Holt, Rinehart & Winston.

Kim, H. S. (2001). Directions for theory development in nursing: For increased coherence in the new century. In N. L. Chaska (Ed.), *The nursing profession: Tomorrow and beyond* (pp. 273-285). Thousand Oaks, CA: Sage.

Lauden, L. (1984). *Science and values.* Berkeley: University of California Press.

Lenz, E. R., Suppe, F., Gift, A. G., Pugh, L. C., & Milligan, R. A. (1995). Collaborative development of middle-range nursing theories: Toward a theory of unpleasant symptom. *Advances in Nursing Science, 17*(3), 1-13.

Levine, M. E. (1995). The rhetoric of nursing theory. *Image: Journal of Nursing Scholarship, 27*(1), 11-14.

Liehr, P., & Smith, M. J. (1999). Middle range theory: Spinning research and practice to create knowledge for the new millennium. *Advances in Nursing Science, 21*(4), 81-91.

Mitchell. (1997). Have disciplines fallen? Nursing Science Quarterly, 10, 110-111.

Meleis, A. I., & Im, E. (2001). From fragmentation to integration in the discipline of nursing: Situation-specific theories. In N. L. Chaska (Ed.), *The nursing profession: Tomorrow and beyond* (pp. 881-891). Thousand Oaks, CA: Sage.

Merton, R. K. (1967). *On theoretical sociology.* New York: Free Press.

Morgan, G. (1983). *Beyond method: Strategies for social research.* Newbury Park, CA: Sage.

National Institute of Nursing Research. (2005). *Strategic planning for the 21st century: Prologue from the NINR director.* Retrieved on May 23, 2005, from http://ninr.nih.gov/ninr/about/strategic.html

National Institutes of Health Office of Budget. (2005). The National Institutes of Health Current Operating Year, Fiscal Year 2005. Retrieved October 10, 2005, from http://officeofbudget.od.nih.gov/UI/CurrentYear.htm

Parker, M. (2006). *Nursing theories and nursing practice* (2nd ed). Philadelphia: F.A. Davis.

Peterson, S. J., & Bredow, T. (2004). *Middle-range theories: Application to nursing research.* Philadelphia: Lippincott Williams & Wilkins.

Pettengill, M. M., Gillies, D. A., & Clark, C. C. (1994). Factors encouraging and discouraging the use of nursing research findings. *Image: Journal of Nursing Scholarship, 26*(2), 143-147.

Phenix, P. H. (1986). *Realms of meaning: A philosophy of the curriculum for general education.* New York: McGraw Hill.

Polkinghorne, D. (1983). *Methodology for the human sciences: Systems of inquiry.* Albany: State University of New York.

Rawnsley, M. M. (1999). Polarities in nursing science: The plight of the emerging nurse scholar. *Nursing Science Quarterly, 12,* 277-282.

Reed, P. G. (1995). A treatise on nursing knowledge development for the 21st century: Beyond postmodernism. *Advances in Nursing Science, 17*(3), 70-84.

Rizzuto, C., & Mitchell, M. (1988). Research in service settings: part I. Consortium project outcomes. *Journal of Nursing Administration, 18*(2), 32-37.

Schumacher, K. L., & Gortner, S. R. (1992). (Mis)conception and reconceptions about traditional science. *Advances in Nursing Science, 14*(4), 1-11.

Schwab, J. (1962). The concept of the structure of a discipline. *The Educational Record, 43,* 197-205.

Silva, M. C., & Sorrell, J. M. (1992). Testing of nursing theory: Critique and philosophical expansion. *Advances in Nursing Science, 14*(4), 12-23.

Smith, M. J., & Liehr, P. R. (2003). *Middle-range theory for nursing.* New York: Springer.

Stark, J. S., & Lattuca, L. R. (1997). *Shaping the college curriculum: Academic plans in action.* Boston: Allyn & Bacon.

Tanner, D., & Tanner, L. (1975). *Curriculum development: Theory into practice.* Basingstoke Hampshire, England: Macmillan.

Titler, M. G. (1997). Research utilization: Necessity or luxury. In J. C. McCloskey & H. K. Grace (Eds.), *Current issues in nursing* (5th ed., pp. 104-117). St. Louis, MO: Mosby.

Titler, M. G. (2001). Research utilization and evidence-based practice. In N. L. Chaska (Ed.), *The nursing profession: Tomorrow and beyond* (pp. 423-437). Thousand Oaks, CA: Sage.

Tripp-Reimer, T., Woodworth, G., McCloskey, J. C., & Bulechek, G. (1996). The dimensional structure of nursing interventions. *Nursing Research, 45,* 10-17.

University of Adelaide Library Guides. (2005). *Nursing journal contents.* Retrieved May 23, 2005, from http://www.library.adelaide.edu.au/guide/med/nursing/nursjnl.html

Waltz, C., & Bausell, R. B. (1981). *Nursing research: Design, statistics and computer analysis.* Philadelphia: F.A. Davis.

Watson, J. (1995). Postmodernism and knowledge development in nursing. *Nursing Science Quarterly, 8,* 60-64.

Standardized Terminologies and Integrated Information Systems

Building Blocks for Transforming Data Into Nursing Knowledge

SUZANNE BAKKEN ◆ LEANNE M. CURRIE

The premises of this chapter are twofold. First, nursing theory, nursing research, and nursing practice must be related integrally in order to foster the development of nursing knowledge. Second, building blocks for the development of nursing knowledge include standardized terminologies for patient problems (e.g., nursing diagnoses, medical diagnoses, and symptoms), nursing interventions, and nursing-sensitive patient outcomes, as well as integrated information systems to support the acquisition, storage, transformation, and presentation of data relevant to nursing. The discussion supporting these premises is organized around three questions:

◆ Why have traditional nursing information systems not fostered the development of nursing knowledge?

◆ How can standardized terminologies and integrated information systems foster the development of nursing knowledge?

◆ What informatics competencies are required to complement the technological building blocks of standardized terminologies and integrated information systems?

WHY HAVE TRADITIONAL NURSING INFORMATION SYSTEMS NOT FOSTERED THE DEVELOPMENT OF NURSING KNOWLEDGE?

Although various types of nursing information systems have been in place for several decades, these systems for the most part have failed to foster the development of nursing knowledge. Several reasons can be posited for this void, including the traditional role of the nursing record as a transaction log rather than as an evolving repository of practice-based nursing knowledge; limited incorporation of standardized terminologies in

information systems in a manner that facilitates data reuse; and application-specific rather than integrated information systems.

Nursing Record as a Transaction Log

In his discussion of a framework for the transition from nursing records to a nursing information system, Turley (1992) notes that storage of the transaction log (what the nurse does when) is not likely to add to the understanding of the patient's condition and problems. Turley states,

> Alone, transaction logs do not reflect the evolvement of patient status, condition resolution, or expected long-term outcomes. All those lost data represent the forfeiture of documented nursing knowledge and will critically affect the development of decision support components of any nursing information system. (p. 178)

This thought is consistent with the recommendations by the Institute of Medicine (Dick & Steen, 1991; Dick, Steen, & Detmer, 1997) reports on the computer-based patient record, which identified the documentation of the logical bases for all diagnoses or conclusions and the clinical rationale for decisions about the management of the patient's care as essential attributes of computer-based patient record systems, and the recent Institute of Medicine (Committee on Data Standards for Patient Safety, 2004) report on data standards for patient safety. In addition, these attributes are critical to knowledge development in health care.

Standardized Health Care Terminologies

Standardized health care terminologies—that is, the set of terms representing a system of concepts—are necessary to reliably and validly describe, support, and analyze health care processes and outcomes (Clark & Lang, 1992). During the last several decades, development of standardized health care and nursing terminologies has been extensive (Beyea, 2000; Huff et al., 1998; International Council of Nurses, 2005; Johnson, Maas, & Moorhead, 2000; Martin, 2004; McCloskey & Bulechek, 2000; NANDA International, 2005; Ozbolt, 1998; Saba, 2004; SNOMED International, 2005). Table 15-1 summarizes the content of selected terminologies related to aspects of the nursing process.

Given the obvious need for the information provided by and the availability of multiple terminologies, one might ask, "Why are standardized terminologies not universally implemented in computer-based systems?" A number of organizations and terminology experts have proposed criteria or standards related to suitability of terminologies for incorporation into computer-based systems (American Nurses Association, 1999b; Chute, Cohn, & Campbell, 1998; Cimino, 1998). Evaluation studies of standardized terminologies against these criteria provide some answers to this question.

The evaluation criteria can be conceptualized broadly into two categories. The first category is composed of criteria that focus on the content of a terminology in relationship to the needs of a particular domain. These criteria include breadth of coverage and depth of clinical

detail (e.g., nursing diagnoses versus individual tasks). In contrast, the second set of criteria (e.g., concept permanence and formal definitions) focuses on the extent to which a terminology is represented in an information system in a manner that supports computer processing for data manipulation and reuse.

Historically, the primary focus of nursing terminology development appropriately has been on the collection and categorization of nursing concepts. Consequently, evaluations of content coverage suggest broad coverage for nursing diagnoses, nursing interventions, and nursing-sensitive outcomes (Henry, Warren, Lange, & Button, 1998; Parlocha & Henry, 1998) and also demonstrate the utility of nonnursing terminologies for representing nursing concepts (Griffith & Robinson, 1992, 1993; Henry, Holzemer, Reilly, & Campbell, 1994). More recently, efforts have focused on integration of nursing terminologies into larger health care terminologies (Bakken, Cashen, Mendonca, O'Brien, & Zieniewicz, 2000; Bakken, Warren, et al., 2002; Matney, Bakken, & Huff, 2003). Nursing diagnoses, interventions, and outcomes from a number of terminologies (Table 15-1) have been integrated into SNOMED Clinical Terms (SNOMED International, 2005), which is freely available for use in the United States through a federal license. The Logical Observation Identifiers, Names, and Codes (LOINC)

TABLE 15-1

Standardized Terminologies for Representing Concepts Relevant to the Nursing Domain			
Terminology	Assess	Diagnose	Intervene
NURSING			
Clinical Care Classification (formerly Home Health Care Classification)*† (Saba, 2004)	●	●	●
International Classification of Nursing Practice (International Council of Nurses, 2005)	●	●	●
NANDA Taxonomy II* (NANDA International, 2005)		●	
Nursing Interventions Classification* (McCloskey & Bulechek, 2000)			●
Nursing Outcomes Classification* (Johnson, Maas, & Moorhead, 2000)	●		
Omaha System*† (Martin, 2004)	●	●	●
Patient Care Data Set† (Ozbolt, 1998)	●	●	●
Perioperative Data Set* (Beyea, 2000)	●	●	●
HEALTH CARE			
International Statistical Classification of Diseases and Related Health Problems: 10th Revision (World Health Organization, 2003)		●	
Logical Observation Identifiers, Names, and Codes (LOINC) (Huff et al., 1998)	●		
Current Procedural Terminology (American Medical Association, 2005)			●
SNOMED Clinical Terms (SNOMED International, 2005)	●	●	●

*Included in SNOMED Clinical Terms.
†Included in LOINC.

database includes nursing assessments and goals status statements and is also available for use without fees (Matney et al., 2003).

Regarding representing nursing concepts in a manner that maximizes the capacity for data sharing, manipulation, and reuse, under the auspices of the International Standards Organization an international standard was developed for nursing diagnoses and nursing actions (Bakken, Coenen, & Saba, 2004). Other groups are working on harmonizing the nursing terminology efforts with those of the Health Level 7 standards organization (Danko et al., 2003; Ozbolt, 2003).

Although a number of challenges remain, significant progress has been made during the last decade to facilitate incorporation of nursing concepts into clinical information systems (Cho & Park, 2003; Hardiker & Bakken, 2004; Hardiker, Bakken, Casey, & Hoy, 2002). In addition, some schools of nursing are integrating standardized nursing terminologies into information systems used by their undergraduate and/or advanced practice nurse students. For example, nurse practitioner students at the Columbia University School of Nursing document their clinical encounters in a personal digital assistant student clinical log (Figure 15-1) that incorporates nursing diagnoses and interventions from the Clinical Classification System and medical diagnoses from the International Classification of Diseases—Clinical Modification and diagnostic tests and procedures from the Current Procedural Terminology (Bakken, Cook, et al., 2004).

Challenge of Information Systems Integration

Systems integration is still a major challenge in most health care organizations, thereby limiting the potential of information systems to influence the quality of nursing practice and also providing a barrier to nursing knowledge development. Historically, stand-alone, application-specific information systems have constrained the relationships that can be examined among various types of data and the transformation processes applied to the data.

Great strides made during the last decade have the potential to decrease the technological barriers to using information systems as facilitators of knowledge development. Most significant among these are the growth of the Internet and resources available on the World Wide Web and the evolution of standards for data exchange among systems. Recently, activity has heightened toward the development of a National Health Information Infrastructure (Thompson & Brailer, 2004). In addition, the move toward tailored (e.g., user-specific) views to a shared data repository rather than to separate information systems has broadened the types of data available. The primary barriers to integrating data from information systems from different organizations are not technical (Committee on Data Standards for Patient Safety, 2004). To maximize knowledge development and use within the context of integrated systems, future efforts must include enhancing the understanding of human-computer interactions at the individual user and organizational level.

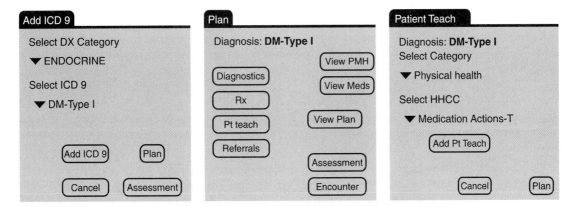

FIGURE 15-1   Gerontology nurse practitioner students enter clinical encounter data using standardized terminologies including International Classification of Diseases—Clinical Modification, Current Procedural Terminology, and Clinical Care Classification. This study was funded by a National Institute of Nursing Research grant.

HOW CAN STANDARDIZED TERMINOLOGIES AND INTEGRATED INFORMATION SYSTEMS FOSTER THE DEVELOPMENT OF NURSING KNOWLEDGE?

Framework for Design Characteristics for Nursing Information Systems

Nursing informatics integrates nursing science, computer science, and information science to manage and communicate data, information, and knowledge in nursing practice and facilitates the integration of data, information, and knowledge to support patients, nurses, and other providers in their decision-making in all roles and settings. This support is enabled by information structures, information processes, and information technology (American Nurses Association, 2001).

The role of nursing informatics in fostering knowledge development in nursing will be discussed using the framework for design characteristics of a nursing information system provided by the National Commission on Nursing Implementation Project Task Force on Nursing Information Systems (Zielstorff, Hudgings, Grobe, & National Commission on Nursing Implementation Project Task Force on Nursing Information Systems, 1993). The framework includes three categories of information required to support professional nursing practice. Patient-specific data are about a particular person and may be acquired from a variety of data sources (e.g., provider observations and interventions, and self-reports of functional status). Domain information and knowledge are specific to the discipline of nursing or to health care in general (e.g., bibliographical literature, clinical practice guidelines, and comparative databases). The National Commission on Nursing Implementation Project framework also delineates four types of information system processes that relate to the three categories of information. Data acquisition is the set of methods by which data become available to the information system (e.g., monitoring devices, entry of symptom data by the patient via the World Wide Web, and keyboard or voice entry of data by the health care provider). Data storage includes the methods, programs, and structures used to organize data for subsequent use and reuse (e.g., data structures and databases). Data transformation or processing comprises the methods (e.g., calculation, abstraction, production rules, and data mining algorithms) by which data or information is "acted upon" according to the needs of the end user. Presentation encompasses the forms in which information is delivered to the end user after processing. These forms include simple textual and graphic and multimedia presentations

(Starren & Johnson, 2000). For example, vital signs or functional status might be best displayed as a line chart in order to examine trends over time, whereas the defining characteristics of altered oral mucous membrane—which include leukoplakia, hyperemia, and hemorrhagic gingivitis—could be presented most effectively using video images.

Transforming Data Through Standardized Terminologies and Information System Processes

The following examples illustrate the dynamic interaction among types of information and system processes.

Fall and Injury Risk Assessment and Management. Inpatient falls are an ongoing patient safety problem and have been identified as 1 of 10 nursing-sensitive quality indicators monitored by the National Database of Nursing Quality Indicators (American Nurses Association, 1999a). As with other nursing sensitive indicators such as pressure ulcers and pain management, adequate nursing assessment and management for fall and injury prevention are critical to a patient's safety during hospitalization.

Standardized fall risk instruments, which represent evidence-based nursing knowledge, have been developed over the past 3 decades (Myers, 2003). Such instruments typically have been integrated into clinical information systems; unfortunately, the integration often has failed to take advantage of the benefits of the computer technologies. Rather the computer-based instrument replicates the paper documentation process in which data are not supported by standardized terminologies, are not represented in a data dictionary, and thus cannot be reused or linked to corollary nursing diagnoses or associated interventions.

New York Presbyterian Hospital has developed a Fall-Injury Risk Assessment instrument that has been integrated into the clinical information system. The instrument was developed via evidence-based methods and includes five elements for fall risk and two elements for injury risk (Currie, Mellino, Cimino, & Bakken, 2004). When fall risk and injury risk are combined, a patient's fall-injury risk can be determined. The instrument is part of a fall and injury prevention and management policy used to guide the characteristics of the computer-based instrument, including stratified nursing interventions per risk level and fall-injury risk assessment by additional members of the care team.

Figure 15-2 illustrates the dynamic interaction among information related to fall and injury risk assessment in an integrated information system. Standardized terminologies provide a foundation by which domain-specific

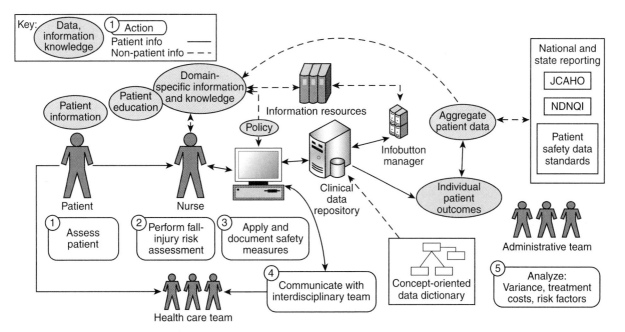

FIGURE 15-2 Illustration of using standardized terminologies and integrated information systems to support fall and injury risk assessment and management. Individual-level patient data not only is used for patient care but also is aggregated and analyzed locally to assess variance, treatment costs, and risk factors. Aggregate data also is reported externally to groups such as the Joint Commission on Accreditation of Healthcare Organizations and National Database of Nursing Quality Indicators. This study was funded by a National Institute of Nursing Research grant.

information and patient data are transformed iteratively for local use, aggregate use, and domain knowledge generation. In this figure the ovals represent data, information, or knowledge; the numbered, rounded rectangles represent actions; and the lines represent pathways of patient and nonpatient data, information, and knowledge transmission.

First, the nurse obtains information from the patient. This information also might be derived from the patient's existing information in the system (e.g., medications and gender). Second, the nurse uses the patient information to perform a standardized assessment for fall-injury risk. Because the Fall-Injury Risk Assessment instrument is integrated into the system, all data are stored in the clinical data repository in a standardized format. Each term has a unique identifier in the concept-oriented data dictionary, thus facilitating data reuse; for example, the ability to view results from previous patient assessments. Third, once the assessment is complete, the nurse exercises his or her clinical judgment to apply the appropriate safety measures and then documents the safety measures in the information system. These data also can be reused. For example, the nurse may want to view the previous nursing interventions applied by nursing colleagues, and administrators may wish to examine which interventions are more effective for a certain group of patients.

At the second or third point in this description, the nurse may want additional information. The Infobutton Manager, described in the next section, is an example of an application that provides links to context-specific information resources. Types of information that may be accessed by the nurse include the policy, patient education materials, or information related to any aspect of the assessment or treatment process. Real-time access to such information can streamline and support the decision-making process.

Fourth, interdisciplinary communication can be facilitated because the Fall-Injury Risk Assessment is located in a centrally accessible location in the information system in which all relevant members of the care team can document and view results. The underlying policy places the patient at the center of the information exchange, thus ensuring that the patient risk data are accessible to other members of the care team.

Fifth, the administrative team can reuse individual or aggregate patient data to examine any of several aspects of the patient's care; for example, a snapshot of risk levels for all patients on a given unit at a certain time. The data also can be reused to report to national benchmarking databases such as the National Database of Nursing Quality Indicators, to document compliance with patient safety goals as required by the Joint Commission on Accreditation of Healthcare Organizations, or to document and report patient safety data to other agencies.

Integration of a standardized risk assessment instrument into a clinical information system provides a method by which data can be collected, manipulated, and stored for efficient reuse. In addition, standardized risk assessments such as the Fall-Injury Risk Assessment instrument can be stored in a section of the computer-based record where the data can be viewed and contributed to by all members of the care team, making the patient the center of the care record. As national patient safety quality indicators increasingly are being standardized, the structure by which to build systems in which data can be reused is increasingly available. In addition, use of standardized terminologies facilitates regional and national benchmarking.

Validation of Nursing Diagnoses. Probabilistic data transformation approaches have been applied to medical diagnostic reasoning for several decades, resulting in the development of medical diagnostic decision support systems such as Iliad (Warner et al., 1988) and DXplain (Barnett, Cimino, Hupp, & Hoffer, 1987). Nursing research and theory have generated defining characteristics and labels for nursing diagnoses (e.g., see Mallick & Whipple, 2000; and NANDA International, 2005). Databases containing nursing diagnoses, predicted defining characteristics, and patient-specific data have the potential to serve as the infrastructure for large-scale validation studies (Delaney, Reed, & Clarke, 2000; Maas & Delaney, 2004). Wide-scale implementation of information systems containing nursing diagnoses and patient attributes will facilitate not only the validation of nursing diagnoses, but also the deployment of decision support systems that are based on empirical data rather than exclusively on predicted relationships.

Linking of Diagnoses, Interventions, and Outcomes. Publications have proposed linkages among diagnoses, interventions, and outcomes (e.g., see McCloskey & Bulechek, 2000). In addition, a number of efforts are focused on implementing standardized terminologies

for nursing diagnoses, interventions, and outcomes in information systems at the enterprise, national, and international level. Prophet, Dorr, Gibbs, and Porcella (1997) described the incorporation of the Nursing Interventions Classification and Nursing Outcomes Classification for online care planning and documentation at the University of Iowa Hospitals and Clinics. The Omaha System has been incorporated into the clinical information system supporting the faculty practices at the University of Pennsylvania School of Nursing (Marek, Jenkins, Westra, & McGinley, 1998). At the national level the criteria used in the information system "recognition" process by the Nursing Information and Data Set Evaluation Center of the American Nurses Association includes a standard related to terminology to document all phases of the nursing process (American Nurses Association, 1997). Some efforts in Europe have centered on the Telenurse Project and its demonstrations of the use of the International Classification of Nursing Practice within electronic patient records (Mortensen, 1999). At the international level, the International Classification of Nursing Practice project is making tremendous progress toward an information infrastructure to examine health care phenomena, nursing activities, and outcomes globally. Hardiker and Bakken (2004) and Hardiker et al. (2002) have used the context of the International Classification of Nursing Practice to focus on formalization of nursing terminologies, on the mediation among conceptual structures required for information systems, and on the functional requirements of tools to assist with structured, electronic data entry in a manner consistent with the clinical nursing process.

Knowledge Discovery in Databases. As large repositories of health care data are developed, it becomes possible to apply data mining and knowledge discovery in databases techniques to answer questions that were not hypothesized at the time of data collection. Similarly to the machine learning techniques applied in the artificial intelligence research of the 1980s, knowledge discovery in databases uses pattern recognition and matching, classification or clustering schemas, and other algorithms to examine relationships in data in order to "discover" answers to the questions posed by that investigator (Fayyad, Piatetsky-Shapiro, Smyth, & Uthurusamy, 1996). Recently, these techniques have been applied in several nursing informatics projects. Abbott, Quirolgico, Manchand, Canfield, and Adya (1998) examined the ability of data elements in the long-term care minimum data set to predict admissions to acute care facilities. Goodwin et al. (1997) reported on an international collaborative nursing informatics research project focused on predicting adult respiratory distress syndrome risk in critically ill patients using data from clinical databases. As data of relevance to nursing become more ubiquitous, such techniques have tremendous potential for knowledge development through empirical research and theory testing (Goodwin, VanDyne, Lin, & Talbert, 2003).

Retrieval and Application of Heterogeneous Sources of Knowledge. In the domain of health care in general, the Unified Medical Language System, a linked collection of source terminologies developed by the National Library of Medicine, has been used to retrieve heterogeneous sources of knowledge for application in patient care settings (Humphreys, Lindberg, Schoolman, & Barnett, 1998). For example, MedWeaver (Detmer, Barnett, & Hersh, 1997) allows the user to move among three types of domain knowledge sources: (1) bibliographic (Medline); (2) diagnostic decision support system (DxPlain); and

(3) Web resources (CliniWeb). Infobuttons (Figure 15-3) provide context-specific access to relevant information on demand at the point of care; for example, cholesterol treatment guidelines when reporting laboratory results (Cimino et al., 2004). PatCIS provides the infrastructure to use patient-specific data from the clinical information system to tailor domain information and knowledge presented to patients (Cimino et al., 2000). Another approach to retrieval and presentation of tailored information is the Heart Care project (Brennan et al., 2001) in which a nursing assessment after coronary artery bypass graft surgery is used to create individualized Web access to a set of information resources.

Translation of Research Protocols Into Standardized Terminologies. A number of investigations have demonstrated the utility of standardized terminologies to abstract narrative records from nursing research studies

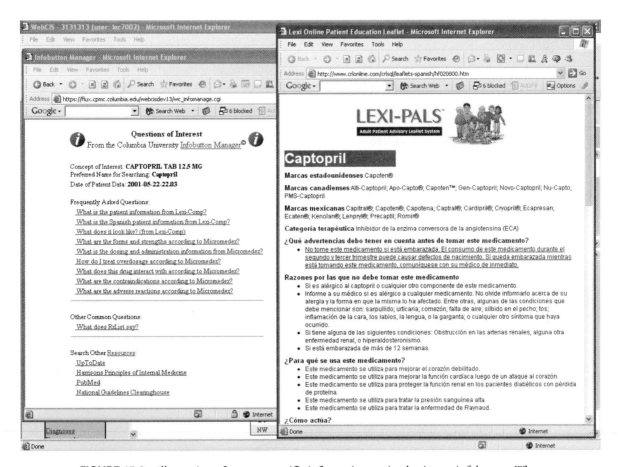

FIGURE 15-3 Illustration of context-specific information retrieval using an infobutton. When the user clicks the infobutton next to a medication list, a list of questions appears. Selecting the question "What is the Spanish patient information from Lexi-Comp?" retrieves the information in Spanish. This study was funded by a National Institute of Nursing Research grant.

(Bowles, 2000; Holzemer et al., 1997; Naylor, Bowles, & Brooten, 2000). The translation of research protocols a priori into standardized terminologies that also are used in practice settings has the potential to expedite not only the collection of research data at the point of care but also the retrieval and application of the research findings into practice. For example, Bakken, Holzemer, et al. (2005) incorporated terms from the Home Health Care Classification (Saba, 1992) for structured data entry and documentation of the Client Adherence Profiling and Intervention Tailoring intervention, a nurse case manager–delivered medication adherence intervention for home care patients receiving highly active antiretroviral therapy. Their results demonstrated the ability of using a standardized terminology to document the dose and the individualization (i.e., tailoring) of the Client Adherence Profiling and Intervention Tailoring intervention. Nurse researchers in general, however, have yet to embrace the incorporation of standardized terminologies into research protocols.

WHAT INFORMATICS COMPETENCIES ARE REQUIRED TO COMPLEMENT THE TECHNOLOGICAL BUILDING BLOCKS OF STANDARDIZED TERMINOLOGIES AND INTEGRATED INFORMATION SYSTEMS?

Technological building blocks such as standardized terminologies and integrated information systems are necessary but not sufficient to realize the promise of using information systems to facilitate the development of nursing knowledge and to link theory, research, and practice. These building blocks must be complemented by informatics competencies. The informatics competencies necessary for knowledge-intensive professions such as nursing go beyond computer literacy.

Staggers, Gassert, and Curran (2001, 2002) published a set of informatics competencies for nurses at four levels of practice: beginning nurse, experienced nurse, informatics specialist, and informatics innovator. Building upon this work and others, the American Nurses Association (2001) published the *Scope and Standards of Nursing Informatics Practice,* which describes informatics competencies for beginning and experienced nurses and for specialists. Other researchers (Tanner, Pierce, & Pravikoff, 2004) have focused on information literacy, a component of informatics competency based on a set of knowledge and skills related to information retrieval that was proposed by the library community in 1989 (American Library Association, 1989), was updated in 1998 (National Forum on Information Literacy, 1998), and is closely tied to evidence-based practice (Sackett, Richardson, Rosenberg, & Haynes, 1998). These include active learning to include the the following processes (American Library Association, 1989):

- Knowing when they have a need for information
- Identifying information needed to address a given problem or issue
- Finding needed information and evaluating the information
- Organizing the information
- Using the information effectively to address the problem or issue at hand

Incorporation of such competencies into all levels of nursing education programs and into nursing practice is essential to foster the development and use of nursing knowledge. However, research suggests that, with a few exceptions, these competencies are not incorporated widely into nursing education or practice (McNeil, Elfrink, & Pierce, 2004; Tanner et al., 2004).

SUMMARY

This chapter has described the vital role of standardized terminologies and integrated information systems as building blocks for the development of nursing knowledge. Examples have illustrated the manner in which these building blocks can facilitate the interrelationships among nursing theory, nursing research, and nursing practice. As the building blocks are broadly implemented, new questions will evolve, such as the following:

- How will definitions of nursing expertise evolve as sources of domain information and knowledge become more accessible at the point of care?
- What are the ways in which interventions built upon standardized terminologies and integrated information systems can and should serve as an extension of the nurse?
- Will standardized terminologies and integrated information systems assist in the delineation of a distinct body of nursing knowledge, or will the boundaries of discipline-specific knowledge blur?
- How will standardized terminologies and integrated information systems affect patient safety?

REFERENCES

Abbott, P. A., Quirolgico, S., Manchand, R., Canfield, K., & Adya, M. (1998). Can the U.S. minimum data set be used for predicting admissions to acute care facilities? [Part 2] *MedInfo, 9,* pp. 1318-1321.

American Library Association. (1989). *Presidential committee on information literacy. Final report.* Chicago, IL: Author.

American Medical Association. (2005). *CPT 2005.* Retrieved February 9, 2005, from http://www.ama-assn.org/

American Nurses Association. (1997). *NIDSEC standards and scoring guidelines.* Washington, DC: American Nurses Publishing.

American Nurses Association. (1999a). *Nursing-sensitive quality indicators for acute care settings and ANA's safety & quality initiative.* Retrieved February 9, 2003, from http://www.nursing-world.org/readroom/fssafe99.htm

American Nurses Association. (1999b). *Recognition criteria for data sets, classification systems and nomenclatures.* Washington, DC: Author.

American Nurses Association. (2001). *Scope and standards of nursing informatics practice.* Washington, DC: American Nurses Publishing.

Bakken, S., Cashen, M. S., Mendonca, E. A., O'Brien, A., & Zieniewicz, J. (2000). Representing nursing activities within a concept-oriented terminological system: Evaluation of a type definition. *Journal of the American Medical Informatics Association, 7*(1), 81-90.

Bakken, S., Coenen, A., & Saba, V. (2004). ISO reference technology model: Nursing diagnosis and action models look to testing for practical application. *Healthcare Informatics, 21*(9), 52.

Bakken, S., Cook, S., Curtis, L., Desjardins, K., Hyun, S., Jenkins, M., et al. (2004). Promoting patient safety through informatics-based nursing education. *International Journal of Medical Informatics, 73*(7-8), 581-589.

Bakken, S., Holzemer, W. L., Portillo, C. J., Grimes, R., Welch, J., & Wantland, D. (2005). Utility of a standardized nursing terminology to evaluate dosage and tailoring of an HIV/AIDS adherence intervention. *Journal of Nursing Scholarship, 37*(3), 251

Bakken, S., Warren, J. J., Lundberg, C., Casey, A., Correia, C., Konicek, D., et al. (2002). An evaluation of the usefulness of two terminology models for integrating nursing diagnosis concepts into SNOMED clinical terms. *International Journal of Medical Informatics, 68*(1-3), 71-77.

Barnett, G. O., Cimino, J. J., Hupp, J. A., & Hoffer, E. P. (1987). DXplain. An evolving diagnostic decision-support system. *Journal of the American Medical Association, 258*(1), 67-74.

Beyea, S. C. (Ed.). (2000). *Perioperative nursing data set.* Denver, CO: Association of Operating Room Nurses.

Bowles, K. (2000). Patient problems and nursing interventions during acute care and discharge planning. *Journal of Cardiovascular Nursing, 14*(3), 29-41.

Brennan, P., Moore, S., Bjornsdottir, G., Jones, J., Visovsky, C., & Rogers, M. R. (2001). HeartCare: An Internet-based information and support system for patient home recovery after coronary artery bypass graft (CABG) surgery. *Journal of Advanced Nursing, 35*(5), 699-708.

Cho, I., & Park, H. A. (2003). Development and evaluation of a terminology-based electronic nursing record system. *Journal of Biomedical Informatics, 36*(4-5), 304-312.

Chute, C. G., Cohn, S. P., & Campbell, J. R. (1998). A framework for comprehensive terminology systems in the United States: Development guidelines, criteria for selection, and public policy implications. ANSI Healthcare Informatics Standards Board Vocabulary Working Group and the Computer-Based Patient Records Institute Working Group on Codes and Structures. *Journal of the American Medical Informatics Association, 5*(6), 503-510.

Cimino, J. J. (1998). Desiderata for controlled medical vocabularies in the twenty-first century. *Methods of Information in Medicine, 37*(4-5), 394-403.

Cimino, J., Li, J., Allen, M., Currie, L., Graham, M., Janetzki, V., et al. (2004). Practical considerations for exploiting the World Wide Web to create infobuttons. *Medinfo,* pp. 277-281.

Cimino, J., Li, J., Mendonca, E., Sengupta, S., Patel, V., & Kushniruk, A. (2000). An evaluation of patient access to their electronic medical records via the World Wide Web. *Proceedings of the American Medical Informatics Association Annual Fall Symposium,* pp. 151-155.

Clark, J., & Lang, N. M. (1992). Nursing's next advance: An international classification for nursing practice. *International Nursing Review, 39,* 109-112.

Committee on Data Standards for Patient Safety. (2004). *Patient safety: Achieving a new standard for care.* Washington, DC: Board on Health Care Services, Institute of Medicine.

Currie, L., Mellino, L., Cimino, J., & Bakken, S. (2004). Development and representation of a falls-injury risk assessment calculator in an electronic health record. *MedInfo,* pp. 721-725.

Danko, A., Kennedy, R., Haskell, R., Androwich, I. M., Button, P., Correia, C. M., et al. (2003). Modeling nursing interventions in the act class of HL7 RIM Version 3. *Journal of Biomedical Informatics, 36*(4-5), 294-303.

Delaney, C., Reed, D., & Clarke, M. (2000). Describing patient problems & nursing treatment patterns using nursing minimum data sets (NMDS & NMMDS) & UHDDS repositories. *Proceedings of the American Medical Informatics Association Symposium,* pp. 176-179.

Detmer, W. M., Barnett, G. O., & Hersh, W. R. (1997). MedWeaver: Integrating decision support, literature searching, and Web exploration using the UMLS Metathesaurus. *Proceedings of the American Medical Informatics Association Annual Fall Symposium,* pp. 490-494.

Dick, R. S., & Steen, E. B. (Eds.). (1991). *The computer-based patient record: An essential technology for health care.* Washington, DC: National Academy Press.

Dick, R. S., Steen, E. B., & Detmer, D. E. (Eds.). (1997). *The computer-based patient record: An essential technology for health care.* Washington, DC: National Academy Press.

Fayyad, U., Piatetsky-Shapiro, G., Smyth, P., & Uthurusamy, R. (1996). *Advances in knowledge discovery and data mining.* Cambridge, MA: MIT Press.

Goodwin, L., Saville, J., Jasion, B., Turner, B., Prather, J., Dobousek, T., et al. (1997). A collaborative international nursing informatics research project: Predicting ARDS risk in critically ill patients. In U. Gerdin, M. Tallberg, & P. Wainwright (Eds.), *NI97* (pp. 247-250). Stockholm: IOS Press.

Goodwin, L., VanDyne, M., Lin, S., & Talbert, S. (2003). Data mining issues and opportunities for building nursing knowledge. *Journal of Biomedical Informatics, 36*(4-5), 379-388.

Griffith, H. M., & Robinson, K. R. (1992). Survey of the degree to which critical care nurses are performing current procedural terminology-coded services. *American Journal of Critical Care, 1,* 91-98.

Griffith, H. M., & Robinson, K. R. (1993). Current Procedural Terminology (CPT) coded services provided by nurse specialists. *Image: Journal of Nursing Scholarship, 25,* 178-186.

Hardiker, N. R., & Bakken, S. (2004). Requirements of tools and techniques to support the entry of structured nursing data. *Medinfo,* pp. 621-625.

Hardiker, N. R., Bakken, S., Casey, A., & Hoy, D. (2002). Formal nursing terminology systems: a means to an end. *Journal of Biomedical Informatics, 35*(5-6), 298-305.

Henry, S. B., Holzemer, W. L., Reilly, C. A., & Campbell, K. E. (1994). Terms used by nurses to describe patient problems: can SNOMED III represent nursing concepts in the patient record? *Journal of the American Medical Informatics Association, 1*(1), 61-74.

Henry, S. B., Warren, J. J., Lange, L., & Button, P. (1998). A review of major nursing vocabularies and the extent to which they have the characteristics required for implementation in computer-based systems. *Journal of the American Medical Informatics Association, 5*(4), 321-328.

Holzemer, W. L., Henry, S. B., Dawson, C., Sousa, K., Bain, C., & Hsieh, S. F. (1997). An evaluation of the utility of the home health care classification for categorizing patient problems and nursing interventions from the hospital setting. *Studies in Health Technology & Informatics, 46,* 21-26.

Huff, S. M., Rocha, R. A., McDonald, C. J., De Moor, G. J. E., Fiers, T., Bidgood, W. D., Jr., et al. (1998). Development of the LOINC (Logical Observation Identifier Names and Codes) vocabulary. *Journal of the American Medical Informatics Association, 5*(3), 276-292.

Humphreys, B. L., Lindberg, D. A. B., Schoolman, H. M., & Barnett, G. O. (1998). The Unified Medical Language System: An informatics research collaboration. *Journal of the American Medical Informatics Association, 5*(1), 1-11.

International Council of Nurses. (2005). *ICNP International Classification for Nursing Practice—Beta 2.* Retrieved February 9, 2005, from http://www.icn.ch/icnp.htm

Johnson, M., Maas, M., & Moorhead, S. (Eds.). (2000). *Nursing Outcomes Classification (NOC)* (2nd ed.). St. Louis, MO: Mosby.

Maas, M. L., & Delaney, C. (2004). Nursing process outcome linkage research: issues, current status, and health policy implications. *Medical Care, 42*(2 Suppl.), 40-48.

Mallick, M. J., & Whipple, T. W. (2000). Validity of the nursing diagnosis of relocation stress syndrome. *Nursing Research, 49*(2), 97-100.

Marek, K. D., Jenkins, M., Westra, B. L., & McGinley, A. (1998). Implementation of a clinical information system in nurse-managed care. *Canadian Journal of Nursing Research, 30*(1), 37-44.

Martin, K. S. (2004). *The Omaha System: A key to practice, documentation, and information management* (2nd ed.). St. Louis, MO: Elsevier.

Matney, S., Bakken, S., & Huff, S. M. (2003). Representing nursing assessments in clinical information systems using the logical observation identifiers, names, and codes database. *Journal of Biomedical Informatics, 36*(4-5), 287-293.

McCloskey, J. C., & Bulechek, G. M. (2000). *Nursing Interventions Classification (NIC)* (3rd ed.). St. Louis, MO: Mosby.

McNeil, B., Elfrink, V., & Pierce, S. (2004). Preparing student nurses, faculty and clinicians for 21st century informatics practice: Findings from a national survey of nursing education programs in the United States. *Medinfo,* pp. 903-907.

Mortensen, R. A. (Ed.). (1999). *ICNP and telematic applications for nurses in Europe: The Telenurse experience* (Vol. 61). Amsterdam: IOS Press.

Myers, H. (2003). Hospital fall risk assessment tools: A critique of the literature. *International Journal of Nursing Practice, 9*(4), 223-235.

NANDA International. (2005). *Nursing diagnoses: Definitions and classification 2005-2006.* Philadelphia: Author.

National Forum on Information Literacy. (1998). *A progress report on information literacy: An update on the American Library Association Presidential Committee on Information Literacy—Final report.* Retrieved December 21, 2005, from http://www.ala.org/ala/acrl/acrlpubs/whitepapers/progressreport.htm

Naylor, M., Bowles, K., & Brooten, D. (2000). Patient problems and advanced practice nurse interventions during transitional care. *Public Health Nursing, 72*(2), 94-102.

Ozbolt, J. G. (1998). *Ozbolt's Patient Care Data Set, Version 4.0.* Nashville, TN: Vanderbilt University.

Ozbolt, J. (2003). The Nursing Terminology Summit Conferences: a case study of successful collaboration for change. *Journal of Biomedical Informatics, 36*(4-5), 362-374

Parlocha, P. K., & Henry, S. B. (1998). The usefulness of the Georgetown Home Health Care Classification system for coding patient problems and nursing interventions in psychiatric home care. *Computers in Nursing, 16*(1), 45-52.

Prophet, C. M., Dorr, G. G., Gibbs, T. D., & Porcella, A. A. (1997). Implementation of standardized nursing languages (NIC, NOC) in on-line care planning and documentation. In U. Gerdin, M. Tallberg, & P. Wainwright (Eds.), *NI97* (pp. 395-400). Stockholm: IOS Press.

Saba, V. K. (1992). Home health care classification. *Caring Magazine, 11*(4), 58-60.

Saba, V. (2004). *Clinical care classification.* Retrieved October 14, 2004, from http://www.sabacare.com

Sackett, D. L., Richardson, W. S., Rosenberg, W., & Haynes, R. B. (1998). *Evidenced-based medicine: How to practice & teach EBM.* Edinburgh, Scotland: Churchill Livingstone.

SNOMED International. (2005). SNOMED clinical terms. Retrieved February 9, 2005, from http://www.snomed.org/

Staggers, N., Gassert, C. A., & Curran, C. (2001). Informatics competencies for nurses at four levels of practice. *Journal of Nursing Education, 40*(7), 303-316.

Staggers, N., Gassert, C. A., & Curran, C. (2002). A Delphi study to determine informatics competencies for nurses at four levels of practice. *Nursing Research, 51*(6), 383-390.

Starren, J., & Johnson, S. B. (2000). An object-oriented taxonomy of medical data presentations. *Journal of the American Medical Informatics Association, 7*(1), 1-137.

Tanner, A., Pierce, S., & Pravikoff, D. (2004). Readiness for evidence-based practice: Information literacy needs of nurses in the United States. *Medinfo,* pp. 936-940.

Thompson, T., & Brailer, D. (2004). *The decade of health information technology: Delivering consumer-centric and information-rich health care. Framework for strategic action.* Washington, DC: Office of the National Coordinator for Health Information Technology. U.S. Department of Health and Human Services.

Turley, J. P. (1992). A framework for the transition from nursing records to a nursing information system. *Nursing Outlook, 40,* 177-181.

Warner, H. R., Haug, P. J., Lincoln, M., Warner Jr., H. R., Sorenson, D., & Fan, C. (1988). Iliad as an expert consultant to teach differential diagnosis. *Twelfth Symposium on Computer Applications in Medical Care,* pp. 371-376.

World Health Organization. (2003). *International Statistical Classification of Diseases and Related Health Problems: 10th Revision.* Retrieved February 1, 2005, from http://www3.who.int/icd/vol1htm2003/fr-icd.htm

Zielstorff, R. D., Hudgings, C. I., Grobe, S. J., & National Commission on Nursing Implementation Project Task Force on Nursing Information Systems. (1993). *Next-generation nursing information systems: Essential characteristics for nursing practice.* Washington, DC: American Nurses Publishing.

Electronic Information and Methods for Improving Education

Realities and Assumptions

JO ELAND

Microwave ovens, remote controls for televisions, cruise control on automobiles, thermostats that control our air-conditioning and furnaces, and cellular telephones are examples of technology that, for the most part, makes our lives easier. Computers allow us instantly to send greetings to children at college, shop on eBay, or order a mother's birthday present with the click of a mouse. When discussion of technology turns to the use of computers in nursing education, many faculty do not view technology in the same frame of mind. Computer technology was supposed to make nurses' lives easier, but in nursing education it has done little more than fill nurses' e-mail in-boxes with hundreds of messages and creates challenges that nurses are ill-equipped to face. The purpose of this chapter is to identify some of the challenges and opportunities facing those involved in nursing education in the area of using online learning to provide quality education. Nurse educators have a marvelous opportunity to engage learners in new ways if they just know what can be done, learn it, and use it to allow learners to approach material in unique ways.

ELECTRONIC LEARNING PREPARATION

Most faculty members have adapted to the reality that e-mail and some World Wide Web usage is a way of life, but that does not prepare them to teach in an online environment. Faculty preparation often has been limited to an orientation to various course management software packages (Blackboard [Blackboard Inc., Washington, D.C.] WebCT [WebCT, Inc., Lynnfield, Massachusetts], or Desire2Learn [Desire2Learn Inc., Ontario, Canada]) with little or no introduction to the actual teaching strategies that can be used. The faculty members faced with the reality that they may have little or no choice about whether to teach online may have three levels of concern: (1) their own limited computer experience, (2) their unfamiliarity with different teaching and learning strategies in an online environment, and (3) the need to understand the basics of the course management software package.

To teach successfully in the online environment, there must be three levels of support structures for teacher and learners. First, professors need support to help them recognize the potential of an online environment, including what can be accomplished that is parallel to classroom teaching, what cannot be accomplished, and the opportunities that exist in an online environment that do not exist in a traditional classroom setting. Second, teachers need technical support in the preparation of the materials and in uploading them to the course management software. Finally, the faculty need timely in-house support to fix any hardware or software problems that arise with their own computer.

Students require, at least, a tour of the course management software so that they can interact with the software successfully to complete their course requirements. Students must have an e-mail account where they receive important messages regarding their course work, which is often a part of the course management software, and must be reminded to check that specific account for messages. Students often prefer to use their personal accounts located on Yahoo (Yahoo! Inc., Sunnyvale, California) or HotMail (Microsoft Corporation, Redmond, Washington) for their e-mail and may be unaccustomed to checking their official university accounts. Students also need to be aware of any additional software their machine needs to have installed, such as Adobe Acrobat (Adobe Systems Inc. San Jose, California), QuickTime (Apple Computer, Inc., Cupertino, California), or RealPlayer (Real Player Inc, Seattle, WA).

Additionally, if they are complete novices at downloading and installing software, they also may require someone to assist them with that task. Students also require technical support for the maintenance of their own computers because their computer is an essential tool to their education. In most university settings that support is provided outside of the university setting but is necessary because of the continuing onslaught of viruses and worms that can render their computers unusable.

DO'S AND DONT'S

Technology should never be used for technology's sake. Placing a syllabus online and recording grades in an online grade book is not online learning, although it might be the first step for a complete novice. Posting hundreds of pages of reading on a Web site also may be a bad idea from two perspectives. Many individuals do not like reading numerous pages on the computer screen or downloading a large syllabus to print. In a similar vein, posting hundreds of Microsoft PowerPoint slides for students to review may prove equally frustrating because of the amount of time required to download and print the files and the cost of ink and paper. Faculty need to ask a simple question of themselves as they prepare to teach an online course: Could the information being delivered to the student be printed and delivered as a guided correspondence course? If the answer to that question is yes, then use the printed version and do not require computers in an online experience because it makes students angry and resentful of technology.

Using syllabus posting, online grading, and PowerPoint slides only touches the surface of what is possible in an online environment. Online learning should be rich in content of the day and should use technology to create a truly unique online experience. Specifically, color photos, video clips, audio lectures, live video chat rooms, and online discussions present opportunities that can create a virtual classroom that is far more interesting than printed text. The electronic libraries of today also provide an opportunity that is unlike anything ever witnessed before: the opportunity to search the world for relevant content that is critical to one's understanding of almost any aspect of human life.

From a more global perspective, if universities truly recognize the potential of online education, students should be allowed to create plans of study that include courses from experts in the field at distant universities. This is particularly exciting when one's area of interest is narrow. Allowing students to meet degree requirements by taking relevant courses from other universities

makes good use of faculty resources, enriches student learning, and is cost-effective.

THE SIZE OF THE PIPE

One of the basic concepts that faculty need to understand in online education is what the author chooses to call the "size of the pipe." This refers to the speed of an Internet connection. Rather than talk about baud or bit rate in the delivery of online materials, it is easier to talk about the diameter of an ordinary pipe. If one compares the diameter of a small water pipe to a kitchen sink (1-inch diameter) to a culvert used for drainage on major roads (8-foot diameter), one can make a comparison that is readily understandable.

A fast Internet connection such as a T1 line (like most work settings have), fiber-optic, DSL, or cable modem can be classified as a big pipe, whereas telephone-based modems are the one-inch kitchen sink pipe, or little pipes. Content for widespread dissemination on the Internet has to be able to be delivered on the lowest common denominator: the kitchen sink pipe (the telephone modem). Until everyone involved has a large pipe (T1, fiber optic, DSL, or cable modem), the critical question to ask in delivering course materials is, How big of a pipe is necessary to deliver a specific type of content? There is no question in my mind that in the not so distant future, the size of the pipe will be larger for all who can afford it and it probably will be available wirelessly via satellite. A second question is, What is the size of the pipe that the students are using to access course materials? In many areas of the country, students do not have access to a big pipe, regardless of the cost, and until that is remedied, course content must be delivered at the lowest common denominator, the kitchen sink pipe (the telephone modem).

USING VIDEO OVER THE WORLD WIDE WEB

Delivery of full-screen live video over the Internet will become a reality, but for the time being, video can be delivered only in small screens much like the movie trailers of the latest movies one can view online. If full-screen video could be delivered to the masses, those who distribute movies certainly would make that an immediate reality for all because the industry could profit by that type of delivery.

If learners have telephone-based modems as stated previously, video lectures are reduced to 3 × 4-inch movies on their computer screen that *severely* limits what can be viewed. The small size of the current viewing screen reduces most classroom lectures to mere "talking heads" with tiny unreadable text or images in a PowerPoint lecture as a backdrop.

Polycom (Polycom, Inc., Pleasanton, California) allows live, high-quality video interaction to take place in a number of locations, and the on-site classroom students can communicate with distant members of the class interactively. A minimal Polycom system can be set up with cameras costing approximately $400 for each site. Depending on the available resources, the video from those sessions can be saved and viewed as QuickTime movies on a Windows (Microsoft) or Macintosh (Apple) operating system. The QuickTime process compresses the video so that it can be delivered over big pipes, but often one has difficulty when viewing the video over small pipes because the video files are huge. An appropriate analogy would be to attempt to stuff a bed pillow through a 1-inch pipe. It would take forever to stuff it in the pipe, and if one finally got it through the pipe, it would not come out in good shape at the other end.

Before investing in Polycom, one must evaluate whether the various institutional security firewalls and virus protection will allow the video signal to be transmitted from the originating site to the student's location. Although one ordinarily is considering where the student is located in the online environment, another advantage to Polycom is that faculty members could be teaching from anywhere in the world where they had a camera, a big pipe, and a computer.

AUDIO FILES

Because audio files are much smaller and can fit through small pipes if compressed, online audio lectures are a realistic choice for lecture delivery. The inflection of the human voice, the enthusiasm, and the passion are reproduced accurately in the audio files. One of the most popular audio compression formats available is MP3 or MP4, which is what the popular portable music players (i.e., iPods [Apple]) are using. These small files also can be listened to on a house, car, or portable stereo. An MP3 or MP4 file format can make a professor's lectures truly portable, and a learner can listen to them on the morning commute, while doing dishes, or while painting the house. When audio files are combined with lecture notes, the result is more like a typical classroom. If the learner is going to use a computer for online courses at a place of employment, another important consideration of using audio files may arise. Many work settings have prevented the download of audio files because of employees downloading music illegally. If this

is an issue, audio files may be burned to a CD-ROM and mailed to the student.

Some professors choose Microsoft Producer to combine audio that is synchronized with PowerPoint slides; however, the question again becomes, "How big is the pipe?" If the pipe is a telephone-based modem, the student's frustration created by the time required to view the class may outweigh the benefit of this format when the content can be delivered using MP3 audio and separate PowerPoint outlines. If the PowerPoint slides are words on a colorful background, then exporting only the outlines will allow all learners to have essential content more readily. If the content has a key graphic or photograph, the graphic can be saved as a separate JPG image and made available for downloading.

PowerPoint slide presentations that have relevant photographs or diagrams included make the learners who have small pipes wait as long as 60 minutes to download them. Students who have telephone-based modems also are plagued by service providers who may disconnect them when downloading files because their server may sense the downloading as inactivity. The learner then is faced with reconnecting to the Internet provider and starting the process again only to lose the connection. This predictably makes learners dislike technology. If a faculty member cannot be convinced to export outlines, PowerPoint slides can be converted to the Adobe Acrobat format, which creates smaller files that will download more quickly.

USE OF DIGITAL PHOTOGRAPHS

With the ease of digital photography and scanning, it is now possible to share color images much more easily than previously; however, there are "pipe" considerations for images as well. Today's computer screens can "see" only 75 dots per inch (dpi) compared with the 1200 dpi images viewed in magazines. With only 75 dpi as opposed to 1200 dpi, the file sizes are much smaller. If students are expected routinely to view images, the images should be at 75 to 150 dpi, and if possible kept to a size around 4 × 6 inches. The ability to resize images is a resource that needs to be available to faculty, either for the task to be completed for them or for the faculty to be taught how to do it. The majority of images printed at 75 dpi look grainy and pixelated (boxy), so if a student chooses to print these images, the images will not look impressive on paper.

If professors have images that they do not wish to have downloaded, those images can be placed on the World Wide Web using a program called Flash (Macromedia,

San Francisco, California). Documents created with Flash cannot be downloaded; however, that does not prevent a clever student from using a screen capture program to have a copy of the image. Recognize that it will be a low-resolution image that will appear normal on the computer screen but less than adequate if it is printed.

ELECTRONIC TEXTBOOKS

In the not so distant future, one can hope that all textbooks will be totally online and available on a subscription basis. For a fee, students would have access to the text during the semester they are taking the course. Authors could keep the content current and updated almost effortlessly, and there would be no more outdated textbooks. Current medical and nursing news could be included in an update section with the insights of the authors. For example, if a cure for acquired immunodeficiency syndrome has been found and is well publicized over the national media, the online authors could point out to the students that, yes, a cure had been found, but the research sample was a small one with individuals in the early stages of the disease and that the findings need to replicated in other settings. Electronic texts would be ecologically friendly, saving trees and preventing back strain from carrying the texts around in backpacks. Online subscriptions also could be available to graduates who then could always have a current text at their fingertips.

ONLINE JOURNALS

One of the most exciting realities of the current electronic world is the availability of publications, especially magazines, online. The world library is available to those institutions that have paid the large amounts of money required to maintain the service. For many online courses the use of the online library of a particular university is a part of the course registration fee. Such options make the world available as long as the learner (and the faculty for that matter) knows how to use them. Gone is the joy of wandering through the physical library and discovering new knowledge; however, the trade-off allows a learner to go beyond the normal parameters and truly search the literature. If national or international students are enrolled, they too have access to the world's libraries by virtue of their enrollment. A nurse who lives hundreds of miles from a traditional library now truly can search the literature and download articles without ever leaving the computer.

DROWNING IN A SEA OF E-MAIL

A useful tip for sending course-related e-mail to students is to put the name of the course in the subject line of the e-mail along with the topic of the e-mail. That way, the student is less likely to ignore the e-mail during sorting. If professors set a filter and corresponding mailbox for the course in their own e-mail account, when students hit the "reply" button to one of the professor-initiated e-mails, the program will sort it into the specific course mailbox.

The use of e-mail stationery, for common responses to student questions, also eases faculty's pain of responding to the same questions over and over. If faculty members invest a small amount of time to create e-mail stationery that addresses common student questions, they need only bring up the stationery, put it in the student's e-mail address and send it. Common faculty-generated e-mails can include (1) clarification of assignments, (2) course grading policy, or (3) extra credit options.

ONLINE DISCUSSIONS

Unlike traditional classroom discussions, online discussions require that all students be prepared to discuss the topic and thoughtfully reply to questions posed by the faculty or other students. The faculty member introduces a topic for discussion and posts an article related to the topic; students respond to the questions posed by faculty or other classmates; and after 1 or 2 weeks, the faculty member closes and summarizes the discussion. Unlike traditional classroom discussions, all students have to be prepared because many faculty make participation in discussions mandatory and evaluate the quality of student responses. Shy students who might not participate in traditional classroom discussions have their opinions heard, and those students who might be inhibited in face-to-face presentation of opposing views are less inhibited. Faculty members can encourage students respectfully to engage each other when they hold opposing views, which is an important part of professional socialization. In the online learning environment, students need to be reminded that because they cannot see their classmates' facial expressions, their comments and responses in print can be interpreted from many perspectives.

GROUP PROJECTS

Most course management software offers group learning opportunities including group chat and group drop boxes where students working on a group project can keep their project online for others to view and update. The group itself may never meet physically, but the current draft of their project is available to work on 24-7.

EXAMINATIONS AND EVALUATION

Online examinations present problems with no easy solution because the learner is not in a classroom with the professor present. If an online examination is posted, nothing can prevent a student from inviting over five friends to answer the examination together. An examination could be posted with a specific time limit to take the examination, and the examination itself could be posted only for 1 hour. This too is problematic because students may not be available during the time chosen to post the examination, and if students are residing in a different time zone, it is even more problematic.

Take-home essay examinations are an option that many use, but of course students can still work on them together. Some universities have specific testing sites where students go to take examinations, whereas others use private settings for online testing. To avoid these testing difficulties, professors have used other forms of evaluation besides testing.

SUMMARY

Electronic education creates new challenges for professor and student that can be overcome to reveal unique opportunities that do not exist in traditional classrooms. The challenge for the faculty is to reframe their expertise to fit the online environment. With appropriate institutional support the online environment can meet the needs of professor and learner in exciting new ways.

Web-Based Education

DIANE J. SKIBA

In nursing, many schools of nursing use Web-based education as a means to provide access to learning opportunities for nurses. "Thousands of online courses are now available, and an increasing number of on-campus courses possess a technology component" (National Postsecondary Education Cooperative, 2004, p. ix). The move from traditional face-to-face classroom teaching to an online environment is not without controversy. Administrators often view online learning as an opportunity to increase the size of the student population. Some faculty readily embrace the concept and have converted their courses from traditional to online. Some faculty believe that nursing as a clinical practice discipline can be taught only in a face-to-face environment. Students are also on both sides of the controversy. But regardless of the controversy, a recent report sponsored by the Sloan Center for Online Education stated that "online enrollments continue to grow at rates faster than for the overall student body and there is no evidence that the enrollments have reached a plateau" (Allen & Seaman, 2004, p. 1).

The purpose of this chapter is twofold: to provide evidence that supports the growth of online learning and to summarize the best practices in Web-based education. The first purpose provides current evidence (1) to address the growth and viability of online learning in higher education as a long-term strategy and (2) to examine satisfaction and quality of online courses. The review of best practice serves as a solid foundation for schools of nursing to create Web-based education programs. This review also provides students with criteria to assess the quality of Web-based educational programs before selecting an online course or degree program.

DEFINITIONS

A multitude of terms are used to describe Web-based education. For example, such education can be called Web-based, online, virtual, distance-based, or Internet learning or education. To clarify, the Sloan Center for Online Education provides definitions and guidelines (Table 17-1). For this chapter, the focus is Web-based education in which the majority of the courses are available online and that does not use traditional face-to-face delivery methods.

GROWTH OF WEB-BASED EDUCATION

Universities and colleges face many challenges with the changing landscape of higher education. With the growing popularity of the Internet, higher education seized the opportunity to provide learning opportunities to a changing student population. The student population now includes older adults who must juggle family, work, and school responsibilities. A large part-time student population now is taking college courses. The growing student population also reflects the diversity of many ethnic and cultural backgrounds. According to National Center for Education Statistics (2002), three quarters of all undergraduate students are "non-traditional." Nontraditional students attend part time, work full time, are financially independent, have dependents, and may be single parents. To further complicate the landscape, Oblinger (2003) identified three different generations of students—Boomers, Gen-Xers, and the Millennials—who are part of the changing student population.

A recent survey by the Sloan Center for Online Education (Allen & Seaman, 2004) examined the state of online education in U.S. higher education. Their survey, directed to chief academic officers of the 3068 institutions of higher education, had a response rate of 38.1%, and 43% of these respondents were from accredited schools. The survey focused on four major questions related to the extent and quality of online education. The survey represented data for the 2003 academic year. Previous data from 2002 academic year provided a basis for comparison over time.

TABLE 17-1

Definitions and Guidelines for Online Education		
Type of Course	**Delivery Method**	**Use of Online/Web/Internet**
Traditional	Course is delivered in a face-to-face environment.	None
Web-facilitated or Web-enhanced	Course is delivered in a face-to-face environment.	Course materials such as syllabus, handouts, or slides are provided on the Web.
Blended or hybrid	Course is delivered in face-to-face and online environments.	From 30% to 79% of course is delivered online or via the Web.
Web/online/ Internet	Course is delivered in an online environment without face-to-face contact.	Eighty percent or more of a course is available online or via the Web.

Modified from Allen, I. E., & Seaman, J. (2004). *Entering the mainstream: The quality and extent of online education in the United States, 2003 & 2004.* Needham, MA: Sloan Center for Online Education.

The first question investigated the growth of online enrollments. The following are some of their findings. More than 1.9 million students are taking online courses as of fall 2003, and growth of 24.8% is projected for fall 2004. "Schools expect the number of online students to grow to over 2.6 million by the fall of 2004" (Allen & Seaman, 2004, p. 1). According to the report, predictions by schools have been accurate. Associate's degree–granting institutions have the "largest number of students taking at least one online course, representing about half of all the students studying online" (p. 12).

A second question investigated whether students were as satisfied with online courses as they were with traditional face-to-face courses. Chief academic officers reported that students are "at least as satisfied with their online courses" (Allen & Seaman, 2004, p. 2). Differences were evident across size of schools, with smaller colleges (under 1500 enrollments) being the least positive. Associate- and graduate-level schools were more positive than specialized or baccalaureate schools.

Chief academic officers also were asked whether online learning was part of their long-term strategy, and the majority (54%) "agreed that online education is critical to their long term strategy" (Allen & Seaman, 2004, p. 2). If the school was large public or a private for-profit school, it was more likely to state that online education was a critical component of the long-term strategy. Lastly, the majority of chief academic officers reported that the quality of online education is equal to or superior to traditional face-to-face instruction. Again, this belief was more associated with larger public institutions.

The last question examined the chief academic officers' perception of the quality of online education. One myth is that online education is of lesser quality than the traditional classroom instruction. Three quarters of the respondents stated that online learning was equal to or superior to face-to-face traditional instruction. Again, a positive correlation was found between size of the institution and positive perception of quality.

The striking results indicate that online learning will continue to grow and in many cases outpace the number of new students entering schools. Higher educational institutions consider online learning crucial to their long-term strategy. Students are satisfied with courses, and the administrators perceive the quality of online courses to be equal to or superior to traditional classroom courses.

BEST PRACTICES

Best practices are the gold standard against which current practice can be judged. Best practices are documented strategies that are perfected within an organization. These best practices are supported by data that demonstrate desired outcomes. Over the last decade, many best practices were defined by a variety of organizations. Some of the best practices were developed through a consensus method by a designated group of knowledgeable members of various communities. Other best practices were defined by synthesizing research results.

An excellent example of a consensus model to establish best practices is the Western Cooperative for Educational Telecommunications (2003) article "Balancing Quality and Access: Principles of Good Practice for Electronically Offered Academic Degree and Certificate Programs." Representatives from higher education regulating agencies, higher education institutions, and the regional accrediting community in the western states created these principles to balance access and quality among electronically offered programs. Each of the principles serves as a measure of quality for electronically offered degree or certificate programs. Their focus is on programs rather than individual courses.

These principles focus on three major components: curriculum and instruction, institutional context and commitment, and evaluation and assessment. The curriculum and instruction principles are as follows:

◆ Each program of study results in learning outcomes appropriate to the rigor and breadth of the degree or certificate awarded.
◆ An electronically offered degree or certificate program is coherent and complete.
◆ The program provides for appropriate real-time or delayed interaction between faculty and students and among students.
◆ Qualified faculty provide appropriate oversight of the electronically offered program.

For students and faculty, an important note is the principle that highlights the interaction between students and faculty. This is an important consideration because many believe the myth that Web-based courses are merely correspondence courses and do not require continuous interaction between students and faculty. This point also is important when one is assessing Web-based courses because many are designed to have students interacting with content and not with each other or the faculty.

The institutional context and commitment principles are divided into several subsections: role and mission, faculty support, resources for learning, students and student support, and commitment to support. One must remember that an electronically offered degree program must fit within the role and mission of the institution and that the technology is appropriate to meet program objectives. Faculty must be provided support services and training in the use of technology. Faculty evaluation mechanisms also must include consideration of teaching and scholarship related to electronically offered degree programs. Any electronically offered program must provide necessary learning resources such as online full-text journal articles to students. The institution must provide sufficient resources to allow all students to complete their degree. Students and student services were particularly emphasized and are listed next:

◆ The program provides students with clear, complete, and timely information on the curriculum, course and degree requirements, nature of faculty/student interaction, assumptions about technological competence and skills, technical equipment requirements, availability of academic support services and financial aid resources, and costs and payment policies.

◆ Enrolled students have reasonable and adequate access to the range of student services appropriate to support their learning.
◆ Accepted students have the background, knowledge, and technical skills needed to undertake the program.
◆ Advertising, recruiting, and admissions materials clearly and accurately represent the program and the services available.

Sue Day-Perroots, dean of extended learning at West Virginia University, created a basic assessment inventory based on the best practices. Her *Guidelines for Electronically Delivered Programs* (2001) is available at the Western Cooperative for Educational Telecommunications Web site (http://www.wcet.info/resources/accreditation).

In 1997, three schools of nursing (Indiana University, University of Kansas Medical Center, and University of Colorado at Denver and Health Sciences Center) partnered with a consultant from the Flashlight Program to develop, implement, and evaluate an instrument to assess outcomes of Web-based nursing courses. The Flashlight Program is a core program of the Teaching, Learning, and Technology affiliate of the American Association of Higher Education (http://www.tltgroup.org/programs/flashlight.html). Through this collaboration the Evaluating Educational Uses of the Web in Nursing (EEUWIN) Benchmarking Project was begun.

The goal of the EEUWIN Benchmarking Project is to help nurse educators begin to evaluate the effectiveness of Web-based courses. The EEUWIN Project helps schools of nursing evaluate their uses of Web-based education and enables them to learn from best practices identified at their own or other institutions. This project uses benchmarking as a method to establish quality outcomes. Identification of best practices is an outcome of the benchmarking process. Benchmarking also provides information on how one ranks compared with the best performance and reveals performance gaps, positive and negative, in an organization.

Given this benchmarking framework, the EEUWIN goals are as follows:

◆ To help schools of nursing evaluate the educational effectiveness of their Web-based programs
◆ To identify a set of best practices for using the Web to deliver nursing programs
◆ To provide schools of nursing with a means to compare their Web-based programs with similar programs at other schools of nursing
◆ To identify the type of person who is participating in Web-based nursing programs and help schools of nursing identify ways of reaching a more diverse learner population.

Billings (2000) developed a framework that served as a conceptual basis for the benchmarking study. The framework incorporated three major components (use of technology, educational practices, and outcomes). Other variables under study included student support. Although faculty support is acknowledged, it is not a performance measure at this time. Under educational practices, six of seven best practices identified by Chickering and Gamson (1991) were included. These educational practices are active learning, peer-to-peer interactions, interactions between faculty and students, time on task, respect for diverse learning, and prompt feedback. Outcomes include variables such as convenience, satisfaction, preference for face-to-face, connectedness, professionalism, and computer proficiency.

The EEUWIN project team has conducted several studies based on the benchmarking data set. An early focus was the validation of the model and how data from benchmarking studies could be used to improve Web-based learning (Billings, Connors, & Skiba, 2001; Skiba, Billings, & Connors, 2003a; Skiba, Billings, & Connors, 2003b; Billings, Connors, Skiba, & Zuniga, 2003). Reliability estimates (Chronbach alphas) for the benchmarking tool have ranged from 0.90 to 0.94 and from 0.73 to 0.93 for subscales. Successive testing over the past 4 years has demonstrated positive correlations between educational practices and Web-based outcomes.

A recent study investigated differences in perceptions of undergraduate and graduate students' experiences in Web-based courses. Comparisons across educational levels were examined for variables related to use of technology, support for technology, educational practices, and outcomes. This study characterized the first of many comparisons that are possible from the existing benchmarking data set. Relatively few studies have examined differences between two educational levels of learners. The results continue to demonstrate that educational practices shape outcomes (Billings, Skiba, & Connors, 2005). The two groups did not differ on many variables. Differences were found on the variables, faculty-student interactions, and time factors that included time on task and time spent in course (Billings, Skiba, & Connors, 2005). In terms of outcomes, the only differences were related to computer proficiency and connectedness. Undergraduates felt more connected and reported having more student-faculty interactions and spending less time on task and in the course. Examination of the generational differences among students and between students and faculty in Web-based courses is an area that demands further research.

Another source of best practices is the Effective Practices project of the Sloan Consortium. The purpose of this project was to share best practices to make quality online education affordable and accessible. The framework consists of five pillars for achieving quality (Moore, 2004). Effective practices must demonstrate evidence of effectiveness in the pillars. Table 17-2 provides the five pillars and a sample of the goals associated with each pillar. For a complete listing, go to http://www.sloan-c.org/effective. Effective practices are nominated and must meet specific criteria. The criteria are innovation, replicability, potential impact, supporting documentation, and evidence and scope.

SUMMARY

Despite the controversy, Web-based education is becoming firmly entrenched in the higher education landscape. Chief academic officers reinforce the notion that online learning is considered an essential piece of

TABLE 17-2

Effectiveness Pillars for Online Education	
Pillar	**Sample Goals**
Learning effectiveness	Interaction is key: with instructors, classmates, the interface, and via vicarious interactions. Online course design takes advantage of capabilities of the medium to improve learning.
Cost-effectiveness	Institutions continuously improve services while reducing costs. Tuition and fees reflect cost of services delivery.
Access	Learner-centered courseware is provided. Feedback from learners is taken seriously and is used for continuous improvement.
Faculty satisfaction	Faculty are rewarded for teaching online. Faculty satisfaction metrics show improvement over time.
Student satisfaction	Students are successful in leaning online. Discussion and interactions with instructors and peers is satisfactory.

From Moore, J. (2004, August). *A synthesis of Sloan-C Effectives Practices.* Needham, MA: Sloan Consortium.

their long-term strategy. Several key resources highlight the quality indicators of a successful Web-based course and also a successful online program. Best practices have been identified clearly in terms of Web-based courses, effectives practices, and electronically offered programs.

If you are a student considering taking an online course or seeking an online degree program, the following are some questions you should ask while investigating your options.

Web-Based Course Questions

- How is the course designed?
- Is the course designed to take advantage of the Web-based medium?
- Is the course designed using a particular learning framework (situated learning, constructivism)
- Is the course based on active learning strategies?
- Does the course provide frequent opportunities to interact with the faculty and my peers?
- Is the course designed to be a repository to disseminate knowledge (text-driven pages, slides, and links) and not foster interactions?
- Do I have access to library resources such as full-text journals and interlibrary loans?
- How do I get my books?
- Does the course respect diverse styles of learning?
- What are the time requirements?
- How often do I need to log into the course per week?
- Does the instructor provide prompt feedback?
- Is the instructor accessible?
- Have students been satisfied with this online course?
- Are there technical supports available to help me?
- Is there a prerequisite course that can help me with the course management platform?

Web-Based Degree Programs

- Are the requirements for program clearly explicated? Are there times I am expected to be on campus?
- Is every course needed in the program available online? If so, how often?
- Does the institution provide some assurance that program will be in operation so I can complete my degree in a reasonable time frame?
- What student support services are available?
- Can I register online?
- Can I receive financial aid?
- How are programs evaluated?
- Are faculty trained to teach online?
- Are there sufficient supports to help faculty with online courses?
- Are there technical supports available to students?
- Is the help desk open 24-7?

- Are students satisfied with the program?
- What is the retention rate for the program?
- What supports does the school provide to create a learner-centered environment for students?
- Are there any fees or other costs associated with Web-based learning?
- How does the online program compare on student outcomes with traditional programs at the institution?

REFERENCES

Allen, I. E., & Seaman, J. (2004). *Entering the mainstream: The quality and extent of online education in the United States, 2003 & 2004*. Needham, MA: Sloan Center for Online Education.

Billings, D. (2000). Framework for assessing outcomes and practices in web-based courses in nursing. *Journal of Nursing Education, 39*(2), 60-67.

Billings, D., Connors, H., & Skiba, D. (2001). Benchmarking best practices in web-based nursing courses. *Advances in Nursing Science, 23*(3), 41-52.

Billings, D., Connors, H., Skiba, D., & Zuniga, R. (2003, September). Benchmarking: undergraduate vs. graduate online courses. Paper presented at the National League for Nursing Summit, San Antonio, TX.

Billings, D. M., Skiba, D. J., & Connors, H. R. (2005). Best practices in web-based courses: Generational differences across undergraduate and graduate nursing students. *Journal of Professional Nursing, 21*(2), 126-133.

Chickering, A. W., & Gamson, Z. F. (Eds.). (1991). *Applying the seven principles for good practice in undergraduate education: New directions in teaching and learning* (No. 47). San Francisco: Jossey-Bass.

Moore, J. (2004). *A synthesis of Sloan-C Effective Practices*. Needham, MA: Sloan Consortium.

National Center for Educational Statistics. (2002). The condition of education, 2002. Retrieved February 1, 2005, from http://nces.ed.gov/pubsearch/pubsinfo.asp?pubid=2002025

National Postsecondary Education Cooperative. (2004). *How does technology affect access in postsecondary education? What do we really know?* (NPEC 2004-831), prepared by Ronald A. Phipps for the National Postsecondary Education Cooperative Working Group on Access-Technology. Washington, DC: U.S. Department of Education.

Oblinger, D. (2003). Boomers, Gen-Xers, and Millennials: Understanding the new students. *Educause Review, 38*(4), 36-47.

Skiba, D., Billings, D., & Connors, H. (2003a). Benchmarking web-based courses in nursing: The EEUWIN Project. In H. deFatima Marin, E. Pereira Marques, E. Hovenga, & W. Goossen (Eds). *Proceedings of the Eighth International Congress in Nursing Informatics: E-health for all: Designing nursing agenda for the future*. Rio de Janeiro, Brazil: E-papers Servicos Editoriais Ltd.

Skiba, D., Billings, D., & Connors, H. (2003b). The EEUWIN (Evaluating Educational Uses of the Web in Nursing)

Benchmarking Project. *Proceedings of the International Medical Informatics Association: Education Work Group Symposium: Teach globally, learn locally. Innovations in health and biomedical informatics education on the 21st century.* Portland, Oregon: Oregon Health & Sciences University.

Western Cooperative for Educational Telecommunications (2003). *Balancing quality and access: Principles of good practice for electronically offered academic degree and certificate programs.* Retrieved February 1, 2003, from http://wcet.info/projects/balancing/principles.asp

CHANGING PRACTICE

A Nurse Is Not a Nurse Is Not a Nurse

PERLE SLAVIK COWEN ◆ SUE MOORHEAD

The changes and issues in practice are presented in this section by specialty area. Although all nurses share certain perspectives and experiences, the chapters in this section reflect that nurses working in different specialties have a wide range of skills and are faced with different issues. Communicating these differences with each other helps nurses understand the vast profession that they share. This year we have added chapters focused on pediatric nursing, forensic nursing, and disease management. We hope to continue expanding this section to include a wide range of specialties. We found these to be interesting additions. If you would like to see other new specialties added to the next edition, we hope you will take the time to share your ideas by completing the form included at the back of the book.

Joel provides an elegant debate chapter about home care and includes issues developing as this arena of care delivery assumes more importance. Slowly, home care is moving to a functional social model suitable to the needs of some, but not all, consumers. Joel begins her chapter by describing the history of home care in the United States. Although nursing traditionally has dominated the home care scene, this care environment is changing. Individual consumers of home care want more say, but home care is dictated by public policy and overall public preference. The definition and philosophy of home care are being challenged by new consumer groups such as the disabled. Joel addresses many questions: To what extent should providers and consumers be able to exercise choice in the selection of a setting for care? Does the consumer have the right to choose home care regardless of cost, or only as the least costly option? Joel frames the debate statement as to whether the recipients of in-home services should have increased autonomy and responsibility in making decisions about their care. On the pro side is a strong consumer lobby complicated by the need to make policy decisions about reimbursement. On the con side are the opinions of providers, especially physicians, who

are returning to home care, driven by economics and need, and the issues related to supervision of assistive personnel. The debate is only beginning. Joel's chapter helps nurses understand the current situation as the issues continue to emerge and take shape. This is a well-written, informative chapter that all nurses should read.

According to Grindel and Banks, an aging population living with chronic illness creates the need for rapid change and attainment of solutions in adult health nursing. Other universal issues such as the nursing shortage, an aging nursing workforce, a mandate for patient safety initiatives, and a lack of leadership complicate the challenges to provide quality patient care. This chapter explores the interrelationships of these universal and intraagency issues and their impact on the practice of adult health nursing. The authors also provide an important discussion of the high risk of increased role turmoil with the clinical nurse leader and doctor of nursing practice proposals and describe current role reversals for nurse practitioners and clinical nurse specialists. Grindel and Banks note that the "the clinical nurse specialist may be employed in a primary care site, whereas the nurse practitioner may work in acute care." They contend that if this trend continues, "nursing education programs will be challenged to develop curricula that support the needed knowledge and skills for these blended roles."

The next chapter in this section is not about a particular specialty but about a trend that affects nurses in all specialties. Eliopoulos discusses the growing and extensive use of alternative and complementary therapies, defined as practices outside the dominant system of managing health and disease taught in American medical schools. Although the rest of the world has long used these therapies, their use is relatively new in the United States. The Office of Alternative Medicine was established in 1992 at the National Institutes of Health and became freestanding in 1998 as the National Center for

Complementary and Alternative Medicine. Eliopoulos discusses the factors that contribute to the rapid growth of complementary and alternative therapies in the United States. She states that the introduction of these new therapies offers nurses an opportunity to reclaim the role of healer. New opportunities for nurses in the areas of aromatherapy, herbal medicine, homeopathy, acupuncture, therapeutic touch, guided imagery, massage therapy, and others are emerging. Nurses can use these therapies to enhance traditional care or to establish private practices. Challenges also are emerging, including the risk that physicians will seek the gatekeeper role to the use of these therapies, licensure issues, and safe use of the therapies. Eliopoulos urges nurses and nursing to find a strong voice that will help integrate these therapies with traditional medicine.

Androwich and Haas provide a detailed review of the definition, standards, mission, and practice standards of ambulatory care nursing and discuss numerous practice issues. The authors use the Ambulatory Care Nursing Conceptual Framework to organize "mega" issues under the ambulatory nursing roles of clinical nursing role, organizational/systems role, and professional role. A few of these issues are disease management, syndromic surveillance, diversity of practice settings, need to incorporate technology and evidence-based practice precepts, educational preparation, delegation and supervision, the rapid pace of care, preparation for telephone communication, need for multistate licensure, and the difficulty of maintaining a common culture across various settings. Despite the issues, the authors believe nurses have a number of opportunities and many rewards in this specialty. This chapter provides an excellent overview of ambulatory nursing and intricately describes these issues for nurses in this specialty.

Some specialties focus on setting, others on the age of the population. Persons older than 65 compose 12% of the U.S. population but account for more than 33% of the country's health care expenditures. Although the aging population is growing rapidly, the number of nurses specializing in gerontology remains small. In their chapter, Zwygart-Stauffacher and Rantz provide an overview of the issues related to the care of the aging population. Increasingly, the elderly are using services across the continuum, and new roles for caregivers are emerging as a result. The authors point out that within the new reimbursement systems, gerontological nurses often must assume tough gatekeeping functions about what services will be provided. They discuss the role of the gerontological clinical specialist compared with that of the gerontological nurse practitioner. They also discuss

the qualifications of faculty, adequacy of associate's degree programs to prepare nurses to work in nursing homes, the need for specialty gerontological content in master's practitioner programs, and the need for more research. In this chapter the authors wrestle with many of the issues related to this specialty that will be helpful to others working in the area.

Another specialty that includes care of a number of elderly and other age-groups is hospice and palliative care, the topic of the next chapter. Martinez begins her chapter with a historical overview of hospice and palliative care. The first hospice in the United States was established in New Haven, Connecticut, in 1974. During the 1980s and 1990s, hospice programs sprang up across the United States. She details the dovetailing of the nursing specializations in these two areas with the culmination of the National Board for Certification of Hospice and Palliative Nurses in 1999. Continuing definitional issues involving major organizations are reviewed with the resultant collaboration of five major organizations and the publication of the *Clinical Practice Guidelines for Quality Palliative Care* in May 2004. Still, definitional and regulatory issues exist between hospice and nonhospice palliative care services, and these issues are deftly explored in this chapter.

Parish nursing began in 1984 and was recognized by the American Nurses Association as a specialized area of practice in 1997. In her chapter, Solari-Twadell defines parish nursing as the combination of ministry and nursing. The nursing role component is health promotion and disease prevention. The author describes her research, which identified the top 30 core NIC (Nursing Interventions Classification) interventions and the interventions most frequently used by the parish nurse in caring for clients. Current issues include the development of a standardized curriculum, the need for role clarity, the development of certification for the specialty, and the financing of the role. Solari-Twadell wants the role of the parish nurse to be fully integrated into the congregation and to have the nurse be a visible member of the ministerial team. The final issue discussed in this interesting chapter is the need for documentation of services rendered. The author discusses some recent efforts to accomplish this using the standardized languages of NANDA International, Nursing Interventions Classification, and Nursing Outcomes Classification.

Hockenberry, Bryant, and Rodgers observe that the goal of pediatric nursing of improving the quality of health care for all children faces numerous obstacles, including single-parent families, poverty, and increasing cultural diversity. More than 72 million children under age 18 live in the United States and represent 25% of the entire population. In 2003, only 68% of children in the United States lived with both parents, down from 77% in 1980; and in 2002, just over one third (34%) of all births in the United States were to unmarried women. The number of children living in families with income below the poverty threshold rose from 11.2 million in 2001 to 11.7 million in 2002. The authors note that pediatric nurses must understand the influence of culture, race, and ethnicity on the development of social and emotional relationships; child-rearing practices; and attitude and beliefs toward health, illness, and treatment practices. This excellent chapter details many emerging pediatric problems including obesity, type II diabetes, injuries, violence, substance abuse, and emotional and mental health problems during adolescence and identifies the preventive health care needs of children. The authors note that caring for the increasing number of children with chronic illnesses and implementing innovative nursing care in the face of emerging technology are major priorities for the future of pediatric nursing. The authors conclude with a thorough review of the changing roles, future needs, and opportunities of pediatric nursing. This is a must-read chapter for anyone interested in pediatric nursing.

The specialty of perinatal nursing is discussed next by Simpson. Perinatal nurses care for mothers and babies during pregnancy, labor, birth, and the postpartum and newborn period. Few health care events are more joyous than attendance at the birth of a healthy baby. Given that this is a normal event in the lives of most women, a reader might think that the specialty would have few issues, but the opposite is true. The changes in the health care delivery system that favor the financial bottom line and convenience have resulted in several challenges for those practicing in this specialty. Simpson does an excellent job of presenting several issues: the continued medicalization of labor and birth, increased use of technology for healthy women, the ongoing conflict between usual practice versus evidence-based care, errors by health care providers, increasing nurse/patient ratios, the proliferation of convenience as the foundation for care, lack of education about the impact of the convenience philosophy among childbearing women, and the forces challenging nurse-midwives as providers. Even though a pregnant woman plans and prepares for a low-tech childbirth, she often agrees during labor to interventions that are unnecessary and have the potential for injury. The use of drugs to stimulate labor contractions artificially has increased 110% since 1989. This and other practices in many perinatal units are done more for convenience, for the provider and patient, rather than allowing the normal process of birth to occur. Unfortunately, adverse outcomes happen related to these convenient practices. Simpson urges perinatal nurses to be advocates for pregnant women and to give them the necessary information they need to make the important decisions during labor and birth. This is a stimulating chapter that is a must-read for anyone interested in this area of practice.

Perioperative nursing, a specialty that is currently under siege, is the topic of the next chapter. Girard addresses the issues in perioperative nursing related to the many changes in surgery. For example, more older adults with more comorbidities are undergoing surgery; more surgery is done in ambulatory care and office settings with minimally invasive technologies; and enhanced imaging devices and robotic technologies have improved the diagnosis and treatment of numerous conditions. These changes and others have challenged the traditional roles of nurses in operating rooms. Surgical technologists have replaced nurses in the traditional scrub role, and new legislative measures in many states are allowing semiskilled technicians to take over the role of the circulator and the scrub person. The author notes that "Hospital administrators quickly accepted the surgical technologist in this role because of the decreased availability of qualified surgical nurses and the lower costs associated with unlicensed personnel in this role." The development of surgical technology programs in hospitals and in technical colleges has produced an increased number of ancillary personnel who are assuming the scrub role and who may assume a circulator role. A new role of registered nurse first assistant whereby nurses with master's degrees, who are an integral part of a surgeon's practice, provide preoperative and postoperative assessment and management has emerged. The perioperative nurse role in the ambulatory setting is highly diversified, and within the operating room, it is highly specialized. The recent name change of the specialty organization from Association of Operating Room Nurses to Association of PeriOperative Registered Nurses reflects many of the changes in the specialty. One of the most serious nursing shortages is in this specialty. The author worries that unless there are effective ways of recruiting students and nurses to the surgical setting, this specialty nursing practice may approach extinction.

Psychiatric nursing is the subject of the next chapter by Stuart, who begins by listing several areas of vulnerability that nurses in this specialty face: fewer nurses are attracted to the specialty; psychiatric nurses often are viewed as expensive workers who can be replaced; few outcome studies document the nature and effectiveness of care delivered by psychiatric nurses; and graduate nursing programs have less course work in psychiatric illness. Stuart gives an overview of the changes that have occurred in five areas: role, activities, models of care, treatment settings, and evidence-based practice. She first reviews the history of psychiatric nursing and how the role has evolved since the emergence of the specialty in the 1950s. Next, she lists psychiatric practice activities in three groups: direct care, communication, and management. She says that communication and management activities need to be integrated better in the current role of the psychiatric nurse. In the area of model of care she outlines four stages of treatment and gives an overview of the goal, assessment, intervention, and outcome for each. This is a helpful model because hospital length of stay continues to decrease and much of psychiatric treatment is now in community-based settings. She then discusses the expansion of mental health treatment settings and the challenges and opportunities provided by the change. Finally, she urges psychiatric nurses to articulate the nature of their care and collect data on the outcomes that they achieve. This is an informative chapter about a specialty that is undergoing a number of changes and is challenged to respond or else.

In a cutting-edge chapter, Lynch introduces forensic nursing through a review of the global evolution of forensic nursing, its relationship with the various specialties in the forensic sciences, and the current and future application of forensic nursing science. She also provides an opportunity to explore innovative pathways that will affect the manner in which victims and perpetrators of criminal violence are processed through the health and justice systems in the new millennium. As an emerging discipline, forensic nursing assumes a mutual responsibility with the forensic medical sciences and the criminal justice system in concern for the loss of life and function caused by human violence and the liability-related issues. Lynch notes that the concept of a nurse investigator represents one member of an alliance of health care providers, law enforcement officials, and forensic scientists in a holistic approach to the study and treatment of victims and perpetrators of physical, psychological, and sexual violence. This chapter details what is perhaps one of the most interesting of all nursing specialties and will be a real joy to all the sleuths among us.

In the final chapter, Howe announces that the disease management industry has opened the door for nurses to use their clinical knowledge and teaching skills in ways not possible in other settings. Disease management is defined as "the product of a standardized nursing intervention with a preidentified chronically ill person over time." The aim of the intervention is always to improve quality of care, understanding that the intervention should lead to optimal clinical, financial, and overall quality of life outcomes. Although no hard data support the number of current and available nursing positions, disease management is a rapidly growing phenomenon, and nurses are the central agents that create its value. Howe briefly describes the disease management industry, identifies common core competencies needed to perform disease management, and provides innovative strategies for preparing nurses for this demanding new profession. This chapter definitely will generate discussion.

As the chapters in this section demonstrate, nurses in all specialties are challenged to keep up with many health care system changes. As nurses attempt to streamline their care to save unnecessary steps and cost, they also must continue to provide enough time to attend to the tasks of caring for people. Nurses need to be vocal about the services that must be retained to ensure safety and quality. Nurses also need to help others to see that nurses are not interchangeable. The nursing profession is large and is composed of a vast array of individuals with differing skills and knowledge. Nurses need to acknowledge their similarities and differences as they move forward amid the turmoil of overwhelming change.

CHAPTER 18

Moving the Care

From Hospital to Home

LUCILLE A. JOEL

The trend toward community-based services, or more correctly alternatives to institutional settings, was set into motion by the growing demand for health care in the face of economic pressures to curtail escalating costs. Demographics had become the destiny with rapidly growing numbers of the aged, disabled, and chronically ill; family caregivers were less readily available; and technological advancement made the movement of sophisticated medical diagnostics and therapeutics out of the hospital possible. The initial presumption was that community-based services would be less costly.

Home care has been an active participant and passive respondent in this transition. Home care has been aggressive in the use of telecommunications to extend its capability (Kling, 2001), developing community-based primary care programs for special populations, and conceptualizing the community as client to tailor personal care service to a geographic area (Joel, 2003). Home care has always thrived on creativity and ingenuity. In turn, home care has been shaped and reshaped by the fortunes of government funding and internal competition. The result was two dominant home care markets: the post–acutely ill and the disabled and chronically ill with varying degrees of restorative potential.

CONTEXT OF CARE IN THE NEW MILLENNIUM

Senge (1990) states that success depends on tracking the patterns of social trends so that one may strategically position to create one's own preferred future. This statement is not an oxymoron but truth which is so basic as to be frightening. These trends are set in motion by the society and are not debatable (assuming that they are interpreted correctly), yet they are broad enough so that stewards of the society can be creative in their response. The challenge is to rise above self-interest, the temptation to protect a field of work, and natural caution about change. Once we have faced our own biases, the world looks more logical, if not more acceptable.

The American public is intrigued by high technology, specialization, freedom of choice, and fierce individualism. Applying these qualities, many would best define the American ethic toward health as "A basic package of services for everyone, but the guarantee that those who have the resources can obtain more for themselves and their own." In contrast, countries with more socialized systems would say, "The greatest good for the most people." This interpretation may answer a lot of questions about why Americans act as they do.

Many expect health to be a personal responsibility. Because most of us suffer a minor amount of serious illness in our lives, this makes good sense. However, the progress of medical science has created a cohort of the frail and vulnerable who continue to have primary health care needs, but those needs take on a new meaning. The frail elderly, disabled and chronically ill, persons with acquired immunodeficiency syndrome, and low-birth-weight babies are among those whose health becomes a public concern and creates serious liabilities should it be ignored. Homelessness, poverty, the absence of family, and environmental pollution are also by-products of industrial and scientific progress, complicating the picture more and generating more need for personal health services.

The financial burden of health care has become substantial for Americans. They continue the search for efficiencies that will allow them to honor a commitment to the needy yet maintain some control over the total number of dollars spent. Americans are not proud or complacent about the fact that 18% or 45 million of the population under the age of 65 had no guaranteed access to health care in 2003 (Kaiser Commission on Medicaid and the Uninsured, 2005).

The search to produce access has begged the question of a defined standard in health care and has focused almost irrationally on cost. Hospitals were targeted as the major offender, given their association with high-tech and aggressive and defensive diagnostics and therapeutics. Rather than searching for programmatic options that promise a better use of resources, the years since 1982 (beginning of the Medicare hospital prospective payment system) have held a flurry of public policy activities with the obvious goal of preserving the status quo in the health care industry to whatever extent possible. Antics included reducing reimbursement for services to the poor so far below cost that few providers would care for them, increasing the copayments and deductibles under Medicare to the extent that seniors pay more out-of-pocket today than before the program was established, and cross-subsidizing public entitlement programs and the medically indigent through private sector payers, a practice that has since been declared illegal in many states. Over the years, generations of statistical equations have been developed (DRGs, CPTs, RBRVSs, RUGs, MDS, MDS2, MDS+, OASIS, HHRG) with the ultimate goal of controlling cost through the prediction of resource use by case mix methodology. Each of these case mix methodologies has been gamed by the industry. Americans continue to pursue technical solutions to political problems. Some of the most hopeful programmatic redesigns have surfaced from private sector: home respite services to ease caregiver burden, case management, a focus on self-care, sensitivity to consumer preference, and seamless programs that give individuals access to all services through a single point of entry. These eventually became part of public entitlement programs but can trace their roots to private sector.

Despite final defeat in the fall of 1994, the Health Security Act of 1993 served as a landmark and a wake-up call for the public conscience. The bill included many of the programs that since have offered some response to public discontent. Clear distinctions between levels of care are becoming common: intensivist, critical care, acute, subacute, skilled, intermediate, custodial, ambulatory, home care, independent, and assisted living. Assisted-living programs with a broad range of on-site and in-home services are popular and gradually are becoming an integral part of public entitlement programs. The Health Security Act bill also proposed movement away from the medical model and toward functional ability as a major indicator for defining the need for home care services. Broader definitions of home and community care included companion and chore services. In its vision this bill was often brilliant, even if its process was politically naive.

HOME CARE INDUSTRY

A definable sequence of events over the past 40 years has shaped modern home care and generated the dilemmas this segment of the industry faces today. Titles 18 and 19 of the Social Security Acts created Medicare and Medicaid. Within those entitlements home care was recognized as reimbursable, but not at first mandatory. Subsequent legislation in 1971 made home health services mandatory as a covered benefit under these programs, in 1972 expanded service to the disabled, and in 1978 expanded service to patients with end-stage renal disease. Elimination of the prior hospitalization requirement and a more flexible redefinition of the term *homebound* followed over time and brought home care into its own. The Medicare hospital prospective payment system of 1982 heightened the use of this segment of the industry. Incentives were offered to hospitals for the early discharge of patients. Referral to home care was the natural consequence.

Certified home health agencies vary in their structures, sponsorship, and auspices. The major types of agencies are the Visiting Nurse Associations (freestanding, nonprofit), public agencies (governmental), hospital-based (operating unit of a hospital), and proprietary agencies (freestanding, for-profit). In 2003, Visiting Nurse Associations numbered 439 and represented about 6% of all agencies, whereas public home health agencies numbered 888 for about 12% of the national total. Visiting Nurse Associations and public agencies have experienced significant decline in recent years. In 1975, they were 23% and 55% of the home care market, respectively. Freestanding proprietary (47%) and hospital-based agencies (24%) have grown the most in recent years, until 1998 when all of these traditional agency types showed a decline (National Association for Home Care, 2001) (Table 18-1).

Home care agencies depend on governmental funding, with almost 61% of revenue coming from Medicare (32%) and Medicaid and other local and state government funds (29%) in 1996 (National Association for Home Care, 2001) (Table 18-2).

Subsequently the Balanced Budget Act of 1997 imposed new restrictions designed to reduce the growth in Medicare home care expenditures. An interim payment system created new beneficiary limits and caused a 34% decrease in Medicare spending for home care during the fiscal years of 1998 to 2000 (National Association for Home Care, 2001). The Balanced Budget Act rules and regulations further decimated the home care industry by designating 1994 as the base

TABLE 18-1

Number of Medicare-Certified Home Care Agencies by Auspice, for School Years 1967-2000

Year	Freestanding Agencies							Facility-Based Agencies		TOTAL
	VNA	COMB	PUB	PROP	PNP	OTH	HOSP	REHAB	SNF	
1967	549	93	939	0	0	39	133	0	0	1,753
1975	525	46	1,228	47	0	109	273	9	5	2,242
1980	515	63	1,260	186	484	40	359	8	9	2,924
1985	514	59	1,205	1,943	832	4	1,277	20	129	5,983
1990	474	47	985	1,884	710	0	1,486	8	101	5,695
1991	476	41	941	1,970	701	0	1,537	9	105	5,780
1992	530	52	1,083	1,962	637	28	1,623	3	86	6,004
1993	594	46	1,196	2,146	558	41	1,809	1	106	6,497
1994	586	45	1,146	2,892	597	48	2,081	3	123	7,521
1995	575	40	1,182	3,951	667	65	2,470	4	166	9,120
1996	576	34	1,177	4,658	695	58	2,634	4	191	10,027
1997	553	33	1,149	5,024	715	65	2,698	3	204	10,444
1998	460	35	968	3,414	610	69	2,356	2	166	8,080
1999	452	35	918	3,192	621	65	2,300	1	163	7,747
2000	436	31	909	2,863	560	56	2,151	1	150	7,157

From Centers for Medicare & Medicaid Services, Center for Information Systems, Health Standards and Quality Bureau. Retrieved January, 2004, from http://www.cms.hhs.gov/researchers.

MB, Combination agencies are combined government and voluntary agencies. These agencies are sometimes included with counts for VNAs.

HOSP, Hospital-based agencies are operating units or departments of a hospital. Agencies that have working arrangements with a hospital, or perhaps even owned by a hospital but operated as separate entities, are classified as freestanding agencies under one of the other categories.

OTH, Other freestanding agencies that do not fit one of the other categories for freestanding agencies.

PNP, Private not-for-profit agencies are freestanding and are privately developed, governed, and owned nonprofit home care agencies. These agencies were not counted separately before 1980.

PROP, Proprietary agencies are freestanding, for-profit home care agencies.

PUB, Public agencies are government agencies operated by a state, county, city, or other unit of local government having a major responsibility for preventing disease and for community health education.

REHAB, These are agencies based in rehabilitation facilities.

SNF, These are agencies based in skilled nursing facilities.

VNA, Visiting Nurse Associations are freestanding, voluntary, nonprofit organizations governed by a board of directors and usually financed by tax-deductible contributions and by earnings.

TABLE 18-2

Sources of Payment for Home Health Care, 2002 and 2003*

Source of Payment	2002 Amount (in billions)	Percent of Total	2003 Amount (in billions)	Percent of Total
Total	$36.1	100.0	$38.3	100.0
Medicare	$11.4	31.6	$12.2	31.9
Medicaid[†]	$4.8	13.3	$5.1	13.3
State and local governments[‡]	$5.7	15.8	$6.0	15.7
Private insurance	$6.7	18.6	$6.9	18.0
Out-of-pocket	$6.5	18.0	$6.9	18.0
Other	$1.1	3.0	$1.1	2.9

From Centers for Medicare & Medicaid Services, Office of the Actuary, National Health Care Expenditures, 1990-2012. (February 2004).

*Data for 2003 is projected. Percentages may not total to 100.0% because of rounding.

[†]Medicaid figures do not include expenditures for non-health services (i.e., personal support services). They represent only the federal share of Medicaid.

[‡]State and local governments include state portion of Medicaid.

year for rate setting, turning back the clock to a period when cost-consciousness was less common among home health agencies. Meanwhile, those agencies that had begun to monitor costs and institute efficiencies early on were penalized for their good business practices. This entire regulatory scene limited the profitability of home care and created a situation in which care was given to public entitlement recipients at a price less than cost. The severest effects of the Balanced Budget Act fell on the sickest and highest-cost patients, in fact forcing them to opt for higher-cost skilled nursing facilities or hospital care (Mackin & Forester, 1999). And the future bodes no better circumstances as home care is costed on a prospective payment system model with OASIS (Outcome and Assessment Information Set) as the clinical data set and the HHRG (Home Health Resource Group) as the case mix methodology. Being more optimistic, the best hope for the industry may be the prospective payment system with its capitated rates. Such arrangements could provide the opportunity to distance home care from the medical model, allowing dollars to be used for personal assistance to normalize living. Whether offered through managed care or case mix methodology, packages of services would be integrated and financially bundled, hopefully allowing the agency or the case manager to make decisions that are personalized and hold the best promise for quality of life (Landi et al., 1999). Economic survival and quality of life can coexist peacefully only where providers have the freedom to be creative in partnership with the recipient of services, new technologies are called into play to improve the human condition, and atypical support systems are encouraged when they contribute to the desired outcomes. This flexibility will require not only a change in reimbursement strategies but also a major reformation of public policy.

Despite a great dependency on public dollars, those dollars have not been extensive. In 2003, freestanding home health services accounted for only 3% of total personal health expenditures in this country, whereas hospital and clinical services offered by physicians and other providers was 61%. One should note that hospital-based home care is included with hospital expenditures (Heffler et al., 2004). The number of Medicaid home care recipients has continued to increase steadily, whereas Medicare numbers only began to rebound slowly in 2001 (National Association for Home Care, 2001).

By 1998, 90% of home care agencies were estimated to have costs that exceeded revenue by 32% for services to Medicaid recipients. Visiting Nurse Associations and hospital-based agencies were the most dependent on government funds, with 80% of their revenues coming from this source. In comparison, only 55% of the revenue of for-profit organizations came from public entitlements. In fact, since the Balanced Budget Act, the number of Medicare clients served through home care and the number of visits per Medicare client have decreased, while this population has increased in skilled nursing and subacute facilities. Whereas between 1996 and 2000 the number of Medicaid recipients receiving home care has more than doubled (National Association for Home Care, 2001).

These figures are important and allow us to make some predictions about the future of home care. Medicare serves clients with episodic problems, where there is a need for skilled nursing services and the client is expected to return to self-care through rehabilitative efforts. Many potential Medicare home care recipients have been redirected into nursing homes, rehabilitation facilities, and subacute care, where treatment can be more vigorous and progress monitored more closely. If the Medicare home care market continues to be overshadowed by Medicaid growth, long-term patients will dominate the market.

This situation would be the natural course of events; however, consumer preferences are poised to intervene. The American Association of Retired Persons is moving forward briskly in support of public entitlement programs where "money follows the person," as opposed to the "person following the money." Opinion polls of the American Association of Retired Persons membership show that most elderly Americans prefer to age in place, spending their declining years in their own homes, if the services and dollars to do so are available. Data on appropriation of state Medicaid monies are not readily available, but taking New Jersey as an example, in 2002 almost 85% of public long-term care dollars went to nursing homes contrasted with about 15% to home care and community-based services. Though this distinction is startling, it represents progress from 1997 when nursing homes received almost 93% and community services slightly more than 7% (Auerbach, 2004).

Progress has been incremental but deliberate and state based. Policy changes include fast-track processing of clients for home care and community service eligibility and a single entry point for institutional and community-based services (Washington and Colorado); options-based counseling that reveals all of the choices open to a client and supports their personal decisions (Wisconsin); a global budget holding funds for community and institutional care to minimize governmental competition, and cash given directly to the consumer in lieu of services, allowing more flexibility in the choices needed for community living (Oregon); and senior foster care and counseling to help nursing home residents to transition back to the community (New Jersey). Arkansas, Florida, and New Jersey have been part of a Cash and Counseling Demonstration Program that provides Medicaid recipients with a cash allowance based on the need for community or home care along with assistance to manage these funds. A control group receives traditional Medicaid services. Preliminary results show a much higher satisfaction with the overall care arrangements in the experimental group compared with how individuals in the control group were spending their lives. The Independent Choices Program in Oregon is comparable, except that it assumes that the participants have the ability to manage their own finances without a fiscal intermediary. Similar strategies have been implemented in Texas, Arizona, Vermont, and Michigan (Auerbach, 2004). These are only a few of the programs that promise a robust future for home care but require the design of new products and services and an active role for home care advocates in lobbying the legislature and educating the government and the consumer about what is possible. A Money Follows the Person Rebalancing Initiative is pending before the current Congress and has been included in the President's 2005 budget.

The caregivers in home care are formal and informal. Unpaid help, especially family members, are the backbone of home care in the United States. Because the Bureau of Labor Statistics and the Centers for Medicare and Medicaid Services count workers in different ways, much of the data is imprecise. However, the general nature of the workforce and the inevitable problems are clear. The largest numbers of workers are home care aides and registered nurses. Between 1998 and 2002 the numbers of full-time equivalent home care aides decreased by 35%. The Centers for Medicare and Medicaid Services records a decrease of 156,394 full-time equivalents in home care personnel from December 1997 to December 2003. In summary, a workforce growth of 8.7% annually from 1993 to 1997 was followed by an overall decline of 10% from 1997 to 2000 (National Association for Home Care, 2001).

The profile of the home health aide is remarkably consistent. Studies describe a middle-aged female, disproportionately minority workforce with low education, low pay, and a high degree of part-time employment. No consistent federal rule exists for the education of home health aides comparable with the standard that exists for nursing assistants in skilled nursing facilities,

and requirements vary from state to state. Whereas registered nurses once were more highly paid in home care than in hospital nursing, this is not the current case. However, registered nurses have always expressed particular satisfaction with the high degree of professional autonomy in home care practice.

The case for home care often is based on arguments of cost-effectiveness. The hospital per diem charge or subacute/skilled nursing daily rate is compared with the charge for a home visit. This logic is specious, given the fact that these are not comparable services. However, specific clinical situations have been analyzed carefully and inclusively and have been found to be particularly suited to home care. These situations include low-birth-weight babies, ventilator-dependent adults, oxygen-dependent children, chemotherapy in children, intravenously administered antibiotics for osteomyelitis and cellulitis, congestive heart failure, and psychiatric care. In these situations, significant dollar savings occurred by moving treatment to the home, or more expensive institutional care was shortened or readmissions were averted when home care was provided.

THE ISSUES

The issues in home care do not stand alone but are affected immensely by other aspects of the health care industry and consumer choice.

Whether movement of health care services into the community is a response to the declining use of hospitals or primarily is due to other factors, it is a trend that seems irreversible. The hospital length of stay continues to decrease, but at a slower pace: 1996 (5.5 days), 1997 (5.3), 1998 (5.3), 2002 (4.9) (National Center for Health Statistics, 2004). Even when hospital-based subacute care is factored into the calculations, only a modest increase in the length of stay and a continuing pattern of decline occur.

Community-based service in the form of home care and the public health have long and proud traditions. These services are not newcomers but took on new significance with the social pressure to curtail cost, and they favor those service settings that seem to be less expensive. Some original presumptions have proved to be naive. Where medical intensity is great or functional ability is so seriously compromised as to require continuous care, home care can be costly. Subacute care has appeared to fill some of these gaps. At the other end of the spectrum, the less needy have chosen assisted living, which does not always eliminate the presence of home care. With these new levels of care as options, the arguments for personal choice and humane and compassionate care are gaining in prominence. Home care is best suited to reinforce and complement the care provided by family, friends, and community resources. It can be the optimum venue for the preservation of dignity and independence. The home continues to be the best place to maintain control over one's own care.

Confusion over roles and responsibilities will be part of any transition from the medical to a social model. New patterns of accountability and authority are not only inevitable but also necessary to do the most with the least for the most needy. And this seems to be the manner in which public policy is reshaping this segment of the industry. Questions will arise about who has the right to authorize services; where the quality controls are, and how quality will be defined; and who is responsible for the practice of nonprofessionals who provide 80% of the hands-on care. Note that this percentage may decrease if more skilled nursing patients choose subacute options in hospitals and nursing homes. Most especially, the supervisory issues around home health aides have become public and frightening.

Nursing has long dominated the home care scene. The roots of many of the most illustrious leaders can be traced to home care. The home often has been touted as the setting that provides the best showcase for nursing practice: autonomy, equality, and respect. The pioneering home care agencies were nurse managed and nurse controlled and were built on a social model that went far beyond the diagnosis and treatment of illness. Can this tradition be recaptured and sustained as home care responds to governmental policy and public preference?

The wild card in the equation continues to be the consumer, or just as often consumer advocates. Consumerism has become militant, and the reaction is no longer new or unexpected. Recipients of care have become uncomfortable with deferring to professionals. The historic practice of "protecting the public from themselves" has been seriously called into question as consumers have access to more information. Direct access to diagnostics and therapeutics is growing. Consumer satisfaction and dissatisfaction as expressed to insurers, particularly in managed care plans, are a driving determinant in who does what and which providers and facilities will be included in a network. The goodwill of plan members is necessary if they are to continue their subscriptions. Medicaid is moving rapidly toward managed care through state waiver programs; Medicare is moving at a slower but deliberate pace.

Chiefly deriving from consumers and their advocates, a broad definition of home care is becoming popular and is receiving much favor in managed care plans where functional ability and quality of life can be addressed with more latitude. Case management is a natural complement to this "social" approach, monitoring abuses and educating the recipient of care to the pros and cons of choices. In 1993 the President's recommendations to the Congress for long-term care entitlements included personal assistance provided to persons with functional impairment where they live, where they recreate, where they work, and where they do business. The intent was to normalize life through personal assistance suited to the preference of the individual (White House Domestic Policy Council, 1993). The extreme application of this principle to nursing homes could involve separating personal care and nursing services from nontherapeutic and hotel services so that the client or client's agent, usually the family, may choose what suits the client best, thereby controlling resources—the ultimate weapon. It suffices to know that this broader vision of home care and in-home services exists, has been proposed for public policy, and enjoys growing support.

Issues of Control

As the home and community become the prevailing sites for care, the control of the medical establishment declines, and this includes nurses. Some may say that consumer demand for more control was the catalyst in this reformation and not its by-product. Consumer allegations of forced dependence on entering the health care system and frequent distrust of provider professionals should have been an anticipated consequence of specialization and high technology. As the personal relationship between the provider and patient began to erode, and the vulnerable easily came to feel victimized.

The position of the consumer is strengthened further by the growing trend to have public entitlement recipients (Medicare, Medicaid, Tricare, and the Federal Employees' Health Benefit Plan) use their resources to "buy" into a managed care plan of their choice. This ability to choose is compromised where managed care plans may be designed primarily for the poor, and choice often is limited to providers and facilities that cannot attract a middle class or private payer client base. To avoid this situation, many state laws require that plan subscribers must include a mix of Medicaid and non-Medicaid recipients.

Discussion inevitably leads to issues of "turf protection," and the public patience has worn thin on this topic. A medicalized system has concentrated services in settings where the balance of power weighs in the direction of the industry and provider professionals.

Public dissatisfaction with this paradigm was slow coming, but long building. The issue is who defines the nature and context of services? The Agency for Healthcare Research and Quality (formerly Agency for Health Care Policy and Research), the Patients' Bill of Rights, Final Directives, and the Patient Protection Bill are examples of public policy intended to guarantee the ability of consumers to make their own informed choices. The dramatic growth of the complementary health market is another consumer strategy to avoid medicalization. Though the migration to home care was motivated primarily by cost, what it will be is based on public preference.

The frail and chronically ill have been the major recipients of home care, and they frequently have been poor. Today they are joined by those in a recuperative mode, who are in a position to demand more and different services including having access to more personal resources, private insurance, and workplace benefits. In addition, younger disabled persons object to the terms *home* and *care* because of the connotations that have become associated with them in this society. They prefer to reserve the term *care* for relationships of intimacy and affection and note that assistive services should not be limited to the home in the usual sense of the word. Rather, services that allow one to maintain a home in the community should help one to live and to flourish wherever that is. Rather than promoting a "caring in place" philosophy, services should follow a person from the home to places where one can be productive, recreate, socialize, or do business such as it is. Advocates of the disabled, this often younger and more militant constituency contends that the recipient of services should be able to select those in an assistive capacity to them and decide whether family is an option. This is contrary to the traditional view, which bases the authorization of services on the potential for rehabilitation or the need for skilled nursing as determined by professionals. The expanded definition of *homebound* was a breakthrough, but rigid interpretation still prevails. More latitude has been observed in state-funded or Medicaid waiver programs where personal assistance and functional impairment are the priority. This also has been the response in programs created to substitute for nursing home confinement.

The ability of home care personnel to provide some rather technically complex care and the frequency and immediacy of supervision, if any, are controversial issues. Many arguments for the increased use of nonprofessional personnel hinge on the ability of the disabled to direct their own care, thereby maintaining control.

One such situation is the creation of a category of worker called the home care medication aide. The proposal is that the medication aide should be able only to help cognitively intact home care patients who are able to recognize their medications and understand their use and side effects. Other controversy focuses on the delegation of specific activities by the professional, notably the nurse. In Oregon, non-nurses may perform nursing functions if they have been taught by a nurse on a patient-specific and procedure-specific basis (Oregon Department of Human Services, 2005).

THE DEBATE

Statement: The recipients of in-home services should have increased autonomy, flexibility, and commensurate responsibility in making determinations about their care.

Pro

The medical model is increasingly out of step with the restructuring delivery system. Primary health care, integrated systems, and community-based services begin to move toward a new paradigm that values self-care, personal responsibility, prudence in resource use, and increased commitment to the common good, the true test of community. The frail elderly, one major market for in-home services, are most concerned with functionality and their perception of their own health than they are with illness. Illness only becomes a priority when it gets in the way of living. The Clinton administration report on health care reform in 1993 recommended eligibility for assisted-living arrangements and home health services based on measurable functional impairments as opposed to medically defined problems and a shift to personal, client-directed care with the standard being that the persons providing service, to the extent possible, be selected, trained, supervised, and evaluated by the recipient (White House Domestic Policy Council, 1993). This same flavor is present in the more recent restructuring of long-term care discussed previously, home care being one dimension.

Realistically, a fence may have to be put around the liberties and choices allowed within the context of home care, especially where public dollars are used. A cap on the total amount of funding available in a preestablished period is one approach. Caution would have to be taken that inadequate funding does not violate the spirit of flexibility and choice. Withholding funding is a common backdoor strategy to reach a goal without the unpleasant policy decisions that would be required with a more forthright approach. Examples abound, but two should suffice, given their familiarity to the reader. Few if any restrictions are placed on the services provided to Medicaid recipients. However, the fees paid to the provider are so low that few providers accept these patients. Abortion is legal, but the poor are denied the public dollars to access the procedure.

The tough policy decisions to allow the consumer to retain maximum control will be slow in coming. The first challenge requires the honesty to separate the control and funding aspects. Though only a finite number of dollars may be available to an individual, allowing decisions about the use of those dollars could honor the spirit of consumer choice. Allowing flexibility may lead to some creative options. Pooling resources in a setting such as a group residential home may pay for more services and consequently more freedom; for the more acutely ill or those recovering from acute illness, fluid movement between levels of care including the home, can be within a predetermined spending cap. This could be accomplished through managed care plans with the proper policies and benefit structure. In many ways, this is the broader application of the "true" hospice concept. The consumer most comfortably makes these decisions if case management, at best independent case management, supports them. A case manager engaged by the payer could be subject to conflict of interest: the need to hold a job versus advocate for the client.

Con

Consumer militancy and the growing political influence of the elderly and younger disabled persons has led to a gradual restructuring of home care to distance it from the mainstream of health care, broaden the definition of home care and in-home assistance, and increase consumer's right to engage and dismiss services.

A first wave of consumerism predated the dramatic onslaught of acute and subacute clinical situations into the home. With the appearance of this new clinical population in the home, more justification appeared for medicalization. Physicians who once abandoned home practice are returning to that setting, some out of economic motivation and others as a response to consumer need. The federal government has approved Medicare reimbursement to physicians for their supervision of the medical regimen in home care, based on the observation that much of home care has become so medically dependent that close supervision is not only justified but also necessary.

Putting aside the apparent medical needs in home care, there remain the chronically ill, frail, and disabled. These populations traditionally have used significant amounts of nonprofessional and assistive services in the home. Surveys indicate that home health agencies rely on part-time, temporary workers and have been assigning heavier case loads with resultant alienation of the workforce. A high turnover rate is common among home health aides and can lead to a lack of reliability and inconsistency of services. Observable quality of care problems follow, such as incomplete work, inadequate skills even for simple activities, failure to carry out orders, client injury or abuse, exploitation of the client, theft, and absenteeism. Given the frequency of such incidents and the basic vulnerability of many home care recipients, closer professional controls can be justified. Little state-to-state consistency exists in maintaining records on disciplinary actions, requiring criminal background checks, or imposing any standard for training or competency testing of home health aides.

Despite the outcry for consumer empowerment, the American public has always found comfort in the medical establishment and the assurance that professionals would act in their best interest. A clear distinction in home care exists between those situations where medical necessity drives the use of resources and others where functional ability and basic services to compensate for functional deficits are needed. Just such a distinction differentiated Medicare and Medicaid, episodic versus continuing care. Whether these distinctions should be perpetuated and how they should, if at all, be recognized in the process of authorizing services for the public is a serious question, more rooted in philosophy than financial expedience.

BEYOND DEBATE

Home care, not unlike other segments of the health care industry, is experiencing a struggle over "consumer control and choice": the definitions to describe it, the public policy to allow it, the dollars to fund it, the economic models to distribute those dollars, and the provider systems to actually make it happen. And this observation forces many issues:

◆ What are the appropriate criteria for maintaining a patient in the home, putting aside economic motivation?

◆ To what extent should providers and consumers be able to exercise choice in the selection of a setting for care?

◆ How appropriate is the medical model to the home care population?

◆ If home care is a cost-efficient proxy for the hospital or nursing home, how is the break-even point identified and what happens once it is reached?

- Does the consumer have the option to choose home care regardless of cost, or only as the less costly option?
- Who is responsible for the supervision of volunteers in the home, including family members, if they undertake medical or nursing activities?
- Are family members supervised or are they the supervisors?
- To what extent can activities be delegated?
- The expanded use of volunteers and family caregivers raises questions of caregiver burden and new categories of reimbursable services, either through dollars paid or tax credits allowed?
- The many relatively unskilled in-home services create a market for new categories of work: such as companion care and chore care. Who supervises this work? This list is not exhaustive.

SUMMARY

The dispute over turf ownership in home care or any sector of health care pits the consumer against the government and its agents, the industry, and the professions. Slowly over time home care and in-home services are moving to a functional/social model that is more suitable to the needs of some, whereas a large constituency of the acutely ill have a real need for continuing medical expertise in the home and are confronted with decisions beyond the capability of most laypeople. The challenge will be to see the distinctions and accommodate them. This was the original premise for the division between the Medicare and Medicaid populations. So there may be something nurses can learn from past practice, including when past practice has outlived its usefulness.

REFERENCES

Auerbach, R. (2004, March). *Rebalancing long term care in New Jersey.* Portland, OR: Auerbach Consulting, Inc. Unpublished manuscript.

Heffler, S., Smith, S., Keehan, S., Clemens, M. K., Zezza, M., & Truffer, C. (2004). Health spending projections through 2013. *Health Affairs.* Retrieved February 27, 2005, from http://content.healthaffairs.org/cgi/reprint/hlthaff.w4.79v1

Joel, L. (2003). *Kelly's dimensions of professional nursing* (9th ed). New York: McGraw-Hill.

Kaiser Commission on Medicaid and the Unisured. (2004). *The uninsured: A primer.* Retrieved February 22, 2005, http://www.kff.org/uninsured/7216.cfm

Kling, B. (2001). *Telehealth as an everyday tool.* Paper presented at the 2001 Symposium NLM National Telemedicine Initiative: Telemedicine and Telecommunications: Options for the New Century. Retrieved January 10, 2005, from http://collab.nlm.nih.gov/tutorialspublicationsandmaterials/Telesymposiumcd/1-1.pdf

Landi, F., Gambassi, G., Pola, R., Tabaccanti, S., Cavinato, T., Carbonin, P. U., et al. (1999). Impact of integrated home care services on hospital use. *Journal of the American Geriatric Society, 47*(12), 1430-1434.

Mackin, A. L., & Forester, T. M. (1999). Home health at the crossroads. *Caring, 18*(9), 12-13, 15.

National Association for Home Care. (2001). *Basic statistics about home care.* Retrieved January 10, 2005, from http://nahc.org/Consumer/hcstats.html

National Center for Health Statistics. (2004). *Hospital utilization (in non-Federal short-stay hospitals).* Retrieved March 1, 2005, from http://www.cdc.gov/nchs/fastats/hospital.htm

Oregon Department of Human Services. Oregon Health Plan, 2005. Retrieved October 18, 2005, from http//www.dhs.state.or.us/healthplan/overview.html

Senge, P. (1990). *The fifth discipline: The art and practice of the learning organization.* New York: Doubleday Currency.

White House Domestic Policy Council. (1993). *The President's health security plan.* New York: Times Books.

Adult Health Medical-Surgical Nursing Practice

Recent Changes and Current Issues

CECELIA GATSON GRINDEL ◆ NOEL KERR

Within the complex health care environment, many forces affect the practice of adult health nursing. Universal issues initiate intraagency dynamics within a variety of practice settings that complicate the achievement of goals for a healthier America. An aging population living with chronic illness creates the backdrop of the need for rapid change and attainment of solutions. Other universal issues such as the nursing shortage, an aging nursing workforce, a mandate for patient safety initiatives, and a lack of leadership complicate the challenges to provide quality patient care. This chapter explores the interrelationships of these universal and intraagency issues and their impact on the practice of adult health nursing. The ultimate goal is to provoke discussion and problem solving among nursing and other health care professionals who shoulder the burden of these issues.

THE AGING POPULATION

The reality of the aging population in the United States is not news. However, a closer look at these statistics give some perspective of the health care needs of the future and the impact those needs will have on the need for health care services. In the year 2000 the number of citizens age 65 or over was approximately 35 million (12.6% of the population); those 85 years or older numbered approximately 3 million. Projections for 2030 suggest that the 65 years and older population will reach more than 70 million, whereas the 85 years and older group will double, reaching approximately 6 million citizens. Although a large majority of those over age 65 report good to excellent health (Federal Interagency Forum on Aging Related Statistics, 2004), their health care needs will increase and the demand for adult health nurses will grow as primary health and acute patient care services are needed by these elders.

Exploring mortality and morbidity statistics provides insight into the future health care needs of the elderly. The leading causes of death among those 65 years and older in 2000 included heart disease, cancer, cerebrovascular disease, chronic lower respiratory diseases, influenza, pneumonia, and diabetes mellitus. Technologies and advances in pharmaceutical agents have improved patient outcomes for cardiovascular disease mortality, whereas the death rates for the other diseases have remained relatively stable over the last 2 decades. However, the elderly frequently encounter chronic illness. Using data from 2001-2002, the Centers for Disease Control and Prevention reported on the percentage of those age 65 years and older who had specific chronic diseases. Leading the list of these diseases were hypertension, arthritis, heart disease, and cancer. Reports of difficulty in performing certain physical tasks increased after age 65. Moderate or severe memory impairment increases with age, and approximately 32% of those 85 years and older are limited by mental impairment (Federal Interagency Forum on Aging Related Statistics, 2004). An increasing need for health care resources, including the services of adult health nurses, will be required to meet the demand for care for the ever-growing elderly population.

NURSING SHORTAGE

Several factors influence the nursing shortage. Most notable are the aging workforce and the many and varied career options for young men and women. Associated with these career options are working conditions that do not include working weekends, holidays, and night shifts. The nursing shortage is a public issue. Media and legislative attention has been given to this ongoing and ever-intensifying crisis. As a result, schools of nursing have seen increased enrollment limited only by the shortage of nursing faculty and clinical nursing instructors and sufficient resources for clinical experiences. Even with legislative and media attention that has drawn more applicants into nursing programs, evidence suggests that the current nursing shortage will continue to be a significant factor well into the future.

Aging Workforce

Amid financial constraints in health care, hospital restructuring, work redesign, and recruitment and retention issues, the aging of the nursing workforce (including those in academic roles) has contributed to the escalating shortage of nurses. The nursing workforce is projected to peak at 2.3 million in 2012 and shrink to 2.2 million by 2020 when the Health Resources and Services Administration forecasts a need of 2.8 million registered nurses in the workforce (Steefel, 2004). A factor contributing to this impending crisis in the United States will be the retirement of a large number of nurses. The average age of today's nurse is 46 years, with the age of nursing faculty averaging 54 years. After many years of dedication to the nursing profession, these nurses will leave the workforce to enjoy the pleasures of retirement. Currently, nurses under 30 years of age account for approximately 30% of the nursing workforce, a decline of about 40% since 1980 (Buerhaus, Staiger, & Auerbach, 2000). This percentage of younger nurses will need to be bolstered by greater numbers of new nurses to offset the expected deficit. Because medical-surgical nursing is the largest specialty in nursing, adults in need of nursing care will be most affected by this deficit.

Recruitment and Retention

Since 2001 an increase of 185,000 hospital-employed nurses has been realized, yet this increase has not eliminated the current nursing shortage (Buerhaus, Staiger, & Auerbach, 2004a). Supporting this reality are the results of two recent national surveys of registered nurses and physicians conducted in 2004. Researchers found that a clear majority of these nurses (82%) and doctors (81%) perceived shortages of registered nurses in the hospitals in which they worked (Buerhaus et al., 2004b; Konelan et al., 2004).

Buerhaus et al. (2004a) examined the demographics of new nurses entering the workforce in 2003. A significant number of these new nurses were older women

and to a lesser extent, foreign-born registered nurses. Two new demographic groups also joined this workforce: younger individuals, particularly women in their early 30s, and men.

The real challenge with recruitment lies in attracting young persons who are committed to providing care to individuals, families, and communities. Currently, applicants come into nursing seeking a career that offers job security. However appealing job security is, the desire to care for others should be the attraction of nursing. Clearly the nursing profession fails to market the exciting challenges of providing care, problem solving patient care issues, leading change that enhances patient outcomes and using lifesaving technologies to monitor patients' progress. Rather, nurses talk about working holidays and weekends, nursing shortages, heavy workloads, and poor management. This picture of the nursing workplace surely will not draw dynamic young men and women to the nursing profession.

Private-sector initiatives have resulted in strong registered nurse employment growth over the last few years (Buerhaus et al., 2004a). Although these initiatives have been effective, a sustained effort to attract men and women into the nursing profession must be achieved. Employment opportunities in the developing world of technology, international business, marketing, and many other professional fields are endless. The challenge is to create a vision of nursing as a profession that is stimulating and challenging, offering opportunities for professional growth and development and personal satisfaction. Reaching out to young children to share this vision is essential for stimulating future interest in nursing.

Decreasing Employer Loyalty

The trend toward outsourcing for services and away from employer loyalty (Shaffer, 2000) was inspired by the large-scale corporate downsizing of the late 1980s that provided the impetus for a "guerilla" workforce comprised of deal-hungry professionals conditioned to signing bonuses, stock options, and higher-than-scale salaries. Over the last decade, the intensifying nursing shortage has created a highly competitive and lucrative market for new graduate nurses. Employers eager to fill open positions have resorted to offering huge sign-on bonuses and creative benefit packages to attract applicants from a pool of potential employees that is inadequate to meet staffing needs regionally or nationally. Employers lose out when new graduate nurses "game" the system by accepting positions; receiving incentives, bonuses, and initial orientation and training; and then leaving after 1 year only to obtain employment with another employer willing to provide similar incentives. New graduate nurses entering the workforce today expect to be "courted" by clinical agencies.

Until recently, clinical agencies have focused on recruitment of nurses rather than retention of their experienced staff. Significant sign-on and retention bonuses are being offered to lure new graduates and experienced nurses to employment sites. Most agencies have come to realize that an experienced nursing staff is invaluable and thus have initiated strategies to retain these knowledgeable and committed nurses. Many have implemented strategies to create and maintain a positive workplace environment, which is key ingredient for the retention of experienced nurses. These trends inadvertently have created a trend away from employer loyalty where the employer is valued only for the short-term financial gains offered the new employee rather than the long-term benefits and opportunity to grow in a mentorship environment.

Travel nursing also contributes to a sense of decreased employer loyalty. Agencies desperate for nursing services contract with travel nurses to employ registered nurses for 3 to 6 months at a time. Travel nursing has become such an accepted phenomenon that professional journals devote specific sections or supplements to the interests and needs of the traveling nurse and the employers who hire them. For many, travel nursing is an attractive option. "Travelers" make more money, have the flexibility of setting their own schedule, enjoy the alternatives to the traditional 8-hour shift, and like being removed from the distractions of policy committees and other ancillary projects (Ostroski, 2004). At the same time they have no long-term commitment to the employing agency nor the community that it serves.

PATIENT SAFETY, PATIENT OUTCOMES, AND THE WORKPLACE ENVIRONMENT

Much has been written about patient safety and outcomes in recent years. Although some improvements have been made in the last decade, barriers to adequate and effective change toward enhanced patient safety and outcomes in the environment are numerous. These barriers include a punitive environment in hospitals, physicians' denial of the scope of the problem, a lack of national leadership to effect change, and a lack of systems thinking (Buerhaus et al., 2004b). A health care delivery system that is decentralized and fragmented also contributes to unsafe conditions for patients (Kohn, Corrigan, & Donaldson, 2000). Threats to patient safety emerge from organizational management practices, workforce deployment practices, work design, and organizational culture (Institute of Medincine, 2004).

The primary role of adult health nurses is to provide quality care that results in positive patient outcomes. Evidence that supports the relationship of nursing care to patient outcomes is documented in the literature. Researchers (Kahn et al., 1990; Mitchell & Shortell, 1997; Rubenstein, Chang, Keeler, & Kahn, 1992) have noted that better patient outcomes are related directly to nursing actions such as ongoing patient monitoring. Yet obstacles such as staffing, entry-into-nursing education, and increased workloads limit patient safety and positive outcomes. In an international study in adult acute care hospitals in the United States, Canada, England, and Scotland, researchers Aiken, Clarke, Sloane, and the International Hospital Outcomes Research Consortium (2002) found that organizational/managerial support for nursing had a profound effect on nurse satisfaction. In addition, organization support for nursing and nurse staffing were related directly to nurse-assessed quality of care. These researchers concluded that key elements to improving quality patient care, diminishing nurse job dissatisfaction and burnout, and improving nurse retention in hospitals include adequate nurse staffing and organizational/managerial support for nursing.

The workload of the adult health nurse has been affected acutely by the nursing shortage and the increase in patient condition severity. As a result, patient safety is threatened by factors such as inadequate nurse staffing, high patient-to-nurse ratios, and extended working hours. In a study that explored nurse-to-patient ratios in 168 adult general hospitals in Pennsylvania, Aiken, Clarke, Sloane, Sochalski, and Silber (2002) determined that an additional patient per nurse was associated with a 7% increase in the likelihood of dying within 30 days of admission and a 7% increase in the odds of failure to rescue, after adjusting for patient and hospital characteristics. In addition, each additional patient per nurse was associated with a 23% increase of the odds of burnout and a 15% increase in the odds of job dissatisfaction. Extended working hours also affect patient safety. Rogers, Hwang, Scott, Aiken, and Dinges (2004) concluded that the risks of making errors were significantly increased when work shifts were longer than 12 hours, when nurses worked overtime, or when they worked more than 40 hours per week.

In 1999, California became the first state in the United States to require mandatory safe licensed nurse-to-patient ratios in all units of acute care facilities

(Shindul-Rosthschild et al., 2003) at a time when no evidence for a specific minimum nurse-to-patient ratio in acute care hospitals existed (Lang, Hodge, Olson, Romano, and Kravitz, 2004). More recent research suggests that a range of four to six patients per nurse in the acute care hospital setting will improve outcomes (Curtain, 2003). Lower nurse-to-patient ratios are associated with lower failure-to-rescue rates, lower inpatient mortality, and shorter lengths of stay (Lang et al., 2004; Aiken, Clarke, Sloane, Sochalski, et al., 2002). Furthermore nurse staffing or individual nurse workload has a definite and measurable impact on patient outcomes such as nosocomial infections and length of stay, medical errors, nurse retention, and patient mortality. The hours of patient care made possible by staffing practices has been shown to be a significant predictor in the rate of patient falls, development of pressure ulcers, respiratory and urinary tract infections, and patient and family satisfaction (Yang, 2003). An important note, however, is that lower nurse-to-patient ratios do not correct system inefficiencies, downtime, or ineffective organizational skills. Ratios must be modified by staff skill mix, organizational characteristics, and the quality of interaction between and among physicians, nurses, and administrators (Duchene, 2002).

Lack of Leadership

Over the past decade, restructuring and reengineering initiatives have been undertaken to decrease costs and increase productivity, yet the results of these initiatives have not always had positive results. Increased patient condition severity and nurse responsibilities have expanded the workload of nurses in hospitals in ways that may affect patient outcomes (Aiken, Clarke, & Sloane, 2001). Nursing leadership was reduced at many levels, including nurse managers who were given oversight of multiple patient care units and staff that included nurses, housekeepers, and dietary aides (Aiken et al., 2001; Sovie & Jawad, 2001). As a result of these restructuring initiatives, nurses perceived a decline in the power and authority of chief nurse officers (Aiken, Clarke, & Sloane, 2000) and have lost trust in hospital administration (Decker, Wheeler, Johnson, & Parsons, 2001; Ingersoll, Fisher, Ross, Soja, & Kidd, 2001). A lack of strong nursing leaders fosters an environment in which the focus is on managing daily activities rather than on creating an efficient, effective environment that emphasizes patient safety, quality care, and positive patient outcomes. Adult health nurses working in fragmented health care delivery systems feel powerless to initiate effective change and thus the voice of nurses

in patient care is diminished (Institute of Medicine, 2004).

No one really doubts the valuable contributions of adult health nurses to the well-being of patients. Strides are being made in health care systems to enhance patient care by improving the work environment of nurses but the reality is that these improvements are not happening as quickly as they should. One can speculate that several factors enter into the slow progression of change and systems improvement. The scarcity of creative leaders who can envision a new direction and have the skills to direct change restricts progress. Organizational structures that place nurses in line positions that do not allow input into the direction of the institution smother even the best nursing leaders. Resources may not be available to initiate creative health care delivery systems that improve patient outcomes and satisfaction. Overcoming these barriers is not an easy task, nor is it area that adult health nurses feel they can or should tackle. Thus they continue to work in inadequate patient care environments until burnout or job dissatisfaction leads them to leave nursing or choose other nursing employment.

From a positive perspective, the nursing profession is heralding quality nursing care and describing essential elements that support that nursing care. The Nursing Organization Alliance recently identified the essential elements of a healthful work environment for nurses (Grindel, in press): (1) a collaborative practice culture; (2) a communication rich culture; (3) adequate numbers of qualified nurses; (4) recognition of the value of nursing contributions; (5) expert, credible, and visible nursing leadership; (6) a culture of accountability; (7) professional development opportunities; and (8) shared decision making at all levels within the agency. These elements are broad, allowing for interpretation within the context of each health care agency. Research is needed to establish whether they do indeed foster a healthful work environment across a variety of agencies. In the meantime, these elements can guide administrators and adult health nurses in assessing the "healthiness" of their workplace environment.

The bright star in heralding excellence in nursing care is the Magnet Movement. The American Nurses Credentialing Center, a subsidiary of the American Nurses Association, recognizes health care delivery institutions that have the structure and processes that support the best in nursing care. The designation of Magnet status informs nurses and consumers about the quality of care within a given health care organization and has been linked with attracting and retaining professional nurses (Lash & Munroe, in press). A select group of health care institutions have achieved Magnet status. Many more are in the process of implementing strategies to meet the criteria for this recognition. Other agencies will never apply for Magnet status because they lack resources to meet the criteria. Legitimate questions can be pondered about the Magnet movement, however. Will patient care in non-Magnet institutions be compromised by the attraction of nurses to Magnet agencies? What criteria can non-Magnet institutions meet to demonstrate that the quality of nursing care in their agency is good even though they lack Magnet recognition?

Although strides have been made in creating work environments that are conducive to quality nursing care, much remains to be done. A decade has passed since hospital restructuring to increase productivity and decrease cost changed the delivery of services. The initiatives of the early 1990s had a negative impact on patient outcomes, patient safety, and nursing practice. To turn these negative outcomes around takes time, but time is of the essence when patient care is compromised.

ROLE TURMOIL IN NURSING

For decades, nursing has struggled with the diversity of entry-into-nursing education programs. In 1964 the ANA declared that the baccalaureate degree should be the entry level of education for nurses. This goal has never been reached. Although there has been a marked decrease in the number of diploma programs, more than 70 diploma schools of nursing are training nurses in the United States today. The associate's degree programs prepare approximately 60% of the nurses entering the workforce, and the remainder of new nurses earns baccalaureate degrees in nursing. The demand for nurses in the workforce is keeping enrollments high in all of these education programs. The dilemma lies in the fact that research is providing evidence that educational preparation can make a difference in patient outcomes. Aiken, Clarke, Cheung, Sloane, and Silber (2003) found that in hospitals with higher proportions of nurses educated at the baccalaureate level or higher, surgical patients experienced lower mortality and failure-to-rescue rates. These results raise several questions. What components of a baccalaureate nursing education foster better patient outcomes? Because it is not practical to eliminate diploma and associate's degree programs, what is the educational mix of nurses that will ensure positive patient outcomes? Is there a ratio of baccalaureate nurses to associate's degree/diploma–prepared nurses that supports better patient outcomes? In this age of high patient condition severity, heavy workloads, and the aging nursing workforce, exploration of the best mix of nurses with different educational backgrounds may contribute to positive patient outcomes.

Lack of Clinical Leadership

An Institute of Medicine report (2004) noted that clinical nursing leadership has been reduced at multiple levels. Leadership models are needed that will assist staff nurses and nurse managers to balance high-tech with "high touch" successfully in today's technological age of health care delivery (Bathrick et al., 2002). New skill sets and behaviors including innovation and leadership are required of nurses entering practice. The definition to what it means to "care" for patients is new; the paradigm of "caring" has shifted from a "do everything" mentality to that of transferring the skills of self-care to patients and their significant others/support systems. Nurses must accept the mandate for patient teaching and skill set transfer in their practice and focus on getting patients out of the hospital and on their own as quickly as possible (Porter-O'Grady, 2003).

With nursing practice now being defined by a service portability, the profession needs leaders within the clinical setting who are able to shift the culture and entrenched view of nurses who practice with a residency-based mode of service delivery. Some nurses remain focused on task and are disheartened by not being able to get all the previously expected work done in today's health care delivery models of shorter lengths of stay and greater condition severities (Porter-O'Grady, 2003). Direct patient care cannot be the only facet of patient care that is valued by the staff nurse; an infrastructure that supports the new self-care paradigm for the practice of nursing (i.e., system improvement activities such evidence-based practice and implementation of policy and standards of care) must be developed and strengthened to ensure excellence in nursing care.

Some nursing leaders are discussing the fact that nursing is in need of staff nurses who are willing to take leadership roles on the unit (C. G. Grindel, personal communication, summer 2004). Staff nurses are not always willing to lead self-governance activities, direct evidence-based practice initiatives, or even serve as charge nurse. This lack of unit-based leadership is of great concern because quality care and positive patient outcomes do not happen without leadership within nursing staff. This phenomenon deserves exploration. Is it a lack of preparation to assume leadership roles or is it a characteristic of the current generation of nurses to avoid such opportunities? A better understanding of this lack of leadership at the staff level is essential to develop strategies that foster leadership within the workplace.

Recently the American Association of Colleges of Nursing (AACN) presented the clinical nurse leader role (AACN, 2005b). The CNL role focuses on effective coordination, management and evaluation of care for groups of patients in complex health systems in the hopes of achieving better patient and nurse outcomes (Long, 2004). Although the roles and responsibilities of the CNL imply that this nurse can provide the leadership necessary to achieve improve nursing outcomes, the description of the role implies a graduate-level educational preparation, leaving one to wonder why the new role is being introduced. The role of the clinical nurse specialist easily could fill this role and eliminate the addition of yet another nurse role.

In the early 1990s the emphasis on primary care and the downsizing of acute care agencies resulted in a new trend in nursing education. The role of the clinical nurse specialist was eliminated from many hospitals as a cost-saving strategy. Now the need for the clinical nurse specialist in acute care settings is beginning to be recognized once again. In anticipation of the need for nurse practitioners in the community, nursing education programs developed curricula for nurse practitioner programs in family, adult, pediatric, women's health, and psychiatric/mental health specialties. Since that time the proliferation of nurse practitioners has abounded to the point that many new nurse practitioners cannot find employment in this role. The employment patterns for nurse practitioners and clinical nurse specialists are changing. Today the clinical nurse specialist may be employed in a primary care site, whereas the nurse practitioner may work in acute care. If this trend continues, nursing education programs will be challenged to develop curricula that support the needed knowledge and skills for these blended roles.

Practice-focused doctoral degree programs are not a recent development in nursing, yet recently the AACN (2005a) developed a position statement to clarify the doctor of nursing practice (DNP) role in nursing. The focus of this terminal degree is practice rather than the research focus of traditional doctorates (doctor of philosophy, doctor of nursing science, doctor of education). Most interesting is the recommendation that the DNP be the graduate degree for advanced nursing practice preparation, including the four current advance practice roles: clinical nurse specialist, nurse practitioner, nurse anesthetist, and nurse-midwife. Many questions arise. What advantage does this degree hold for the nurse? The public generally understands the practice roles for the clinical nurse specialist, nurse practitioner, nurse anesthetist, and nurse-midwife. Will the public understand the DNP? State nurse practice acts for advanced practice nurses recognize the current advanced practice roles. Will confusion be introduced with the DNP? The AACN position statement recommends that DNP candidate be encouraged to take extra courses to become nurse educators. Will they be prepared to meet the criteria for tenure in research-focused colleges and universities? Will the DNP decrease the number of nurses who enter research doctoral programs? If so, who will carry on the advancement of nursing science?

Change is a sign of progression. These new advance practice roles may truly advance nursing practice and patient care. However, the risk of increased role turmoil is high. Are the benefits to the nursing profession significant enough to justify these new roles?

IMPLICATIONS FOR ADULT HEALTH NURSES

Ensuring quality health care for the American public is the responsibility of consumers, health care providers, legislators, health care systems, and insurers. Adult health nurses are faced with many challenges as they strive to do their part in ensuring quality health care as demonstrated by positive patient outcomes, yet these nurses can make a difference in patient outcomes and in the workplace. Expert nurses caring for adult populations must do the following:

◆ Be on the cutting edge of practice through continuous professional development.
◆ Maintain a focus on the skills, abilities, and contributions of nurses to the well-being of the public.
◆ Assume leadership roles within the workplace
◆ Test patient care delivery models to enhance patient safety and efficiency and promote better patient outcomes.
◆ Test strategies to improve the workplace environment.
◆ Market an image of nursing that highlights the challenges and excitement of a career in nursing, with a focus on young children.
◆ Implement health promotion strategies for healthier American citizens, particularly the elderly.
◆ Conduct research on the effect of quality nursing care on patient outcomes.
◆ Be politically active to ensure legislation that supports health promotion and health maintenance for the American public.

Nursing education can contribute to the advancement of adult health nursing practice by the following means:

◆ Exploring employment trends for adult health nurses to adjust nursing education programs as needed
◆ Strengthening the development of leadership skills in nursing education programs at all levels
◆ Educating nursing students to provide care within the new self-care paradigm of the delivery of patient care: transferring the skills of self-care to patients and their significant others/support systems
◆ Focusing on research from the perspective of evidence-based practice, outcomes measurement, and program evaluation.

To serve adult patients and their families in the midst a changing health care environment, adult health nurses must be active participants in the change. Their knowledge and skills must incorporate the latest in health care practices. They must have a voice in the implementation of patient care by taking leadership roles in the workplace. The specialty organizations for adult health care must support their constituents by presenting them with the latest developments in medical-surgical patient care and by keeping them abreast of the evolution of new practice models, the latest research on adult patient outcomes, and legislation affecting health care. These adult health specialty organizations must promote excellence in patient care by providing their members professional development opportunities related to nursing care, leadership, and research. The health care of America's adults depends on it.

REFERENCES

Aiken, L. H., Clarke, S. P., & Sloane, D. M. (2000). Hospital restructuring: Does it adversely affect care and outcomes? *Journal of Nursing Administration, 30*(10), 457-463.

Aiken, L. H., Clarke, S. P., & Sloane, D. M. (2001). Hospital restructuring: Does it adversely affect care and outcomes? *Journal of Health and Human Services Administration, 23*(4), 416-442.

Aiken, L. H., Clarke, S. P., Sloane, D. M., & International Hospital Outcomes Research Consortium. (2002). Hospital staffing, organization, and quality of care: Cross-national findings. *International Journal of Quality Health Care, 14*(1), 5-13.

Aiken, L. H., Clarke, S. P., Sloane, D. M., Sochalski, J., & Silber, J. H. (2002). Hospital nurse staffing and patient mortality, nurse burnout, and job dissatisfaction. *JAMA: The Journal of the American Medical Association, 288*(16), 1988-1993.

Aiken, L. H., Clarke, S. P., Cheung, R. B., Sloane, D. M., & Silber, J. H. (2003). Educational levels of hospital nurses

and surgical patient mortality. *JAMA: The Journal of the American Medical Association, 290*(12), 1617-1623.

Association of American Colleges of Nursing. (2005a). *AACN position statement on the practice doctorate in nursing, October 2004.* Retrieved on February 9, 2005, from http://www.aacn.nche.edu/DNP/pdf/DNP.pdf

Association of American Colleges of Nursing. (2005b). *The clinical nurse leader.* Retrieved on January 15, 2005, from http://www.aacn.nche.edu/CNL/index.htm

Bathrick, T., Kramer, S. M., Lohre, J. B., Norton, M. A., Scherger, D., Walkes, M. C., et al. (2002). Leadership in the digital age: A framework to balance high touch with high tech. *Seminars for Nurse Managers, 10*(2), 120-129.

Buerhaus, P. I., Staiger, D. O., & Auerbach, D. I. (2000). Why are shortages of hospital RNs concentrated in specialty care units? *Nursing Economics, 18*(3), 111-116.

Buerhaus, P. I., Staiger, D. O., & Auerbach, D. I. (2004a). *Trends: New signs of a strengthening U.S. nurse labor market?* Retrieved January 30, 2005, from http://content.healthaffairs.org/cgi/reprint/hlthaff.w4.526v1

Buerhaus, P., et al. (2004b). *Physicians assess the nursing shortage.* Unpublished manuscript. Nashville, TN: Vanderbilt University.

Curtain, L. (2003). An integrated analysis of nurse staffing and related variables: Effects on patient outcomes. *Online Journal of Issues in Nursing, 8*(3), 9.

Decker, D., Wheeler, G., Johnson, J., & Parsons, R. (2001). Effect of organizational change on the individual employee. *The Health Care Manager, 19*(4), 1-12.

Duchene, P. (2002). Staff ratios: Just about numbers? *Nursing Management, 33*(7), 10.

Federal Interagency Forum on Aging Related Statistics. (2004). *Older Americans 2004: Key indicators of well-being.* Retrieved January 30, 2005, from http://www.agingstats.gov/chartbook2004/slides.html

Grindel, C. G. (in press). Guidelines to support a healthful work environment for nurses. *Med-Surg Nursing.*

Ingersoll, G., Fisher, M., Ross, B., Soja, M., & Kidd, N. (2001). Employee response to major organizational redesign. *Applied Nursing Research, 14*(1), 18-28.

Institute of Medicine. (2004). *Keeping patients safe: Transforming the work environment of nurses.* (Page, A., Ed.). Retrieved January 25, 2005, from http://www.nap.edu/openbook/0309090679/html/1.html

Kahn, K., Rogers, W., Rubenstein, L., Sherwood, M., Reinisch, E., Keeler, E., et al. (1990). Measuring quality of care with explicit process criteria before and after implementation of the DRG-based prospective payment system. *JAMA: The Journal of the American Medical Association, 264*(15), 1965-1973.

Kohn, L., Corrigan, J. M., & Donaldson, M. S. (Eds.). (2000). *To err is human: Building a safer health system.* Retrieved January 25, 2005, from http://www.nap.edu/openbook/0309068371/html/1.html

Konelan, M., et al. (2004). *Nurses assess the nursing shortage and the hospital workplace climate.* Unpublished manuscript. Nashville, TN: Vanderbilt University.

Lang, T. A., Hodge, M., Olson, V., Romano, P. S., & Kravitz, R. L. (2004). Nurse patient ratios: A systematic review on the effects of nurse staffing on patient, nurse employee and hospital outcomes. *Journal of Nursing Administration, 34*(7/8), 326-337.

Lash, A. A., & Munroe, D. (2005). Magnet status: A communique to the profession and the public about nursing excellence. *Med-Surg Nursing, 14,* S7.

Long, K. A. (2004). Preparing nurses for the 21st century: Re-envisioning nursing education and practice. *Journal of Professional Nursing, 20*(2), 82-88.

Mitchell, P., & Shortell, S. (1997). Adverse outcomes and variations in organization of care delivery. *Medical Care, 35*(11 Suppl.), NS19-NS32.

Ostrowski, M. (2004). Meet the travelers: Four nurses tell us why they decided to become travelers and what they've learned along the way. *RN Career Search 2005: Directory of Nursing Opportunities, 67*(12), 47-50.

Porter-O'Grady, T. (2003). Innovation and creativity in a new age for health care. *Journal of the New York State Nurses Association, 34*(2), 4-8.

Rogers, A. E., Hwang, W. T., Scott, L. D., Aiken, L. H., & Dinges, D. F. (2004). The working hours of hospital staff nurses and patient safety. *Health Affairs (Millwood), 23*(4), 202-212.

Rubenstein, L., Chang, B., Keeler, E., & Kahn, K. (1992). Measuring the quality of nursing surveillance activities for five diseases before and after implementation of the drug-based prospective payment system. In *Patient Outcomes Research: Examining the Effectiveness of Nursing Practice.* Proceedings of the State of the Science Conference, Bethesda, MD, National Institutes of Health, National Center for Nursing Research. Washington DC: U.S. Government Printing Office.

Shaffer, F. A. (2000). Outsourcing: A managerial competency for the 21st century. *Nursing Administration Quarterly, 25*(1), 84-88.

Shindul-Rosthschild, J., Fontaine, D., Furillo, J., Malloch, K., Pinkham, J., & Blakeney, B. A. (2003). Mandatory nurse/patient ratios: A good idea or not? *Nursing 2003, 33*(10), 46-48.

Sovie, M., & Jawad, A. (2001). Hospital restructuring and its impact on outcomes. *Journal of Nursing Administration, 31*(12), 588-600.

Steefel, L., (2004). *Shortage relief in sight? New study adds up the number of RNs entering the workforce.* Retrieved January 30, 2005, from http://www.nurseweek.com/news/Features/04-11/NursingShortage_print.html

Yang, K. (2003). Relationships between nurse staffing and patient outcomes. *Journal of Nursing Research, 11*(3), 149-157.

Alternative and Complementary Therapies

Recent Changes and Current Issues

CHARLOTTE ELIOPOULOS

Be it the woman using ginger to control morning sickness, a senior citizen group that wants to reduce the risk of falls by establishing a daily tai chi routine, or the surgical patient who asks for therapeutic touch to be performed postoperatively to speed the elimination of anesthesia, clients in virtually all practice settings are challenging nurses with the use of complementary and alternative medicine (CAM).

Nearly one in four Americans is using CAM, and most of these individuals are doing so without the knowledge or advice of their health care provider (Barnes, Powell-Griner, McFann, & Nahin, 2004). Consumers are demonstrating their support of new CAM modalities not only philosophically but also financially, spending as much for these therapies as they do for all out-of-pocket physician expenditures (Eisenberg et al., 1998). The consumer-driven growth of CAM poses interesting possibilities for nurses if they are ready to meet the challenge. A proactive approach is essential to promoting quality in the use of new modalities and ensuring a strong role for nursing in the integration of CAM into conventional practice settings.

GROWTH OF COMPLEMENTARY AND ALTERNATIVE MEDICINE

By definition, CAM consists of practices outside of the dominant system for managing health and disease that have not been taught in American medical schools or practiced in U.S. hospitals (Barnes et al., 2004). Although nearly 90% of the world population uses what Americans consider CAM as their primary source of medical care and were doing so for centuries before America was discovered, CAM is relatively new to the United States (Box 20-1). Just in 1992 the National Institutes of Health established the Office of Alternative Medicine for the purpose of evaluating the growing use of CAM. The Office of Alternative Medicine became a freestanding center within the National Institutes of Health in 1998 and was renamed the National Center for Complementary and Alternative Medicine. The center has categorized CAM into five major categories of practice (Box 20-2):

◆ Alternative medical systems
◆ Mind-body interventions
◆ Biologically based therapies
◆ Manipulative and body-based methods
◆ Energy therapies

Many factors are responsible for the increasing use of CAM, not the least of which is consumers' dissatisfaction with the experience of using conventional medicine. During the same period in which conventional care has become characterized by skyrocketing costs, abbreviated hospital stays, and 5-minute impersonal office visits, CAM practitioners have created practices in which the consumer is treated with a holistic, nonrushed approach in an appealing environment (i.e., pleasant scents, sights, and sounds versus the cold sterility of the usual conventional practice setting).

In addition to being a "feel good" experience, CAM has proved to be effective in treating many conditions without the side effects or risks of medications and other conventional treatments. Today's increasingly well-informed, health-conscious consumers desire interventions that can promote wellness and stimulate the healing capabilities of their own bodies rather than merely treat symptoms. They appreciate an active role in their health care and to be empowered to affect their own health status.

The baby boomers have played a role in the popularity of CAM. This generation, like no other, has demonstrated an interest in diet, exercise, and other health-promoting measures and is unwilling to accept disease and disability as expected outcomes of aging. They desire that which is natural, appreciate the mind-body connection, and have heightened sensitivity to their spiritual dimensions.

BOX 20-1

Alternative and Complementary Therapies: Facts About the Use of Complementary and Alternative Medicine in the United States

- Nearly 40% of Americans use alternative therapies.
- Highest use was among the following:
  - Women
  - Older adults (a direct correlation was found between the use of mind-body therapies and age)
  - Well-educated individuals
  - Persons who had been hospitalized within the past year
  - Former smokers
  - African-American adults, when megavitamin therapy and prayer were included in the definition of complementary and alternative medicine
- Individuals use these therapies for the following reasons:
  - They believed that when combined with conventional care, complementary and alternative medicine would help their condition (54.9%).
  - They had curiosity or interest in these therapies (50.1%).
  - They thought that conventional medicine alone would not help them (28%).
  - They received a recommendation from a conventional practitioner (26%).
  - They saw these therapies as less expensive options to conventional care (13%).
- The most common problems that complementary and alternative medical therapies were used to treat were the following:
  - Back pain or problems
  - Neck pain or problems
  - Joint pain or stiffness
  - Anxiety
  - Depression

Data from Barnes, P., Powell-Griner, E., McFann, K., & Nahin, R. (2004). Complementary and alternative medicine use among adults: United States, 2002. In *Advance data from vital and health statistics, 343.* Gaithersburg, MD: National Center for Complementary and Alternative Medicine.

Unlike previous generations that showed a blind obedience to the medical establishment, baby boomers have challenged authority and redefined professional-client relationships. Natural, holistic therapies that empower and actively engage individuals in activities to promote health and well-being are well received by this group.

NURSING AND COMPLEMENTARY AND ALTERNATIVE MEDICINE

Nurses historically have been identified as healers; this was the foundation on which the profession was built. As the profession grew, there was a legitimate need for nursing to become more science based, and it did so rather successfully. But nurses now must question whether the pendulum has swung too far in the direction of science and technology. In many settings, nurses can recite a patient's laboratory results, yet know nothing of that patient's unique life story; provide a treatment to the patient, yet have their minds and hearts elsewhere;

sense that the patient could benefit from their presence, yet retreat to the desk to satisfy documentation requirements.

Complementary and alternative medicine offers an exciting arena for nurses to reclaim their role as healers. The basic principles that are woven through CAM are consistent with the nursing views of health and healing (Eliopoulos, 1999):

The body has the ability to heal itself. Florence Nightingale promoted this principle when she wrote that medicine and surgery can remove obstructions, but nature alone cures (Nightingale, 1859). Nursing has long assisted individuals in getting their bodies and minds in optimal states for healing to occur.

Health and healing are related to a harmony of mind, body, and spirit. Long before CAM was recognized in the United States or the term *holistic* was used commonly, nursing attended to the needs of the whole person. Whole-person care is the thread woven through the nursing process.

BOX 20-2

Categories of Complementary and Alternative Therapies

1. Alternative medical systems

   Alternative medical systems are built on complete systems of theory and practice. Often these systems have evolved apart from and earlier than the conventional medical approach used in the United States. Examples of alternative medical systems that have developed in Western cultures include homeopathic medicine and naturopathic medicine; examples that have developed in non-Western cultures include traditional Chinese medicine and Ayurveda.

2. Mind-body interventions

   Mind-body medicine uses a variety of techniques designed to enhance the capacity of the mind to affect bodily function and symptoms. Some techniques that were considered complementary and alternative medicine (CAM) in the past have become mainstream (for example, patient support groups and cognitive-behavioral therapy). Other mind-body techniques are still considered CAM, including meditation, prayer, mental healing, and therapies that use creative outlets such as art, music, or dance.

3. Biologically based therapies

   Biologically based therapies in CAM use substances found in nature, such as herbs, foods, and vitamins. Some examples include dietary supplements, herbal products, and the use of other so-called natural but as yet scientifically unproven therapies (for example, using shark cartilage to treat cancer).

4. Manipulative and body-based methods

   Manipulative and body-based methods in CAM are based on manipulation and/or movement of one or more parts of the body. Some examples include chiropractic or osteopathic manipulation and massage.

5. Energy therapies

   Energy therapies involve the use of energy fields. They are of two types:
   - *Biofield therapies* are intended to affect energy fields that purportedly surround and penetrate the human body. The existence of such fields has not yet been scientifically proved. Some forms of energy therapy manipulate biofields by applying pressure and/or manipulating the body by placing the hands in, or through, these fields. Examples include therapeutic touch, Reiki, and qi gong.
   - *Bioelectromagnetic-based therapies* involve the unconventional use of electromagnetic fields, such as pulsed fields, magnetic fields, or alternating current or direct current fields.

From National Center for Complementary and Alternative Medicine. (2002). *Get the facts: What is complementary and alternative medicine (CAM)?* Retrieved February 1, 2005, from http://nccam.nih.gov/health/whatiscam/index.htm.

Basic, good health practices build the foundation for healing. In most practice settings, nurses are the primary professionals responsible for assessing and planning for all aspects—physical, emotional, socioeconomic, spiritual—of the individual. Nurses educate, counsel, and coach individuals in diet, exercise, safe medication use, lifestyle modifications, and other practices that promote good health.

Healing practices are individualized. Learning about the uniqueness of each patient through comprehensive assessment and planning and implementing care that is tailored to fit the patient are basic nursing standards of practice that foster individualized care.

Clients are responsible for their own healing. The promotion of self-care and maximum independence are highly valued foundations of nursing practice.

As can be seen, the principles embraced in CAM are consistent with those long advanced by nursing. These basic principles of healing that guide CAM offer nursing an opportunity to highlight nurses' historical and special role as healers in this new arena.

Complementary and alternative medicine offers nurses the potential for innovative practice models. Increasing numbers of nurses are obtaining training in aromatherapy, herbal medicine, homeopathy, acupuncture, acupressure, therapeutic touch, guided imagery, massage therapy, and other modalities. Advanced preparation or certification in a specific modality can enable nurses to offer a wider range of services to clients in traditional care settings, as witnessed when a nurse in a primary care setting helps an individual correct incontinence with the use of biofeedback or when a nurse in an intensive care unit assists a patient in controlling pain with the use of therapeutic touch and guided imagery. These new skills also can enable nurses to establish private practices in which clients contract directly with nurses for specific therapies (e.g., therapeutic touch and stress reduction classes), wellness counseling, coaching for effective living with a chronic condition, or guidance in the integration of CAM and conventional therapies.

CHALLENGES

Exciting new opportunities within the realm of CAM can be accompanied by new problems for nurses to address. Although many of the interventions used within CAM are healing modalities that nurses are competent to practice independently, the risk exists that physicians will seek a gatekeeper role that requires that CAM therapies be ordered and managed through them. The medical model is the paradigm in which physicians have been socialized, thus it is understandable that they would gravitate toward a physician-led and physician-controlled approach to CAM. Furthermore, it is understandable that the health care system would support a physician-led model for reimbursement of CAM services (i.e., CAM therapies would require a physician's order to qualify for reimbursement). The implications could be that a qualified nurse in a conventional practice setting would be restricted from doing therapeutic touch, recommending an herbal alternative, or performing acupuncture—or obtaining reimbursement for these activities—without a physician's order. Because most CAM therapies are not medical procedures, the wisdom of a physician-directed paradigm is questionable.

Rather than a physician-directed paradigm, nurses could be working in settings that are directed by nonphysician CAM practitioners. For example, a healing center that offers the services of an acupuncturist, a homeopath, and a hypnotherapist may employ a nurse. Confusion may arise related to delegation, direction, and supervision of the nurse. Strong role models of nursing will be needed to work in collaboration with CAM practitioners without allowing them to determine nursing practice or delegate inappropriately to nurses.

Licensure issues could develop for nurses who practice CAM. The area of massage therapy exemplifies the potential complications that could arise. How much of a massage can a nurse perform in caregiving before it becomes a therapeutic massage requiring licensure as a massage therapist? Would a nurse who is a licensed massage therapist and works exclusively doing massage therapy meet state practice requirements to maintain a nursing license? These questions already are surfacing in various states and are likely to be compounded as nurses increasingly practice CAM modalities.

Nurses may need to assume leadership in helping consumers use CAM safely. As mentioned before, most consumers are using CAM without the knowledge of their conventional practitioners. Many consumers are influenced and make decisions regarding their use of CAM by advertising claims and testimonials. They may see a television commercial describing an herbal preparation that can "melt pounds away" or have a neighbor who is a distributor for a magnet company advise them of the benefits of magnets for pain control. Consumers could be tempted to self-diagnosis and seek CAM remedies without the benefit of a comprehensive evaluation, thereby delaying the diagnosis and treatment of medical conditions; they also could use CAM therapies that could prove harmful to them, as could happen with herb-drug interactions. A strong advocacy role by nurses will be essential to protecting consumers in this new arena.

Nurses need to play an important role in developing the new paradigm that emerges as CAM therapies become more accepted and are used in the conventional health care system. Complementary and alternative medicine, although widely used in holistic practices, does not equate to holistic care. Substituting a medical technology with a CAM modality without identifying the interrelationships and factors affecting the bio-psycho-social-spiritual dimensions of the person is not holistic care. Rather, such care is a continuation of a fragmented system of health care delivery using a different set of treatment modalities. Nursing must be a strong voice in promoting a holistic model that integrates the best from CAM and conventional medicine.

REFERENCES

Barnes, P., Powell-Griner, E., McFann, K., & Nahin, R. (2004). Complementary and alternative medicine use among adults: United States, 2002. In *Advance data from vital and health statistics, 343*. Gaithersburg, MD: National Center for Complementary and Alternative Medicine.

Eisenberg, D. M., Davis, R. B., Ettner, S. L., Appel, S., Wilkey, S., Van Rompay, M., et al. (1998). Trends in alternative medicine use in the United States, 1990-1997: Results of a follow-up national survey. *JAMA: The Journal of the American Medical Association, 280*, 1569-1575.

Eliopoulos, C. (1999). *Integrating alternative and conventional therapies: Holistic care of chronic conditions* (pp. 76-77). St Louis, MO: Mosby.

Nightingale, F. (1859). *Notes on nursing*. London: Harrison and Sons.

Ambulatory Care Nursing

Challenges for the Twenty-First Century

SHEILA A. HAAS ◆ IDA M. ANDROWICH

The ambulatory care setting offers numerous opportunities for nurses to practice in a variety of roles. Of the 209,324 registered nurses identified as employed in ambulatory care settings, approximately 16% are managers, 51% are staff nurses, and 21% are in advanced practice roles such as midwife, nurse practitioner, certified nurse anesthetist, or clinical nurse specialist. Of the remaining 12%, approximately 1% are identified as researchers, educators, consultants, and private duty, with 8% identified as "other" (USDHHS, 2000). Ambulatory care nurses report the highest levels of satisfaction with their jobs despite salaries below the mean for every type of position for nurses employed in ambulatory care settings. Staff nurses in ambulatory care earn 86% of the salary of staff nurses in hospitals.

Other than nurses practicing in long-term care, ambulatory care nurses have the lowest percentage of preparation at the baccalaureate or higher-degree level and are the most likely of any group to be employed part-time. Next to hospital nurses, ambulatory care nurses are the youngest of nurses, with 44.3 years as the average age. The expanded life expectancy of the U.S. population coupled with increases in incidence of chronic illnesses has led to movement of care out of hospitals and an expanded demand for ambulatory care nurses. Forecasts for future full-time equivalent nurse demand between the years 2000 and 2020 indicate a 70% anticipated increase in the need for nurses in outpatient settings, second only to the demand for home health care nurses.

Statistics at the national level demonstrate nearly 4.9 million health care workers are employed in ambulatory care in the year 2004 (U.S. Department of commerce, 2004) (http://www.stat-usa.gov). Exact figures are difficult to get for nursing because of the tremendous growth in primary care settings. Thus given the size, growth, and importance of the field, defining the practice would appear straightforward.

This is not the case. In fact, Stavins (1993) claims that one of the most difficult challenges facing ambulatory nursing is "defining our role." This chapter focuses on the definitional aspects of the ambulatory care nursing role and identifies and discusses several of the issues facing nurses in this practice field.

DEFINING AMBULATORY CARE NURSING

Verran (1981) is credited with an early interest in delineation and definition of ambulatory care nursing. In her seminal study, she used a Delphi methodology and ambulatory care nurses' expert opinions to delineate seven "responsibility areas" in the ambulatory care nurse role. Other researchers have continued this effort (Haas & Hackbarth, 1995a; Hackbarth, Haas, Kavanagh, & Vlasses, 1995; Hastings & Muir-Nash, 1989; Hooks, Dewitz-Arnold, & Westbrook, 1980; Joseph, 1990; Parrinello, & Witzel, 1990; Pinkney-Atkinson & Robertson, 1993).

In *Administration and Practice Standards* the American Academy of Ambulatory Care Nursing (1993) states that ambulatory care nursing operationally is defined as "nursing practice in an ambulatory care setting. Nursing care provided to patients with institutional episodes of care of less than 24 hours" (p. 19). Unfortunately, although this definition delineates nursing practice by the environment in which the nurse practices and the amount of time the nurse spends with a patient, it is not useful in capturing essential characteristics and role elements.

This need to depict ambulatory nursing as it is today for practicing nurses, other health care providers, policy makers, and the public led the American Nurses Association (ANA) and the American Academy of Ambulatory Care Nursing (1997) to establish a joint task force to write a monograph on ambulatory care nursing: *Nursing in Ambulatory Care: The Future is Here.* As part of this charge, the task force developed a conceptual definition of ambulatory care nursing. In the absence of a rich and recent literature from which to cull the universal characteristics of ambulatory care nursing, members of the task force were asked to assemble focus groups in their ambulatory care organizations. Each focus group responded to the question "What are the universal characteristics of ambulatory care nursing?" Commonly occurring themes in the reports assisted the task force in the evolution of a conceptual definition of ambulatory care nursing.

Using the American Nurses Association *Social Policy Statement* (1995) as a foundation, the fask force developed the following definition:

> Professional ambulatory care nursing includes those clinical, management, educational, and research activities provided by registered nurses for and with individuals who seek care for health-related problems or concerns or seek assistance with health maintenance and/or health promotion. These individuals engage predominantly in self-care and self-managed health activities or receive care from family and significant others outside an institutional setting.
>
> Ambulatory care nursing services are episodic, less than 24 hours in duration, and occur as a single encounter or a series of encounters over days, weeks, months, or years. Ambulatory nurse-patient encounters take place in health care facilities as well as in community-based settings, including schools, workplaces or homes.
>
> They occur as personal visits or as encounters using the telephone and other communication devices. Ambulatory care nursing services focus on cost-effective ways to maximize wellness; prevent illness, disability, and disease; minimize symptoms of acute minor ailments; and support patients in the management of chronic disease to effect more positive health states throughout the life span up to and including a peaceful death (American Nurses Association & American Academy of Ambulatory Care Nursing, 1997, pp. 13-14).

The American Academy of Ambulatory Care Nursing (AAACN) is "the association of professional nurses who identify ambulatory care nursing as essential to the continuum of high quality, cost-effective patient care." The mission of the AAACN is to advance the art and science of ambulatory nursing (AAACN, 2000). The AAACN was established in 1978 by a group of nursing directors and supervisors in ambulatory care who recognized the need for well-prepared nurse administrators in the expanding arena of ambulatory care. The AAACN originally was named the American Academy of Ambulatory Nursing Administration, and the name was changed in 1993 to reflect the commitment of the organization to the development of all nurses working in ambulatory care. As part of this commitment, the AAACN publishes and updates standards for ambulatory care nursing.

The sixth edition of the *Ambulatory Care Nursing Administration and Practice Standards* (AAACN, 2004, p. 6) reflects seven core ambulatory care nursing values:

1. Responsible health care delivery for individuals and communities
2. Visionary and accountable leadership
3. Productive partnerships and alliances
4. Innovative and responsible risk taking
5. Responsive member services
6. Diverse and committed membership
7. Continual advancement of professional ambulatory care nursing practice

The nine *Ambulatory Care Nursing Administration and Practice Standards* are designed to "promote consistent, thoughtful, effective management of increasingly complex nursing roles and responsibilities in a changing ambulatory care environment" (AAACN, 2004, p. 4). The standards are designed to be used with specialty practice nursing organization standards such as those promulgated by the American Nurses Association. The standards address issues such as the structure and organization of ambulatory care nursing, staffing, competency of nursing staff, nursing practice, continuity of care, ethics and patient rights, environment, research, and performance improvement. Each standard includes a rationale for the standard and criteria by which to measure the contribution of nursing. The AAACN standards are presented as recommendations and are intended to be adapted to fit many diverse ambulatory care settings. Because ambulatory care practice is ever expanding and changing, the AAACN is committed to revising, updating, and promulgating its standards. Examples of diversity in practice roles are beginning to appear in the literature in response to challenges presented by managed care and an aging chronically ill population. Schroeder, Trehearne, and Ward (2000a) define and justify an expanded role for the nurse clinician in managed care and delineate (2000b) the impact of this role on costs, quality, and provider and on patient satisfaction.

CURRENT ISSUES IN AMBULATORY CARE NURSING

Along with the need for definitional clarity of the ambulatory nursing role are also several issues or concerns relating to ambulatory care nursing. The Ambulatory Care Nursing Conceptual Framework (Figure 21-1) is used to organize these current issues. Several ambulatory care nursing "mega" issues (Futch & Phillips, 2003)

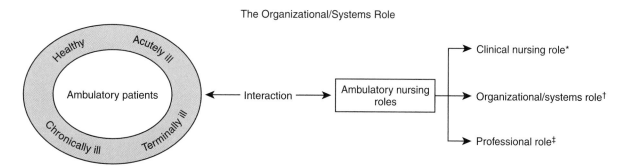

The Organizational/Systems Role

*CLINICAL NURSING ROLE	†ORGANIZATIONAL/SYSTEMS ROLE	‡PROFESSIONAL ROLE
Patient education	Practice/office support	Evidence-based practice
Advocacy (compassion, caring, emotional support)	Healthcare fiscal management (reimbursement and coding)	Leadership inquiry and research
Care management	Collaboration/conflict management	Utilization
Assess, screen, triage	Informatics	Clinical quality improvement
Telephone practice	Context of care delivery/models	Staff development
Collaboration/resource Identification and referral	Care of the caregiver	Regulatory compliance (risk management)
Primary, secondary, and tertiary prevention	Priority management/delegation/ supervision	Provider self-care
Clinical procedures, independent/ interdependent/dependent	Ambulatory culture/cross cultural Competencies	Ethics
Communication/documentation	Ongoing political/entrepreneurial skills	
Outcome management	Structuring customer-focused systems	
Protocol development/usage	Workplace regulatory compliance (EEOC, OSHA)	
	Advocacy interorganizational and in community	
	Legal issues	
	Workload	

FIGURE 21-1 Ambulatory nursing roles.
(From Haas, S. [1998]. Ambulatory care nursing conceptual framework. *AAACN Viewpoint, 20*[3], 16-17. Reprinted with permission of the publisher, American Academy of Ambulatory Care Nursing, East Holly Avenue, Box 56 Pitman, NJ, 08071-0056; Phone 800-AMB-NURS; Fax 856-589-7463.)

fall under each of the ambulatory nursing roles. Under the clinical nursing role are the following issues:

1. Patient preferences and privacy
2. Disease management
3. Syndromic surveillance
4. Documentation challenges in nursing practice leading to limited understanding of ambulatory nursing practice
5. Telephone practice

Under the organizational/systems role are the following issues:

1. Diversity of practice in ambulatory care settings, including the use of varied conceptual models of health and evolving issues with costs of ambulatory care for the individual patient

2. The need to incorporate technology, compliance programs, and evidence-based practice precepts into the delivery of care
3. Time management and the rapid pace of ambulatory patient encounters
4. The increased need for delegation and supervision of unlicensed assistive personnel

Under the professional role are the following issues:

1. The nursing shortage and the limited number of nurses with baccalaureate or advanced academic preparation practicing in ambulatory care
2. The need for a multistate compact for professional nurses and attention paid to other legislative regulation issues that have an impact on ambulatory nursing practice

Under the clinical nursing role are patient preferences and privacy. In a climate of concern for patient safety and the public recognition that quality and efficacy of all medical care is not equal, patients are assuming increased roles in managing or comanaging their health care. Many states, such as Illinois, have passed legislation to support consumers in their evaluation of health care options. The governor of Illinois recently signed a consumers right-to-know bill into law that requires health care organizations to make price and performance information for outpatient procedures available to consumers ("Law Gives Illinoisans," 2005). In 2003, 294,355 ambulatory surgeries were performed. Seventy-five percent of Illinois registered voters said posting of charges and performance information would affect decisions, thus creating competition and potentially lowering prices and improving quality. The Illinois Department of Public Health posts mean charges for 30 outpatient ambulatory surgery procedures.

Most of the literature that focuses on patient safety is hospital based and is concerned with medication errors, yet little work has been completed on error outside of the hospital setting. Wakefield (2000) urges nurses in outpatient settings to evaluate their practice for sources of error and to participate in initiatives designed to improve patient safety.

Disease Management

Along with the increasing life expectancy in the population is an increase in the number of individuals who suffer from medically complex chronic disease and disorders resulting from unhealthful lifestyle choices. Consequently, an ever-increasing part of the role of the nurse in ambulatory care is to guide patients as they make choices about their health care options. This requires skill in assessment of patients' information needs and the ability to elicit preferences and convey factual information in a manner useful to patients in decision making. Although case management has been used for many years to focus on public health issues, more recently institutions such as Carondelet–St. Mary's in Tucson, Arizona, have used it as a mechanism to control costs (Martin, 1999). More recently the concept of population-based management has been used to convey approaches that focus on populations identified by disease, payer, geographic location, or other demographic characteristic. Nurses in ambulatory care settings increasingly are involved in identifying inclusion criteria, interventions to be provided, and outcomes to be measured and tracked for these various populations.

Syndromic Surveillance

The term *syndromic surveillance* applies to surveillance using health-related data (typically symptom clusters) that precede a given diagnosis and signal a sufficient probability of a number of cases or a potential population outbreak that would warrant further response. Though historically the syndromic surveillance has been used to target the investigation of potential cases, public health officials increasingly are exploring the usefulness of syndromic surveillance methods in detecting outbreaks associated with bioterrorism. This has implications for ambulatory nursing practice because ambulatory care nurses are often in settings where patients would show early symptoms. They are in a position to evaluate syndromic surveillance systems for early detection of outbreaks and to provide guidance to communities in defining their needs and priorities for these systems, particularly in response to the threat of terrorism.

Documentation Challenges in Practice

The nature of ambulatory practice, with its relatively rapid pace for patient encounters, high patient volume, and scheduled time constraints, does not contribute to comprehensive documentation of nursing care. The use of the nursing elements of the Nursing Minimum Data Set (Werley & Lang, 1988) in ambulatory practice remains limited. Unfortunately, with no documentation trail, paper or electronic, justifying the value of nursing is problematic, and the care rendered by nurses in these settings becomes invisible. Documentation concerns identified a decade ago remain today (Androwich & Phillips, 1992). These concerns include limited use of the standardized nursing terminology (Nursing Minimum Data Set) in practice settings, documentation systems designed primarily for physicians, no classification scheme for interventions or outcomes, and limited use of the problem list. When nursing interventions are documented, the assessment data leading to the individual nursing judgment often are omitted; thus the link to patient outcome remains unknown. In addition, no generally accepted methods of measuring productivity, nursing intensity, or patient condition severity exist in the ambulatory setting, nor have nurses defined the concept of *episode of care* in a manner that could link visits within an episode of care to determine the effectiveness of specific interventions in achieving outcomes. Documentation needs to be captured in an automated patient record in order to link encounters in a meaningful, retrievable manner. This inability to link visits into meaningful units is an issue when goals are set over a period of time. Many of the nursing interventions that are identified for a pregnant woman occur over the duration of the pregnancy and into the postpartum period. When the single visits are documented, but not linked to related visits, there is an inability to demonstrate an effective outcome related to nursing care. As nurses move increasingly to automated documentation in ambulatory care, they will need to determine the best method conceptually to examine and capture an entire episode of care. Unless ambulatory care nurses assume a leadership role in the selection and implementation of clinical information systems, the documentation needs of the practice likely will not be addressed.

Telephone Nursing Practice

The telephone communication dimension (Haas & Hackbarth, 1995a; Hackbarth et al., 1995) of the ambulatory care nurse role is an aspect that is unique to ambulatory nursing practice. Ambulatory care nurses also have concerns about this role dimension. Some of these concerns are related to the amount of education that they receive regarding telephone communication, particularly telephone triage and telephone advice, both of which have a high liability risk potential. Assessment of the client over the telephone requires a high level of assessment skills, including the ability to identify nuances in each situation, well-developed communication and decision-making skills, and proficiency in documentation. Nurses in ambulatory settings need to collaborate with physicians and other members of the health care team in establishing protocols that include health promotion and disease prevention and treatments for symptoms. Finally, nurses need to be educated that all telephone communication must be documented appropriately. The AAACN has developed and promulgated the *Telephone Nursing Practice Administration and Practice Standards* (1997) and in 2004 offered a third edition of these standards, *Telehealth Nursing Practice Administration and Practice Standards,* and a Telephone Nursing Practice Core Course, which is a manual that focuses on essential competencies to prepare ambulatory care nurses to do telephone nursing practice (American Academy of Ambulatory Care Nursing, 2004). National certification in telephone nursing practice (TNP) is available through the National Certification Corporation. Haas and Androwich (1999) used the Nursing Intervention Classification to enhance understanding of the breadth and depth of nursing practice via communication devices. They proposed four telephone interventions to reflect the complexity of TNP: telephone consultation; telephone follow-up; surveillance: telephone; and triage: telephone. These telephone interventions can be used to educate nurses regarding telephone practice and to evaluate performance of telephone practice nurses.

Telephone nursing practice has faced many challenges related to difficulties with securing reimbursement for this practice. In managed care organizations, TNP prevents unnecessary patient visits to the primary care office or emergency room and thus conserves resources for the managed care plan. In a predominantly fee-for-service or preferred provider organization, there are incentives to encourage patient visits especially to the primary care practice. Therefore in this environment there is no way to pay for TNP or to carve out specific practice time for TNP. This is also the kind of environment in which nurses may end up doing TNP on the run without the education necessary to do TNP and also without the protocols. Greenberg (2000) found in a follow-up survey of pediatric clinic callers (approximately 85% were managed care clients) that respondents were satisfied with their interaction with the nurse and 80% reported that without this interaction, they would have sought medical care elsewhere. Telephone nursing practice was performed by "specially trained and experienced registered nurses using approved, written clinic-specific protocols" (p. 117). This study also documented cost savings for the pediatric clinic.

Demand management is a term given to a method of care delivery and a marketing initiative. Once used predominantly by managed care organizations, demand management is now common in many types of ambulatory care organizations. Kastens (1998) defines *demand management* as "the provision of health information to consumer, creating an educated and empowered member who accesses and participates in medical decisions to assure that the right kind of care is provided at the right time" (p. 321). Kastens maintains that demand management is essential for managing the well population and acute or chronically ill patients. Demand management centers include nurse triage and advice and physician referral. Many demand management centers use established protocols for nurse triage and advice.

ORGANIZATIONAL/SYSTEMS ROLE

Diversity in Practice

A marked diversity exists in the types of settings where ambulatory care is delivered. Among the major private sector ambulatory care settings are university hospital outpatient departments, community hospital outpatient departments, physician group practices, health maintenance organizations (HMOs), physician offices, and nurse-managed centers. Ambulatory care settings that are publicly funded include community health clinics; Indian Health Service; and Community, Migrant Worker Health Centers. Within each of these distinct settings the philosophy of care and the model of care delivery may have a different model of health as a foundation. Smith (1981) defines four such models of health: the clinical model, the role-performance model, the adaptive model, and the eudaimonistic model, any of which could be operative in a given setting.

Not surprisingly, the clinical model, or medical model, is frequently the driving force in physician group practices and even in university hospital ambulatory care and community hospital ambulatory care. However, somewhat surprisingly, the clinical model predominates in many HMOs (Haas, Hackbarth, Kavanagh, & Vlasses, 1995). Health maintenance organizations, by definition, should be more focused on health promotion and disease prevention.

Diversity in types of settings, models of health, and the consequent models of care delivery is an issue for nursing when nurses who work in a setting find that they have difficulties working under the prevailing model and philosophy. Furthermore, they may have difficulty identifying this lack of congruence in values as the root of the problem. Nurses will say, "I want to have time to do health promotion with my clients, yet I have so much paperwork and clerical work that I just can't get to it"; "I want to work with the vast array of patient/family problems, but all I have time for is their physical ailments"; or, "I want to work as a colleague with the physicians and really get into health promotion." Operative in each of these situations is a clinical model of health driving the practice model; consequently, the scheduling of patient visits and the provider's time are dictated by this view of health.

Solutions to this issue involve educating nurses about the many and various types of ambulatory care settings, educating nurses and physicians about multiple models of health with their practice implications, and enhancing the care provider's ability to determine operative models of health in different settings. The optimal outcome would be health care professionals who will choose a practice setting for employment where there is a good fit between their professional goals and the mission, philosophy, model of health, and care delivery model of the organization. If there is not a good fit, at least the professional enters the organization with an understanding and awareness of the model currently operating and, if needed, the wherewithal to initiate change.

As more acquisitions and mergers occur, health care networks will encompass multiple health care organizations and agencies. Conceivably, networks will include several different types of ambulatory care agencies. For example, an academic health center may have in its network one or more HMOs, a university hospital outpatient center, a community hospital outpatient center, and two or more physician group practices. Ambulatory patients will move between these settings. Patients may receive primary care in an HMO or physician group practice or the community hospital outpatient center and then be referred to the university hospital outpatient center for consultation with specialists. Referrals may be made from the university hospital outpatient center back to the original primary care referral source. Ambulatory care nurses working in each of these agencies will need excellent negotiation skills, and furthermore, they will need to be expert at assessing the cultures in each of the agencies with which they interact. A "seamless system of care" demands that the culture and requisite practices of each agency not impede a patient's progress. At this point in time, nurses are but neophytes in understanding organization culture. The survival of evolving health care networks will depend on management and blending of multiple organizational cultures with and among settings.

Incorporating Technology and Evidence-Based Practice

Nurses are surrounded with an overwhelming increase in technological capabilities: Web-based information retrieval and storage, telehealth delivery modes for patient education, and clinical decision support systems that automate care processes. Teich and Wrinn (2000) describe systems in which results review, electronic records, referral processing, secure messaging, order entry for prescriptions, and tests and decision support in the form of alerts are possible—all using a Web-based portal. The development and use of these systems likely will affect the role elements of the nurse in ambulatory care settings. With many of the coordination of care activities that would normally belong to the registered nurse becoming automated, how will the ambulatory care registered nurse of the twenty-first century reshape the role? Kerfoot (2000) identifies a technical intelligence quotient as a survival skill for the new millennium. She defines technical intelligence quotient as not merely being aware of how a specific technology works but as understanding the relationships among the technology, the users, and the affected systems and how they interact to produce outcomes.

This leads to a discussion of evidence-based medicine or nursing. The standard definition of evidence-based medicine (or nursing) is "The conscientious, explicit and judicious use of the current best evidence in making decisions about the care of individual patients." The goal of evidence-based medicine is to provide rigorous answers for simple questions. If I am a patient, What is my "best" care option? If I am a provider, How am I doing? How am I doing compared to others? Inside the system? Outside the system? For the profession, How can we improve what we are doing? Nurses know that measures of quality require accurate, timely, relevant data. Consequently, nurses need information on health outcomes, clinical outcomes, consequences of care, utilization data, and processes of care.

Time Management and the Rapid Pace of Care in Ambulatory Care Settings

The high volume of patients with which the nurse must interact affords a limited time for each patient. This means that the nurse must make rapid assessments, plan nursing care, and execute that plan in quick order. This leads to a continuing tension between the available time in an encounter and the ideal time needed for a complete nursing assessment. The nurse has difficulty being the patient's advocate if there is no time to spend in understanding what the patient's needs, values, and preferences are. Added to this is the demand that nurses in ambulatory care multitask. Nurses may do higher-level care and at the same time find that they cannot spend as much time on teaching, referrals, and care coordination when they also have to do the work of nursing assistants in some clinics.

Continuity of care, the extent to which the same provider is seen during a sequence of encounters, has been given attention, with the number of physician providers seen as a determinant of quality of primary care (Spooner, 1994). If nursing care can affect patient outcomes in ambulatory practice, then it is necessary to develop models of care delivery to ensure similar continuity. Dickey (1998) recommends visit planning in ambulatory care. "The primary purpose of visit planning is to improve recognition, and ultimately treatment of patients' major health needs regardless of when or how the patient presents" (p. 89). Steps in visit planning include the following:

1. Twenty-four to 48 hours before seeing a patient, an experienced ambulatory care nurse previews the chart, updates the problem list, and makes a preliminary visit plan.

2. During the visit, the nurse obtains a clear, concise understanding of the reasons for the visit and develops a final visit plan based on the patient's needs.
3. Throughout the process the nurse manages the patient flow and serves as a patient advocate.
4. Exit visit planning occurs at the conclusion of the provider's portion of the visit.

In the exit interview the nurse has the opportunity to go over the visit with the patient, assessing learning needs and correcting any misapprehensions the patient may have with respect to future therapeutic plans, medications, and educational needs. Hartley (2002) recommends use of the patient-administered Primary Care Assessment Survey (Safran et al., 1998) while patients are waiting to be seen. Results of this survey can be used to improve ambulatory care outcomes such as accessibility, continuity and comprehensiveness of care, integration of care patient-provider interaction, and patient trust of providers. Oermann, Masserang, Maxey, and Lange (2002) did a quasi-experimental design research intervention study in which they provided education about the patients' health problem via videotape while the patients were waiting to be seen. Patients who received the taped education while waiting were significantly more satisfied with education received during their visit. Findings such as these have potential to leverage nurses' time as educators and coordinators of patient care in ambulatory settings.

Frequently, nurses in ambulatory care are used to leverage the physician's practice, and little value is placed on the dimensions of the nursing role or the nursing interventions themselves. A number of differentiated nursing practice models can be used to address this (Hermann, 1993; Schroeder et al., 2000a). In the model described by Hermann, nursing practice is diversified to incorporate registered nurses with differing educational preparation and practice experience. The three levels of nursing are the staff registered nurse (usually associate's degree or diploma prepared), who typically supervises unlicensed personnel, provides basic triage patient education, and administers medications; the registered nurse II (bachelor of science in nursing [BSN]) who functions with a broader yet still limited scope; and the clinical nurse specialist–nurse practitioner.

Delegation and Supervision

Nonlicensed assistive workers traditionally have been used in ambulatory care settings. As in inpatient settings, there is a push in ambulatory care to maximize the use of assistive personnel. A movement even exists to remove all professional nurses from some ambulatory care organizations, based on the misinformed assumption that "nursing care" in ambulatory settings is strictly technical care and can be provided by technicians at a lower cost. This movement is reinforced further by the fact that there are limited ways to calculate nursing intensity in ambulatory care and to predict the level of nursing staff needed (Haas & Hastings, 1998).

Patient care delivery roles are available for assistive personnel and professional nurses in ambulatory care. Assistive personnel should be doing lower-level nursing activities that do not require discretionary judgment or critical thinking. Nurses working in ambulatory care want to delegate many activities that fall under the dimensions of enabling operations and technical procedures (Haas & Hackbarth, 1995a). Delegation of these dimensions would allow the professional nurse time for higher-level activities in dimensions such as teaching, care coordination, and community outreach. Nurses working in ambulatory care also need time to delegate and supervise assistive personnel. Currently, no empirical data give direction as to the optimal number of assistive personnel that one nurse can supervise in the ambulatory setting. Many nurses working today grew up under primary nursing in hospitals. They have little experience with delegation and supervision of assistive workers, and many have mistaken notions about how assistive workers are "working on their license." Consequently, these nurses are reluctant to delegate to assistive personnel for fear of what may happen not only to the patient but also to their license and livelihood.

As more assistive workers are incorporated in delivery models in ambulatory care organizations, nurses will need to be educated regarding delegation and supervision, and evaluation studies will be necessary to identify optimal staffing ratios, including optimal spans of control. Haas and Gold (1997) recommend effective supervision strategies:

1. Know your assistive workers, role expectations for them, and their level of competency (in ambulatory care there is marked confusion and/or blurring of scopes of practice between licensed practical nurses, nurse's aides, and medical assistants).
2. Allocate time for supervision, rounding, and evaluating care delivery.
3. Develop open communication channels.
4. Adhere to patient care and work performance standards.

5. Give timely feedback, positive and negative, and make time for sharing improvement strategies.

A need also exists for nursing intensity indexes and systems in ambulatory care so that client demands for nursing care can be tracked and appropriate staffing can be planned and budgeted (Haas & Hackbarth, 1995b; Hastings, 1992; Verran, 1986). Cusack, Jones-Wells, and Chisholm (2004) provide an excellent review of current thinking in condition severity/intensity tools and outline the process used in one oncology setting to develop an ambulatory intensity system. Jones, Cusack, and Chisholm (2004) delineate implementation of ambulatory intensity system in an ambulatory oncology center; and Cusack, Jones, and Chisholm (2004) find that the process of applying the ambulatory intensity system tool daily supports making conscious decision about delegation to nonnursing personnel. Caveats to consider regarding assistive workers are that assistive workers are more costly than professional nurses when there is insufficient work to occupy their time for an entire shift. When assistive workers are in a delivery model, a significant portion of professional nursing time will be consumed in delegation and supervision; thus when the bulk of the care needs are higher-level care, hiring a nurse who can do all care and who does not require supervision may be more cost-effective. For example, there will be more activities that can be assigned to assistive workers in high-volume clinics such as general surgery or ophthalmology and perhaps less work for assistive workers in an oncology clinic where chemotherapy is being given and emotional support, care planning, and education needs are many.

PROFESSIONAL ROLE

The nursing shortage and the level of educational preparation of ambulatory care nurses pose significant challenges. The U.S. Department of Labor predicts a million vacant nursing positions by 2020. In addition, a significant nursing faculty shortage exists, so nurse educators cannot prepare all the persons who aspire to be nurses today. This will adversely affect ambulatory care where nurses typically are recruited from acute care after years of experience. If one waits to recruit, there may be few or no nurses available in years to come. In addition, significant numbers of nurses currently working in ambulatory care have many years of nursing and ambulatory care experience; however, many also have less than baccalaureate preparation as their highest level of nursing education (Hackbarth et al., 1995). With expansion of ambulatory nursing roles comes increasing expectations that ambulatory care nurses coordinate care within the health care network and the community. Yet nurses without baccalaureate preparation have not had formal course work or clinical experiences with community health nursing. Adding to this problem is the fact that significant numbers of currently practicing ambulatory care nurses do not belong to any professional nursing organizations (Haas & Hackbarth, 1995a). Therefore continuing education through programs, newsletters, and collegial information sharing is less available to ambulatory care nurses who are not members of professional organizations. A short-term solution has been the push to have ambulatory care nurses get certified by the American Nurses Credentialing Center. Preparation for certification has been an initiative of the AAACN. However, to provide for the future, current ambulatory care nurses must work with educators in baccalaureate nursing programs to develop hands-on student clinical experiences in ambulatory care and to develop ambulatory care nurses as preceptors for baccalaureate students.

The issue of basic nursing preparation and continuing education for nurses practicing ambulatory care presents a challenge. Yet without ongoing education, it is becoming increasingly difficult for the non–master's prepared nurse to compete with master of business administration degree holders for management positions in the ambulatory setting. Creative mechanisms are needed to provide incentives for nurses to enhance their formal educational preparation and to keep current with regional and national practice issues and trends. Clinical ladders or professional nursing advancement programs offer mechanisms that provide incentives and rewards for nurses who seek educational opportunities to enhance their practice. Distance learning through videoconferencing and online computer course work offer opportunities for formal for-credit course work and continuing education. Learning through distance education formats provides accessibility and flexibility for nurses no matter the size or location of their practice environment. The challenge is to get sufficient credible distance learning programming prepared in a timely fashion. The need for more BSN nurses to work in ambulatory care organizations has been identified, yet there is currently no way to provide entreé to employment of new BSN graduates in ambulatory care.

Ambulatory care organizations might be more willing to hire new nurse graduates if they were educated about nursing practice in ambulatory care. For example, BSN students should have parallel ambulatory care clinical experiences. Students should spend as much

time caring for pediatric, obstetric, mental health, and elderly clients in ambulatory settings as they do in hospital settings. As patients with increasingly complex problems are cared for in ambulatory care settings, nurses must be concerned about patient outcomes. Linda Aiken has demonstrated that the presence of BSN-prepared nurses in acute care enhances patient outcomes (Aiken, Clarke, Cheung, Sloane, & Silber, 2003).

Need for the Intrastate Nurse Licensure Compact

As TNP became more and more prevalent, it became obvious that there were potential violations of state Nurse Practice Acts by nurses who were consulting, providing surveillance, triaging, or following up with patients who reside across state lines if the nurse is not licensed to practice nursing in the state where the patient resides. The AAACN developed a position statement regarding multistate licensure in an effort to inform nurses of the risks to their license and took this position statement to the National Federation of Specialty Nursing Organizations so that those organizations could have the opportunity to endorse the position statement if they so wished and could begin to educate their members as to the risks.

The current licensure system does not address issues that have come about as a result of health care restructuring, technological advances, and increasing consumerism (Hutcherson & Williamson, 1999):

1. Increases in multistate and national health care systems
2. Movement toward community-based care
3. Increases in managed care, use of telephone triage, and telephone consultation
4. Increases in use of automated monitoring of patients and telehealth modalities in the delivery of care
5. Growing expectations by consumers of inclusion in health care decision making

Legal authority for practice is a concern for any professional nurse who provides care for clients in a state in which the nurse is not currently licensed, such as nurses working in integrated delivery systems, nurses working in tertiary referral health care systems, telephone practice nurses, flight nurses, and nursing faculty. Current state licensure laws do not address adequately whether states have authority to regulate practice of a nurse who is located physically in another state. The nurse licensure compact allows a nurse to have one license (in his or her state of residency) and to practice in others states that have enacted the compact, as long as the individual acknowledges that he or she is subject to the practice laws and discipline of each state. Under the compact, practice across state lines would be allowed, whether physical or electronic, unless the nurse is under discipline or a monitoring agreement that restricts practice across state lines. To achieve mutual recognition, each state would have to enter into an *interstate compact* that allows nurses to practice in more than one state (National Council of State Boards of Nursing, 2005). "An interstate compact is an agreement between two or more states established for the purpose of remedying a particular problem of multistate concern" (*Black's Law Dictionary*). An interstate compact supersedes state laws and may be amended by all party states agreeing and then changing individual state laws (National Council of State Boards of Nursing, 2004).

The National Council of State Boards of Nursing believes that the *mutual recognition model of nurse licensure* enacted through the interstate compact is the preferred regulatory model because it (1) maintains state-based regulatory system, (2) can be implemented incrementally on a state-by-state mode, (3) can be implemented without uniform requirements for licensure in each state, (4) meets demands of integrated delivery systems, (5) meets the challenges of technological advances in telehealth, and (6) meets the need of the public for access to nursing care. The benefits of the interstate compact include the following:

1. It enhances nurse's mobility.
2. It maintains a state-based system of licensure and discipline.
3. It does not change practice laws in each state and allows each state Nurse Practice Act to maintain the authority to regulate nursing practice in the individual state.
4. It deals only with licensure issues.
5. It expands consumer access to qualified nurses.

By the year 2005, 18 states had adopted the interstate compact. Legislation is pending in other states. With the nursing shortage, many states are considering the compact to make it easier for nurses to move quickly into other states. The interstate compact requires that nurses obtain only one license in the state of residency (domicile, IRS tax status), that nurses agree to abide by the state Nursing Practice Act in their home state and states where clients are resident at the time care is provided, and that if an incident occurs, the home state and remote state can take disciplinary action, and the compact will enable exchange of investigative information. Advantages of the one license concept include reduced barriers to interstate practice for nurses, cost-effectiveness and simplicity for the licensee, unduplicated listing of licensed nurses (national data on the nursing population would be accurate), improved tracking for disciplinary purposes, and increased interstate commerce.

Some nursing organizations have concerns about mutual recognition and the interstate compact. The issues include lack of uniform requirements for licensure in each state; confidentiality and information sharing particularly in terms of discipline issues (however, less than 1% of all licensed registered and practical nurses experience final disciplinary actions in a given year [National Council of State Boards of Nursing, 2004]); the potential that the compact could facilitate strike breaking; access to laws, rules, and other practice-related information; licensure linked to state of residence; and the need for a separate compact and time line for advanced practice nurses. In the latter, so much variability exists between states in the scope of practice for advanced practice nurses that a separate compact is being devised for their practice.

Challenges with the interstate compact begin with informing all nurses of the need for and benefits of the time line for enactment of the interstate compact. Current information is available on the National Council of State Boards of Nursing Web site (http://www.ncsbn.org). The American Organization of Nurse Executives also has information on multistate licensure, as does the American Academy of Ambulatory Care Nurses (http://www.inurse.com).

SUMMARY

Although concerns and challenges abound in the rapidly evolving world of ambulatory care nursing, they also provide multiple opportunities for nursing. Experienced ambulatory care nurses say that they would work in no other field of nursing. The opportunities to provide primary health care and build long-term relationships with patients, families, and health care colleagues are but a few of the rewards of working in ambulatory care nursing.

REFERENCES

Aiken, L. H., Clarke, S. P., Cheung, R. B., Sloane, D. M., & Silber, J. H. (2003). Educational levels of hospital nurses and surgical patient mortality. *JAMA: The Journal of the American Medical Association, 290*, 1617-1623.

American Academy of Ambulatory Care Nursing, Standards Revision Task Force. (1993). *Ambulatory care nursing administration and practice standards*. Pitman, NJ: Jannetti.

American Academy of Ambulatory Care Nursing, Standards Revision Task Force. (2000). *Ambulatory care nursing administration and practice standards.* Pitman, NJ: Jannetti.

American Academy of Ambulatory Care Nursing, Telephone Practice Standards Task Force. (1997). *Telephone nursing practice administration and practice standards.* Pitman, NJ: Jannetti.

American Academy of Ambulatory Care Nursing, TNP Standards Review Task Force. (2004). *Telehealth nursing practice administration and practice standards.* Pitman, NJ: Jannetti.

American Academy of Ambulatory Care Nursing. (2004). *Ambulatory care nursing administration and practice standards.* Pitman, NJ: Jannetti.

American Nurses Association. (1995). *Social policy statement.* Washington, DC: Author.

American Nurses Association & American Academy of Ambulatory Care Nursing Task Force. (1997). *Ambulatory care nursing: The future is here.* Washington, DC: Author.

Androwich, I., & Phillips, K. (Eds.). (1992). *The use of the minimum data set in ambulatory nursing, American Academy of Ambulatory Nursing Administration.* Pitman, NJ: Janetti.

Cusack, G., Jones, A., & Chisholm, L. (2004). Patient intensity in an ambulatory oncology research center: A step forward for the field of ambulatory care—Part III. *Nursing Economics, 22*(4), 193-195.

Cusack, G., Jones-Wells, A., & Chisholm, L. (2004). Patient intensity in an ambulatory oncology research center: A step forward for the field of ambulatory care. *Nursing Economic$, 22*(2), 58-63.

Dickey, L. (1998). Outpatient visit planning: Turning episodic care into comprehensive care. *Nursing Economic$, 16*(2), 88-90.

Futch, C., & Phillips, R. (2003). The mega issues of ambulatory care nursing. *Nursing Economic$, 21*(3), 140-142.

Garner, B. A. (Ed.). (2004). *Black's law dictionary.* Eagan, MN: ThomsonWest.

Haas, S., & Androwich, I. (1999). Telephone consultation. In G. Bulecheck & J. McCloskey (Eds.), *Nursing interventions: Effective nursing treatments.* Philadelphia: Saunders.

Haas, S., & Gold, C. (1997). Supervision of unlicensed assistive workers in ambulatory care. *Nursing Economic$, 15*(2), 57-59.

Haas, S., & Hackbarth, D. (1995a). Dimensions of the staff nurse role in ambulatory care: Part III. Using research data to design new models of nursing care delivery. *Nursing Economic$, 13*(3), 230-241.

Haas, S., & Hackbarth, D. (1995b). Dimensions of the staff nurse role in ambulatory care: Part IV. *Nursing Economic$, 13*(4).

Haas, S., Hackbarth, D., Kavanagh, J., & Vlasses, F. (1995). Dimensions of the staff nurse role in ambulatory care: Part II. Comparison of role dimensions in four ambulatory settings. *Nursing Economic$, 13*(3), 152-165.

Haas, S., & Hastings, C. (1998). *Getting your foot in the ambulatory care door.* Presented at the American Nurses Association 1998 Biennial Convention Workshop in San Diego, CA.

Hackbarth, D., Haas, S., Kavanagh, J., & Vlasses, F. (1995). Dimensions of the staff nurse role in ambulatory care: Part I. Methodology and analysis of data on current staff nurse practice. *Nursing Economic$, 13*(2), 89-98.

Hartley, L. A. (2002). Perspectives in ambulatory care: Using the primary care assessment survey in an ambulatory setting. *Nursing Economic$, 20*(5), 235-236, 248.

Hastings, C. (1992). Classification issues in ambulatory care nursing. *Journal of Ambulatory Care Management, 10*(3), 50-64.

Hastings, C., & Muir-Nash, J. (1989). Validation of a taxonomy of ambulatory nursing practice. *Nursing Economic$, 7,* 142-149.

Hermann. (1993). Diversified nursing practice in ambulatory care. *Nursing Economic$, 11*(3), 176-179.

Hooks, M., Dewitt-Arnold, D., & Westbrook, L. (1980). The role of the professional nurse in the ambulatory care setting. *Nursing Administration Quarterly, 4*(4), 12-17.

Hutcherson, C., & Williamson, S. H. (1999). Nursing regulation for the new millennium: The mutual recognition model. Online Journal of Issues in Nusing. Retrieved January 3, 2006 from, http://www.nursingworld.org/ojin/topic9/topic9_2.htm

Jones, A., Cusack, G., & Chisholm, L. (2004). Patient intensity in an ambulatory oncology research center: A step forward for the field of ambulatory care—Part II. *Nursing Economic$, 22*(3), 120-123.

Joseph, A. (1990). Ambulatory care: An objective assessment. *Journal of Nursing Administration, 20*(11), 18-24.

Kastens, J. (1998). Integrated care management: Aligning medical center and nurse triage services. *Nursing Economic$, 16*(60), 320-322, 329.

Kerfoot, K. (2000). TIQ (Technical IQ): A survival skill for the new millenium. *Nursing Economic$, 18*(1), 29-31.

Law gives Illinoisans greater access to information about health care costs. (2005, June 15). *Suntimes News.* Retrieved July 1, 2005, from http://www.suntimesnews.com/2/news_archive/june_05/0615law.htm

Martin, C. (1999). Nursing case management: How the current model is evolving. *AAACN Viewpoint, 21*(6), 1-4.

National Council of State Boards of Nursing. (2005). Nurse licensure contract. Retrieved July 1, 2005, from http://www.ncsbn.org/nlc/index.asp

Oermann, M., Masserang, M., Maxey, M., & Lange, M. P. (2002). Perspectives in ambulatory care: Clinic visit and waiting: Patient education and satisfaction. *Nursing Economic$, 20*(6), 292-295.

Parrinello, K., & Witzel, P. (1990). Analysis of ambulatory nursing practice. *Nursing Economic$, 8,* 322-328.

Pinkney-Atkinson, V., & Robertson, B. (1993). Ambulatory nursing: The handmaiden/specialist dichotomy. *Journal of Nursing Administration, 23*(9), 50-57.

Safran, D., Kosinski, M., Tarlov, A., Rogers, W., Taira, D., Liberman, N., et al. (1998). The primary care assessment survey: Tests of data quality and measurement performance. *Medical Care, 36*(5), 728-739.

Schroeder, C., Trehearne, B. B., & Ward, D. (2000a). Expanded role of nursing in ambulatory managed care: Part I. Literature, role development, and justification. *Nursing Economic$, 18*(1), 14-19.

Schroeder, C., Trehearne, B., & Ward, D. (2000b). Expanded role of nursing in ambulatory managed care: Part II. Impact on outcomes of costs, quality, provider and patient satisfaction. *Nursing Economic$, 18*(2), 71-78.

Smith, J. (1981). The idea of health: A philosophical inquiry. *Advances in Nursing Science, 3*(3), 43-50.

Spooner, S. A. (1994). Incorporating temporal and clinical reasoning in a new measure of continuity of care. *Proceedings of the Annual Symposium on Computer Applications in Medical Care.* pp. 716-721.

Stavins, M. (1993). Ambulatory nursing: Facing the future. *Journal of Ambulatory Care Management, 16*(4), 67-71.

Teich, J., & Wrinn, M. (2000). Clinical decision support systems come of age. *MD Computing, 17*(1), 43-46.

United States Department of Health and Human Services (USDHHS). (2000). The registered nurse population, March 2000. Findings from the national sample survey of registered nurses.

Verran, J. (1981). Delineation of ambulatory care nursing practice. *Journal of Ambulatory Care Management, 4*(2), 1-13.

Verran, J. A. (1986). Patient classification in ambulatory care. *Nursing Economic$, 4*(5), 347-351.

Wakefield, M. (2000). Research urgently needed on mistakes in outpatient settings. *AAACN Viewpoint, 22*(5), 3-4.

Werley, H. H., & Lang, N. M. (Eds.). (1988). *Identification of the Nursing Minimum Data Set.* New York: Springer.

Gerontological Nursing

Recent Changes and Current Issues

MARY ZWYGART-STAUFFACHER ◆ MARILYN J. RANTZ

For more than 30 years the aging of America was known to be occurring and that there would be an explosion of older adults in America. The twenty-first century finds Americans facing this aging explosion with increased knowledge about the aging process and evidence-based research to guide the care for the elderly, yet there continues to be a limited number of adequately prepared professional nurses to address this potentially serious deficit in health care delivery for the elders of the United States and internationally. For decades, gerontological nurse experts have stated, "The time is here, the time is now, and the elderly population projections for the twenty-first century are staggering," yet Americans remain woefully unprepared.

Cost implications for caring for the elderly are equally staggering. Costs are associated not only with vast increases in numbers of elderly but also in the complexity of the multiple chronic diseases and acute exacerbations that occur. Persons 65 and older compose approximately 12.4% of the population and therefore one out of every eight Americans. By 2030, the number will be about twice that, or about 20% of the population (Administration on Aging, 2004), with those 85 and older being statistically the fastest growing subset of the elderly population. The elderly of America also are becoming more diverse, with elders reflecting the increased diversity of the U.S. population.

Although those 65 and older account for only about 12% of the population, they account for well over one third of the country's personal health care expenditures. As the older population grows, so will their use of services. In 1990, about 1.5 million impaired persons over the age of 65 used some type of community service at least once. By the year 2020, 2.4 million impaired older persons will use community services (U.S. Senate Special Committee on Aging, 1991). To understand the scope of the costs of these services, in 1992, more than $60 billion was spent on long-term care and home and community care for the elderly (Cohen, Kumar,

McGuire, & Wallack, 1992). In comparison, the cost of these services increased substantially by 1996, when $125.5 billion was spent on nursing home and home health care for the elderly. Additionally, the Medicare Hospital Insurance and Supplementary Medical Insurance program financed $203.1 billion in spending for health care of the aged and disabled, bringing the total spent on those over 65 years of age to $326.6 billion (Levit et al., 1997).

Considering the costs and needs for services for older persons today and in the future, one must ask, Does the nation have the nursing workforce to address the needs of gerontological clients? This question is even more ominous with the nursing shortage and is compounded by the nursing faculty shortage: Who will educate the future nurses and help nurses licensed today to care for the complexity of care and service issues in the face of an unprecedented aging workforce and seniors? Can today's workforce adjust to work effectively in changing delivery systems? How can nurse educators better prepare the gerontological nursing workforce of tomorrow? These are major issues confronting gerontological nursing today.

CHANGING DELIVERY SYSTEMS

Older adults are using services across the continuum of care; they no longer depend on hospitalizations, which are coupled with ongoing supervision from their primary care physician, to manage their chronic conditions. Older adults are using a multitude of community-based home care and social services, residential care, assisted living, and subacute care and long-term care services. Despite nurses' generalized lack of knowledge about geriatric care; the past 20 years has seen the development of exciting new nursing models in the delivery of care to older adults (Mezey, Boltz, Esterson, Mitty, 2005). Yet as the number of elderly increase, the shortcomings of the present long-term care paradigm will become a more serious and costly problem. Though there are diverse options for some elderly, depending on regional variation and ability to pay, for many elderly and their families, choice is limited at best. The new paradigm of care must be holistic with an array of strategies that meet the needs of the older adult (Maas, 2004).

Nurses have been underused and some would say less than creative in approaching this new care crisis. New roles are emerging, however, as nurses assist seniors to navigate the continuum of care. The nurse becomes the person who helps seniors navigate those uncertain waters as they try to use services from multiple settings across multiple agencies funded from a variety of sources. Yet advanced practice nurses are underused in long-term care, notwithstanding evidence of their positive influence on resident outcome and cost-effectiveness (Rantz et al., 2001). New nursing roles are not without dilemmas. Gerontological nurses now must make decisions that are not only client-focused but also economic-focused. Seldom before have nurses played such integral roles in the allocation of resources. Nurses in the past cared for seniors without concerns regarding cost implications. Today, as nurses assume case management or care coordination roles, they must consider cost. Moreover, nurses must make tough decisions about allocation of resources for the client. This is a new era for gerontological nurses. Nurses must be aware of what services cost and help seniors make wise, cost-effective choices while ensuring that they receive the services they need. Yet gerontological nurses, like other health care providers, are dually challenged because they may not identify needs consistent with those of their clients (Zwygart-Stauffacher, Lindquist, & Savik, 2000).

As seniors use a variety of services across the continuum of care, funding of services via managed care contracts becomes a tremendous challenge for gerontological nursing. When funded via managed care contracts, services must be provided within a capitated budget. This means that the fee is set for *all* services that individuals will use, and nurses must assume gatekeeping functions and make tough decisions about which type of services seniors will receive. Capitation is a different approach than the fee-for-service, in which costs of services are totaled and billed at the end. As managed care is implemented fully for Medicare recipients, as is proposed by the Centers for Medicare and Medicaid Services, limits on acute care use and hospitalization will become apparent. No longer will seniors with multiple chronic illnesses primarily use multiple hospitalizations for the management of their illnesses. As much as possible, they will be managed on an outpatient basis, and some

tough decisions will have to be made about when to stop treatment.

The elderly use more hospital care, with greater than 3 times as many individuals more than 65 years of age being discharged from the hospital than those 45 to 64 years of age (Administration on Aging, 2004). The elderly receiving acute care services are requiring the most complex care with multiple system disorders or illnesses, requiring a tremendous depth and breadth of knowledge for care of that older adult. The nurse in the community will be part of a health care team that will be making some tough decisions not to hospitalize some very sick individuals with complex illnesses and allow them to die at home, in a nursing home, in a subacute unit, or in an assisted-living setting.

ADVANCED PRACTICE NURSE IN GERONTOLOGICAL NURSING

With the evolution of managed care and complex care delivery systems, the gerontological nurse prepared at the graduate level is being viewed as the appropriate provider or coordinator of care services. Therefore an increase in the number of individuals prepared with graduate degrees in gerontological nursing is required. Historically, the advanced practice gerontological nurse is a master's-prepared individual with a clinical specialization in gerontological nursing.

In the 1970s only a few programs at the master's level were preparing gerontological nurse practitioners; this education was not embraced by the nursing community until the mid to late 1980s. Now, two advanced clinical practice roles exist in which gerontological specialization are developed: the gerontological clinical nurse specialist and the gerontological nurse practitioner. Yet even with the expansion of two graduate preparation options, the numbers of individuals prepared with gerontological nursing specialization have not been realized. The number of certified gerontological nurse practitioners has risen from 1570 in 1993 (American Nurses Credentialing Center, 1994) to 3240 as of January 2000 (American Nurses Credentialing Center, personal communication, 2000). Another 847 nurses are certified as gerontological clinical nurse specialists. In 2002 only 42 nurses nationally were certified by the American Nurses Credentialing Center as advanced practice geriatric nurses. Can this limited number of advanced practice geriatric nurses exert more than a minimal impact on the health care needs of the majority of older adults (Mezey & Fulmer, 2002)? Interestingly, not even half as many advanced practice nurses are certified as are pediatric nurse practitioners, whose numbers exceed 10,000 (National Certification Board of Pediatric Nurse Practitioners and Nurses, personal communication, 2000).

Though the literature in the 1990s supported the merger of these two roles (nurse practitioner and clinical nurse specialist) and the emergence of a single advanced practice gerontological nurse preparation (Fulmer & Mezey, 1994; Schuren, 1996), that has not come to fruition. Although the roles have similarities, the differences have been little discussed in the nursing community (Page & Arena, 1994). At issue is whether one individual can be prepared who can integrate the competencies of both these roles when minimal research has been conducted to compare these roles (Fenton & Brykczynski, 1993; Lyons, 1996). These roles traditionally have been setting-specific, with the nurse practitioner providing ambulatory and primary care services and the clinical specialist providing services to special patient populations in long-term care and acute care settings and staff education or development. If a blending of these roles can occur, the resulting issue becomes, Can nurse educators prepare clinically competent individuals in a blended role who can meet the demands of the role expectations successfully across settings? Nurse practitioners have been prepared with a variety of primary care skills targeted specifically to allow them to direct the primary care of older adults. That has not been the case for clinical nurse specialists. These nurses have received information and education targeted to managing nursing problems older adults present, not assuming responsibility for directing with the client the management of their health care. These two role functions are distinct. Historically, the individuals who have merged both role functions have done so with a clinical nurse specialist master's followed with a post-master's specialization for nurse practitioner.

Another key issue is whether family nurse practitioners or adult nurse practitioners will be viewed as having the knowledge and experience necessary to work with the elderly in their health care management. Technically, individuals prepared as family or adult nurse practitioners were allowed to sit for the American Nurses Credentialing Center certification as gerontological nurse practitioners until 1996, when the center instituted the policy that allowed only individuals who have been prepared in a gerontological nurse practitioner program to sit for the gerontological nurse practitioner examination. No longer is the crossover from family and adult nursing to gerontological nursing allowed. Given the complexity of gerontological clients and the complexity of the knowledge base that is required for successfully managing the role functions of the gerontological nurse practitioner, clearly the formal gerontological education needs to be the foundation for gerontological certification and clinical practice.

An additional issue related to preparing individuals at the advanced practice level is the need to restructure curricula in academic institutions in light of cost containment. The trend is to minimize specialization content in an effort to try to include more students in all courses. These cost-containment efforts are likely to affect specialized courses such as gerontological courses. The cost-containment efforts likely will make those courses options for students because it is more costly and time consuming to arrange specialized didactic and clinical components. Some presume that one can obtain the knowledge that is necessary for delivering gerontological care by simply completing clinical practicum with older adults without specialized didactic content within the graduate program. This is a disturbing trend.

The benefits of advanced practice nurses in long-term and acute care are well supported in the literature for enhancing quality care in a cost-effective manner (Institute of Medicine, 2001; Kane et al., 1988; Naylor et al., 1999; Ryden et al, 2000). Only 3% of all advanced practice nurses specialize in geriatrics, yet older adults compose more than 85% of nursing home residents and nearly 50% of hospitalized patients (Hamric, Spross, & Hanson, 2000). Cost-effective care also cannot occur with many advanced practice nurses not understanding cost of care delivery. Nurse educators can no longer afford to teach students how care should be delivered without an understanding of what that care would cost. Nursing research must be cognizant of the cost of care and differentiated outcomes of care related to cost.

To help address the undereducation of advanced practice gerontological nurses, the American Association of Colleges of Nursing and the John A. Hartford Institute have joined forces to develop geriatric competencies and curriculum materials for all baccalaureate nursing programs and core competencies of the adult and family nurse practitioner as related to gerontological content (Hartford Foundation Institute for Geriatric Nursing, n.d.). The goal is that all advanced practice nurses would have increased competency in caring for the elderly, with clear guidelines for the appropriate point of referral to the geriatric advanced practice nurse.

Aside from the content issues of what is an appropriate knowledge base for all nurses and nurses specializing in nursing care of the elderly, qualifications of the faculty are at issue. Already in the early 1990s there was a call of alarm, as reflected in a report of the planning committee for the White House Conference on Aging that revealed that an alarming 40% of the nursing faculty teaching in graduate-level gerontological nursing programs had *no* formal gerontological preparation. Compounding this concern was that greater than three fourths (77%) of all clinical preceptors and instructors in all programs in nursing have no formal preparation working with the elderly (Dye, 1992). In 1995, Mezey had advised that failure to produce adequate number of faculty to teach gerontology had affected adversely the care of the elderly. And now in the early twenty-first century the faculty shortage is even greater than had been anticipated only a decade ago. How can gerontological advanced practice nurses be prepared by faculty without gerontological preparation? With the nationwide crisis of nursing faculty shortage, where will the next generation of nursing faculty with gerontological nursing expertise come from?

UNDERGRADUATE NURSING EDUCATION

Based on our experience, we concur with Fulmer and Mezey (1994) that traditionally, basic nursing programs have included little geriatric nursing content and that most faculty lack preparation in geriatric nursing. Without course work in geriatric nursing, the faculty lacks preparation in geriatric nursing to be qualified to teach those courses. Yurchuck and Brower (1994) reported that only 12% of undergraduate faculty has specific gerontological preparation. Minimal progress has been seen since these initial reports. Rosenfeld, Bottrell, Fulmer, and Mezey (1999) examined the geriatric content in the baccalaureate curriculum of 80% of university programs in 1997. Of the respondent nursing programs, only 40% reported at least one full-time faculty member certified in geriatrics by the American Nurses Credentialing Center. (The American Nurses Credentialing Center is the only body certifying gerontological nurses.) Twenty percent of the part-time faculty was reported to be certified. How can a school of nursing hope to achieve the standard proposed by Rosenfeld et al. "that the nursing community assure that every nurse graduating from a baccalaureate nursing program have a defined level of competency." When one considers the approach to undergraduate nursing education, clearly nurse educators would not be put in the position of teaching pediatric or obstetrical nursing without preparation in those fields. Why have nurse educators been allowed to teach gerontological nursing without a knowledge base or practice base for their instruction? Because of the sheer numbers of older adults using the health care delivery system and the complexity of the

clinical problems that they present, it is imperative that faculty be prepared clinically and theoretically to teach these courses. Simply having "taken care of elders" is not sufficient preparation.

Sister Rose Therese Bahr (1994) said it so well: "What's wrong? Despite the amount of money made available for post-doctoral study, few faculty are taking advantage of the opportunity to upgrade their knowledge and gerontological nursing. I would hazard a guess that the attitude problems of students not wishing to choose gerontological nursing as a career starts with the faculty who also have an attitude problem. To be based in reality means that all of us are on the continuum of aging. All persons will get old unless a traumatic event occurs that ends life much earlier. What are faculty afraid of that they shy away from content and clinical experience that evolves around the care of the aged?" (p. 38).

Issues surrounding undergraduate nursing education must include grappling with the problem of associate's degree education. Most of the registered nurses working in nursing homes are prepared at the associate's degree level. Many associate's degree curricula do contain content concerning gerontological nursing; however, most do *not* contain a specialized gerontological nursing course. These curricula also lack content and practica in nursing leadership and advanced health assessment. How can nurses prepared at this level be expected to assume a supervisory level position or coordinate comprehensive assessments as are required in nursing homes and hospitals across the nation.

The Institute of Medicine and Committee on Nursing Home Regulations (1986) has recommended that "Nursing homes should place their highest priority on recruitment, retention, and support of adequate numbers of professional nurses who are trained in gerontology and geriatrics to insure an adequate number and appropriate mix of professional and non-professional nursing personnel to meet the needs of all types of residents in each facility." However, many nursing homes have received waivers from even the minimal increases in staffing standards required by the Omnibus Reconciliation Act (Francese & Mohler, 1994). These homes claim that shortages of registered nurses and inadequate reimbursement to pay their salaries are the reasons that they cannot meet their staffing standards. Nursing must become involved to correct these delivery system problems. What creative strategies will nurse administrators conceive to address the shortage of adequate staffing during the present workforce issues that are facing the United States?

Additionally, nursing must deal with the issue of how much preparation a student can receive in a 2-year program to be able to deal with complex problems of elderly in nursing homes and other settings. However, it must be acknowledged that one of the major providers of nursing services in nursing homes are licensed practical nurses prepared with even less formal education. How can this level of educational preparation equate with quality, when clear evidence is available that outcomes of acute care are enhanced with a greater percent of nurses prepared at the baccalaureate or master's level?

Home care is an exploding source of services for seniors. Most nurses working in the home care arena are prepared at the associate's degree level. Traditionally, public health or community-based services were to be provided by baccalaureate-prepared nurse, but this is no longer the case. Nurses are going into homes, a complex environment, to care for individuals with complicated clinical problems, and these nurses have minimum formal nursing education and often have limited experience. At some point, nursing must address this issue and establish the baseline for professional gerontological nursing and general nursing practice at the baccalaureate level. And what will the newly created clinical nurse leader's role be in the future of gerontological nursing? What should it be?

Is it in fact the time to reconsider curriculum development in nursing programs based on the changing society and health care needs. Quinn et al. (2004) challenge nurse educators to consider four areas on which to base curricular changes: the increasing number of older adults, condition severity versus chronicity care issues, population-based policy developments, and the need for education for nurses to work with ever-changing health care needs. What would the nursing curriculum look like, and how might future nurses be prepared if these aspects were used as themes/threads for curricular development and revisions?

CURRENT CLINICAL AND SYSTEMS ISSUES

To identify the current and changing clinical and systems issues of gerontological nursing discussed in gerontological literature, the table of contents of the journals listed in Box 22-1 for the years 1992 to 1995 and 1995 to 2000 were analyzed using qualitative methods. The trends in order of frequency of publication are identified for these two periods and are listed in Boxes 22-2 and 22-3.

BOX 22-1

Journals Selected for Table-of-Contents Analysis (1992-1995 and 1995-2000)

Journal of Gerontological Nursing
Geriatric Nursing
The Gerontologist
Journal of the American Geriatrics Society
Journals of Gerontology
Journal of Long-Term Care Administration
IMAGE: The Journal of Nursing Scholarship
Nursing Research
Research in Nursing and Health
Nursing Outlook

When one compares the trends in the gerontological nursing literature from 1992 to 1995 and 1995 to 2000 with trends identified from a literature review from 1980 to 1990 for a report to the Institute of Medicine (Lang, Kraegel, Rantz, & Krejci, 1990), some new issues have surfaced. Although during the early 1990s, the emergence of dementia special care units and subacute units was paramount, with controversy surrounding these special care programs and units, this was less of an issue by the late 1990s. Some have seen these units as options for long-term care agencies to improve their financial position, whereas others are concerned whether the agencies can provide the level of clinical expertise that these more acutely ill elderly need. By the later 1990s the literature reflected the expansion of services to the elderly from a community/residential care focus for those with dementia. This effort to delay nursing home admission provides another exciting role for the nurse: manager of care for elders residing in these new facilities. The minimum data set (MDS) assessment instrument mandated for use in all nursing homes in 1990 was an issue at the beginning of the 1990s, though its use and usefulness were being addressed by the end of the century. Controversy continues to surround the MDS instrument and the data that are collected. Some were concerned about pursuing research activities using MDS data, raising concerns about validity and reliability. Others were concerned about how regulators would interpret aggregated assessment information from MDS data, how payment mechanisms may be designed using the data, and how comparisons would be made across agencies. By 2004 the federal government was using MDS data. The government also created and is publishing another measure called quality measures on the Center for Medicare and Medicaid Services Web site (http://www.medicare.gov) to compare nursing homes.

BOX 22-2

Trends in Gerontological Research Literature: Clinical Issues

TRENDS IDENTIFIED FROM 1992 TO 1995

Reminiscence
Restraints
   Problems associated with restraints
   Efforts to reduce use of restraints
Disruptive/aggressive behavior
   Nursing strategies to manage such behavior
Wandering
Functional status
   Maintaining function
   Measurement of functional status
   Using functional status to predict illness
Activities of daily living
Elderly response to hospitalization
Use of life-sustaining or lifesaving procedures
Tube feedings
   Positive and negative aspects of use
   Ethical dilemmas of use
Relocation stress
Urinary incontinence
Failure to thrive
Substance abuse
Depression
Alzheimer's
Elder abuse
Wellness promotion

TRENDS IDENTIFIED FROM 1995 TO 2000

Assessment issues
Wellness
   Promotion
   Disease prevention
Alzheimer's
Functional status
Urinary incontinence and other issues
Disruptive/aggressive behavior
   Nursing strategies to manage such behavior
Restraints
   Problems associated with restraints
   Efforts to reduce use of restraints
Activities of daily living
Falls
Depression
Relocation stress
Sustaining/saving life
Wandering
Elder abuse

BOX 22-3

Trends in Gerontological Research Literature: Systems Issues

TRENDS IDENTIFIED FROM 1992 TO 1995

Dementia special care units
   Resource use
   Regulation of units
   Effectiveness of units
Subacute care units
Discharge from acute care settings
Family caregiving
   Collaboration between facilities and families
   Stress associated with caregiving
Community-based services
   Continuum of care
   Financing
   Gaps in home health coverage
Life-care community developments
Advanced directives and self-determination
Delaying nursing home placement
Financing long-term care
Staffing issues in nursing homes
   Use of nurse practitioners and clinical nurse
     specialists
   Retention of staff and training issue
Minimum data set for nursing homes
   Validation of and research using the minimum
     data set
Health care reform
Financing of acute care

TRENDS IDENTIFIED FROM 1995 TO 2000

Evidenced-based practice
   Practice guidelines
   Research utilization
   Family caregiving
   Collaboration between facilities
   Stress associated with collaboration
Community based services; assisted living
Staffing issues
Dementia special care units
   Resource use
   Effectiveness of units
Discharge from acute care settings
   Assisted living
   Aging in place
Self-determination
Financing of long-term care
Financing of acute care
Minimum data set
   Quality indicators
   Quality measures
Subacute care units
   Residential care facilities
   Quality improvement teams/processes
Health care reform
Life-care community developments
Delaying of nursing home placement

By the late 1990s, issues surrounding assessment, wellness, and functional status were represented more frequently in the gerontological literature. Possibly, this is a result of the emergence of advanced practice roles and the use of this provider in all types of settings, but particularly the nursing home setting.

In the early 1990s the number of studies related to advanced directives and the use of life-sustaining procedures greatly increased. Possibly the Patient Self-Determination Act of 1991 is raising these issues for discussion, or perhaps public debate surrounding health care reform and costs of services is bringing these issues forward. Elder abuse in the current survey is represented more clearly in the nursing gerontological literature. This development likely is related to increased public and professional awareness of the problem and attention by nurse researchers. The issues of restraints and behavioral issues were more prominent at the end of the century, possibly related to the effect of Omnibus Reconciliation Act of 1987 and new Health Care Financing Administration and Joint Commission on Accreditation of Healthcare Organization guidelines for restraint usage for clients in nursing homes and hospitals.

The development of community-based services across the continuum of care has been cited more frequently in the nursing literature, as has the development of life-care communities for older adults. These services are considered by many authors to be significant trends for the future of gerontological care delivery. Aging in place is a concept that is all too overdue and one that allows for nurses to focus and develop these new models of care (Rantz et al., 2005). Other trends for the future identified in the literature are delivery of acute care services in long-term care facilities and an increased emphasis on research about care delivery and care needs of older adults. These trends could hold much promise for improving the quality of care and quality of life of long-term care residents.

WHERE GERONTOLOGICAL NURSING NEEDS TO GO NEXT

With the complexity and diversity of clinical problems, clearly gerontological nursing education must be enhanced so that nurses working with older adults are prepared educationally to deal with their complex problems. Additionally, nurses need to be prepared to address the complex systems issues that permeate the complicated delivery systems that older persons must traverse. Gerontological nursing education must prepare professionals not only to deal with these complex issues

but also to shape the future of care delivery for older adults.

A threat to the present successful trajectory of gerontological nursing research is the dearth of gerontological nursing students entering nursing doctoral programs, which is a direct result of the small numbers of students in master's programs in gerontological nursing (Whall, 2004). Nursing must have nurse researchers who have gerontological nursing experience to guide research that is relevant and clearly addresses the issues of older adults. Gerontological nurse researchers who are grounded in clinical experience with older adults can direct relevant research that truly adds to improving the quality of care that older adults receive or improves the education that nurses receive for gerontological nursing. Additionally, nurse researchers who are out of touch with the realities of clinical service systems are not prepared to ask relevant questions that will make significant differences for older adults. With shrinking research dollars and increased competition for resources for research activity, the true relevance of the topic under investigation and the impact it will have on clinical practice and patient outcomes must be clear. Researchers who are educated formally and are experienced in the care of the elderly are crucial to the future of gerontological nursing. Will the newly proposed doctor of nursing practice, as supported by the American Association of Colleges of Nursing, encourage more nurses to pursue clinical doctoral education and possibly result in an even greater decrease in those interested in pursuing a doctor of philosophy?

Recruitment of individuals into gerontological nursing practice who have a true commitment to the elderly and the services that they need is important. Gerontological services are in a growing market with growing opportunities. As with any expanding market, whether individuals are motivated to choose gerontological nursing because they are truly interested in caring for older adults or whether job and economic security are the prime motivators is not always clear. This motivation clearly can affect the outcome of care and the individualization of the care provision.

Nurses who have a commitment to gerontological nursing need to embrace this time of health care reform and configure systems of care, determine and refine what appropriate care outcomes will be, and pursue building those service delivery systems. Now is the time for gerontological nurses to design the future, not react to someone else's designs. Now is the time for gerontological nurses to designate what the critical outcomes of gerontological nursing should be and design a path to achieve the outcomes. Now is the time for the nursing profession to make those decisions to change nursing education, care delivery systems, and care outcome determinates that will enhance quality care to all elders in the future and sustain nurses in their careers as gerontological specialists. Nurse educators are up to challenge, but only if they all embrace the challenge.

REFERENCES

Administration on Aging. (2004). *A profile of older Americans: 2003.* Retrieved June 20, 2005, from http://www.aoa.gov/prof/statistics/profile/2003/profiles2003.asp

American Nurses Credentialing Center. (1994). *Credentialing catalog.* Silver Spring, MD: American Nurses Association.

Bahr, R. T. (1994). Response to "Issues facing faculty in long-term care." In E. L. Middy (Ed.), *Mechanisms of quality in long-term care: Education* (pp. 37-41). New York: National League for Nursing Press.

Cohen, M. A., Kumar, N., McGuire, T., & Wallack, S. S. (1992). Financing long-term care: A practical mix of public and private. *Journal of Health Politics, Policy, and Law, 17*(3), 403-423.

Dye, C. A. (1992). *Education and training.* Report of the White House Conference on Aging Planning Committee, Washington DC: U.S. Government Printing Office.

Fenton, M., & Brykczynski, K. (1993). Qualitative distinctions and similarities in practice of clinical nurse specialist and nurse practitioners. *Journal of Professional Nursing, 9*(6), 313-326.

Francese, T., & Mohler, M. (1994). Long-term care nurse staffing requirements: Has OBRA really helped? *Geriatric Nursing, 15*(3), 139-141.

Fulmer, T., & Mezey, M. (1994). Contemporary geriatric nursing. In W. R. Hazard, J. P. Blass, J. B. Halter, J. G. Ouslander, & M. Tinetti (Eds.), *Principles of geriatric medicine and gerontology* (3rd ed., pp. 249-258). New York: McGraw-Hill.

Hamric, A., Spross, J., & Hanson, C. (2000). *Advanced nursing practice* (2nd ed.). Philadelphia: W.B. Saunders.

Hartford Foundation Institute for Geriatric Nursing. (n.d.). *Education.* Retrieved December 21, 2005, from http://www.serve.com/Hartford/resources/index.html

Health Care Financing Administration. (1996). Baltimore, MD: Bureau of Data Management and Strategy, Office of Health Care Information Systems.

Institute of Medicine. (2001). *Crossing the quality chasm: A new health system for the 21st century.* Washington, DC: National Academy Press.

Institute of Medicine & Committee on Nursing Home Regulations. (1986). *Improving the quality of care in nursing homes.* Washington, DC: National Academy Press.

Kane, R., Kane, R., Arnold, S., Garrard, J., McDermott, S., & Kepferle, L. (1988). Geriatric nurse practitioners as nursing home employees: Implementing the role. *The Gerontologist, 28*(4), 469-477.

Lang, N. M., Kraegel, J. M., Rantz, M. J., & Krejci, J. W. (1990). *Quality of care for older people in America.* Kansas City, KS: American Nurses Association.

Levit, K. R., Lazenby, H. C., Braden, B. R., Cowan, C. A., Sensenig, A. I., McDonnel, P. A., et al. (1997). National health expenditures. *Health Care Review, 19*(1), 161-200.

Lyons, B. L. (1996). Meeting societal needs for the CNS competencies: Why the CNS and NP roles should not be blended in master degree programs. *Online Journal of Issues in Nursing.* Retrieved June 20, 2005, from http://www.nursingworld.org/ojin/tpc1/tpc1_3.htm

Maas, M. (2004). Long-term care for older adult: Advocating for a new health care paradigm. *Journal of Gerontological Nursing, 30,* 3-4.

Mezey, M. (1995). Why good ideas have not gone far enough: Improving gerontological nursing education. In T. Fulmer & M. Matzo (Eds.), *Strengthening gerontological nursing education* (pp. 3-19). New York: Springer.

Mezey, M., Boltz, M., Ester, J., & Mitty, E. (2005). Evolving models of geriatric nursing care. *Geriatric Nursing, 26*(1), 11-15.

Mezey, M., & Fulmer, R. (2002). The future history of gerontological nursing. *The Journals of Gerontology. Series A, Biological Science and Medical Sciences, 57*(7), M438-M441.

Naylor, N., Brooton, D., Campell, R., Jacobsen, B. S., Mezey, M. D., Pauly, M. V., et al. (1999). Comprehensive discharge planning and home follow-up of hospitalized elders: A randomized clinical trial. *JAMA: The Journal of the American Medical Association, 281*(7), 613-620.

Page, N., & Arena, D. (1994). Rethinking the merger of the clinical nurse specialist and the nurse practitioner. *Image: The Journal of Nursing Scholarship, 26*(4), 315-318.

Quinn, M., Berding, C., Daniels, E., Gerlach, M. J., Harris, K., Nugent, K., et al. (2004). Shifting paradigms: Teaching gerontological nursing from a new perspective. *Journal of Gerontological Nursing, 30*(1), 21.

Rantz, M., Marek, K., Aud, A., Tyrer, H., Skubic, M., Demiris, G., et al. (2005). A technology and nursing collaboration to help older adults age in place. *Nursing Outlook, 53*(1), 40-45.

Rantz, M., Popejoy, L., Petroski, G., Madsen, R., Mehr, D., Zwygart-Stauffacher, M., et al. (2001). Randomized clinical trail of a quality improvement intervention in nursing homes. *The Gerontologist, 41*(4), 525-545.

Rosenfeld, P., Bottrell, M., Fulmer, T., & Mezey, M. (1999). Gerontological nursing content in baccalaureate nursing programs: Findings from a national survey. *Journal of Professional Nursing, 15*(2), 84-94.

Ryden, M., Snyder, M., Gross, C., Savik, K., Pearson, V., Krichbaum, K., et al. (2000). Value-added outcomes: The use of advanced practice nurses in long-term car facilities. *The Gerontologist, 40,* 654-662.

Schuren, A. W. (1996). The blended role of the clinical nurse specialists and the nurse practitioner. In A. B. Hamrick, J. A. Spross, & C. M. Hanson (Eds.), *Advanced nursing practice: An integrative approach.* Philadelphia: W.B. Saunders.

U.S. Senate Special Committee on Aging. (1991). *Aging America: Trends and projections* [DHS# (FCoA) 91-28001]. Washington, DC: U.S. Department of Health and Human Services.

Vladeck, B. C, Miller, N. A., & Clauser, S. V. (1993). The changing face of long-term care. *Health Care Financing Review, 14*(4), 5-23.

Whall, A. (2004). Looking past and looking forward to the preferred gerontologic nursing future: 2003 Doris Schwartz Award Presentation. *Journal of Gerontological Nursing, 30*(4), 4-6.

Yurchuck, E., & Brower, H. (1994). Faculty preparation for gerontological nursing. *Journal of Gerontological Nursing, 20*(1), 17-24.

Zwygart-Stauffacher, M., Lindquist, R., & Savik, K. (2000). Development of health care delivery systems that are sensitive to the needs of stroke survivors and their caregivers. *Nursing Administration Quarterly, 24*(3), 33-42.

CHAPTER
23
Hospice and Palliative Care
Recent Changes and Current Issues

JEANNE M. MARTINEZ

Palliative care has emerged over the past 25 years as an area of specialty practice for nursing and medicine. In the United States the origins of palliative care began in the form of hospice programs in the 1970s, often referred to through the 1980s as the "hospice movement" with its underpinnings of the "hospice philosophy." Hospice became a reimbursable benefit under Medicare in 1983, within a managed care type of structure. Beginning in the 1990s, a revolution in palliative care outside of hospice programs has evolved, spurred in large part by the interests of major funding organizations such as the Soros Open Society Institute (Project on Death in America) and the Robert Wood Johnson Foundation. These organizations poured vast resources into research and other end-of-life and palliative care initiatives. Nursing has been at the forefront of developing and defining hospice and nonhospice palliative care principles and practices, moving the knowledge base of palliative care forward, and expanding and integrating its availability to many care settings.

Currently, a split exists among some palliative care specialists about the definition of palliative care, along with an uneasy sense of competition between many hospice and nonhospice palliative care programs and leaders. One major concern is that one or both types of care may not continue as a viable option for patients in the future. The answer may lie in part in the resolve of palliative care and hospice stakeholders to strengthen forces, with increased collaboration between palliative and hospice care providers. This collaboration is needed to maximize optimal patient care along the trajectory of illness and across all health settings, especially given the growing population of the elderly, chronically ill, and those at the end of life.

MODERN EVOLUTION IN CARE OF THE DYING

In the 1960s, two major forces occurring across an ocean from each other initiated and ultimately provided the basis for hospice and palliative care practice. Elisabeth Kübler-Ross published *On Death and Dying* (1969), her landmark book describing the death-denying culture in the United States. Kübler-Ross brought the issue of dying to the attention of the American lay public and created a framework for describing the dying experience. Around the same time in England, Dame Cicely Saunders provided physician leadership in establishing St. Christopher's Hospice, the first modern hospice in the world created to care exclusively for the dying. Many of the standards of care developed at St. Christopher's remain the hallmarks of palliative care today. Dame Saunders began her interest in the dying as a volunteer, became a nurse, and received a degree in social work before studying to become a physician (Martinez & Wagner, 2000). This unusual background may have situated her uniquely to understand the essential need for an interdisciplinary team to provide optimal palliative care.

The current application of the term *palliative care* to describe the concept of holistic care with a focus on symptom management for the terminally ill is attributed to Dr. Balfour Mount, who established the first integrated palliative care unit in a North American hospital in 1974 at the Royal Victoria Hospital in Montreal, Canada. Nursing leadership in hospice care began with Dr. Florence S. Wald, with her desire to bring the principles of Dame Saunders work to America. Dr. Wald's research, "A Nurse's Study of Care for Dying Patients" (USPHS Grant NU 00352), was instrumental in the development of Hospice Incorporated in Branford, Connecticut, the first hospice in the United States (Corless, 1983). Established in 1974, and now named Connecticut Hospice, the inpatient facility remains one of the few buildings architecturally designed for care of the dying (Chan, 1976).

In the 1990s the Robert Wood Johnson Foundation identified the improvement of end-of-life care as one major focus of its foundation, funding many large initiatives, such as the following:

◆ The Center to Advance Palliative Care—a program to promote palliative care in hospitals, with its administrative base at Mount Sinai Hospital in New York.

◆ The EPEC Project (Education for Physicians on End-of-life Care*)—a national train-the-trainer initiative established under the auspices of the American Medical Association to provide educational training for physicians and other health care providers in practice. This program now is located at Feinberg School of Medicine, Northwestern University, Chicago.

◆ ELNEC (End-of-Life Nursing Education Consortium)—a national train-the-trainer initiative for nursing educators and nurses in practice. Originally based in Washington, D.C., ELNEC now is administered by the Hospice and Palliative Nurses Association national office in Pittsburgh.

◆ Last Acts—a national coalition established with the mission to improve care and caring near the end of life. Many other smaller initiatives in end-of-life care around the country have been funded by the Robert Wood Johnson Foundation, primarily in hospitals and medical schools. Many of these initiatives and their outcomes were reflected in the "Means to a Better End: A Report on Dying in America Today," published by Last Acts in November 2002 (Robert Wood Johnson Foundation, 2005).

The Soros Foundation Open Society Institute, Project on Death in America, has completed its grant making but in the past decade has distributed $45 million over 9 years to "transform the culture and experience of dying and bereavement." Awards were granted for professional and public education, the arts, research, clinical care, and public policy projects related to the dying experience (Open Society Institute, 2005).

The Hospice Nurses Association, the first professional organization dedicated to promoting excellence in hospice nursing, was formed in 1987. Out of that group the National Board for Certification of Hospice Nurses was established in 1992, offering the first specialty certification examination in hospice nursing in 1994. In 1997 the Hospice Nurses Association changed its name to the Hospice and Palliative Nurses Association, recognizing the similarity between (nonhospice) palliative care and hospice practice (Sheldon, Dahlin, & Zeri, 2000). This consistent base of practice was confirmed by a 1998 Role Delineation Study conducted by the National Board for Certification of Hospice Nurses and provided the scientific basis for the examination to include nonhospice palliative nursing practice (Anderson, Raudonis, & Kirschling, 1999). In 1999 the National Board for Certification of Hospice Nurses became the National Board for Certification of Hospice and Palliative Nurses to reflect the applicability of the examination to nonhospice palliative practice.

THE DEFINITION CONTROVERSY

Several major definitions of palliative care are used. The current World Health Organization (2005) definition of palliative care is the following:

> Palliative Care is an approach that improves the quality of life of patients and their families facing the problems associated with life-threatening illness, through the prevention and relief of suffering and of early identification and impeccable assessment and treatment of pain and other problems, psychosocial and spiritual. Palliative Care:
>
> ◆ Provides relief from pain and other distressing symptoms;
> ◆ Affirms life and regards dying as a normal process;
> ◆ Intends neither to hasten or postpone death;
> ◆ Integrates the psychological and spiritual aspects of patient care;
> ◆ Offers a support system to help patients live as actively as possible until death;
> ◆ Offers a support system to help the family cope during the patient's illness and in their bereavement;
> ◆ Uses a team approach to address the needs of patients and their families, including bereavement counseling, if indicated;
> ◆ Will enhance quality of life, and may also positively influence the course of illness;
> ◆ Is applicable early in the course of illness, in conjunction with other therapies that are to prolong life, such as chemotherapy or radiation therapy, and includes those investigational … Needed to better understand and manage distressing clinical complications.

The current World Health Organization definition offers a distinct change from the 1990 definition that defined palliative care as "The active total care of patients

---

*In 2004 the EPEC acronym meaning was changed to Education in Palliative and End-of-life Care.

VIEWPOINTS

whose disease is not responsive to curative treatment." The revised definition has moved away from defining palliative care only for those with end-stage illness.

The Hospice and Palliative Nurses Association (1999) still maintains this definition:

> Hospice and palliative nursing practice is the provision of nursing care for the patient and their family with the emphasis on their physical, psychosocial, emotional and spiritual needs at the end of life. This is accomplished in collaboration with an interdisciplinary team in a setting that provides 24-hour nursing availability, pain and symptom management and family support.

The underlying controversy reflected in these definitions is perhaps in part due to the fundamental issue of confronting dying. Some practitioners feel that care for the dying needs to remain explicit in any definition of palliative care and that not doing so returns the profession to the time before Kübler-Ross, when discussion of dying was not open and honest. Conversely, others believe that the term *palliative* is a preferable antidote to the hospice word because *hospice,* synonymous with dying, is too confrontive and creates a major barrier to hospice care.

Another view is that palliative care must be integrated into the care of all those who are seriously ill, regardless of prognosis, and should not be linked exclusively with end-stage care.

A positive step in bringing these various viewpoints together occurred in the creation of the National Consensus Project, a coalition group of five major organizations representing hospice and palliative care interests. The goal of the coalition was to develop comprehensive palliative care guidelines, given the lack of regulation and consistency of palliative specialty practice. The *Clinical Practice Guidelines for Quality Palliative Care* was published in May 2004. The guidelines are organized into eight domains (Box 23-1) and largely reflect standards similar to hospice program guidelines (National Consensus Project, 2004). These standards can be applied to any patient care setting, are not limited to treatment of those identified as terminally ill, and are intended to be applied across the health care continuum.

HOSPICE VERSUS PALLIATIVE CARE

Hospice always provides palliative care, but palliative care can be provided outside of hospice (Figure 23-1). Hospice was developed specifically for the dying, ideally to be used at the time an ill person begins to fail, needs

---

BOX 23-1

Clinical Practice Guidelines for Quality Palliative Care

DOMAINS OF PALLIATIVE CARE
1. Structure and processes of care
2. Physical aspects of care
3. Psychological and psychiatric aspects of care
4. Social aspects of care
5. Spiritual, religious, and existential aspects of care
6. Cultural aspects of care
7. Care of the imminently dying patient
8. Ethical and legal aspects of care

From National Consensus Project. (2004). *Clinical practice guidelines for quality palliative care.* Retrieved July 1, 2005, from http://www.nationalconsensusproject.org/Guideline.pdf.

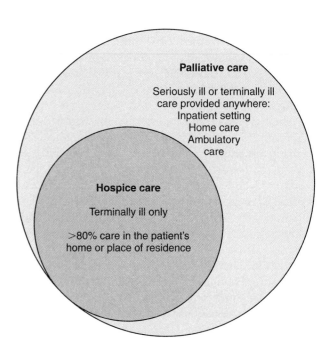

FIGURE 23-1 Hospice versus palliative care. (Note that the figure is *not* intended to indicate the proportion of patients who receive hospice and palliative care; these statistics are known for hospice only.)

care and services, but still can benefit from planning for and experiencing a meaningful end of life. Hospice practitioners are only too aware that life span, prognosis, and time of death are unpredictable even in the face of terminal illness (Christakis & Escarce, 1996).

The Medicare Hospice Benefit criteria of patients needing to be designated to be within 6 months of death is imposed on hospices by government regulation (*Medicare Conditions of Participation for Hospice Care,* 1983).

What often is misunderstood is that the Medicare Hospice Benefit regulation does provide for reasonable accommodations should an individual patient enrolled in hospice exceed the 6-month expected prognosis. Indeed, "outliers" can receive hospice services for a year or more. Patients who continue to decline and need care can remain enrolled in hospice. However, the requirement to inform the patient and family about the 6-month criterion and to have their physician make that determination can make patients, family members, and physicians reluctant to access the Medicare Hospice Benefit (Lynn, 2001).

Nonhospice palliative care services have no such requirement and therefore can see patients earlier in the serious illness, when a patient also needs pain and symptom management and emotional and spiritual support. Earlier in illness, patients also have better opportunity to plan for medical and care decisions they may face in the future and to communicate these to family and physicians. Palliative care is needed for two major populations for which hospice cannot care (Lynn, 2001):

1. Patients who do not desire hospice care but are nonetheless terminally ill. These patients may be unwilling to make the decision to forgo further attempts at curative treatment, which is required by hospice care, and often are seen in acute care settings, particularly in intensive care, emergency room, geriatric, general medicine, and oncology units.

2. Patients with chronic, serious illnesses that eventually will cause their deaths. These patients still may experience periods of medical stability, responding to treatment of illness exacerbations. This makes it even more difficult for physicians to predict prognosis and therefore makes them less sure of the determination of the patient as terminally ill.

Each program, whether hospice or (nonhospice) palliative care, has its advantages and limitations in providing patient care. Both are constrained in different ways in being able to provide continuity of care across all health settings—from physician's office or clinic to hospital to extended care and into the patient's home—which is how the patient receives care. Patients with palliative care needs who receive comprehensive palliative services can have their care plan disrupted, including having their advance care planning overturned, by a trip to the emergency room, a setting that still is not prepared to provide optimal services to an patient at end of life with an emergent problem.

Although hospice and other palliative care programs share underlying principles in their approach to patient care (National Consensus Project, 2004), their differences are largely due to the regulatory mandates governing hospice care (Table 23-1). Hospice is regulated, providing helpful mandates such as an interdisciplinary team that *must* include at a minimum a physician, nurse, social worker, chaplain or other counselor, and volunteers. Although all palliative care ideally is provided by an interdisciplinary team including the members already mentioned, palliative care practice is not required to do so. In fact, some palliative care consultation services currently consist of a single nurse or single physician.

TABLE 23-1

Differences Between Hospice and Palliative Care	
Hospice Care	**Other Palliative Care**
Regulated	Not regulated
Distinct reimbursement benefit, adequate for all patients	Provided as part of other reimbursed care (or not, but not adequate for all patients)
Mostly provided in patient's home	Mostly provided in inpatient, acute care settings
Hospice provided exclusively	Integrated with other care
Mandates interdisciplinary care	Interdisciplinary care recommended but varies widely in practice
Mandates focused on spiritual and psychological	Care often has a medical symptom management social care focus
Only provided to terminally ill	May be provided to seriously chronically ill and in end-stage conditions

Hospice care has a reimbursement system in the form of the Medicare Hospice Benefit. Most states in the United States have a Medicaid Hospice Benefit as well, often providing the same mandates and reimbursement as the Medicare program. Some private insurance benefits provide Hospice Care as well, but the reimbursement and services covered vary greatly. Private benefits cap all of hospice care at a few thousand dollars; others provide the same coverage as the Medicare Hospice Benefit, and still others only offer limited home nursing visits on a fee-for-service basis. This often provides a barrier to hospice care. Hospices also find that even the comprehensive Medicare Hospice Benefit does not provide adequate funding to cover all populations needing hospice care. Most hospice programs today continually must rely on philanthropy to provide needed patient care and to maintain financial viability. Part of the reimbursement issue is that most of hospice care (Medicare and Medicaid) is paid per diem; that is, the hospice is paid a daily fixed rate regardless of the number of services, medications, and durable medical equipment provided. This payment system works well for hospices when the patient's length of stay is such that there is a period of stability in the patient's status, because hospices use most of their resources during the first week and the last week of care. For the past 3 years (2001 to 2003), the national median length of stay in hospice was 21 days (National Hospice and Palliative Care Organization, 2004). Therefore most of the hospice care provided involves patient days when the resource use of the hospice is the highest, with few of the "stable" care days in between the beginning and the end of care. A study published in September 2004 comparing matched hospice and nonhospice Medicare recipients concluded that a hospice length of stay of 2 to 3 months was optimal for clinical and financial outcomes (Pyenson, Connor, Fitch, & Kinzbrunner, 2004). Palliative care services, however, have no distinct reimbursement but usually are reimbursed by the same physician billing mechanisms used for all medical care: inpatient consultation charges for inpatient hospital care, office visit fees in an ambulatory care model, and home visit charges for home services. In some states, nurse practitioners and social workers can bill for services as well. Completely lacking for many palliative care services, however, is specific reimbursement for (non–nurse practitioner) nurses, social work (for which individual billing is not permitted), counselor, and bereavement services. Palliative care teams that do provide these services tend to be funded by research grants, philanthropy, general hospital operations support, or a combination of the these. Because of this lack of reimbursement, palliative care services may not be as comprehensive, particularly in meeting spiritual and psychosocial needs specific to end-stage illness, grieving, and dying. Palliative care services can be self-defining and often focus on addressing pain and other physical symptoms to the detriment of a more holistic approach to patient care. Similarly, emotional support and grief care to families may not be included in services offered by a specific palliative care program, whereas this care to the family system is mandated by hospice regulations.

COMMON (NONHOSPICE) PALLIATIVE CARE MODELS

The most common palliative care service models are inpatient units or a facility dedicated to palliative or end-stage care, a hospital-based palliative care consultation service, and an ambulatory clinic model (Center to Advance Palliative Care, 2005). Other palliative care initiatives include integration of palliative care into the existing health care organization. The following are examples of these:

- Palliative care protocols or standing orders
- Family information on grieving and grief counseling resources
- Bereavement follow-up and services provided directly by the hospital
- Facility design to enhance patient/family comfort and quality of life

CURRENT TRENDS

Hospice programs have proven positive outcomes. In 2003, 50% of hospice patients died at home, with only 9% dying in acute care (nonpalliative care unit) hospitals. This compares favorably with all U.S. deaths in 2003 when 25% died at home and 50% died in acute care hospitals (National Hospice and Palliative Care Organization, 2004). Hospice has a history of high patient/family satisfaction rates. The rule, not the exception, for hospice programs is to receive most of their ongoing philanthropy from grateful patients and families. The most recent study of Medicare costs matching hospice and nonhospice patients determined a range of cost savings for hospice recipients from $1115 to $8879 per patient (Pyenson et al., 2004; Table 23-1).

However, hospice care length of stay needs to increase for the benefit of patients and the viability of programs.

Palliative care programs need to continue to evolve to meet the recommended standards of care for those patients who are not yet terminal but who are in need of symptom management, counseling, care planning, and support, and for those who are dying in acute care settings or who do not have access to or do not desire hospice care. Palliative care services need to ensure that they meet the recommended standard of linking with hospice programs to provide timely referral for hospice care, where possible. Palliative care programs have the opportunity to identify patients for hospice and introduce the concept earlier in illness. To continue to provide this much-needed approach to care, palliative care programs will need to provide continued evidence of strong patient care outcomes and cost-effectiveness.

THE FUTURE

Collaboration is one important mechanism for improving all end-of-life care. The National Board for Certification of Hospice and Palliative Nurses, Hospice and Palliative Nurses Association, and the Hospice and Palliative Nurses Foundation have formally collaborated under an umbrella organization, the Alliance for Excellence in Hospice and Palliative Nurses (Martinez, 2005). This formal link allows these three organizations, each with a unique focus, to support the common mission of moving hospice and palliative care nurses together into the future. An example is the National Board for Certification of Hospice and Palliative Nurses decision to offer specialty examinations in hospice and palliative care to the other nursing team members: licensed practical nurses/vocational nurses and nursing assistants. The Hospice and Palliative Nurses Association supported this initiative by creating new membership categories and providing specific educational offerings to these members of the team. The Hospice and Palliative Nurses Foundation is providing certification scholarships for each of these specialty examinations.

The National Consensus Project provides another example of collaboration and support, bringing to the table nurses, physicians, and program representatives who together defined the quality standards that will affect future palliative patient care.

All of these programs and professionals need each other. Hospice and palliative care programs have collaborated successfully and have found that they can be complementary, not competitive. Together they educate and support one another and work to fill in the needed gaps in patient care.

REFERENCES

Anderson, C. M., Raudonis, B. M., & Kirschling, J. M. (1999). Hospice and palliative nursing role delineation study: implications for certification. *Journal of Hospice and Palliative Nursing, 1*(2), 45-55.

Center to Advance Palliative Care. (2005). *Building a hospital-based palliative care program.* Retrieved July 13, 2005, from http://www.capc.org/building-a-hospital-based-palliative-care-program/

Chan, L-Y. (1976) Hospice: a new building type to comfort the dying. *AIA Journal, 65,* 42-45.

Christakis, N. A., & Escarce, J. J. (1996). Survival of Medicare patients after enrollment in hospice programs. *New England Journal of Medicine, 335,* 172-178.

Corless, I. B. (1983). The hospice movement in North America. In C. A. Corr & D. M. Corr (Eds), *Hospice care principles and practice.* New York, NY: Springer Publishing.

Kübler-Ross, E. (1969). *On death and dying.* New York: MacMillan.

Lynn, J. (2001). Serving patients who may die soon and their families: the role of hospice and other services. *JAMA: The Journal of the American Medical Association, 285,* 925-932.

Martinez, J. M. (2005). The Alliance for Excellence in Hospice and Palliative Nursing. *Journal of Hospice and Palliative Nursing, 7*(1), 1-2.

Martinez, J. M., & Wagner, S. J. (2000). Hospice care. In S. L. Groenwald, M. H. Frogge, M. Goodman, & C. H. Yarbro (Eds.), *Cancer nursing: Principles and practice* (4th ed.). Sudbury, MA: Jones and Bartlett.

Medicare conditions of participation for hospice care [GPO Access CITE: 42CFR418]. (1997). Washington, DC: U.S. Government Printing Office.

National Consensus Project. (2004). *Clinical practice guidelines for quality palliative care.* Retrieved July 1, 2005, from http://www.nationalconsensusproject.org/Guideline.pdf

National Hospice and Palliative Care Organization. (2004). *Hospice facts and figures.* Retrieved July 1, 2005, from http://www.nhpco.org/files/public/Hospice_Facts_110104.pdf

Open Society Institute. (2005). *Project on Death in America.* Retrieved July 12, 2005, from http://www.soros.org/initiatives/pdia

Pyenson, B., Connor, S., Fitch, K., & Kinzbrunner, B. (2004). Medicare costs in matched hospice and non-hospice cohorts. *Journal of Pain and Symptom Management, 28*(3), 200-210.

Robert Wood Johnson Foundation. (2005). Means to a better end report. Retrieved July 1, 2005, from http://www.rwjf.org/files/publications/other/meansbetterend.pdf

Sheldon, J., Dahlin, C., & Zeri, K. (2000). *The Hospice and Palliative Nurses Association statement on the scope and standards of hospice and palliative nursing practice.* Dubuque, IA: Kendall/Hunt Publishing.

World Health Organization. (2005). *WHO definition of palliative care.* Retrieved July 13, 2005, from http://www.who.int/cancer/palliative/definition/en/

Parish Nursing

Recent Changes and Current Issues

P. ANN SOLARI-TWADELL

The ministry of parish nursing practice is 2 decades old. In 1984 the Rev. Granger Westberg, a Lutheran clergyman and conceptualizer of parish nursing, approached Lutheran General Hospital regarding piloting the congregational-based health promotion nursing role with six nurses in six congregations beginning the trial in 1985. Since that time the innovative nursing role has been molded to fit the needs of congregations from most all denominations (Evans, 2002).

The ministry of parish nursing practice is a specialized professional practice distinguished by the following characteristics (Solari-Twadell, 1999, p. 15):

1. Parish nursing holds the spiritual dimension to be central to the practice encompassing the physical, psychological, and social dimension of the person.
2. This congregationally based nursing role balances knowledge with skill, the sciences with theology and the humanities, service with worship, and nursing care functions with some pastoral care functions.
3. The focus of the ministry of parish nursing practice is the local congregation and its ministry. In collaboration with the pastoral staff and members of the congregation, the congregation is transformed over time into a health place in the community.
4. In partnership with other community resources, the ministry of parish nursing practice fosters new and creative responses to health concerns.

RECENT CHANGES

Identification of Core and Most Frequently Used Interventions by Parish Nurses

In most literature the role of the parish nurse is described through seven functions. These functions are integrator of faith and health, health educator, personal health counselor, referral agent and liaison with congregational and community resources, trainer of volunteers, developer of support groups, and health advocate

(Holstrom, 1999, p. 69). These descriptors are simple and to the point; however, they do not detail the complexity of the parish nurse role or represent the diversity of interventions used by the parish nurse. In addition, for research purposes the seven functions are not discrete. In other words, the content of the seven functions of the parish nurse overlap: the function of health counselor can be part of health education; the function of integrator of faith and health could be operational in each of the other six functions of the parish nurse role. A national study involving 2330 parish nurses focused on the ministry of parish nursing practice using the third edition of the Nursing Interventions Classification (NIC) Use Survey (Iowa Intervention Project Research Team, 1996). The NIC captures the interventions used by all nurses (Dochterman McCloskey & Bulechek, 2004, p. x). This study resulted in the identification of the top 30 core interventions (Table 24-1) and the interventions most frequently used by the parish nurse in caring for clients (Table 24-2) (Solari-Twadell, 2002, p. 193). The identification of the core and most frequently used interventions for the ministry of parish nursing practice allows for the work of the parish nurse to be understood more clearly. The NIC system has seven domains. The complexity of the parish nurse role unfolds in reviewing Table 24-1, in which six of the seven domains identified in the NIC system are used by parish nurses in their practice. The only domain for which there were no reported interventions used by the parish nurse in this study is domain two—physiologic complex. The finding that no interventions were used from this domain reflects that the parish nurse does not function using invasive, more medical model–based interventions. Instead, most of the core interventions are included in the behavioral domain that is consistent with the health promotion aspect of the parish nurse role. Use of the NIC system to describe the role of the parish nurse makes the ministry of parish nursing practice

TABLE 24-1

Nursing Interventions Written in by Parish Nurse Respondents as Essential or Core to the Ministry of Parish Nursing Practice by Rank Order*

Intervention	Rank	Domain	Class
Health Education (5510)	1	3. Behavioral	S. Patient Education
Active Listening (4920)	2	3. Behavioral	Q. Communication Enhancement
Spiritual Support (5420)	3	3. Behavioral	R. Coping Assistance
Emotional Support (5270)	4	3. Behavioral	R. Coping Assistance
Presence (5340)	5	3. Behavioral	R. Coping Assistance
Spiritual Growth Facilitation (5426)	6	3. Behavioral	R. Coping Assistance
Caregiver Support (7040)	7	5. Family	X. Life Span Care
Grief Work Facilitation (5290)	8	3. Behavioral	R. Coping Assistance
Hope Instillation (5310)	9	3. Behavioral	R. Coping Assistance
Coping Enhancement (5230)	10	3. Behavioral	R. Coping Assistance
Counseling (5240)	11	3. Behavioral	R. Coping Assistance
Decision-Making Support (5250)	12	3. Behavioral	R. Coping Assistance
Forgiveness Facilitation (5280)	13	3. Behavioral	R. Coping Assistance
Health System Guidance (7400)	14	6. Health System	Y. Health System Mediation
Touch (5460)	15	3. Behavioral	R. Coping Assistance
Support System Enhancement (5440)	16	3. Behavioral	R. Coping Assistance
Humor (5320)	17	3. Behavioral	R. Coping Assistance
Dying Care (5260)	18	3. Behavioral	R. Coping Assistance
Health Screening (6520)	19	4. Safety	V. Risk Management
Religious Ritual Enhancement (5424)	20	3. Behavioral	R. Coping Assistance
Consultation (7910)	21	6. Health System	Y. Health System Mediation
Support Group (5430)	22	3. Behavioral	R. Coping Assistance
Teaching: Disease Process (5602)	23	3. Behavioral	S. Patient Education
Program Development (8700)	24	7. Community	C. Community Health Promotion
Referral (8100)	25	6. Health System	B. Information Management
Anticipatory Guidance (5210)	26	3. Behavioral	R. Coping Assistance
Telephone Consultation (8180)	27	6. Health System	B. Information Management
Documentation (7920)	28	6. Health System	B. Information Management
Family Support (7142)	29	5. Family	X. Life Span Care
Exercise Promotion (0201)	30	1. Physiologic Basic	A. Activity and Exercise Management

*The number listed after each intervention is the code number for that intervention.

more understandable to nurses or other health professionals who are familiar with the NIC system and may be one of the links to integrating this nursing practice more effectively into the continuum of care.

Growth of the Ministry of Parish Nursing Practice

The growth of parish nursing has been consistent and reaches beyond the borders of the United States (Clark & Olson, 2002; Van Loon & Carey, 2002). However, until recently there was little documentation that detailed the development of the ministry of parish nursing practice throughout the United States. Results from a study on parish nursing in the United State reported practicing respondents from all states except Alaska, Vermont, and Rhode Island (Solari-Twadell, 2002, p. 78). Even though there were no parish nurse respondents from these states in this study, parish nurse programs serve congregations in theses states. This substantiated that over the last 20 years the ministry of parish nursing practice has been established within congregations ecumenically in all states within the United States. This reflects significant work on the part of many nurses, clergy, and members of congregations, as well as denominational leaders, to

VIEWPOINTS

TABLE 24-2

Combined Set of Interventions Derived from Nursing Interventions Selected as the Top 30 Interventions Used "Several Times a Day/Daily," "Weekly," and "Monthly"*

Intervention	Daily	Weekly	Monthly
1. Learning Facilitation (5520)	n = 177	n = 212	
2. Learning Readiness Enhancement (5540)	n = 119		
3. Active Listening (4920)	n = 479	n = 316	
4. Presence (5340)	n = 349	n = 341	
5. Touch (5460)	n = 300	n = 289	
6. Spiritual Support (5429)	n = 289	n = 363	
7. Emotional Support (5270)	n = 285	n = 379	
8. Spiritual Growth Facilitation (5426)	n = 257	n = 330	
9. Humor (5320)	n = 201	n = 258	
10. Hope Instillation (5310)	n = 185	n = 292	n = 359
11. Counseling (5240)	n = 173	n = 272	
12. Decision-Making Support (5250)	n = 153	n = 310	n = 389
13. Self-Esteem Enhancement (5400)	n = 137	n = 224	n = 351
14. Support System Enhancement (5440)	n = 136	n = 270	n = 398
15. Religious Ritual Enhancement (5424)	n = 128	n = 246	
16. Self-Awareness Enhancement (5390)	n = 118	n = 208	
17. Truth Telling	n = 117		
18. Values Clarification (5480)	n = 107		
19. Coping Enhancement (5230)	n = 96	n = 269	n = 374
20. Health Education (5510)	n = 260	n = 317	n = 426
21. Teaching: Disease Process (5602)	n = 127	n = 307	n = 447
22. Teaching: Individual (5606)	n = 100	n = 190	n = 358
23. Health Screening (6520)	n = 96		n = 430
24. Vital Signs Monitoring (6680)	n = 91		
25. Caregiver Support (7040)	n = 94	n = 245	n = 447
26. Documentation (7920)	n = 236	n = 228	
27. Telephone Consultation (8180)	n = 175	n = 241	
28. Telephone Follow-up (8190)	n = 132		
29. Consultation (7910)	n = 98	n = 211	n = 430
30. Program Development (8700)	n = 92		n = 442
31. Energy Management (0180)		n = 292	
32. Nutrition Counseling (5246)		n = 209	n = 405
33. Grief Work Facilitation (5290)		n = 224	n = 443
34. Forgiveness Facilitation (5280)		n = 199	n = 353
35. Support Group (5430)		n = 198	n = 361
36. Family Support (7140)		n = 197	n = 395
37. Health System Guidance (7400)		n = 205	n = 459
38. Weight Reduction Assistance (1280)			n = 353
39. Dying Care (5260)			n = 428
40. Anticipatory Guidance (5210)			n = 387
41. Teaching: Prescribed Medication (5616)			n = 424
42. Teaching: Procedure Treatment (5618)			n = 404
43. Teaching: Prescribed Diet (5614)			n = 383
44. Environmental Management: Safety (6486)			n = 369
45. Fall Prevention (6490)			n = 358
46. Family Integrity Promotion (7100)			n = 364
47. Family Involvement Promotion (7110)			n = 393
48. Referral (8100)			n = 370
49. Health Care Information Exchange (7960)			n = 347

*The number listed after each intervention is the code number for that intervention. These interventions are listed in rank order because of the reporting of multiple times frames in one table.

educate members on the benefits of incorporating health ministry in their congregations through developing the ministry of parish nursing practice to serve the health needs of its members and the members of the community at large.

CURRENT ISSUES

Naming

Currently, many names are given to the nurses serving in the ministry of parish nursing practice. Some nurses serving their congregations are called "congregational nurses," others are called "temple nurses," and yet others are called "pastoral care nurses." Currently, no matter what their title, nurses serving their congregations fulfilling the functions of the parish nurse must be practicing within the scope of the practice as designated by the *Scope and Standards for Parish Nurses* published by the American Nurses Association and the Health Ministry Association (1998). These standards are in the final stages of revision. Part of the revision is a move to change the title of these standards to the *Scope and Standards of Faith Community Nursing*. This name change is being considered because the use of the word *parish* is language that is seen as being limited to particular faith traditions, whereas the term *faith community* is understood to present a broader scope of religious communities. It remains to be seen whether the change will occur and, if it does, whether it will result in confusion or clarity.

Sustainability of the Ministry of Parish Nursing Practice

The ministry of parish nursing practice can make a difference in the life of a congregation, the health of its members, and ultimately in the future health of the community only if there is long-term presence of the parish nurse as an integral part of the pastoral team of the congregation and thus in the life of the congregation. One way in which the ministry of parish nursing practice is involved and integrated into the life of the congregation is through the development of a health cabinet/committee. The health cabinet/committee is a part of the organizational structure of the congregation and "is composed of a small group of individuals, usually about five to seven in number, drawn from health professionals and others who are interested in exploring issues of faith and health in a congregational setting" (Patterson, 2003, p. 41). The health cabinet, once educated on the ministry of parish nursing practice and the relationship between faith and health, can be a support to the parish nurse and advocate for the work of the parish nurse to be integrated into all aspects

of congregational life. Once the ministry of parish nursing practice is integrated into the ministry of the congregation, it is less likely to disappear with a change in the pastor or parish nurse.

Financial perspectives of health ministry also may be an issue that integrates the parish nurse into the life of the congregation. Even if the parish nurse chooses not to be paid for services provided to congregational members, it is important that the ministry of parish nursing practice have money dedicated to projects related to the health ministry in the congregation. A ministry that appears in the budget for the congregation has to be understood and valued to be funded. Once funded, the assigning of dollars to the ministry can be debated, but to be debated, the members of the committee need to understand the nature and importance of the ministry to the members of the congregation. This means that the parish nurse must be active in continually educating all members of the congregation as to the services rendered and detailing how these services are valued by the members of the congregation. This often is accomplished best by having members who have experienced the benefit write letters or communicate in other ways the value of the parish nursing services to the members of the congregation and possibly the community at large.

Another way that the parish nurse integrates the ministry of parish nursing practice into the congregation is regular reports or communication (Fuentes, 2003, p. 167). Using the congregation bulletin or newsletter to communicate relevant information can be an effective way for the parish nurse to educate members as to the value of the services provided and the importance of this health ministry to the mission of the congregation.

Sustainability of the ministry of parish nursing practice can be accomplished through recognition of the important role the congregation can play in the health of its members and the community at large. Recognition of the value of the congregation in supporting the health of the community, by the health care system, is one step toward seeing the congregation as part of the continuum of care. This recognition of the congregation in health can be enhanced only by the presence of a ministry of parish nursing practice.

Documentation of Outcomes

Documentation remains an important responsibility for the parish nurse. The parish nurse is a registered professional nurse providing client services. These services must be documented. The fact that the location of the services being provided is one where documentation is not done traditionally or records usually are not kept is not sufficient reason for the professional nurse to abandon practices dictated by the Nurse Practice Act of the state. More importantly, not only do services rendered by the parish nurse need to be documented, but also the impact or outcome of these services needs to be measured. Stakeholders invested in the ministry of parish nursing practice will be interested in the difference the service of the parish nurse is making in the quality of the client's life.

Using documentation systems set up to service the ministry of parish that integrate the standardized nursing languages of North America Nursing Diagnosis Association (NANDA), Nursing Intervention Classification System (NIC) and Nursing Outcome Classification System (NOC) can be one way of measuring the impact or outcomes of the services being offered to members of the faith community. Computerized documentation systems are replacing the familiar paper charts with laptops or palmtop computers (Burkhart, 2005, p. 7). Some parish nurses currently are using electronic documentation systems to report on interventions provided to members of their faith communities. Once this data is reported, it can be aggregated and formulated into a report that gives statistics as to numbers of clients served, the interventions provided, and the outcomes that result from the services offered. This data is important to create value that can contribute to sustainability.

Professionalism of the Providers

The integrity of the ministry of parish nursing practice relies on the integrity of the registered professional nurses who assume the position of parish nurse. Next to integrity of the nurse is the preparation the nurse has received to prepare for the ministry of parish nursing practice. A national study of parish nurses reported that the No. 1 factor in supporting the parish nurse to operationalize the role was participation in the standardized basic preparation course in parish nursing offered through the International Parish Nurse Resource Center by providers across the United States (Solari-Twadell, 2002, p. 178). Presently, no certification for the ministry of parish nursing practice is available. Participation in a basic preparation program in parish nursing is currently one of the best vehicles for exhibiting preparation for the ministry of parish nursing practice.

SUMMARY

Those who have worked hard over the last 20 years to integrate the ministry of parish nursing practice into the life of their congregations are to be commended. In a short period, parish nursing is active in all mainline denominations, is present in all states in the United States, and is growing internationally. The future work of the next 20 years is to integrate the ministry of parish nursing practice into the continuum of care professed by the health care system with recognition of the valuable role the congregation can play in promoting the health of its members through the ministry of parish nursing practice. Parish nursing continues to make contributions to the profession of nursing and the communities served by offering creative responses to the present health care concerns. The real challenge will be continuing to offer these creative solutions while making inroads to the current health care system. Perhaps in making these inroads, the real transformation of the health care system will be initiated.

REFERENCES

American Nurses Association. (1998). *Scope and standards of parish nursing practice* (9806st 4M). Washington, DC: Author.

Burkhart, L. (2005). A click away: Documenting spiritual care. *Journal of Christian Nursing, 1*(22), 6-13.

Clark, M. B., & Olson, J. K. (2002). A partnership that matters: Collaborative interdisciplinary ministry among faith community nurses and faith group leaders. In L. Vandecreek & S. Mooney (Eds.), *Parish nurses, health care chaplains and community clergy: Navigating the maze of professional relationships* (p. 89). New York: Haworth Press.

Dochterman McCloskey, J. C., & Bulechek, G. M. (Eds.). (2004). *Nursing interventions classification (NIC)* (4th ed.). St. Louis, MO: Mosby.

Evans, P. K. (2002). Who are parish nurses? In L. Vandecreek & S. Mooney (Eds.), *Parish nurses, health care chaplains and community clergy: Navigating the maze of professional relationships* (p. 10). New York: Haworth Press.

Fuentes, S. (2003). Program evaluation. In S. D. Smith (Ed.). *Parish nursing: A handbook for the new millennium.* New York: Haworth Press.

Holstrom, S. (1999). Perspectives on a suburban parish nursing practice. In P. A. Solari-Twadell, & M. A. McDermott (Eds.), *Parish nursing: Promoting whole person health within faith communities* (pp. 67-73). Thousand Oaks, CA: Sage Publications.

Iowa Intervention Project Research Team. (1996). *Core interventions by specialty.* Iowa City, IA: Author.

Patterson, D. (2003). *The essential parish nurse: ABC's for congregational health ministry.* Cleveland, OH: Pilgrim Press.

Solari-Twadell, P. A. (1999). The emerging practice of the parish nursing. In P. A. Solari-Twadell & M. A. McDermott (Eds.), *Parish nursing: Promoting whole person health within faith communities* (p. 15). Thousand Oaks, CA: Sage Publications.

Solari-Twadell, P. A. (2002). The differentiation of the ministry of parish nursing practice within congregations

[UMI No. 30564429]. *Dissertation Abstracts International,* *63*(6), 569A.

Van Loon, A. M., & Carey, L. B. (2002). Faith community nursing and health care chaplaincy in Australia: A new collaboration. In L. Vandecreek & S. Mooney (Eds.), *Parish nurses, health care chaplains and community clergy: Navigating the maze of professional relationships* (pp. 143-157). New York: Haworth Press.

Pediatric Nursing

Recent Changes and Current Issues

MARILYN J. HOCKENBERRY ◆ ROSALIND BRYANT ◆ CHERYL RODGERS

The goal for pediatric nursing is to improve the quality of health care for all children. Although most American children are healthy, disparities by race, ethnicity, socioeconomic status, and geography exist. More than 72 million children under age 18 live in the United States and represent 25% of the population (Vessey & Ben-Or, 2000). Pediatric nurses face many challenges related to their ability to provide comprehensive pediatric health care. Numerous obstacles including single-parent families, poverty, and increasing cultural diversity in this country have the potential to affect future children's health outcomes.

SINGLE-PARENT FAMILIES

In 2003, only 68% of children in the United States lived with both parents, down from 77% in 1980 (America's Children 2004, n.d.). Living in two-parent households has long been associated with more favorable health care outcomes for children, independent of higher incomes in these families (Biblarz & Raferty, 1999). In 2002, just over one third (34%) of all births in the United States were to unmarried women (America's Children 2004, n.d.). Managing shortages of money, time, and energy are major concerns for single parents. Examples of resources needed for single-parent families include flexible health services that are open in the evenings and weekends, reliable and safe child care, community programs that enhance parenting skills, and recreational centers that are available for the entire family.

POVERTY

The number of children living in families with incomes below the poverty threshold rose from 11.2 million in 2001 to 11.7 million in 2002 (Wertheimer, 2005). Children living in single-parent households with no father present continue to experience a higher poverty rate than two-parent families: 39.6% compared with 8.5% (America's Children 2004, n.d.). Minority children are more likely to live in poverty. Children living in poverty experience little if any preventive health care, inadequate health maintenance, and limited access to medical treatment. For example, although infant mortality rates have decreased overall, the disparity in infant death rates between white and black babies has widened (Wertheimer, 2005). Poverty has the great potential to affect children's health care outcomes.

DIVERSITY

The United States has more racial, ethnic, and religious minority groups that any other country in the world. One third of Americans less than 18 years of age are classified as a racial or ethnic minority (Lichter, 2005; Villarruel, 2001). Because American culture is becoming more diverse (Murdock, 2005), pediatric nurses must be knowledgeable about the minority groups within their communities and must be able to apply understanding of the various cultures to daily clinical practice. For example, nurses must understand the influence of culture, race, and ethnicity on the development of social and emotional relationships, child-rearing practices, and attitudes and beliefs toward health and illness. Nurses must evaluate cultural beliefs related to the causes of illness and treatment practices when caring for diverse families.

EMERGING PEDIATRIC PROBLEMS

The health of the nation's children continues to improve in many areas, such as lower pregnancy rates for adolescents and expanded vaccine coverage. However, modern society and its influence on the family and the explosion of technology and information systems are a few examples of changes that are influencing the emergence of significant medical problems that affect the future health of children. Examples of emerging pediatric problems include obesity, type 2 diabetes, injuries, violence, substance abuse, and emotional and mental health problems during adolescence.

Obesity and Type 2 Diabetes

Advancements in entertainment and technology such as television, computers, and video games have contributed to the growing childhood obesity problem in the United States. Approximately 63% of the 8- to 18-years-olds have a television in their bedrooms and watch television an average of 4 hours a day (Robinson & Sargent, 2005). The minority populations, especially African American and Hispanic children from low socioeconomic families, watch more than 4 hours of television daily, encouraging sedentary activity with intake of high-caloric, fatty foods (Fitzgibbon & Stolley, 2004). The National Health and Nutrition Examination Survey reported that the prevalence of overweight children doubled and the prevalence of overweight adolescents tripled between 1980 and 2000 (Dietz, 2005).

Childhood obesity is the most common nutritional problem among American children and is increasing in epidemic proportions along with type 2 diabetes (Yensel, Preud'homme, & Curry, 2004). Obesity in children and adolescents is defined as a body mass index at or greater than the 95th percentile for youth of the same age and gender (Dietz, 2005; Covington et al., 2001). Lack of outside physical activity because of unsafe environments and inconvenient facilities for physical activities, combined with easy assess to video games and television within the home, tend to promote obesity among low-income diverse children. Overweight youth, especially of Latino, African American, and Native American descent, have increased risk for developing diabetes, insulin resistance, hypertension, and heart disease (Jackson, 2001; Yensel et al., 2004). A major nursing health prevention focus, consistent with the Healthy People 2010 primary goals, is the reduction of obesity in children aged 6 to 19 years from the current 20% in all ethnic groups to less than 6% (Duderstadt, 2004; National Center for Health Statistics, 2004).

Childhood Injuries

Injuries are the most common cause of death and disability to children in the United States. Unintentional injuries among children 19 and under have dropped to 39%, and the violent death rate has dropped 36 % in the same age bracket; however, the trend now has plateaued (Rivara, 2005). Despite the decrease in injuries to children, motor vehicle–related accidents continue as the most common

cause of death in children older than 1 year of age. As children grow older, the percentage of deaths from injuries increases. The most common types of unintentional injuries in addition to motor vehicle accidents include drowning, burns, and firearm accidents. Many childhood injury fatalities can be avoided. For example, the majority of bicycling deaths are from head injuries. Although helmets reduce the risk of head injury by 85%, few children wear them (National Safety Council, 2000).

Pediatric nurses can be instrumental in reducing childhood injuries and fatalities by implementing preventive measures such as instructing families and children on the benefits of wearing seat belts, using child booster/infant car seats, and using helmets and protective equipment with skateboarding, in-line skating, bicycling, or riding of four-wheelers. Other injury-preventive measures include the safe storage of guns, adequate pool fencing, use of smoke detectors, and safe placement of household toxins and medications.

Violence

Each day, 10 children in the United States are murdered by gunfire, equivalent to approximately 1 child every 2$^{1}/_{2}$ hours. Strikingly higher homicide rates are found among the minority populations, especially in African-American children. Violence permeates American households through television programs, commercials, video games, and movies that tend to desensitize the child toward violence. By the time preschoolers grow up and graduate from high school, they will have viewed more than 200,000 violent acts on television (Groves, 2005). Violence also permeates the schools with the availability of guns, illicit drugs, and the presence of gangs, exemplified by the deadliest school shooting in U.S. history at Columbine High School in Colorado in 1999 (Fisher & Kettl, 2003). Although declines have been observed in serious violent crime victimization of youth and offending (perpetration) by youth (America's Children 2004, n.d.), assessment of high-risk behaviors in American youth must continue to be a major focus of health promotion.

Substance Abuse

Risk-taking behaviors, particularly in males, tend to begin in the first decade of life and continue into adolescence with drinking of alcohol while driving, speeding, carrying a weapon, or using illicit drugs. Alcohol and illicit drug use occurs most commonly between the age of 12 and 17 years and is associated with violence and injury (Jackson, 2001). Alcohol is the drug of choice among adolescents because parents see it as better than illicit drugs, so youth receive limited education on the adverse effects of alcohol. About 10.9 million youths between the ages of 12 and 20 (primarily males) report drinking alcohol, with nearly 19.2% reported as being binge drinkers and 6.1% as being heavy drinkers. Sixty-six percent of youths who drank alcohol heavily and 52% of youths from 12 to 17 years of age who smoked cigarettes daily also were users of illicit drugs (Substance Abuse and Mental Health Services Administration, 2004).

An estimated 2.6 million new marijuana users emerged in 2002, with 69% being under age 18 years. Use of marijuana, the most commonly used illicit drug, declined slightly from 20.6% in 2002 to 19.6% in 2003. During the same period, lysergic acid diethylamide (LSD; 1.3% to 0.6%), Ecstasy (2.2% to 1.3%), and methamphetamine (0.9% to 0.7%) also decreased (National Center for Health Statistics, 2004). The slight decline in American youth's illicit drug use is attributed to education regarding the adverse effect of illicit drugs, parental disapproval, decreased availability of drugs, and consistent participation in church and organized activities such as scouting and sports.

Mental Health and Emotional Problems

Mental health problems affect one out of five school-age children in the United States. Children and adolescents with mental health problems are more likely to drop out of school than are those with other disabilities. One of the most common mental health problems is attention deficit-hyperactivity disorder (ADHD) (Kelleher, 2005). Attention deficit-hyperactivity disorder is characterized by inattentiveness, impulsivity, and at times hyperactivity occurring in children as early as 3 years old (Medd, 2003). ADHD affects every aspect of the child's life but is most obvious in the classroom. Family education, counseling, medication, proper classroom placement, environmental manipulation, and behavior therapy are important management strategies for these children.

Suicide is defined as a self-chosen death and is the third leading cause of death in children ages 10 to 19 (Doucette, 2005). The American Association of Suicidology (2005) estimates that in a typical high school classroom, three students (one boy and two girls) likely have made a suicide attempt in the last year. Suicide is a preventable occurrence, placing a heavy burden on the nurse's ability to identify the at-risk child or adolescent who may display mental health and emotional problems. Nurses caring for children and adolescents with mental health and emotional problems must work closely with the social worker, counselor, psychologist, or psychiatrist to formulate a collaborative individualized treatment plan to promote the child's mental health.

PEDIATRIC PREVENTIVE HEALTH CARE NEEDS

The National Children's Study is the largest long-term study of children's health and development conducted in the United States. The study is designed to follow 100,000 children and their families from birth to age 21 to understand the link between children's environments and their physical health, emotional health, and development (American Academy of Pediatrics, 2004). One can hope that a study of this magnitude will provide innovative interventions for families, children, and health care providers to eradicate childhood obesity, dental caries, and unhealthful diets and bring a significant reduction in violence, injury, substance abuse, and mental health disease among the nation's children. This study supports the Healthy People 2010 primary goals to increase the quality and years of healthful life and eliminate health disparities related to race, ethnicity, and socioeconomic status (Betz, 2002). This national study provides numerous opportunities for pediatric nurses to participate as advocates for providing preventive health care for all children.

Nutritional Maintenance and Dental Prevention

Nutrition is an essential component for healthy growth and development, and its promotion begins at birth. Human milk is the preferred form of nutrition for all infants. Breast-feeding provides the infant with micronutrients, immunological properties, and several enzymes that enhance digestion and absorption of these nutrients (Wilson, 2005). Many working mothers tend to wean their infants early to avoid the hassle of breast pumping during the workday. However, over the past several years, a resurgence in breast-feeding has occurred because of the education of mothers and fathers regarding the benefits of breast-feeding.

Young children tend to establish eating habits during the first 2 to 3 years of life, and the nurse is instrumental in guiding parents with the selection of nutritious foods. During childhood, the eating preferences and attitudes related to food habits are established by family influences and culture. During adolescence, parental influence diminishes as the adolescent makes food choices related to peer acceptability and sociability that may be detrimental to the chronically ill child with diabetes, hypertension, or heart or renal disease.

Unhealthful diets permeate the lower social class, often because of the lack of nutritious fresh fruits and vegetables and adequate milk and protein intake. In addition, the lifestyles of homeless and migrant children place this population at risk for inadequate food intake, causing nutrient deficiencies, developmental and growth delays, depression, hunger, and behavior problems. Nurses work closely with families to incorporate customs, health beliefs, traditions, and values of the various ethnic groups to obtain the acceptance and compliance regarding the benefits of ingesting affordable nutritious foods rather than the perceived cheaper high-caloric foods.

The Healthy People 2010 project reports that nearly one in five children between the ages of 2 and 4 years have visible cavities, primarily in Latino children. The most common form of early dental disease is early childhood caries that may begin at the first birthday and progress to pain and infection within the first 2 years of life. Preschoolers of low-income families are twice as likely to develop tooth decay and only half as likely to visit the dentist (Edelstein, 2005). Because caries is a preventable disease, the nurse plays an essential role in promoting early tooth care by instructing the children and parents on dental hygiene beginning with the first tooth eruption, drinking fluoridated water including bottled water, and instituting early dental preventive care.

Immunizations

The World Health Organization (2004) states that the two public health interventions that have had the greatest impact on world health are clean water and vaccines. An increased number of persons view immunizations as harmful or have religious objections to immunizing their children; therefore the nurse needs to be cognizant of this population of children through early recognition of preventable communicable diseases. Nurses should review the child's immunization record at each clinic visit and instruct the parent to keep immunizations current, reinforcing the plan to establish an immunization registry throughout the United States to attain the 90% goal of vaccinated 2-year-olds as mandated by Healthy People 2010 (National Center for Health Statistics, 2004).

MEDICAL PROGRESS: CREATING CHALLENGES FOR PEDIATRIC NURSES

Although medical progress continues to occur, it does not guarantee equity of health outcomes (Wise, 2005). Social inequities leading to poverty are linked directly to increased childhood illness and suffering. These social inequities create important priorities for pediatric nursing. Despite the challenges, nurses' roles in pediatric nursing must continue to focus on health promotion and disease prevention for all children.

Caring for the increasing number of children with chronic illnesses and implementing innovative nursing care in the face of emerging technology are major priorities for the future of pediatric nursing. Increased survival of very-low-birth-weight infants and the changing role of genetics in disease identification and management are examples of medical progress that are creating unique challenges for pediatric nurses. Increased trends in home-based nursing care are an ongoing priority for the pediatric specialty. Despite advances in medical technology, children still die in this country. A continued challenge for pediatric nurses is to provide the best palliative care possible for children who will not survive.

Chronic Illness

Because of advances in medical technology, more children with chronic illnesses and disabilities are living longer. Each year nearly 500,000 children in the United States with chronic illnesses become adults. In addition, more than 90% of children with severe disabilities survive into adulthood (American Academy of Pediatrics, 2002). Some individuals with disabilities have health insurance, but most rely on Medicaid because of their high rate of unemployment, inability to pay the high health insurance premiums, or lack of availability of employer-based health insurance. Individuals with disabilities may have a difficult time qualifying for Medicaid. Uninsured individuals are more likely to go without needed health care, receive fewer preventive services, and have to pay higher prices for services and drugs (White, 2002). Pediatric nurses play a major role as advocates for their patients with chronic illness by negotiating ways for them to continue to obtain needed health care into adulthood.

Adolescents with special health care needs strive to become independent members of society by seeking an education, job, social interaction, recreation, and health (White, 2002). The ability to achieve successful adult outcomes involves developing strategies to assist with receiving education, training, employment, and community living (Betz, 1999). Growing into an adult with a chronic illness must include transition to an adult health care facility; however, many times the person is reluctant to transfer care. For a young adult with a chronic illness, transitioning from a pediatric to an adult health care center can be a stressful event because differences in practice styles between adult and pediatric centers may exist. In addition, some pediatricians have concerns about the level of care and may not want to "let go" of their patients (Lewis-Gray, 2001). The successful transition requires early planning and a multidisciplinary approach to health care. A well-timed transition allows young adults to optimize their ability to assume adult roles and functioning (American Academy of Pediatrics, 2002).

Pediatric nurses often assume responsibility for implementing transitional care within their specific patient population. Nurses also serve as legislative advocates for the lifelong needs of the chronically ill child and young adult.

Low-Birth-Weight Infants

Forty thousand very-low-birth-weight (VLBW) infants, weighing less than 1500 g at birth, are born every year (McCormick & Richardson, 2002). Because of advanced technology and increased health care expertise, the mortality of these infants has decreased significantly. These improved survival rates create many subsequent health-related issues. Very-low-birth-weight infants often experience general health problems such as recurrent infections, frequent hospitalizations, and poor physical growth (Saigal, Hoult, Streiner, Stoskopf, & Rosenbaum, 2000). In addition, these infants are at increased risk for cognitive and educational impairments (Anderson, Doyle, & Victorian Infant Collaborative Study Group, 2004). As VLBW children grow, they may experience behavioral disorders, attention disorders, and increased academic difficulties. Because of the academic difficulties, VLBW children are more likely to have lower intelligence quotients, resulting in academic difficulties that lead to an increased high school drop out rates (McCormick & Richardson, 2002). Parents, teachers, nurses, and health care professionals must learn to recognize potential deficits for VLBW children so that appropriate assistance can be initiated when needed.

Although VLBW children show a greater potential for cognitive deficits, rates of high-risk behavior such as smoking, alcohol use, or marijuana use are similar to rates found in normal-birth-weight children (McCormick & Richardson, 2002). These researchers found that despite cognitive, behavioral, and health problems, VLBW children had higher ratings of health-related quality of life compared with normal-birth-weight children. Further research is needed to evaluate the multitude of long-term complications and their resultant outcomes of VLBW infants as they grow into adulthood.

Genetics

The Human Genome Project has changed the way health care providers think about genetics and evaluate disease. The Human Genome Project has identified genes that allow for identification of a variety of pediatric-specific diseases (Williams, 2000). The establishment of some diagnoses early in life, such as sickle cell disease, allows for early education and prophylactic treatment to minimize potential complications caused by the disease.

In other diseases, such as Down syndrome or fragile X syndrome, early diagnosis does not assist with any significant treatment benefit (Edgar, 2004). Medical genetic clinics throughout the country now are specializing in pediatrics. Genetic clinics provide a broad range of comprehensive services, including diagnosis, treatment, and management of the full range of genetic disorders. A major focus for these clinics is genetic counseling and education on the prevention of genetic conditions.

Pediatric nurses play important roles within the field of genetics. Nurses provide comprehensive assessments for the evaluation of physical anomalies or morphological features throughout the child's life span that may indicate a genetic disease. When the genetic team is consulted, the pediatric nurse serves as an educator for the family regarding expectations from the consultation. Religious, cultural, and ethical concerns are major issues and should be discussed before the genetic consultation (Bowers, 2002).

Pediatric nurses specializing in genetics assist in developing ethical research policies, contribute to health policies, and assist with identification of genetic health care services. Pediatric nurse educators provide instrumental roles by integrating new knowledge discovered from genetic research findings into their clinical practices (Olsen et al., 2003). Future nursing research regarding genetics is needed to evaluate the impact of a genetic condition on end-of-life decisions, relationships among race, ethnicity, culture, and genetics and identification of disparities of groups using genetic services (Williams & Tripp-Reimer, 2001).

Home Health Care

As more children with chronic illnesses and severe disabilities are living longer, these children need to be cared for in a setting that promotes normal growth and development. Hospitalization can interfere with a child's ability to develop interpersonal family and friend relationships that are an important component of normal growth and development. Caring for a chronically ill child at home can promote quality of life for the child and family while allowing for cost-effective health care to be provided. Careful planning, coordination, and preparation of the family are essential for successful care at home. Chronically ill and disabled children should meet the following criteria to be considered for home care services:

◆ The child's medical condition must be stable.
◆ The family/guardian must want the child at home and have the motivation and ability to learn the child's care.

- The community must have the necessary supportive services available.
- Financial support must be available for the services.

For the pediatric patient, family-centered nursing is essential in the home care setting. Home health nurses collaborate with parents and children to set mutual health goals for the child or adolescent. Home health nursing increases the child's and parent's self-management skills and knowledge of the child's illness (Navaie-Walieser, Misener, Mersman, & Lincoln, 2004). Ongoing assessments evaluate the success of the home care program along with ongoing modifications in the care. The use of advanced medical technology in the home care setting along with parent's comfort level of care provided in the home is assessed continually. Careful analysis, shared experiences, and future research studies are needed to support the appropriateness and cost-effectiveness of home health care pediatric programs.

END-OF-LIFE CARE

Pediatric nurses have always been instrumental in caring for the patient and family throughout all aspects of the illness. The focus of care without cure becomes important when decisions must be made regarding a child's end-of-life care. Many obstacles arise in providing quality palliative care to dying children. Parent's fears and denial of death are common, especially when faced with an acute event leaving the child critically ill.

Palliative care for children brings with it numerous controversies that must be addressed: decisions regarding where the child should die; clarification of do not resuscitate orders; use of medical interventions including nutrition, hydration, and antibiotics; and discontinuation of potentially life-sustaining treatments such as ventilation and dialysis (Lang & Quill, 2004). One may find obstacles to providing good palliative care created by the health care staff. For example, some nurses may be distracted by the ability of advanced technology to sustain life and may be more focused on the tasks involved in maintaining life than on providing optimal end-of-life care. Nurses play major supportive roles for parents who are making important decisions regarding end-of-life care, measures that can or should be withheld or withdrawn, and the type of care that a critically ill child should receive (Marsi, Farrell, & Jacroix, 2000). Pediatric nurses must be able to provide clear communication, demonstrate good listening skills, and have an awareness of the parent's values, including cultural, ethnic, and religious beliefs.

CHANGING ROLES IN PEDIATRIC NURSING

As medical technology advances, the opportunities for nurses specializing in the care of children abound. Continued traditional roles for primary care nursing in urban and rural settings are critical to eliminating health disparities that are most obvious for racial and ethnic minorities in this country. Pediatric nurses in advanced practice roles are greatly needed in communities to support the Healthy People 2010 national health objectives (Jackson, 2001). Primary care pediatric nurses are instrumental in evaluating the barriers that prevent health care access to the minority communities. Awareness of the environments in which the children nurses care for live allows nurses expertly to identify factors that support or prevent health care access in their communities.

Advanced pediatric nursing practice has seen many changes over the past decade. Although primary care continues to be essential in promoting child health outcomes, changes in health care delivery, patient condition severity, and reimbursement are shifting the traditional roles of advanced practice pediatric nursing (Sperhac & Strodtbeck, 2001). The skills of the pediatric clinical nurse specialist and nurse practitioner now are required in many acute care settings. This blended role uses the traditional practitioner emphasis on assessment, diagnosis, and health care management and integrates it with the clinical nurse specialist focus on coordination of care, patient and family education, and psychosocial management (Brady & Neal, 2000). This blending of the two roles supports a more seamless integration of care between inpatient and outpatient settings (Sperhac & Strodtbeck, 2001).

Another new role emerging for pediatric nurses in the past decade is the development of the acute care nurse practitioner (Teicher, Crawford, Williams, Nelson, & Andrews, 2001). The acute care nurse practitioner specializing in pediatrics provides cost-effective, quality care for critically ill children admitted to acute care units. The role is meeting an essential need for health care experts who are knowledgeable in the care of critically ill infants and children. As tertiary settings increase the number of critical care units, the acute care nurse practitioner's role provides a model that allows for an increased workload in critical care facilities.

Another challenge for pediatric nursing roles is the growing number of children living with chronic health problems (Lipman & Hayman, 2000). Children with chronic illnesses require continuity of care and long-term management, often made more difficult in the complex health care delivery systems. Pediatric nurses specializing in the care of children with chronic illness promote optimal care for this group of patients through case management and collaboration. Knowledge of growth and development, health maintenance, and the specifics related to the chronic illness allows the nurse to become the health care provider most instrumental in promoting quality health care outcomes.

Although roles for pediatric nurses continue to emerge in primary and critical care settings and in caring for children with chronic illnesses, opportunities for pediatric nurses continue to increase in research, consultation, and education. In the past 25 years, nurse researchers have made unique contributions to the care of infants and children, adolescents and their families (Lipman & Hayman, 2000). More doctorally prepared pediatric nurses are focusing on research in the clinical settings. Opportunities for joint positions in clinical settings for pediatric nursing experts and as faculty members in schools of nursing continue to create unique ways to blend expert clinical practice with education. The future of continued excellence in the pediatric nursing specialty depends on the collaboration among expert clinicians, educators, and researchers.

REFERENCES

American Academy of Pediatrics. (2002). A consensus statement on health care transitions for young adults with special health care needs. *Pediatrics, 110*(6), 1304-1306.

American Academy of Pediatrics. (2004). *The National Children's Study.* Retrieved December 1, 2004, from http://www.aap.org/family/natlchstudy.htm

American Association of Suicidology. (2005). *About AAS.* Retrieved January 30, 2005, from http://www.suicidology.org/displaycommon.cfm?an=1

America's Children 2004. (n.d.) *Education.* Retrieved December 1, 2004, from http://www.childstats.ed.gov/americaschildren/pdf/ac2004/summlist.pdf

Anderson, P. J., Doyle, L. W., & Victorian Infant Collaborative Study Group. (2004). Executive functioning in school-aged children who were born very preterm or with extremely low birth weight in the 1990s. *Pediatrics, 114*(1), 50-57.

Betz, C. L. (1999). Adolescents with chronic conditions: Linkages to adult service systems. *Pediatric Nursing, 25*(5), 473-476.

Betz, C. L. (2002). Editorial: Healthy Children 2010: Implications for pediatric nurse practice. *Journal of Pediatric Nursing, 17,* 153-156.

Biblarz, T. J., & Raferty, A. E. (1999). Family structure, educational attainment, and socioeconomic success: Rethinking the pathology of matriarchy. *American Journal of Sociology, 105*(2), 321-365.

Bowers, N. R. (2002). Meeting the standard of genetic nursing care. *Journal for Specialists in Pediatric Nursing, 7*(3), 123-126.

Brady, M. A., & Neal, J. A. (2000). Role delineation study of pediatric nurse practitioners: A national study of practice responsibilities and trends in role functions. *Journal of Pediatric Health Care, 14,* 149-159.

Covington, C. Y., Cybulski, M. J., Davis, T. L., Duca, G. E., Farrell, E. B., Kasgorgis, M. L., et al. (2001). Kids on the move: Preventing obesity among urban children. *American Journal of Nursing, 101,* 73-75, 77, 79, 81-82.

Dietz, W. H. (2005). Overweight: An epidemic. In A. G. Cosby, R. E. Greenberg, L. H. Southward, & M. Weitzman (Eds.), *About children: An authoritative resource on the state of childhood today* (pp. 110-113). Elk Grove Village, IL: American Academy of Pediatrics.

Doucette, A. (2005). Youth suicide. In A. G. Cosby, R. E. Greenberg, L. H. Southward, & M. Weitzman (Eds.), *About children: An authoritative resource on the state of childhood today* (pp. 146-149). Elk Grove Village, IL: American Academy of Pediatrics.

Duderstadt, K. G. (2004). Advocacy for reducing childhood obesity. *Journal of Pediatric Health Care, 18,* 103-105.

Edelstein, B. L. (2005). Tooth decay: The best of times, the worst of times. In A. G. Cosby, R. E. Greenberg, L. H. Southward, & M. Weitzman (Eds.), *About children: An authoritative resource on the state of childhood today* (pp. 106-109). Elk Grove Village, IL: American Academy of Pediatrics.

Edgar, D. A. (2004). Advances in genetics: Implications for children, families and nurses. *Paediatric Nursing, 16*(6), 26-29.

Fisher, K., & Kettl, P. (2003). Teachers' perceptions of school violence. *Journal of Pediatric Health Care, 17,* 79-83.

Fitzgibbon, M. L., & Stolley, M. R. (2004). Environmental changes may be needed for prevention of overweight in minority children. *Pediatric Annals, 33,* 45-49.

Greaser, J., & Whyte, J. J. (2004). Childhood obesity: Is there effective treatment? *Consultant,* pp. 1349-1353.

Groves, B. M. (2005). Violence. In A. G. Cosby, R. E. Greenberg, L. H. Southward, & M. Weitzman (Eds.), *About children: An authoritative resource on the state of childhood today* (pp. 26-29). Elk Grove Village, IL: American Academy of Pediatrics.

Jackson, P. L. (2001). Healthy People 2010: The pediatric nursing challenge for the next decade. *Pediatric Nursing, 27,* 498-502.

Kelleher, K. (2005). Mental health. In A. G. Cosby, R. E. Greenberg, L. H. Southward, & M. Weitzman (Eds.), *About children: An authoritative resource on the state of childhood today* (pp. 138-141). Elk Grove Village, IL: American Academy of Pediatrics.

Lang, F. L., & Quill, T. (2004). Making decisions with families at the end of life. *American Family Physician, 70*(4), 720-723.

Lewis-Gray, M. D. (2001). Transitioning to adult health care facilities for young adults with a chronic condition. *Pediatric Nursing, 27*(5), 521-524.

Lichter, D. T. (2005). Families: Diversity and change. In A. G. Cosby, R. E. Greenberg, L. H. Southward, & M. Weitzman (Eds.), *About children: An authoritative resource on the state of childhood today* (pp. 178-181). Elk Grove Village, IL: American Academy of Pediatrics.

Lipman, T. H., & Hayman, L. L. (2000). Celebrating 25 years of pediatric nursing research: Progress and prospects. *American Journal of Maternal/Child Nursing, 25,* 331-335.

Masri, C., Farrell, C. A., & Jacroix, J. (2000). Decision making and end-of-life care in critically ill children. *Journal of Palliative Care, 16*(Suppl.), S45-S52.

McCormick, M. C., & Richardson, D. K. (2002). Premature infants grow up. *New England Journal of Medicine, 346*(3), 197-198.

Medd, S. E. (2003). Children with ADHD need our advocacy. *Journal of Pediatric Health Care, 17,* 102-104.

Murdock, S. H. (2005). Minority child population growth. In A. G. Cosby, R. E. Greenberg, L. H. Southward, & M. Weitzman (Eds.), *About children: An authoritative resource on the state of childhood today* (pp. 182-185). American Elk Grove Village, IL: American Academy of Pediatrics.

National Center for Health Statistics. (2004). *About Healthy People 2010.* Retrieved January 30, 2005, from http://www.cdc.gov/nchs/about/otheract/hpdata2010/abouthp.htm

National Safety Council. (2000). *Injury facts: 2000 edition.* Itaska, IL: Author.

Navaie-Waliser, M., Misener, M., Mersman, C., & Lincoln, P. (2004). Evaluating the needs of children with asthma in home care: The vital role of nurses as caregivers and educators. *Public Health Nursing, 21*(4), 306-315.

Olsen, S. J., Feetham, S. L., Jenkins, J., Lewis, J. A., Nissly, T. L., Sigmon, H. D., et al. (2003). Creating a nursing vision for leadership in genetics. *Medsurg Nursing, 12*(3), 177-183.

Rivara, F. P. (2005). Impact of injury. In A. G. Cosby, R. E. Greenberg, L. H. Southward, & M. Weitzman (Eds.), *About children: An authoritative resource on the state of childhood today* (pp. 122-125). Elk Grove Village, IL: American Academy of Pediatrics.

Robinson, T. N., & Sargent, J. D. (2005). Children and media. In A. G. Cosby, R. E. Greenberg, L. H. Southward, & M. Weitzman (Eds.), *About children: An authoritative resource on the state of childhood today* (pp. 22-25). Elk Grove Village, IL: American Academy of Pediatrics.

Saigal, S., Hoult, L. A., Streiner, D. L., Stoskopf, B. L., & Rosenbaum, P. L. (2000). School difficulties at adolescence in a regional cohort of children who were extremely low birth weight. *Pediatrics, 105*(2), 325-331.

Sperhac, A. M., & Strodtbeck, F. (2001). Advanced practice in pediatric nursing: Blending roles. *Journal of Pediatric Nursing, 16,* 120-126.

Substance Abuse and Mental Health Services Administration. (2004). *2003 National Survey on Drug Use and Health: Results.* Retrieved January 26, 2005, from http://www.drugabusestatistics.samhsa.gov/NHSDA/2k3NSDUH/2k3results.htm

Teicher, S., Crawford, K., Williams, B., Nelson, B., & Andrews, C. (2001). Emerging role of the pediatric nurse practitioner in acute care. *Pediatric Nursing, 27,* 387-390.

Vessey, J. A., & Ben-Or, K. (2000). Pediatric primary care: Preparing for the future. *Pediatric Nursing, 26,* 170-173.

Villarruel, A. M. (2001). Scientific inquiry: Eliminating health disparities for racial and ethnic minorities: A nursing agenda for children. *Journal of the Society of Pediatric Nurses, 6,* 32-34.

Wertheimer, R. (2005). Poverty. In A. G. Cosby, R. E. Greenberg, L. H. Southward, & M. Weitzman (Eds.), *About children: An authoritative resource on the state of childhood today* (pp. 92-95). Elk Grove Village, IL: American Academy of Pediatrics.

White, P. H. (2002). Access to health care: Health insurance considerations for young adults with special health care needs/disabilities. *Pediatrics, 110*(6), 1328-1335.

Williams, J. K. (2000). Impact of genome research on children and their families. *Journal of Pediatric Nursing, 15*(4), 207-211.

Williams, J. K., & Tripp-Reimer, T. (2001). From ecology to base pairs: Nursing and genetic science. *Biological Research for Nursing, 3*(1), 4-12.

Wilson, D. (2005). Health promotion of the newborn and family. In M. J. Hockenberry, D. Wilson, & M. L. Winkelstein (Eds.), *Wong's essentials of pediatric nursing* (pp. 175-221). St Louis, MO: Mosby.

Wise, P. H. (2005). Medical progress and inequalities in child health. In A. G. Cosby, R. E. Greenberg, L. H. Southward, & M. Weitzman (Eds.), *About children: An authoritative resource on the state of childhood today* (pp. 196-199). Elk Grove Village, IL: American Academy of Pediatrics.

World Health Organization. (2004). *Immunization, vaccines and biologicals: The history of vaccination.* Retrieved May 18, 2004, from http://www.who.int/vaccines-diseases/history/history.shtml

Yensel, C. S., Preud'homme, D., & Curry, D. M. (2004). Childhood obesity and insulin-resistant syndrome. *Journal of Pediatric Nursing, 19,* 238-246.

Perinatal Nursing

Recent Changes and Current Issues

KATHLEEN RICE SIMPSON

Every day in the United States approximately 11,200 babies are born to women in the nearly 3000 hospitals that provide perinatal services (Hamilton, Martin, & Sutton, 2004). These mothers and babies are cared for during pregnancy, labor, birth, and the postpartum period by perinatal nurses dedicated to providing a safe and therapeutic environment to promote the best possible outcomes for their patients. Few professional experiences are more rewarding than attendance at the birth of a healthy newborn and sharing the joy with the new mother and her family. Perinatal nursing offers the best of all specialty areas of professional nursing practice and includes the prenatal course, obstetrical triage, and labor, birth, perioperative, postanesthesia, postpartum, and newborn care. Perinatal nurses caring for women with high-risk pregnancies and preterm infants use medical-surgical and critical care nursing knowledge and skills. No other specialty in nursing offers a wider range of activities and opportunities to make a difference in the lives of women, newborns, and their families. The focus of perinatal nursing is on making families and creating our future. Although approximately 4% of registered nurses in the United States are men, perinatal nursing remains predominantly a specialty of nurses who are women. This woman-to-woman connection is powerful for perinatal nurses and patients.

As a specialty, perinatal nurses face many challenges; some are specific to perinatal care, and others are shared with nursing in general. These challenges are related in part to recent changes in health care delivery systems that seem to favor the financial bottom line and convenience for providers over practices that promote patient safety and to the socialization of women to childbearing. Current issues of importance that require assertive actions by perinatal nurses, if significant changes are to occur, are the continued medicalization of labor and birth, increased use of technology for healthy women,

the ongoing conflict between "the way we've always done it" versus evidence-based care, errors by health care providers that contribute to maternal-fetal injuries, increasing nurse/patient ratios, the proliferation of convenience as the foundation for care during labor and birth, lack of education about the impact of this convenience philosophy among childbearing women, and the forces challenging nurse-midwives as the primary care providers for healthy women. Each of these issues is discussed in the context of why perinatal nurses are in this situation and what they can do to make significant changes.

THE MEDICALIZATION OF LABOR AND BIRTH

Unlike other nursing specialties, perinatal nurses care for women during a healthy, natural life event. Labor and birth are natural physiological processes. Most women do well with support and selected minimal intervention. Yet many women in the United States give birth in a high-technology, low-touch environment with electronic devices monitoring every physiological parameter possible (Simpson, 2003). Even when an unmedicated, low-technology childbirth is planned and prepared for extensively, many women who are vulnerable during labor and birth find themselves agreeing to interventions that clearly are unnecessary and have the potential for iatrogenic injuries (Simpson & Atterbury, 2003). When birth occurs in a hospital, there is a tendency to view the process as a medical event. In this setting, birth is controlled and managed; arbitrary time frames rule what is a natural process. Despite a substantial body of evidence to suggest this is not the best approach, if labor is not proceeding according to the "labor curve," interventions routinely are used to hasten the process. For example, amniotic membranes frequently are ruptured artificially to speed labor, which causes a significant increase in umbilical cord compression evidenced by variable fetal heart rate decelerations (Garite, Porto, Carlson, Rumney, & Reimbold, 1993; Goffinet et al., 1997). Convenience for the provider in shortening labor is not worth these risks to the fetus. Amniotomy results in a non–clinically significant decrease in the length of labor of at most up to 1 hour (Fraser, Turcot, Krauss, & Brisson-Carrol, 2000).

The use of drugs to stimulate labor contractions artificially has increased 125% since 1989, the first year these data were collected (Hamilton et al., 2004). Compelling evidence indicates that elective labor induction increases the risk of cesarean birth for nulliparous women (Simpson & Atterbury, 2003). Most women in the United States labor in bed, eliminating the normal physiological advantages of an upright maternal position. Ample data indicate that coached closed glottis pushing beginning immediately at 10 cm cervical dilation when the woman does not yet feel the urge to push increases the risk of nonreassuring fetal heart rate patterns, low umbilical cord pH, fetal acidemia, perineal trauma, and urinary dysfunction (Fraser et al., 2000; Handa, Harris, & Ostergard, 1996; Roberts, 2002; Sampselle & Hines, 1999; Schaffer et al., 2005; Simpson & James, 2005). Yet this practice continues because providers intuitively believe coached pushing will shorten the second stage of labor contrary to the results of multiple randomized trials (Fraser et al., 2000; Hansen, Clark, & Foster, 2002; Mayberry, Hammer, Kelly, True-Driver, & De, 1999; Roberts, 2002).

If the second stage of labor does not proceed within outdated time frames, vacuum extractors using between 400 and 600 mm Hg of pressure often are applied to the fetal head to hasten birth. The U.S. Food and Drug Administration (1998) has issued warnings to health care providers about the risk of fetal injuries with this device; however, use of the procedure is at an all-time high (Hamilton et al., 2004). Although an extensive body of research suggests otherwise, many women in the United States have an episiotomy immediately before birth. This unnecessary procedure is painful, delays recovery, and increases risk of urinary and fecal incontinence for women later in life (Hartmann et al., 2005). Many hospitals in the United States have strict visitor policies based on crowd-control principles that disregard the desires of women to have those she wishes attend birth (Simpson, 2005a).

This medicalization of childbirth continues for many reasons. Hospitals have invested millions in high technology related to the birthing process. That technology, once in place, becomes the part of the routine for caring for women during labor and birth. There was hope that this technology would reduce the incidence of cerebral palsy; however, despite continuous electronic fetal monitoring during labor as the routine in U.S. hospitals since the late 1970s, the incidence of cerebral palsy remains the same as it was before the introduction of this device (American College of Obstetricians and Gynecologists, 2005). There was hope that electronic fetal monitoring would be a factor in reducing professional liability for health care providers and institutions; however, "bad baby" cases instead have increased over the years. Conflict in interpreting the data from electronic fetal monitoring now has become a major part of lawsuits alleging perinatal malpractice. Problems with interrater and intrarater reliability related to electronic fetal monitoring are reality in everyday clinical practice. Thus it is no surprise that experts disagree when asked to offer testimony for the defense and plaintiffs.

Another significant reason for the continued medicalization of childbirth is that perinatal care is provided primarily by physicians, who are educated and trained to monitor and intervene, rather than by nurse-midwives, who believe less is more when it comes to interventions for childbearing women. Nurse-midwives believe in and support the inherent power of women to give birth naturally and with selected interventions as needed. Unfortunately, only 8% of births in the United States are attended by nurse-midwives (Hamilton et al., 2004). Financial and philosophical reasons prohibit or inhibit certified nurse-midwives (CNMs) from getting privileges to attend births in many hospitals. Some areas of the country have more obstetricians-gynecologists than are needed to support the target population. Thus there is an effort to prevent CNMs from effectively entering the market. Healthy women at low risk for complications during pregnancy can be managed by CNMs and have been shown to have similar clinical outcomes and lower costs of care. Increased access to CNMs by this healthy patient population would help to reverse the current trend in making birth a medical event.

INCREASED USE OF TECHNOLOGY

Some argue that the lack of one-to-one nursing care in the United States for women in labor has led to electronic monitors providing much of the maternal-fetal assessment data during labor and birth. Just as likely, the increased use of technology has contributed to the perception by health care administrators that one-to-one nursing care during labor is no longer needed. The latest monitors allow electronic assessment of multiple

VIEWPOINTS

physiological variables that are displayed on a central screen at nurses' stations. In this type of setting, nurses have less need to interact personally with the woman in labor. Consider the following scenario: a healthy woman at term agrees to an induction of labor, which leads to epidural anesthesia, slow progress of labor and attachment of the following nine intervention and monitoring devices: a main intravenous line and additional line with oxytocin, internal fetal scalp electrode, intrauterine pressure catheter, epidural catheter, automatic blood pressure device, cardiac monitor, pulse oximeter, and Foley catheter. An interesting note is that none of these devices or interventions is recommended by the professional associations that promulgate guidelines and standards of care for women in labor—such as the Association of Women's Health, Obstetric and Neonatal Nurses, the American College of Nurse-Midwives, the American College of Obstetricians and Gynecologists, or the American Society of Anesthesiologists—yet they are the routine in many labor and birth units in the United States (Simpson & Atterbury, 2003).

THE "WAY WE'VE ALWAYS DONE IT" VERSUS EVIDENCE-BASED PERINATAL CARE

The lack of integration of evidence-based care for healthy pregnant women contributes to high-technology labor and birth becoming the norm. Perinatal nurses only can be advocates for healthy childbearing women when they have knowledge of current standards and guidelines from their professional associations. Many nurses are unaware of their specialty nursing organization. Of those who are aware, few are members. Although there are 2.5 million registered nurses in the United States, the Association of Women's Health, Obstetric and Neonatal Nurses has approximately 17,000 members. Undoubtedly, there are many more perinatal nurses in the United States. In addition to the awareness of and adherence to professional guidelines and standards of care, perinatal nurses must have knowledge about all areas of their specialty practice. The ability to search computer databases for pertinent literature and critically to evaluate the combined weight of what is known about each intervention is requisite for perinatal nurses in the advocacy role who want to provide safe and effective care. Perinatal nurses must be aware of the body of evidence to suggest that routine interventions during labor and birth lead to iatrogenic injuries. They must be willing to work collaboratively with physician colleagues to make evidence-based perinatal care a reality.

Commitment to practice based on evidence and standards is an ongoing process and may require substantial changes and more professional energy than the usual methods of implementing and evaluating changes in patient care, but it is well worth the additional effort. Discussions about clinical practice that are based on evidence and standards of care rather than hierarchical relationships, personal preferences, and old routines can be helpful in setting the stage for real collaboration. Nurse leaders must promote the "different but equal" contribution nurses make to clinical outcomes. For perinatal nurses to have an equal voice in these discussions about clinical practices, they must make efforts to keep abreast of current evidence and evolving trends that have the potential to enhance maternal-fetal outcomes. However, to be able to evaluate critically the evidence that is available and to present credible recommendations, nurses need knowledge of the research process and skills in critiquing research studies. Unfortunately, according to the latest data, 57% of registered nurses in the United States today do not hold a 4-year college degree (Department of Health and Human Services, 2002). Without the education about the research process that is provided during baccalaureate education, it is difficult for nurses to bring a similar level of understanding and evaluation of the evidence under consideration to a clinical discussion with physician colleagues.

The wide disparity in education between nurses and physicians is one of the contributing factors to the lack of equal partnership in developing and implementing evidence-based clinical interventions. An equal voice in clinical discussions must be the voice of one who has been educated in an institution of higher learning in a manner similar to other members of the health care team (Simpson & Knox, 2001). The lack of college education among the majority of practicing nurses is one of the most significant barriers to enhancing the professional status of nurses and contributes to the present hierarchical relationships between nurses and physicians. Nurses have been debating this issue for too long. The time is now to set a date for requiring the baccalaureate degree as the criterion for entry into professional nursing practice (American Association of Colleges of Nursing, 2000). The profession can grandfather in the current nurses and move forward united in providing consumers with care they deserve, delivered by professionals who have been educated adequately to provide that care (Gennaro & Lewis, 2000). Only with additional education will nurses be able to participate fully in processes that promote evidence-based care for mothers and babies.

ERRORS BY HEALTH CARE PROVIDERS THAT RESULT IN MATERNAL-FETAL INJURIES

Even though use of multiple interventions and sophisticated technologies to monitor maternal-fetal status has become the norm, these techniques and machines have not decreased the risk of maternal-fetal injuries. This is a serious issue facing perinatal nurses today. Along with emergency departments and perioperative services, perinatal units account for most of the claims of patient injuries and death (Simpson & Knox, 2003). The release of the report from the Institute of Medicine *To Err Is Human: Building a Safer Health System* late in 1999 highlighted what risk managers and perinatal care providers already knew: errors by health care providers are an unfortunate common occurrence during inpatient stays (Kohn, Corrigan, & Donaldson, 1999). A preventable adverse outcome for a mother or baby can be tragic, with long-term and even fatal consequences in some cases. Fetal and neonatal injuries are more common than maternal injuries. Six common recurring clinical problems account for most fetal and neonatal injuries (Knox, Simpson, & Townsend, 2003):

1. Inability to recognize or appropriately respond to antepartum and intrapartum fetal compromise
2. Inability to perform a timely cesarean birth (30 minutes from decision to incision) when indicated by fetal or maternal condition
3. Inability to resuscitate a depressed baby appropriately
4. Inappropriate use of oxytocin or misoprostol, leading to uterine hyperstimulation, uterine rupture, and fetal compromise or death
5. Inappropriate use of forceps, vacuum, or fundal pressure, leading to maternal-fetal trauma or preventable shoulder dystocia
6. Mismanagement of the second stage of labor, resulting in maternal-fetal injuries

Many of the clinical problems are interrelated and can be attributed to communication failures and the trend toward provider convenience taking precedence over established professional standards and the latest evidence. In obstetrics, complications leading to death are rare because mothers and infants are generally healthy (Simpson, 2005b). Even care that would be judged by expert peers to be substandard rarely results in injury or death. The odds are always in favor of a good outcome because of the healthy population. These clinical conditions allow some practitioners to disregard practice based on professional standards and rigorous evidence, often without consequences. However, even one preventable injury or death of a mother or infant is one too many.

Perinatal providers must make safety the No. 1 priority to promote the best possible maternal-fetal outcomes. Patient safety, particularly for the most vulnerable populations (mothers and babies), is a matter of integrity. Everyone in the health care system, including administrators, members of the leadership team, and individual providers, has a moral obligation to do everything possible to keep patients safe (Ryan, 2004). Perinatal unit operations and health care provider relationships must be reexamined in the context of implementing a system designed for maternal-fetal safety.

NURSE-TO-PATIENT RATIOS

The increasing trend toward fewer nurses caring for more patients during labor and birth is a major barrier to quality perinatal care. When the nurse has more patients than can be cared for adequately, the constant priority setting and elimination process contribute to shortcuts and provision of only the most basic care (Knox, Kelley, Simpson, Carrier, & Berry, 1999). Unfortunately, for some nurses the basics may be high-tech interventions and documentation, whereas supportive care in labor is considered a luxury. Ample data suggest that more favorable nurse-to-patient ratios improve outcomes and decrease risks of morbidity and mortality (Aiken, Clarke, Sloane, Sochalski, & Silber, 2002; Needleman, Buerhaus, Mattke, Stewart, & Zelevinsky, 2002). However, as costs of care have accelerated, perinatal units have suffered staffing cuts. The increased use of technology to monitor maternal-fetal status during labor, the high rate of epidural anesthesia, and the fact that most women and fetuses are healthy have contributed to the ability of institutions providing perinatal care to "get away with" using fewer nurses in perinatal services (Knox, Simpson, et al., 2003). Nurses are adept at on-the-spot problem solving and work-arounds when they are faced with situations and systems that put patients at risk. However, their ability to keep patients safe under these conditions often allows the hospital and the health care team to avoid investing time and effort to redesign unsafe systems (Needleman & Buerhaus, 2003).

PROLIFERATION OF CONVENIENCE AS THE FOUNDATION FOR LABOR AND BIRTH

Artificial induction of labor is at the highest level in the United States since these data began being collected from birth certificates in 1989 (Hamilton et al., 2004). The incidence of labor induction is most likely much higher than reported because of inaccuracy issues with data retrieved from birth certificates. Multiple factors influence the decision to induce labor (Simpson & Atterbury, 2003). Clearly, not all indications are clinical or are in the best interests of mothers and babies. Increasingly, convenience has become a significant factor in artificial induction of labor. This is a complex issue that involves all participating parties: the pregnant woman, her family, the obstetrician or CNM, the institution, and the perinatal nurse (Simpson & Thorman, 2005). In 1995 the American College of Obstetricians and Gynecologists included "psychosocial indications" as an accepted reason for induction. Previously, the position of the college had been that induction of labor solely for convenience was not recommended (American College of Obstetricians and Gynecologists, 1991). The most likely reason for this change was that routine practices were not consistent with published standards, exposing physicians to liability risks if adverse outcomes resulted from artificial labor induction. The controversial issue is, Who benefits more from this convenience approach to labor induction? Women agree to or choose induction of labor for many reasons. For some women, advance planning and prior arrangements can provide reassurance and a sense of control over an otherwise unpredictable process. Additional factors such as child care for other children, availability of the labor support person or father of the baby, choice of attending physician on call, avoidance of holidays, maternity leave constraints, and even a federal income tax deduction in the preferred year can enter into the pregnant woman's decision to agree to or request an elective induction of labor (Simpson & Thorman, 2005).

If pregnant women are informed fully about the indications for induction, risks and benefits of the proposed method, and possible alternative approaches as recommended by American College of Obstetricians and Gynecologists (1999), the woman's choice should be honored if the appropriate resources are available to induce labor safely. However, many discussions between women and their physician before induction fall short of meeting these criteria. An all-too-common occurrence during admission of a pregnant woman for induction is the realization by the nurse that the woman did not request an induction of labor and is unaware of the indications, potential risks, and alternative approaches (Simpson & Thorman, 2005). Although not well documented in the literature or discussed openly in professional forums, a scheduled induction of labor offers some real convenience advantages to the physician and CNM. Scheduling several women for an induction of labor on the same day starting early in the morning

allows patient management to be done concurrently and increases the likelihood that most women will give birth by the end of the day. When physicians and CNMs schedule inductions routinely, the risk to the women of going into spontaneous labor and giving birth at a time that is inconvenient is avoided. As the number of patients who have scheduled inductions increase, the number of physician and CNM telephone calls and trips to the hospital in the middle of the night and on weekends is likely to decrease (Simpson & Atterbury, 2003).

Another example of provider convenience is shortening the second stage of an otherwise normal labor by application of forceps or a vacuum extractor and cutting an episiotomy (Simpson & Thorman, 2005). Perinatal nurses can help to avoid the temptation by physicians to shorten the second stage when there are no maternal-fetal indications by calling physicians at appropriate times when birth is imminent, so they are not delayed in the hospital when they have an office full of pregnant women waiting to be seen. This requires knowledge of the labor process and keen assessment skills. All interventions for convenience involve some risk of an adverse outcome. Unfortunately, the current culture in many perinatal units supports routine practices for convenience rather than patience and allowing the normal process and progress of birth to occur. In this situation, routine practices for convenience continue until the inevitable adverse outcome occurs.

One way to understand how practices that involve risk can come to be favored over patience and patient safety is provided by Vaughn (1996) in her analysis of the *Challenger* disaster. She found that professional standards of any work group will degrade slowly and incrementally over time. Vaughn termed this progressive degradation in safe practice *the normalization of deviance*. Operational systems and clinical practices that are known to be risky continue because the risk continually is redefined in the context of injuries that do not occur. This phenomenon of human behavior is especially prevalent when the chances of the risk occurring are small. Most mothers and babies are healthy, so care involving increased risk does not usually result in patient injury (Simpson, 2005b). As time goes on, practice becomes increasingly less safe because "they get away with it." Perinatal practices that involve convenience for health care providers should be evaluated in terms of risks and benefits for mothers and babies. Before proceeding, it should be clear who the beneficiary of the convenience is. Women should be informed fully that practices or interventions being considered are for convenience, and they should be allowed to make a decision about whether to go forward (Simpson & Thorman, 2005). Avoiding risk of the normalization of deviance in any perinatal setting is a significant challenge for perinatal nurses but one that can be met if the goal of the best possible outcomes for mothers and babies is ranked higher in priority than convenience. This goal will require physicians and nurses to come to consensus that patient safety is the No. 1 priority and that some may be inconvenienced waiting for nature to take its course.

LACK OF KNOWLEDGE AMONG CHILDBEARING WOMEN ABOUT THE IMPACT OF THE PHILOSOPHY OF CONVENIENCE

Information about pregnancy and birth has never been more available for childbearing women than today. A visit to the local bookstore reveals aisles of books on all sorts of related topics. More than 10,000 Internet sites are devoted to pregnancy and childbirth. Yet many pregnant women seem to be uninformed about the implications of artificial induction of labor, epidural anesthesia, assisted instrumental vaginal birth, and elective cesarean birth on the eventual outcomes of pregnancy. Rarely is a woman admitted for an elective induction of labor who is able to articulate accurately the risks involved. Most women are not involved actively in the decision to use forceps or a vacuum to shorten the second stage of labor or are informed about the risks of the procedure versus waiting for the fetus to descend spontaneously. Few women question the need for an episiotomy when the procedure is imminent. Women put their trust in their health care providers. Trust is a good thing, but not blind trust. A fully informed woman is a partner in the decision-making process. However, even women who are fully informed agree to things they had planned to avoid when they are vulnerable during the process of labor and birth. Perinatal nurses, as advocates for pregnant women, need to make sure that women have the necessary information to make important decisions during labor and birth (Simpson & Thorman, 2005). Unfortunately, this advocacy can be seen by some as interfering with the physician-patient relationship. One way to increase the likelihood that women who are informed and have made choices actually realize care based on those choices is the implementation of a birth plan listing available options. The women can complete birth plans during the prenatal period and make them part of the medical record. The perinatal nurse then can review requests and appropriateness based on the individual clinical situation on admission for childbirth.

The content of prepared childbirth classes should include an objective review of the risks and benefits of commonly used interventions during labor and birth, and this information should be reinforced by nurses who care for women during the intrapartum period.

SUMMARY

Many issues in perinatal care could benefit from the collective efforts of all perinatal nurses to improve the way they routinely care for childbearing women. Much of what nurses do in perinatal care is based on myths, rituals, and "the way we've always done it" (Simpson & Thorman, 2005). Those who are invested in the old ways will resist attempts for significant change. The best hope for change is a firm commitment to providing care based on the combined weight of available evidence. This commitment involves perinatal nurses making an effort to become educated about how to critique these data and apply the evidence to everyday clinical practice. Knowledge is power. This power is within all perinatal nurses who arm themselves with the skills required to have clinical discussions with physician colleagues based on evidence and thus become true partners in determining the best practices for routine perinatal care.

REFERENCES

Aiken, L. H., Clarke, S. P., Sloane, D. M., Sochalski, J., & Silber, J. H. (2002). Hospital nurse staffing and patient mortality, nurse burnout and job dissatisfaction. *Journal of the American Medical Association, 288*(16), 1987-1993.

American Association of Colleges of Nursing. (2000). *The baccalaureate degree in nursing as minimal preparation for professional practice* [Position statement]. Washington, DC: Author.

American College of Obstetricians and Gynecologists. (1991). *Induction of labor* (Tech. Bulletin No. 157). Washington, DC: Author.

American College of Obstetricians and Gynecologists. (1995). *Induction of labor* (Tech. Bulletin No. 217). Washington, DC: Author.

American College of Obstetricians and Gynecologists. (1999). *Induction of labor* (Practice Bulletin No. 10). Washington, DC: Author.

American College of Obstetricians and Gynecologists. (2005). *Intrapartum fetal heart rate monitoring* (Practice Bulletin No. 62). Washington, DC: Author.

Department of Health and Human Services. (2002). *The registered nurse population: Findings from the National Sample Survey of Registered Nurses.* Washington, DC: Author.

Food and Drug Administration. (1998). *FDA public health advisory: Need for caution when using vacuum assisted delivery devices.* Washington, DC: Author.

Fraser, W. D., Turcot, L., Krauss, I., & Brisson-Carrol, G. (2000). Amniotomy for shortening labor. *Cochrane Database of Systematic Reviews, 2,* CD000015.

Garite, T. J., Porto, M., Carlson, N. J., Rumney, P. J., & Reimbold, P. A. (1993). The influence of elective amniotomy on fetal heart rate patterns and the course of labor in term patients: A randomized study. *American Journal of Obstetrics and Gynecology, 168*(6, Pt. 1), 1827-1831.

Gennaro, S., & Lewis, J. (2000). Is the BSN as the criteria for entry in professional nursing practice still worthwhile and realistic? *MCN: The American Journal of Maternal Child Nursing, 25*(2), 62-63.

Goffinet, F., Fraser, W., Marcoux, S., Breart, G., Moutquin, J. M., & Darvis, M. (1997). Early amniotomy increases the frequency of fetal heart rate abnormalities: Amniotomy study group. *British Journal of Obstetrics and Gynaecology, 104*(5), 548-553.

Hamilton, B. E., Martin, J. A., & Sutton, P. D. (2004). Births: Preliminary data for 2003. *National Vital Statistics Reports, 53*(9), 1-18.

Handa, V. L., Harris, T. A., & Ostergard, D. R. (1996). Protecting the pelvic floor: Obstetric management to prevent incontinence and pelvic organ prolapse. *Obstetrics and Gynecology, 88*(3), 470-478.

Hansen, S. L., Clark, S. L., & Foster, J. C. (2002). Active pushing versus passive fetal descent in the second stage of labor: A randomized controlled trial. *Obstetrics and Gynecology, 99*(1), 29-34.

Hartmann, K., Viswanathan, M., Palmieri, R., Gartlehner, G., Thorp, J., Jr., & Lohr, K. N. (2005). Outcomes of routine episiotomy: a systematic review. *JAMA: The Journal of the American Medical Association, 293*(17), 2141-2148.

Knox, G. E., Kelley, M., Simpson, K. R., Carrier, L., & Berry, D. (1999). Downsizing, re-engineering and patient safety: Numbers, newness and resultant risk. *Journal of Healthcare Risk Management, 19*(4), 18-25.

Knox, G. E., Simpson, K. R., & Townsend, K. E. (2003). High reliability perinatal units: Further observations and a suggested plan for action. *Journal of Healthcare Risk Management, 23*(4), 17-21.

Kohn, L., Corrigan, J., & Donaldson, M. (Eds.). (1999). *To err is human: Building a safer health system.* Washington, DC: National Academies Press.

Mayberry, L. J., Hammer, R., Kelly, C., True-Driver, B., & De, A. (1999). Use of delayed pushing with epidural anesthesia: Findings from a randomized controlled trial. *Journal of Perinatology, 19*(1), 26-30.

Needleman, J., & Buerhaus, P. (2003). Nurse staffing and patient safety: Current knowledge and implications for action. *International Journal of Quality Health Care, 15*(3), 275-277.

Needleman, J., Buerhaus, P., Mattke, S., Stewart, M., & Zelevinsky, K. (2002). Nurse-staffing levels and the quality of care in hospitals. *New England Journal of Medicine, 346*(22), 1715-1722.

Roberts, J. E. (2002). The "push" for evidence: Management of the second stage. *Journal of Midwifery and Women's Health, 47*(1), 2-15.

Ryan, M. J. (2004). Patient safety: A matter of integrity. *Journal of Innovative Management, 9*(3), 11-20.

Sampselle, C., & Hines, S. (1999). Spontaneous pushing during birth: Relationship to perineal outcomes. *Journal of Nurse Midwifery, 44*(1), 36-39.

Schaffer, J. I., Bloom, S. L., Casey, B. M., McIntire, D. D., Nihira, M. A., & Leveno, K. J. (2005). A randomized trial of the effects of coached vs uncoached maternal pushing during the second stage of labor on postpartum pelvic floor structure and function. *American Journal of Obstetrics and Gynecology, 192*(5), 1692-1696.

Simpson, K. R. (2003). Labor and birth today: Things have changed. *Journal of Obstetric, Gynecologic and Neonatal Nursing, 32*(6), 765-766.

Simpson, K. R. (2005a). Does practice make perfect? Not always. *MCN: The American Journal of Maternal Child Nursing, 30*(4), 290.

Simpson, K. R. (2005b). Failure to rescue: Implications for evaluating quality of care during labor and birth. *Journal of Perinatal and Neonatal Nursing, 19*(1), 23-33.

Simpson, K. R., & Atterbury, J. (2003). Labor induction in the United States: Trends and issues for clinical practice. *Journal of Obstetric, Gynecologic and Neonatal Nursing, 32*(6), 767-779.

Simpson, K. R., & James, D. C. (2005). Effects of immediate versus delayed pushing during second stage labor on fetal wellbeing: A randomized clinical trial. *Nursing Research, 54*(3), 149-157.

Simpson, K. R., & Knox, G. E. (2001). Perinatal teamwork: Turning rhetoric into reality. In K. R. Simpson & P. A. Creehan (Eds.), *AWHONN's perinatal nursing* (2nd ed., pp. 57-71). Philadelphia: Lippincott Williams & Wilkins.

Simpson, K. R., & Knox, G. E. (2003). Common areas of litigation related to care during labor and birth: Recommendations to promote patient safety and decrease risk exposure. *Journal of Perinatal and Neonatal Nursing, 17*(1), 110-125.

Simpson, K. R., & Thorman, K. E. (2005). Obstetric "conveniences": Elective induction of labor, cesarean birth on demand and other potentially unnecessary interventions. *Journal of Perinatal and Neonatal Nursing, 2*(19), 134-144.

Vaughn, D. (1996). *The Challenger launch decision: Risky technology, culture and deviance at NASA.* Chicago: University of Chicago Press.

Perioperative Nursing

Recent Changes and Current Issues

NANCY GIRARD

The specialty practice area of perioperative nursing is facing many of the same issues nurses in general are facing. The general health care delivery system in the United States today is broken, and no one person or profession can fix it. Changes will require team effort and an increased awareness of the true health care needs of the people of the United States. Many Americans have inadequate or no insurance, care is fragmented and often unattainable even for the insured, third-party payers control the extent of treatment, and faith in the system is declining. In lieu of these national problems, current major issues affecting perioperative nurses can be categorized into four areas: practice/role issues, skill issues, fiscal issues, and professional issues. These categories of issues are interconnected and should be considered factors that affect each other. Some of the variables affecting these factors are the following:

◆ By 2006 the average family health insurance premium will exceed $14,500; premium costs will have increased by more than $5,000 in just 3 years (National Coalition on Health Care, 2004).

◆ In 2002, health care spending in the United States was $1.6 trillion, up 9.3% from 2001 (National Center for Health Statistics, 2004).

◆ Americans' average annual out-of-pocket expenses for health care rose 26% between 1995 and 2001, to $2,182 (National Center for Health Statistics, 2004).

◆ Costs are expected to grow because scientists continually are discovering medicines to treat diseases of aging and individuals are living longer. The elderly population, now 36 million, is expected to reach 70 million by 2030 (Pear, 2003).

◆ The number of Americans without health insurance rose to 43.6 million in 2002 (Simmons, 2003).

◆ Consumers of health care are more knowledgeable and are more aware of their options because of the Internet (Agency for Healthcare Research and Quality, 2005).

◆ Changes in regulatory and legislative mandates require health care institutions and providers continually to evaluate and improve the quality of health care (Joint Commission on Accreditation of Healthcare Organizations, 2005).

◆ Federal mandates related to the computerized patient record and the protection of personal health information will result in closer restrictions and guidelines for patient data collected in and shared by health care facilities (U.S. Department of Health and Human Services, 2005).

◆ Enhanced imaging devices have improved and will continue to improve the diagnosis and treatment (including surgery) of numerous health conditions.

◆ Innovations such as minimally invasive surgery, computerized technology, and robotic surgery (Meadows, 2002) will allow surgery to be done with greater precision, less tissue injury, and improved patient outcomes.

PRACTICE/ROLE ISSUES

Perioperative nurses feel strongly that they, as professional nurses, must remain in the role of patient advocate and caretaker in surgical sites (Association of Perioperative Registered Nurses [AORN], 2002). The major goals of perioperative nursing are to maintain a safe environment, prevent nonsurgical injury, support emotional and psychological needs of the patient and the family, and provide timely and accurate information to all. The nurse assesses, plans, implements, and evaluates nursing care, just as in any other practice site. For anyone who has had surgery recently or who knows someone close to them who had surgery, the influence of a registered nurse (RN) may have made the difference between client satisfaction and dissatisfaction, as well as in minimizing mishaps and inadvertent errors during the procedure.

The traditional perioperative nursing roles are under attack. The question being debated today by many within and outside of nursing is, "Are professional registered nurses needed in the operating room and in areas where surgical interventions are being performed?" If the answer is yes, the next debate is, What will they do? Historically, perioperative nurses had two roles: circulator and scrub nurse. Within the last decade, surgical technicians have taken over the role of scrub person, and nursing has maintained a nebulous hold on the professional circulating role. New legislative measures in many states are allowing semiskilled technicians to take over the role of the circulator and the scrub person. Hospital administrators quickly accepted the surgical technologist in this role because of the decreased availability of qualified surgical nurses and the lower costs associated with unlicensed personnel in this role. The development of surgical technology programs in hospitals and in technical colleges has produced an increased number of ancillary personnel who are assuming the scrub role and who are beginning to assume a circulator role.

Roles of the perioperative nurse are expanding beyond circulating and scrubbing. Additional roles include those of manager, educator, case coordinator, researcher, consultant, informatics specialists, industrial supply company representatives, and advanced practice nurses. Many nurses are obtaining additional education beyond their basic nursing education in order to expand their perioperative practice roles. The most common formal graduate educational degrees for those aspiring to be leaders are master in nursing administration or master in business administration. Perioperative nursing roles are being expanded as nurses become certified registered nurse first assistants (CRNFAs), who work as a hospital employee or with a private physician practice. Some nurses maintain their own business and hire out to surgeons requesting CRNFAs. A CRNFA may or may not have an advanced degree, but the nurse has additional education in first assisting (AORN, 2005). The advanced practice nurse role is becoming more recognized and used in the surgical settings today (AORN, 2004b). Most states identify three advanced practice categories that perioperative nurses are joining by getting graduate education (master of science in nursing): clinical nurse specialists, nurse practitioners, or certified registered nurse anesthetists. These advanced practice nurses are providing care during the whole continuum of the surgical experience, from home to home. They are practicing in the surgical units, clinics, offices, freestanding surgery centers, and the home. As health care delivery continues to change, one must ask whether the major future role of perioperative nursing is beyond the operating room.

Meanwhile, the role of the perioperative nurse in hospitals and ambulatory surgery settings has become highly diversified. What was once a homogenous population of caregivers is now a group that often has little in common except the incidence of a surgical episode. For example, perioperative nurses in ambulatory settings assume responsibility for the care of the patient throughout the entire perioperative period, from preadmission to discharge. Some ambulatory-based perioperative nurses make discharge follow-up calls or visits to the home. Perioperative nurses are separating out into arenas such as gastrointestinal, radiology, endoscopy, orthopedic, cardiovascular, and other surgical subspecialties along with the physicians. These subspecialties often take the perioperative nurse out of the traditional operating room, which has led to a fragmentation of perioperative nursing, and it also draws members away from the AORN as they move to start their own specialty organizations. This movement lends importance to the issue of practice because the perioperative group no longer speaks with one voice and thus is in jeopardy of losing what little political influence it has at the present time.

SKILL ISSUES

The change in skill requirements for perioperative nurses is a big issue today. Technological advances are changing the practice of surgery. Innovations in minimally invasive surgery, virtual reality and robotic technology, computerized technology, gene therapy, and nanotechnology are transforming surgical techniques. Computerized and enhanced imaging devices have and will continue to improve the diagnosis and surgical treatment of numerous health conditions. With the growth in technical and computerized equipment, perioperative nurses are facing continuous updates and training needs. Indeed, many feel as though they should have taken engineering rather than nursing courses in order to cope with all the new equipment. The newest innovations may require certification and specialization to prepare nurses to implement and monitor the patient using the technology in surgical settings. Because of the constant upgrading of existing and new technology, it is impossible for nursing schools to prepare competent new graduates adequately in every skill. This responsibility must be absorbed by the surgical institutions as staff development or on-the-job training.

With the increasingly complex technological aspects of intraoperative care must come training with each piece of technology. Some technology is so detailed that the skills needed are provided by the company that manufactures the product rather than the employer. Hands-on training is essential, and many skills require competency testing and even certification. By one estimate, there could be up to 450 different pieces of equipment in an operating room for just one surgery, so cross-training for everything is impossible. In the past, perioperative nurses, like any other nurse, could be cross-trained to work in all areas of surgery. Today that is impossible. A nurse who is excellent in heart surgery may have no knowledge of brain surgery. Thus perioperative nurses have become as specialized in surgery as physicians and can no longer be available for assignment in every room for every kind of surgery. The general perioperative nurse of the past is gone, and management now must hire for specific skill sets (B. Duffy, AORN president, personal communication, December 12, 2004). A big issue is often the lack of perception of administration and management as to the knowledge and skill needs of these nurses, and many continue to require an all-around practitioner. This is unreasonable. A physician gains more respect and ability as he or she focuses on one aspect of care, whether it is orthopedics or eye surgery. Nurses should have that same respect and opportunity.

The increased skill levels needed by perioperative nurses require the presence of a unit educator to teach and train the nurses in any new technology. Because more new graduates are being recruited into perioperative nursing, basic skill training also still is needed. Nurses assuming educator roles are responsible for the design, implementation, and evaluation of perioperative education programs for staff, patients, and families, as well as in-service education and orientation programs for all members of the surgical team. Advanced practice nurses can assist unit educators as clinical resource persons for these teaching endeavors, although that is not their main role.

One of the first cutbacks in the hospital to decrease costs is the deletion of the educator. As described previously, training is essential in the operating room. Because of the shortage of new perioperative nurses, new graduates are being hired into the operating room. These graduates must be oriented and their competencies must be determined in order to provide safe care. Without a perioperative educator, these tasks can be accomplished only with a longer and more inefficient method.

Finally, mobile computer and communication technology skills are essential for perioperative nurses. The use of personal handheld devices and wireless computers are increasing in surgical areas to provide more efficient workflow and allow documentation and care planning that has the potential to reduce errors. Perioperative nurses today must be computer literate and must have the skills to use all methods of communication technology.

FISCAL ISSUES

The cost of health care in the United States today is driving all aspects of care, including nursing. Great concern exists today about the extent of the benefits given through Medicare and Medicaid programs. National 2006 Medicare budget cuts to hospitals have been estimated to be $740 million, going to $4.7 billion over the next 5 years (American Hospital Association, 2005). These cuts will greatly affect reimbursements to community and nonprofit hospitals, which probably will rethink the workforce needed to be hired by these hospitals. Because Medicaid mainly covers the low-income populations of mothers with children, the elderly, and the disabled, these individuals will seek care in emergency rooms of community hospitals rather than paying the increased copayments being proposed. The costs of caring for the elderly are greatly affecting acute care hospitals as the population ages. Surgery now is being performed on persons up into their late 80s and even into their 90s, which will drive fiscal issues and cost containment further.

Just when advanced practice nurses and CRNFAs are becoming eligible to bill for third-party reimbursement, costs are being cut, particularly those of Medicaid. Community- and state-run health care institutions, such as acute care hospitals, will be affected by any cuts. Salary costs of any business are the major budgetary consideration, so managers will be looking at more cost-effective methods to stay in business. These changes can affect perioperative nurses because to date no empirical evidence justifies having a professional RN in the role of circulator.

Still, an argument to retain advanced practitioners and CRNFAs in the operating room is that they now can bill for third-party reimbursement in many states. This could be considered salary replacement or additional income to those employing them, which might help these nurses retain their positions.

The Health Care Financing Administration proposed a rule change that would allow hospitals and ambulatory surgery centers reimbursed by Medicare and Medicaid to determine their own staffing patterns for surgical services. This proposed rule would replace prescriptive rules that currently state that a physician, osteopathic physician, or RN must supervise an operating room. To date, no final decisions on this proposed rule change have been made, and ongoing debate continues related to this controversial change (Romig, 2000).

Today, more surgeries and minimally invasive procedures are performed outside of traditional hospital operating rooms. In addition to the growth in ambulatory care procedures, office-based surgery is the latest trend in surgery. As more procedures are performed in office settings, the number of surgeries performed in hospital and ambulatory care settings is anticipated to decrease. These changes in clinical settings will continue to drive significant financial changes in the hospital, which will affect the traditional role of the perioperative nurse further. Ambulatory surgical centers were established in an effort to decrease costs and create an efficient process for patient and staff members. Changes in reimbursement, the shift to minimally invasive surgical techniques, cost-containment efforts, and high levels of patient and staff satisfaction further contributed to the expansion of ambulatory surgical settings.

One concern that could be debated is, if surgery can be done outside the operating room, *should* it be done? Although the general public supports this, the trend was started for financial reasons. Surgery is cheaper outside of a hospital. Some major surgeries, such as an abdominal aortic aneurysm repair, now may be done in radiology departments without the assistance of a perioperative nurse (or *any* nurse). Although this may be accepted in some institutions, in others the knowledge the perioperative nurses brings to the practice, such as sterile technique, may be missing, thus increasing the incidence of postprocedure infection.

PROFESSIONAL ISSUES

Professionalism is an issue for nursing in general. Professionalism is a major problem with the identification of perioperative nurses as professionals because of the lack of visibility. Perioperative nurse still, for the most part, remain behind closed doors. In addition, students exposed to the operating room often do not see professional nursing being performed when only observing, or they have a bad experience and do not further consider this as a career choice. Nurses are accountable for this situation. Unfortunately, in many

schools, nursing faculty frequently tell students not to go into the operating room after graduation and discourage interest in the specialty. This has led to a continual decline in RNs in the operating room. Today, new nurses are not entering the perioperative arena in sufficient numbers to replace retiring nurses. In addition, the older perioperative nurse may be having trouble keeping up with the physical activity needed to perform in the operating room, so the impact of retirement is being felt around the country. One measure being used to counteract this loss is to replace RNs with semiskilled and unskilled personnel.

A threat to the professional RN continuing in the operating room is one from the Association of Surgical Technologists (2005), which is developing national legislative and regulatory initiatives that include functions previously only performed by the circulating nurse. As this chapter is being written, a bill is being introduced in the state of Texas that will require hospitals and surgery centers in the state to hire only certified surgical technologists. Senate Bill 930 is available on the Web at http://www.capitol.state.tx.us/tlo/79R/billtext/SB00930I.HTM. If the bill passes, the law takes effect September 2005 in the state of Texas. A comparable bill is being presented at the national level. The nursing profession is opposing this bill vigorously because it provides for broad grandfathering and waivers for education, which may not retain the quality of surgical patient care desired. Although the good intentions of the bill are to provide educated and qualified surgical technicians who perform a valuable and needed service as part of the operating room team, in reality the bill provides less skilled entry to compete with the professional nurse in the operating room, does not meet any current criteria for certification, and allows for minimal education. The bill also potentially could put surgical technicians under the supervision of the surgeon, not the RN, which may further affect the professional role of the RN.

Entry into practice is an ongoing issue with perioperative nurses as with all other nurses. In the recent 2005 Annual Congress of the Association of PeriOperative Nurses, the delegates reapproved the position statement that "AORN believes there should be one level for entry into nursing practice; AORN believes the minimal preparation for entry into the practice of nursing should be the baccalaureate degree" (AORN, 2004a). At the present, an RN who practices in the perioperative setting can have an associate's degree, bachelor of science in nursing, or diploma. Advanced practice nurses must adhere to their state criteria for practice, including obtaining a masters' degree. Some hospitals still call non–masters'-prepared nurses clinical specialists, but these nurses do not have the education or proper certification to practice in this role. This is becoming more important as state boards of nursing now are looking closely at scope of practice to ensure that nurses are not practicing beyond their academic preparation. This scrutiny can affect many acute care institutions that now are hiring family nurse practitioners for surgical areas and even to assist in surgery, rather than acute care nurse practitioners and CRNFAs.

Another professional issue is the continuing discussion about the roles of the certified registered nurse anesthetist and the CRNFA, particularly if they are hired by independent surgeons and are not staff at a hospital. Practice privileges, financial reimbursement, job descriptions, and actual roles are in ongoing development and depend on the state and the institution. Often the ability of these practitioners to perform adequately in their roles depends on their ability to charge for third-party reimbursement. This also varies from state to state.

The majority of health care organizations has been concerned with safety of the patient for several years, and AORN has mandated continually that safety is the ultimate goal for practice in this arena. A major reason to retain the professional nurse in the operating room is to maintain and improve quality of care that is safe and effective (American Hospital Association, 2005).

Perioperative nurses have always focused on safety in all aspects of the surgical patient care because this is one area where the patient has no ability to cope with threatening situations alone. The AORN is working in close collaboration with other health care organizations to provide safe and optimal care. For example, perioperative nurses are promoting a National Time Out. The focus of the 2005 National Time Out Day is "safe medication administration in the operating room."

Physical, emotional, and psychological aspects must be considered to give quality care. Professional nurses have the education and depth of knowledge to provide this care. This degree of nursing care can be provided only by a professional, and if semiskilled or unskilled workers replace the RN in the operating room, the patients may be the ones who suffer from inadequate or insufficient care.

SUMMARY

Practice/roles, skills, fiscal, and professional issues are affecting the perioperative nurse. Debate on every issue is ongoing within the health care arena. These issues are influenced by socioeconomic factors and by the changing demographic characteristics and cultures today.

Perioperative nurses need to continue to demonstrate their contributions to quality care in surgical settings, using evidenced-based outcomes to validate their practice. Although few empirical findings are available to support the roles, practice, and professional concerns, clinical evidence is available. The presence of RNs in the operating room is vital to quality patient care, and this specialty must be supported by nurses and management. The loss of this professional role would be a great loss to future surgical patients and their loved ones.

REFERENCES

Agency for Healthcare Research and Quality. (2005). *Consumers and patients.* Retrieved June 8, 2005, from http://www.ahrq.gov/consumer/index.html#quality

American Hospital Association. (2005). *Protecting the health care safety net.* Retrieved June 8, 2005, from http://www.aha.org/aha/annual_meeting/content/05_Medicare.pdf

Association of Perioperative Registered Nurses. (2002). *Statement on mandate for the registered professional nurse in the perioperative practice setting.* Retrieved June 8, 2005, from http://www.aorn.org/about/positions/mandate.htm

Association of Perioperative Registered Nurses. (2004a). *AORN position statement on entry to practice.* Retrieved June 8, 2005, from http://www.aorn.org/about/positions/pdf/Final%20PS%20on%20Entry%20into%20Practice.pdf

Association of Perioperative Registered Nurses. (2004b). *Definition of perioperative advanced practice nurse.* Retrieved June 8, 2005, from http://www.aorn.org/about/positions/advpractice.htm

Association of Perioperative Registered Nurses. (2005). *AORN official statement on RN first assistants.* Retrieved June 8, 2005, from http://www.aorn.org/about/positions/pdf/POS-RNFA.pdf

Association of Surgical Technologists. (2005). *2005 Prospectus/Media Kit PDF Index* (see Surgical technologist STAT sheet [p. 20]). Retrieved June 8, 2005, from http://www.ast.org/Content/Advertise/2005_Media_Kit.pdf

Joint Commission on Accreditation of Healthcare Organizations. (2005). *Joint Commission announces 2006 National Patient Safety Goals.* Retrieved June 8, 2005, from http://www.jcaho.org/news+room/news+release+archives/06_npsg.htm

Meadows, M. (2002). Robots lend a helping hand to surgeons. *U.S. Food and Drug Administration, FDA Consumer Magazine.* Retrieved June 8, 2005, from http://www.fda.gov/fdac/features/2002/302_bots.html

National Center for Health Statistics. (2004). *Health, United States, 2004: With chartbook on trends in the health of Americans.*

Retrieved June 8, 2005, from http://www.cdc.gov/nchs/data/hus/hus04trend.pdf#exe

National Coalition on Health Care. (2004). *Health insurance coverage.* Retrieved April 20, 2005, from http://www.nchc.org/facts/coverage.shtml

Pear, R. (2003, August 19). Prescription drugs now, day of reckoning later. *New York Times,* p. A19.

Romig, C. (2000). Legislative update. *Surgical Services Management, 6*(1), 49-52.

Simmons, H. E. (2003). *Statement by Dr. Henry E. Simmons, M.D., M.P.H., F.A.C.P., President, National Coalition on Health Care* [Press release]. Retrieved June 8, 2005, from http://www.nchc.org/news/press_releases/2003/2003_09_29.pdf

U.S. Department of Health and Human Services. (2005). *Office for Civil Rights—HIPAA. Medical privacy: National standards to protect the privacy of personal health information.* Retrieved June 8, 2005, from http://www.hhs.gov/ocr/hipaa

Psychiatric Nursing

Recent Changes and Current Issues

GAIL W. STUART

The specialty of psychiatric nursing is challenged by current health care realities as mental health issues have emerged as a major source of disability and morbidity for children, adults, and the elderly. The World Health Organization identified mental illnesses as the leading cause of disability worldwide (World Health Organization, 2001). Specifically, of all health-related disability, the highest proportion (24%) is related to psychiatric/mental health disorders, followed by alcohol and drug use disorders (12%), and Alzheimer's disease and dementia (7%) (Figure 28-1). Thus fully 43% of health-related disability is due to mental health issues. Four out of the 10 leading causes of disability for persons over the age of 5 are mental illnesses. Major depression is the leading cause of disability among developed nations, and manic-depressive illness, schizophrenia, and obsessive-compulsive disorder also rank at the top. Mental illness is a tragic contributor to mortality, with suicide perennially representing one of the leading preventable causes of death in the United States. In fact, worldwide, suicide accounts for more deaths than homicide and war combined.

The U.S. Surgeon General's historic first Report on Mental Health alerted the nation to the fact that more than 54 million Americans have a mental illness in any given year, although fewer than 8 million seek treatment (U.S. Department of Health and Human Services, 1999). One in five Americans, therefore, is living with a mental illness, and if he or she seeks treatment, treatment usually depends on the skills of primary care providers. Furthermore, one half of all visits to primary care providers are estimated to be due to conditions that are caused or exacerbated by mental or emotional problems. At present, parity for mental health care has been enacted at the national level and by many states across the country. Advances in genetics and neurobiology abound, and the field is moving quickly to a paradigm of evidence-based practice. Clearly, mental health is the "trump card" within the health care system because it has been linked to the development of and recovery from a wide variety of medical illnesses.

The case is clear that there is a growing need for psychiatric–mental health nurses. Today, more than 82,000 registered nurses work in mental health organizations in the United States, and more than 17,000 of them have graduate degrees (Manderscheid & Henderson, 2001). However, these numbers are too few to meet the growing need for mental health care, and evidence suggests that psychiatric nurses will age out of the workforce faster than nonpsychiatric nurses (Hanrahan & Gerolamo, 2004; Hanrahan et al., 2003). Now more than ever, psychiatric nurses must face the question of whether they are vulnerable to becoming extinct and replaced by others, or whether they are viewed as valuable, competent clinicians who can function in a world of changing mental health care needs, processes, priorities, and structures. The following are many areas of vulnerability for psychiatric nursing:

- Fewer nurses are being attracted to the specialty of psychiatric nursing in spite of the growing need for mental health care.
- The amount of content devoted to understanding psychiatric illnesses and working with psychiatric patients in nursing educational programs has decreased steadily over the past decade and has been reduced significantly in the 2004 NCLEX-RN test plan.
- Many nursing faculty continue to stress the misguided notion that new graduates should practice in medical-surgical settings before going into psychiatric nursing, when current health care realities suggest that all new graduates should have experience in psychiatric settings to meet the growing mental health needs of medically ill patients and their families.
- The stigma surrounding psychiatric patients permeates to those who provide their care, including psychiatric nurses.

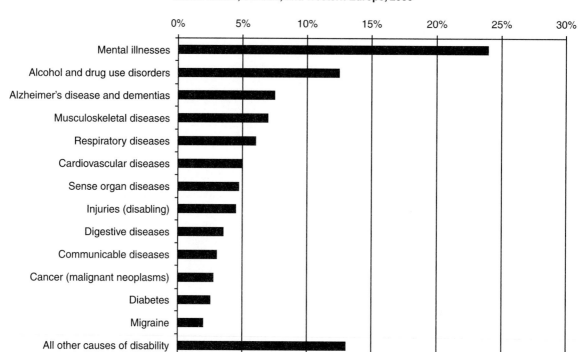

Figure 28-1 Causes of disability*
United States, Canada, and Western Europe, 2000

*Causes of disability for all ages combined. Measures of disability are based on the number of years of "healthy" live lost with less than full health (i.e., YLD: years lost due to disability) for each incidence of disease, illness, or condition. All data shown add up to 100%

FIGURE 28-1 Causes of disability in the United States, Canada, and Western Europe in 2000.

- The biopsychosocial skills and expertise of psychiatric nurses often are poorly delineated and underused in many mental health care systems.
- Psychiatric nurses frequently are viewed as expensive mental health care providers who can be replaced by two or more less costly personnel.
- Threats to nursing autonomy are increasing as State Boards of Nursing and other regulatory bodies delimit master's-prepared psychiatric nurses to practicing in the "extended" role requiring the full supervision of physicians.
- Relatively few outcome studies document the nature, extent, and effectiveness of care delivered by psychiatric nurses.
- Psychiatric nurses continue to experience difficulty receiving direct reimbursement from many third-party payers for the services they provide.

- Role differentiation for psychiatric nurses based on education and experience often is lacking in the position descriptions, job responsibilities, and reward systems of the organizations in which they practice.
- The specialty is struggling with the education and certification of advanced practice psychiatric–mental health nurses in clinical nurse specialist, nurse practitioner, and combined roles. Graduate programs in psychiatric nursing have moved away from the preparation of clinical nurse specialists and toward that of nurse practitioners, often with inadequate didactic and clinical work related to the diagnosis and nonmedication treatment of psychiatric illnesses.
- Advanced practice registered nurses–psychiatric mental health are underused in managed care and primary care delivery systems.

◆ Psychiatric nursing faculty often teach from traditional schools of thought rather than teaching on evidence-based treatments.

These are critical issues for the specialty. Psychiatric nurses need to continue to move into the continuum of care and clearly articulate their skills, functions, and abilities. They also must demonstrate their cost-effectiveness and establish differentiated levels of practice based on education, experience, and credentials (Feldman, Bachman, Cuffel, Friesen, & McCabe, 2003; Reiss-Brennan, Stuart, & Trotter Betts, 2003; Stuart, Worley, Morris, & Bevilacqua, 2000; Wheeler & Haber, 2004). Other survival skills needed by psychiatric nurses include management of negative emotionality, achievement of collegial unity, understanding the nature of transitions, revising career trajectories, and marketing themselves (Thomas, 1999). Such strategies will position psychiatric nurses as visible, interdependent, central, and collaborating professionals who have much to offer a reformed health care system.

Recent changes and current issues are occurring in five discrete areas of psychiatric nursing practice: (1) role, (2) activities, (3) models of care, (4) treatment settings, and (5) evidence-based practice. Each of these areas is explored based on historical perspectives, recent developments, and future challenges in the field.

ROLE

Psychiatric nurses remember the 1950s and 1960s fondly because they mark the emergence of the identity of the specialty. It was an exciting and stimulating time, and the early psychiatric nursing leaders who contributed to this identity formation—Gregg (1954), Mellow (1968), Peplau (1952, 1962, 1978), and Tudor (1952)—will forever remain larger than life for their early contributions to the emerging specialty area. The challenges they faced were to identify and describe the roles and functions for psychiatric nursing specialty practice and to disseminate them widely within the broader community of nurses.

The challenges for psychiatric nurses in the 1970s and 1980s were somewhat different. During these years, nurses worked to define the nature and focus of nursing as a practice discipline and examined aspects of the art and science of nursing. Psychiatric nurses worked parallel to the overall nursing profession and moved psychiatric nursing into the mainstream of nursing practice by helping elaborate psychosocial concepts,

thus further defining the caring and holistic dimensions of professional nursing practice.

Psychiatric nurses in the 1990s faced a new challenge—that of integrating the rapidly expanding bases of psychobiology, the neurosciences, psychopharmacology, and psychotherapy into the holistic biopsychosocial practice of psychiatric nursing (Abraham, Fox, & Cohen, 1992; Babich & Tolbert, 1992; Hays, 1995; McEnany, 1991; Pothier, Stuart, Puskar, & Babich, 1990). Advances in understanding the interrelationships of biology, brain, behavior, emotion, and cognition offered new opportunities for psychiatric nurses. In addition, the taxonomy used to categorize and diagnose mental illnesses was becoming increasingly precise and more interdisciplinary. A final issue to emerge was the importance of sociocultural factors in psychiatric care. Psychiatric nurses saw the need to become realigned with care and caring, which represent the art of psychiatric nursing and give balance to the science and high technology of current mental health care practices (McBride, 1996).

The task for psychiatric nurses today and in the years ahead is to evolve beyond the formative work in the field and enact psychiatric nursing roles and functions based on current realities. For example, the nurse-patient relationship as first described by Peplau (1952) has grown in complexity from its original historical elements. That relationship needs to be reconceptualized in a health care environment in which there is greater consumer responsibility and a broader context of clinician accountability. The concept of the nurse-patient relationship thus has evolved into that of the nurse-patient partnership that incorporates new dimensions of the professional psychiatric nursing role (Figure 28-2).

Enacting the nurse-patient partnership requires expanding the traditional roles of the nurse to include the elements of clinical competence, patient-family advocacy, fiscal responsibility, interdisciplinary collaboration, social accountability, and legal-ethical obligations (Stuart, 2005b). No longer can psychiatric nurses focus exclusively on bedside care and the immediacy of patient needs. Rather, they must broaden the context of their care and the responsibility and understanding they bring to the caregiving situation. Thus the current practice of psychiatric nursing requires greater sensitivity to the social environment and active advocacy for the diverse needs of patients and families of the mentally ill. Current practice also mandates thoughtful consideration of complex legal and ethical dilemmas that arise from a health care system that is embracing the efficiencies of managed care, which often disadvantages and discriminates against those with psychiatric illness. New models of delivering mental health care require greater skill in interdisciplinary collaboration built on the psychiatric nurse's clinical competence and professional self-assertion and balanced by a clear understanding and respect for the cost indexes and financial aspects of psychiatric care in general and psychiatric nursing care in particular. Each of these elements must permeate to a greater degree the education, research, and clinical components of the current state of psychiatric nursing.

ACTIVITIES

The three domains of contemporary psychiatric nursing practice are direct care, communication, and management activities. Within these overlapping domains, the teaching, coordinating, delegating, and collaborating functions of the psychiatric nursing role are expressed. Often the communication and management domains of practice are overlooked, minimized, or discounted in discussions of psychiatric nursing. However, these integrating activities are critically important and time-consuming aspects of the psychiatric nurse's role. These aspects are also valuable in a reformed health care system that places great emphasis on efficient patient assessment, triage, and management. Thus they are critical aspects of contemporary psychiatric nursing practice.

Psychiatric nurses must be able to delineate further the various activities they engage in within each of these domains. Box 28-1 lists the range of specific activities that can be enacted by a psychiatric nurse in each area

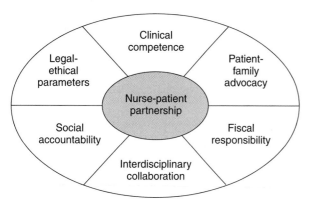

FIGURE 28-2   Nurse-patient partnership.

BOX 28-1

Psychiatric Nursing Activities

DIRECT CARE ACTIVITIES
Activity therapy
Advocacy
Aftercare follow-up
Behavioral treatments
Case consultation
Case management
Cognitive treatments
Community assessment
Community-based care
Community education
Complementary interventions
Compliance counseling
Counseling
Crisis intervention
Discharge planning
Environmental change
Environmental safety
Family interventions
Group work
Health maintenance
Health promotion

Health teaching
High-risk assessment
Holistic interventions
Home health care
Individual counseling
Informed consent acquisition
Intake screening and evaluation
Interpreting diagnostic and laboratory tests
Medication administration
Medication management
Mental health promotion
Mental illness prevention
Milieu therapy
Nutritional counseling
Ordering diagnostic and laboratory tests
Parent education
Patient triage
Physical assessment
Physiological treatments
Play therapy
Prescription of medications
Promotion of self-care activities

(Stuart, 2005b). Although not all psychiatric nurses participate in all of these activities, these activities do reflect the current nature and scope of competent caring by psychiatric nurses. In addition, psychiatric nurses do the following:

◆ Make biopsychosocial health assessments that are culturally sensitive.

◆ Design and implement treatment plans for patients and families with complex health problems and comorbid medical conditions.

◆ Engage in case management activities, such as organizing, accessing, negotiating, coordinating, and integrating services and benefits for individuals and families.

◆ Provide a "health care map" for individuals, families, and groups to guide them to community resources for mental health, including the most appropriate providers, agencies, technologies, and social systems.

◆ Promote and maintain mental health and manage the effects of mental illness through teaching and counseling.

◆ Provide care for the physically ill with psychological problems and the psychiatrically ill with physical problems.

◆ Manage and coordinate systems of care integrating the needs of patients, families, staff, and regulators.

Finally, psychiatric nurses must be able to articulate the general and the specific aspects of their practice to patients, families, other professionals, administrators, and legislators. When such skills and competencies are identified, psychiatric nurses will be able to ensure their

BOX 28-1

Psychiatric Nursing Activities—cont'd

DIRECT CARE ACTIVITIES—cont'd
Provision of environmental safety
Psychiatric rehabilitation
Psychobiological interventions
Psychoeducation
Psychosocial assessment
Psychotherapy
Rehabilitation counseling
Relapse prevention
Research implementation
Social action
Social skills training
Somatic treatments
Stress management
Support of social systems
Telehealth

COMMUNICATION ACTIVITIES
Clinical case conferences
Development of treatment plans
Documentation of care
Forensic testimony
Interagency liaison
Peer review
Professional nurse networking
Report preparation
Staff meetings
Transcription of orders
Treatment team meetings
Verbal reports of care

MANAGEMENT ACTIVITIES
Budgeting and resource allocation
Clinical supervision

Collaboration
Committee participation
Community action
Consultation/liaison
Contract negotiation
Coordination of services
Delegation of assignments
Grant writing
Marketing and public relations
Mediation and conflict resolution
Mentorship
Needs assessment and forecasting
Organizational governance
Outcomes management
Performance evaluations
Policy and procedure development
Practice guidelines formulation
Professional presentations
Program evaluation
Program planning
Publications
Quality improvement activities
Recruitment and retention activities
Regulatory agency activities
Risk management
Software development
Staff and student education
Staff scheduling
Strategic planning
Unit governance
Utilization review

From Stuart, G., & Laraia, M. (2005). *Principles and practice of psychiatric nursing* (8th ed.). St. Louis, MO: Mosby.

appropriate role use, adequate compensation for the nursing care provided, and the most efficient use of scarce human resources in the delivery of quality mental health care. Health care reform, patient and family needs, scientific developments, economic realities, and societal expectations are the forces that will shape the future roles and activities of psychiatric nurses.

MODEL OF CARE

As a result of rising health care costs, changing reimbursement trends, and problems with accessibility of care, there has been a reformulation of the model of care for psychiatric illness in this country. Fifteen years ago, most psychiatric care was provided in hospital units, where the average length of stay for acute inpatient treatment was about 25 days, compared with 19 days in 1991, 10 days in 1995, and 7 days in 2000. Not surprisingly, most psychiatric nurses were employed by inpatient facilities. Now, however, most inpatient psychiatric settings have an average length of stay of 5 days, and inpatient crisis stabilization programs often involve only a 2- or 3-day length of stay. These changes stimulated reciprocal changes in the goals, assessments, interventions, and expected outcomes of psychiatric care. Mental health providers, including psychiatric nurses, need to reevaluate the models of care they use based on the patient's treatment stage, setting, and resources.

One current psychiatric nursing model of care identifies four treatment stages: (1) crisis, (2) acute, (3) maintenance, and (4) health promotion (Stuart, 2005c). These stages reflect the range of the adaptive-maladaptive continuum of coping responses and suggest a distinct set of psychiatric nursing activities. For each stage, the psychiatric nurse identifies the treatment goal, focus of the nursing assessment, nature of the nursing interventions, and expected outcome of nursing care (Figure 28-3).

In the *crisis stage of treatment* the nursing goal is the stabilization of the patient; the nursing assessment focuses on risk factors that threaten the patient's health and well-being; the nursing intervention is directed toward managing the environment to provide safety; and the expected outcome of nursing care is that no harm will come to the patient or others.

In the *acute stage of treatment* the nursing goal is for the patient's illness to be placed in remission; the nursing assessment is focused on the patient's symptoms and maladaptive coping responses; the nursing intervention is directed toward treatment planning with the

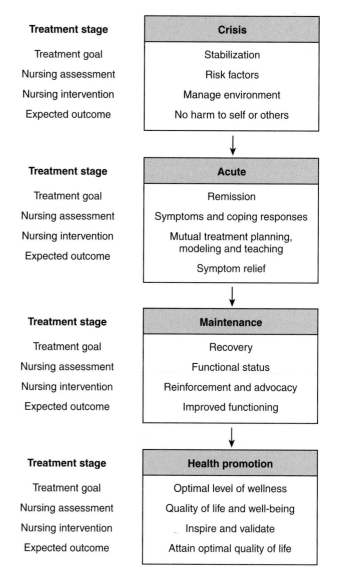

FIGURE 28-3   Stages of psychiatric treatment.

patient and the modeling and teaching of adaptive responses; and the expected outcome of nursing care is symptom relief.

In the *maintenance stage of treatment* the nursing goal is the complete recovery of the patient; the nursing assessment is focused on the patient's functional status; the nursing intervention is directed toward reinforcing the patient's adaptive coping responses and patient advocacy; and the expected outcome of nursing care is improved patient functioning.

In the *health promotion stage of treatment* the nursing goal is for the patient to achieve the optimal level of wellness; the nursing assessment is focused on the patient's quality of life and well-being; the nursing intervention is directed toward inspiring and validating the patient; and the expected outcome of nursing care is that the patient will attain the optimal quality of life.

The maintenance and health promotion treatment stages often have been overlooked by psychiatric nurses because the activities associated with these stages of treatment traditionally have not been valued and reimbursement for providing care in these areas has been limited. With health care reform and the emergence of managed mental health care, however, activities related to these stages are becoming more important aspects of the contemporary psychiatric nursing role.

This model of care also helps to determine how the psychiatric nurse functions in each setting. For example, in previous years most psychiatrically ill patients entered the psychiatric hospital in the acute treatment stage and were able to stay in the hospital until the goal of symptom remission was attained. This created the need for comprehensive treatment plans with long-term interventions for recovery. Today, however, most patients are admitted to inpatient units in the crisis treatment stage and have stabilization as their treatment goal, thus mandating different nursing interventions and expected outcomes. The psychiatric care goals of symptom remission and recovery now most often are pursued in community-based settings, requiring new skills and competencies of psychiatric nurses.

However, one might question whether psychiatric nurses actually have changed their expectations and treatment plans based on the changing nature of inpatient care. It has been suggested that psychiatric nurses have not fully "owned" inpatient care (Delaney, 2002; Mohr & Pumariega, 2004) and that difficulty recruiting and retaining psychiatric nurses in inpatient settings may be directly attributable to a mismatch between traditional nursing expectations and current caregiving and fiscal realities.

TREATMENT SETTINGS

Traditional practice settings for psychiatric nurses have included psychiatric hospitals, community mental health centers, psychiatric units in the general hospital, residential treatment facilities, and private practice. More recently, alternative treatment settings throughout the continuum of mental health care have emerged for psychiatric nurses. Specifically, hospitals are being transformed into integrated clinical systems that provide inpatient care, partial hospitalization or day treatment, residential care, home care, and outpatient or ambulatory care. Psychiatric nurses who continue to work within inpatient units have seen the goals, processes, and structures of care change drastically, reflective of the new models of psychiatric nursing care described earlier (Delaney, Ulsafer-Van Lanen, Pitula, & Johnson, 1995; Maree, 2005). Nurses who staff inpatient units no longer have their responsibilities limited to activities delivered exclusively in the hospital setting. Rather, they are likely to be flexibly assigned daily to other settings in the continuum of mental health care based on fluctuating patient census and organizational need.

The future of psychiatric care resides in the community. Community-based treatment settings have expanded to include foster care or group homes, hospices, visiting nurse associations, emergency departments, nursing homes, shelters, primary care clinics, schools, prisons, industrial settings, homes, managed care facilities, and health maintenance organizations. Psychiatric nurses are moving into the domain of primary care and are working with other nurses and physicians to diagnose and treat psychiatric illness in patients with somatic complaints. Cardiovascular, gynecological, respiratory, gastrointestinal, and family practice settings are appropriate for assessing patients for anxiety, depression, and substance abuse disorders. As health care initiatives continue to move into schools and other community settings, psychiatric nurses are assuming leadership roles in providing expertise through consultation and evaluation.

Psychiatric nurses are well suited to provide comprehensive health care to patients in psychiatric settings and primary care environments. In particular, advanced practice psychiatric nurses acting as consultants to non-psychiatric providers in hospital-based or outpatient clinics are in a unique position to assess and triage these patients based on the immediacy of their needs. Early assessment and triage can minimize the length of time between psychiatric referral and intervention. By identifying patients in crisis and intervening in a timely fashion, they may reduce failed appointments and enhance the efficacy of treatment. In fact, primary care settings may well be the "new frontier" of psychiatric nursing practice.

Psychiatric nurses also provide medical and medication management for selected groups of patients in collaborative practices. For example, patients who are having difficulty being stabilized on their medications or who have comorbid medical illnesses are seen in a psychiatric nursing clinic in which nurses and physicians collaborate to provide high-quality patient care.

Psychiatric nurses who obtain prescriptive authority can expand further the services they provide and deliver cost-effective psychiatric care to communities that do not have access to a psychiatrist.

This widened range of settings maximizes the psychiatric nurse's potential contribution to the delivery of mental health care. The specific role the nurse assumes in any one of these psychiatric treatment settings, however, depends on a number of factors, including the following:

◆ Legal parameters of practice as defined by the Nurse Practice Act in one's state
◆ Clinical competence of the nurse as a consequence of education, experience, and certification in psychiatric nursing
◆ Philosophy, mission, values, goals, and organizational structure of the treatment setting
◆ Needs of the consumers of mental health services
◆ Number of available staff and the services they are able to provide
◆ Consensus reached by the mental health care providers who work together regarding their respective roles, responsibilities, and accountabilities
◆ Resources and revenues available to offset the cost of care needed and provided

The new opportunities for psychiatric nursing practice that are emerging throughout the continuum of mental health care are exciting for the specialty. They allow psychiatric nurses to demonstrate their flexibility, accountability, and self-direction as they move forward into these expanding areas of practice. They also require that psychiatric nurses be proactive in articulating their skills and activities and demonstrate their expertise in designing interventions, planning programs, implementing treatment strategies, managing staff, and collaborating with other health care providers in a variety of traditional and nontraditional treatment settings. Perhaps most important, the expansion of mental health treatment settings is providing psychiatric nurses with the opportunity to implement primary, secondary, and tertiary prevention functions from a holistic, biopsychosocial perspective, thus expanding their base of practice to better meet the mental health needs of individuals, families, groups, and communities.

EVIDENCE-BASED PRACTICE

A final aspect of current psychiatric nursing is the emphasis being placed on evidence-based practice. This includes the identification, description, measurement, and use of data pertaining to the efficacy and effectiveness of the care provided by psychiatric nurses (Newell & Gournay, 2000; Rosswurm & Larrabee, 1999; Stetler et al., 1998). This is the greatest area of challenge for the specialty that has found it difficult to articulate the nature and outcomes of psychiatric nursing care (Barrell, Merwin, & Poster, 1997; Benson & Briscoe, 2003; Jackson & Stevenson, 2000; Merwin & Mauck, 1995; Poster, Dee, & Randell, 1997). This has created problems in justifying the need for psychiatric nurses in various treatment settings and in giving psychiatric nurses the recognition and compensation they deserve based on their actual and potential contributions to the mental health delivery system.

Evidence-based care and clinical effectiveness emphasize the importance of clinical practice, which, when delivered to patients, is effective in achieving expected health outcomes. For example, although more than 110 of the interventions described in the Nursing Intervention Classification codes relate to "psychosocial" care, few of them are supported by a strong research base (Dochterman & Bulecheck, 2004). Psychiatric nurses must be sensitive to the issues of cost and quality and must support their practice with data from outcome studies that reflect clinical, functional, satisfaction, and financial indicators. This is the essence of evidence-based psychiatric nursing practice. The use of measurement or rating scales must be viewed as an essential part of psychiatric nursing practice, and nurses would benefit greatly from mastering the technology that supports this process. Nurses need to research the impact of their activities and control the data set related to nursing outcomes. Finally, nurses need to know how to access, interpret, and use findings from efficacy and effectiveness outcome research (Stuart, 1999).

Outcome data for psychiatric nurses can include health status, functional status, quality of life, the presence or absence of illness, type of coping responses, and satisfaction with treatment. Outcome evaluation can focus on a psychiatric clinical condition, a nursing intervention, or the caregiving process (Coughlin, 2001). The outcomes that need continued examination by psychiatric nurses fall into four categories:

◆ Clinical outcomes: the patient's treatment response
◆ Functional outcomes: the maintenance or improvement in the patient's biopsychosocial functioning
◆ Perceptual outcomes: the patient's and family's satisfaction with the response to treatment, caregiving process, and health care providers
◆ Financial outcomes: costs and resources used to achieve the treatment response

Box 28-2 presents specific indicators related to each of these categories (Stuart, 2005a).

Outcome data documenting the quality, cost, and effectiveness of psychiatric nursing practice are perhaps the most important issue on the psychiatric nursing agenda. More work is needed in this area, and studies must be able to stand up to the scientific review of the broader community of mental health professionals, regulators, and payors by being methodologically sound, empirically grounded, and replicated across the continuum of psychiatric treatment settings (National Advisory Mental Health Council, Clinical Treatment and Services Research Workgroup, 1999). The results of this work then can be used to provide a shared knowledge base, formulate practice guidelines, provide data on clinical course, and better manage mental health care and the way in which it is delivered in this country.

Finally, the need to implement evidence-based practice and critically to evaluate the outcomes of psychiatric nursing care is a task for each psychiatric nurse regardless of role, activity, model of care, or treatment setting. Psychiatric nurse clinicians, educators, administrators, and researchers must assume responsibility for answering the question that is likely to determine the future of psychiatric nursing. What difference does psychiatric nurse caring make? Only a clear and credible answer to this question will position psychiatric nurses as central, visible, competent, interdependent, and collaborating professionals who have much to offer a reformed health care system.

BOX 28-2

Categories of Outcome Indicators

CLINICAL OUTCOME INDICATORS
Coping responses
High-risk behaviors
Incidence reports
Medical complications
Mortality
Number of treatment episodes
Readmission
Recurrence
Relapse
Symptomatology

FUNCTIONAL OUTCOME INDICATORS
Activities of daily living
Family relationships
Functional status
Housing arrangement
Occupational abilities
Quality of life
Social interaction

SATISFACTION OUTCOME INDICATORS
Patient and family satisfaction with the following:
   Caregiving process
   Delivery system
   Organization
   Outcomes
   Providers

FINANCIAL OUTCOME INDICATORS
Cost per treatment episode
Costs related to disability
Length of inpatient stay
Revenue per treatment episode
Use of health care resources

From Stuart, G., & Laraia, M. (2005). *Principles and practice of psychiatric nursing* (8th ed.). St. Louis, MO: Mosby.

REFERENCES

Abraham, I., Fox, J., & Cohen, B. (1992). Integrating the bio into the biopsychosocial: Understanding and treating biological phenomena in psychiatric-mental health nursing. *Archives of Psychiatric Nursing, 6,* 296.

Babich, K., & Tolbert, R. (1992). What is biological psychiatry? How will the trend toward biological psychiatry affect the future of the psychiatric mental health nurse? *Journal of Psychosocial Nursing and Mental Health Services, 30,* 33.

Barrell, L., Merwin, E., & Poster, E. (1997). Patient outcomes used by advanced practice psychiatric nurses to evaluate effectiveness of practice. *Archives of Psychiatric Nursing, 11*(4), 184-197.

Benson, W., & Briscoe L. (2003). Jumping the hurdles of mental health care wearing cement shoes: Where does the inpatient psychiatric nurse fit in? *Journal of the American Psychiatric Nurses Association, 9,* 123.

Coughlin, K. M. (Ed.). (2001). *2000 Behavioral outcomes & guidelines sourcebook.* New York: Faulkner & Gray.

Delaney, K. (2002). Inpatient psychiatric nursing: Set up to stagnate? *Journal of the American Psychiatric Nurses Association, 7,* 39.

Delaney, K., Ulsafer-Van Lanen, J., Pitula, C. R., & Johnson, M. E. (1995). Seven days and counting: How inpatient nurses might adjust their practice to brief hospitalization. *Journal of Psychosocial Nursing, 33*(8), 36-40.

Dochterman, J., & Bulechek, G. (2004). *Nursing Interventions Classifications (NIC)* (4th ed.). St. Louis, MO: Mosby.

Feldman, S., Bachman, J., Cuffel, B., Friesen, B., & McCabe, J. (2003). Advanced practice psychiatric nurses as a treatment resource: survey and analysis. *Administration and Policy in Mental Health, 30,* 479.

Gregg, D. (1954). The psychiatric nurse's role. *American Journal of Nursing, 54,* 210-212.

Hanrahan, N., & Gerolamo, A. (2004). Profiling the hospital-based psychiatric registered nurse workforce. *Journal of the American Psychiatric Nurses Association, 10,* 282.

Hanrahan, N., Stuart, G., Brown, P., Johnson, M., Drucker, C., & Delaney, K. (2003). The psychiatric nursing workforce: Large numbers, little data. *Journal of the American Psychiatric Nurses Association, 9,* 1.

Hayes, A. (1995). Psychiatric nursing: What does biology have to do with it? *Archives of Psychiatric Nursing, 9*(4), 216-224.

Jackson, S., & Stevenson C. (2000). What do people need psychiatric and mental health nurses for? *Journal of Advanced Nursing, 31,* 378.

Manderscheid, R., & Henderson, M. (Eds.). (2001). *Mental health United States, 2000.* Washington, DC: Department of Health and Human Services, Center for Mental Health Services.

Maree, E. (2005). Hospital based psychiatric nursing care. In G. Stuart & M. Laraia (Eds.), *Principles and practice of psychiatric nursing* (8th ed.). St. Louis, MO: Mosby.

McBride, A. (1996). Psychiatric-mental health nursing in the twenty-first century. In A. McBride & J. Austin (Eds.), *Psychiatric-mental health nursing: Integrating the behavioral and biological sciences.* Philadelphia: Saunders.

McEnany, G. (1991). Psychobiology and psychiatric nursing: A philosophical matrix. *Archives of Psychiatric Nursing, 5,* 255.

Mellow, J. (1968). Nursing therapy. *American Journal of Nursing, 68,* 2365.

Merwin, E., & Mauck, A. (1995). Psychiatric nursing outcome research: The state of the science. *Archives of Psychiatric Nursing, 9*(6), 311-331.

Mohr, W., & Pumariega, A. (2004). Level systems: Inpatient programming whose time has passed. *Journal of Child and Adolescent Psychiatric Nursing, 17,* 113.

National Advisory Mental Health Council, Clinical Treatment and Services Research Workgroup. (1999). *Bridging science and service.* Rockville, MD: National Institutes of Health, National Institute of Mental Health.

Newell, R., & Gournay, K. (2000). *Mental health nursing: An evidence-based approach.* London: Churchill Livingstone.

Peplau, H. (1952). *Interpersonal relations in nursing.* New York: GP Putnam's Sons.

Peplau, H. (1962). Interpersonal techniques: The crux of psychiatric nursing. *American Journal of Nursing, 63,* 53.

Peplau, H. (1978). Psychiatric nursing: Role of nurses and psychiatric nurses. *International Nursing Review, 25,* 41.

Poster, E., Dee, V., & Randell, B. (1997). The Johnson behavioral systems model as a framework for patient outcome evaluation. *Journal of the American Psychiatric Nurses Association, 3*(3), 73-80.

Pothier, P., Stuart, G., Puskar, K., & Babich, K. (1990). Dilemmas and directions for psychiatric nursing in the 1990s. *Archives of Psychiatric Nursing, 4,* 284.

Reiss-Brennan, B., Stuart, G., & Trotter Betts, V. (2003). Commentary from the field. *Administration and Policy in Mental Health, 30,* 492.

Rosswurm, M., & Larrabee, J. (1999). A model for change to evidence-based practice. *Image: The Journal of Nursing Scholarship, 31*(4), 317-322.

Stetler, C., Brunell, M., Giuliano, K., Morsi, D., Prince, L., & Newell-Stokes, V. (1998). Evidence-based practice and the role of nursing leadership. *Journal of Nursing Administration, 28*(7/8), 45-53.

Stuart, G. (1999). Mental health services research. In C. Shea, L. Pelletier, E. Poster, G. Stuart, & M. Verhey (Eds.), *Advanced practice nursing in psychiatric and mental health care.* St. Louis, MO: Mosby.

Stuart, G. (2005a). Evidence-based psychiatric nursing practice. In G. Stuart & M. Laraia (Eds.), *Principles and practice of psychiatric nursing* (8th ed.). St. Louis, MO: Mosby.

Stuart, G. (2005b). Roles and functions of psychiatric nurses: Competent caring. In G. Stuart & M. Laraia (Eds.), *Principles and practice of psychiatric nursing* (8th ed.). St. Louis, MO: Mosby.

Stuart, G. (2005c). A stress adaptation model of psychiatric nursing care. In G. Stuart & M. Laraia (Eds.), *Principles and practice of psychiatric nursing* (8th ed.). St. Louis, MO: Mosby.

Stuart, G., Worley, N., Morris, J., & Bevilacqua, J. (2000). Role utilization of nurses in public psychiatry. *Administration and Policy in Mental Health, 27*(6), 423-441.

Thomas, S. (1999). Surrounded by banana peels: Is psychiatric nursing slipping? *Journal of the American Psychiatric Nurses Association, 5*(3), 88-96.

Tudor, G. (1952). Sociopsychiatric nursing approach to intervention in a problem of mutual withdrawal on a mental hospital ward. *Psychiatry, 15,* 193.

U.S. Department of Health and Human Services. (1999). *Mental health: A report of the surgeon general.* Rockville, MD: Substance Abuse and Mental Health Services Administration, Center for Mental Health Services, National Institutes of Health, National Institute of Mental Health.

Wheeler, K., & Haber, J. (2004). Development of psychiatric-mental health nurse practitioner competencies: Opportunities for the 21st century. *Journal of the American Psychiatric Nurses Association, 10,* 1291.

World Health Organization. (2001). *The World Health Report 2001: Mental health: New understanding, new hope.* Geneva, Switzerland: Author.

Forensic Nursing

Recent Changes and Current Issues

VIRGINIA A. LYNCH

INTRODUCTION TO FORENSIC NURSING

Health care around the world is provided through many diverse public and private mechanisms. However, the primary responsibilities of public health are carried out through laws, policies, and programs promulgated, implemented, and enforced by or for the state. In many cases, the department of health and human services or the ministry of health oversees national health care policy. Central to all programs of health care delivery and promotion (physical, psychological, and social well-being) is the concept of prevention, which involves three levels of care: primary prevention, secondary prevention, and tertiary care (World Health Organization, 1978). In a similar framework the forensic nursing model addresses the interfaces of body, mind, spirit, and now, the law.

FORENSIC NURSING SCIENCE

One of the most compelling dilemmas facing the health and justice systems today concerns the ability to keep pace with the rapid advances in medicine, scientific technology, and legislative issues pertaining to patient care. In a milieu of continuously changing scientific requirements, these advances affect traditional standards of care, explicitly where health care interfaces with the law. The process of change affects the practice of nurses, specifically those who specialize in caring for victims of violence, and the suspect in or perpetrator of criminal acts (Campbell & Lynch, 2006).

Crime and violence bring together the two most powerful systems that affect the lives of people throughout the world—*health care* and *justice*. The need for policies to address critical issues related to violence and its associated trauma is a multidisciplinary issue concerning physicians, nurses, attorneys, judges, sociologists, psychologists, social workers, forensic and political scientists, advocates and activists, and criminal justice practitioners. Effective management of forensic cases is an area previously lacking in sufficient policy and legislation to ensure protection of the patient's legal, civil, and human rights.

This chapter reviews the global evolution of forensic nursing, its relationship with the various specialties in the forensic sciences, and the current and future application of forensic nursing science. The chapter also provides an opportunity to explore innovative pathways that will influence the manner in which victims and perpetrators of criminal violence are processed through the health care and justice systems in the new millennium. As an emerging discipline, forensic nursing assumes a mutual responsibility with the forensic medical sciences and the criminal justice system in concern for the loss of life and function caused by human violence and liability-related issues. The concept of a nurse investigator represents one member of an alliance of health care providers, law enforcement officials, and forensic scientists in a holistic approach to the study and treatment of victims and perpetrators of physical, psychological, and sexual violence. Forensic nurses do not compete with, replace, or supplant other practitioners; rather, they fill voids by accomplishing selected forensic services concurrently with other health and justice professionals. This role provides a uniquely qualified clinician, blending biomedical knowledge with the basic principles of law and human behavior. The forensic nurse examiner provides the traditional nursing associate that has been historically absent in forensic medicine.

EMERGING DISCIPLINE

The genesis of a new specialty in nursing is emerging in response to criminal violence as we have moved inexorably into the twenty-first century. As a specialty practice, forensic nursing unites health care systems and the law in a joint concern for social justice. The American Academy of Forensic Sciences was the first formally to recognize the scientific role of the forensic nurse as an essential partner to other forensic specialists in the clinical investigation of trauma involving the living and the dead. In 1992 the International Association of Forensic Nurses was founded, providing a forum for nurses who practice their specialties within the arena of the law. The American Nurses Association Congress of Nursing Practice accorded forensic nursing a formal specialty status in 1995. The Standards and Scope of Forensic Nursing Practice were approved and published in 1997. Concurrently, the American Nurses Association recognized forensic nursing as one of the four dominant areas for nursing development in the twenty-first century (Marullo, 1997). This new perspective provides a vital link in policy with the criminal justice system in a shared responsibility in the legal and social dimensions of crime.

Forensic nursing is multidimential in definition, addressing issues related to health care and the law. In the clinical environs this role is defined as the "application of clinical and scientific knowledge to questions of law related to the civil and criminal investigation of trauma in the survivors of traumatic injury and patient treatment involving court-related issues" (Lynch, 1995). Forensic nursing is defined further as "the application of the nursing process to public or legal proceedings; the application of the forensic aspects of health care in the scientific investigation of trauma and/or death related issues involving abuse, violence, criminal activity, liability concerns and traumatic accidents" (Lynch, 1991).

As an emerging discipline, forensic nursing assumes a distinctive role in cases that require essential forensic knowledge and skills. Where inadequate numbers or lack of forensically skilled physicians presents a threat to public health and safety, the forensic nurse examiner represents a new approach to forensic health care. Forensic nurses also work with government leaders who formulate national health policy and apply their expertise to help provide a greater measure of effectiveness in forensic health services.

FORENSIC VS. FORENSICS

Contemporary forensic nursing has broadened its scope of practice to include the investigation of trauma in clinical and community-based institutions and legal agencies. Forensic nurses are embracing new employment opportunities in public and private facilities, establishing independent practice roles, and serving in national, state, and local government agencies in which the concept of a clinical investigator provides a new perspective in the investigation of *crimes against persons*. The nurse's clinical education and experiential background is a major

strength in forensic investigation that has provided important analytical and observational skills, allowing nurses to venture beyond the traditional role of the nurse. Vision, commitment, and endurance are strengths that have achieved new and challenging roles for forensic nurses and sustain their capacity for performance in this field. Collaboration and innovation are two significant qualifications of the forensic nurse to implement positive change in antiquated health care and justice systems. Prevention is a major goal of the forensic nurse that parallels the major purpose of traditional medicine and nursing. These qualities help to prevent needless human tragedy and to advance progress in this field of specialization.

With the support of the national and international bodies of nursing, forensic specialists in medicine and science, and the advent of this new nursing specialty, new roles and educational programs are being defined that until now have not existed. Inclusion of forensic nursing as an accepted discipline for membership in the American Academy of Forensic Sciences has provided a vital resource for education and experience unavailable in traditional health care practice. The academic application of forensic science to nursing practice has revealed a wider role in the clinical investigation of crime and in the legal process.

HISTORICAL PERSPECTIVE

Although nursing had not yet evolved as a discipline, midwives filled the caregiver role until the days of Florence Nightingale. Thus aspects of forensic nursing are noted before the French Revolution in the fourteenth century, where court testimony concerning sexual assault and proof of pregnancy was limited to the midwife practitioner (Camp, 1976). Yet the inclusion of nurses in contemporary clinical forensic practice has been met with some resistance. Furthermore, from the beginning of medical specializations, physicians have had their skilled nursing associates in every medical specialty with the exception one: forensic medicine. Currently, the forensic nurse examiner is providing that missing component of professionalism and efficacy for the forensic medical practitioner that has been afforded to medical clinicians.

For some unidentified reason, the preferred assistant to the forensic physician in clinical practice and forensic pathology has been the individual with a law enforcement background. Employment of individuals with medical or health care skills, education, and expertise, thus separating the medical investigation from the criminal investigation, now is recognized as making intuitive sense to ensure effective medical investigation. Separation of the components of investigation also individualizes the objectives and responsibilities of each respective discipline to the investigator with an appropriate knowledge base. Because trauma is the central issue in the prosecution of *crimes against persons,* one should consider that issues of trauma are not a component skill of law enforcement training or in the education of judicial law. Issues of trauma, however, are a central cognate in nursing education.

The forensic nurse investigator was recognized first in 1975 as a specialty within the forensic sciences as one who worked for forensic pathologists assessing the investigation of questioned death at the scene of crime. Since that time, forensic nursing has undergone a significant paradigm shift to include clinical forensic practice. The clinical investigation of trauma was brought to the attention of professional nursing in 1986, based on the role of the police surgeon of the United Kingdom, a role generally lacking throughout North America. However, forensic nursing has been recognized as a globally significant resource in forensic psychiatric practice and in the management of incarcerated patients throughout the past century.

Nurses practicing in this forensic role became the first to be referred to informally as *forensic nurses* because of the services they provided to a forensic patient population within a forensic facility. These nurses were taught the unique and necessary skills required to assess and manage the accused in custody and the offenders of social crimes as they worked with this patient population. No formal training yet existed; no formal specialty titled them as forensic nurse examiners. In the last 3 decades, numerous institutions of higher education have developed specific curricula for the forensic psychiatric nurse and correctional or custody nurse who practice within the judicial and correctional systems.

The forensic psychiatric nurse works with the accused before adjudication and provides, among other services, court-ordered mental health evaluations. This role is differentiated from the correctional/custody nurse when the patient is found guilty of a crime and is incarcerated in a jail or prison system. Both nurses must have specialized forensic education and training to be identified as a forensic specialist in nursing. The establishment of the International Association of Forensic Nurses has provided identified and approved specific titles based on specialized education and clinical skills that entitle one to be called a forensic nurse examiner.

The respected opinion of well-known forensic pathologists in the United States has indicated that it is preferable to teach investigative techniques to nurses rather than to teach medical concepts to police officers. To limit a law enforcement officer's perspective to the medical objectives when the officer has been "computerized" and objectified by training to function as a criminal investigator is considered difficult. Thus each discipline should remain separate in responsibility: the medical investigator provides the medical cause and manner of death, and the criminal investigator determines whether a crime was committed and, if so, who committed the crime. Too often, a conflict of interest may result where education and training are not specific to the objectives of the discipline. Considering that the clinical forensic nurse has evolved from the role of the clinical forensic medical practitioner, one should expect that this new forensic expert would be embraced as an extension of professional growth and development.

Traditionally, the title of the clinical forensic physician has been the police surgeon, district surgeon, district medical officer, or most contemporarily, the forensic medical examiner who has assumed the legal responsibilities required by the judicial system to provide the clinical investigation of trauma. This role differs from that of the forensic pathologists whose primary focus is the medical investigation of death. However, a shortage of forensically skilled physicians has long been recognized worldwide, often presenting a serious problem in the accurate evaluation of abuse and neglect, crime-related injury, and human rights violations.

Clinical forensic physicians are not generally on staff in the emergency department and must be notified to respond to the hospital to assess the patient, or the patient often is transferred to a forensic facility. If those who are the first to admit the patient for trauma assessment are lacking in forensic skills, the subtle indications of abuse in the patient may go unrecognized and unreported. Under these circumstances the forensic physician may not be notified to assess the injury. Studies indicate that the average victim of interpersonal violence is admitted and released 7 to 9 times before anyone in the clinical setting recognizes that the person is a victim of crime. Too often the patient is treated and released without adequate forensic evaluation and is released back into the care of the perpetrator of interpersonal violence who brought the patient to the hospital.

With a heightened awareness of victimology in clinical and community health care, crime-related trauma and collection of evidence has become a major concern in clinical nursing. The nurse is most frequently among the first to see the patient and to recognize injury and the nonverbal indicators of abuse. Thus clinical forensic nursing is recognized as an essential component of current health care delivery in many countries today. One can reasonably expect that clinical forensic nursing will become a requirement for emergency/trauma nurses within the next 5 to 10 years. Because no clinical forensic physician routinely exists within the United States health care system, and with the continual influx of medicolegal patients involving forensic case management, the assistance of the forensic nurse examiner helps relieve an unnecessary workload on the medical staff, provides a more timely patient response, and ensures the careful documentation of injury and collection and security of evidence that often is lost or destroyed by nonforensic personnel.

In many countries, the absence of a forensic physician who is resident in the emergency department has long been noted to delay forensic patient services and thus emergency medical treatment. Patients often are transferred to other clinical facilities for forensic intervention, delaying treatment and increasing the risk of losing highly fragile and perishable biological evidence. Delay and transfer not only increase hazards to evidence recovery but also are psychologically harmful to the emotionally traumatized patient.

In an article titled "Death by Red Tape" published in *Dawn,* a leading Pakistani news source cited cases of patients in Pakistan who were refused forensic services upon admission to the casualty department and were transferred to other locations where access to a medicolegal officer was available. This article further admonished the forensic system because of the loss of lives during long waits and transfer of patients. In most hospital facilities in many countries, when the medicolegal officer does respond, the officer does not provide emergency treatment but rather documents the forensic injury and evidence, leaving lifesaving intervention or trauma care to the staff physicians and surgeons. With a forensic nurse examiner on staff, this unnecessary loss of dignity, emotional trauma, and death could be avoided. As these needs are identified and filled by nurses, the formal recognition of forensic nurse examiner has been recognized as a direct response of the health care profession to violence.

VIOLENCE AND PUBLIC HEALTH

Social violence presents a constant threat to public health and safety. Violence is defined as stimuli that evoke a nonaccidental act involving intrapersonal or interpersonal actions resulting in physical or psychological injury to one or more individuals (Stanhope & Lancaster, 1996). A pernicious epidemic of human violence indicates that crime-related trauma is the major health care issue most frequently associated with violence and the law. Trauma ranks higher than heart disease or cancer for reasons of hospital admissions. The need for standardized protocol and clinical specialists specifically responsible for the care and treatment of crime-related injury and death is now essential. Internationally, a coordinated effort to ensure that these cases receive comprehensive medical attention, evidentiary examinations, emotional support, and referral information has been addressed through the evolution of a forensic specialist in nursing.

NURSING AND LAW ENFORCEMENT

Role development of the forensic specialist in nursing practice represents a multidisciplinary team of health care providers, law enforcement agencies, and forensic science operatives uniting in a common concern for the plight of victims of human violence and those accused of criminal acts. Forensic nursing represents a partnership between nurses and the legal agencies in the community. This involves nurses working together with police officers, the correctional and judicial system, and forensic psychiatric patients, who often are considered a component of evil in society. Unfortunately, this relationship often has been one of friction and distrust for both parties. Nurses historically have displayed fear, guilt, and lack of confidence in cooperating with police officers during the investigation of criminal violence. Nurses have cited several reasons for their reaction when police request medical records or ask specific questions regarding a patient:

♦ Lack of clear understanding of the law in the nurse-patient relationship and concerning the police
♦ Fear of incriminating the patient
♦ Fear of self-incrimination
♦ Fear of intimidation during cross-examination in court
♦ Lack of confidence in medicolegal documentation
♦ Concern for staff involvement in potential legal issues
♦ Lack of confidence where nurses must seek physician approval
♦ Perception by the patient of participating in perceived police abuses
♦ Lack of understanding the rules of reasonable search and seizure
♦ Fear of disciplinary actions for involving the hospital in legal issues

These reasons are generally not without justification. The nursing literature cites numerous instances in which a lack of interagency coordination and cooperation has led to serious conflict with the police. Reports by nursing staff also cite instances in which they were told not to get involved with police cases because it would involve the hospital or physician in addressing legal issues or require court appearances. This can be frustrating for the police during the investigation of a crime; lack of cooperation also may result in a miscarriage of justice for the patient.

In other circumstances, failure to cooperate with police may occur in countries where the police are seen as the arm of the government or a political body that practices summary executions and government-sanctioned torture. The nurse may feel that any information given to the police regarding the patient will be misused and that an innocent individual may be arrested without just cause. Through the implementation of forensic nursing specialists as an institutional liaison to law enforcement agencies, this problem is being resolved. Police investigators indicate that they find the availability of a forensic nurse to bridge the gap between clinical staff, patient and patient's families, and the medical records department has improved the flow of critical information and security of evidence and has eliminated unnecessary confrontations. Where the multidisciplinary team approach is applied, the motivated and skilled forensic nurse can be an invaluable resource for the criminal justice system and for the hospital and the patient.

However, once the police agencies and the courts become familiar with the benefits of clinical forensic nurses that specialize in sexual assault evaluations and death investigation, forensic nurses become accepted members of the alliance of clinical and criminal investigators. Police officers who work with forensic nurse investigators consider them to be invaluable to the forensic system. The following statement represents one example of a police officer's perspective for forensic nurse examiners:

Before entering a law enforcement profession, I worked 10 years in the medical profession. I spent a lot of time in the emergency trauma area and watched the interaction between law enforcement and the emergency department. I have worked 24 years in law enforcement and have many stories to tell about the law enforcement/emergency department relationship. Within any group of people, you have different views on civil liberties, crimes, and people in uniform. Compounding the issue is that hospitals get their advice from private attorneys who often have an anti-police attitude and discourage the hospitals from interaction

with police. "If they want the evidence, they can get a search warrant." "You are not obligated to answer any questions." These are common responses that I have heard over the years. The unfortunate side is that the patient has to go back into the community after he or she has received treatment and needs to go back into a safe environment.

The advent of the forensic nurse has opened the door to a new era in criminal justice. We now have someone at the hospital who knows the laws and understands their role in the community. It begins with having a designated person to serve as a liaison for the patrol officer: someone to talk with about a patient or their injuries; someone who can document injuries or collect critical sexual assault evidence. Just knowing how long semen may be detectable in the vaginal vault already exceeds the knowledge of a patrol officer. Special examination rooms with forensic nurse examiners help to decrease an unnecessary wait for the patient and the patrol officer in a victim-friendly environment, away from the emergency department or police department. From here a decision can be made about how to collect important evidence that may lead to the apprehension of a dangerous person or the exoneration of an innocent person.

The value of the forensic nurse extends outside the medical facility. Attorneys need someone who can read medical reports and tell them what is there. The strength or weakness of the medical evidence is also important. From here the diversity of expertise expands in many directions. Elder abuse, child abuse, mental health, questioned deaths—all need assistance from the forensic nurse. When a senior citizen has suspicious bedsores, a nurse from outside the care facility is the best qualified to determine whether this constitutes abuse and to work with local law enforcement to get the problem resolved.

In our community, a forensic nurse is active in death determinations, crime scene response, domestic violence cases, and training to law enforcement. Nursing is about service to others through medicine. Law enforcement is about service to others through protection. Forensic nursing is about service through building bridges between medicine and law enforcement for the long-term benefit of others within their community.

Officer Jim Pex
Coos County Police Department
Coos County, Oregon, USA
August 20, 2004

RESPONSIBILITIES OF THE CLINICIAN

Medicolegal and psychosocial interaction is a new and important role for nurses that requires a combination of knowledge where human behavior interfaces with the law. Because the current policies of advocacy programs mandate the inclusions of criminal justice and health care providers, it is especially timely to propose that the forensic nursing examiner be placed in the trauma treatment environs to serve as a valuable link in interagency cooperation, ensuring that human needs and medicolegal interests are served. Most emergency personnel and prehospital care providers ordinarily have only secondary interests in forensic matters. The responsibility of the trauma team is to provide lifesaving intervention that requires concentration on details unrelated to forensic evidence. Yet enlightened legal systems call for the recognition and reporting of crime-related trauma and the collection and security of evidence. Because the nurse is among the first to evaluate the patient, to document injury, or to recognize nonverbal indicators of abuse that require investigation, forensic nursing is essential to contemporary health care.

INVESTIGATION OF TRAUMA

The forensic nurse examiner serves a vital role in the investigation of crime-related trauma. Because of the increasing caseload of patients who present to the emergency department with medicolegal-related injuries, the need for a forensic clinician has been recognized. Fatal or near-fatal injuries resulting from intentional or unintentional acts involving criminality or civil actions constitute forensic cases. Although a forensic case can involve any patient admitted to the hospital with liability-related injuries, specific categories include sexual assault, domestic violence, abuse, neglect, motor vehicle and pedestrian trauma, attempted suicide, job-related injuries, malpractice, drug abuse or tampering, and environmental hazards (Lynch, 1995, p. 490). These cases necessitate attention to forensically significant evidence. In addition, there are growing concerns for sensitivity to the victims and their families.

ROLE AND RELEVANCE OF THE FORENSIC NURSE

Role specificity includes the following:

Clinical forensic nurse: Provides care for the survivors of crime-related injury and deaths that occur within the health care institution. This specialist has a duty to defend the patient's legal rights through the proper collection and documentation of evidence that represents access to social justice.

Forensic nurse investigator: Employed in a medical examiner or coroner's jurisdiction and represents the decedent's right to social justice through a scientific investigation of the scene and circumstances of death.

Forensic nurse examiner: Provides an incisive examination and evaluation of trauma related to forensic cases: any type of interpersonal violence such as child abuse, domestic violence, elder abuse, or injury resulting from lethal weapons, torture, or police brutality.

Forensic psychiatric nurse: Specializes in the care and treatment of criminal defendants and patients in legal custody who have been accused of a crime or have been ordered by the court to receive a psychiatric evaluation.

Legal nurse consultant: Provides consultation and education to judicial, criminal justice, and health care professionals in areas such as personal injury, product liability, and malpractice, among other legal issues related to health care. Each of these primary roles and other subspecializations of the forensic nurse is investigative and requires specific knowledge of the law and the skill of expert witness testimony.

NATURE AND IMPORTANCE OF THE PROBLEM

The emergency department nurse is often the first person in a position to note the types of trauma present when a patient arrives for treatment. Even if police officers are involved in the incident, uniformed officers are not trained in the legal aspects of trauma, nor are they usually in a position to observe wound characteristics accurately because of various obstacles such as contamination of the injury, clothing, and poor lighting. Although prompt and effective patient care is paramount in the treatment of victims of trauma, recognition of the forensic implications of injury is of the utmost importance.

The Joint Commission on Accreditation of Healthcare Organizations has emphasized guidelines for written policies and procedures that require appropriate staff to be trained in the identification of crime victims and procedures needed to work with abuse survivors. These standards include criteria to identify possible abuse victims of physical assault, rape, or sexual molestation of spouses, partners, and children. Specific guidelines regarding procedures for patient evaluation include patient consent, examination, and treatment. A mandate that unequivocally provides for the role of the forensic clinician is set forth in the hospital policy regarding responsibility in collection, retention, and safeguarding of specimens, photography, and other trace and physical evidence. Medical record documentation to include examinations, treatment referrals to other care providers and community-based family violence agencies, and required notification of authorities are among the responsibilities of the care provider. Yet the need to establish specific guidelines for the facilitation of adult and child victims of suspected abuse or neglect has brought about little change in the majority of hospitals nationwide.

Research indicates that these issues remain a significant problem in hospital emergency departments. Attention to the problem was accentuated when the Family Violence Prevention Fund in San Francisco and the San Francisco Injury Center for Research and Prevention (1992) conducted a study to evaluate the circumstances of cases of domestic violence against patients admitted to California emergency departments. This survey, the first of its kind in the nation, found that only 5% of adult victims of domestic violence were identified.

Reasons cited for the failure to meet Joint Commission on Accreditation of Healthcare Organizations standards for dealing with this category of crime victims were (1) time constraints, (2) lack of training, and (3) reluctance by the medical worker and the victim to talk about domestic violence. This landmark 1992 survey of the 397 emergency departments revealed that as few as 1 in 5 emergency departments are meeting the national hospital accreditation requirements on this issue. Only 59 of those emergency departments reporting had specific forensic policies, and only 8 were addressing identification, treatment, and intervention adequately. Although response rate indicated that health care professionals were enthusiastic about helping these victims, few had programs developed to do so. California was not alone in facing violence and its associated trauma. Where time constraints interfere with the ideal clinical intervention in such cases, having forensic specialists in nursing can ease the workload of the physician and better meet the needs of the victim of domestic violence, the criminal justice system, and other medicolegal agencies.

IDENTIFICATION OF WOUND CHARACTERISTICS

The investigation of trauma often begins with the evaluation of wound pattern characteristics. Detailed documentation of the appearance of the wound may be the identifying factor in determining the type of weapon used to inflict the injury. Wound characteristics constitute evidence that may be obscured by emergency trauma care. Therefore where the emergency department nurse may be the first to have the opportunity to observe traumatic injury closely, the nurse also may be the only person to observe such trauma in its original state.

Nurses who become involved in the investigation of traumatic injuries have a responsibility beyond the immediate treatment environment that includes issues related to the patient's right to know, the public right to know, and the administration of justice.

The nurse's documentation should include the location of the injury and approximate measurements of sharp, blunt, and fast force injuries, as well as uniquely patterned injuries such as bite marks. Diagrams, body maps, or photography are helpful in reconstructing injury patterns in subsequent investigations or at autopsy. For patients who survive or whose wound is excised or extended surgically, later reconstruction of the injury is not possible. The specific importance of reconstruction is magnified when the patient lives for an indefinite period of time and later dies as a result of the injury. Treatment procedures and the natural healing process alter the condition of the wound, thus eliminating the possibility of determining, for example, whether the wound was inflicted with a single- or double-edged knife or whether the gunshot wound was an entrance or exit wound.

Nurses should have an accurate knowledge of the types of injuries generally resulting in medicolegal cases and should be familiar with the appropriate terminology required to describe them. Failure to recognize and describe injuries has confounded the testimony of victim and perpetrator as a defense strategy in the courtroom. The nurse not only will be made to appear unprofessional, but a serious crime may go unpunished and could result in the release of a dangerous offender.

INVESTIGATION TECHNIQUE

Nurses are recognized as an invaluable resource to prosecutors who often have little or no knowledge of trauma. Yet the majority of cases prosecuted are crimes against persons, and they involve traumatic injury. Valuable notations such as recording of the names and addresses of witnesses, monitoring of the procedures or events before treatment, and safeguarding of clothing and other personal effects should be documented in the charting. Personal property may constitute forensic evidence and should never be released to the family without permission of the police. By implementing forensic protocol that emphasizes cooperation with the criminal justice sector, nurses are initiating a critical link in trauma systems that will provide for increased coordination and services.

Implementation of the role of clinical forensic nurse would provide a uniquely skilled and qualified forensic professional whose responsibilities would be (1) to develop the appropriate forensic protocols in compliance with accreditation standards; (2) to triage patients at risk for forensic injuries; (3) to report to proper legal agencies; (4) to document, collect, and preserve evidence; (5) to secure evidence and maintain the chain of custody; and (6) to serve as a liaison between the health care institution and law enforcement agencies and the medical examiner/coroner and to make referrals when medical treatment and/or crisis intervention is required.

The forensic nurse liaison could initiate significant constructive changes as one essential component of a network of medicine, nursing, law, and social services. The implementation of regular in-service programs on the forensic aspects of health care would be a primary responsibility of the forensic nurse specialist. This would serve to advise the medical and nursing staff and other first responders on the legal requirements of trauma care. Forensic standards also serve as a means to transmit developing knowledge in technical and social interventions. Those who are among the first to come in contact with victims of suspected abuse must understand the application of forensic policies to emergency medical services.

THE INVESTIGATION OF DEATH

Societal need to understand the disease mechanisms and biomechanical factors associated with death is essential to systems of public health and the administration of justice. The processes that help to determine precise precipitating factors and causes of death not only benefit medical science but also serve the general welfare by ensuring that accidental and crime-related fatalities are investigated systematically for cause, manner, and mechanism of death. Regardless of the circumstances of death, typically there are acute emotional reactions of significant others and inherent legal consequences. For example, the precise way individuals die and the events that surround the dying process can determine the execution of last wills and testaments, life insurance distributions, and rights of survivorship. Death cannot be viewed apart from the consideration of civil and criminal laws and social justice principles that govern human existence from a social, moral, and religious perspective (Campbell & Lynch, 2006).

NURSE CORONERS AND DEATH INVESTIGATORS

Sudden and unexpected deaths associated with crime-related trauma demand a legal investigation that remains

a complicating factor. When the shock of death is compounded by violence, the reaction of survivors is often a complex multidimensional scenario of shock, anguish, and despair. The interface with the next of kin is a delicate situation that requires a balance of empathy and objectivity.

Although forensic nursing is a new concept in clinical practice, it has been a respected practice in death investigation for the past 30 years. Forensic nursing, as a scientific discipline, originally defined its role as a medical examiner's investigator in the field of death investigation. To clarify the scope of forensic nursing practice, a direct application to clinical nursing and an interrelationship to the living and the deceased have been established (Lynch, 1993b).

John C. Butt (1993), chief medical examiner of Alberta, Canada, was the first to recognize that the registered nurse represented a valuable resource to the scientific investigation of death. As early as 1975, Butt established a program using registered nurses as death scene investigators, citing nurses' biomedical education and interpersonal communication skills as their most important qualifications. Butt further emphasized their knowledge of medical terminology, pharmacology, and familiarity of natural disease processes as an invaluable resource to the medical examiner. He also cited nurses' experience in public relations as a major priority: representing him at the scene, handling confidential material, and being comfortable relaying sensitive information to bereaved family members.

Because as much as 65% to 72% of the U.S. medical examiner's caseload is natural deaths requiring no high investigative profile involving law enforcement, the use of nurse investigators in these cases allows police officers to devote more time to criminal investigation (Lynch, 1993a). Butt stressed the importance of teamwork between criminal and biomedical investigative personnel. He expressed concern that medically untrained officers often disregarded medical evidence, maintained poor sensitivity, and were noncommunicative with grieving families. Conversely, by nature of their education in forensic health science, nurses recognize the importance of the integrity of criminal evidence, the suspect interview, and the investigation of leads. A nurse's skill in clinical documentation, strict guidelines regarding confidentiality, and sterile technique to prevent cross-contamination of specimens provides the foundation for a unique clinician in death investigation.

However, human consolation is not the primary objective of criminal investigation, and families often feel that police officers treat them in less than an empathic and compassionate manner in the immediate postdeath period. Whether the death occurs at the crime scene or in the emergency department, police often rely on the nurse to facilitate the notification of death with the next of kin.

Although every unexpected death has actual or potential medicolegal aspects, most unattended deaths are the result of a terminal illness or other natural causes. Where deaths often occur in isolation without the attendance of a physician or those skilled in emergency services, families may resent the dramatic intrusion of the police during the investigation process. Where forensic nurse investigators are part of the medical examiner and law enforcement team, the nurse provides a holistic approach to the scientific investigation of death. As trends in crime and violence change, new anti-violence legislation is being implemented; consequently, new personnel resources are required to ensure that these legislative mandates are meeting the needs of society effectively.

As the health and justice systems worldwide prepare for the challenges of this century, the trend of using forensic nurse investigators has moved across Canadian provinces and into the United States. Most recently, departments of legal medicine in South Africa and Singapore have appointed forensic nurses as death investigators. Forensic pathologists who employ nurse investigators stress the importance between criminal and biomedical investigative personnel. They express concern that medically untrained officers often disregard medical evidence, maintain poor sensitivity, and are noncommunicative with grieving families. Because the unexpected death is often responsible for arousing suspicion in the clinical and community environment in which there is a shortage of forensic pathologists or clinical forensic physicians, the forensically trained nurse provides a previously untapped resource to medicolegal agencies.

The forensic nurse death investigator has an advantage in providing investigative skills through their familiarity with natural disease processes and the subtle indications of trauma associated with abuse and neglect. Their ability to document correctly the patterned injuries, medications, and surgical interventions and to interpret medical records is of great benefit to the forensic pathologists and to the police officers.

Although individuals hired as death investigators traditionally have had extensive background in law enforcement, recent advances in forensic science indicate that investigators require stronger backgrounds in

pharmacology, anatomy and physiology, medical and nursing terminology, and legal issues. Medical examiners and coroners who endorse the employment of forensic nurse investigators find that the nurse who is cross-trained in criminalistics and legal issues provides a collaborative practice approach that is beneficial to forensic professionals A forensic specialist in nursing represents a revolutionary concept for using traditional nursing abilities in an area of human services not previously explored by nurses but which is making significant contributions to the area of death investigation and service to law enforcement and to the community.

The nurses' expertise in death investigation is recognized in enlightened communities where lay officiators of death have been outdated in today's concerned society. Nurses are being elected as coroners in communities that recognize the need to provide a more professional approach to the scientific investigation of death. In the United States, where the law does not require the coroner to be a physician, no longer is the unskilled, untrained, non-medically oriented (often politically driven) lay officiator of death preferred when the option is a qualified, licensed, credentialed, or certified forensic nurse educated in the biomedical sciences and experienced in the principles and philosophies of forensic medicine. Such a professional contributes to the overall quality of community life.

FORENSIC RESPONSIBILITIES

Forensic nurse death investigators provide community services to the bereaved families of those taken by sudden, catastrophic death through crisis intervention and grief counseling, often reviewing the autopsy report in the family's home to assist them in a caring and empathic setting. Experience with death and dying brings a unique understanding of the wide range of behavioral response by victims in crisis. When one considers the impact of unresolved grief on stress-related diseases, the care given in the immediate postdeath period is crucial.

A prototype position description representing one role of the forensic clinical nurse specialist has been defined. A number of individual roles—such as an elder abuse specialist, child abuse specialist, death investigator, or other separately identified role—would evolve from this basic list of role functions. As the health and justice systems prepare to move into the next century, forensic nursing provides a missing link between the forensic physician and the nursing assistant.

EXPECTATIONS

The preparation of the forensic clinical nurse specialists provides the knowledge base and clinical skills appropriate for the role of a coroner or medical examiner's investigator involved in the scientific investigation of questioned deaths. The forensic clinical nurse specialist is prepared to do the following:

1. Use principles and skills in communication, interviewing, and physical assessment for making appropriate nursing interventions with the decedent's family and with relevant persons in the community.
2. Synthesize and apply skills of physical assessment and knowledge of biomedical investigation to assess, plan, provide, and evaluate nursing interventions with and on behalf of the deceased, the family, and the community.
3. Participate effectively on the multidisciplinary medical examiner's team to plan and provide direct and supportive nursing care; to assess needs for and make referral to other health care services, and to counsel individuals and families throughout periods of stress.
4. Participate in investigations, under the direction of the medical examiner, to determine circumstances surrounding sudden death. This includes the following:
   ◆ Visiting the scene of death and working with the police
   ◆ Independently identifying and developing health details and collecting medical evidence related to the cause of death in criminal and noncriminal cases
   ◆ Interpreting the client's health history and circumstances before the death
   ◆ Researching health records and preparing case history summaries to facilitate death investigations
   ◆ Interviewing physicians and other health care providers to help establish cause and manner of death
   ◆ Providing direction in handling the body and personal effects of the deceased
   ◆ Arranging transportation of the body if necessary
   ◆ Conducting interviews with persons reporting deaths and with other persons as appropriate
5. Plan and implement forensic educational programs for nurses, other health care providers, and the community; for example, in child abuse, in child safety, grief counseling, and in health maintenance, promotion, and prevention programs for persons at risk for major health problems.
6. Assume accountability as a forensic nurse specialist by accepting responsibility as a nurse clinician, recognizing one's own abilities and limitations, and consistently seeking guidance, counseling, direction, and learning experiences that promote professional and personal development.
7. Demonstrate a leadership role in forensic nursing—including innovation, consultation, advocacy, accountability and responsibility—to improve services to the family, the community, and as appropriate, the criminal justice system in cases of sudden death.

Although every unexpected death has actual or potential medicolegal aspects, most unattended deaths are the result of a terminal illness or other natural causes. Where deaths often occur in isolation without the attendance of a physician or those skilled in emergency services, families may resent the dramatic intrusion of the police during the investigation process. Where forensic nurse investigators are part of the medical examiner and law enforcement team, the nurse provides a holistic approach to the scientific investigation of death.

ADVANCES IN FORENSIC AND NURSING SCIENCE

In combating increasingly sophisticated crime, new and improved identification procedures can help revolutionize the ability to bring to justice those who commit criminal violence, particularly the serial sexual offender and murderer. Clinical professional support for law enforcement is imperative in this quest to transmit developing knowledge through improved treatment and services that include forensic intervention.

BIOTECHNICAL ADVANCEMENT

With the advent of the twenty-first century, forensic science is on the threshold of an explosion of biotechnical advancement. This knowledge requires responsibilities of health care professionals previously unrecognized as forensic nursing and forensic health science. The forensically educated nurse will be a critical component in the recognition and proper collection of forensic evidence in complex criminal cases. With the emerging application of DNA profiling, virtually any genetic evidence—such as semen, blood, or tissue—may provide the crucial answer to the identification and apprehension (or elimination) of a perpetrator.

SEXUAL ASSAULT NURSE EXAMINER

Because of the universal lack of qualified forensic physicians skilled in the clinical evaluation of sexual assault patients in most areas of the world, the need for increased numbers of specialists to conduct the forensic examination within the strict guidelines of current standardized care has been identified. Many physicians also are lacking the ability to provide expert witness testimony and have insufficient interpersonal skills. Critical to recovery, psychological interventions contribute continuity of care from the crime scene to clinical facilities and courts of law.

The forensic nurse who specializes in the care and treatment of the sexual assault patients is known as a sexual assault nurse examiner. This specialist is a registered nurse who has received advanced education in the area of sexual assault evaluation. The sexual assault nurse examiner, as a forensic nurse examiner, provides an independent forensic examination that includes the identification of trauma, the collection of evidence, and testimony as an expert witness. Each team of sexual assault nurse examiners works under the director of clinical forensic medicine and maintains a collaborative relationship with the medical staff.

VICTIMOLOGY

Nursing involvement in public service activities covers a wide range of activities related to community education, program development, and defining of policies and protocol that affect and involve victims of violence and abuse. Nurses often have been the first to recognize the need for a rape crisis program in a rural areas where resources for victims were nonexistent. Education of law enforcement officials regarding the dynamics of sexual offenders and their victims, essential victim rights, and victim needs also currently is being better achieved. Sexual violence requires the support of an advocate who not only can provide emotional stabilization but also can serve as a liaison with police, judges, juries, and the victim's immediate family in a knowledgeable and professional manner.

The forensic nurse examiner generally works within the framework of a Sexual Assault Response Team (SART) that provides a multidisciplinary approach to the investigation and treatment of sexual assault cases. The team is comprised of members of the law enforcement agencies, advocates, and sexual assault nurse examiners. By using this approach, members are able to initiate a forensic interview, expedite the forensic examination, and provide the much needed information for community referrals, advocacy, and criminal justice services for the victims of sexual assault.

EDUCATION AND TRAINING

Advanced preparation is required for nurses who provide sexual assault evaluations. The International Association of Forensic Nurses, Council of Sexual Assault Nurse Examiners, has defined the Standard of Care and Educational Guidelines for nurses who provide these services for law enforcement agencies. Certification examination for the sexual assault nurse examiner previously has been sponsored by individual state agencies; however, in 2002 the first national certification credentialing examination was implemented through the International Association of Forensic Nurses for nurses in North America.

GENERAL GUIDELINES FOR THE FORENSIC NURSE

The forensic nurse should understand what constitutes human abuse and should be prepared to describe accurately specific acts in proper terms. Intimate partner abuse can be characterized by physical, sexual, and emotional abuse. Rarely do physical injuries occur without precedents of emotional abuse, neglect, and exploitation. Note that these definitions are broad and may be applied to children, women, the elderly, and other vulnerable subjects.

◆ Human abuse is the willful infliction of injury, unreasonable confinement, or cruel punishment of another individual. Acts that cause mental or emotional injuries or that negatively affect growth, development, or psychological functioning are also acts of human abuse.

◆ Neglect is the failure on the part of a caregiver to provide the goods or services that are necessary to avoid physical harm, mental anguish, or mental illness for someone under his or her care or to leave that person in a situation where he or she could be exposed to serious harm.

◆ Exploitation is the illegal or improper act or process of using the resources of an adult, child, elderly, dependent, or disabled person for monetary or personal benefit.

For nurses to become emotionally involved with patients who have been abused and to want to assume a protective role in their behalf is not uncommon. However, the nurse must guard against trying to rescue the victim while reassuring the person that there is help. As a concerned ally, the nurse should not judge or preach to the victim. Admonishment or patronizing behaviors are counterproductive. Remaining objective, providing appropriate nursing and safety interventions, and displaying a professional caring demeanor help to build trust between the nurse and the victim.

Primarily the nurse must be aware of the signs and symptoms of abuse. The nurse should take action and say something such as, "I see you have a lot of bruises. You can talk to me about how they happened." The nurse must listen carefully and express concern for the abused victim's safety and welfare. The nurse should explore whether children are in the household too, because they also may be victims. The nurse should provide telephone numbers of local resources (e.g., hotlines and shelters) even though the individual may be reluctant to take them. A discreet card that can be hidden in a wallet or a shoe is appropriate.

Nurses often feel that intimate violence between adults "is their own concern." The principles and philosophies of forensic nursing compel nurses to take an active role in domestic violence by careful interviews and assessments and by generating the required report forms. The philosophies of a caring nursing practice will guide the interaction and the relationship that is being established. No emergency/casualty department exists in any hospital in any country that does not come into contact with domestic violence victims. Many women seeking to escape from interpersonal violence turn to health care professionals for help. In the United States, victims of intimate partner violence visit their doctors 8 times more often than women who are not abused; yet only about 10% of these women are identified as abused ("Stalking 101," 2001). This statistic can be attributed to the health care professional's lack of information and education and the reluctance to ask the right questions. Health care workers often hesitate to get involved in intimate partner violence.

The Emergency Nurses Association and the Joint Commission on Accreditation of Healthcare Organizations have set forth recommendations for instituting protocols in facilities to manage victims of domestic violence. In the United States the Healthy People 2010 objectives include goals such as reducing the rate of physical assault by former or current intimate partners, reducing the annual rape or attempted rape rates, and reducing physical assaults. Forensic nursing can have a direct effect in achieving these goals. Detailed screenings,

interviews, referrals, and treatment of injuries may be tedious and time consuming, especially considering the intense workload in the emergency/casualty department. Some survivors of intimate violence have reported they felt twice victimized, once by the abuser and again by the health care workers who tend to treat the injuries and ignore the cause. Screening for intimate partner violence and providing help for victims through referral processes are ways to interrupt the cycle of violence, thus reducing further injury or even death for thousands of victims. Important concepts for the forensic nurse examiner when dealing with victims of intimate partner violence are confidentiality, safety, objectivity, caring, and the documentation of injury and collection of evidence.

COURT ROOM RESPONSIBILITIES

A nurse expert witness is defined as a nurse qualified by education, experience, occupation, present position, degrees held, publications, and professional organization membership that establish the credibility as an expert to give opinions as to whether the nursing care administered met the an acceptable standard of care. As nurse expert witnesses are increasingly used in courts (specifically in sexual assault and domestic violence cases, as medical examiner's investigators or nurse coroners), the expanded role of the nurse provides unique and vital services involving a distinct body of knowledge not found in the practice of any other profession. Establishing the appropriate standard for nurses who practice in advanced nursing roles and encompass court testimony is critical to protect the legal rights of victims and professional nurses. Educational requirements and courtroom standards currently are held admissible under the foregoing definition.

Individual state or provincial penal codes ultimately define the criteria for the court to qualify a witness as one who may state only facts or opinion based on reasonable certainty. Briefly put, forensic nursing links the nursing profession to the criminal justice system by providing forensic expertise where the victim or perpetrators most often have the first point of contact after a crime: a hospital. The forensic specialist in nursing is taught to maintain a high index of suspicion and is skilled in the identification of injuries consistent with weapons, interviewing of victims, collection and preservation of evidence, and service as a liaison with the police and the medical examiner. Later in the process, forensic nurses are recognized as effective expert witnesses. As trends in crime and violence change, new antiviolence legislation is being implemented; consequently, new personnel resources are required to ensure that these legislative mandates are meeting the needs of society effectively.

HUMAN RIGHTS

The application of nursing science to the process of human rights investigation now is recognized as one aspect of the legal and ethical responsibilities of the nurse. The forensic nursing specialist has a vital role in the identification of victims of human rights abuse and the investigation of violations of humanitarian law. Forensic nursing as a clinical subspecialty provides an important resource to clinical forensic medicine and the human rights community. As an emerging discipline, forensic nursing assumes a mutual responsibility with forensic scientists and the criminal justice system concerning the loss of human life and function because of the intimidation, domination, and control of political, religious, cultural, and interpersonal oppressors. The unique skill of nurses educated in forensic technique enhances investigative capabilities and forensic functions.

In addition to traditional professional nursing care, nurses specializing in the care and treatment of victims of pernicious human behavior offer the complex skills of assessment of covert and latent patterned injuries, recognition and collection of human bite mark evidence, photographic documentation, recovery and preservation of genetic evidence, and provision of crucial intervention in emotional trauma associated with human rights violations. A forensic specialist in nursing is ideally qualified to assist in initiatives designed to address forensic guidelines that provide accurate assessment and documentation and to address the educational needs of staff to ensure compliance with forensic details. These distinct responsibilities include the role of assessor, educator, and therapist often required when caring for individual, family, and community survivors of cruel and inhumane treatment. The forensic nurse also assists institutional staff members with critical incident stress debriefing.

Sexual assault is a violent act that results in serious physical and emotional sequelae that are inflicted continually upon victims of social and political torture. The forensic nurse as a sexual assault examiner provides the advanced physical assessment and stabilization of the victim's emotional state, collection of forensic evidence, and courtroom testimony in cases where no medical treatment is required. Many forensic nurses specializing in the scientific investigation of death assist forensic pathologists questioned death cases. Participation in

this area includes investigation at the crime scene, postmortem examinations in the autopsy laboratory, exhumations, and disaster site recovery. Other nurses practice their forensic skills in forensic mental health nursing, as hostage negotiators, and as nurse attorneys or legal nurse consultants.

The academic and professional development of the forensic clinical nurse specialist provides an incisive exploration of the principles and philosophies of the forensic sciences that include the following: the structure and function of institutions of legal medicine, forensic psychopathology, signs and legal aspects of death, certification of death, bioethics, victimology, traumatology, sexual and domestic violence, forensic pathology, organ/tissue recovery, medicolegal documentation, and rules of evidence. Forensic education prepares nurse clinicians with excellent observation, assessment, clinical, and communication skills and in prevention and rehabilitation issues essential to caring for individuals who have been violated by government institutions and domestic terrorists.

Current nursing theories and practices support the development of forensic intervention in response to the complex, sensitive needs of survivors of human torture and human rights violations. Nurses can bring empathy, compassion, and respect for human rights victims. Forensic specializations in the biomedical and social sciences incorporate emergency and advocacy interventions while providing scientific knowledge to combat destructive social and political conditions. Because of its holistic orientation, forensic nursing helps provide a humanistic approach to the application and protection of internationally recognized human rights standards. This new *health and justice* specialist provides a uniquely qualified clinical professional, blending biomedical knowledge with the basic principles of law and of human behavior in caring for survivors of torture.

UNIVERSAL NEED

The need to promote the image of police as defenders of the innocent and as being proactive in the apprehension of those who have violated the law is universal. In many countries, law enforcement agencies are viewed with suspicion because the government currently is using or previously has used the police to carry out government-sanctioned torture or punitive measures. For example, in South Africa the aftermath of apartheid has left a bitter relationship with the health care professional who recalls the fear of being charged with terrorism for treating any patient with any injury from a lethal weapon. Under the new constitution, this is no longer a concern of health care professionals, yet only time and trial will establish a close working relationship with the South African police force.

With the current approach to restructuring of forensic services, South Africa has entered into an era in which the culture of human rights is being nurtured. In the shadows of a time where claims of evidence tampering, fabrication, and other professional improprieties threatened the legal, civil, and human rights of the accused, improved forensic services and victim management will extend humanitarian rule of law. In response to the overwhelming need to create positive change for more competent, accessible forensic services and to provide a system of support to forensic physicians in South Africa, the Northern Cape Province took a bold and direct approach. Through their vision for new and improved medicolegal services, the forensic physicians established the first forensic nursing practice in Kimberley, Republic of South Africa, in 1997. This innovative approach emanated from the concerted efforts of Dr. Tromp Els, chief forensic medical officer; the National Restructuring Committee for Forensic Services; Office of the Attorney General–Northern Cape Province; Henrietta Stockdale College of Nursing, University of the Orange Free State; and the Department of Health, Welfare, and Environmental Affairs.

In the aftermath of apartheid, interpersonal violence is recognized as the major cause of injury and death and poses a serious threat to public health and safety in this area of the world. As forensic professionals in South Africa search for solutions to an identified problem, forensic nursing has been acknowledged as one mechanism to assist in combating the impact of crime. The struggle of South Africa in transition to a democratic society requires assistance and specialized training within the health and justice systems in order to deliver effective services. In response to this important opportunity to aid the republic in providing intervention to victims of human violence and the development of antiviolence strategies came a select group of professionals, a team of forensic specialists who were willing to share their unique knowledge, resources, and skills to prevent serious abuses of individual human rights.

In a collaborative endeavor, several members of the American Academy of Forensic Science and the International Association of Forensic Nurses came together to promote and establish the practice of forensic nursing in the Republic of South Africa. These individuals represented the mission of their professional organizations and the tenets of their respective disciplines.

The International Liaison Committee on Forensic Health Science in Nursing, established by the president of the American Academy of Forensic Sciences in 1996, represented a united endeavor to improve the quality of forensic services, the treatment of victims, the prosecution of sexual assault and domestic violence cases, and the advancement of human rights.

A MODEL PROGRAM

The project in the Republic of South Africa, initiated on May 18, 1997, provided 240 contact hours of didactic instruction in the principles and philosophies of clinical forensic evaluation and the scientific investigation of death. Clinical supervision in sexual assault examination, use of colposcopic magnification and postmortem procedures, and field experience in crime scene search, evidence collection, courtroom testimony, and forensic photography completed the curriculum. A 6-month internship is required under the direction of the chief forensic medical officer of the province and regional district surgeons in specific areas where the forensic nurse examiners are located. Candidates in the initial course were composed of 13 nurses and 2 police officers who successfully completed the requirements of the course. This cadre of forensic nurses offers a new resource in the clinical management of cases of child abuse, sexual assault, and other crime-related injuries, as well as in the investigation of questioned deaths. In the interest of justice, forensic nurses will afford a new perspective in scientific knowledge, professionalism, and evidentiary principles that will assist existing medicolegal specialists to inform, educate, and safeguard public health and safety. The legal and regulatory process will be better equipped to prevent atrocities of the past and to provide fundamental rights and freedoms to the next generation of children.

THE FUTURE OF FORENSIC NURSING

Forensic science is an important but often neglected area in emergency practice. Violence has a profound influence on the public health system and affects all areas of the health care institution. Identification of the subtlest signs of abuse and subsequent intervention are important responsibilities for nurses. Traditionally, these responsibilities were relegated specifically to law enforcement agencies. However, the support of criminal justice has provided an impetus that has served as a driving force to involve nurses in forensic role behavior.

The forensic nursing specialist has a vital role in the emergency department or trauma center because of the increasing caseload of patients who have medicolegal-related problems. Fatal or near-fatal injury resulting from intentional or unintentional acts involving criminality or civil action brings health care professionals into the arena of the law that constitutes forensic cases. These cases necessitate attention to forensically significant evidence. In addition, there are growing concerns for sensitivity to victims of violence and their families or significant others.

Medicolegal and psychosocial interaction is a new and important role for nurses that requires knowledge where human behavior interfaces with the law. Because the current policies of advocacy programs mandate the inclusions of criminal justice and health care providers, it is especially timely to propose that the forensic nursing specialist be placed in the trauma treatment environs to serve as a valuable link in interagency cooperation, ensuring that human needs and medicolegal interests are served. Because most emergency personnel and prehospital care providers ordinarily have only secondary interests in forensic matters, the motivated and skilled forensic nurse can be an invaluable resource for the criminal justice system, the hospital, and the patient.

THE EVOLUTION OF A GLOBAL NETWORK OF FORENSIC NURSING

Along with the new millennium came extraordinary challenges and opportunities available to the nursing profession worldwide—challenges in defining the way nurses care for patients, conduct research, teach students, address antiquated laws and policies, and participate in the global enterprise of health care. These challenges will not cease; they will require continuous quality improvement, innovative educational programs, and the realization that the framework for forensic nursing science must remain an ever-evolving work. The dynamics of culture, tradition, and religious practices will continue to pose a threat to the most vulnerable subjects in each society, affecting the way nurses practice nursing. Nurses must prepare graduates and reeducate practicing nurses to face the changing health care delivery system of the future.

Nursing students in the United States who are participating in forensic nursing programs often appear to be surprised that there is a need to study human rights and international law, the broader focus on transcultural nursing, and the recognition of indicators of torture. Yet the United States receives a greater number of immigrants and refugees than any other country in the world, bringing with it survivors of war and torture and victims of cultural practices that have maimed and crippled many. Where centers of justice, immigration laws, and deportation pertaining to the legal residence of these populations are established, one also will find large communities of immigrants and refugees seeking to combine their resources, support, and strategies for survival. These peoples also are seeking comfort, understanding, and protection in a new, strange environment that threatens their understanding of the laws, causes fear of accusation of wrongdoing, and inhibits their desire to be accepted. The fear of being judged for their traditions, cultural practices, and worship of religious practices remains a covert concern, often driving their beliefs into secrecy and their customs underground.

Nurses must learn to understand the impression that may be left with these individuals recently arriving from their country of origin where doctors, nurses, and police may have participated in their imprisonment, mutilation, and evaluation of the extent of punishment or torture they may receive without causing death. An awareness of cultural and traditional practices such as female genital mutilation, the practice of honor killings, bride burning, dowry deaths, child prostitution, incarceration of rape victims rather than the perpetrator, and the poverty and lack of education for women must become a part of nursing education in today's multicultural, dissimilar population subject to the often ethnocentric and confined perspective of American health care services.

Nurses must strive to include in their strategic plan for nursing the issues that have been identified as having the highest priority by the World Health Organization, not limiting their concerns to their state and national agendas. Nursing research, curricula, and practice must address prevention of human immunodeficiency virus and acquired immunodeficiency syndrome and the direct connection to sexual assault, prevention of disease and death related to the lack of early detection and management of chronic conditions of the immigrant and refugee populations transferred from their countries of origin, the reduction of abuse against women and children in a culturally competent and sensitive manner, the reduction of infant mortality among this group, and the risk factors from a contaminated environment that they have not experienced before.

ACHIEVING AN INTERNATIONAL FOCUS

Canada was the first to join with the International Association of Forensic Nurses at the initial founding meeting to establish the bond between the United States and forensic nursing that today has directed the expansion of this mission into other areas of the world.

Those who have reached out to developed and developing countries in need of a new resource to address violence and its associated trauma have discovered that the similarities of interpersonal crime (crimes against women, children, and the elderly) are basically the same everywhere. The major commonality linking each of these countries in health beliefs, cultural differences, societal values, and nursing care is the impact of domestic violence, child abuse, crimes against the elderly, and most specifically, sexual assault. Other commonalties include homicide, alcohol abuse, and suicide. As in any country, culture, or society, children are those most violated by mistreatment, neglect, brutality, sexual abuse, and war.

For forensic nurses to understand better the necessary approach to assist in the forensic assessment and management of medicolegal cases requires the incorporation of transcultural nursing perspectives, the ethical and moral dimensions of human care, health care practices of diverse cultures, and a review of the law—local, national, and international, as well as an in-depth knowledge of the United Nations Declaration of Human Rights. A strong working knowledge of the law not only promotes the interaction with local law enforcement agencies and helps to develop an accurate approach to forensic nursing interventions but also may protect the nurse practicing outside his or her own national boundaries. An increased awareness of the law also enables the nurse to present informed, appropriate lectures and an awareness of how the current standards of nursing practice differ.

The establishment of the International Association of Forensic Nurses in 1992 has promoted the education and implementation of forensic nursing roles worldwide. The vision of this founding group was to develop an organization that would encompass a wide and diverse body of those who practice nursing within the arena of the law. Nurses who apply concepts and strategies of forensic science in their specialty practice include death investigators, sexual assault nurse examiners, forensic psychiatric nurses, correctional nurse specialists, legal nurse consultants, forensic geriatric and pediatric specialists, nurse attorneys, forensic clinical nurse specialists, and other forensic nursing roles as they evolve. With the establishment of graduate and undergraduate education programs, role development in forensic nursing in the United States and abroad is recognized as one important component in antiviolence strategies.

To meet the health care needs of an increasingly diverse population of patients with forensic assessment needs in the United States, the International Association of Forensic Nurses determined to maintain and encourage a worldwide focus in membership, Scope and Standards of Practice, and a commitment to establish practices internationally. The International Association of Forensic Nurses recognizes membership of more than 2500 in 11 countries and territories. Institutions of higher learning are offering formal and informal curricula in Australia, Canada, England, Scotland, Singapore, Brunei, Central America, India, Italy, South Africa, Turkey, Zimbabwe, and Japan. South Africa has become the first country in which the minister of health has designated forensic nursing as a National Priority Program. Through advanced technology, forensic nursing has entered the World Wide Web via digital distance delivery. Internet education and information connects this new frontier in forensic health care with the global community.

SUMMARY

The development of a new field of practice is a challenging experience that brings together professionals who recognize a mutual benefit through collaborative practice, an exchange of knowledge, and shared successes in order to reach common goals. Nurses must remain concerned with improving the health care of at-risk populations and with advancing the information technologies that are revolutionizing forensic nursing research, clinical care, and forensic education. Nurses must find a clinical partnership with nurses from other countries with similar interest to address specific concerns and threats to health and justice. In the near future, developed and developing countries will be served by nurses prepared in the basic principles and philosophies of forensic nursing science.

REFERENCES

Barber, J. (1991). Frontiers and challenges in critical care: Foreword. *Critical Care Nursing Quarterly, 14*(3), 3.

Bays, J., & Lewman, L. (1992). Toluidine blue in the detection at autopsy of perineal and anal lacerations in victims of sexual abuse. *Archives of Pathology Laboratory Medicine, 116*(6), 620-621.

Besant-Matthews, P. (1994). Personal communication.

Birk, S. (1992). Emerging specialties: Expanded opportunities. *The American Nurse, 24,* 7-9.

Brigham and Women's Hospital. (1994). *Know with the insiders know: Domestic violence: A manual for healthcare providers.* Boston: Author.

Butt, J. (1993). *Sudden death and police investigation* (2nd ed.). Calgary, Alberta, Canada.

Campbell, J., & Lynch, V. (2006). Violence against women. In V. Lynch (Ed.), *Forensic nursing* (chap. 6). St. Louis, MO: Mosby.

Camp, S. (1976). *Gradwald's legal medicine* (3rd ed.). Chicago: Yearbook Medical.

Duval, J. (1995). *Role of the forensic nursing specialist in an urban trauma center* [Abstract D 44, p. 101]. In Proceedings of the 47th Annual Meeting of the American Academy of Forensic Sciences, Seattle, WA.

Eckert, W. G., Bell, J. S., Stein, R. J., Tabakman, M. B., Taff, M. L., & Tedeschi, L. G. (1986). Clinical forensic medicine. *American Journal of Forensic Medicine and Pathology, 7*(3), 182-185.

Family Violence Prevention Fund in San Francisco, San Francisco Injury Center for Research and Prevention. (1992).

Filer, D., & Filer, L. (1993). *Whither or wither forensic in the United Kingdom* [Abstract 33]. In Programs and Abstracts of the 3rd World Meeting of Police Medical Officers, Harrogate, England.

Freeman, A. (1988). Gunshot wounds: Initial assessment and management. *The Australian Nurses' Journal, 10*(1), 40-45.

Jezierski, M. (1994). Abuse of women by male partners: Basic knowledge for emergency nurses. *Journal of Emergency Nursing, 20*(5), 361-372.

Joint Commission on Accreditation of Health Care Organizations. (1994). *AMH accreditation manual for hospitals.* Oakbrook, IL: Author.

Kopser, K., Horn, P. B., & Carpenter, A. D. (1994). Successful collaboration within an integrative practice model. *Clinical Nurse Specialist, 8*(6), 330-333.

Lynch, V. (1988). Biomedical investigation as a mental health nursing role. In J. Lancaster (Ed.), *Adult psychiatric nursing* (3rd ed.). New Hyde Park, NY: Medical Examination Publishing.

Lynch, V. (1991). Forensic nursing in the emergency department: A new role for the 1990's. *Critical Care Nursing Quarterly, 14*(3), 69-86.

Lynch, V. (1993a). Forensic aspects of health care: New roles, new responsibilities. *Journal of Psychosocial Nursing and Mental Health Services, 31*(11), 5-6, 46-47.

Lynch, V. (1993b). Forensic nursing: Diversity in education and practice. *Journal of Psychosocial Nursing and Mental Health Services, 31*(11), 7-14.

Lynch, V. (1995, April). Forensic nursing: an essential element in managing society's violence and its victims. *ASTM Standardization News.*

Lynch, V. (1995). *Role of the forensic nurse specialist in the identification of sexual assault trauma* [Abstract D 43, p. 100]. In Proceedings of the 47th Annual Meeting of the American Academy of Forensic Sciences, Seattle, WA.

Marullo. (1997). Key note address. Kansas City, MO: International Association of Forensic Nurses.

Smock, W., Ross, C., & Hamilton, F. (1994). Clinical forensic medicine: How ED physicians can help with the sleuthing. *Emergency Legal Briefings, 5*(1), 1-8.

Stanhope, M., & Lancaster, J. (1996). *Community health nursing: Promoting health of aggregates, families, and individuals.* St Louis: Mosby.

World Health Organization. (1978, September 12). *Declaration of Alma-Ata: Health for all. Series No. 1.* Geneva, Switzerland: Author.

CHAPTER
30

Disease Management

Are Nurses Ready?

RUFUS HOWE

The disease management industry has opened the door for nurses to use their clinical knowledge and teaching skills in ways not possible in other settings. Although there are no hard data to support the number of current and available nursing positions, disease management is a rapidly growing phenomenon, and nurses are the central agent that creates its value. The value of this role to nurses is demonstrated clearly in the unusually low turnover rate compared with other traditional nurse roles. Nurses are interviewing all over the country for disease management positions at local hospitals, health insurance companies, and independent vendors.

What at first seems like an opportunity for a nonhospital or clinic position, however, may be a significant stressor because of the nontraditional nature and requirement for new skills necessary to perform well in this new role. The purpose of this chapter is to describe briefly the disease management industry, identify common core competencies needed to perform disease management, and determine strategies for preparing nurses for this demanding new profession.

DISEASE MANAGEMENT

At its most basic level, disease management is the product of a standardized nursing intervention with a preidentified chronically ill person over time. The aim of the intervention is always to improve quality of care, understanding that the intervention should lead to optimal clinical, financial, and overall quality of life outcomes. Key elements of disease management include program key clinical and financial indicators, identification strategies, population stratification, clinical evidence and assessment, and behavior change interventional techniques.

Program Key Clinical and Financial Indicators

Because disease management is an intervention that is subject to outside scrutiny, a limited number of clinical and financial markers are used to determine the success factors of the program. Clinical indicators for a heart failure program may include the rate of patients who are weighing themselves daily, who are taking an angiotensin-converting enzyme inhibitor, or who can recount the warning signs for worsening clinical status. Financial indicators may include the rate of emergency or hospital admissions and differences in total medical cost from baseline to a time in the future. Disease managers use these indicators to focus their efforts during each encounter.

Identification Strategies

Disease management programs traditionally require some form of identification mechanism. Health insurance plans use medical or pharmacy claims to identify disease management participants. Other programs may use self or physician referral strategies. The challenge with any disease management program is the nature and accuracy of the source of the data that identify the patient.

Population Stratification

Once identified, the target population is sorted into groups using stratification rules. In disease management, stratification is synonymous with encounter frequency. The rules are meant to gauge the clinical status in order to determine the urgency and possibly the qualification level of nurse who should see a given patient. The data used for stratification almost always are gleaned during the first conversation with the disease manager. Some rudimentary programs also use stratification to propose clinical interventions. Segmentation is another form of stratification and is used to presort a population into groups based only upon clinical and financial data located in health-related databases. Rules-based or neural net predictive models are applied to the patient data to determine relative risk levels that then are used to assign risk categories or values. The result of segmentation is the ability to contact the right patient at the right time with the right "level" of disease manager.

Clinical Evidence and Assessment

Disease management programs are the manifestation of the best clinical evidence available: clinical guidelines operationalized. Clinical content drives many elements of a disease management program, from key clinical indicators to stratification to assessment and even behavior change techniques. Assessments contain important clinical data necessary for the best understanding of the patient's situation and form the basis for proposing potential interventions that will close gaps in care and ultimately improve the quality of life for the patient. Clinical evidence is not the same as evidence-based medicine. Evidence-based medicine is best defined as the "the conscientious, explicit, and judicious use of current best evidence in making decisions about the care of individual patients" (Sackett, Haynes, Guyatt, & Tugwell, 1991). This definition makes it clear that evidence-based medicine is much more than research. Evidence-based medicine is the process of applying best practices to a patient and astute clinician (disease manager in this case) to propose and carry out interventions.

Behavior Change Interventional Techniques

Disease management depends on patients and physicians making changes to their usual practices. Behavior change is a phenomenon that is elusive, even magical. What causes a behavior change is largely unknown. Well-known behavior change techniques, when applied correctly, are able to accomplish this seemingly impossible task to enough patients and physicians to make a difference across the population. No matter what technique is applied, the common requirements are that there is a triggering issue and a method for bringing the issue to the forefront, identifying strategies to influence the issue, and tracking whether the technique is working.

DESCRIPTION OF THE DISEASE MANAGEMENT INDUSTRY

The disease management industry as it exists today began around 1994. The early entrants were large pharmaceutical and hospital systems or other large health-related businesses. Today, independent disease management companies, health insurance plans, or pharmaceutical companies provide disease management services. Each entity has a business model based on creating clinical and financial value. Value is expressed as a positive clinical status change, improved cost, or a return on investment.

Disease management in hospitals or outpatient clinics is considered a service business that seeks to make a profit on behalf of its sponsors.

The competitive landscape has caused a rapid evolution into more effective and efficient disease management models. This evolution has spawned a trade organization, the Disease Management Association of America (http://www.dmaa.org). The Disease Management Association of America has taken on the task of bringing competitors together for the good of a maturing industry, has proposed a definition of disease management holds regular trade and educational conferences, and supports legislation that favors disease management.

Accreditation organizations such as the Utilization Review Accreditation Commission, National Committee for Quality Assurance, and Joint Commission on Accreditation of Healthcare Organizations (JCAHO) have embraced disease management by providing certification standards that can be applied across practice settings. The certifications have resulted in a normalization of how disease management is delivered and are a useful yardstick for those who are purchasing disease management.

From a nursing professional organization standpoint, little exists today that supports disease managers. Organizations such as the Case Management Society of America (http://www.cmsa.org) recognize the emergence of disease managers and are providing separate conference tracks and Web-based clinical communities. However, organizations such as the American Nurses Association and the National League of Nursing have done little to nothing to further professional certification or development of disease managers.

Early attempts have been made to incorporate disease management into nursing degree programs. One university has submitted a grant to offer a master's-level disease management program. That other opportunities to hold a disease management graduate nursing degree will arise in the next 6 to 8 years is entirely possible.

Several dedicated texts have highlighted various aspects of disease management. In their book, Nash and Todd (2001) describe the disease management industry and offer strategies to implement such a program. I have written *The Disease Manager's Handbook* (Howe, 2005). This book covers the body of knowledge necessary to practice disease management and is intended for use in disease manager training. Another book, by Huber (2005), called *Disease Management: A Guide for Case Managers* is written to describe disease management in the context of case management. The practice or work approach differences between case and disease management have been the subject of debate and inquiry, and rightly so.

DISEASE MANAGEMENT ROLE

A view into the Web-based career sites (i.e., http://www.monster.com) using "disease management" as search criterion reveals a wealth of information. At any given time, hundreds of job opportunities are available in many settings. A distillation of common disease manager role expectations follows.

The primary duties for nurses are the following:

♦ Performs administrative duties to include engaging patients, explaining program details, conducting and scheduling patients, and ensuring that contact information is current
♦ Conducts clinical assessments
♦ Forms care plans, perhaps across one or many conditions
♦ Provides interventions to patients and their families that may include goal setting care coordination with primary care provider or case manager and provision of relevant written material
♦ Creates documents interactions that are helpful for other care team members and are consistent with quality tracking mechanisms
♦ Refers appropriate patients to other health team members when the opportunity arises
♦ May participate in ongoing training of fellow disease managers
♦ May be asked to obtain certifications or specialized training that is consistent with the disease management program objectives

Other knowledge, skills, and abilities the disease manager must have are these:

♦ Knowledge of managed care, disease management principles, and how these two create value for each other
♦ Experience with educating adult learners
♦ Ability to communicate effectively with health care team members such as physicians, case managers, family members, and others who may be involved with the care of the patient
♦ Experience with being a member of a health care team
♦ Ability to participate in quality management programs (The nurse should have a basic understanding of how quality metrics are used for program improvement.)
♦ Experience in telephonic or call centers (a plus)
♦ Multitasking ability in a high-volume environment (a key skill)

♦ Strong computer skills, which are essential for programs that require that the interaction be tracked with a clinical information system
♦ Flexibility to work in a rapidly changing environment
♦ Fluency in another language (Some programs have specific language requirements, especially Spanish.)

These requirements describe a nurse who is working within a disease management workflow that is like and unlike a more traditional environment. Of note is the implication that the disease manager practices in a dynamic, somewhat stressful, and demanding role. Taken on this level, this is not that different from the medical-surgical nurse who cares for 20 to 50 patients at a time. The difference is that the nurse is trained specifically in skills required for inpatient settings: medication administration, hygiene-related care, patient teaching around typical inpatient scenarios, and nurse care planning. As will be illustrated later in the chapter, other new skills are necessary, skills that have a far different emphasis in disease management practice.

Academic Preparation

One major issue for disease management is the academic preparation of nurses as it relates to disease management requirements. A seminal study, "Trends in Registered Nurse Education Programs: A Comparison Across Three Points in Time—1994, 1999, 2004" (Adams, Valiga, Murdock, McGinnis, & Wolfertz, 2004), seems to support the notion that nurses are prepared partially for disease management practice. The purpose of the study was to compare how nursing education has changed from 1994 to 2004. The investigators state that "Over the past decade, demands on nurse educators altered secondary to increased health services delivery in community-based settings, changing population demographics, and technological changes in educational and health services delivery. Coupled with the current shortage of registered nurses (RNs), the alterations generated calls—from both inside and outside of the nursing profession—for nurse educators to experiment with different teaching/learning modalities and to initiate innovative nursing education practices. In other words, nurse educators were challenged to think 'outside of the box' when educating tomorrow's nurses ... to make the evolutionary and revolutionary alterations in nursing education processes and outcomes needed to keep pace with today's complex, unpredictable healthcare environment."

Twelve nursing programs completed a 16-page questionnaire that examined nursing education across various domains. Of the several interesting results from this study, the following list of nursing education topics was the most germane to the disease management training discussion. This list represents the items emphasized more in 2004 than in 1994, and all items are relevant to disease management practice:

◆ Case management
◆ Informatics/computers
◆ Patient care outcomes
◆ Health care cost/finance/financial management
◆ Critical thinking
◆ Evidence-based practice
◆ Prevention
◆ Alternative therapies/holistic approaches to care
◆ Collaborative partnerships
◆ Health promotion/wellness care
◆ Community-based care in nontraditional settings

Additional skills are required but are not normally addressed in nursing undergraduate training programs. These additional skills normally are covered by formal on-the-job training programs offered by each disease management sponsor. These skills are highlighted next.

Telephone Sales

Unlike usual nursing settings, disease managers often are required to "sell" their service, even though the service is almost always free and voluntary. Nurses are expected to memorize opening scripts that compel a patient to listen, absorb, and agree to participate in the program within seconds of the first interaction. Ideally, the patient is aware that a registered nurse will be calling them and that the service is endorsed by their primary care provider and health insurance plan. This foreknowledge is sometimes not present, and the call becomes a "cold call" that produces anxiety for the nurse and the patient. Training in this area is critical for nurses who are in a nurturing, not sales, profession.

Motivational Interviewing

Motivational interviewing is a technique used by trained practitioners to support and maintain behavior change efforts. Training covers interviewing techniques under a wide variety of circumstances and entails role-play as a central feature of the learning process. Although motivational interviewing is part of some nursing education programs (for instance, the School of Nursing at Oregon Health Sciences University; Nurs 507f, Introduction to Motivational Interviewing; Susan Butterworth, professor), it is not emphasized to the degree necessary to support robust disease management interventions.

Treatment-Based (Physician) Care Planning

Disease management requires the nurse to understand the form and function of physician care planning over and above nursing care plans. This represents a level of critical thinking, analysis, and orientation not normally covered in nursing programs. The primary transition point for new disease management nurses is the role of diagnostics in the formulation of the treatment plan. Treatment plans are discussed in the same way the physician would discuss them with the patient, making the conversation feel foreign to the nurse.

Medication Management

Medication management has two distinct aspects for the disease management nurse. First is the selection and dosing of the appropriate agent given the context of the patient's clinical picture. Nurses are not trained to prescribe medications and thus are not used to thinking in this fashion. Secondly, medication compliance strategies are important in disease management and are not normally an issue for inpatient nurses. Ambulatory-based nurses have an advantage in this area because they often are dealing with issue from a community health perspective.

Health Risk Appraisal

The health risk appraisal in its purest form gauges the cardiovascular or cancer risk of a patient via a risk score. The patient responses may guide awareness of risky issues that become discussion points for future behavior change initiatives. The area of health risks is not new to nurses, but the notion of a risk score and how that applies to risk is sometimes elusive from the population management perspective. To understand the health risk scoring clearly, nurses are trained in basic health-related epidemiology principles, including predictive modeling and relative risk.

Behavior Change

Behavior change is well covered in some nursing programs, but application of behavior change theories and techniques are not emphasized to the degree necessary for disease managers. This may be because nursing training focuses primarily on episodic rather than longitudinal care relationships. Disease management programs tend to hang their hat on a few dominant and proven behavior change techniques and train accordingly. Accomplishing true behavior change remains one of the most challenging aspects of a disease manager's role.

Shared Decision Making

Shared decision making is a method by which a clinician presents treatment options, explains the benefits and risks of each, and leads the patient to a mutually agreed upon conclusion. In some respects, nurses are well suited for this process by virtue of their orientation to patient advocacy. The real issue is in acquiring the knowledge necessary to guide the member through the many options put before a patient when confronted with such choices. Disease management programs have a list of common shared decision-making conversations and train specifically to the content related to each.

Appointment-Based Practice (Pacing)

The unsaid aspect of disease management practice is the ability to speak with large numbers of patients per day while creating the illusion of ample time spent with each one. Primary care providers (physicians, physician assistants, and nurse practitioners) are used to this because of the way their appointment schedules are organized. Nurses, however, typically do not have the training or work experience that would expose them to the pacing and guided discussion approach necessary to work their way through the day. This aspect of practice is handled through call or encounter metrics that track numbers of patients and perhaps time per encounter.

Generalist Approach

Today, most disease management programs demand a generalist approach rather than a narrow, condition- or disease-based approach. At issue is the transition of many nurses from narrowly focused practice settings such as maternity wards, intensive care units, and orthopedic clinics. Disease management nurses are trained to be deeply conversant in as many as 50 different conditions. This aspect of the training is daunting and requires ongoing monitoring and clarification.

Business Considerations

A disease management nurse must embrace several business considerations. First, as was mentioned earlier in this chapter, the nurse is the agent of value, not a liability. Although this relationship change is a positive one, it takes time getting used to it. In disease management the frontline person is responsible for the success or failure of the program, and this is highly evident. This may introduce new or different feelings of responsibility or accountability not felt in prior settings.

Second, because the nurse is the creator of value, the onus on the nurse is to think critically about the business-related aspects of the role. For example, nurses realize that not reaching certain behavior change goals may negatively affect contractual savings promises and thus may threaten the program credibility and market presence. Lastly, and probably the hardest business concept to embrace, is population management techniques that provide "good enough" care across many people, rather than the "cover-all-the-issues" tendency that many nurses have. To leave lower-priority clinical issues alone is difficult once a relationship is formed, but that is the nature of how disease management works.

STRATEGIES FOR NURSING IN DISEASE MANAGEMENT

This chapter covers a variety of issues faced by nurses who choose to participate in disease management programs. The issues are simple by themselves but complex taken as a whole. One way to view future strategies may be to think of disease management nursing as an emerging profession. In this view, strategies would include provision of more directed undergraduate and graduate training programs, distinct professional nursing certification, professional journals for nursing research purposes, and professional forums or organizations dedicated to disease management. None of these exist today for nurses, and although this may seem dim, the opportunities are there for the aspiring school, nursing, and professional organization.

Another way of tackling these issues may be through a commercial effort to provide training to disease managers. Independent companies provide such training today. The issue at hand is that disease management is performed largely in proprietary settings, and outside training initiatives will go only so far.

Whatever the mechanism, the disease management industry has amassed the fundamental knowledge set and the best training practices for disease managers. The best solution to preparing nurses to become better disease managers probably lies in a combination of market pressure, patient demand, and the natural evolution of nursing education.

REFERENCES

Adams, C., Valiga, T., Murdock, J., McGinnis, S., & Wolfertz, J. (2004). *Trends in registered nurse education programs: A comparison across three points in time—1994, 1999, 2004.* Retrieved

January 4, 2006 from http://www.nln.org/aboutnln/nursetrends.htm

Howe, R. (2005). *The disease manager's handbook.* Boston: Jones and Bartlett.

Huber, D. (2005). *Disease management: A guide for case managers.* Philadelphia: W.B. Saunders.

Nash, D., & Todd, W. (2001). *Disease management: A systems approach to improving patient outcomes.* San Francisco: Jossey-Bass.

Sackett, D. L., Haynes, R. B., Guyatt, G. H., & Tugwell, P. (1991). *Clinical epidemiology. A basic science for clinical medicine* (2nd ed.). Boston: Little, Brown.

QUALITY IMPROVEMENT

Role of Nursing in Achieving Quality Health Care Systems

KATHRYN J. DOLTER, GUEST EDITOR

The U.S. health care system is facing cost, quality, and access challenges in the twenty-first century. It has higher health care expenditures yet poorer quality and less access than other developed nations. In a recent study published by the World Health Organization, the U.S. health care system ranked thirty-seventh out of 191 countries. The ranking was based on several dimensions: overall level of population health, distribution of health in the population, responsiveness, distribution of financing, and fairness of financial contribution. The cost of health care in the United States exceeded $1.7 trillion in 2004. The approximately $4200 per capita health care spending in the United States exceeds the per capita health expenditures of all other Organization of Economic Cooperation and Development countries, with U.S. health per capita health care expenditures being 2 to 3 times that of most those nations. Health care dollars in the United States are not spent on preventive services, with 75% of health care dollars being spent on the care of chronic illness. Compared with similar Organization of Economic Cooperation and Development countries—Australia, Canada, France, Germany, and the United Kingdom—the United States appears to offer lower quality of care despite having the highest per capita spending rate, and approximately 43 million persons—including 8.5 million children—do not have health insurance.

After documenting the "serious and pervasive nature" of the quality issues facing the U.S. health care system, the Institute of Medicine produced two reports: *To Err Is Human* (1999) and *Crossing the Quality Chasm* (2001). These reports outlined the quality issues in U.S. health care and made recommendations for addressing identified problems. The report *To Err Is Human* cited estimates of hospital deaths caused by iatrogenic injuries ranging from 44,000 to 98,000 per year and identified that the number of errors in hospitals exceeded the number from the eighth leading cause of death in America. Nursing has a key role in ensuring patient safety. The report *Crossing the Quality Chasm* concluded that the American health care delivery system is lacking in each of the six dimensions of quality defined within the report. Specifically, the report charges that U.S. health care is not (1) safe—avoiding injuries to patients from the care that is intended to help; (2) effective—providing services based on scientific knowledge; (3) patient-centered—providing care that is respectful and responsive; (4) timely—reducing waits and harmful delays; (5) efficient—avoiding waste, including waste of supplies, ideas, and energy; and (6) equitable—providing care that does not vary in quality because of personal characteristics such as geographic location and socioeconomic status.

The report *Crossing the Quality Chasm* identified that health care in America not only is unsafe as identified in *To Err Is Human* but also is ineffective: care defined by the best evidence is not occurring. Though the United States spends $32.4 billion on health care research, that evidence is not getting translated into practice. This ineffectiveness has two extremes: overuse and underuse of health care technologies. Nurses must become aware of the *Crossing the Quality Chasm* report and recommendations and of the pivotal role nursing has in the ultimate achievement of the six aims of quality health care within the systems of care that exist in the United States. Nurses must take part in the redesign of the U.S. health care system to ensure quality patient care.

In the debate chapter, Hinshaw, one of the nurse members of the expert panel authoring the Institute of Medicine series report *Keeping Patients Safe: Transforming the Work Environment of Nurses,* describes the pivotal role of nurses in patient safety and the quality of care in the U.S. health care system. Hinshaw summarizes the key points of the Institute of Medicine reports and describes how nurses must be involved in organizational, local, and national political change processes in order to meet the challenge of transforming the Institute of Medicine reports into reality.

With safety one of the six aims of a quality health care system, Nelson and Powell-Cope describe their framework for patient safety, which focuses on the health care system and nursing process redesign to reduce error in health care. Nelson is currently the director of the Veterans Administration Patient Safety Center of Inquiry; Powell-Cope is the associate director, Diffusion of Innovations, at the center. Nelson and Powell-Cope describe the hazard condition inputs (patient factors, unintentional unsafe acts by providers, situational factors, and latent factors); safety defense processes (patient, provider, technical, and organizational safety defenses), and outcomes (intermediate patient, process, and systems outcomes of cost, error types and rates, and patient and provider satisfaction) that affect patient safety. With their framework, they explain why adverse events occur in nursing and provide an overview about what can be done to reduce the incidence and severity of adverse events.

In *Priority Areas for National Action* (2003), the Institute of Medicine makes a case for focusing on specific conditions in an effort to have a greater impact on achieving visible health care quality improvement. Specific conditions for focus were identified based on the criteria of impact (extent of the total economic, mortality, and disability burden of a disease or condition on the U.S. population); improvability (extent of the gap in the care of that disease or condition for which evidence-based interventions could effect change in one or more of the six aims identified in the *Crossing the Quality Chasm* report); and inclusiveness (broad application to all segments of the U.S. population regarding gender, race, and socioeconomic status). Priority conditions were identified in the major topic areas of preventive care, behavioral health, chronic conditions, inpatient/surgical care, children and adolescents, and end of life. End-of-life areas identified included frailty and pain control in cancer.

With prevention, a major category of the priority conditions focus, Allen, who is currently a nurse member of the U.S. Preventive Services Task Force, makes the case for nurse involvement in preventive activities. She provides an overview of the need for prevention; the focus of the federal government on prevention via its Healthy People 2000 and Healthy People 2010 initiatives; and the work of U.S. Preventives Services Task Force in identifying and delineating the evidence-base of preventive interventions. Allen then provides examples of nurse involvement in evidence-based prevention guideline implementation.

Nurse involvement in the transformation of care related to chronic conditions is addressed by Davis, who served as associate director for clinical improvement at Improving Chronic Illness Care from 1998 to 2005. Davis defines how nurses can improve care for the chronically ill in their population. Given the aging of Americans, this is an important area for nurses to address.

Lunney, an expert in end of life and frailty, provides an overview of the role of nursing in the care of the frail elder, a focus of improvement in the priority condition end-of-life category. Lunney describes the demographics of aging and the various end-of-life trajectories but focuses on frailty at the end of life, its definition and demographics, and the assessment and identification of the frail elder. Describing the unpredictability of death in the frail elder, Lunney describes the challenges of striking the right balance between palliative care and rehabilitation in this population and assisting frail elders prepare for death while still keeping their focus on living.

Leadership by Example (2003) contains the Institute of Medicine recommendations that the federal government and federal health care systems demonstrate leadership in developing systems of care that epitomize quality. Dolter describes federal initiatives that provide support to the provision of quality health care at the unit and organizational level, as well as federal health system programs that provide examples of how to implement programs directed toward achieving the six aims of quality. Dolter emphasizes the need to use already developed quality tools so as to avoid the "reinvention of the wheel" that often characterizes health care improvements, reinventions that promulgate the development of local "pet rocks." With personnel being the most expensive budget item in any health care system, use of the already developed quality improvement tools developed by the federal government and other respected entities decreases time to implementation and eliminates wasted personnel efforts that could be directed toward implementation.

The challenge for nurses is to become aware of the Institute of Medicine's *Crossing the Quality Chasm* report and to participate in the implementation of each recommendation in the report. Only with the involvement of frontline nurses will the vision of transformation of health care into a system of care that is safe, effective, efficient, timely, patient-centered, and equitable be achieved. This section is important for all nurses to read to begin to understand and solve the issues associated with these Institute of Medicine reports. Much room for improvement exists in this area as nurses strive to enhance quality care. The following section provides a reading list of related publications for nurses who want to read further in this area.

INSTITUTE OF MEDICINE SERIES BOOKS AND EXECUTIVE SUMMARY WEB SITES

To Err Is Human: Building a Safer Health System (1999)
http://books.nap.edu/execsumm_pdf/9728.pdf
Crossing the Quality Chasm: A New Health System for the 21st Century (2001)
http://books.nap.edu/execsumm_pdf/10027.pdf
Envisioning the National Health Care Quality Report (2001)
http://books.nap.edu/execsumm_pdf/10073.pdf
Fostering Rapid Advances in Health Care: Learning from System Demonstrations (2002)
http://books.nap.edu/execsumm_pdf/10565.pdf

Leadership by Example: Coordinating Government Roles in Improving Health Care Quality (2002)
http://books.nap.edu/execsumm_pdf/10537.pdf
Health Professions Education: A Bridge to Quality (2003)
http://books.nap.edu/execsumm_pdf/10681.pdf
Priority Areas for National Action: Transforming Health Care Quality (2003)
http://books.nap.edu/execsumm_pdf/10593.pdf
Keeping Patients Safe: Transforming the Work Environment of Nurses (2004)
http://books.nap.edu/execsumm_pdf/10851.pdf
Patient Safety: Achieving a New Standard for Care (2004)
http://books.nap.edu/execsumm_pdf/10863.pdf
1st Annual Crossing the Quality Chasm Summit: A Focus on Communities (2004)
http://www.nap.edu/execsumm_pdf/11085.pdf

Institute of Medicine Recommendations

Can We Meet the Challenges?

ADA SUE HINSHAW

In April 1986 the National Center of Nursing Research was established at the National Institutes of Health (NIH) after a 2-year legislative process. A major argument used during that relatively short process was to quote an Institute of Medicine (IOM) recommendation from the 1983 report *Nursing and Nursing Education: Public Policy and Private Actions* suggesting that "it was important to establish an entity for nursing research in the mainstream of scientific investigation" (Hinshaw, 2004, p. 112). Such a recommendation does not result in action without major strategic planning and effort by interested and invested individuals and organizations even when they are given by a prestigious body such as the IOM, which is the health advisor to the nation and specifically to the U.S. Congress and federal agencies. Unification of the general nursing professional organizations such as the American Nurses Association and more than 75 specialty nursing organizations plus collaborative groups acted on the IOM recommendation on nursing research in two separate legislative processes and successfully established the National Center of Nursing Research in 1986, as well as redesignating it to the National Institute of Nursing Research (NINR) in 1994. Although the creation of the NINR was important to the nursing profession, it has been ultimately valuable for changing health practice and leading to positive health outcomes. Thus this is an exemplary example of the ability of the nursing profession to meet the challenge of turning IOM recommendations into important programs that improve health for the American public.

A new series of IOM studies focused on improving the quality of care in U.S. health systems confronts the nursing profession with a current and future set of challenges. Can nursing build on multiple sets of recommendations to change the status quo of American health care and enhance the quality of care provided?

INSTITUTE OF MEDICINE: QUALITY OF CARE INITIATIVE

In 1998 the IOM launched an initiative to study the quality of care in the health systems of the country and provide recommendations from experts in the health professions addressing the issues. This was accomplished by forming the Committee on the Quality of Care in America. A series of reports would be published from this group's review, analysis, and synthesis of multiple bodies of research resulting in numerous recommendations for change in the American health care system. Why would recommendations from such an organization be important, and could they actually motivate action by health care professionals and organizations and other stakeholders?

The IOM is an organization of major experts from the various health professions in the United States including physicians, nurses, dentists, pharmacists, social workers, and public health practitioners. In addition, experts from law, social policy, corporate health care, health administrators, ethicists, and others who bring valuable perspectives to health care are involved. The IOM was created legislatively to provide expert advice to the U.S. Congress and federal agencies regarding health and health care for the American public. The IOM is part of the National Academies of Science. Over the years the IOM has earned a strong reputation for providing critical recommendations on health care because of its consistent policy of basing the suggestions on research and expert interpretation of such research.

The IOM provides a variety of reports on health and health care issues raised by the U.S. Congress, one of the federal agencies, or a health professional group. These reports are the result of a systematic review and critique process done by study panels of health and health-related experts from multiple disciplines. In the reviews, relevant research from a number of disciplines related to the health issue under study is critiqued and analyzed, and a thoughtful set of recommendations is generated. Every report and set of recommendations then is critiqued through an independent process conducted through another section of the National Academies of Science by a second group of experts in the field. Through these processes the IOM has earned the reputation of a prestigious organization the work of which is highly respected and trusted. The IOM has earned its status as "advisor to the nation to improve health."

As reports from the IOM initiative on the improvement of the quality of care began to be published, the various health professions and organizations began to strategize for the implementation of the recommendations. A series of reports have highlighted major issues and concerns with the American health care systems.

To Err Is Human: Building a Safer Health System (Kohn et al., 2000) was the initial report, and it created a major crisis for hospital systems. The report suggested that up to 98,000 individuals died each year because of errors in the care provided in hospitals. The report adopted a different approach to health care errors, placing emphasis on the system factors that perpetrate such errors and on health professional responsibility. The major thesis was that most errors resulted from system pressures and processes, not individual health care provider problems. The recommendations addressed the need for change in health system processes with particular emphasis on monitoring and reporting health care errors.

Most hospitals in the country immediately implemented new policies on examining medical and health care errors, instituted patient safety committees, and reviewed all major life-threatening errors in detail with suggestions for change in system processes and with hospital trustees receiving planned reports on patient safety outcomes. These are examples of hospital response to the first quality of care report. Accrediting bodies such as the Joint Commission on the Accreditation of Healthcare Organizations (JCAHO) have integrated a number of the IOM report recommendations into their regulations. Nurses have been an integral part of the various strategies; for example, leading the development of unit patient safety committees and hospital-wide safety committees and participating on hospital executive boards.

The *To Err Is Human* report (Kohn et al., 2000) has been particularly important to nurses and the nursing profession. Because nurses are often the health provider at the point of care, they are also often the individuals committing the final step in an error process. For example, medication errors often result from a rushed physician writing a hurried order, a pharmacist who is filling multiple orders, and a nurse who has worked too many hours with too many patients not checking closely enough before delivering the medicine. Taking a systems approach to such errors does not relieve the responsibility of the nurse but does provide important support for understanding the error in context. Changing the system to provide several checkpoints for intercepting such errors is expected to be a more effective method for decreasing the incidence of mistakes.

Crossing the Quality Chasm: A New Health System for the 21st Century (Institute of Medicine, 2001, p. 1) essentially suggested that the "American health care system is in need of fundamental change." This report suggested an agenda for crossing the chasm through a national commitment by health professionals, policy makers, purchasers, regulators, health care trustees, health administrators, consumers, and other stakeholders to six aims for improving the quality of care over the next 10 years. The six aims recommended that health care should be safe, effective, patient-centered, timely, efficient, and equitable. Thirteen recommendations suggested improving health care under several major headings; that is, formulating new rules to redesign and improve care, building organizational supports for change, and establishing a new environment for health care.

The *Crossing the Quality Chasm* (Institute of Medicine, 2001) report also adopted a health systems approach and specifically provided recommendations at the organizational level, including changes in safety processes and informational technology for facilitating care. In addition, the report focused on the payment and incentive system, recommending the alignment of payment policies with the improvement of care.

This report was particularly of interest to the nursing profession because the focus of nurses' practice is the patient, so facilitating "patient-centered" care drew heavily on nurse members in the subsequent IOM committees to implement this concept in health care (Dr. Joan Shaver, personal communication, 2005). The other five aims are also values of the nursing profession and thus goals that the professional nursing organizations could embrace. However, although *Crossing the Quality Chasm* (Institute of Medicine, 2001) provided the broad context for the series of quality of care reports, the recommendations were more difficult to implement because they were more macro and less specific in terms of providing direction.

Another IOM study focused heavily on patient safety and achieving positive patient outcomes through improving and changing the work environment of nurses—a major health challenge in terms of improving quality of care. Enhancing the quality of nursing care is complicated by the shortage of nurses, and the focus on work environment was meant to provide recommendations for the recruitment and retention of nurses in work environments and to show how strong environments would facilitate nurses' ability to provide high-quality care resulting in positive patient outcomes.

The report *Keeping Patients Safe: Transforming the Work Environment of Nurses* (Page, 2004) was charged with identifying the key aspects in the work environment that have an impact on patient safety and to suggest potential improvements for working conditions that could increase patient safety. The report reviewed numerous bodies of research from nursing, health services, organizational psychology, organizational sociology, design, and architecture to identify unsafe workforce deployment, unsafe work and work space design, and punitive organizational cultures that hinder the prevention and reporting of errors. Eighteen recommendations were given in four areas: (1) leadership and management practices, (2) work processes, (3) workforce capability, and (4) organizational culture.

Implementing the recommendations of the *Keeping Patients Safe* (Page, 2004) report poses unique and interesting challenges to the nursing profession. It is important for nursing to provide leadership in responding to the report recommendations in partnership with other health professionals, health care administrators, and other stakeholders. The response strategies must be careful not to accept sole responsibility for the issues raised in the report but to be true to the systems approach taken in this and the other quality of care reports. Conferences held by the University Hospital Consortium Nurse Executives and the American Organization of Nurse Executives specifically have focused on evolving strategies for addressing the recommendations. The recommendations also need to influence regulations such as those for hospital accreditation. A representative for JCAHO was a member of the IOM study committee for this report, and the president of

JCAHO talked with the committee several times. Hopefully, such interactions will influence the implementation of the recommendations.

Another major IOM report addressed the quality of health care in America: *Unequal Treatment: Confronting Racial and Ethnic Disparities in Health Care* (Smedley, Stith, & Nelson, 2003, p. 1). In considering the health care provided to racial and ethnic minorities, the study committee was charged with examining the influence of health professionals and the health care systems in which care is delivered. Essentially, the committee suggested the following:

> [T]hey found evidence that stereotyping, biases and uncertainty on the part healthcare providers can all contribute to unequal treatment. The conditions in which many clinical encounters take place—characterized by high time pressure, cognitive complexity, and pressures for cost containment—may enhance the likelihood that these processes will result in care poorly matched to minority patients' needs. Minorities may experience a range of other barriers to accessing care, even when insured at the same level as whites, including barriers of language, geography, and cultural familiarity. Further, financial and institutional arrangements of health systems, as well as the legal, regulatory, and policy environment in which they operate, may have disparate and negative effects on minorities' ability to attain quality care. (p. 1)

This report has generated a number of research agendas for the NIH, the NINR, and the Agency for Healthcare Research and Quality. A number of the National Institutes of Health have specific agendas for funding and reporting health disparities research (NIH, 2001). For example, the National Institute of Environmental Health Sciences has a specific initiative for funding health disparities research focused on the interrelationships of poverty, environmental pollution, and health (NIH, 2001). The NINR (2005) has a specific "Strategic Plan on Reducing Health Disparities." Health disparities are a high priority for funding according to the strategic plan. Major studies have been funded to investigate ways of improving such health disparities.

The health disparities information also is influencing nursing education. For example, undergraduate and graduate students are being exposed to the *Unequal Treatment* report in order to sensitize young professionals to the obvious biases embedded in health care and how to counter them (Guthrie & Hinshaw, 2005; Sampselle et al., 2000). A number of nurse scholars have been engaged in national policy discussions to lead change for health care in this area; for example, Dr. Martha Hill co-chaired the IOM study report on *Unequal Treatment*

(Smedley et al., 2003), and Dr. Antonia Villarruel is part of a Centers for Disease Control and Prevention panel and an additional study on minority health with the IOM (Institute of Medicine, study panel member, personal communication, 2004-2006). The translation of the information from the *Unequal Treatment* report into professional practice is one the major challenges nursing now faces.

Several of the quality of care studies recommend that the suggestions being outlined in the reports can be realized only if the health care disciplines work together. Interdisciplinary education across the health professions was a specific recommendation of the *Crossing the Quality Chasm* (Institute of Medicine, 2001) report suggesting that "an interdisciplinary summit be held to develop next steps for reform of health professions education in order to enhance patient care quality and safety" (p. 1). The multidisciplinary summit, held in June 2002, included allied health, nursing, medical, and pharmacological educators and students in addition to many other stakeholders. The summit report *Health Professions Education: A Bridge to Quality* (Greiner & Knebel, 2003) provides an important basic vision for the future: "All health professionals should be educated to deliver patient-centered care as members of an interdisciplinary team, emphasizing evidence-based practice, quality improvement approaches, and informatics" (p. 3).

The *Health Professions Education* report (Greiner & Knebel, 2003) recommendations targeted educational processes and institutions, curriculum and core competencies, accreditation systems, and credentialing processes across all the health professions. The American Association of Colleges of Nursing and the National League for Nursing have implemented discussions and initiatives regarding interdisciplinary professional education. The position statement from American Association of Colleges of Nursing (1995) on interdisciplinary education and practices states that "While each discipline has its own focus, the scope of health care mandates that health professionals work collaboratively and with other related disciplines. Collaboration emanates from an understanding and appreciation of the roles and contributions that each discipline brings to the care delivery experience. Such professional socialization and ability to work together is the result of shared educational and practice experiences." Some universities have generated special curricular projects to provide interdisciplinary education for health care providers; for example, the University of Washington (Mitchell et al., 2000).

The IOM study *Priority Areas for National Action: Transforming Health Care Quality* (Adams & Corrigan, 2003) grappled with the question of "where" does the health care field begin to improve the quality of health care. The expert members of this study panel outlined several criteria for determining priority areas for health care, suggesting that the priorities be those that do the following:

◆ Influence the health needs of the U.S. population across the entire life span
◆ Involve the total dimension of health care from keeping individuals well and optimizing health to being concerned with the cure and care of individuals experiencing disease and illnesses

The criteria essentially involved the impact, improvability, and inclusiveness of the American people in terms of health and illness. A list of 20 priorities was recommended that focused on a number of diverse areas; for example, care coordination, self-management, and conditions such as asthma, cancer, and diabetes. Other priorities were children with special needs, end-of-life care, frailty associated with old age, and obesity.

The Institute for Healthcare Improvement (2005) systematically searches for initiatives that are generated from the IOM Quality of Care Program and sets of report recommendations. This search recently traced 120 endeavors that have been published or presented. Although these efforts are exciting and motivating, obviously a number of challenges remain in terms of translating the report recommendations into professional practice and education and in using them to shape health policy.

SHAPING HEALTH POLICY AND PROFESSIONAL PRACTICE

Milio (1984), in her classic article, addressed the fact that research only does not ensure that the information will influence health policy or professional practice. The IOM reports pose the same challenge. How can the information that is synthesized and systemically analyzed, resulting in a set of carefully considered recommendations by experts in the field of study, be translated into professional practice or used to shape health policy?

The field of health policy has a defined body of knowledge consisting of models and processes that guide the use of research in shaping policy and thus professional practice (e.g., Longest, 1996; Richmond & Kotelchuck, 1983). Nursing has drawn on these models and has adapted them to the discipline as nursing research has been used to influence health policy (Feetham & Meister, 1999; Fawcett & Russell, 2001). Mason, Leavitt, and Chaffee (2002) address the inter-relationship of policy to politics in their text *Policy and Politics in Nursing and Health Care.*

In adapting Richmond and Kotelchuck's classic model (1983) for using research to influence health policy, Feetham and Meister (1999) outline three components basic to the translation process:

◆ Knowledge base that includes the accrued research and experience about the subject and the methods and processes for generating the information

◆ Political will that involves the hopes, concerns, willingness to act, and aspirations of multiple groups who have a stake in and are committed to the subject under study

◆ Social strategies that include plans and programs for shaping policy or changing practice based on the knowledge base and political will

Feetham and Meister's model (1999) is consistent with the more detailed policy cycle conceptualization developed by Shamian, Skelton-Green, and Villeneuve (2003) that embeds information and research into an eight-stage process. The eight stages consist of values and beliefs, emergence of problems and issues, knowledge and development of research, public awareness, political engagement, interest group activation, public policy deliberation, and adoption, as well as regulation, experience, and revision.

According to Shamian et al. (2003), there are two major parts to the cycle. Phase 1 is Getting to the Policy Agenda; that is, moving from values and beliefs to public awareness. This phase outlines the importance of the individuals valuing and believing in the policy they are attempting to formulate and implement. In addition, it is critical that the public, when they become involved, value the issue. Often the public is represented by elected local city council officials, state representatives, and congressional representatives and senators. For example, when the NINR was being considered legislatively, nursing highly valued the need for research for professional practice, whereas the policy makers valued nurses and their contribution to health care.

The model by Shamian et al. (2003) illustrates the manner in which research and information is embedded in the policy-making process. Values and beliefs have to be combined with research that substantiates the policy issue and its importance to the public. Research alone will not be sufficient to motivate policy makers. The exception to this principle is when the research is overwhelming and the issue addressed is critical to the health and well-being of the American people. The development of policies about smoke-free environments and smoking cessation is an excellent example of overwhelming research evidence that ultimately convinced policy makers and the public of the value of such policies. This policy legislation required a number of years and many legislative attempts because of the major business lobbies invested in tobacco in this country. The policy process also requires making the public aware of the issue and its value and engaging in political activity to involve multiple groups who are interested in the issue.

Phase II, Moving into Action, involves political engagement and progresses to regulation and revision. Political engagement means that the issue needs to be introduced to policy makers, usually in some form of city council proposal or state or national legislation. Shamian et al. (2003) suggest that the issue must have been "softened up." This refers to the idea that stakeholders in the issue and policy makers have to become familiar with the issue so that support and involvement can be obtained. For example, with the NINR, during the initial year one legislation, the nursing professional associations and major nursing leaders had to be convinced that placing a nursing research entity at the NIH was important. A number of major leaders believed the profession and its nurse scientists were not "ready" for this step. The policy makers in Congress were more convinced that the NINR was a valuable idea because they were committed to nursing and women's issues and did not understand nursing research but believed it would be important to nurses and the public. The initial round of legislation allowed the nursing profession to become unified around the idea of the NINR and to move the second round of legislation into law. This step was done through interest group discussions and forming of coalitions with multiple groups that valued nursing such as the American Association of Retired People. The second round of legislation allowed for the steps of public policy deliberation and adoption to regulation, experience, and revisions. Extensive deliberation in congressional committees, presidential compromise, and ultimately overriding of a presidential veto were part of the legislation process authorizing the NINR to be established at the NIH (Hinshaw, 2004).

Fawcett and Russell (2001) elaborate on Hinshaw's early conceptualization (1988, 2001) of using nursing research to shape health policy. These models address how research influences health policy at multiple levels; that is, the health care organization with individuals and families, the community, or local health policies and at the state, national, and international levels. Fawcett and Russell outline how the environment affects each level and the important nursing health policy outcomes that are desired with each level.

Several examples illustrate the use of research and the IOM recommendations at various policy-making levels. The quality of care reports *To Err Is Human* (Kohn et al., 2000), *Crossing the Quality Chasm* (Institute of Medicine, 2001), and *Keeping Patients Safe* (Page, 2004) provide multiple recommendations for implementation at the health care organizational level. The formation of patient safety committees at the hospital organization and patient unit levels are examples of this implementation. Communities adopting smoke-free environments and smoking cessation policies for restaurants and other public places are examples of city council policy actions based on other IOM reports; for example, *Clearing the Smoke: The Science Base for Tobacco Harm Reduction* (2001). At the state level, a number of states have instituted patient safety committees as part of opening the deliberations about additional laws needed to enhance patient safety in health care organizations. Nationally, the quality of care reports are being used to shape regulations for health care organizations (JCAHO) and guide the development and implementation of hospital improvement for patient care projects. The Institute for Healthcare Improvement has numerous such projects initiated, such as the following:

◆ "Patient Safety/Quality Improvement Clerkship, University of Tennessee, College of Medicine" (n.d.)
◆ "Transforming Care at the Bedside: Sparking Innovation and Excitement on the Hospital Unit" (n.d.)
◆ "Improvement Report: An Integrated Approach to Improving Patient Care" (n.d.)

CAN THE CHALLENGES BE MET?

The Feetham and Meister (1999), Shamian et al. (2003), Fawcett and Russell (2001), and Hinshaw (1988, 2001) models provide guidance as to how the recommendations given in the IOM reports can be translated into professional practice and health policy. This is the major challenge confronting the profession. If the recommendations are not considered carefully and explicit decisions are not made and leadership is not taken by nurses in health care organizations and professional associations, critical information from the IOM reports will not be implemented.

The nursing profession was highly successful in translating the recommendation of the *Nursing and Nursing Education: Public Policy and Private Action* (Institute of Medicine, 1983) report into the implementation of the National Center of Nursing Research, referred to currently as the NINR, within a relatively short 2-year legislative process. Political will was a major component of that success. The nursing professional organizations, general and specialty associations, unified to work with champions in the U.S. Congress and other coalition friends to translate the recommendation into a social strategy or action—the establishment of the NINR. All nurses understood the value of generating a science base through research that could improve professional practice and optimize quality outcomes for individuals, families, and communities. Generating political will through unification of all nursing professional associations, identifying and consistently supporting a series of champions in the House of Representatives and the Senate, forming coalitions with nonnursing stakeholders, educating policy makers on the value of a research base for nursing practice, and taking advantage of a timely congressional moment when the policy makers needed a strong women's issue to show support for this constituency resulted in major policy support for the legislation to establish the NINR at the NIH in the mainstream of health research.

Using this example, how can the nursing profession meet the challenge of implementing the major recommendations from the series of IOM reports on quality of care? Several initiatives have been undertaken to use these recommendations in health care organizations and to change the behavior of health professionals. This is only a beginning, however. The report *Crossing the Quality Chasm: A New Health System for the 21st Century* (Institute of Medicine, 2001) calls for drastic fundamental change that is patient-centered and is led by health professionals functioning in interdisciplinary teams as a number of high-priority areas of health and illness are improved. The approach focuses on changing health care systems, such as transforming the work environment of nurses and other health professionals and building interdisciplinary educational processes and thus changing the practice of health care providers. These recommendations obviously call for fundamental change in the health care systems and the way in which health professionals are educated in this country.

Can nursing meet the challenge of implementing the IOM quality of care report recommendations, working with other disciplines? History suggests that nursing successfully has confronted this challenge before and has the knowledge and experience to do so again.

REFERENCES

Adams, K., & Corrigan, J. M. (Eds.). (2003). *Priority areas for national action: Transforming health care quality.* Quality Chasm Series. Washington, DC: National Academies Press.

American Association of Colleges of Nursing. (1995). *Interdisciplinary education and practice* [AACN position statement]. Retrieved June 21, 2005, from http://www.aacn.nche.edu/Publications/positions/interdis.htm

Fawcett, J., & Russell, G. (2001). A conceptual model of nursing and health policy. *Policy, Politics and Nursing Practice 2*(2), 108-116.

Feetham, S., & Meister, S. (1999). Nursing research of families: State of the science and correspondence with policy. In A. S. Hinshaw, S. L. Feetham, & J. L. F. Shaver (Eds.), *Handbook of clinical nursing research* (pp. 251-264). Thousand Oaks, CA: Sage Publications.

Greiner, A. C., & Knebel, E. (Eds.). (2003). *Health professions education: A bridge to quality.* Washington, DC: National Academies Press.

Guthrie, B., & Hinshaw, A. S. (2005). N295 Honors Seminar, University of Michigan, Ann Arbor, Fall 2004.

Hinshaw, A. S. (1988). Using research to shape health policy. *Nursing Outlook, 36*(1), 21-24.

Hinshaw, A. S. (2001). Shaping health policy through nursing research and scholarship. *Nursing Leadership Forum, 5*(3), 87-89.

Hinshaw, A. S. (2004). Chapter 6: Ada Sue Hinshaw. In E. Houser & K. N. Player (Eds.), *Pivotal moments in nursing: Leaders who changed the path of a profession* (pp. 105-127). Indianapolis, IN: Sigma Theta Tau International.

Institute for Healthcare Improvement. (n.d.). *Improvement report: An integrated approach to improving patient care.* Retrieved June 21, 2005, from http://www.ihi.org/IHI/Topics/ChronicConditions/AllConditions/ImprovementStories/ImprovementReportAnIntegratedApproachtoPatientCare.htm

Institute for Healthcare Improvement. (n.d.). *Patient safety/quality improvement clerkship: University of Tennessee College of Medicine.* Retrieved June 21, 2005, from http://www.ihi.org/IHI/Topics/HealthProfessionsEducation/EducationGeneral/EmergingContent/PatientSafetyQualityImprovementClerkshipUniversityofTennesseeCollegeofMedicine.htm

Institute for Healthcare Improvement. (n.d.). *Transforming care at the bedside: Sparking innovation and excitement on the hospital unit.* Retrieved June 21, 2005, from http://www.ihi.org/IHI/Topics/MedicalSurgicalCare/TransformingCare/ImprovementStories/TransformingCareattheBedsideinitiativePrototypephase.htm

Institute of Medicine. (1983). *Nursing and nursing education: Public policy and private action.* Washington, DC: National Academies Press.

Institute of Medicine. (2001). *Clearing the smoke: The science base for tobacco harm reduction.* Retrieved June 21, 2005, from http://www.iom.edu/Object.File/Master/4/145/0.pdf

Institute of Medicine. (2001). *Crossing the quality chasm: A new health system for the 21st century.* Washington, DC: National Academies Press.

Kohn, L. T., Corrigan, J. M., & Donaldson, M. S. (Eds.). (2000). *To err is human: Building a safer health system.* Washington, DC: National Academies Press.

Longest, B. B. (1996). *Seeking strategic advantage through health policy analysis.* Chicago, IL: Health Administration Press.

Mason, D. J., Leavitt, J. K., & Chaffee, M. W. (2002). *Policy and politics in nursing and health care* (4th ed.). Philadelphia: Saunders.

Milio, N. (1984). Nursing research and the study of health policy. *Annual Review of Nursing Research, 2*(3), 291-306.

Mitchell, P. H., Crittenden, R., Howard, E., Lawson, B. Z., Root, R., & Schaad, D. C. (2000). Tools and systems for improved outcomes: Interdisciplinary clinical education: Evaluating outcomes of an evolving model. *Outcomes Management for Nursing Practice, 4*(1), 3-6.

National Institutes of Health. (2001). *Health disparities research.* Retrieved June 21, 2005, from http://www.niehs.nih.gov/oc/factsheets/disparity/home.htm

National Institute on Nursing Research. (2005). *Strategic plan on reducing health disparities.* Retrieved June 21, 2005, from http://ninr.nih.gov/ninr/research/diversity/mission.html

Page, A. (Ed.). (2004). *Keeping patients safe: Transforming the work environment of nurses.* Washington, DC: National Academies Press.

Richmond, J. B., & Kotelchuck, M. L. (1983). Political influences: Rethinking national health policy. In C. H. McGuire, R. P. Foley, A. Gorr, R. W. Richards, & Associates (Eds.), *Handbook on health professions education* (pp. 386-404). San Francisco: Jossey-Bass.

Sampselle, C. M., Wyman, J. F., Thomas, K. K., Newman, D. K., Gray, M., Dougherty, M., et al. (2000). Continence for women: A test of AWHONN's evidence-based protocol in clinical practice. *JOGNN: Journal of Obstetrics, Gynecologic, & Neonatal Nursing, 29*(1), 18-26.

Shamian, J., Skelton-Green, J., & Villeneuve, M. (2003). Policy is the lever for effecting change. In M. McIntyre & E. Thomlinson (Eds.), *Realities of Canadian nursing: Professional, practice and power issues* (pp. 83-104). Philadelphia: Lippincott Williams & Wilkins.

Smedley, B. D., Stith, A. Y., & Nelson, A. R. (Eds.). (2003). *Unequal treatment: Confronting racial and ethnic disparities in healthcare.* Washington, DC: National Academies Press.

Nursing Care Priority Area

CHAPTER
32

Patient Safety

AUDREY NELSON ◆ GAIL POWELL-COPE

Murphy's Law: You can't make anything foolproof because fools are so ingenious.

M urphy's Law is meaningful when nurses think about how to make health care safer for their patients. For decades, nursing has been part of a health care system that hides mistakes, blames individuals for errors, and ignores the role of complex systems in producing errors. Nursing has a responsibility to play an active role in reshaping health care to make it safer for patients and their families. The intent of this chapter is to provide an overview of the problem of patient safety and ground it in a conceptual framework and to highlight ways that nurses can make health care safer. Evidence-based approaches are identified, including recommendations outlined in three critical patient safety reports: *To Err Is Human* (Institute of Medicine, 2000), *Crossing the Quality Chasm* (Institute of Medicine, 2001), and *Keeping Patients Safe* (Page, 2004).

BACKGROUND

The explicit purpose of health care is continually to reduce the burden of illness, injury, and disability and to improve the health and functioning of the people in the United States (Institute of Medicine, 2001, p. 6). Medical errors and preventable adverse effects jeopardize this purpose. Errors and adverse events potentiate illness or injury, delay rehabilitation, impede healing, and compromise patient safety. They also can result in deleterious effects on patient functional status and quality of life. Patients at highest risk for errors or adverse events have been identified as elderly in poor health, persons with chronic disabling conditions, and persons hospitalized for long periods (Perper, 1994).

Over the past decade, health care has undergone a significant transformation. The shift from predominantly acute, episodic care to care across the continuum for chronic conditions has changed the patient population

and length of stay significantly. Health care costs have increased substantially in large part because of the aging population, increased patient demand for new services, technologies, and drugs, as well as inefficient use of resources and medical errors. The current highly fragmented health care system is lacking in basic clinical information systems, resulting in poorly designed care processes characterized by unnecessary duplication of services and long wait times and delays. The growing complexity of science and technology, increase in chronic conditions, a poorly organized delivery system, and constraints on exploiting the revolution in information technology combine to increase the risk of errors and related adverse events. These systems failures set up individual providers to fail, regardless of how dedicated they are or how hard they try (Institute of Medicine, 2001). Nursing structures and processes as components of the health care system can pose significant barriers or can be facilitators to nursing errors depending on their design and use:

◆ Nursing processes are overly complex, requiring multiple steps and handoffs that slow down the process and decrease, rather than improve, safety. These processes waste resources, leave unaccountable gaps in coverage, result in loss of information, and fail to build on the strengths of care providers (Institute of Medicine, 2001).

◆ The relationship between nursing interventions and patient outcomes often is delayed and is less precise compared with non–health care technical systems, such as those used in aviation and nuclear power (Ternov, 2000). This makes it difficult for nurses to anticipate risk and learn from errors.

◆ Nursing care is organized within groups of registered nurses, licensed practical nurses/licensed vocational nurses, and nurses aides, each having a unique role, culture, and rules. Lines of authority are not always clear, and communication breakdowns negatively affect patient safety. Further, nurses work within interdisciplinary teams in which similar issues with lines of authority and communication arise.

◆ Patients are admitted for diverse problems; many are elderly and have multiple comorbidities, increasing risks for adverse events. The stress of an acute illness, traumatic injury, or coping with a chronic illness/disability over time can interfere with the patient's ability to adhere to treatment plans, further increasing risk for adverse events.

◆ Patients are transferred not only across care settings (e.g., from emergency room to medical intensive care to a general neurology unit and finally to long-term care) and within nursing but also across shifts, causing opportunities for errors and loss of information during these handoffs.

◆ In many health care facilities, patient safety goals have been sacrificed in favor of goals related to productivity and cost containment. Providers are expected to care for more patients, who are more acutely ill, in shorter time. These workload demands contribute to adverse events.

◆ Lengths of inpatient stays have been reduced dramatically over the past decade, transferring the risk for adverse events from the hospital setting to the home, where adverse events can go undetected and result in more serious consequences for the patient.

THEORETICAL UNDERPINNINGS OF PATIENT SAFETY

Patient safety is defined as freedom from accidental injury. Although not all errors cause injury, accidental injury can result from errors. An *error* is failure of a planned action to be completed as intended or use of a wrong plan to achieve an aim (Institute of Medicine, 2001). Errors can lead to an *adverse event,* defined as an unintentional error that results in negative consequences for the patient, including falls, fall-related injuries (e.g., hip fracture), or pressure ulcers. More than 70% of adverse events are thought to be preventable, with 24% unpreventable, and the remaining 6% viewed as potentially preventable (Leape, 1994).

Human-system interface errors, or active errors, show up immediately and are committed by providers working at the "sharp end" (Reason, 1994); that is, providers who have direct contact with patients. Nurses with direct patient care responsibilities function at the sharp end, placing them as the last line of defense in protecting the patient from harm. Because nurses and other clinicians are at this sharp end, they as individuals have been blamed for errors and mistakes. Clinicians and their actions are more visible than are underlying systems.

Blaming nurses for commission of errors is a universal, natural, emotionally satisfying, and legally convenient response. However, blaming leads to countereffective measures such as disciplinary actions, exhortations to "be more careful," or retraining. Blaming is not effective in reducing adverse events and focuses attention on the last and probably least remedial link in the accident chain—the provider (Reason, 1994). This "shame and blame" mentality continues to be pervasive in health care, but it is slowly changing. Albert Wu (2000) described this cycle of blame and victimization related to errors and adverse events in health care:

> Although patients are the first and obvious victims of medical mistakes, doctors are wounded by the same errors; they are the second victims. Nurses, pharmacists and other members of the healthcare team are also susceptible to error and vulnerable to its fallout. Given the hospital hierarchy, non-physician providers have little latitude to deal with their mistakes; they often bear silent witness to mistakes and agonize over conflicting loyalties to the patient, institution and team. They too are victims. (Wu, 2000)

Most contemporary experts view patient safety within a systems perspective. From this perspective, errors are the result of the interaction among complex systems (Perrow, 1984). Figure 32-1 depicts the framework for patient safety, explaining why adverse events occur in nursing and what can be done to reduce the incidence and severity of adverse events.

Risk Factors

Risk factors for adverse events address the underlying causes related to the *patient, provider, technology,* and *organization.* Normal accident theory posits that accidents are inevitable and the likelihood of accidents increases in organizations that exhibit complexity and tight coupling of processes (Perrow & Langton, 1994). Different sources of error interact with latent risk factors to produce accidents (Rasmussen, 1990, 1994). Latent failures are delayed-action consequences of decisions about the design, maintenance, operation, or organization taken by upper management of an organization or system. Latent failures relate to the design and construction of the environment and equipment, the structure of the organization, planning and scheduling, training and selection of staff, forecasting, information management, budgeting, and allocation of resources. These risks may

VIEWPOINTS

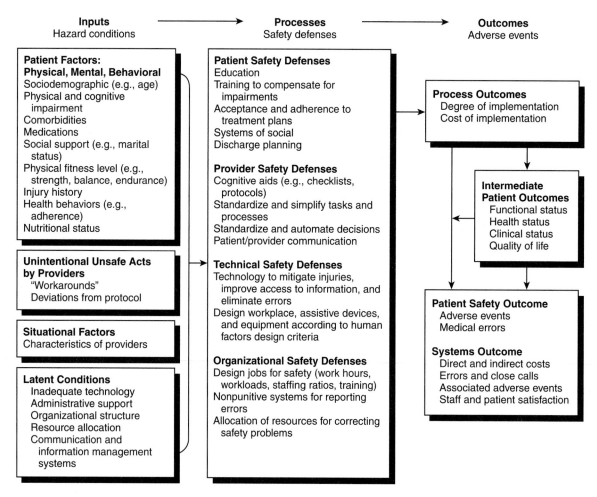

FIGURE 32-1 Conceptual framework.

lie dormant for a long time until activated by more apparent actions in the system (Bogner, 1994; Feldman & Roblin, 2000). The number of latent factors embedded in organizational systems can align and result in accidents (Reason, 1990, 1997, 2000). Moreover, the link between latent risk factors and an error is more difficult to prove compared with the more obvious link between proximal actions of a person at the sharp end of errors (Reason, 1994).

Patient Risk Factors. *Patient risk factors* can contribute to errors and subsequent adverse events. These risk factors include type and severity of illness or disability, physiological signs and symptoms, psychosocial factors (e.g., lack of compliance and depression), comorbidities, and age. Patient risk factors can facilitate or impede safety barriers and have a direct effect on situational risk factors. Understanding the epidemiology related to

adverse events in subpopulations is critical for identifying patients at high risk, designing models for predicting adverse events, designing screening tools, and for designing primary and secondary prevention strategies. For example, from research, nurses know that risk of a person falling increases dramatically as the number of risk factors increases, ranging from a probability of 0.27 with zero or one risk factor to 0.78 for those with four or more risk factors (Institute of Medicine, 2001). In one study, the probability of fractures ranged from 0 with no identified predictors to 0.129 with all six predictors present (Nguyen, Eisman, Kelly, & Sambrook, 1996). The injury susceptibility in older adults stems from a high prevalence of comorbid diseases (e.g., osteoporosis) and age-related decline (e.g., slowed reflexes), which can make even a mild fall dangerous. A multitude of risk factors for falling has been reported, including lower extremity weakness, gait and balance disorders, previous falls, functional impairment, visual deficits, cognitive impairment, depression, polypharmacy, and stroke (American Geriatrics Society, 2001; Nevitt, 1997; Rubenstein, Josephson, & Robbins, 1994; Rubenstein, Powers, & MacLean, 2001; Yates, Lai, Duncan, & Studenski, 2002). A few studies have identified specific risk factors for injurious falls (Alexander, 1996; Dargent-Molina et al., 1996; Hale, Delaney, & McGaghie, 1992; Hill, Schwartz, Flicker, & Carroll, 1999; Lord et al., 1994; Luukinen, Koski, Laippala, & Kivela, 1997; Nevitt, 1997; Nguyen, Eisman, et al., 1996; Nguyen, Sambrook, et al., 1994; Rubenstein, Josephson, et al., 1994; Tinetti, Mendes de Leon, Doucette, & Baker, 1994; Tinetti & Williams, 1998; Tromp, Smit, Deeg, Bouter, & Lips, 1998; Trueblood & Rubenstein, 1991); however, the relative contribution of each risk factor has not been determined adequately. Risk factors also can be categorized as nonmodifiable (e.g., age and gender) or modifiable. The advantage of grouping risk factors into nonmodifiable and modifiable risk factors is that it allows for the identification of clinical interventions to decrease risk, such as review and modification of risky medication regimens.

Situational Risk Factors. *Situational risk factors* are characteristics of the nurse, such as years of experience or familiarity with patient or the interactions of clinicians given the circumstances of a situation or their interaction with patients. Situational risk factors affect and are affected by patient risk factors and latent risk factors. Situational factors play an important role by triggering the dormant latent failures into activity. Cognitive sciences provide a way to identify and understand situational risk factors for adverse events. These sciences, based on a variety of disciplines—such as artificial intelligence, neuroscience, philosophy, and psychology—focus on perception, learning, memory, language, concept formation, problem solving, and thinking as factors that contribute to errors and adverse events (Bogner, 1994).

Latent Risk Factors. *Latent risk factors* are organizational structures and processes of patient care that can contribute to errors such as ineffective management (e.g., erroneous administrative decisions, inadequate staffing or scheduling, and excessive workload demands), human behavior (poorly performed procedures, lack of training), technology (e.g., outdated equipment and negligent maintenance), and physical environment (e.g., physical barriers that limit access to the environment for a person with a disability) (Wagenaar, Hudson, & Reason, 1990). These factors may have a delayed impact on how well the system resists errors, prevents adverse events, or mitigates injuries to the patient (Feldman & Roblin, 1997).

For example, managers and administrators, who have no direct contact with patients, can create dilemmas and shape trade-offs among competing goals for persons at the sharp end of clinical practice. The competing organizational goals of patient safety usually focus on productivity, cost, and service (Cook & Woods, 1994). A pattern to accidents in complex systems includes one or more latent risk factors that caused the adverse event. Latent risk factors act as error traps; they impede problem solving or delay error detection. In the case of falls, the physical environment plays a role in predisposing a person to falling. Research has shown, for example, that indoor falls and fractures are more common than those occurring outdoors in home-dwelling elders (Luukinen, Herala, et al., 2000). Additionally, self-perceived safety of residence was linked to hip fracture (Haentjens, Autir, & Boonen, 2002), and change in residence was linked to recurrent falls (Luukinen, Koski, Kivela, & Laippala, 1996).

Safety Barriers

High reliability theory posits that accidents can be prevented through organizational design and management decisions and actions (Bigley & Roberts, 2001; Roberts & Rousseau, 1989). General systems theory posits that the entity under examination, such as a hospital unit, is defined as a system with interrelated subsystems (Bogner, 1994). Safety barriers are forces that intervene to prevent an active failure from progressing to an error with a bad outcome, or they can be planned interventions that target identified risk factors, thus reducing the likelihood of an adverse event. Flaws in the system safety barriers almost always can be demonstrated; however, interventions to prevent adverse events involve designs to create or strengthen safety defense barriers. These interventions can be directed toward the patient, provider, technology, or the organization. Safety barriers can be weak or strong, multidimensional or focused, and can involve ability to absorb the effect of or prevent active failures.

Patient Safety Defenses. *Patient safety defenses* are aimed at changing modifiable patient risk factors through psychoeducational efforts ultimately to reduce the occurrence and severity of adverse events. For example, several studies are demonstrating the health benefits of tai chi, particularly for older adults. Wang, Collet, and Lau (2004), in a systematic review of reports on the physical and psychological effects of tai chi on various medical conditions, found benefits in balance and strength, cardiovascular function, flexibility, immune system, symptoms of arthritis, muscular strength, and psychological effects. Seven clinical trials (two randomized and five nonrandomized) reported significantly improved balance, flexibility, and strength of knee extension, and reduced occurrence of falling in community-dwelling elders. Unfortunately, many of the studies lacked comparison groups and lacked detailed information for evaluating the validity of the studies. Patient-focused strategies are supported by a range of social psychological theories such as social learning theory (Bandura, 1986), transtheoretical model of change (Prochaska, 1997), and theory of planned behavior (Madden, Ellen, & Ajzen, 1992).

Provider Safety Defenses. *Provider safety defenses* focus on overcoming human limitations imposed by memory, practice variations, complex processes, and provider-patient communication. Examples include clinical tools such as standardized protocols, clinical practice guidelines, and simplifying complex processes. Recently, the Veterans Health Administration National Center for Patient Safety released a falls toolkit for reducing practice variation and improving falls prevention in outpatient settings. The toolkit includes tools for clinicians such as screening tools, guidelines for functional assessment, and patient education videos on falls prevention and the use of hip protectors, which when used should facilitate prompt identification of individuals at risk and effective strategies for patient evaluation and treatment to reduce risk (toolkit available at http://www.patientsafetycenter.com). Provider safety defenses are supported by diffusion theory that addresses the spread of new knowledge or innovation to a defined population, over time, through specific channels (Rohrbach, Graham, & Hansen, 1993) and multidimensional models for implementing evidence-based practice (Grimshaw et al., 2001a, 2001b; Grol, 1997; Grol & Grimshaw, 1999).

Technology Safety Defenses. *Technology safety defenses* focus on overcoming technology limitations imposed by equipment or lack of proper equipment. For example, our research has shown that if nurses are provided with accessible lifting equipment, they are much more likely to use it. In the case of falls, hip protectors are showing promise to prevent hip fractures by shunting the energy of a fall away from the greater trochanter or absorbing the impact, thereby protecting the greater trochanter from fracturing (Kannus et al., 2000; Rubenstein, 2000). Evidence supports the use of hip protectors to prevent hip fractures, if they are worn at the time of fall (Becker, Walter-Jung, & Nikolaus, 2000; Cameron, 2002; Parkkari, Heikkila, & Kannus, 1998). A human factors perspective based on ergonomics, applied experimental psychology, and human factors engineering supports finding ways in which human performance can be improved, thus reducing adverse events, by focusing on the interface between human beings and machines (Bogner, 1994). Effective implementation of technology is not always an intuitive process. Individuals must have the knowledge and skills to use technology safely or it could pose additional safety risks.

Organizational Safety Defenses. *Organizational safety defenses* are aimed at changing organizational structures and processes that contribute to adverse events. Recent research suggests that the number of registered nurse hours and the proportion of care provided by registered nurses are linked to adverse events in acute care, such as urinary track infections, gastrointestinal bleeding, pneumonia, shock or cardiac arrest, and "failure to rescue," defined as death from pneumonia, shock or cardiac arrest, upper gastrointestinal bleeding, sepsis, or deep venous thrombosis in medical patients. In surgical patients, registered nurse staffing variables were linked to urinary tract infections and failure to rescue (Needleman, Buerhaus, Mattke, Stewart, & Zelevinsky, 2002). Aiken, Clarke, Sloane, Sochalski, and Silber (2002) found that in hospitals with high patient-to-nurse ratios, surgical patients experienced higher risk-adjusted 30-day mortality and failure-to-rescue rates. Moreover, patient-to-nurse staffing ratios were linked to burnout and job dissatisfaction.

Outcomes

As with other conceptual models of health conditions, outcomes can include process and intermediate and long-term outcomes. Process evaluation assists in determining how and why the safety barrier resulted in the intermediate and ultimate outcomes. Process evaluation contributes to determining external validity and thus the reproducibility and application of findings of research to other settings and populations, the understanding of causal mechanisms and thus theory building, and the building of more efficient interventions (Sidani & Braden, 1998). Much clinical research has been limited because nurses do not understand the mechanisms of interventions and how interventions affect outcomes. Intermediate outcomes represent the more direct impact of interventions on patients, providers, and organizations compared with ultimate outcomes that are markers of effectiveness and the more traditional health services outcomes such as quality and cost. In the case of nurses, nurses ultimately are concerned with improving quality of care by decreasing adverse events and injuries associated with adverse events, improving the work environment and retaining a high-quality and productive workforce, and in developing high-performing organizations that embrace a positive culture of safety.

CHARACTERISTICS OF ENVIRONMENTS THAT PROMOTE PATIENT SAFETY

Creating a culture of safety is a necessary step toward patient safety. No universally agreed upon definition of a safety culture exists, yet many have written on the topic and describe attributes of a positive culture of safety. These attributes include leadership that allocates resources for improving safety, public leadership support for reducing errors and improving patient safety, reporting systems that are nonpunitive (Weeks & Bagian, 2000), systems in which nurses learn from mistakes (Marx, 2001), accountability at all levels of an organization (O'Hara, 2001), and open communications about errors (Manasse, Turnbull, & Diamond, 2002). Turning to the anthropological literature, two anthropologists examined more than 150 definitions of culture and stated that "Culture is explicit and implicit patterns of behavior that are acquired and transmitted by symbols created by humans, including their embodiments in artifacts. The essential core of culture consists of traditional ideas and their attached values. Culture is a product of action, and a condition of further action" (Kroeber & Kluckhorn, 1952). This definition implies that culture is multifaceted and includes behaviors, attitudes, values, artifacts (e.g., health care technology and equipment), language, social interaction (e.g., communication), social organization (e.g., the structures of hospitals and health care workforce, policies, and roles of individuals in the organization), and material life (e.g., how resources and funding are allocated to safety initiatives). Implied in this definition is that a culture of safety is learned and therefore can be changed.

Two key characteristics of environments promote patient safety: seamlessness and transparency. *Seamlessness* is defined as promoting interdependent persons and technologies to perform as a unified whole, especially at points of transition between and among nurses and other health care providers, across sites of care, and over time (Institute of Medicine, 2001, p. 45). Handoffs that occur when there is a transfer of care for a patient from one person or group to another is a work process known to compromise patient safety (Institute of Medicine, 2001, pp. 11-12). Failure to communicate important clinical information or the communication of misinformation during handoffs has been implicated in communication breakdowns potentially leading to adverse events. Handoffs most commonly affect nurses because

shift reports occur during the transfer of patient care responsibilities between nurses when one group ends its work shift and another group begins. As handoffs, nursing shift reports are a source of error because they create opportunities for gaps in the continuity of patient care through loss of information or interruptions in care delivery (Cook, Render, & Woods, 2000; Institute of Medicine, 2004). Handoffs are recognized as high-risk work processes because they occur on every acute care unit 3 times per day in all health care settings and have a high probability of error because of interruptions, high environmental noise levels, interaction among multiple nurses, poorly designed work stations, and the transmission of large amounts of information critical to patient care (Ferraco & Spath, 2000). Despite the fact that every inpatient unit uses nursing shift reports, there is no standard evidence-based process (e.g., face-to-face, audiotape recorded, or walking rounds) or content (e.g., overview of patient status or problem focus). *Transparency* is defined as being visible to outsiders, with no attempt to conceal (Institute of Medicine, 2001, p. 45). Transparent organizations foster confidential care but make great efforts never to keep a secret from the patient. Nurses have a critical role in developing delivery systems that foster seamlessness and transparency.

Fostering patient safety is a laudable goal. Efforts to create nursing environments that promote patient safety include one of five proactive approaches in the way nursing care delivery is designed (Reason, 1997, p. 125; Spath, 2000a, p. xxvii). Nursing care delivery systems should be designed to do the following:

1. Eliminate errors
2. Reduce the numbers of errors
3. Catch errors before harm occurs, eliminating injuries
4. Contain errors to mitigate adverse outcomes associated with errors
5. Review errors and learn from them (Spath, 2000b; Box 32-1)

CHALLENGES IN CREATING FAIL-SAFE WORK ENVIRONMENTS FOR NURSES

Creating reliable environments that promote patient safety is challenging, particularly in health care settings where nurses work. Health care environments are complex, with thousands of error-prone patient care processes that need to be evaluated and redesigned. Once a reliable system is designed, any one of a number of things can happen to sabotage efforts; for example, nursing turnover, new equipment, short staffing, or some other factor could get in the way of providing safe patient care.

BOX 32-1

Approaches to Create Fail-Safe Nursing Environments

- *Eliminate errors:* You can eliminate some errors completely through "forcing functions" that only allow you to perform the task safely. For example, the size and fitting at the end of a tube will prevent you from inserting it in the wrong outlet.
- *Reduce the numbers of errors:* It is not always possible to eliminate errors, so the goal may be to decrease the number of errors by adding backup functions. For example, two persons need to check to see that the patient receives the right blood. Another strategy might be to have IVs mixed centrally instead of on the unit where interruptions and distractions could contribute to errors.
- *Catch errors before harm occurs:* Because not all errors can be prevented, it is wise to develop strategies to detect errors before an injury occurs. For example, protocols that require nurses to monitor vital signs every 15 minutes after certain drugs are administered are a way to detect problems before serious adverse events occur.
- *Contain errors to mitigate error-related adverse outcomes:* You can reduce the severity of error-related injuries by designing protocols for timely and effective responses once an error has been discovered. For example, if the wrong eye drops are administered, quickly flushing the eyes could prevent serious harm.
- *Review errors and learn from them:* Recognizing that errors are inevitable, creating a work culture that encourages nurses to report and talk about errors can create a learning environment that prevents others from making the same mistake or allows others to design a solution so that the error is not repeated.

Modified from Spath, P. L. (2000). Reducing errors through work system improvements. In P. L. Spath (Ed.), *Error reduction in health care* (pp. 199-234). San Francisco: Jossey-Bass.

The following are some of the challenges:

1. Historically, the discipline of nursing has tended to emphasize the individual as the target of care activities. Creating a positive culture of safety, however, requires nurses to view patient care as a complex undertaking that occurs within complex systems of care. Continued efforts to focus on the individual patient may be counterproductive to a systems approach to ensure safe and reliable care.

2. Nurses also try hard to work within the limited resources they have available. Nurses are notorious for work-arounds; that is, shortcuts that avoid technology or other systems that were designed for safety. For example, bar code medication administration was implemented in the Veterans Administration and lauded for the potential to reduce medication errors significantly. However, when the equipment is not working or is cumbersome, nurses will find ways to circumvent it. For example, the process for bar code medication administration requires that the nurse locate the patient and scan the identification band. Scanning the band allows the nurse to access the patient's medication drawer, and the medications scanned must match the patient identification. However, nurses found that scanning the identification bracelets was difficult because the scanner was connected to the medication cart with a wire, and often they could not maneuver the cart close enough

to the bedside to reach the identification bracelet with the scanner. As a work-around, nurses made duplicate identification bands for all patients, attached them with a ring, and kept them on the medication cart. This way, the nurse could scan the identification at the medication cart without ever having to check the identification bracelet on the patient, thus opening up a situation for an error to occur by scanning the wrong bracelet for the wrong patient.

3. In nursing the direct link between a nursing action and the patient outcome is rarely clear or precise (Ternov, 2000). For this reason, it is more difficult to isolate unsafe practices and more challenging to redesign work (because which approach is best is not always evident). The evidence base for nursing practice is growing, but so are technological advances and changes in the way health care is delivered. For this reason, no clear agreement exists on precise approaches for safe nursing practice.

4. Although nursing care is critical and can contribute to life and death, nursing practice often relies on outmoded systems of work. Most hospitals do not have access to technologies to promote patient safety. Solutions such as electronic medical records, computerized order entry, bar code medication administration, ceiling-mounted patient lifts, and other devices are commercially available to promote safer work environments, but few hospitals purchase

these devices. Nurses performing in these technology-deprived systems are "set up to fail," regardless of how hard they try or how dedicated they are (Institute of Medicine, 2001, p. 4).

Many approaches to building a safe working environment seem counterintuitive and contradict the professional belief systems of nursing. Redesigning nursing practice is not easy because nursing care delivery is complex. Systematic implementation of sophisticated new technologies, powerful new drugs, or new nursing procedures poses a significant challenge. Add the unique combination of diverse patients, multiple processes, organizational goals stressing "do more with less," and interdisciplinary teams, and one has a human factors engineering nightmare (Spath, 2000a, p. xxvii).

Change is never easy, and the resistance should not be underestimated when one is redesigning nursing practice to promote patient safety. Barriers to change include individual beliefs about roles, professional cultural values, and organization culture that discourage nurses from collaborating freely in shaping an organizational culture that firmly supports systems to identify and reduce errors and preventable adverse events (Jones, 2002).

RECOMMENDATIONS

Patient safety defenses include processes or structures to reduce the risk of adverse events related to exposure to medical care across a range of diagnoses or conditions (Shojania, Duncan, McDonald, Wachter, & Markowitz, 2001). So where to start? The Institute of Medicine (2001) identified six areas to enhance patient safety:

1. Design care processes that more effectively address the needs of chronically ill patients: coordinate seamless care across settings and clinicians and over time.
2. Make effective use of information technologies to automate clinical information.
3. Enhance the knowledge base and competencies of providers.
4. Improve coordination of care across patient conditions, services, and settings, over time.
5. Promote the effectiveness of health care teams.
6. Incorporate process and outcome measures into daily work.

A high-risk process is defined as any health care delivery activity that (1) has a high probability of error, (2) occurs with sufficient frequency, and (3) would result in severe patient injury if an error were made (Ferraco & Spath, 2000, pp. 17-95). Examples of high-risk processes are the following:

◆ Diagnostic and therapeutic decision making
◆ Patient assessment/observation
◆ Transfer of patient care responsibilities between caregivers and facilities (handoffs)
◆ Communication (among nursing staff, between nurses and other health care providers, and between caregivers and patients)
◆ Monitoring of patients during and immediately following high-risk interventions (e.g., restraints)
◆ Medication administration (prescribing, preparing, dispensing) and monitoring the effects of the medication

Efforts to redesign nursing care delivery systems should focus on eliminating or reducing errors, mitigating the effect of errors by catching them quickly so as to eliminate or reduce injuries associated with errors, and creating systems to review errors and learn from them (Reason, 1997, p. 125; Spath, 2000a, p. xxvii). General work system improvement principles have been delineated for enhancing patient safety and are included in Box 32-2. Box 32-3 describes examples of redesign efforts that use the foregoing principles.

SUMMARY

Nursing practice does not occur in a vacuum. Nursing is a complex endeavor embedded within complex organizations and systems of care. To promote patient safety, all disciplines must work together to redesign care processes most fraught with human error or those likely to cause injurious adverse events. Nursing can and should take the lead in preventing nurse-sensitive adverse events, such as iatrogenic pressure ulcers, patient falls, elopements, and pain.

A major barrier to improving patient safety is budgetary constraints and an organizational emphasis on productivity. Even where budget is not a major concern, recruitment and retention of qualified nurses is a limitation. In this context, it is difficult to conceptualize how to spend more time and money on safety. To be successful, policies with financial incentives are needed in health care.

Nursing should declare the promotion of patient safety a serious goal with creative operational plans and clearly defined executive responsibility. Now is the time to progress away from the "shame and blame" mentality, away from the retrospective review of errors, and away from the feeling of powerlessness to change work systems.

BOX 32-2

Work System Improvement Principles for Enhancing Patient Safety

Simplify the process; reduce handoffs. Streamline the number of steps; for example, use hospital-wide transfer templates when transferring patients from critical care to step-down or general units.

Reduce reliance on memory. Use checklists, protocols, clinical pathways, preprinted physician orders, and computerized decision aids.

Standardize. Reduce unnecessary variation in practice; for example, implement clinical practice guidelines that address patient problems commonly encountered by nurses, such as pain, pressure ulcers, and falls.

Improve information access. Ensure that all staff have good information; for example, mark the right leg to avoid wrong site surgery.

Design for errors. Design to detect errors and correct them; for example, institute double checks for high-risk processes such as blood or insulin administration.

Adjust work schedules. Reduce workload and fatigue that impairs decision-making abilities.

Adjust the environment. Reduce/eliminate noise, poor lighting, glare-producing surfaces, clutter, electrical interference, humidity, and moisture; consider layout, equipment, supplies, and procedures in workplace design, such as wheelchair locks, repositioning of call lights, and raised toilet seats to decrease falls.

Improve communication. Avoid indirect communication, and decrease the number of communications per task; for example, a policy that prohibits verbal orders for medications.

Decrease reliance on vigilance. Involve family and patient.

Provide adequate safety training. Make staff are aware of hazards relevant to their jobs and the strategies to avoid them.

Choose the right staff for the job. Ensure staff have the ability and competencies necessary to perform their jobs; ensure that staff have adequate resources; for example, rapid deployment of competent personnel when labor-intensive events occur.

Automate. Acquire computerized order entry, access to patient information, clinical decision support, and expert systems. Automation works best when it pauses when an error is detected.

Modified from Spath, P. L. (2000). Reducing errors through work system improvements. In P. L. Spath (Ed.), *Error reduction in health care* (pp. 199-234). San Francisco: Jossey-Bass.

BOX 32-3

Efforts to Enhance Patient Safety

- Develop computer-aided decision support tools to assist nurses and patients in applying research to practice in real time.
- Design jobs for safety, addressing issues related to fatigue, job stress, workload, staffing ratios, training, and constant sources of distraction.
- Avoid having nurses rely on memory and vigilance; rather, use reminder systems, checklists, protocols, and color coding while eliminating look-alike/sound-alike products.
- Promote use of electronic medical record or some version of automated clinical data.
- Standardize and automate certain decisions; for example, use of fall risk assessment tools and fall precaution protocols.
- Reduce the number of patient handoffs and unnecessary transfers of patients.[1,2]
- Design strategies to enhance communication between and among nurses at all levels, patients, and other health care providers.
- Nurses have little control over their workload, and this problem is exacerbated by nursing shortages. This environment creates safety risks for patients because nursing ability to monitor, conduct surveillance, and rescue is diminished. Two ways to redesign the hospital system to match staffing and workload demands are (1) system redesign to increase nurses' control of their workload and (2) development of systems for rapid deployment of staff when workload swells. One documented example of how nurses took control of patient flow in emergency rooms and intensive care units was shown to improve access to care, optimize

Continued

BOX 32-3

Efforts to Enhance Patient Safety—cont'd

patient outcomes by enabling timely diagnostic and therapeutic interventions, and decrease wasting of resources.[3] Another example is the traffic light approach, by which nurses are empowered to accept, delay, or prevent a transfer or admission to their units with a red, yellow, or green light system.[4]

- Design nursing care delivery systems that build in redundancies or backup plans. For example, what happens if the wound care specialist is off? When using electronic medical records, how do you access laboratory data or document patient care if the computer system is down?

- Develop a proactive system for evaluating root causes of errors and adverse events, also known as anticipatory failure analyses. Examples include Hazop (hazard and operability study), FMEA (failure mode and effect analysis), HACCP (hazard analysis and critical control point), and FTA (fault tree analysis).[5]

- Differentiate the need for specification/standardization versus customization in patient care. Generally, situations lacking certainty and clinical agreement require customization, whereas situations with clear science should be standardized.[6] For example, standardize data displays so that all are expressed in the same units, consistently locate off/on switches, and consistently locate supplies. Overspecification can result in too many handoffs, unnecessary steps, and a lack of ability to customize. A useful engineering principle is to "design for usual but be prepared for unusual."

- Color-code supplies to decrease errors.

- Use smart cards for storage of patient medical records in a wallet-size card with embedded chips that can be accessed with a card reader. A CD-ROM can be used to store patient information such as digital images of radiographs. This decreases the likelihood of errors when admitting a patient and can reduce repetition of tests.

- Redesign procedures, job designs, equipment, communication, and information technology to respect human factors and to decrease the stress associated with nursing practice. For example, put electrical outlets at waist height and use fast electric beds, ceiling-mounted patient lifts, and ergonomically sound computer stations and chairs.

- Support a culture of safety that permeates all aspects of the organization. For example, if you are supervisor, do not blame an individual nurse for an error but commit to examining the system that allowed the error and correcting the system errors so that the error does not happen again. A culture of safety includes (1) strong, clear, and visible attention to safety, (2) nonpunitive systems for reporting errors, (3) incorporation of safety principles, such as standardization and simplification, (4) team training, and (5) transparency in communicating errors to patients.

- Mitigate harm from errors, have antidotes and up-to-date information available, equipment designed to default to least harmful mode, and teams trained in crisis response, not only for cardiopulmonary resuscitation but also for management of disturbed behavior, elopement management for elderly confused patients, and management of other high-risk patient crises.

[1]Leape, L. (1994). Error in medicine. *JAMA: The Journal of the American Medical Association, 272*(23), 4.
[2]Cook, R. I., and Woods, D. D. (1994). Operating at the sharp end: The complexity of human error. In M. S. Bogner (Ed.), *Human error in medicine* (pp. 255-310). Hinsdale, NJ: Lawrence Erlbaum.
[3]Rozich, J. D., & Resar, R. K. (2002). Using a unit assessment tool to optimize patient flow and staffing in a community hospital. *Journal on Quality Improvement, 28*(1), 31-41.
[4]Institute for Healthcare Improvement Hospital Flow Strategy Team presentation in Boston, January 2002, cited in Rozich, J. D., & Resar, R. K. (2002). Using a unit assessment tool to optimize patient flow and staffing in a community hospital. *Journal on Quality Improvement, 28*(1), 31-41.
[5]Feldman, S. E., & Roblin, D. W. (2000). Accident investigation and anticipatory failure analysis in hospitals. In P. L. Spath (Ed.), *Error reduction in health care* (pp. 139-154). San Francisco: Jossey-Bass.
[6]Institute of Medicine. (2001). *Crossing the quality chasm* (p. 64). Washington, DC: National Academies Press.

Nurses need to move toward a culture of safety and prospective evaluation of hazardous conditions to redesign nursing care delivery systems to fix underlying system problems to prevent future occurrences. Nurses need proactive approaches for monitoring and analyzing high-risk nursing tasks and processes to identify where additional safeguards are needed to reduce the likelihood of errors or adverse events (Spath, 2000a, p. xxv).

In summary, it is time to take action. Patient safety is not free, but costs will vary. Many high-risk nursing tasks can be redesigned with little or no cost, whereas some of the technological solutions will require substantial fiscal resources. The benefits of work redesign to promote patient safety are significant and likely to result in other advantages related to improvements in nurse recruitment/retention, quality of care, patient satisfaction, and potential cost savings.

REFERENCES

Aiken, L. H., Clarke, S. P., Sloane, D. M., Sochalski, J., & Silber, J. H. (2002). Hospital nurse staffing and patient mortality, nurse burnout, and job dissatisfaction. *JAMA: The Journal of the American Medical Association, 228*(16), 1987-1993.

Alexander, N. B. (1996). Gait disorders in older adults. *Journal of the American Geriatric Society, 44*(4), 434-451.

American Geriatrics Society. (2001). Guideline for the prevention of falls in older persons. American Geriatrics Society, British Geriatrics Society and American Academy of Orthopedic Surgeons panel on falls prevention. *Journal of the American Geriatrics Association, 49*(5), 664-672.

Bandura, A. (1986). *Social foundations of thought and action.* Englewood Cliffs, NJ: Prentice Hall.

Becker, C., Walter-Jung, B., & Nikolaus, T. (2000). The other side of hip protectors. *Age and Aging, 29*(2), 186.

Bigley, G. A., & Roberts, K. H. (2001). Structuring temporary systems for high reliability. *Academy of Management Journal, 44*, 1281-1300.

Bogner, M. S. (1994). Introduction. In M. S. Bogner (Ed.), *Human error in medicine* (pp. 1-11). Hillsdale, NJ: Lawrence Erlbaum Associates.

Cameron, I. (2002). Hip protectors: Prevent fractures but adherence is a problem. *BMJ, 324*(7334), 375-376.

Cook, R., Render, M., & Woods, D. (2000). Gaps in the continuity of care and progress on patient safety. *British Medical Journal, 320*(7237), 791-794.

Cook, R. I., & Woods, D. D. (1994). Operating at the sharp end: The complexity of human error. In M. S. Bogner (Ed.), *Human error in medicine* (pp. 255-310). Hillsdale, NJ: Lawrence Erlbaum Associates.

Dargent-Molina, P., Favier, F., Grandjean, H., Baudoin, C., Achott, A. M., Hausherr, E., et al. (1996). Fall-related factors and risk of hip fracture: The EDIPOS prospective study. *Lancet, 348*(9021), 145-149.

Feldman, S. E., & Roblin, D. W. (1997). Medical accidents in hospital care: Applications of failure analysis to hospital quality appraisal. *Joint Commission Journal on Quality Improvement, 23*(11), 569.

Feldman, S., & Roblin, D. (2000). Accident investigation and anticipatory failure analysis in hospitals. In P. L. Spath (Ed.), *Error Reduction in Health Care* (pp. 139-154). San Francisco: Jossey-Bass.

Ferraco, K., & Spath, P. L. (2000). Measuring performance on high risk processes. In P. L. Spath (Ed.), *Error reduction in health care* (pp. 17-95). San Francisco: Jossey-Bass.

Grimshaw, J., Shirran, L., Thomas, R., Mowatt, G., Fraser, C., Bero, L., et al. (2001a). Changing provider behavior: An overview of systematic reviews of interventions. *Medical Care, 39*(8, Suppl. 2), II-2–II-45.

Grimshaw, J., Shirran, L., Thomas, R., Mowatt, G., Fraser, C., Bero, L., et al. (2001b). Changing provider behavior: An overview of systematic reviews of interventions to promote implementation of research findings by healthcare professionals. In A. Haines & C. Silagy (Eds.), *Evidence based practice in primary health care.* London, United Kingdom: BMJ Books.

Grol, R. (1997). Beliefs and evidence in changing clinical practice. *British Medical Journal, 315*(7105), 418-421.

Grol, R., & Grimshaw, J. (1999). Evidence-based implementation of evidence-based medicine. *Journal of Quality Improvement, 25*(10), 503-512.

Haentjens, P., Autir, L., & Boonen, S. (2002). Clinical risk factors for hip fracture in elderly women: A case-control study. *Journal of Orthopaedic Trauma, 16*(6), 379-385.

Hale, W. A., Delaney, M. J., & McGaghie, W. C. (1992). Characteristics and predictors of falls in elderly patients. *Journal of Family Practice, 34*(5), 577-581.

Hill, K., Schwartz, J., Flicker, L., & Carroll, S. (1999). Falls among healthy, community-dwelling older women: a prospective study of frequency, circumstances, consequences and prediction accuracy. *Australian & New Zealand Journal of Public Health, 23*(1), 41-48.

Institute of Medicine. (2000). *To err is human: Building a safer health system.* Washington: National Academies Press.

Institute of Medicine. (2001). *Crossing the quality chasm.* Washington, DC: National Academies Press.

Institute of Medicine. (2004). *Keeping patients safe: Transforming the work environment of nurses.* Washington, DC: National Academies Press.

Jones, B. (2002). Nurses and the code of silence. In M. Rosenthal & K. Sutcliffe (Eds.), *Medical error* (pp. 84-100). San Francisco: Jossey-Bass.

Kannus, P., Parkkari, J., Niemi, S., Pasanen, M., Palvannen, M., Jarvinen, M., et al. (2000). Prevention of hip fractures in elderly people with the use of a hip protector. *New England Journal of Medicine, 343*(21), 1506-1513.

Kroeber, A. L., & Kluckhorn, C. (1952). *Culture: A critical review of concepts and definitions.* Cambridge, MA: Harvard University.

Leape, L. L. (1994). The preventability of medical injury. In M. S. Bogner (Ed.), *Human error in medicine* (pp. 13-26). Hillsdale, NJ: Lawrence Erlbaum Associates.

Lord, S. R., Sambrook, P. N., Gilbert, C., Kelly, P. J., Nguyen, T., Webster, I. W., et al. (1994). Postural stability, falls, and fractures in the elderly: Results from the Dubbo Osteoporosis Epidemiology Study. *Medical Journal of Australia, 160*(11), 684-685.

Luukinen, H., Herala, M., Koski, K., Honkanen, R., Laippala, P., & Kivela, S. L. (2000). Fracture risk associated with a fall according to type of fall among the elderly. *Osteoporosis International, 11*(7), 631-634.

Luukinen, H., Koski, K., Kivela, S. L., & Laippala, P. (1996). Social status, life changes, housing conditions, health, functional abilities and life-style as risk factors for recurrent falls among the home-dwelling elderly. *Public Health, 110*(2), 115-118.

Luukinen, H., Koski, K., Laippala, P., & Kivela, S. L. (1997). Factors predicting fractures during falling impacts among community-dwelling older adults. *Journal of the American Geriatrics Society, 45*(11), 1302-1309.

Madden, T., Ellen, P., & Ajzen, I. (1992). A comparison of the theory of planned behavior and the theory of reasoned action. *Personality and Social Psychology Bulletin, 18*(1), 3-9.

Manasse, H. R., Turnbull, J. E., & Diamond, L. H. (2002). Patient safety: Review of the contemporary American experience. *Singapore Medical Journal, 43*(5), 254-262.

Marx, D. (2001). *Patient safety and the "just culture": A primer for health care executives.* Unpublished manuscript, the Trustees of Columbia University, New York.

Needleman, J., Buerhaus, P., Mattke, S., Stewart, M., & Zelevinsky, K. (2002). Nurse-staffing levels and the quality of care in hospitals. *New England Journal of Medicine, 346*(22), 1715-1722.

Nevitt, M. C. (1997). Falls in the elderly: risk factors and prevention. In J. C. Masdeu, L. Sudarsky, & L. Wolfson (Eds.), *Gait disorders in aging*. Philadelphia: Lippincott-Raven.

Nguyen, T. V., Eisman, J. A., Kelly, P. J., & Sambrook, P. N. (1996). Risk factors for osteoporotic fractures in elderly men. *American Journal of Epidemiology, 144*(3), 255-263.

Nguyen, T., Sambrook, P., Kelly, P., Jones, G., Lord, S., Freund, J., et al. (1994). Prediction of osteoporotic fractures by postural instability and bone density. *British Medical Journal, 308*, 274-275.

O'Hara, P. (2001). *Nuclear safety culture: An organizational development model*. Unpublished manuscript.

Page, A. (Ed.). (2004). *Keeping patients safe: Transforming the work environment of nurses*. Washington: National Academies Press.

Parkkari, J., Heikkila, J., & Kannus, P. (1998). Acceptability and compliance with wearing energy-shunting hip protectors: a 6-month prospective follow-up in a Finnish nursing home. *Age and Aging, 27*, 225-229.

Perper, J. A. (1994). Life-threatening and fatal therapeutic misadventures. In M. S. Bogner (Ed.), *Human error in medicine* (pp. 27-52). Hillsdale, NJ: Lawrence Erlbaum Associates.

Perrow, C. (1984). *Normal accidents: Living with high risk technologies*. New York: Basic Books.

Perrow, C., & Langton, J. (1994). The limits of safety: The enhancement of a theory of accidents. *Journal of Contingency Management, 2*, 212-220.

Prochaska, J. O., Redding, C. A., & Evers, K. E. (1997). The transtheoretical model and stages of change. In K.Glanz, F. M. Lewis, & B. K. Rimer (Eds.), Health Behavior and Health Education (2nd ed., pp. 60-84). San Francisco: Jossey-Bass Publishers.

Rasmussen, J. (1990). Human error and the problem of causality in analysis of accidents. *Philosophical Transactions of the Royal Society of London Series B: Biological Science, 327*(1241), 449-460.

Rasmussen, J. (1994). Afterword. In M. S. Bogner (Ed.), *Human error in medicine* (pp. 385-393). Hillsdale, NJ: Lawrence Erlbaum Associates.

Reason, J. T. (1990). *Human error*. New York: Cambridge University Press.

Reason, J. T. (1994). Forward. In M. S. Bogner (Ed.), *Human error in medicine*. Hillsdale, NJ: Lawrence Erlbaum Associates.

Reason, J. (1997). *Managing the risks of organizational accidents* (p. 125). Brookfield, VT: Ashgate.

Reason, J. T. (2000). Human error: Models and management. *British Medical Journal, 320*, 768-770.

Roberts, K. H., & Rousseau, D. M. (1989). Research in nearly failure-free, high reliability systems: Having the bubble. *IEEE Transactions on Engineering Management, 36*(2), 132-139.

Rohrbach, L. A., Graham, J. W., & Hansen, W. B. (1993). Diffusion of a school-based substance abuse prevention program: Predictors of program implementation. *Preventive Medicine, 22*(2), 237-260.

Rubenstein, L. (2000). Hip protectors: a breakthrough in fracture prevention. *New England Journal of Medicine, 343*(21), 1562-1563.

Rubenstein, L. Z., Josephson, K. R., & Robbins, A. S. (1994). Falls in the nursing home. *Annals of Internal Medicine, 121*(6), 442-451.

Rubenstein, L. Z., Powers, C. M., & MacLean, C. H. (2001). Quality indicators for the management and prevention of falls and mobility problems in vulnerable elders. *Annals of Internal Medicine, 135*(8, Pt. 2), 686-693.

Shojania, K. G., Duncan, B. W., McDonald, K. M., Wachter, R. M., & Markowitz, A. J. (Eds). (2001). *Making health care safer: A critical analysis of patient safety practices.* (Evidence Report/Technology Assessment No. 43, AHRQ Pub. No. 01-E058). Rockville, MD: Agency for Healthcare Research and Quality.

Sidani, S., & Braden, C. (1998). *Evaluating nursing interventions: A theory-driven approach.* Thousand Oaks, CA: Sage Publications.

Spath, P. L. (Ed.). (2000a). *Error reduction in health care* (p. xxvii). San Francisco: Jossey-Bass.

Spath, P. L. (2000b). Reducing errors through work system improvements. In P. L. Spath (Ed.), *Error reduction in health care* (pp. 199-234). San Francisco: Jossey-Bass.

Ternov, S. (2000). The human side of medical mistakes. In P. L. Spath (Ed.), *Error reduction in health care* (pp. 109-110). San Francisco: Jossey-Bass.

Tinetti, M. E., Mendes de Leon, C. F., Doucette, J. T., & Baker, D. I. (1994). Fear of falling and fall-related efficacy in relationship to functioning among community living elders. *Journal of Gerontology, 49*(3), M140-M147.

Tinetti, M. E., & Williams, C. S. (1998). The effect of falls and fall injuries on functioning in community-dwelling older persons. *Journal of Gerontology: Medical Sciences, 53*(2), M112-M119.

Tromp, A. M., Smit, J. H., Deeg, D. J., Bouter, L. M., & Lips, P. (1998). Predictors for falls and fractures in the

Longitudinal Aging Study Amsterdam. *Journal of Bone and Mineral Research, 13*(12), 1932-1939.

Trueblood, P. R., & Rubenstein, L. Z. (1991). Assessment of instability and gait in elderly persons. *Comprehensive Therapy, 17*(8), 20-29.

Wagenaar, W. A., Hudson, P. T., & Reason, J. Y. (1990). Cognitive failures and accidents, *Applied Cognitive Psychology, 4*(4), 273-294.

Wang, C., Collet, J. P., & Lau, J. (2004). The effect of tai chi on health outcomes in patients with chronic conditions. *Archives of Internal Medicine, 164,* 493-501.

Weeks, W., & Bagian, J. (2000). Developing a culture of safety in the Veterans Health Administration. *American College of Physicians—American Society of Internal Medicine, 3*(6), 270-276.

Wu, A. W. (2000). The doctor who makes mistakes needs help too. *British Medical Journal, 320,* 726-727.

Yates, J. S., Lai, S. M., Duncan, P. W., & Studenski, S. (2002). Falls in community-dwelling stroke survivors: An accumulated impairments model. *Journal of Rehabilitation Research and Development, 39,* 385-393.

Leadership by Example

Resources for Nurses Involved in Health System Process Improvements

KATHRYN J. DOLTER

The *Crossing the Quality Chasm* report (Institute of Medicine, 2001) concluded that the American health care delivery system is lacking in each of the six aims of quality as defined within the report. Specifically the report charges that U.S. health care is not the following:

◆ Safe: avoiding injuries to patients from the care that is intended to help
◆ Effective: providing services based on scientific knowledge
◆ Patient-centered: providing care that is respectful and responsive
◆ Timely: reducing waits and harmful delays
◆ Efficient: avoiding waste, including waste of supplies, ideas, and energy
◆ Equitable: providing care that does not vary in quality because of personal characteristics such as geographical location and socioeconomic status

Crossing the Quality Chasm (Institute of Medicine, 2001) then recommends that the U.S. health care system processes need to be redesigned in accordance with the rules delineated in Box 33-1.

In a follow-on report, *Leadership by Example: Coordinating Government Roles in Improving Health Care Quality,* the Institute of Medicine (Corrigan, Eden, & Smith, 2003) proposes that the federal government, as the primary regulator, largest purchaser ($512.6 billion), largest single provider (100 million people), and sponsor of applied health services research, should take the leadership in health care process redesign. The underlying theme of the recommendations from this report are that the federal government needs to lead the U.S. health care system in the development of best practices, health care performance measurements, informatics, and transparency of health services so as to avoid the opportunity costs associated with reinvention of the wheel. The large

influence of the federal government is exerted through health care programs such as Medicare, Medicaid, the Veterans Health Administration, the Department of Defense TRICARE, the Indian Health Service, and the State Children's Health Insurance Program. With the enormous influence exerted by these programs, nurses in all U.S. health care systems, whether civilian or governmental, will be affected by the implementation of the recommendations of this report.

This chapter identifies safety, effectiveness, performance measurement, and transparency resources and initiatives that the federal government has developed—whether in response to the Institute of Medicine *Leadership by Example* report or serendipitously—to facilitate health care system achievement of the six aims of a quality health care system. Frontline nurse awareness of strategic initiatives related to quality often appears lacking. Awareness and use of strategic federal quality imitative resources will support frontline nurse involvement in health care process redesign at the local level. Only through change at the local level can the health care system truly be transformed. Frontline nurse involvement in system process redesign will be essential to the transformation of U.S. health care system into a system of care that is safe, effective, efficient, timely, patient-centered, and equitable.

FEDERAL PATIENT SAFETY RESOURCES/INITIATIVES

With an estimated 98,000 patients dying from iatrogenic errors in U.S. hospitals alone every year (Kohn, Corrigan, & Donaldson, 1999), the first aim of a quality health care system is to be safe. Federal government resources and initiatives that promote the provision of safe patient care include those from Medicare, Medicaid,

BOX 33-1

Crossing the Quality Chasm Rules for Health System Process Redesign

1. *Care based on continuous healing relationships.* Patients should receive care whenever they need it and in many forms, not just face-to-face visits. This rule implies that the health care system should be responsive at all times (24 hours a day, every day) and that access to care should be provided over the Internet, by telephone, and by other means in addition to face-to-face visits.
2. *Customization based on patient needs and values.* The system of care should be designed to meet the most common types of needs but have the capability to respond to individual patient choices and preferences.
3. *The patient as the source of control.* Patients should be given the necessary information and the opportunity to exercise the degree of control they choose over health care decisions that affect them. The health system should be able to accommodate differences in patient preferences and encourage shared decision making.
4. *Shared knowledge and the free flow of information.* Patients should have unfettered access to their own medical information and to clinical knowledge. Clinicians and patients should communicate effectively and share information.
5. *Evidence-based decision making.* Patients should receive care based on the best available scientific knowledge. Care should not vary illogically from clinician to clinician or from place to place.
6. *Safety as a system property.* Patients should be safe from injury caused by the care system. Reducing risk and ensuring safety require greater attention to systems that help prevent and mitigate errors.
7. *The need for transparency.* The health care system should make information available to patients and their families that allows them to make informed decisions when selecting a health plan, hospital, or clinical practice or choosing among alternative treatments. This should include information describing the performance on safety, evidence-based practice, and patient satisfaction of the system.
8. *Anticipation of needs.* The health system should anticipate patient needs, rather than simply react to events.
9. *Continuous decrease in waste.* The health system should not waste resources or patient time.
10. *Cooperation among clinicians.* Clinicians and institutions should collaborate and communicate actively to ensure an appropriate exchange of information and coordination of care.

Reprinted with permission from *Crossing the quality chasm: A new health system for the 21st century.* © 2001 by the National Academy of Sciences, Courtesy of the National Academies Press. Washington, DC.

---

the Agency for Health Care Research and Quality (AHRQ), the Veterans Health Administration (VHA), the Department of Defense (DoD), and the Indian Health Service.

Agency for Health Care Research and Quality

The AHRQ provides many key patient safety resources (Table 33-1). Key resources include online publication of evidence reports, online journals, and downloadable provider and patient fact sheets. In its online evidence report, *Making Health Care Safe: A Critical Analysis of Patient Safety Practices,* AHRQ (2001b) identified evidence-based safety practices. This report identified, evaluated, and prioritized for implementation patient safety practices by strength of evidence and cost of implementation, providing an excellent starting point for selection of local patient safety initiatives (Table 33-2). Another AHRQ report, *Advances in Patient Safety: From Research to Implementation* (2005a), identified federal patient safety initiatives that have occurred in the 5 years since the Institute of Medicine report *To Err Is Human* (Kohn et al., 1999). The AHRQ *Patient Safety Network* is an online newsletter that can be delivered to any e-mail account. The newsletter provides updates on patient safety journal articles, press releases, newspaper and magazine articles, and meetings and conferences. The AHRQ also has *Web M&M: Morbidity and Mortality Rounds Online,* which contains case presentations of patient safety incidents with the possibility of continuing education units, forums for discussion, and slide shows for local use of spotlight cases. Provider fact sheets from AHRQ regarding patient safety include *30 Safe Practices for Better Health Care* (2005g); patient fact sheets include *20 Tips to Help Prevent Medical Errors: Patient Fact Sheet* (2000) and *20 Tips to Help Prevent Medical Errors in Children* (2003b).

The AHRQ also has funding programs to increase the development and implementation of evidence-based patient safety practices. Recent and current

TABLE 33-1

Federal and Other Organization Patient Safety Quality Improvement Resources/Initiatives Web Sites

Resource/Initiative	Web Site
AGENCY FOR HEALTHCARE RESEARCH AND QUALITY	
• Main "Medical Errors & Patient Safety" page	http://www.ahrq.gov/qual/errorsix.htm
• Evidence reports	
Making Health Care Safer	http://www.ahrq.gov/clinic/ptsafety/
Advances in Patient Safety: From Research to Implementation	http://www.ahrq.gov/qual/advances/
• Patient Safety Network	http://psnet.ahrq.gov/
• Web M&M	http://www.webmm.ahrq.gov/
• Fact sheets	
Provider (example):	http://www.ahrq.gov/qual/30safe.htm
30 Safe Practices for Better Health Care	
Patient (example):	http://www.ahrq.gov/consumer/20tips.htm
20 Tips to Help Prevent Medical Errors	
• Funding programs	
Patient Safety Challenge Grants	http://www.ahrq.gov/qual/ptsfchall.htm
AHQR Partnerships in Implementing Patient Safety	http://www.ahrq.gov/qual/pips.htm
Patient Safety Improvement Corps	http://www.ahrq.gov/about/psimpcorps.htm
• Patient Safety Task Force	http://www.ahrq.gov/qual/taskforce/psfactst.htm
• Centers for Education and Research on Therapeutics (CERTS)	http://www.certs.hhs.gov/centers/index.html
University of Arizona CERT	http://www.arizonacert.org/
QT Drug List	
Education Tool Box	
Medicine Cabinet	
Duke University CERT	http://dukecerts.dcri.duke.edu/patients/heart/hf _resources.html
Heart failure resources	
VETERANS HEALTH ADMINISTRATION	
National Center for Patient Safety	http://www.patientsafety.gov/
• Falls Toolkit	http://www.patientsafety.gov/SafetyTopics/fallstoolkit/ index.html
• VHA Hand Hygiene Information and Tools	http://www.patientsafety.gov/SafetyTopics/HandHygiene/ index.html
• *Ensuring Correct Surgery* (patient brochure)	http://www.patientsafety.gov/SafetyTopics/CorrectSurg/ CorrSurgPt.pdf
• Cognitive aids	http://www.patientsafety.gov/SafetyTopics/CogAids/ RCA/index.html
Falls prevention	
Root cause analysis	
Health failure mode and effect analysis	
DEPARTMENT OF DEFENSE	
• Patient Safety Program	https://patientsafety.satx.disa.mil/
Patient Safety Library	https://patientsafety.satx.disa.mil/Library/
• Patient Safety Center	http://www.afip.org/PSC/index.html
Patient Safety Center links	http://www.afip.org/PSC/links.html
• *Journal of Nursing Risk Management*	http://www.afip.org/Departments/legalmed/jnrm.html
• Army Medical Department	http://www.qmo.amedd.army.mil/ptsafety/pts.htm
Patient Safety Web site	
• 2004 Eisenberg Winner	https://139.161.100.52/jcaho/
Patient Safety Video Clips	

Continued

TABLE 33-1—cont'd

Federal and Other Organization Patient Safety Quality Improvement Resources/Initiatives Web Sites

Resource/Initiative	Web Site
OTHER U.S. GOVERNMENT RESOURCES	
• Food and Drug Administration	
Medwatch	http://www.fda.gov/medwatch/
Public Health Notifications	http://www.fda.gov/cdrh/safety.html
OTHER: INTERNATIONAL GOVERNMENTAL	
• Australian Council for Safety and Quality in Health Care	http://www.safetyandquality.org/
• United Kingdom National Health Service, National Patient Safety Agency	http://www.npsa.nhs.uk/
OTHER: PRIVATE ORGANIZATIONAL	
• Institute for Healthcare Improvement	http://www.ihi.org/IHI/Topics/PatientSafety/
• Institute for Safe Medication Practices	http://www.ismp.org/
• Joint Commission on the Accreditation of Healthcare Organizations	
General	http://www.jcaho.org/
National Patient Safety Goals	http://www.jcaho.org/accredited%2Borganizations/patient%2Bsafety/npsg.htm
Patient Safety Speak Up Initiatives (Wrong Site Surgery, Infection, Medication Errors)	http://www.jcaho.org/accredited%2Borganizations/speak%2Bup/speak+up+initiatives.htm
• National Patient Safety Foundation	http://www.npsf.org/html/resources_links.html
State Resources Section	http://www.npsf.org/html/state_resources.html

funding programs include the AHRQ Partnerships in Implementing Patient Safety (2005b)—AHRQ and health organization partnerships; Patient Safety Challenge Grants (2004b)—shared-cost grants supporting the translation of patient safety innovations into practice; and the Patient Safety Improvement Corps (2005d)—an AHRQ/VHA partnership to improve patient safety through patient safety knowledge and skills education of designated state and state hospital partner teams.

The AHRQ also has established seven Centers for Education and Research on Therapeutics (CERTs). The purpose of CERTs is to conduct research and provide education that will advance the optimal use of drugs, medical devices, and biological products. The CERTs are located at the University of Arizona, HMO Research Network, Duke University, the University of Pennsylvania, the University of Alabama at Birmingham, the University of North Carolina at Chapel Hill, and Vanderbilt University Medical Center (http://www.certs.hhs.gov/centers/index.html). The CERT sites are selected via a competitive peer review process. Each CERT maintains a Web site that contains resources such as the QT syndrome toolbox and interactive medicine cabinet at the University of Arizona (http://www.arizonacert.org/) and the heart

failure patient resources at Duke University (http://dukecerts.dcri.duke.edu/patients/heart/hf_resources.html), which includes a brochure, video, and patient tips.

Additionally, the AHRQ is a member organization of the Patient Safety Task Force, the goals of which are to "coordinate integrating data collection on medical errors and adverse events; coordinate research and analysis efforts; and promote collaboration on reducing the occurrence of injuries that result from medical errors" (AHRQ, 2005a). The task force currently includes the Centers for Disease Control and Prevention, the Food and Drug Administration, and the Centers for Medicare and Medicaid Services. The task force will be expanded in the future to include other public and private sector organizations (AHRQ, 2005b). Table 33-1 lists the AHRQ patient safety resource Web sites.

Veterans Health Administration

The VHA is definitely a leader in the patient safety arena. Through its National Center for Patient Safety, the VHA focuses "on prevention not punishment, applying human factor analysis and the safety research of high reliability organizations (aviation and nuclear power) targeted at identifying and eliminating system

TABLE 33-2

Patient Safety Practices With the Greatest Strength of Evidence Regarding Their Impact and Effectiveness

Item	Patient Safety Problem	Patient Safety Practice	Implementation Cost/Complexity
1	Venous thromboembolism	Appropriate prophylaxis (Chap. 31*)	Low
2	Perioperative cardiac events in patients undergoing noncardiac surgery	Use of beta-blockers perioperatively (Chap. 25)	Low
3	Central venous catheter–related bloodstream infections	Use of maximum sterile barriers during catheter insertion (Chap. 16.1)	Low
4	Surgical site infections	Appropriate use of antibiotic prophylaxis (Chap. 20.1)	Low
5	Missed, incomplete, or not fully comprehended informed consent	Asking that patients recall and restate what they have been told during informed consent (Chap. 48)	Low
6	Ventilator-associated pneumonia	Continuous aspiration of subglottic secretions (Chap. 17.2)	Medium
7	Pressure ulcers	Use of pressure-relieving bedding materials (Chap. 27)	Medium
8	Morbidity caused by central venous catheter insertion	Use of real-time ultrasound guidance during central line insertion (Chap. 21)	High
9	Adverse events related to chronic anticoagulation with warfarin	Patient self-management using home monitoring devices (Chap. 9)	High
10	Morbidity and mortality in postsurgical and critically ill patients	Various nutritional strategies (Chap. 33)	Medium
11	Central venous catheter–related bloodstream infections	Antibiotic-impregnated catheters (Chap. 16.2)	Low

From Agency for Healthcare Research and Quality. (2001). *Making health care safer: A critical analysis of patient safety practices.* Retrieved June 29, 2005, from http://www.ahrq.gov/clinic/ptsafety.
*Chapter numbers refer to chapters of the source document.

vulnerabilities" (VA National Center for Patient Safety, 2005). The National Center for Patient Safety Web site includes resources that can assist other health care organizations, including hazard summaries, tools and toolkits, health care failure mode and effect analysis tools, cognitive aids, and links to other governmental and nongovernmental patient safety resources.

Hazard summaries are provided on the topics such as anticoagulation, oxygen cylinders, and magnetic resonance imaging. In the hazard summaries a system wide issue identified by "close calls and adverse events" at private and VHA hospitals identifies root causes and suggested recommendations to decrease/eliminate hazards. The health care failure mode and effect analysis tools include a PowerPoint presentation, worksheets, and references. Tools and toolkit topics include hand hygiene and falls prevention tools and references.

Tools vary by topic but include posters, links to other sites, training resources, references, and policies that can provide a "straw-man" for local policy development efforts. The cognitive aids, online interactive educational patient safety assessment, and analysis tools with practical application to real clinical situations are especially helpful. Table 33-3 lists the cognitive aids available on the National Patient Safety Center Web site. Embedded within the Web site are links to other private, governmental, and international patient safety–related Web sites. The international links include those to the Australian Council for Safety and Quality in Health Care *(http://www.safetyandquality.org/)* and to the United Kingdom National Health Service, National Patient Safety Agency *(http://www.npsa.nhs.uk/).* Both of these sites include strategic and local-level tools to effect patient safety improvements.

TABLE 33-3

List of Cognitive Aids	
Tool	**Veterans Health Administration Descriptor**
Triage Cards™ http://www.patientsafety.gov/SafetyTopics/Cog Aids/Triage/index.html	"Presents questions RCA teams need to know the answer to when completing RCAs and describes how to use the 5 Rules of Causation when developing causation statements."
Fall Prevention and Management http://www.patientsafety.gov/SafetyTopics/Cog Aids/FallPrevention/index.html	"Tips and suggestions on how to initiate and implement fall prevention interventions and strategies."
Escape and Elopement Management http://www.patientsafety.gov/SafetyTopics/Cog Aids/EscapeElope/index.html	"Tips and suggestions on interventions that may be used to prevent patients from escaping and eloping."
The Healthcare Failure Mode Effect **Analysis Process** http://www.patientsafety.gov/SafetyTopics/Cog Aids/HFMEA/index.html	"Provides tips, hints, and directions on how to complete a proactive risk assessment using the NCPS developed model."
Root Cause Analysis Tools http://www.patientsafety.gov/SafetyTopics/Cog Aids/RCA/index.html	"Provides tips, hints and directions on how to complete an RCA using the NCPS developed analysis process including use of Event Flow and Cause and Effect diagramming."

From Veterans Health Administration, VA National Center for Patient Safety. *Patient safety topics.* Retrieved December 29, 2005, from http://www.patientsafety.gov/SafetyTopics.html#Aids
NCPS, National Center for Patient Safety; *RCA,* root cause analysis.

Department of Defense

The DoD has been involved in the implementation of system wide patient safety initiatives since its involvement in the Quality Interagency Coordination Task Force (QuIC) formed following a presidential directive resulting from the release of the Institute of Medicine report *To Err Is Human* (Kohn et al., 1999). "The purpose of the QuIC was to ensure that all Federal agencies involved in purchasing, providing, studying, or regulating health care services were working in a coordinated manner toward the common goal of improving quality care" (AHRQ, 2005f). Other federal partners in the Quality Interagency Coordination Task Force include the VHA and the Department of Health and Human Services.

Following participation in the Quality Interagency Coordination Task Force, DoD developed a systemwide patient safety program for its health care systems (Army, Navy, and Air Force), including a DoD database to assist in the analysis of actual and close-call patient safety events maintained by the Armed Forces Institute of Pathology (http://www.afip.org/PSC/index.html). Besides DoD-specific policies, the main Web site contains a patient safety library that includes universally relevant tools such as downloadable dangerous abbreviation posters; team training manuals on how to develop a culture of safety; health care failure mode and effect analysis and root cause analysis references; teamwork references, a patient safety organization assessment tool; and myriad of other patient safety–specific tools. The Armed Forces Institute of Pathology Web site also contains a link to the *Journal of Nursing Risk Management* (http://www.afip.org/Departments/legalmed/jnrm.html). The journal, published annually with recent issues available online, provides up to 21.3 contact hours in nursing continuing education through the Maryland Nurses Association. These continuing education units are free to all military and full-time federal health care providers and are only $10 for nonfederal providers.

The Army Medical Department patient safety Web site contains systemwide policies but also contains some implementation tools such as posters, brochures, and reporting tools that might be adapted for local use. The Army site also links to a patient safety video series developed by Major Danny Jaghab, a dietician formerly stationed at the Brooke Army Medical Center. The 36-part series training program titled "2003/2004 JCAHO National Patient Safety Goals" received a 2004 John M. Eisenberg Patient Safety and Quality Award. Dr. Eisenberg was a health care quality leader who led the Agency for Health Care Research and Quality before his death in 2002. The series was developed to provide mandatory Joint Commission on Accreditation of Healthcare Organizations patient safety and medical center–specific process improvement training for Brooke Army Medical Center staff. The video clips were sent out as a link via e-mail for staff to view at their convenience and were placed on the intranet of the medical center. Though the clips were developed in 2003/2004, they have current information and serve as an example of what can be achieved at a local medical center level. Table 33-1 lists DoD resources.

Private Organizations

Though the federal government has provided great leadership in the patient safety arena, other national organizational leaders include the Institute for Safe Medication Practices (ISMP), the National Patient Safety Foundation, the Joint Commission on Accreditation of Healthcare Organizations, and the Institute for Healthcare Improvement. Locally relevant ISMP tools include patient safety brochures; posters; a medication safety solution toolkit; a medication patient safety pocket guide; a free online subscription to the *ISMP Medication Safety Alert! Nursing Edition;* medication hazard alerts; lists of error-prone abbreviations, symbols, and dose designations; and medication safety videos from the U.S. Food and Drug Administration and ISMP. One ISMP tool is the list of high-alert medications (Box 33-2). The ISMP also is addressing safety issues associated with computerized physician order entry.

Just one of the major highlights of the National Patient Safety Foundation Web site is its resource section, which includes links to online fact sheets and brochures (including those in Spanish), a state-by-state listing of patient safety resources, patient- and family-specific patient safety resources, and nursing-specific patient safety resources. The Joint Commission on Accreditation of Healthcare Organizations, besides providing direction for national patient safety through its accreditation efforts to focus hospital patient safety improvement via its National Patient Safety Goals, also provides support of local patient safety initiatives through its Speak Up initiative brochures and other tools. The Speak Up initiative focuses on partnering with patients to conquer patient safety problems. The Institute for Healthcare Improvement, a major leader of health care patient safety and quality improvement, recently has initiated its 100K Lives Campaign designed to "implement changes in care that have been proven to prevent avoidable deaths" (Institute for Healthcare Improvement, 2005).

BOX 33-2

Institute for Safe Medication Practices List of High-Alert Medications

CLASS/CATEGORY OF MEDICATIONS

Adrenergic agonists, IV (e.g., epinephrine)
Adrenergic antagonists, IV (e.g., propranolol)
Anesthetic agents, general, inhaled and IV (e.g., propofol)
Cardioplegic solutions
Chemotherapeutic agents, parenteral and oral
Dextrose, hypertonic, 20% or greater
Dialysis solutions, peritoneal and hemodialysis
Epidural or intrathecal medications
Glycoprotein IIb/IIIa inhibitors (e.g., eptifibatide)
Hypoglycemics, oral
Inotropic medications, IV (e.g., digoxin and milrinone)
Liposomal forms of drugs (e.g., liposomal amphotericin B)
Moderate sedation agents, IV (e.g., midazolam)
Moderate sedation agents, oral, for children (e.g., chloral hydrate)
Narcotics/opiates, IV and oral (including liquid concentrates and immediate- and sustained-release formulations)
Neuromuscular blocking agents (e.g., succinylcholine)
Radiocontrast agents, IV
Thrombolytics/fibrinolytics, IV (e.g., tenecteplase)
Total parenteral nutrition solutions

SPECIFIC MEDICATIONS

Amiodarone, IV
Colchicine injection
Heparin, low molecular weight, injection
Heparin, unfractionated, IV
Insulin, subcutaneous and IV
Lidocaine, IV
Magnesium sulfate injection
Methotrexate, oral, nononcological use
Nesiritide
Nitroprusside, sodium, for injection
Potassium chloride for injection concentrate
Potassium phosphates injection
Sodium chloride injection, hypertonic, more than 0.9% concentration
Warfarin

From Institute for Safe Medication Practices. *ISMP's List of High-Alert Medications.* Retrieved December 29, 2005, from http://www.ismp.org/Tools/highalertmedications.pdf.

BOX 33-3

List of Agency for Healthcare Research and Quality Evidence-Based Practice Centers

Blue Cross and Blue Shield Association, Technology Evaluation Center
Duke University*
ECRI*
Johns Hopkins University
McMaster University
Oregon Health & Science University†
RTI International—University of North Carolina
Southern California
Stanford University—University of California, San Francisco
Tufts University—New England Medical Center*
University of Alberta, Edmonton, Canada
University of Minnesota, Minneapolis
University of Ottawa, Canada

From Evidence-based Practice Centers. (2004, September). *Synthesizing scientific evidence to improve quality and effectiveness in health care.* Rockville, MD: Agency for Healthcare Research and Quality. Retrieved December 29, 2005, from http://www.ahcpr.gov/clinic/epc/#Centers.
*Evidenced-based Practice Centers that focus on technology assessments for Centers for Medicare and Medicaid Services.
†Evidenced-based Practice Center that focuses on evidence reports for the U.S. Preventive Services Task Force.

FEDERAL EFFECTIVENESS RESOURCES/INITIATIVES

Agency for Healthcare Research and Quality

The AHRQ has led the effort in development of evidence-based clinical information and transition of evidence-based information into practice in the United States. As the former Agency for Health Care Policy and Research, the agency developed evidence-based clinical practice guidelines. In 1997 the agency transitioned to conducting "systematic, comprehensive analyses of the scientific literature to develop evidence reports and technology assessments on clinical topics that are common, expensive, and present challenges to decisionmakers" (AHRQ, 2001a) via its Evidence-based Practice Centers. The goal of the Evidenced-based Practice Center initiative is "to promote evidence-based practice in everyday care" (Evidence-based Practice Centers, 2004). Currently, 13 Evidenced-based Practice Centers are located throughout the country (Box 33-3). As of June 2005, 125 evidence reports have been published and are available online for topics as diverse as *Economic Incentives for Preventive Care* (Kane, Johnson, Town, & Butler, 2004) to *Pharmacological and Surgical Treatment of Obesity* (Shekelle et al., 2004) and *Use of Episiotomy in Obstetrical Care: A Systematic Review* (Viswanathan et al., 2005). The Evidenced-based Practice Centers also publish technical reviews, which have included *Closing the Quality Gap: A Critical Analysis of Quality Improvement Strategies* (AHRQ, 2004a). The second and third volumes in this series critically analyze quality improvement strategies that focus on diabetes (AHRQ, 2004b) and hypertension (Shojania, McDonald, Wachter, & Owens, 2005), respectively. All Evidenced-based Practice Center reports are available on the Internet.

The AHRQ National Guideline Clearinghouse is a "comprehensive database of evidence-based clinical practice guidelines and related documents." The goal of the National Guideline Clearinghouse (2004) is

> to provide physicians, nurses, and other health professionals, health care providers, health plans, integrated delivery systems, purchasers and others an accessible mechanism for obtaining objective, detailed information on clinical practice guidelines and to further their dissemination, implementation and use.

Features of the National Guideline Clearinghouse are listed in Box 33-4 and include a tool that allows online comparison of two or more guidelines; ability to download guidelines to a PDA or Palm device; already developed guideline comparisons from the National Guideline Clearinghouse; a listserv to discuss guidelines-related topics; and a database of guideline-related annotated bibliographies. The guideline clearinghouse can be browsed or queried. Subscribers can receive automatic notification of new guidelines.

The development of evidence-based recommendations regarding preventive services is also sponsored by the U.S. Preventive Services Task Force (USPSTF). The USPSTF is "an independent panel of experts in primary care and prevention that systematically reviews the evidence of effectiveness and develops recommendations for clinical preventive services" (AHRQ, 2005h). The USPSTF recommendations are published on the Web in the *Guide to Clinical Preventive Services, 2005* (AHRQ, 2005c). Recommendations are downloadable to a Palm device or PDA. Notification of USPSTF guidelines updates can be obtained automatically via subscription to the USPSTF listserv. The AHRQ also provides support to the implementation of prevention guidelines through its Putting Prevention into Practice program. Resources include a step-by-step implementation guide for primary care practices (AHRQ, 2002), downloadable worksheets, presentations, consumer

National Guideline Clearinghouse Features

- "Palm-based PDA Downloads of the Complete NGC Summary for all guidelines represented in the database"
- "A Guideline Comparison utility that gives users the ability to generate side-by-side comparisons for any combination of two or more guidelines"
- "Unique guideline comparisons called Guideline Syntheses prepared by NGC staff, compare guidelines covering similar topics, highlighting areas of similarity and difference. NGC Guideline Syntheses often provide a comparison of guidelines developed in different countries, providing insight into commonalities and differences in international health practices."
- "An electronic forum, NGC-L for exchanging information on clinical practice guidelines, their development, implementation and use"
- "An Annotated Bibliography database where users can search for citations for publications and resources about guidelines, including guideline development and methodology, structure, evaluation, and implementation"

From National Guideline Clearinghouse. (2004). *About NCG*. Retrieved December 29, 2005, from http://www.guideline.gov/about/about.aspx.

brochures in English and Spanish, and fact sheets (AHRQ, 2005e).

Besides development of evidence via its Evidenced-based Practice Centers and the USPSTF and dissemination of evidence through its guideline clearinghouse, AHRQ has a major focus on the implementation of evidence in practice. This not only occurs in its Putting Prevention into Practice efforts but also is realized in its research program, Translating Research into Practice. This research program is designed to identify evidence-based implementation strategies for getting research into practice.

Other AHRQ effectiveness initiatives include programs focused on outcomes and technology assessments. Table 33-4 lists AHRQ effectiveness Web sites.

Veterans Health Administration and Department of Defense Effectiveness Efforts

The VHA has been involved in the development and implementation of clinical practice guidelines since 1992 as part of its External Review Program in an effort to increase the percentage of care delivery in the Veterans Administration facilities based on evidence. From the

development of the first guideline on ischemic heart disease, the Veterans Administration transitioned from directing implementation of locally selected guidelines assessed via self-report through directed implementation of nationally developed guidelines assessed by systematic performance measures. Through this effort, the Veterans Administration has led the way in health systemwide guideline implementation, demonstrating remarkable improvements in guideline-based performance measurement.

In 1998 the Veterans Administration partnered with the DoD to develop DoD/VHA clinical guidelines for implementation across the Veterans Administration, Army, Navy, and Air Force health systems. From the initial consensus-based development, the process transitioned to formalized, systematic, rigorous guideline development. Developed guidelines were selected based on high-volume, high-cost, high-risk conditions within the VHA and DoD health systems.

Although the VHA was able to achieve implementation of guideline evidence into practice via its systematic External Review Program, the DoD, because of its inability to obtain patient-level data, focused its implementation efforts on strategic support of local guideline implementation efforts while developing its electronic metric measurement capabilities. To this end, the DoD developed guideline-specific implementation toolkits; panels of DoD and Veterans Administration frontline providers designed patient-, provider-, and system-level tools that then were piloted and refined before incorporation into a toolkit focused on the "making the best way the easiest way" in support of local implementation teams. The DoD worked closely with the RAND Corporation to develop a systematic guideline implementation process; the Army Medical Department/RAND guideline implementation guide developed from this partnership is downloadable from http://www.qmo.amedd.army.mil/general%20documents/rand_document_4_01.pdf (Nicholas, Farley, Vaiana, & Cretin, 2001).

The DoD/VHA guidelines, provider tools, and performance measures are located on the VA/DoD Clinical Practice Guidelines Web site. The full DoD/VHA guideline toolkits, including patient self-management and system tools and guideline-specific annotated Web site directories can be found at the Army Medical Department Web site (Table 33-4).

Other Federal and Private Organization Effectiveness Initiatives

Other federal effectiveness implementation initiatives include the Centers for Disease Control and Prevention

TABLE 33-4

Federal Patient and Other Organization Effectiveness Quality Improvement Resources/Initiatives Web Sites

Resource/Initiative	Web Site
AGENCY FOR HEALTHCARE RESEARCH AND QUALITY	
Evidence-Based Practice Centers	http://www.ahcpr.gov/clinic/epcindex.htm
National Guideline Clearinghouse	http://www.guideline.gov/
U.S. Preventive Services Task Force	http://www.ahrq.gov/clinic/uspstfix.htm
• *Guide to Clinical Preventive Services, 2005: Recommendations of the U.S. Preventive Services Task Force*	http://www.ahrq.gov/clinic/pocketgd.htm
• AHRQ's Prevention Program LISTSERV	http://www.ahcpr.gov/clinic/prev/prevlistserv.htm
• Put Prevention into Practice	http://www.ahrq.gov/clinic/ppipix.htm
• Outcomes and Effectiveness	http://www.ahrq.gov/clinic/outcomix.htm
• Technology Assessments	http://www.ahrq.gov/clinic/techix.htm
• Translation of Research into Practice (TRIP)-II	http://www.ahrq.gov/research/trip2fac.htm
VETERANS HEALTH ADMINISTRATION/DEPARTMENT OF DEFENSE	
Clinical Practice Guidelines	http://www.oqp.med.va.gov/cpg/cpg.htm
DEPARTMENT OF DEFENSE	
Army Medical Department guidelines and condition-specific guideline toolkits	http://www.qmo.amedd.army.mil/pguide.htm
Army/RAND guideline implementation manual	http://www.qmo.amedd.army.mil/general%20 documents/rand_document_4_01.pdf
OTHER FEDERAL GOVERNMENT AGENCIES	
Centers for Disease Control and Prevention	http:www.cdc.gov
Guide to Community Preventive Services	http://www.thecommunityguide.org/default.htm
OTHER PRIVATE ORGANIZATIONS	
Institute for Clinical Systems Improvement	http://www.icsi.org/knowledge/

Guide to Community Preventive Services: Systematic Reviews and Evidence-Based Recommendations providing graded evidence reviews by topic regarding implementation intervention. Among the many private organizations in the effectiveness arena, the Institute for Clinical Systems Improvement provides free access to its provider guidelines. Its Web site also has readily accessible patient and family guidelines, guideline impact studies, order sets, and patient education resources (Table 33-4).

FEDERAL PERFORMANCE MEASUREMENT AND TRANSPARENCY RESOURCES/INITIATIVES

Essential to any quality improvement is the development and use of evidence-based performance measurement and transparency of measurement efforts. The AHRQ has a quality measure clearinghouse and Web-based introductory-level education on quality measurement

and published the first national quality report in 2003 assessing progress toward quality improvement goals (AHRQ, 2003a). The VHA has had an evidence-based performance measurement system in place that has been driving change since the mid-1990s. However, the recent effort of the Centers for Medicare and Medicaid Services Hospital and Nursing Home Compare programs actually integrate performance measurement with transparency. With Hospital Compare one can identify the extent to which hospitals within a user-selected radius of a given location or zip code are meeting evidence-based condition-specific metrics. This Web-based provision of provider-specific quality of care information is expected someday to influence consumer choice of providers and further drive health provider quality improvement efforts. Hospital Compare measures include eight related to heart attack care, four related to heart failure care, and five related to pneumonia care. Nursing Home Compare measures are

TABLE 33-5

Federal Patient and Other Organization Measurement and Transparency Quality Improvement Resources/Initiatives Web Sites	
Resource/Initiative	Web Site
AGENCY FOR HEALTHCARE RESEARCH AND QUALITY	
Quality Tools (clearinghouse for quality measures and tools)	http://www.qualitytools.ahrq.gov/
Understanding Quality Measurement	http://www.ahrq.gov/chtoolbx/understn.htm
CENTERS FOR MEDICARE AND MEDICAID SERVICES	
Quality Initiatives	http://www.cms.hhs.gov/quality/
Hospital Compare	http://www.hospitalcompare.hhs.gov/
Home Care Compare	http://www.vnavt.com/home_care_compare.htm
Nursing Home Compare	http://www.medicare.gov/NHCompare/Include/Data Section/Questions/SearchCriteria.asp?version= default&browser=IE%7C6%7CWinXP&language= English&defaultstatus=0&pagelist=Home
VETERANS HEALTH ADMINISTRATION OTHER PRIVATE ORGANIZATIONS	http://www1.va.gov/Health_Benefits/
National Quality Forum	http://www.qualityforum.org/

directed toward long-term and short-term stays. Table 33-5 lists federal and other organization measurement and transparency initiatives and their corresponding Web sites.

SUMMARY

With the Institute of Medicine recommendations that the federal government and federal health care systems demonstrate leadership in developing systems of care that epitomize its *Leadership by Example* report (Corrigan, Eden, & Smith, 2003), federal initiatives can provide support to the provision of quality health care at the local level. Nurses must use these already developed resources to decrease time to implementation of evidence-based quality improvements and avoid increased costs of improvements that reinvention would entail. Reinvention of the wheel in health care quality improvement is costly in term of dollars and in terms of lives.

REFERENCES

Agency for Healthcare Research and Quality. (2000). *20 tips to help prevent medical errors.* Retrieved June, 28, 2005, from http://www.ahrq.gov/consumer/20tips.htm

Agency for Healthcare Research and Quality. (2001a). *AHRQ profile: Advancing excellence in health care.* Retrieved December 29, 2005, from http://www.ahcpr.gov/about/profile.htm

Agency for Healthcare Research and Quality. (2001b). *Making health care safer: A critical analysis of patient safety practices.* Retrieved June 29, 2005, from http://www.ahrq.gov/clinic/ptsafety

Agency for Healthcare Research and Quality. (2002). *A step-by-step guide to delivering clinical preventive services: A systems approach.* Retrieved June 29, 2005, from http://www.ahrq.gov/ppip/manual/

Agency for Healthcare Research and Quality. (2003a). *National healthcare quality report.* Retrieved October 10, 2004, from http://www.qualitytools.ahrq.gov/qualityreport/browse/browse.aspx

Agency for Healthcare Research and Quality. (2003b). *20 tips to help prevent medical errors in children.* Retrieved June 29, 2005, from http://www.ahrq.gov/consumer/20tipkid.htm

Agency for Healthcare Research and Quality. (2004a). *Closing the quality gap: A critical analysis of quality improvement strategies: Volume 1—Series overview and methodology.* Retrieved June 28, 2005, from http://www.ahrq.gov/clinic/tp/qgap1tp.htm

Agency for Healthcare Research and Quality. (2004b). *Patient safety challenge grants.* Retrieved June 28, 2005, from http://www.ahrq.gov/qual/ptsfchall.htm

Agency for Healthcare Research and Quality. (2005a). *Advances in patient safety: From research to implementation* (Vols. 1-4). Retrieved June 28, 2005, from http://www.ahrq.gov/qual/advances

Agency for Healthcare Research and Quality. (2005b, June). *AHRQ partnerships in implementing patient safety.* Retrieved June 28, 2005, from http://www.ahrq.gov/qual/pips.htm

Agency for Healthcare Research and Quality. (2005c, June). *Guide to clinical preventive services, 2005: Recommendations of* the *U.S. Preventive Services Task Force* (AHRQ Pub. No. 05-0570). Rockville, MD: Author. Retrieved December 29, 2005 from http://www.ahrq.gov/clinic/pocketgd.htm

Agency for Healthcare Research and Quality. (2005d). *Patient safety improvement corps: An AHRQ/VA partnership.* Retrieved June 28, 2005, from http://www.ahrq.gov/about/psimpcorps.htm

Agency for Healthcare Research and Quality. (2005e). *Put prevention into practice.* Retrieved December 29, 2005 from http://www.ahrq.gov/clinic/ppipix.htm#tools

Agency for Healthcare Research and Quality. (2005f). *Quality Interagency Coordination (QuIC) Task Force.* Retrieved December 29, 2005 from http://www.quic.gov/

Agency for Healthcare Research and Quality. (2005g). *30 Safe Practices for Better Health Hare.* Retrieved June 28, 2005, from http://www.ahrq.gov/qual/30safe.htm

Agency for Healthcare Research and Quality. (2005h). *U.S. Preventive Services Task Force (USPSTF).* Retrieved December 29, 2005, from http://www.ahcpr.gov/clinic/uspstfix.htm

Corrigan, J. M., Eden, J., & Smith, B. M. (Eds.). (2003). *Leadership by example: Coordinating government roles in improving health care quality.* Washington, DC: National Academy Press.

Evidence-based Practice Centers. (2004). *Synthesizing scientific evidence to improve quality and effectiveness in health care.* Rockville, MD: Agency for Healthcare Research and Quality. Retrieved December 29, 2005 from http://www.ahcpr.gov/clinic/epc/

Institute for Healthcare Improvement. (2005). *100K lives campaign.* Retrieved August 3, 2005, from http://www.ihi.org/IHI/Programs/Campaign/

Institute of Medicine. (2001). *Crossing the quality chasm: A new health system for the 21st century.* Washington, DC: National Academies Press.

Kane, R. L., Johnson, P. E., Town, R. J., & Butler, M. (2004). *Economic incentives for preventive care.* (Evidence Report/Technology Assessment: Number 101). Retrieved June 29, 2005, from http://www.ahrq.gov/clinic/epcsums/ecincsum.htm

Kohn, L. T., Corrigan, J. M., & Donaldson, M. S. (Eds.). (1999). *To err is human: Building a safer health system.* Washington, DC: National Academy Press.

National Guideline Clearinghouse. (2004). *About NCG.* Retrieved December 29, 2005, from http://www.guideline.gov/about/about.aspx

Nicholas, W., Farley, D. O., Vaiana, M. E., & Cretin, S. (2001). *Putting practice guidelines to work in the Department of Defense medical system: A guide for action.* Santa Monica, CA: RAND.

Shekelle, P. G., Morton, S. C., Maglione, M., Suttorp, M., Tu, W., Li, Z., et al. (2004). *Pharmacological and surgical treatment of obesity.* (Evidence Report/Technology Assessment: Number 103). Retrieved June 29, 2005, from http://www.ahrq.gov/clinic/epcsums/obesphsum.htm

Shojania, K. G., McDonald, K. M., Wachter, R. M., & Owens, D. K. (Series Eds.). (2005). *Closing the quality gap: A critical analysis of quality improvement strategies. Volume 3—Hypertension care.* Retrieved June 29, 2005, from http://www.ahrq.gov/clinic/tp/hypergap3tp.htm#Report

VA National Center for Patient Safety. (2005). *National Center for Patient Safety (NCPS).* Retrieved December 29, 2005, from http://www.patientsafety.gov/

Viswanathan, M., Hartmann, K., Palmieri, R., Lux, L., Swinson, T., Lohr, K. N., et al. (2005). *The use of episiotomy in obstetrical care: A systematic review.* (Evidence Report/Technology Assessment: Number 112). Retrieved June 29, 2005, from http://www.ahrq.gov/clinic/epcsums/epissum. htm

Nursing Care Priority Area

Prevention

JANET D. ALLAN

WHY PREVENTION

Lifestyle-related behaviors are a leading cause of preventable disease and death in the United States (Box 34-1). Consider that more than 67% of adult Americans are overweight or obese and 23% smoke (Fine, Philogene, Gramling, Coups, & Sinha, 2004). Unhealthy lifestyles are estimated to account for more than 50% of preventable deaths in the United States (Fine et al., 2004; Whitlock, Orleans, Pender, & Allan, 2002), yet interventions to address such behaviors and immunizations and screening for risk factors for disease are underused in health care settings. For example, a recent national survey reported that 67% of adults in long-term care and nursing homes never received a pneumococcal vaccination (Kelley et al., 2004), and less than 42% of overweight adults were advised to lose weight (Allan, 2004). Without making health promotion and disease prevention a part of all health care, the health of the nation will continue to decrease. Despite the fact that for more than 2 decades Healthy People 2010 (U.S. Department of Health and Human Services, 2000) has set broad national goals for improving health, only 5% percent of the $1.4 trillion spent on health care in the United States is allocated to preventing disease and promoting health (Kelley et al., 2004). In a recent report the Institute of Medicine also established priority areas for prevention (Adams & Corrigan, 2003). Prevention activities that target changing the health behaviors of Americans in particular offer the greatest potential of any current approach for decreasing morbidity/mortality, for improving the quality of life, and for reducing health care costs (Kelley et al., 2004; Whitlock et al., 2002). As stated in the 2001 Institute of Medicine report *Crossing the Quality Chasm*, such prevention activities must be based on the best available scientific evidence.

Agreement is strong that practice should be based on evidence (Jennings, 2004). Nurses should and can take the leadership in integrating and institutionalizing evidence-based preventive services into the care of all patients. Focusing on health promotion and disease

prevention is a basic tenet of nursing practice. Nurse clinicians, particularly advanced practice and community health nurses, can play a critical role in leading the needed paradigm shift to evidence-based nursing to provide the highest quality preventive care.

This chapter has three general purposes:

1. To describe the Healthy People 2010 goals and targeted lifestyle factors
2. To discuss the mission, methods, and products of the U.S. Preventive Services Task Force (Task Force) as related to prevention interventions
3. To describe evidence-based practice and the role of the nurse in prevention through the implementation of evidence-based nursing practice

THE CHALLENGE OF HEALTHY PEOPLE 2010

Healthy People 2010, which provides a vision and plan for health services in the next decade, established two major goals for the United States: (1) to increase quality and quantity of healthy life and (2) to eliminate health disparities among different segments of the population (U.S. Department of Health and Human Services, 2000). Critical to achieving these goals is the necessity for health care systems and providers to promote healthy lifestyles through well-planned preventive services among the populations they serve and to make policy changes to integrate such services into the health care systems.

The greatest potential for improving the health of the nation and improving quality of life is to focus on changing lifestyle-related health behaviors of Americans. Healthy People 2010 identified five critical lifestyle factors as health indicators by which to track progress in improving the health of the nation over the next decade (U.S. Department of Health and Human Services, 2000). The five critical lifestyle behaviors are tobacco use, overweight/obesity (unhealthy eating), physical inactivity, substance abuse (includes risky drinking), and risky sexual behavior (Table 34-1). Unhealthy eating combined with physical inactivity results in overweight/obesity that accounts for most of the deaths

BOX 34-1

The Case for Prevention

Unhealthy lifestyles such as unhealthy diet, physical inactivity, substance abuse, tobacco use, and risky sexual behaviors account for more than 50% of preventable deaths in the United States.

Only 7% of U.S. adults have no risky lifestyle behaviors, whereas 41% have two risky behaviors.

Only 5% of the $1.4 trillion spent on health care is allocated to preventing disease and promoting health.

Sixty-seven percent of adults in long-term care and nursing homes did not receive a pneumococcal vaccination.

Only 42% of overweight U.S. adults have been advised to lose weight by their health care provider.

TABLE 34-1

Healthy People 2010 Lifestyle Health Indicators

Health Indicator	1997 Baseline	2010 Goals
Tobacco use (%)		
Cigarette smoking, adults	24	12
Overweight and obesity (%) (A)		
Obesity in adults (>20 yr)	23	15
Overweight/obesity in children and teens (6-19 yr)	11	5
Physical activity (%) (B)		
No leisure time physical activity (>18 yr)	40	20
Moderate physical activity		
Adults (>18 yr)	15	30
Adolescents (grades 9-12)	20	30
Substance abuse (C)		
Proportion of adults exceeding low-risk drinking		
Females	72	50
Males	74	50
Binge drinking (%)		
Adolescents (12-17 yr)	8.3	3
High school seniors	32	11
College students	39	20
Adults	16	6
Responsible sexual behavior (%)		
Unmarried females (18-44 yr) whose partners did not use condoms	77	50

A. Adult obesity (BMI >30); children/teens (>95th percentile of gender and age-specific BMI from year 2000 U.S. growth charts).
B. Moderate activity of 30 minutes a day, >5 days a week.
C. Males: >14 drinks/week or >4 drinks/occasion: females: >7 drinks/week or >3 drinks/occasion.
Source: From *Healthy People 2010* (USDHHS, 2000). Adapted from public domain document.

from unhealthy lifestyle behaviors. A 2001 national survey reported that 66% of the adult population was sedentary and 21% engaged in risky drinking. In fact, most adults had multiple risky lifestyle-related behaviors, 41% had two risky behaviors, and 14% had three (Fine et al., 2004). Because economically and socially disadvantaged populations have higher proportions of risky health behaviors, improving health behaviors is also one approach to reducing health disparities (Whitlock et al., 2002).

Health Promotion and Disease Prevention

Clearly a focus on reducing unhealthy behaviors may hold the most promise for improving health. In addition, nurses must address health promotion and disease prevention. The body of literature related to health, health promotion, and disease prevention is vast (see Pender, Murdaugh, and Parsons [2002] for a detailed discussion of theories and models related to health promotion and disease prevention). In this chapter, the classic public health definition of *levels of prevention* based on the concept of the natural history of disease is used (Shamansky & Clausen, 1980). *Primary prevention* as applied to individuals is defined as interventions that promote healthier lifestyles or reduce the risk of disease in otherwise healthy individuals (Box 34-2). Primary prevention can involve immunizations (measles, pertussis, influenza) to prevent infectious diseases, use of fluoride to prevent cavities in children, and implementation of interventions that promote health (counseling about physical activity or healthy diet or not to smoke). *Secondary prevention* as applied to individuals is defined as interventions that identify risk factors for disease (screening for elevated blood pressure or hyperlipidemia in healthy adults) and screening to detect disease among individuals at risk for disease (screening for chlamydial infection in young, sexually active women, for smoking, for dementia, or for developmental delay).

Prevention Activities and Evidence-Based Practice

Nurse clinicians and other health professionals have a major role in primary and secondary prevention. Nurse clinicians, especially advanced practice nurses and

BOX 34-2

Levels of Prevention

PRIMARY PREVENTION

Promote healthier lives (counseling on healthy diet, breast-feeding, not to smoke).

Prevent disease (immunizations; fluoride to prevent cavities in children).

SECONDARY PREVENTION

Identify risk factors (screening for elevated blood pressure, lipids, osteoporosis).

Implement early disease detection (screening for breast cancer, cervical cancer, dementia).

BOX 34-3

Definition of Evidence-Based Practice

Evidence-based practice embodies the integration of the best research evidence with clinical expertise, patient values and preferences to make decisions about patient care.

From Sackett, D., Straus, S., Richardson, W., Rosenberg, W., & Haynes, R. (2000). *Evidence-based medicine: How to practice and teach EBM.* London: Churchill Livingstone.

BOX 34-4

Scope of the U.S. Preventive Services Task Force

TYPES OF RECOMMENDATIONS

Screening (dementia)

Counseling (breast-feeding)

Immunizations (influenza)

Chemoprevention (hormone therapy)

TARGET POPULATIONS

Asymptomatic and at-risk infants to elders

PRACTICE SETTINGS

Primary care, school-based clinics

Emergency rooms, family planning clinics, nursing homes

community health nurses, currently counsel patients on physical activity, smoking, and diet; deliver immunizations and screen for modifiable risk factors such as high blood pressure and high cholesterol; and provide screening tests for early detection of cancer, infectious diseases, and other chronic illnesses. Nurses can and should do more.

Do nurses or other health professionals deliver prevention interventions consistent with Healthy People 2010 targets? Are these interventions based on the best available evidence? Studies suggest mixed results with better adherence to Healthy People 2010 targets than to evidence-based guidelines (Burns, Camaione, & Chatterton, 2000; Lawvere et al., 2004; McMenamin et al., 2004; Melynk & Fineout-Overholt, 2005; Yarnall, Pollack, Ostbye, Krause, & Michener, 2003). To deliver needed and effective preventive care, nurses and other health professionals need knowledge of primary and secondary prevention interventions based on high-quality scientific evidence and practice sites that support the delivery of preventive care. In other words, for nurses to provide prevention interventions effectively, they must develop an evidence-based practice (Box 34-3). Such a practice is based on using the best scientific evidence and clinical expertise integrated with

patient values to make care decisions (Sackett, Straus, Richardson, Rosenberg, & Hayes, 2000). The Task Force is the major national group to provide evidence-based recommendations for preventive services and is an invaluable source of practice guidelines for nurses.

THE U.S. PREVENTIVE SERVICES TASK FORCE AND EVIDENCE-BASED PRACTICE

The Task Force was established in 1984 to develop evidence-based recommendations for comprehensive clinical preventive services for the United States (Woolf & Atkins, 2001). Amazingly, just 20 years ago, most prevention recommendations were based not on a rigorous review of the scientific evidence for a particular prevention intervention but on consensus panels that used "practice wisdom" and advocacy for certain interventions by professional groups. Thus the creation of the Task Force acknowledged the need for evidence-based prevention interventions for the nation and marked the beginning of the *movement* for evidence-based practice.

The two most critical missions of the Task Force are to evaluate the scientific evidence of effectiveness of individual clinical preventive services for asymptomatic and at-risk populations across the life span and then to issue age and risk factor recommendations. The Task Force reviews the evidence for effectiveness of four types of clinical preventive services: screening, counseling, immunizations, and chemoprevention that could be delivered by clinicians in primary care settings (Box 34-4).

The primary audiences for Task Force recommendations are primary care clinicians (nurse practitioners, physicians, and physician assistants).

The Task Force represents a successful public-private partnership to translate research findings into better preventive care with multidisciplinary membership consisting of 12 to 20 experts in primary care and prevention research. The first Task Force had one nurse member, the second no nurse member, and the third and now permanent Task Force has two nurse members. Until 2002 when federal legislation authorized a permanent Task Force, each Task Force (there have been three) met for 4 years, reviewed the evidence on a wide range of prevention topics, and then developed and published a series of recommendations. For example, the first Task Force published a series of journal articles on individual interventions and in 1989 released the *Guide to Clinical Preventive Services* (U.S. Preventive Services Task Force, 1989) that reviewed evidence for 169 screening tests, counseling interventions, immunizations, and chemopreventive regimens. Subsequent Task Forces have continued to review the evidence on a wide range of topics and issue recommendations. The Agency for Healthcare Quality and Research currently houses and staffs the Task Force.

Clinicians are the primary audience for Task Force recommendations. However, as the credibility and reputation of the Task Force has grown over the past 20 years, other groups have become major users of Task Force products. Such groups include provider organizations, health plans/insurers including Medicare, purchasers, quality monitoring organizations, and policy makers. For example, Task Force recommendations have become the foundation for performance measures such as HEDIS (health employer data and information set), which is used to judge quality like those measures designed and used by the National Center for Quality Assurance.

FROM TOPIC SELECTION TO RECOMMENDATION: THE THIRD TASK FORCE AS A MODEL FOR DEVELOPING EVIDENCE-BASED PREVENTION RECOMMENDATIONS

Topic Selection

The Third Task Force used a deliberative process to select topics for review over a 4-year period. More than 40 topics (new and needing update from the 1996 Task Force) suggested by members, federal agencies, consumers, and other groups were selected based on two major criteria: burden of suffering and evidence for the effectiveness of the intervention (Harris et al., 2001). For example, updating screening for lipid disorders in adults was selected because of the large number of adults at risk for hyperlipidemia (burden of suffering); counseling for breast-feeding, a new topic, was selected because of evidence of the effectiveness of counseling interventions in promoting breast-feeding; and breast cancer screening was selected to review evidence that women could be screened at 40 not at 50.

Review of the Evidence and Development of Recommendations

Once a topic is selected for review, Task Force members focus the literature review of that topic on the questions and evidence most critical to making a recommendation. Diagrams called analytic frameworks are used to make explicit the populations, diagnostic or therapeutic interventions, and the health outcomes to be considered in the literature review. For each section of the analytic framework, key questions are developed to guide the literature search. The Task Force then uses the results of the literature search to evaluate the quality of the evidence and to categorize the net benefit (benefits minus harms) of implementing the preventive intervention. The Task Force uses its assessment of the evidence and the magnitude of net benefit of using an intervention (screening, counseling, or chemoprevention) to make a recommendation, which is coded as a letter: *A* (strongly recommended) to *D* (recommend against). An *I* recommendation is given to topics in which the evidence is insufficient to determine the net benefit of using the intervention (see Harris et al. [2001] for a detailed account of Task Force methods).

Screening and Treatment of Obesity as an Example

The literature review on the screening and treatment of obesity was guided by the analytic framework illustrated in Figure 34-1 and the key questions. The analytic framework depicts the linkage of steps from the population of interest, adults 18 and older without disease, to screening for obesity, to interventions for those determined to be obese or overweight, to the intermediate (lowered blood pressure) and health outcomes (sustained weight loss). Key questions included (1) Is there a reliable and valid screening test for obesity? and (2) Do any interventions lead to sustained weight loss?

The literature review reported that a valid and reliable screening test, the body mass index, was available; that counseling and behavioral, pharmacological, and surgical interventions were effective; that weight loss effected intermediate outcomes (lowered blood pressure and lipids); and that evidence of effects on health outcomes

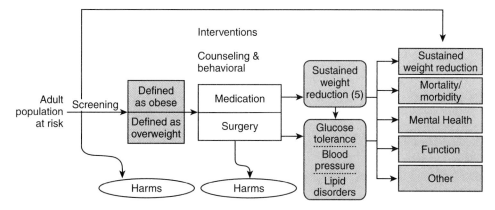

FIGURE 34-1   Screening and treatment for obesity.

was limited (Allan, 2004; McTigue et al., 2003; U.S. Preventive Services Task Force, 2003c). Based on the evidence and the determination of a net benefit from the intervention, three recommendations were approved. The following is an example of one of the approved recommendations:

> The USPSTF recommends that clinicians screen all adult patients for obesity and offer intensive counseling and behavioral interventions to promote sustained weight loss for obese adults. *B Recommendation* (U.S. Preventive Services Task Force, 2003c).

This recommendation for obesity screening and treatment is only one of the more than 40 recommendations issued by the Third Task Force. Box 34-5 illustrates the age, gender, and scope of the evidence-based prevention interventions issued by the Third Task Force.

Dissemination and Sources of Evidence-Based Interventions

Once recommendations are approved, the Task Force uses a variety of means to disseminate the recommendations for a particular topic and evidence review on that topic. For every set of recommendations, the Task Force publishes a "Recommendation and Rationale Statement" in a medical journal (with a reprint in four nursing journals) or posts it on the Agency for Healthcare Quality and Research Web site. The obesity recommendations, implications for clinicians and a detailed discussion of the evidence can be found in "Screening for Obesity: Recommendations and Rationale" (U.S. Preventive Services Task Force, 2003c). Reprints of all Task Force recommendations can be found in the following four nursing journals: *American Journal of Nursing, Nurse*

BOX 34-5

Third U.S. Preventive Services Task Force Recommendations Across the Life Span

SCREENING
Bacterial vaginosis in pregnancy
Breast cancer
Cervical cancer
Chlamydial infection
Colorectal cancer
Dementia
Depression
Developmental delay
Diabetes
Family and intimate partner violence
Gestational diabetes
High blood pressure
Lipid disorders
Newborn hearing
Osteoporosis
Prostate cancer
Skin cancer
Vision in children

CHEMOPREVENTION
Aspirin for the primary prevention of cardiovascular events
Breast cancer chemoprevention
Hormone replacement therapy
Vitamin supplementation

SCREENING AND COUNSELING
Obesity
Risky drinking

COUNSELING
Breast-feeding
Healthy diet
Physical activity

Practitioner, Journal of the American Academy of Nurse Practitioners, and *American Journal of Nurse Practitioners.*

Numerous other sources of evidence-based prevention guidelines exist. The Guide to Community Preventive Services (Community Guide) housed in the Centers for Disease Control and Prevention issues evidence-based population interventions to improve health in communities, workplace, schools, and health care organizations (Briss, Brownson, Fielding, & Zaza, 2004). For example, the Community Guide has issued recommendations on the effectiveness of physical activity interventions in school and strategies to reduce tobacco use. These recommendations are particularly helpful to nurses who work in occupational, community, and school health settings (http://www.thecommunityguide.org). Other sources of clinical guidelines include the National Guideline Clearing House at the Agency for Healthcare Quality and Research and the Association of Women's Health, Obstetric & Neonatal Nurses. The Agency for Healthcare Quality and Research recently created a nursing Web site (http://www.ahrq.gov/about/nursing) to provide information about research and training opportunities for nurses at the agency. (See Box 34-6 for a listing of Web-accessible resources for evidence-based prevention recommendations.)

EVIDENCE-BASED PRACTICE AND THE ROLE OF THE NURSE IN PREVENTION

Use of evidence-based practice is one of the five core competencies requisite for all health professionals to meet the challenges of a twenty-first century health care system (Greiner & Knebel, 2003). Basing clinical practice on the best possible evidence is becoming the standard for care for nursing and other disciplines (Taylor-Seehafer, Abel, Tyler, & Sonstein, 2004). Use of an evidence base for practice, specifically health promotion and disease prevention, is essential to improve the health of the public. The evidence of the effectiveness of behavior change interventions is increasing. The strongest evidence that clinician counseling to patients to change risky lifestyle behaviors is effective has been shown in the areas of encouraging smoking cessation, reducing problem drinking, losing weight, and modifying diet-associated cardiovascular risk factors (McTigue et al., 2003; U.S. Preventive Services Task Force, 2003a, 2003b, 2003c; Whitlock, Polen, & Green, 2004).

As stated previously, evidence-based practice is based on using the best scientific evidence and clinical expertise integrated with patient values to make care decisions (Sackett et al., 2000). This implies that clinicians/nurses

---

BOX 34-6

Resources for Evidence-Based Prevention Interventions

- Agency for Healthcare Quality and Research: U.S. Preventive Services Task Force Recommendations
  - Preventive services: http://www.preventiveservices.ahrq.gov
  - "Men: Stay Healthy at Any Age" (pdf): http://www.ahrq.gov/clinic/ppipix.htm
  - "Women: Stay Healthy at Any Age" (pdf): http://www.ahrq.gov/clinic/ppipix.htm
  - Nursing: http://www.ahrq.gov/about/nursing
- Community Guide: http://www.thecommunityguide.org
- Healthy People: http://www.healthypeople.gov
- BestBets (evidence-based clinical answers): http://www.bestbets.org
- National Guideline Clearinghouse: http://www.guideline.gov
- Tobacco Cessation Resources
  - Quitting resources: http://www.ahrq.gov/consumer/index.html#smoking
  - Material for clinicians: http://www.ahrq.gov/path/tobacco/htm
  - Smokefree.gov: http://www.smokefree.gov
  - QuitNet.com: http://www.quitnet.com
  - Centers for Disease Control and Prevention: http://www.cdc.gov/tobacco
  - Toll-free quit line: 1-800-784-8669
- Association of Women's Health, Obstetric and Neonatal Nurses: http://www.awhonn.org

---

must know how to find, critically appraise, and use the best evidence to provide care. The following are examples:

◆ If you are caring for an adult smoker, would you not want to know the most effective intervention to help him or her stop smoking?

◆ If you are taking care of a new mother who wants to breast-feed, would you want to know the most effective interventions to help her be successful?

◆ If you are working in a community prenatal clinic, would you want to use the most effective screening and behavioral interventions to reduce alcohol misuse?

Implementing an evidence-based practice involves examining the presence or absence of an evidence base for interventions used in nursing practice, determining areas that are not evidenced, collecting and appraising the evidence on those interventions, and integrating that evidence with one's expertise and the patient's values and preferences. Melynk and Fineout-Overholt's recent book *Evidence-Based Practice in Nursing & Healthcare* (2005) provides an excellent primer on the aforementioned process. Ideally, nurses should be evaluating their current practice and using this process to develop the evidence base for their practice.

To increase evidence-based prevention activities in one's practice without implementing the whole process of developing an evidence-based practice (Melynk & Fineout-Overholt, 2005; Taylor-Seehafer et al., 2004), nurses individually or as a group can do the following:

1. Step One: Assess your current practice for the use of interventions that address the five Healthy People 2010 risky lifestyle behaviors. If not all five are addressed, move to the next step. If all five are addressed, select one and review for currency of evidence and appropriateness for practice.

2. Step Two:
   ◆ Select one risky lifestyle behavior evidence-based intervention to implement within your practice.
   ◆ Use the Web-available resources listed in Box 34-6 to provide the evidence-based prevention intervention.
   ◆ Implement the evidence-based risky lifestyle behavior intervention in your practice and evaluate the results on patient outcomes.

Implementing a Smoking Cessation Intervention as an Example

Tobacco use is the leading preventable cause of death in the United States, causing more than 440,000 deaths annually (U.S. Preventive Services Task Force, 2003b). Evidence shows that brief counseling of 3 minutes or less and the use of pharmacotherapeutic agents such as the nicotine patch, gum, or nasal spray or sustained-release bupropion are effective in helping individuals stop smoking (Bialous & Sarna, 2004; U.S. Preventive Services Task Force, 2003b.) The Task Force recommended that clinicians screen all adults and pregnant women for tobacco use and provide tobacco cessation counseling interventions for those who smoke (U.S. Preventive Services Task Force, 2003b). The following five A's (*ask, advise, assess, assist,* and *arrange*) behavioral counseling framework is a useful and proven framework to implement a smoking cessation intervention in practice (Bialous & Sarna, 2004; Rice & Stead, 2004; U.S. Preventive Services Task Force, 2004).

Five Steps to a Smoking Cessation Intervention

Use the following five steps to implement a smoking cessation intervention:

1. Ask patient about tobacco use (record smoking status annually, years smoking and cigarettes/day, and quit history).

2. Advise patient to quit (discuss benefits and risks of smoking).

3. Assess willingness of patient to quit (assess interest in quitting; if not ready, give information about cessation and bring up topic on another visit).

4. Assist patient to quit (develop a plan to quit—quit date, use of medications, and identification of triggers to relapse such as stress and food patterns; and develop a plan to address relapse).

5. Arrange follow-up and support (schedule follow-up visit, have patient enlist support of friends, and refer patient to informational Web sites and telephone quit lines).

This smoking cessation intervention can be implemented in primary and tertiary care settings. This intervention is probably one of the most effective and easiest evidenced-based interventions to implement in practice. This intervention is a way to launch an evidenced-based practice. The nurse must overcome the barriers: patients do want to quit, and nurses have the time to provide a smoking cessation intervention. Many resources for patients and providers related to tobacco use are available. The newest are the U.S. Department of Health and Human Services toll-free tobacco quit line (1-800-784-8669) and a Web site for information and advice (www.smokefree.gov). (See Box 34-6 for other resources.)

SUMMARY

Focusing on prevention, especially lifestyle-related behaviors, offers the greatest potential for decreasing morbidity and mortality, improving quality of life, and decreasing health care costs. Many nurses currently are involved in delivering health promotion and disease prevention interventions. Nurses can and should do more to implement in their practices this long-standing tenet of the profession. By taking the leadership in implementing prevention interventions with individuals and communities, nursing can make a major contribution to the health of the public. Such interventions must be evidence-based. Nurses must support the paradigm shift to evidence-based nursing practice.

REFERENCES

Adams, K., & Corrigan, J. M. (Eds.). (2003). *Priority areas for national action: Transforming health care quality.* Washington, DC: National Academies Press.

Allan, J. (2004). Rampant obesity: What can you do? *Sexuality, Reproduction and Menopause, 2,* 195-198.

Bialous, S., & Sarna, L. (2004). Sparing a few minutes for tobacco cessation. *American Journal of Nursing, 104,* 54-60.

Briss, P., Brownson, R., Fielding, J., & Zaza, S. (2004). Developing and using the guide to community preventive services: Lessons learned about evidence-based public health. *Annual Review of Public Health, 25,* 281-302.

Burns, K., Camaione, D., & Chatterton, C. (2000). Prescription of physical activity by adult nurse practitioners: A national survey. *Nursing Outlook, 48,* 28-33.

Greiner, A. C., & Knebel, E. (Eds.). (2003). *Health professions education: A bridge to quality.* Washington, DC: National Academies Press.

Harris, R., Helfand, M., Woolf, S., Lohr, K., Mulrow, C., Teutsch, S., et al. (2001). Current methods of the U.S. Preventive Services Task Force: A review of the process. *American Journal of Preventive Medicine, 20*(3S), 21-35.

Institute of Medicine. (2001). *Crossing the quality chasm: A new health system for the 21st century.* Washington, DC: National Academies Press.

Jennings, M. (2004). Translational research: Disrupting the status quo. *Nursing Outlook, 52,* 66.

Kelley, E., Moy, E., Kosiak, B., McNeill, D., Zhan, C., Stryer, D., et al. (2004). Prevention health care quality in America: Findings from the first national healthcare quality and disparities reports. *Preventing Chronic Disease: Public Health Research, Practice and Policy, 1,* 1-5.

Lawvere, S., Mahoney, M., Symons, A., Englert, J., Klein, S., & Mirand, A. (2004). Approaches to breast cancer screening among nurse practitioners. *Journal of the American Academy of Nurse Practitioners, 16,* 38-43.

McMenamin, S., Schmittdiel, J., Halpin, H., Gillies, R., Rundall, T., & Shortell, S. (2004). Health promotion in physician organizations: Results from a national study. *American Journal of Preventive Medicine, 26,* 259-264.

McTigue, K., Harris, R., Hemphil, B., Lux, L., Sutton, A., & Lohr, K. (2003). Screening and interventions for obesity in adults: Summary of the evidence for the U.S. Preventive Services Task Force. *Annals of Internal Medicine, 139,* 933-949.

Melynyk, B., & Fineout-Overholt, E. (2005). *Evidence-based practice in nursing & healthcare.* Philadelphia: Lippincott Williams & Wilkins.

Pender, N., Murdaugh, C., & Parsons, M. (2002). *Health promotion in nursing practice* (4th ed.). Upper Saddle River, NJ: Prentice Hall.

Rice, V., & Stead, L. (2004). Nursing interventions for smoking cessation. *Cochrane Database Systematic Reviews, 1,* CD001188.

Sackett, D., Straus, S., Richardson, W., Rosenberg, W., & Haynes, R. (2000). *Evidence-based medicine: How to practice and teach EBM.* London: Churchill Livingstone.

Shamansky, S., & Clausen, C. (1980). Levels of prevention: Examination of the concept. *Nursing Outlook, 28,* 104-108.

Taylor-Seehafer, M., Abel, E., Tyler, D., & Sonstein, F. (2004). Integrating evidence-based practice in nurse practitioner education. *Journal of the American Academy of Nurse Practitioners, 16,* 520-525.

U.S. Department of Health and Human Services. (2000). *Healthy people 2010.* Washington, DC: U.S. Government Printing Office.

U.S. Preventive Services Task Force. (1989). *Guide to clinical preventive services: An assessment of the effectiveness of 169 interventions.* Baltimore: Williams & Wilkins.

U.S. Preventive Services Task Force. (2003a). Behavioral counseling in primary care to promote a healthy diet. *American Journal of Preventive Medicine, 24,* 93-100.

U.S. Preventive Services Task Force. (2003b). Counseling to prevent tobacco use and tobacco-caused disease. Retrieved June 1, 2005, from http://www.ahrq.gov/clinic/3rduspstf/tobacccoun/tobcounrs.htm

U.S. Preventive Services Task Force. (2003c). Screening for obesity in adults: Recommendations and rationale. *Annals of Internal Medicine, 139,* 930-932.

U.S. Preventive Services Task Force. (2004). Screening and behavioral counseling interventions in primary care to reduce alcohol misuse. *Annals of Internal Medicine, 140,* 555-557.

Whitlock, E., Orleans, T., Pender, N., & Allan, J. (2002). Evaluating primary care behavioral counseling interventions: An evidence-based approach. *American Journal of Preventive Medicine, 22,* 267-284.

Whitlock, E., Polen, M., & Green, C. (2004). Behavioral counseling interventions in primary care to reduce risky/harmful alcohol use by adults: summary of the evidence for the U.S. Preventive Services Task Force. *Annals of Internal Medicine, 140,* 558-569.

Woolf, S., & Atkins, D. (2001). The evolving role of the prevention in health care: Contributions of the U.S. Preventive Services Task Force. *American Journal of Preventive Medicine, 20*(Suppl. 3), 13-20.

Yarnall, K., Pollack, K., Ostbye, T., Krause, K., & Michener, J. (2003). Primary care: Is there enough time for prevention? *American Journal of Public Health, 93,* 635-641.

Nursing Care Priority Area

Chronic Conditions

CONNIE DAVIS

> Ultimately, the secret of quality is love. You have to love your patients, you have to love your profession, you have to love your God. If you have love, you can work backward to monitor and improve the system.
>
> **Donabedian, 2001, p. 140**

SCOPE OF THE PROBLEM

Chronic illness dominates health care today. More than half of all Americans over age 18 have a chronic condition. More than 80% of those over age 65 have one or more chronic illnesses. Eighty-one percent of hospitalizations can be attributed to chronic illness. Even among children, 35% live with a chronic respiratory condition, and 15% have a chronic emotional or behavioral disorder. These chronic conditions account for 83% of all health care spending (Partnership for Solutions, 2004). In 2003 the cost of heart disease in the United States was estimated to be $351 billion, including the cost of lost productivity ($142 billion) (National Center for Chronic Disease Prevention and Health Promotion, "Preventing," Costs section, ¶1). A 2002 study done for the American Diabetes Association showed similar estimates for the cost of diabetes in the United States at $132 billion in indirect and direct costs (National Center for Chronic Disease Prevention and Health Promotion, "National Estimates," Cost of diabetes in the United States section, ¶1)

The Institute of Medicine report *Crossing the Quality Chasm* (2001) described six dimensions of focus for improvement activities: safety, effectiveness, timeliness, efficiency, patient-centeredness, and equity. When these dimensions are used to measure the processes and outcomes of chronic illness care, American health care comes up woefully lacking. In a large survey of adults living in the United States, McGlynn et al.* (2003) found

that around 50% of the time, patients are not receiving the care they should receive. Patients report waiting for services and results (Schoen et al., 2004). Quality indicators in primary care vary by up to 13% for patients of different races, and patients state that they feel uninformed by their providers (Partnership for Solutions, 2004).

The *Crossing the Quality Chasm* report is slowly influencing health care delivery. In follow-up to the report, the Institute of Medicine identified priority areas for addressing quality. Chronic conditions are the focus of the priority areas because they are present across the life span; affect health care institutions of all types; and represent an excessive burden in disability, mortality, and cost and because there are examples of solutions to quality problems (Adams & Corrigan, 2003). The *Crossing the Quality Chasm Summit* emphasized the special role of communities in addressing quality of care and highlighted successful programs that addressed the priority areas (Adams, Greiner, & Corrigan, 2004).

The *Crossing the Quality Chasm* report also has influenced the Centers for Medicare and Medicaid Services and the Joint Commission on Accreditation of Healthcare Organizations. The Centers for Medicare and Medicaid Services (2005) is urging the adoption of disease management and is conducting demonstration projects. The Joint Commission on Accreditation of Healthcare Organizations (2005) has a program for accreditation of disease-specific care.

CLOSING THE GAP

The need to close these gaps in quality of care can be organized around three themes:

1. Patient-centered care
2. Evidence-based methods
3. Population focus

The agenda for interactions with chronically ill patients has two goals: the delivery of effective clinical

---

*I would like to thank Gwendolyn Davis and Susan Bennett for help in the preparation of this manuscript.

care and the support of self-management efforts, a major component of patient-centered care. When these two goals are met for all patients, good chronic illness care is assured. This chapter explores each of these themes in more detail.

Patient-Centered Care

The Institute of Medicine (2001) denotes key characteristics of patient-centered health care as creating working partnerships with patients and their families; ensuring that decisions respect and honor patient's wants, needs, and preferences; providing patients with the education and support they need to make informed treatment decisions; and enabling patients to be the central resource in their own health and/or the health of their family. Patients with chronic illness are the primary providers of their own care. They constantly make health decisions: when and what to eat, what kind and how much activity to pursue, whether to take medications, and how much medication to take. Efforts at quality improvement must be geared to this reality: patients (along with their families and caregivers) determine the care they ultimately receive.

Extensive literature describes the self-management support needs of patients with chronic illness. Through interviews with patients with many different chronic conditions, Corbin and Straus (1988) described the three tasks of living with a chronic condition. The first task is taking care of the illness. This task encompasses activities such as taking medications and learning to monitor symptoms or physiological control, such as pain, fatigue, blood pressure, or blood glucose. The second task, learning to adapt daily life, means balancing the demands and events of daily life with caring for the condition. A worker on the night shift who has diabetes determines how to schedule medication and eating into a challenging routine. A diagnosis of chronic illness often brings emotional changes. Coping with these changes is the third task. Common emotions are anger, fear, and frustration. Individuals with chronic illness have a higher rate of depression at the outset or as a result of living with a chronic condition (Gagnon & Patten, 2002).

These tasks can form the agenda of health care interactions with chronically ill patients and the content of patient education and self-management training programs. Because the tasks are common to any condition, successful programs include patients with a variety of illnesses (Lorig et al., 1999, 2001). Condition-specific programs may serve informational and specific skill needs (such as the use of a peak flow meter) but also may discourage successful daily self-management if comorbidities and common tasks across conditions are not considered. A patient who sees a specialist physician, nurse, or care manager for each condition—such as diabetes, chronic heart failure, and depression—may be internalizing a message that specialist expertise is required in the daily management of the condition.

Effective support for patients with chronic illness focuses on building self-efficacy, or self-confidence. Lorig and Holman (2003) describe methods found to increase self-efficacy. They include performance mastery (learning new skills), modeling (seeing others in similar situations manage their conditions), reinterpretation of symptoms (such as attributing fatigue to deconditioning instead of arthritis, thereby encouraging the patient to become more physically active), and social persuasion (such as working in groups). The specific activities common to successful self-management programs are referred to as the five A's: *assessment* of self-management status (including confidence), *advice* tailored to the patient, *agreement* on a self-management goal, *assistance* with making action plans and problem solving to meet the goal, and *arranging* follow-up and resources (Glasgow et al., 2002). These methods and activities can be incorporated into individual and group interactions.

Informed treatment decisions necessitate using language that patients and colleagues understand. Clinical terminology and nursing diagnoses do not promote communication with patients. One simple technique to clarify understanding is "closing the loop" by asking patients to repeat what they have heard. In studies with physicians, patients with diabetes had improved outcomes when providers closed the loop (Schillinger et al., 2003).

Patient-centered care results in a patient-derived care plan. One example of effective communication is the Shared Care Plan (found at http://www.patient-powered.org). The Web-based Shared Care Plan resides on a secure server and records crucial information for patient care, such as current medication lists, allergies, and less traditional information such as learning style and the patient's life goals. With the patient's permission, the care plan can be viewed (and edited) by emergency room personnel, primary care teams, care managers, and the patient's caregivers. The care plan is in the patient's language and is understandable to all who refer to it.

Patient-centered care requires communication and collaboration as demonstrated by the Shared Care Plan. For patients with chronic illness, the most effective type of collaboration includes working with an interdisciplinary team. Multiple studies have demonstrated the success of interdisciplinary team care for chronic illness (Dietrich et al., 2004; Shortell et al., 2004; Sperl-Hillen et al., 2000; Taplin, Galvin, Payne, Coole, & Wagner, 1998; Wagner, 2000). To work effectively in a team, all team members focus on the patient's needs and divide roles and responsibilities to best meet those needs. Everyone on the health care team should be working at his or her highest capability but also should be willing to assist in any capacity when need dictates. Everyone in the health care setting can assist in chronic illness care. For example, volunteers, laboratory technicians, housekeepers, and receptionists can use and teach skills such as goal setting, problem solving, and action planning. Trained peer educators have been found to be as effective as professionals for patients with chronic illness (Lorig, Feigenbaum, et al., 1986).

Evidence-Based Methods

For chronic illness care, the evidence base typically refers to clinical trials of effective drug therapy, an essential but overemphasized contributor to outcomes. Nurses who are familiar with clinical guidelines, monitor medication use, and assist patients in understanding and evaluating their medications can increase the chance that patients are receiving evidence-based care. An emerging evidence base describes effective self-management support techniques, as noted under Patient-Centered Care.

Two additional kinds of evidence that frequently are left unconsidered are the evidence base for quality improvement methods and the evidence base for system redesign. Quality improvement methods now can be grounded in evidence. Langley, Nolan, Nolan, Norman, and Provost (1996) developed the model for improvement (Figure 35-1) through work with multiple organizations and describe a successful method for testing and implementing change. The model for improvement begins by asking three questions:

1. What are we trying to accomplish?
2. How will we know that a change is an improvement?
3. What change can we make that will result in an improvement?

An aim statement answers the first question, a measurement strategy answers the second, and the clinical and system design evidence base can answer the third.

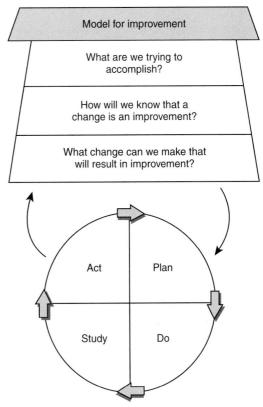

FIGURE 35-1   Model for improvement.
From Langley, G. J., Nolan, K. M., Nolan, T. W., Norman, C. L., & Provost, L. P. (1996). *The improvement guide: A practical approach to enhancing organizational performance* (p. 10). San Francisco: Jossey-Bass.

These three questions are coupled to activity: the plan-do-study-act cycle (Figure 35-2). The plan-do-study-act method directs those involved in improvement to start with small tests of new ideas to build the improved system instead of spending time designing improvements in the absence of experience. An example of using a plan-do-study-act is found in the Box 35-1. These test cycles remove many of the barriers found in historical quality improvement methods. Small tests decrease the risk of large-scale failure, allow hesitant staff members to observe change before participating in it, create confidence and data to demonstrate that the changes are useful, and point out any consequences or factors that should be considered when making a change. Cycles of testing lead to cycles of implementation, and the change is made permanent (Figure 35-3).

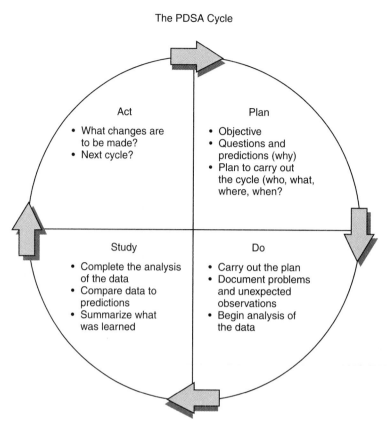

FIGURE 35-2   Plan-do-study-act detail.
From Langley, G. J., Nolan, K. M., Nolan, T. W., Norman, C. L., & Provost, L. P. (1996). *The improvement guide: A practical approach to enhancing organizational performance* (p. 60). San Francisco: Jossey-Bass.

The second new type of evidence base is system design. Don Berwick (1996), a leading figure in quality improvement, says, "Every system is perfectly designed to achieve the results it achieves" (p. 619). Following this reasoning, the current health care system is perfectly designed to deliver substandard clinical care, inequities in health care, and uninformed patients. In the past, health care workers or patients have been blamed for quality shortcomings. A more helpful way to solve these problems and change outcomes is to redesign the system that created them.

The chronic care model (Figure 35-4) serves as the evidence base for system redesign in chronic illness care. This model was developed by reviewing effective clinical trials, interviewing successful chronic illness programs, and visiting nationally recognized programs that deliver outstanding care (Bodenheimer, Wagner, & Grumbach, 2002; Wagner, Davis, Schaefer, Von Korff, & Austin, 1999).

In this model, improved outcomes result from productive interactions between a prepared health care team and an informed, activated patient. The model then describes six categories of design principles that promote patient activation and team care: self-management support, delivery system design, decision support, clinical information systems, the organization of health care, and community resources and policies. Box 35-2 gives the principles in detail.

The principles form the basis for tests of change (plan-do-study-act cycles). For example, a nurse who wants to use effective self-management support techniques might decide to test goal setting in an interaction. A nurse practitioner might test the same principle by holding a group visit for patients with chronic illness. Each principle is the basis for many unique but evidence-based ways to improve care.

By using these two evidence-based methods, the model for improvement and the chronic care model,

BOX 35-1

Plan-Do-Study-Act Example

PLAN

Objective: Determine whether making an action plan is feasible in our family practice clinic.

Questions and predictions: Does the office nurse have enough time? Will patients like making an action plan? We predict that patients will like it but that it will bog down our flow.

Specifics: Dr. B will send the first patient with hypertension that we see on Tuesday to Nurse A after the visit. Nurse A will use the action planning form with the patient.

DO

Nurse A did the plan and noted unexpected occurrences. Nurse A timed the interaction, and Medical Assistant C kept track of patient flow.

STUDY

The action planning took 7 minutes. The next patient had to wait for 5 minutes for an immunization. The patient was a little surprised about the new part of the medical visit and needed some background information about goal setting. The patient liked making an action plan.

ACT

Try again tomorrow but have a handout for patients about goal setting to review while waiting for the doctor.

an organization can redesign its system to be more effective. Both models have been used widely throughout the United States and Canada. The two models often are combined in collaborative improvement projects involving multiple organizations or sites within an organization (Daniel et al., "Case Studies," 2004; Daniel et al., "A State-Level," 2004; Fulton, Penney, & Taft, 2001; Glasgow et al., 2002; Quinn et al., 2001; Wagner et al., 2001).

Population Focus

"It is important that an aim never be defined in terms of activity or methods. It must always relate directly to how life is better for everyone" (Deming, 1994, p. 52).

Improvements in chronic illness care will not be achieved unless the improvements target everyone in need of care. This requires the use of public health approaches such as population surveillance and outreach.

Outside of public health settings these approaches commonly are called population-based care. Population-based care can be defined as the effective and efficient delivery of evidence-based services to a distinct group of patients. The population is determined by a variety of factors such as geography, organizational affiliation, or care site. A nurse working in a long-term care facility might serve a population of patients on a floor, a home care nurse might consider a caseload the population, the home care agency would consider all the patients it serves as the population, and a nurse working in a primary care clinic might serve a population based on the care team. Further division into subpopulations targets interventions to those who will benefit. For example, an office practice might decide to target care management for patients who do not have good clinical control and are not confident self-managers, or a community agency might offer smoking cessation classes to clients who smoke and have indicated that they prefer learning in groups.

Most current practices in outpatient settings rely on patients to seek care. Quality improvement for population-based care is designed around an assessment of the needs of the population and the current quality indicators. The quality indicators should reflect the patients' needs for clinical care and self-management support. Measures such as self-confidence (Lorig, Stewart, et al., 1996), quality of life and activation (Hibbard, Stockard, Mahoney, & Tusler, 2004) should be considered. Systematic provision of services (following a framework such as the chronic care model) for all members of the population will contribute to better health.

SUMMARY

To improve chronic illness care, care must be patient-centered, evidence-based, and delivered to everyone in the population. Patient-centeredness requires a new emphasis on collaboration, communication, and cooperation. Using the evidence base means moving beyond clinical guidelines and into improvement methodology and system redesign. Population-based care necessitates changing the care of every patient. The challenge of improving chronic illness care can be met by an adequately prepared collegial workforce concerned with patient needs. Nurses can help meet this challenge by maintaining the focus on the patient, using the evidence for quality improvement and system redesign, and ensuring that all patients benefit from improvement.

Repeated Use of the PDSA Cycle

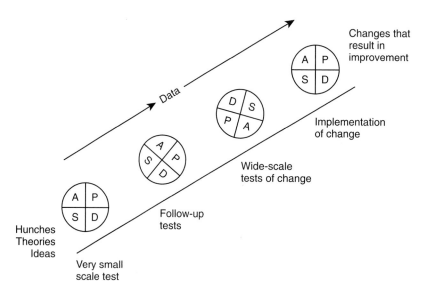

FIGURE 35-3 Improvement ramp.
From Langley, G. J., Nolan, K. M., Nolan, T. W., Norman, C. L., & Provost, L. P. (1996). *The improvement guide: A practical approach to enhancing organizational performance* (p. 9). San Francisco: Jossey-Bass.

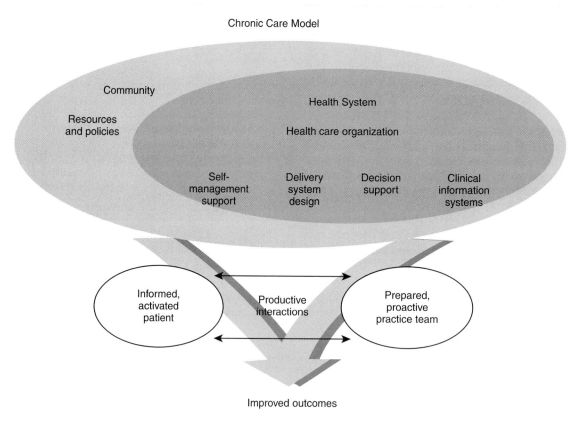

FIGURE 35-4 The chronic care model.
From Wagner, E. H. (1998). Chronic disease management: What will it take to improve care for chronic illness? *Effective Clinical Practice, 1,* 3.

BOX 35-2

Principles of Chronic Care Model

Self-management support: Empower and prepare patients to manage their health and health care.
- Emphasize the patient's central role in managing his or her health.
- Use effective self-management support strategies that include assessment, goal setting, action planning, problem solving, and follow-up.
- Organize internal and community resources to provide ongoing self-management support to patients.

Delivery system design: Ensure the delivery of effective, efficient clinical care and self-management support.
- Define roles and distribute tasks among team members.
- Use planned interactions to support evidence-based care.
- Provide clinical case management services for patients with complex conditions.
- Ensure regular follow-up by the care team.
- Give care that patients understand and that fits with their cultural background.

Decision support: Promote clinical care that is consistent with scientific evidence and patient preferences.
- Embed evidence-based guidelines into daily clinical practice.
- Integrate specialist expertise and primary care.
- Use proven provider education methods.
- Share evidence-based guidelines and information with patients to encourage their participation.

Clinical information system: Organize patient and population data to facilitate efficient and effective care.
- Provide timely reminders for providers and patients.
- Identify relevant subpopulations for proactive care.
- Facilitate individual patient care planning.
- Share information with patients and providers to coordinate care.
- Monitor performance of practice team and care system.

Health care organization: Create a culture, organization, and mechanisms that promote safe, high-quality care.
- Visibly support improvement at all levels of the organization, beginning with the senior leader.
- Promote effective improvement strategies aimed at comprehensive system change.
- Encourage open and systematic handling of errors and quality problems to improve care.
- Provide incentives based on quality of care.
- Develop agreements that facilitate care coordination within and across organizations.

COMMUNITY: MOBILIZE COMMUNITY RESOURCES TO MEET NEEDS OF PATIENTS
- Encourage patients to participate in effective community programs.
- Form partnerships with community organizations to support and develop interventions that fill gaps in needed services.
- Advocate for policies to improve patient care.

From Improving Chronic Illness Care. (n.d.). *The chronic care model.* Retrieved December 29, 2005, from http://www.improvingchroniccare.org/change/model/components.html

REFERENCES

Adams, K., & Corrigan, J. M. (Eds). (2003). Executive summary [Electronic version]. In Committee on Identifying Priority Areas for Quality Improvement, *Priority areas for national action: Transforming health care quality.* Washington: National Academy of Sciences.

Adams, K., Greiner, A. C., & Corrigan, J. M. (Eds.). (2004). Executive summary [Electronic version]. In *First Annual Crossing the Quality Chasm Summit: A Focus on Communities.* Washington, DC: National Academy of Sciences.

Berwick, D. M. (1996). A primer on leading the improvement of systems. *British Medical Journal, 312,* 619.

Bodenheimer, T., Wagner, E. H., & Grumbach, K. (2002). Improving primary care for patients with chronic illness: The chronic care model, Part 2. *JAMA: The Journal of the American Medical Association, 288,* 1909-1914.

Centers for Medicare and Medicaid Services. (2005). *Demonstration projects and evaluation reports.* Retrieved March 25, 2005, from http://www.cms.hhs.gov/researchers/demos/

Corbin, J., & Straus, A. (1988). *Unending work and care: Managing chronic illness at home.* San Francisco: Jossey-Bass.

Daniel, D. M., Norman, J., Davis, C., Lee, H., Hindmarsh, M. F., McCulloch, D. K., et al. (2004). Case studies from two collaboratives on diabetes in Washington State. *Joint Commission Journal on Quality and Safety, 30,* 103-108.

Daniel, D. M., Norman, J., Davis, C., Lee, H., Hindmarsh, M. F., McCulloch, D. K., et al. (2004). A state-level application of the chronic illness breakthrough series: Results from two collaboratives on diabetes in Washington State. *Joint Commission Journal on Quality and Safety, 30*(2), 69-79.

Deming, W. E. (1994). *The new economics for industry, government, education* (2nd ed.). Cambridge, MA: MIT Press.

Dietrich, A. J., Oxman, T. E., Williams, J. W., Jr., Schulberg, H. C., Bruce, M. L., Lee, P. W., et al. (2004). Re-engineering systems for the treatment of depression in primary care: Cluster randomised controlled trial. *British Medical Journal, 329,* 602.

Donabedian, A. (2001). A founder of quality assessment encounters a troubled system firsthand. Interview by Fitzhugh Mullan. *Health Affairs (Millwood), 20,* 137-141.

Fulton, T. R., Penney, B. C., & Taft, A. (2001). Exploring a chronic care model in a regional healthcare context. *Health Management Forum, 14,* 6-24.

Gagnon, L. M., & Patten, S. B. (2002). Major depression and its association with long-term medical conditions. *Canadian Journal of Psychiatry, 47,* 149-152.

Glasgow, R. E., Funnell, M. M., Bonomi, A. E., Davis, C., Beckham, V., & Wagner, E. H. (2002). Self-management aspects of the improving chronic illness care breakthrough series: Implementation with diabetes and heart failure teams. *Annals of Behavioral Medicine, 24,* 80-87.

Joint Commission on Accreditation of Healthcare Organizations. (2005). *Disease-specific care certification.* Retrieved March 25, 2005, from http://www.jcaho.org/dscc/dsc/dsc.htm

Hibbard, J. H., Stockard, J., Mahoney, E. R., & Tusler, M. (2004). Developing the patient activation measure (PAM): Conceptualizing and measuring activation in patients and consumers. *Health Services Research, 39,* 1005-1026.

Institute of Medicine. (2001). *Crossing the quality chasm: A new health system for the 21st century.* Washington, DC: National Academy Press.

Langley, G. J., Nolan, K. M., Nolan, T. W., Norman, C. L., & Provost, L. P. (1996). *The improvement guide: A practical approach to enhancing organizational performance.* San Francisco: Jossey-Bass.

Lorig, K., Feigenbaum, P., Regan, C., Ung, E., Chastain, R. L., & Holman, H. R. (1986). A comparison of lay-taught and professional-taught arthritis self-management courses. *Journal of Rheumatology, 13,* 763-767.

Lorig, K. R., & Holman, H. (2003). Self-management education: history, definition, outcomes, and mechanisms. *Annals of Behavioral Medicine, 26,* 1-7.

Lorig, K. R., Ritter, P., Stewart, A. L., Sobel, D. S., Brown, B. W., Jr., Bandura, A., et al. (2001). Chronic disease self-management program: 2-year health status and health care utilization outcomes. *Medical Care, 39*(11), 1217-1223.

Lorig, K. R., Sobel, D. S., Stewart, A. L., Brown, B. W., Jr., Bandura, A., Ritter, P., et al. (1999). Evidence suggesting that a chronic disease self-management program can improve health status while reducing hospitalization: a randomized trial. *Medical Care, 37*(1), 5-14.

Lorig, K., Stewart, A., Ritter, P., Gonzalez, V., Laurent, D., & Lynch, J. (1996). *Outcome measures for health education and other health care interventions.* Thousand Oaks, CA: Sage Publications.

McGlynn, E. A., Asch, S. M., Adams, J., Keesey, J., Hicks, J., DeCristofaro, A., et al. (2003). The quality of health care delivered to adults in the United States. *New England Journal of Medicine, 348,* 2635-2645.

National Center for Chronic Disease Prevention and Health Promotion. (2005). *National diabetes fact sheet: National estimates on diabetes.* Retrieved March 25, 2005, from http://www.cdc.gov/diabetes/pubs/estimates.htm

National Center for Chronic Disease Prevention and Health Promotion. (2005). *Preventing heart disease and stroke.* Retrieved March 25, 2005, from http://www.cdc.gov/nccdphp/ bb_heartdisease/

Partnership for Solutions. (2004). *Chronic conditions: Making the case for ongoing care. September 2004 Update.* Retrieved December 2, 2004, from http://www.partnershipforsolutions,org/DMS/files/chronicbook2004.pdf

Quinn, D. C., Graber, A. L., Elasy, T. A., Thomas, J., Wolff, K., & Brown, A. (2001). Overcoming turf battles: Developing a pragmatic, collaborative model to improve glycemic control in patients with diabetes. *Joint Commission Journal on Quality Improvement, 27,* 255-264.

Schillinger, D., Piette, J., Grumbach, K., Wang, F., Wilson, C., Daher, C., et al. (2003). Closing the loop: Physician communication with diabetic patients who have low health literacy. *Archives of Internal Medicine, 163*(1), 83-90.

Schoen, C., Osborn, R., Huynh, O. T., Doty, M., Davis, K., Zapert, K., et al. (2004, October 28). *Primary care and health system performance: Adults' experiences in five countries.* Retrieved December 2, 2004, from http://content.healthaffairs.org/cgi/reprint/hlthaff.w4.487v1

Shortell, S. M., Marsteller, J. A., Lin, M., Pearson, M. L., Wu, S. Y., Mendel, P., et al. (2004). The role of perceived team effectiveness in improving chronic illness care. *Medical Care, 42,* 1040-1048.

Sperl-Hillen, J., O'Connor, P. J., Carlson, R. R., Lawson, T. B., Halstenson, C., Crowson, T., et al. (2000). Improving diabetes care in a large health care system: an enhanced primary care approach. *Joint Commission Journal on Quality Improvement, 26,* 615-622.

Taplin, S., Galvin, M. S., Payne, T., Coole, D., & Wagner, E. (1998). Putting population-based care into practice: Real option or rhetoric? *Journal of the American Board of Family Practice, 11,* 116-126.

Wagner, E. H. (2000). The role of patient care teams in chronic disease management. *British Medical Journal, 320,* 569-572.

Wagner, E., Davis, C., Schaefer, J., Von Korff, M., & Austin, B. (1999). A survey of leading chronic disease management programs: Are they consistent with the literature? *Managed Care Quarterly, 7,* 56-66.

Wagner, E. H., Glasgow, R. E., Davis, C., Bonomi, A. E., Provost, L., McCulloch, D., et al. (2001). Quality improvement in chronic illness care: A collaborative approach. *Joint Commission Journal on Quality Improvement, 27*(2), 63-80.

Nursing Care Priority Area

Frailty, Palliative, End of Life

JUNE R. LUNNEY

A third of all health care provided in this country is provided to those aged 65 or older (Lubitz, Beebe, & Baker, 1995), and a significant proportion of that care is provided in the last year of life (Hogan, Lunney, Gabel, & Lynn, 2001). The Institute of Medicine has delineated frailty associated with old age as one of the 20 priority areas for improvement in health care quality (Adams & Corrigan, 2003). As the average life expectancy increases, nurses more and more will find themselves providing care to frail elders who are approaching the end of life. The quality of that care thus will be a significant reflection on overall nursing care quality.

GROWTH AND CHANGE AHEAD

The changing demography of the United States will have a profound impact on health care. First, the absolute number of elderly persons will increase, especially in the number of those older than 80 years of age. Since 1900 the U.S. population has tripled, but the number of older adults has increased elevenfold. Demographers estimate that the number of persons aged 80 years or more will more than double in the next 30 years (Centers for Disease Control and Prevention, 2003).

The second important aspect of this change in demography relates to the proportion of elderly. The increase in ratio of elderly to younger members of society means that there will be an increase in social dependency— fewer workers to pay bills for health care—and an increase in family dependency, or fewer younger family members to care for elders (Callahan, 1987). The issue of fewer family members to care for their older loved ones is compounded further by changes in family lifestyles, especially the increased likelihood that grown children, men and women alike, will have full-time employment outside of the home. Nurses play an important role in helping the elderly to meet their personal care needs, and this change will affect how nurses can provide for this assistance.

In addition to the demographic shift, changes are ongoing in the health of elders as they end their lives. The average American born in 2001 will die at the age of 77 (Kochanek, Murphy, Anderson, & Scott, 2004), largely because the leading causes of death in 1900 (injury and infection) no longer threaten Americans. In 2000 the top three causes of death were heart disease, cancer, and stroke, accounting for 60% of deaths (Centers for Disease Control and Prevention, 2004). "Today we die by inches instead of miles" (Webb, 1997).

TRAJECTORIES OF DYING

With the change in leading causes of death, there is more diversity developing in how life ends. Conceptualizing the end of life as a trajectory helps to provide a framework to describe this diversity. In a 1968 ethnographic study of how people die, Glaser and Strauss (1968) described three different trajectories of dying: abrupt, surprise deaths; expected deaths (short-term and lingering); and entry-reentry deaths, where individuals slowly decline but return home between stays in the hospital. More recently, these ideas have come to be expressed commonly as functional trajectories (Institute of Medicine, 1997; Lynn, 2001).

Some die suddenly, progressing from normal functioning to death in a brief time. These decedents usually have little forewarning and often little or no interaction with the health care system before dying. Sudden deaths include those resulting from myocardial infarction or massive stroke. Others die after a distinct terminal phase of illness, which is most typical of cancer patients. Cancer patients may function reasonably well with their illness for some time before their illness becomes overwhelming and nonresponsive to treatment. Researchers have found that most cancer patients then decline rapidly, usually dying within a 6-week terminal phase (Morris, Suissa, Sherwood, Wright, & Greer, 1986).

A third group, mostly those who have a serious and eventually fatal organ system failure such as congestive heart failure or chronic obstructive pulmonary disease, experience gradually diminishing functional status with periodic dramatic exacerbations of their illness. Each exacerbation could cause death, but usually a person has many such episodes. The prognosis for survival remains ambiguous. For example, half of the patients with heart failure who die from their disease do so within 1 week of the point at which a multivariable prognostic model would assign them at least a 50% probability of living longer than 6 months (Lynn, Harrell, Cohn, Wagner, & Connors, 1997).

Members of the frailty group experience an even slower decline with steadily progressive disability before dying from complications such as those associated with advanced frailty of old age, stroke, or dementia. These individuals may experience functional dependency, requiring assistance with instrumental and fundamental activities of daily living for years before they die.

The distribution of decedents among these various trajectories is not certain. An estimate derived from a study of the Medicare payments for a population-based sample of elderly decedents suggests that nearly half of those who die after the age of 65 will do so after a period of frail health (Lunney, Lynn, & Hogan, 2002). In this study, 47% of the deceased Medicare beneficiaries had had at least one Medicare claim in the last year of life associated with a diagnosis of stroke, Alzheimer's disease, dementia, acute delirium, Parkinson's disease, hip fracture, incontinence, pneumonia, dehydration, syncope, or leg cellulitis. Each of these conditions generally is associated with frailty and advanced old age.

To admit that people could simply die of old age is not politically correct (Nuland, 1995). That possibility does not fit with that societal notion that all disease is open to systematic biomedical attack—that we can "do away" with even cancer and heart disease. Yet some have argued that even healthy, very elderly persons who do not develop an acute or chronic life-threatening disease eventually undergo an irreversible fatal decline (McCue, 1995). Furthermore, even in the presence of one or more pathological conditions, death among very old persons might be considered to be somewhat "opportunistic," the particular final cause of death almost a random event occurring on top of an older person's more generalized disease processes (Havlik & Rosenberg, 1992). The focus of this chapter is on those elderly persons who die after the age of 80 years, with or without a diagnosed life-threatening illness. The fact of their increasing frailty, whether existing with chronic illness or not, has tremendous implications for nursing care at the end of life.

FRAILTY

The term *frailty* rarely was used before the 1980s (Hogan, MacKnight, & Bergman, 2003), but as more attention became focused on the health issues of an older population, a need emerged to differentiate groups within the heterogeneous group of persons over the age of 65. Early on, frailty was viewed as a "failure to thrive" (Braun, Wykle, & Cowling, 1988; Egbert, 1993; Palmer, 1990) and as a pathological condition open to reversal. Yet although the syndrome may be improved with treatment and even forestalled or prevented to some degree, it is widespread and progressive in advanced old age. Broadly defined, frailty is a state of increased vulnerability to stressors, a condition in which decreased reserve can result in the failure to manage acute insults such as exacerbations of a chronic disease, acute illness, or injury (Fried et al., 2001; Hogan, MacKnight, et al., 2003; Morley, Perry, & Miller, 2002). Some research has focused on the physical changes that occur as elders become frail (Fried et al., 2001), but investigators also acknowledge the complex interaction of medical and social problems that contribute to the decreased ability to respond to stress (Jones, Song, & Rockwood, 2004; Studenski et al., 2004; Winograd et al., 1991).

Ongoing theoretical and empirical work is contributing to a more refined definition of frailty. Studenski et al. (2004) point out that frailty as a physical state should be distinguished from the consequences of frailty. The physical state of frailty includes losses of strength, endurance, immune function, balance, body weight, and mobility. The consequences include changes in functional independence, social roles, and psychosocial factors and an increased risk of falling, increased length of hospital stays, and greater need for long-term care.

Among the total population of persons 65 years of age and older, approximately 6% to 7% would be classified as physically frail, but that proportion increases to 25.7% to 36.6% of those 85 years of age and older (Bradley, Fried, Kasl, & Idler, 2001; Puts, Lips, & Deeg, 2005; Rockwood, Howlett, et al., 2004). In general, women experience frailty more frequently (Fried et al., 2001; Puts et al., 2005). Men tend to live less long than women and to die more suddenly. Blacks, those who are less well-educated, and persons experiencing poorer health also experience frailty more frequently (Fried et al., 2001). As the number of indicators of frailty increase, the likelihood of death also increases (Mitnitski, Graham, Mogilner, & Rockwood, 2002; Puts et al., 2005; Rockwood, Staknyk, et al., 1999).

Frailty is significantly associated with age, yet it is a better predictor of death than is chronological age. Frailty also is associated with, but is not the same as, disability and comorbidity. This is an important distinction because the nature of the health care services required by each of the three groups—frail elders, disabled elders, and elders with multiple comorbid conditions—differs (Fried et al., 2001). As Fried et al. point out, care of those with two or more chronic diseases needs to focus on coordinating care among multiple providers and settings, as well as paying particular attention to interactions of treatments that may cause adverse outcomes. Persons with disability most need rehabilitative and supportive services, with particular attention to minimizing the risk for social isolation. Frail elders need special consideration because of their vulnerability to the stressors associated with hospitalization and medical procedures, but they also need attention to ensure that reversible underlying causes of frailty are treated and that secondary prevention strategies are put in place to minimize complications. Fried's research team also has investigated the degree of overlap among the three groups. Nearly half of a population-based sample of elderly reported two or more health problems, but only 10% of this subgroup met the criteria for physical frailty. Among the total sample, 7% were classified as physically frail, and 7% were disabled; but only 27% of the frail elders were also disabled, and only the same proportion of disabled were also frail. Keeping these distinctions in mind is important as nurses consider clinical screening tools and other indicators to use to identify frailty among older persons.

Indicators of Frailty

Given the complexity of the syndrome of frailty, not surprisingly, many different ways of assessing it are available. The physical symptoms of frailty generally are agreed to involve involuntary weight loss, self-reported fatigue or exhaustion, increased weakness, moving more slowly, and decreased physical activity (Bortz, 2002; Fried et al., 2001; Hamerman, 1999; Morley et al., 2002). These physical changes are associated with a number of metabolic indicators, including decreased serum albumin, increased creatinine clearance, and increased cytokines (particularly interleukin-6). Finally, because the physical state of frailty has many potential negative consequences, a wide variety of clinical problems are highly suggestive of frailty, such as fractures resulting from falls, incontinence resulting directly from muscle weakness but also from the decreased ability to toilet in a timely way, and pressure sores triggered from inactivity, decreased body mass, and altered protein metabolism.

Cognitive impairment frequently coexists with frailty in the oldest old and therefore often is treated as an indicator of frailty. Yet the relationship between the two disorders needs further research. Most of the available research investigates the relationship between cognitive impairment and disability, not frailty. As indicated before, disability—especially when measured as dependency in activities of daily living—is often a consequence of frailty but is not synonymous with it. Investigators have observed a high prevalence of dependency in activities of daily living among the cognitively impaired (Aguero-Torres et al., 1998; Artero, Touchon, & Ritchie, 2001; Mehta, Yaffe, & Covinsky, 2002), but cognitive impairment is not an independent predictor of disability (Kempen & Ormel, 1998) or frailty (Rockwood, Howlett, et al., 2004).

Many clinical indexes exist to help identify frail elders. Examples include the Clinical Targeting Criteria, a list of 15 clinical conditions that frequently are associated with frailty and can be used with medical records to screen a clinic or inpatient population. These conditions include confusion, falls, impaired mobility, polypharmacy, and pressure sores. Other indexes are based on patient interviews or examinations, such as the Clinical Global Impression of Change in Physical Frailty (Studenski et al., 2004) or Groeningen Frailty Indicator (Schuurmans, Steverink, Lindenberg, Frieswijk, & Slaets, 2004). These indexes generally include questions about mobility, disability, nutrition, perceived health, cognition, and psychosocial factors. A third type of index is based on a set of markers derived from other health data (Gray, Smyth, Palmer, Zhu, & Callahan, 2002; Puts et al., 2005). Indicators such as weight loss or abnormal metabolic values, such as low serum albumin or high creatinine, form the basis of these indexes. Nurses caring for older patients should be alert to these indicators of frailty and incorporate the information in their care planning.

Identifying the End of Life for Frail Elders

Identifying the last phase of life for the frail elderly is a unique challenge. Experts recently evaluated the research evidence about end-of-life care and concluded that "the evidence does not support a definition of the interval referred to as the end of life" (National Institutes of Health, 2005). They further acknowledged that although older age and frailty may be surrogates for life-threatening illness, evidence is insufficient for understanding these variables as components of end of life. Indeed, much work needs to be done to understand better the complexity of dying for those who reach advanced old age.

By definition, the frail elderly have diminished physiological reserve. Dr. Joan Teno used the phrase "tightrope walker" and likened the stochastic event such as pneumonia, a fall, or hip fracture that leads to death in a frail elder as a "sudden gust of wind" (Teno, Goldstein, &

Walter, 2004). Many frail elders function with gradually reducing capacity until this "gust of wind" overwhelms them. For these elderly, the transition to end of life is bimodal: a long period of gradually diminishing capacity ending with a short period of rapid decline. Indeed, the last months of life for the frail elderly may include characteristics from any of the four functional trajectories of dying: a precipitous drop caused by a crisis such as an infection superimposed on low function; a sharp, short decline to death caused by a triggering event such as a hip fracture; or an erratic course associated with multiple exacerbations of underlying chronic illnesses. Figure 36-1 represents the trajectories of dying adapted to illustrate the various ways that life could end among already frail elders.

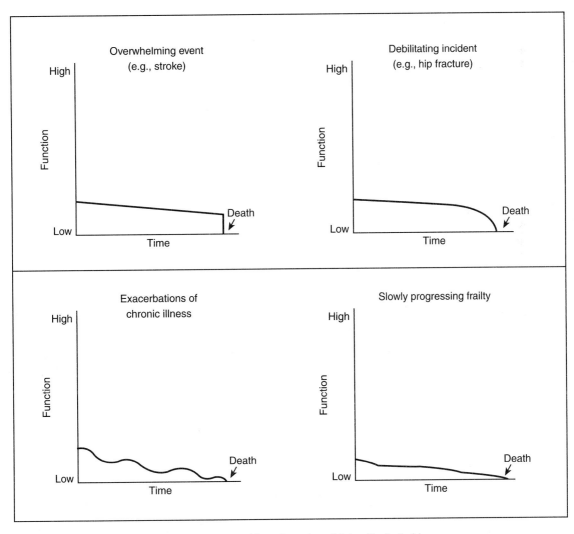

FIGURE 36-1 Possible trajectories of dying for frail elders.

As depicted in Figure 36-1, for some frail elders the last year of life may follow a long period of gradually diminishing capacity, and although patient, family, and health care providers recognize that the end of life is near, no one may be able to describe the point at which "failing" becomes "dying." Some have noted that death is often imminent when frail elders begin to make statements about approaching death, start saying good-byes, report dreams or visions of persons from the past, or begin to withdraw socially and spend more time in inward reflection (Kesler, Mowers, Griffie, & Prochnow, 2003). Symptoms, signs, and problems that nursing home physicians evaluate as indicative of a short life expectancy include little or no nutritional or fluid intake, somnolence, episodes of delirium, and worsening pressure ulcers (Brandt et al., 2005). However, Brandt's group also found that by the time nursing home residents were classified as having a limited life expectancy, they had a median duration of survival of only 3 days. Defining a precise period as the end of life for frail elders may never be possible with the clarity and certainty that many seek to have. Yet that lack of precision does not preclude the usefulness of acknowledging the need for changes in health care goals as elders become physically frail in advanced old age.

Important End-of-Life Issues for Frail Elders

Implications of the unpredictability of death for frail elders are profound. Because physical frailty includes potentially reversible components, such as poor nutritional intake, decreased strength and endurance, and emotional detachment, striking the right balance between rehabilitation and palliative care is key and yet also challenging. Regular physical activity is important to maintain joint mobility and improve functional capacity for any elder, especially the frail. Providing encouragement to stay physically active without piling guilt on those who have begun "taking to bed" (Clark, Dion, & Barker, 1990) requires keen insight into the individual client and well-honed negotiating skills on the part of the clinician.

Closely related to this issue is the need to recognize the difference between the emotional detachment that is part of ending life for many frail elders and clinical depression, which is common but reversible. Depression screening questions that may help in this discernment process relate to assessing negative emotions such as "feeling like a failure," "finding no meaning in life," and "not being able to laugh or see the funny side of things." Nondepressed frail elders may respond negatively to these items but still report that they are too tired to do

anything, have lost interest in other people, and have lost interest in books, radio, or television shows. Allowing frail elders to begin an emotional detachment from life without suffering needlessly from reversible depression requires nurses to listen carefully and probe gently to ascertain mood accurately.

Equally challenging is the task of helping to prepare high-risk elders for death while still keeping their focus on living. Discussions about older adults' preferences for the end of life should begin before they are too ill or cognitively impaired to voice their opinions (Vig, Davenport, & Pearlman, 2002). Much has been written about the shortcomings of advanced directives (Fagerlin & Schneider, 2004), but the more interactive process of advance care planning remains an important component of caring for those of advanced age (Emanuel, 2004). Researchers have shown that the elderly can be surprised and mildly discomfited when their health care providers bring up the topic of end-of-life decision making when they are not ill, but they still express appreciation for the opportunity to begin the discussion (Finucane, Shumway, Powers, & D'Alessandri, 1988; Kellogg, Crain, Corwin, & Brickner, 1992). Research is less clear about the likelihood that preferences regarding decisions in various hypothetical situations change much between a discussion held in advance of serious illness and an actual life-threatening event (Carmel & Mutran, 1999; McParland, Likourezos, Chichin, Castor, & Paris, 2003).

Experts have uncovered important aspects of communication to consider when raising end-of-life issues with frail elders who are not imminently dying. Elderly patients want different kinds of information from health care providers than clinicians expect. They want information on how to cope with their health problems, not what kinds of negative events might occur in the future and involve health care decisions (Hines, Babrow, Badzek, & Moss, 2001). Chronically ill elderly persons have been found to engage readily in preparing for certain aspects of death, such as completing wills and making funeral arrangements, but at the same time, they are less likely to plan for future serious illness (Carrese, Mullaney, Faden, & Finucane, 2002). In fact, a recent book about "navigating the emotional terrain of our elders" cautions that the current older generation lived through a different time in history and speaks a different emotional language. Having weathered the Great Depression and World War II in their youth, the current elderly generation may be more inclined to stoic acceptance of untoward events such as death and not seek to "process" the event the way their younger caregivers and care providers may expect (Pipher, 1999).

Cognitive function in the frail elderly plays an especially important role at the end of life. The prevalence of dementias such as Alzheimer's disease and vascular dementia increases sharply in advanced old age (Jorm & Jolley, 1998; Kukull & Ganguli, 2000). Many of those who live until their late 80s will lose the ability to direct their own care before reaching the end of life.

Considerable research has focused on dementias involving memory loss, but other forms of cognitive impairment also influence how those of advanced old age cope with the end of life (Park, Polk, Mikels, Taylor, & Marshuetz, 2001; Royall, Chiodo, & Polk, 2003; Royall, Palmer, Chiodo, & Polk, 2004). Executive control functions are cognitive processes that orchestrate relatively simple ideas or actions into complex goal-directed behavior. Impairments in these functions are becoming more common as the population ages (Workman et al., 2000). Pronounced age declines also occur in effortful cognitive processing and processing speed (Brown & Park, 2003). An elder may demonstrate good recall and have considerably more stored knowledge and experience compared with a younger adult but may be somewhat slow to take in new information. Although these impairments are not uncovered in the common clinical screening tools such as the Mini-Mental State Examination, they do have an important influence on an elder's autonomy for the purpose of health care decision making and for living independently (Bell-McGinty, Podell, Franzen, Baird, & Williams, 2002; Royall, Cabello, & Polk, 1998; Workman et al., 2000).

To provide quality care, nurses must assess and consider the full range of cognitive abilities. A frail elder with mild cognitive impairment may be overwhelmed easily by the complex healthcare system as the elder's health declines, but he or she still may be able to input into decision making if given time and assistance to process new information (Allen et al., 2003). With current medical advances the time and circumstances of death increasingly have become areas of decision making, and society places a stigma on "giving up" too soon (Kaufman, Shim, & Russ, 2004). As family members assume increasing responsibility for interactions with health care providers and health decisions for their overwhelmed older loved ones, nurses can help them seek feedback from the elderly person at the level at which that loved one can understand and respond to choices appropriately (Barron, Duffey, Byrd, Campbell, & Ferrucci, 2004). This is especially important when family members are afraid to let go without some signal from their loved one that the time has come.

Delirium adds to the complexity related to cognitive impairment at the end of life. Unlike with dementia, symptoms of delirium are often dramatic, appearing suddenly in a short time and fluctuating hourly (Arnold, 2004). Because delirium is associated with a physical or medical condition such as infection, dehydration, drug toxicity, and renal failure, the primary goal is to uncover the contributing factors. Episodes of delirium at the end of life are especially disconcerting to the family members of nondemented elders, who hoped for a peaceful death for their loved one who is instead agitated, fearful, and confused. Skilled assessment and management of delirium greatly enhances the quality of nursing care of the frail elderly.

Managing the symptom burden of this population at the end of life is made particularly complex by the likelihood of multiple underlying causes, altered pharmacokinetics, and a diminished tolerance of treatment regimens. Yet older adults are just as likely as their younger counterparts to experience pain, breathlessness, loss of appetite, depression, vomiting, and dry mouth (Derby & O'Mahony, 2001). Pain management is one example of how this population presents challenges distinct from younger adults. Studies repeatedly have documented the problem of inadequate pain assessment in the elderly. The elderly may be less inclined to report pain because they expect pain to occur as part of the aging process or because they do not want to cause distress in their family caregivers. Furthermore, pain assessment for cognitively impaired elders is a special problem. In addition to underreporting of pain, inadequate analgesia is a significant problem among the elderly. Adequate pain relief requires special considerations in managing the side effects of analgesia for frail elders because of their declining metabolism and altered health habits. For example, managing constipation from the slowing of peristalsis that accompanies opioids is a particular challenge with the decreased fluid intake common among frail elderly.

PALLIATIVE CARE: CLOSING THE GAP WITH END OF LIFE

Good symptom management and supportive care are central to the concept of hospice care, which was introduced to this country by an exchange between Dame Cicely Saunders and Florence Wald of the Yale School of Nursing in the mid-1960s. Hospice care gathered momentum in the following decades and was recognized as a way to provide more humane care for Americans dying of terminal illness while possibly reducing costs. Eventually the Medicare hospice benefit facilitated the widespread adoption of hospice as a model of care but at the same time limited its ultimate growth by requiring certification of a prognosis of 6 months or less and cessation of curative treatments. More recently, the concept of palliative care has become popularized as supportive care appropriate from the day of diagnosis of a life-threatening illness, gradually increasing in emphasis to become the predominant mode of care at the end of life. Although in reality palliative care tends to be implemented at the very end of life, it has the potential to be an approach and a model of care with broader implications for those with serious illness because it complements rather than replaces curative treatment.

The original definition of palliative care developed by the World Health Organization included the concept of a "debilitating condition" along with that of a "life-threatening illness." Although the language about debilitating conditions is no longer part of the definition (World Health Organization, 2005), it is acknowledged in the *Clinical Practice Guidelines for Quality Palliative Care* published by the National Consensus Project (2004). These guidelines include persons with frailty among the population to be served by palliative care, listing frailty as one of the progressive chronic conditions that fits the palliative care criteria of being persistent or recurring and adversely affecting daily function or reducing life expectancy (p. 4). Yet just as hospice care first took hold among terminally ill cancer patients, the concept of palliative care to date has been recognized most often as appropriate for those with a life-threatening illness, such as cancer or acquired immunodeficiency syndrome. Extension of this philosophy or model of care to frail elders who do not have a clear terminal illness requires broadening the prevailing concept of end of life. For those who reach advanced age and develop indications of increasing physical frailty, death may not be clearly within sight, but it is figuratively around the corner. To accommodate the complex and unpredictable ways in which older persons die, supportive care should be offered simultaneously with rehabilitation and treatment throughout advanced age. Figure 36-2 illustrates the potential for palliative care to close the gap with end of life by more readily including the elderly who reach advanced age without a clear life-threatening diagnosis.

Nurses are particularly well equipped to lead this effort to improve the quality of care provided to the frail elderly at the end of life by seamlessly integrating

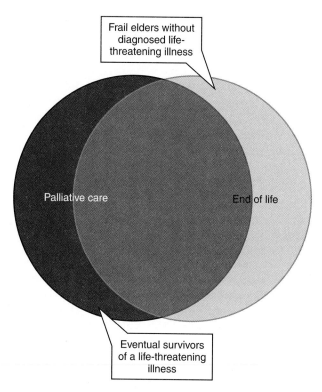

FIGURE 36-2 Current relationship of palliative care and care provided at the end of life.

the precepts of palliative care. Good symptom management and psychosocial support are key ingredients of quality nursing care and also of palliative care. The challenge for nurses caring for this subgroup of elders is the unpredictability of death. By developing more comfort with the uncertainty and complexity that accompanies the end of life for this population, nurses can help frail elders to be prepared for death at the same time that they maintain a good quality of life and enjoy living.

REFERENCES

Adams, K., & Corrigan, J. M. (Eds.). (2003). *Priority areas for national action: Transforming health care quality.* Washington, DC: National Academies Press.

Aguero-Torres, H., Fratiglioni, L., Guo, Z., Viitanen, M., von Strauss, E., & Winblad, B. (1998). Dementia is the major cause of functional dependence in the elderly: 3-year follow-up data from a population-based study. *American Journal of Public Health, 88*(10), 1452-1456.

Allen, R. S., DeLaine, S. R., Chaplin, W. F., Marson, D. C., Bourgeois, M. S., Dijkstra, K., et al. (2003). Advance care planning in nursing homes: correlates of capacity and possession of advance directives. *Gerontologist, 43,* 309-317.

Arnold, E. (2004). Sorting out the 3 D's: delirium, dementia, and depression. *Nursing, 34,* 36-42.

Artero, S., Touchon, J., & Ritchie, K. (2001). Disability and mild cognitive impairment: A longitudinal population-based study. *International Journal of Geriatric Psychiatry, 16,* 1092-1097.

Barron, J. S., Duffey, P. L., Byrd, L. J., Campbell, R., & Ferrucci, L. (2004). Informed consent for research participation in frail older persons. *Aging Clinical and Experimental Research, 16,* 79-85.

Bell-McGinty, S., Podell, K., Franzen, M., Baird, A. D., & Williams, M. J. (2002). Standard measures of executive function in predicting instrumental activities of daily living in older adults. *International Journal of Geriatric Psychiatry, 17,* 828-834.

Bortz, W. M. (2002). A conceptual framework of frailty: a review. *The Journals of Gerontology: Series A Biological Sciences and Medical Sciences, 57,* M283-M288.

Bradley, E. H., Fried, T. R., Kasl, S. V., & Idler, E. (2001). Quality-of-life trajectories of elders in the end of life. In M. P. Lawton (Ed.), *The end of life: Scientific and social issues* (Vol. 20, pp. 64-96). New York: Springer.

Brandt, H. E., Deliens, L., Ooms, M. E., van der Steen, J. T., van Der Wal, G., & Ribbe, M. W. (2005). Symptoms, signs, problems, and diseases of terminally ill nursing home patients: A nationwide observational study in the Netherlands. *Archives of Internal Medicine, 165*(3), 314-320.

Braun, J. V., Wykle, M. H., & Cowling, W. R., III. (1988). Failure to thrive in older persons: A concept derived. *Gerontologist, 28,* 809-812.

Brown, S. C., & Park, D. C. (2003). Theoretical models of cognitive aging and implications for translational research in medicine. *Gerontologist, 43,* 57-67.

Callahan, D. (1987). *Setting limits: Medical goals in an aging society.* New York: Simon & Schuster.

Carmel, S., & Mutran, E. J. (1999). Stability of elderly persons' expressed preferences regarding the use of life-sustaining treatments. *Social Science & Medicine, 49,* 303-311.

Carrese, J. A., Mullaney, J. L., Faden, R. R., & Finucane, T. E. (2002). Planning for death but not serious future illness: qualitative study of housebound elderly patients. *British Medical Journal, 325,* 125-127.

Centers for Disease Control and Prevention. (2003). Public health and aging: Trends in aging. *Morbidity and Mortality Weekly Report, 52,* 101-106.

Centers for Disease Control and Prevention, Gerontological Society of America, & Merck Institute of Aging & Health. (2004). *The state of aging and health in America 2004.* Washington, DC: Merck Institute of Aging & Health.

Clark, L. P., Dion, D. M., & Barker, W. H. (1990). Taking to bed: Rapid functional decline in an independently mobile older population living in an intermediate-care facility. *Journal of the American Geriatrics Society, 38,* 967-972.

Derby, S., & O' Mahony, S. (2001). Elderly patients. In B. R. Ferrell & N. Coyle (Eds.), *Textbook of palliative nursing* (pp. 435-449). New York: Oxford University Press.

Egbert, A. M. (1993). 'The dwindles': Failure to thrive in older patients. *Postgraduate Medicine, 94,* 199-201.

Emanuel, L. L. (2004). Advance directives and advancing age. *Journal of the American Geriatrics Society, 52,* 641-642.

Fagerlin, A., & Schneider, C. E. (2004). Enough: The failure of the living will. *Hastings Center Report, 34,* 30-42.

Finucane, T. E., Shumway, J. M., Powers, R. L., & D'Alessandri, R. M. (1988). Planning with elderly outpatients for contingencies of severe illness: a survey and clinical trial. *Journal of General Internal Medicine, 3,* 322-325.

Fried, L. P., Tangen, C. M., Walston, J., Newman, A. B., Hirsch, C., Gottdiener, J., et al. (2001). Frailty in older adults: evidence for a phenotype. *The Journals of Gerontology: Series A Biological Sciences and Medical Sciences, 56*(3), M146-M156.

Glaser, B., & Strauss, A. L. (1968). *Time for dying.* Chicago: Aldine Publishing.

Gray, L. K., Smyth, K. A., Palmer, R. M., Zhu, X., & Callahan, J. M. (2002). Heterogeneity in older people: Examining physiologic failure, age, and comorbidity. *Journal of the American Geriatrics Society, 50,* 1955-1961.

Hamerman, D. (1999). Toward an understanding of frailty. *Annals of Internal Medicine, 130,* 945-950.

Havlik, R. J., & Rosenberg, H. M. (1992). The quality and application of death records of older persons. In R. B. Wallace & R. F. Woolson (Eds.), *The epidemiologic study of the elderly* (pp. 262-280). New York: Oxford University Press.

Hines, S. C., Babrow, A. S., Badzek, L., & Moss, A. (2001). From coping with life to coping with death: Problematic integration for the seriously ill elderly. *Health Communication, 13,* 327-342.

Hogan, C., Lunney, J., Gabel, J., & Lynn, J. (2001). Medicare beneficiaries' costs of care in the last year of life. *Health Affairs, 20*(4), 188-195.

Hogan, D. B., MacKnight, C., & Bergman, H. (2003). Models, definitions, and criteria of frailty. *Aging Clinical and Experimental Research, 15,* 1-29.

Institute of Medicine. (1997). *Approaching death: Improving care at the end of life.* Washington, DC: National Academy Press.

Jones, D. M., Song, X., & Rockwood, K. (2004). Operationalizing a frailty index from a standardized comprehensive geriatric assessment. *Journal of the American Geriatrics Society, 52,* 1929-1933.

Jorm, A. F., & Jolley, D. (1998). The incidence of dementia: A meta-analysis. *Neurology, 51,* 728-733.

Kaufman, S. R., Shim, J. K., & Russ, A. J. (2004). Revisiting the biomedicalization of aging: Clinical trends and ethical challenges. *Gerontologist, 44,* 731-738.

Kellogg, F. R., Crain, M., Corwin, J., & Brickner, P. W. (1992). Life-sustaining interventions in frail elderly persons: Talking about choices. *Archives of Internal Medicine, 152,* 2317-2320.

Kempen, G. I., & Ormel, J. (1998). The impact of physical performance and cognitive status on subsequent ADL disability in low-functioning older adults. *International Journal of Geriatric Psychiatry, 13,* 480-483.

Kesler, T. C., Mowers, R., Griffie, J., & Prochnow, J. (2003). Assessment of dying. *American Journal Nursing, 103,* 52-53.

Kochanek, K. D., Murphy, S. L., Anderson, R. N., & Scott, C. (2004). Deaths: Final data for 2002. *National Vital Statistics Report, 53,* 1-115.

Kukull, W. A., & Ganguli, M. (2000). Epidemiology of dementia: Concepts and overview. *Neurologic Clinics, 18,* 923-950.

Lubitz, J., Beebe, J., & Baker, C. (1995). Longevity and Medicare expenditures. *New England Journal of Medicine, 332,* 999-1003.

Lunney, J. R., Lynn, J., & Hogan, C. (2002). Profiles of older Medicare decedents. *Journal of the American Geriatrics Society, 50,* 1108-1112.

Lynn, J. (2001). Perspectives on care at the close of life. Serving patients who may die soon and their families: The role of hospice and other services. *JAMA: The Journal of the American Medical Association, 285,* 925-932.

Lynn, J., Harrell, F., Jr., Cohn, F., Wagner, D., & Connors, A. F., Jr. (1997). Prognoses of seriously ill hospitalized patients on the days before death: Implications for patient care and public policy. *New Horizons, 5,* 56-61.

McCue, J. D. (1995). The naturalness of dying. *JAMA: The Journal of the American Medical Association, 273,* 1039-1043.

McParland, E., Likourezos, A., Chichin, E., Castor, T., & Paris B. (2003). Stability of preferences regarding life-sustaining treatment: A two-year prospective study of nursing home residents. *Mount Sinai Journal Medicine, 70*(2), 85-92.

Mehta, K. M., Yaffe, K., & Covinsky, K. E. (2002). Cognitive impairment, depressive symptoms, and functional decline in older people. *Journal of the American Geriatrics Society, 50,* 1045-1050.

Mitnitski, A. B., Graham, J. E., Mogilner, A. J., & Rockwood, K. (2002). Frailty, fitness and late-life mortality in relation to chronological and biological age. *BMC Geriatrics, 2,* 1.

Morley, J. E., Perry, H. M., III, & Miller, D. K. (2002). Editorial: Something about frailty. *The Journals of Gerontology: Series A Biological Sciences and Medical Sciences, 57,* M698-M704.

Morris, J. N., Suissa, S., Sherwood, S., Wright, S. M., & Greer, D. (1986). Last days: a study of the quality of life of terminally ill cancer patients. *Journal of Chronic Diseases, 39,* 47-62.

National Consensus Project. (2004). *Clinical practice guidelines for quality palliative care.* Brooklyn, NY: Author.

National Institutes of Health. (2005). *Improving end-of-life care: State-of-the-science conference statement.* Bethesda, MD: Author.

Nuland, S. B. (1995). *How we die: reflections on life's final chapter.* New York: Vintage Books.

Palmer, R. M. (1990). 'Failure to thrive' in the elderly: Diagnosis and management. *Geriatrics, 45,* 47-55.

Park, D. C., Polk, T. A., Mikels, J., Taylor, S. F., & Marshuetz, C. (2001). Cerebral aging: integration of brain and behavioral models of cognitive function. *Dialogues in Clinical Neuroscience, 3,* 151-165.

Pipher, M. (1999). *Another country: Navigating the emotional terrain of our elders.* New York: Riverhead Books.

Puts, M. T., Lips, P., & Deeg, D. J. (2005). Sex differences in the risk of frailty for mortality independent of disability and chronic diseases. *Journal of the American Geriatrics Society, 53,* 40-47.

Rockwood, K., Howlett, S. E., MacKnight, C., Beattie, B. L., Bergman, H., Hebert, R., et al. (2004). Prevalence, attributes, and outcomes of fitness and frailty in community-dwelling older adults: Report from the Canadian study of health and aging. *The Journals of Gerontology: Series A Biological Sciences and Medical Sciences, 59,* 1310-1317.

Rockwood, K., Stadnyk, K., MacKnight, C., McDowell, I., Hebert, R., & Hogan, D. B. (1999). A brief clinical instrument to classify frailty in elderly people. *Lancet, 353,* 205-206.

Royall, D. R., Cabello, M., & Polk, M. J. (1998). Executive dyscontrol: An important factor affecting the level of care received by older retirees. *Journal of the American Geriatrics Society, 46,* 1519-1524.

Royall, D. R., Chiodo, L. K., & Polk, M. J. (2003). Executive dyscontrol in normal aging: Normative data, factor structure, and clinical correlates. *Current Neurology and Neuroscience Reports, 3,* 487-493.

Royall, D. R., Palmer, R., Chiodo, L. K., & Polk, M. J. (2004). Declining executive control in normal aging predicts change in functional status: The freedom house study. *Journal of the American Geriatrics Society, 52,* 346-352.

Schuurmans, H., Steverink, N., Lindenberg, S., Frieswijk, N., & Slaets, J. P. (2004). Old or frail: what tells us more? *The Journals of Gerontology: Series A Biological Sciences and Medical Sciences, 59,* M962-M965.

Studenski, S., Hayes, R. P., Leibowitz, R. Q., Bode, R., Lavery, L., Walston, J., et al. (2004). Clinical global impression of change in physical frailty: Development of a measure based on clinical judgment. *Journal of the American Geriatrics Society, 53*(5), 1560-1566.

Teno, J. M., Goldstein, M. K., & Walter, L. C. (2004). AGS meeting highlight: Health care screening and older adults: For how long and on whom? *Annals of Long-Term Care, 12*(3), 33-34.

Vig, E. K., Davenport, N. A., & Pearlman, R. A. (2002). Good deaths, bad deaths, and preferences for the end of life: a qualitative study of geriatric outpatients. *Journal of the American Geriatrics Society, 50,* 1541-1548.

Webb, M. (1997). *The good death.* New York: Bantam Books.

Winograd, C. H., Gerety, M. B., Chung, M., Goldstein, M. K., Dominguez, F., Jr., & Vallone, R. (1991). Screening for frailty: criteria and predictors of outcomes. *Journal of the American Geriatrics Society, 39,* 778-784.

Workman, R. H., Jr., McCullough, L. B., Molinari, V., Kunik, M. E., Orengo, C., Khalsa, D. K., et al. (2000). Clinical and ethical implications of impaired executive control functions for patient autonomy. *Psychiatric Services, 51,* 359-363.

World Health Organization. (2005). *WHO definition of palliative care.* Retrieved August 1, 2005, from http://www.who.int/cancer/palliative/definition/en/

GOVERNANCE

Challenges to Nursing Leadership in a Changing Nursing Practice World

PERLE SLAVIK COWEN ◆ SUE MOORHEAD

The structures in which nursing has been practiced through the years sometimes have been a constraint to the ability of professional nurses to govern their own practice. In the changing terrain of health care at the turn of the millennium the entire field is shifting, offering unusual challenges for nursing to play a more prominent role in governance issues. The pressures for cost control push nursing leaders to be experts not only in the domain of quality of patient care but also in the economic underpinnings of the field. Use of less costly personnel to provide patient care has emerged through the years as one way of addressing cost problems. Although on the one hand nursing is diminished somewhat in some aspects in institutional settings; on the other hand, in areas outside of hospital nursing the role of nursing is expanding and becoming progressively more independent. Increasingly, the dichotomy between nursing education and nursing practice is narrowing. As nursing educational programs become more involved in the provision of services, the lines between funding for educational programs and funding for service become blurred. As nursing moves toward more independence, governance models for nursing centers and community-based practices are beginning to emerge. One of the hallmarks of a profession is that of being able to govern one's domain. In nursing this has always been in question, with boundary problems an issue vis-à-vis medicine and institutional controls within hospital settings. This section provides a wonderful overview of the complexities of nursing and its governance in a changing health care environment.

In the opening debate chapter, Zimmermann addresses the question of the use of unlicensed assistive personnel: Do they erode the quality of care or make more appropriate use of professionally prepared nurses? Zimmerman states, "the *unlicensed assistive personnel* term comprises at least 50 different job titles of workers who are not highly skilled or otherwise credentialed."

One can argue that the use of unlicensed assistive personnel is a necessary part of cost control because the average wage for a professional nurse is 144% higher than that for a unlicensed assistive personnel. However, this figure does not take into account fringe benefits, which are the same for both types of employees, the costs of training, the lack of stability (turnover) of the staff, and the costs of supervision. More recent research suggests that hiring of more registered nurses does not decrease profits. Zimmermann argues that there is a need to determine the skill mix necessary to provide quality care. Nurses need to know what can be delegated and what cannot. In concluding the chapter, Zimmermann goes back to Florence Nightingale's admonition to "do the sick no harm." Obviously, the final answer for safe, effective, quality care and staffing involves many aspects of the situation. Clearly, one essential component of this question concerns who the staff are, including their experience, education, training, credentials, and qualifications.

In the next viewpoint chapter, Goode and Boyle focus on leadership in acute care hospitals. New challenges are on the horizon for nurse leaders who work in acute care hospitals. These organizations need to prepare for growth because of the aging of the baby boomer generation, new technology, and a shortage of health care workers. Nurse leaders must be prepared to take on these challenges and to lead the nursing profession to better outcomes than have been achieved in the past, according to these authors. Today, greater emphasis is placed on quality of care and safety than has ever been experienced in the past. The chapter focuses on quality and patient safety, technology, patient-centered care, hospital margins, the work environment, evidence-based practice, diversity (patients and workforce), and the learning organizations. The authors conclude that "nurse leaders must embrace a personal obligation to create a positive, healthful work environment for their staffs."

This chapter clearly articulates the many challenges faced by nurse leaders in acute care settings.

In the next viewpoint chapter, Clancy and Abrams discuss three of the challenges nurses face in today's health care system: mandatory overtime, staffing ratios, and unions. Mandatory overtime as defined by the Fair Labor Standards Act is time as hours worked more than 40 hours per week or more than 80 hours for a 2-week period. This does not include hours for which a staff member has volunteered. Mandatory overtime is the staffing vehicle of last resort according to the American Organization of Nurse Executives. The chapter highlights the threats to patient safety and individualized care brought about by mandatory overtime. Currently, 10 states have addressed this issue in a variety of ways. The second focus of this chapter, staffing ratios, is a greatly debated topic. Recent years have seen a movement toward mandating the number of patients for which a nurse in a given discipline can care for over a given time. The chapter highlights the debate on this issue and suggests the positive and negative potential outcomes of pro and con viewpoints on the issue of staffing ratios. Unions, the third focus, are a growing force in nursing and provide a mechanism for nurses to influence the practice environment collectively. As Clancy and Abrams suggest, "self-organization reflects groundswell support for better representation of nurses' collective interests." When threats of unionization arise, they usually are based on an underlying atmosphere of mistrust, miscommunication, and feelings of helplessness. Registered nurse union membership has increased nearly 80% in the last decade. This chapter is a must read for all nurses today—whether they are at the bedside or the boardroom.

Shifting back to more traditional governance roles, Specht and Maas discuss shared governance models in nursing. They conclude that one of the hallmarks of a profession is self-governance of practice. Nursing history tells a story of nursing in institutional settings being governed predominantly by the institution rather than by the profession. In stark contrast to this picture is medicine, which has been practiced in institutional settings but has retained control of its practice. The authors note that interest in self-governance in nursing fluctuates with the ebb and flow of nurse shortages. At times of shortage, self-governance becomes more predominant. Some of the inherent issues that complicate self-governance are (1) the lack of clearly defined criteria for self-governance, (2) the mixed motives in instituting such systems, and (3) disagreements about how self-governance models should be implemented. Nurses, as employees, need to accommodate the organization and the profession. Noting that considerable confusion exists about participation in decision making and shared governance, the authors advocate that nurses participate in shared governance for the whole system, not nursing as a part of the system. The authors conclude that top-down and bottom-up approaches have been used but that the unit approach is most desirable because of the buy-in of nurses to this model and their true participation at that level.

The nursing leadership roles of the future undoubtedly will be more challenging than those of the past. The revolutions in the scientific realm, the explosion of information, and the movement of care from institutional to home and community settings, coupled with the ever-present concerns for cost control, place nursing leadership in a most interesting position. How nurses rise to the challenge likely will determine how far nursing will travel from being a pawn in the game of health care to controlling its own destiny. Governance of practice continues to be a key focus for staff nurses and nurse administrators.

Who Should Provide Nursing Care?

POLLY GERBER ZIMMERMANN

IS NURSING BY ANY ROLE THE SAME?

Unlicensed assistive personnel (UAP) and other assistive licensed or credentialed health care providers (emergency medical technicians, paramedics, and licensed practical nurses [LPNs] and licensed vocational nurses) constitute a sizable presence in today's acute care hospital environments. The term *unlicensed assistive personnel* covers at least 50 different job titles of workers who are not highly skilled or otherwise credentialed. Other positions, such as an emergency medical technician or LPN, do have more formal training and requirements, but their educational preparation, skills, and responsibilities are not as extensive as that for a registered nurse (RN).

The American Nurses Association (1992) defines UAP as unlicensed employees who are trained to function in an assistive role under the professional registered nurse in the provision of patient/client activities. Activities performed by UAP are delegated by and under the supervision of the professional registered nurse. Position statements of professional nursing organizations allow a place for such assistive roles in direct nursing and indirect nonnursing patient care activities, provided the RN determines, delegates, and oversees the process in the hospital setting.

Is the increasing use of these roles for nursing care today's answer for efficient, affordable, quality patient care solutions? The debate for that answer must weigh financial considerations, quality of care, the RN shortage, patient safety, use and standardization of these roles, and the definitions of nursing and effective staffing.

BACKGROUND

Initially, the nursing shortage of World War II created team nursing, a sharp demarcation of routine tasks under a skill mix ratio of 70% auxiliary workers and 30% RNs. In the 1970s and 1980s, however, primary care by RNs with undivided responsibility dominated.

This change was attributed to the interest of the administrations in nurses' abilities for increased productivity and to the professionalization of nursing (Brannon, 1990). Unlicensed assistive personnel were used mainly in the 1980s because of a shortage of nurses.

As health care costs were rising, many hospitals embraced "reengineering" of health care in the 1990s. This fundamental rethinking of processes often included hiring less-skilled, cheaper auxiliary workers as a way to cut labor expenses, a cost that typically consumes 55% of the budget. Currently, 97% of hospitals employ UAP with the skill mix at about 70% RNs nationwide. However, in California, the LPN counts as a "nurse" in the mandated nurse/patient staffing ratios.

FINANCIAL CONSIDERATIONS

Unlicensed Assistive Personnel/Lesser-Qualified Staff Are a Necessary Aspect of Cost Controls

Inpatient hospital care accounts for about one third of the $1.6 trillion the nation spends annually on health care (Appleby, 2004). Hospitals remain under significant pressure to control costs because of significant Medicare and Medicaid payment shortfalls, price competition, and managed care. Some areas, such as emergency departments, have significant chronic overcrowding related to the uneven distribution of the health care "safety net" for society. The Centers for Disease Control and Prevention (2005) reported that 36% of the emergency departments serve a high volume of the "safety net" patients, generally uninsured, low-income patients in a high population density area and some rural areas.

Nursing labor represents about 23% of the hospital workforce, traditionally the single largest labor cost for hospitals. Registered nurses' wages are significantly higher than for other assistive personnel roles. To have more people available is better than to insist on "Cadillac care" of only RNs for the lesser-skilled tasks.

Unlicensed Assistive Personnel/Lesser-Qualified Personnel Are NOT an Essential Aspect of Cost Control

Looking only at the wage expense is too narrow of a perspective. Hiring and benefit costs (which typically run about 30%) are the same for all categories of workers. However, additional training and supervision expenses now are incurred for the assistive roles. With the increased use of assistive roles, RNs have more patients for nursing functions and spend more time supervising (Manuel & Alster, 1994; Shindul-Rothschild, Berry, & Long-Middleton, 1996; Ventura, 1999). In one survey, after more assistive personnel were added, 67.5% of RNs reported increased patient loads and 35.8% said they were spending more time supervising (Shindul-Rothschild et al., 1996).

Productivity varies between these types of workers. One study found that UAP have 40% downtime, whereas the RNs only have 12% (Curry, 1992). Gardner (1991) found costs actually were reduced when care was structured using primary nursing compared with team nursing. One emergency department attempted to increase productivity by adjusting the skill mix to a higher technician percentage. Only higher-level trained personnel, such as emergency medical technicians and paramedics, were hired into the structured technician role. Although morale was improved, the per patient number of hours worked actually went up, and the profit margin decreased. These results were attributed to the high mobility of the technician population, which then required constant training, and the high patient condition severity, which required more advanced assessments and skills (Jones, 1999).

Research shows that hiring more RNs does not decrease profits. McCue, Mark, and Harless (2003) found that a 1% increase in the number of full-time RNs increased operating expenses by about 0.25%. However, the increase had no effect on the profit margin. By contrast, a 1% increase in nonnurse personnel (such as administrative and operational support staff) increased the operating costs by 0.18% and diminished profits by 0.21%. The better staffing at Magnet hospitals does not cost more because Magnet hospitals have shorter lengths of stay, reduced nurse turnover, and fewer needlestick injuries. Besides, Press Ganey Associates (2005) found that there is 60% likelihood that if employees are satisfied, the patients are satisfied.

Many other larger health care cost drivers occur in the areas of malpractice, capital expenditures, regulation, and administration, and medication. For instance, the growth in drug expenditures is predicted to continue to outpace the growth in overall health care expenditures and the growth of the U.S. economy. The average cost now to develop one approved drug is considered $2 billion (Hoffman, Shah, Vermeulen, Hunkler, & Hontz, 2004). Future cost saving is predicted to occur through consolidation of health systems rather than cutting labor costs.

Overall, *Futurescan: Health Trends and Implications, 2005-2010* (American College of Healthcare Executives, 2005) indicates the concept of health care organizations competing on value, which includes cost *and* quality dimensions, has become a reality. In the end, the question that may drive the debate is what *should* the spending priorities of a hospital be?

QUALITY OF CARE

The process of determining the exact effect of varying the total number and ratio in the skill mix of RNs is not as easy as it first seems. The number of patient contacts is not the same as what is accomplished when a contact occurs, such as adherence to infection control protocols or ongoing assessment. Overall, Sovie (1995) recommends at least a 70% RN staff for medical-surgical units and an 80% RN staff for intensive and intermediate care units. Blegen, Goode, and Reed (1998) found that the benefit from increasing RNs in the staff ratio was verified up to a staff mix of 87.5% RNs (Emergency Nurses Association, 1999).

California's mandatory patient/staff ratios require a 5:1 ratio on a medical-surgical unit. Many are concerned with the ramifications of "artificial" number guidelines because unit staffing often must be flexible. An unpredictable patient deterioration suddenly could require 2:1 staffing for safe care. The first hours after a patient's admission, discharge, and transfer require nurse time-intensive work, regardless of the patient's diagnosis. Overall, unit staffing should be adjusted according to the (1) skill and knowledge level of the nursing staff, (2) accessibility of the ancillary service personnel, (3) practice behaviors of physicians, (4) patient condition severity, (5) complexity and intensity of the care, and (6) work environment (American Nurses Association, 1999; Rockey, 2000).

Using Lesser-Qualified Personnel Does NOT Affect the Quality of Care

Health care personnel in assistive roles are a reality that is here to stay. The question is really not "if" but "how" best to manage the use of these roles. Nursing needs to

DEBATE

consider ways to increase the effective use of UAP as part of the team. Properly used, assistive personnel can result in the RN having more time for the higher-level professional nursing responsibilities and tasks.

One study found that 71% of the responding RNs said that UAP do provide the extra hands they need to get the work done, and 59% said that UAP add to the quality of patient care (Ventura, 1999). In one program that used nursing students as RN extenders, the RNs spent 8% more time on assessment, teaching, and family support (Davis, 1994). A survey of hospital-based RNs found that 59% felt that UAP added to quality of patient care and only 18% indicated that UAP detracted from quality of patient care (Ventura, 1999).

Using Lesser-Qualified Personnel Does Affect the Quality of Care

Decreases in RN staffing have coincided with a rise in hospital errors, infection rates, and readmissions. Earlier studies often showed more unambiguous relationships between staffing and outcomes because many factors that affect morbidity and mortality outcomes were not considered. Some of these factors include the care from other disciplines, the severity and complexity of the patient's condition, patient characteristics (e.g., elderly or immunosuppressed), and the work environment (Blegen et al., 1998). For instance, many emergency departments notice a need for more staff for the same census after their space is enlarged, in part because it takes more time to travel the distance to accomplish the same tasks.

A growing body of studies show that a higher ratio of RNs to non-RNs improves patient care outcomes. Even more specifically, the studies are beginning to indicate more that it is the RN hours of care per patient per day that may be among the most meaningful figures to consider in the evaluation of patient care.

Results from some of these studies follow:

- Lower mortality rates were related to several factors, including a higher RN skill mix (Hartz et al., 1989).
- Thirteen studies have found that patient morbidity and mortality are affected adversely by changing the total number of RNs on staff and the RN component in the skill mix (Aiken & Lake, 1992).
- For Magnet hospitals, a statistically significant result was that the higher the nurse staffing, the lower the mortality rate (Aiken, Smith, & Lake, 1994).
- The percentage of hours of care delivery by RNs and the RN skill mix were related inversely to the unit rates of medication errors, decubitus ulcers, and patient complaints (Blegen et al., 1998).
- An inverse relationship was found between RNs providing care and postsurgical complications of urinary tract infections, pneumonia, and thrombosis (Kovner & Gergen, 1998).
- An extensive study comparing team nursing and primary care nursing models demonstrated that quality was better and that costs were reduced with primary care (Gardner, 1991).
- In a study that looked at the effects of staffing in 80% of the nation's acute care hospitals, Bond, Raehl, Pitterle, and Franke (1999) found that as the number of RNs per occupied hospital bed increases, mortality rate decreases. This study, completed by three pharmacists and a biostatistician, also found that as the numbers of LPNs and hospital administrators increases, mortality rate increases.
- Using the 10 American Nurses Association quality indicators for nursing care in acute care institutions, the single most consistent and significant predictor was the percentage of RNs in the nursing staff caring for the patients. As the percentage of the RNs increased, so did the patients' perception of satisfaction with care, pain management, education, and overall care. The higher nurse staffing per condition severity–adjusted day was correlated highly with shorter lengths of stay and a significant inverse relationship to preventable conditions: pressure sores, pneumonia, postoperative infections, and urinary tract infections (American Nurses Association, 1997; Moore, Lynne, McMillen, & Evans, 1999).
- A study from the Agency for Healthcare Research and Quality reported that one additional hour of RN care cuts a patient's risk of pneumonia by 8% and the chance of urinary tract infection by nearly 10% (Kennedy, 2000a, 2000b).
- A review of the medical records of 118,940 Medicare patients hospitalized with acute myocardial infarction found that a higher RN staffing level was associated with lower mortality rates, whereas higher LPN staffing levels were associated with higher mortality rates. These results, after adjustments were made for numerous variables, were not accounted for in previous studies, including hospital volume, teaching status, and nursing skill mix (Person et al., 2004).
- Hospitals with low nurse staffing levels tend to have higher rates of poor patient outcomes such as pneumonia, shock, cardiac arrest, and urinary tract infections (Stanton & Rutherford, 2004).
- Paulson (2004) found a triage system using nurses provided more services (antipyretics for fevers, ordered radiographs and laboratory tests per standing orders, transported patients to radiology) during triage and yet were associated with a decreased wait

time (by 73 minutes) and a decreased likelihood of patients leaving without being seen (by 85%) compared with a triage system using UAP. The Emergency Nurse Association Comprehensive Standard VII is that safe, effective, and efficient triage can be performed only by a professional registered nurse who is educated in the principles of triage and who has a minimum of 6 months' experience in emergency nursing.

NURSING SHORTAGE

Lesser-Qualified Workers Are Part of the Answer to the Nursing Shortage

Today's nursing shortage (average vacancy rate of 13%) is only predicted to worsen. The U.S. Bureau of Labor Statistics indicates that RNs top the list of occupations with the largest projected job growth in the years 2002 to 2012. Job openings are anticipated to increase to 623,000 by the year 2012 (e.g., a total of 2.9 million, up from 2.3 million RNs employed in 2002). The reality is that somebody doing something is better than no one.

Lesser-Qualified Workers Are NOT Part of the Answer to the Nursing Shortage

The current working conditions left over from reengineering is a contributing factor to today's nursing shortage. With the options available today, nurses no longer will tolerate inadequate work conditions. Although 2.7 million nurses are licensed in the United States, only about 59% work in hospitals. Better staffing numbers and qualifications will result in higher nurse satisfaction and better hospital recruitment and retention.

PATIENT SAFETY

The November 1999 Institute of Medicine original report estimated that up to 98,000 preventable deaths occurred each year because of medication and diagnosis errors, failure to apply critical preventive precautions (e.g., failure to rescue), and other preventable errors. The Health Grades 2004 study now estimates that previous Institute of Medicine estimates were too low and that medical errors in U.S. hospitals actually contribute up to 195,000 patient deaths a year (Davies, 2004).

Lesser-Qualified Workers Do NOT Affect Patient Safety

In a survey of physicians and the general public, about a third of both groups indicated they had experienced a medical error directly or through a family member. In the survey, 50% of physicians and 70% of the general public blamed the medical errors on overworked, stressed, or fatigued health care workers (Blendon et al., 2002).

The who of patient safety is not as important as the working conditions. Rogers, Hwang, and Scott (2004) support the role of regular time breaks to prevent errors. They found that longer breaks/meals seemed to safeguard against errors and help control the accumulation of risk associated with prolonged work tasks. Others also have found support for the safety effects of controlling the length of shifts, total hours worked, and adequate sleep (Lockley et al., 2004).

Lesser-Qualified Workers DO Affect Patient Safety

The Joint Commission for Accreditation of Healthcare Organizations (2005) reviews sentinel events—for example, any unexpected occurrence involving death or serious physical or psychological injury—or the risk thereof. Operative and postoperative complications are third on the list (12.3%), and medication errors are fourth (11%). Self-identified root cause analyses of organizations (e.g., what organization system or process can be altered to reduce the likelihood of human error) found some of the most common causes of error are orientation/ training, patient assessment, and staffing.

New technologies and declining average length of stay have resulted in higher patient acuity. About 43% of surveyed workers said their workload hindered their ability to keep patients safe, and about two thirds of them worried at least once a day about making a mistake that could injure a patient (Weingart, Karbstein, Davis, & Phillips, 2004).

- Facilities with more favorable staffing levels had lower rates of employee injury (Yassi et al., 2004)
- Blendon et al. (2002) found that 51% of physicians and 69% of the general public respondents listed increasing the number of nurses in hospitals as a solution for errors.

For example, take the act of administering medication. Superficially, administration of medication looks simple enough to pick up a matching pill and watch a patient swallow it. In reality, many highly intellectual processes are occurring to ensure that the medication is the right drug in the right dose to the right patient at the right time. Assessments are needed to determine the patients' responses.

Pharmacology "decision support," computer assistance to prevent drug errors, was anticipated to prevent a quarter of adverse drug events (Landro, 2005). However, these programs were not able to provide the more sophisticated interventions needed regarding drug dosages and patient-monitoring strategies that could avert harm. In a 20-week study, more than half of the studied patients experienced an "adverse drug event" (Nebeker, Hoffman, Weir, Bennett, & Hurdle, 2005). Experts warn that even the most sophisticated computer systems cannot create a culture of safety and replace the needed critical thinking by the nurse.

ROLE STANDARDIZATION IN UTILIZATION

If assistive personnel are here to stay, should the emphasis then be on proper training, credentialing, and standardization of these roles? Is the answer more legitimization and acceptance?

Yes, Focus on Role and Personnel Development

Currently, no universal federal standards have been developed for many assistive roles, and personnel in these roles tend to have a high turnover rate. Some extended care facilities report a UAP turnover rate of 100%. Employers tend to be reluctant to invest training monies for questionable long-term benefit. Ventura (1999) found that RNs reported that 55% of their hospitals gave UAP 3 weeks or less of job training: half did not feel the UAP with whom they worked had adequate training. Another study found that 59% of hospitals offered less than 20 hours of classroom orientation and 41% provided less than 40 hours of on-the-job training (Barter & Furmidge, 1994).

No, the Development Will Not Make an Essential Difference

The ingrained difficulty in team nursing is the frequent blurring or informal violations of the assigned distinct task delineations and responsibilities as a result of the ever-changing nature of patient needs and interactions. On-the-spot decisions, requiring a depth of knowledge and trained critical thinking are made at the bedside during "routine" care. Much of the ongoing observations and conclusions made (even often subconsciously) are not readily apparent, such as the patient is "stable" or the patient looks "sick."

Many RNs feel frustration at being responsible for care they do not even witness or at being required to delegate what they are not comfortable delegating but what their employer insists they must delegate. The sponsors of the California patient ratio law also included a prohibition of using unlicensed, minimally trained personnel to perform procedures normally done by nurses. These tasks included medication administration, venipuncture, intravenous therapy, parenteral or tube feedings, invasive procedures (including insertion of nasogastric tubes, catheters, or tracheal suctioning), patient assessment or education, and postdischarge care.

The envelope, however, keeps getting "pushed." Some emergency department fast-track staff have only an LPN in the physically separated area to do all nursing actions, yet assume an RN located elsewhere will cosign all charts for the assessment and discharge teaching of the "supervisor." The American Medical Association has proposed the solution of an assistive registered care technologist reporting to physicians. In 2005, nurses in Illinois spearheaded the defeat of proposed legislation for a "medication technician" role to administer drugs in long-term care facilities.

No state Nurse Practice Act allows even LPNs to perform an independent nursing assessment. No distinction is made between the patient's condition severity; for example, a stable clinic patient with a stubbed toe versus an acute care patient with a gunshot wound. Legal experts warn that plaintiffs are beginning to add causes of actions to their complaints that the staff was inadequate or was not qualified (Brous, 2004).

Only a nurse can do nursing. To take the inherent complexity of the profession for granted is easy because it is so familiar. But there is a reason that years of preparation are required to be an RN. Florence Nightingale maintained that nursing is an art; and if it is to be made an art, it then requires as exclusive a devotion and as hard a preparation as any painter's or sculptor's work. She believed that one cannot compare dealing with dead canvas or cold marble with a living body, the temple of God's spirit. The answer is not to legitimize and regulate any new roles to substitute for the education and expertise of an RN.

DEFINING NURSING

An overarching aspect of this debate is what does "nursing" as a verb entail? Is nursing a list of tasks that can be prioritized, delegated, and supervised? Or is nursing an embodied art and skill that incorporates the whole of patient care knowledge, assessment, prioritization, and discernment into something bigger than the sum of its parts? Can protocols or care tracks be developed for others systematically to "nurse," or does it require hands-on involvement?

What often is not included in definitions of nursing is the aspect of the ever-changing nature of these processes applied to *this* individual patient. Application involves critical thinking of a more qualified individual.

Nursing protocols are designed as "expert systems"; for example, the parts require the experience, interpretation, and decision-making capabilities of an RN. For instance, is the patient's rash purpura? Is the pulse thready? Standard systems can guide, and minimize the risk of omissions by, the nurse but not eliminate the need for a nurse.

Nursing also involves holistic approach beyond the "cookbook approach" that transcribes just what a patient says or rotely carries out a physician's orders. Nursing uses interpersonal skills to hear what is not being said. For instance, the patient presents a request for medication for a headache. The nurse skillfully detects key physical and behavioral signs that lead into astute follow-up questions to discover the presence of domestic violence.

WHAT IS SAFE, EFFECTIVE, ADEQUATE STAFFING?

The answer to this essential global question includes many various aspects:

◆ The Joint Commission on the Accreditation of Healthcare Organizations (2005) indicates that the answer is combination of human resource/administrative indicators and clinical/service indicators, not one single factor. Human resource indicators include nursing care hours per patient date, direct/indirect, on-call or per diem use, overtime, sick time, staff injuries, staff satisfaction, staff turnover rate, staff vacancy rate, and understaffing compared with the staffing plan. Commission clinical indicators include patient falls, injuries to patients, length of stay, medication events, patient/family complaints, pneumonia, postoperative infections, pressure ulcers, shock/cardiac arrest, upper gastrointestinal bleeding, and urinary tract infection. The commission also holds that an analysis of indicators is required at the level most effective for planning staffing needs within the organization, reflecting its unique characteristics, specialties, and services and the service area. For example, falls may be an effective indicator for a medical-surgical unit but not a postpartum unit.

◆ Labor Management Institute consultants Cavouras and Suby (2004) specifically recommend considering measures such as overtime because of scheduled shifts compared with end-of-shift overtime, supplemental staffing compared with core staffing as a percentage of total worked hours (core staffing should meet 85% of schedule needs), length of time positions remain vacant, family medical leave time as a percentage of total worked hours, and a nursing turnover rate of 10% or less.

◆ The Institute of Medicine report *Keeping Patients Safe: Transforming the Work Environment for Nurses* (Page 2005) includes the design of nurses' work, their staffing levels, hours, and management and culture of health care organizations.

◆ Nursing leadership traditionally uses objective indicators such as vacancy and turnover, nursing care hours/patient/day, patient condition severity indexes, and skill mix. Staff nurses' perception of the adequacy of staffing includes these traditional objective aspects but also is affected typically by other factors. These factors include competence of co-workers, how well staff members work together, computerized order entry, number of new graduates and float nurses, degree of autonomy permitted, adequacy of support and ancillary services, and type of care delivery system.

SUMMARY

Obviously, the final answer for safe, effective, quality care and staffing involves many aspects, rather than an exclusive focus. However, clearly one essential component to include is *who* the staff is, including experience, education, training, credentials, and qualifications. Nothing in life is risk-free. Another aspect involves answering the value question of how much risk does society want to tolerate based on who the caregiver is. Patients implicitly trust nurses to be their advocate: 79% percent of the public considers nurses the top profession for being the most honest and ethical (Jones, 2002). Nurses need to take the reins in shaping the preferred future of human health care. Nursing has the responsibility to be the keeper of its professional standards. It is time to consider the full implications of Florence Nightingale's admonition (1859) to "do the sick no harm." Fulfilling that axiom includes more than nurses' individual practice. Fulfillment involves making strategic and tactical choices based on all the relevant issues for the number and composition of staffing that best and most responsibly meets the patients' needs.

REFERENCES

Aiken, L., & Lake, E. (1992, December). *Summary of empirical literature on the relationship between nursing skill mix or RN-to-patient ratio and hospital mortality.* Philadelphia: Center for Health Services and Policy Research, School of Nursing, University of Pennsylvania.

Akin, L. H., Smith, H. L., & Lake, E. T. (1994). Lower Medicare mortality among a set of hospitals known for good nursing care. *Medical Care, 32*(8), 771-787.

American College of Healthcare Executives & Society for Healthcare Strategy and Market Development. (2005, March). *Futurescan: Health trends and implications, 2005-2010.* Chicago, IL: Author.

American Nurses Association. (1992). *Position statement on registered nurse utilization of unlicensed assistive personnel.* Washington, DC: Author.

American Nurses Association. (1997). *Implementing nursing's report card: A study of RN staffing, length of stay and patient outcomes.* Washington, DC: Author.

American Nurses Association. (1999). *Principles for nurse staffing.* Washington, DC: Author.

Appleby, J. (2004, July 26). Cutting nurses' patient loads boost care, costs. *USA Today.*

Barter, M., & Furmidge, M. (1994). Unlicensed assistive personnel: Issues related to delegation and supervision. *Journal of Nursing Administration, 24*(4), 36-40.

Blegen, M. A., Goode, C. J., & Reed, L. (1998). Nursing staffing and patient outcomes. *Nursing Research, 47*(1), 43-50.

Blendon, R. J., DesRodies, C. M., Brodie, M., Berson, J. M., Rosen, A. B., Schneder, E., et al. (2002). Views of practicing physicians and the public on medical errors. *New England Journal of Medicine, 347*(24), 1933-1940.

Bond, C. A., Raehl, C. L., Pitterle, M. E., & Franke, T. (1999). Heath care professional staffing, hospital characteristics, and hospital mortality rates. *Pharmacotherapy, 19*(2), 130-138.

Brannon, R. (1990). The reorganization of the nursing labor process: From team to primary nursing. *International Journal of Health Services, 20*(3), 511-524.

Brous, E. (2004). LPNs and fast-track staffing. In P. G. Zimmermann (Ed.), Managers forum. *Journal of Emergency Nursing 30*(3), 260-261.

Cavouras, C. A., & Suby, C. M. (2004). What is effective staffing? *CMS: The Journal of Clinical Systems Management, 6*(12), 11-13.

Centers for Disease Control and Prevention. (2005). *National Hospital Ambulatory Medicine Care Survey: 2002 ED Summary.* Retrieved July 23, 2005, from http://www.cdc.gov

Curry, J. (1992). Bridge over troubled waters: ED nurses share strategies regarding use of prehospital care providers in the emergency department. *Journal of Emergency Nursing, 18*(6), 30A-35A.

Davies, P. (2004, July 27). Fatal medical errors said to be more widespread. *The Wall Street Journal,* p. D5. Retrieved July 27, 2004, from http://www.tmit1.org/downloads/Fatal_Medical_Errors_WSJ_07_27_04.pdf

Davis, D. (1994). Effective utilization of a scarce resource: RNs. *Nursing Management, 25*(2), 78-80.

Emergency Nurses Association. (1999). *Standards of emergency nursing practice* (4th ed.). Des Plaines, IL: Author.

Gardner, K. (1991). A summary of findings of a five-year comparison study of primary and team nursing. *Nursing Research, 40*(2), 113-117.

Hartz, A. J., Krakauer, H., Kuhn, E. M., Young, M., Jacobsen, S. J., Gay, G., et al. (1989). Hospital characteristics and mortality rates. *New England Journal of Medicine, 321,* 1720-1725.

Hoffman, J. M., Shah, N. D., Vermeulen, L. C, Hunkler, R. J., & Hontz, K. M. (2004). Projecting future drug expenditures—2004. *American Journal of Health-System Pharmacy, 62,* 145-158.

Institute of Medicine. (1999). To error is human: Building a safer health system. Retrieved January 5, 2005 from http://www.iom.edu/Object.File/Master/4/117/toErr-Spager.edu

Joint Commission on Accreditation of Healthcare Organizations. (2005). *Accredited organizations—fast track.* Retrieved July 23, 2005, from http://www.jcaho.org/accredited+organizations

Jones, C. (1999). Staffing standards. In P. G. Zimmermann & B. Pierce (Eds.), Manager's forum. *Journal of Emergency Nursing, 25*(3), 221-223.

Jones, J. M. (2002). *Effects of year's scandals evident in honesty and ethics ratings.* Retrieved December 17, 2002, from www.gallup.com/poll/releases/pr021204asp

Kennedy, M. S. (2000a). News: A medical error wake-up call. *American Journal of Nursing, 100*(2), 21.

Kennedy, M. S. (2000b). News: Study shows link between nursing care and improved patient health and safety. *American Journal of Nursing, 100*(2), 21.

Kovner, C., & Gergen, P. J. (1998). Nurse staffing levels and adverse events following surgery in U.S. Hospitals. *Image: The Journal of Nursing Scholarship, 30*(4), 314-321.

Landro, L. (2005, December 1). The informed patient. *The Wall Street Journal,* p. D1. Available July 22, 2005, from http://www.healthgrades.com/PressRoom/index.cfm?fuseaction=InNews&rowno=1&re_fuseaction=InNews

Lockley, S. W., Cronin, J. W., Evans, E. E, Cade, B. E., Lee, C. J., Landrigan, C. P., et al. (2004). Effect of reducing interns' weekly work hours on sleep and attentional failures. *New England Journal of Medicine, 351*(18), 1829-1837.

Manuel, P., & Alster, K. (1994). Unlicensed personnel no cure for an ailing health care system. *Nursing & Health Care, 15*(1), 18-21.

McCue, M., Mark, B. A., & Harless, D. W. (2003). Nurse staffing, quality, and financial performance. *Journal of Health Care Finance, 29*(4), 54-76.

Moore, K., Lynn, M. R., McMillen, B. J., & Evans, S. (1999). Implementation of the ANA report card. *Journal of Nursing Administration, 29*(6), 48-54.

Nebeker, J. R., Hoffman, J. M., Weir, C. R., Bennett, C. L., & Hurdle, J. F. (2005). High rates of adverse drug events in a highly computerized hospital. *Archives of Internal Medicine, 165,* 1111-1116.

Nightingale, F. (1859). *Notes on hospitals.* London: Parker & Sons.

Page, A. (Ed.). (2004). *Keeping patients safe: Transforming the work environment of nurses.* Washington, DC: National Academies Press.

Paulson, D. L. (2004). A comparison of wait times and patients leaving without being seen when licensed nurses versus unlicensed assistive personnel perform triage. *Journal of Emergency Nursing, 30*(4), 307-311.

Person, S. D., Allison, J. J., Kiefe, C. I., Weaver, M. T., Williams, O. D., Centor, R. M., et al. (2004). Nurse staffing and mortality for Medicare patients with acute myocardial infarction. *Medical Care 42*(1), 4-12.

Press Ganey Associates. (2005). *HCAHPS news.* Retrieved July 23, 2005, from http://www.pressganey.com/scripts/news.php?news_ie=84

Rockey, L. (2000, January 19). Nurse-patient ratios: RNs demand adequate staffing to ensure quality of care. *The Chicago Tribune, NursingNews,* p. 1.

Rogers, A. E., Hwang, W. T., & Scott, L. D. (2004). The effect of work breaks on staff nurse performance. *Journal of Nursing Administration, 34*(11), 512-524.

Shindul-Rothschild, J., Berry, D., & Long-Middleton, E. (1996). Where have all the nurses gone? Final results of the AJN patient care survey. *American Journal of Nursing, 96*(11), 24-30.

Sovie, M. D. (1995). Tailoring hospitals for managed care and integrated health systems. *Nursing Economics, 13*(2), 2-83.

Stanton, M. A., & Rutherford, M. K. (Eds.). (2004). *Hospital nurse staffing and quality of care. Research in Action,* Issue 14 (AHRQ Pub. No. 04-0029). Rockville, MD: Agency for Healthcare Research and Quality.

Ventura, M. J. (1999). Staffing issues. *RN, 62*(2), 26-31.

Weingart, S. N., Karbstein, K., Davis, R. B., & Phillips, R. S. (2004). Using a multi-hospital survey to examine the safety culture. *Joint Commission Journal on Quality and Safety, 30*(3), 125-132.

Yassi, A., Cohen, M., Cvitkovich, Y., Park, I. H., Ratner, P. A., Ostry, A. S., et al. (2004). Factors associated with staff injuries in intermediate care facilities in British Columbia, Canada. *Nursing Research, 53*(2), 87-98.

Leadership in Transition in Acute Care Hospitals

COLLEEN J. GOODE ◆ KATHY A. BOYLE

"Far and away the best prize that life offers is the chance to work hard at work worth doing."

Theodore Roosevelt

Nurse leaders who work in acute care hospitals will be facing new challenges as health care prepares for growth because of the aging of the baby boomer generation, new technology, and a shortage of health care workers. It is essential that nursing have nurse leaders who are prepared to take on these challenges and lead the nursing profession to better outcomes than have been achieved in the past. Nurses are transitioning to a time when greater emphasis will be placed on quality of care and safety than has ever been experienced. Evidence indicates that hospital margins will continue to be a challenge, and nursing will compete with other needs as hospitals strive to grow, to fund capital needs, and to care for many patients who do not have insurance. The United States is rapidly facing a shortage of all workers, including health care workers. Recruitment will be difficult, and retention will be essential. Providing a positive, healthy work environment will be a necessity. The patients for whom nurses are privileged to care will be more involved in their care, and patient-centered care will be the norm. Evidence-based clinical practice and evidence-based management practice will take on new meaning. Instead of being a "nice" thing to do, these practices will be an expected. Education of all nurses will need to increase, competencies for practice will change, and residency programs for nurses will become commonplace. Health care organizations will need to establish themselves as learning organizations because change will be constant. Hard work will be required to be a great leader, but the journey will be exciting, for it will be possible to influence greatly the quality of care and enjoyment of work for the staff. This chapter addresses each of these transitions and the skills needed for nurses to transition to leadership excellence.

QUALITY AND PATIENT SAFETY

The Institute of Medicine reports *To Err Is Human* (Kohn, Corrigan, & Donaldson, 2000) and *Crossing the Quality Chasm* (Institute of Medicine, 2001) have propelled the U.S. health care industry into a focused effort to address the rate of medical errors, which are causing up to 98,000 preventable deaths per year. In addition, the Joint Commission on Accreditation of Healthcare Organizations published standards for improving safety through the National Patient Safety Goals, and all hospitals are struggling to meet these standards. Several national patient safety coalitions, such as the National Coordinating Council on Medication Error Reporting, the Medication Error Coalition, the National Patient Safety Foundation, and the National Quality Forum, are working to promote quality care and patient safety initiatives.

Fortune 500 companies and other large private and public organizations that provide health benefits for their employees have emphasized patient safety and quality care through the Leapfrog initiatives. This volunteer program is aimed at maximizing employer purchasing power by seeking health care for employees at only those hospitals that meet their evidence-based quality standards. New safety measures such as hospital-acquired infection rates, failure-to-rescue rates, death rates, and wrong-side surgery are emerging as the leading indicators of quality (Futurescan, 2004). Acute care hospital quality measures are being reported publicly, and some third-party payers are basing payment on quality outcomes. Future nurse leaders face the challenge of being knowledgeable regarding quality of care and patient safety, as well as operationalizing measurement of quality and safety outcomes and performance improvement initiatives in their own health care organizations.

Meaningful change cannot take place within an organization without a fundamental change in the culture of patient safety. Nurse leaders play a fundamental role in the development of this culture. The practice of patient safety exists through the connections of organizational elements such as (1) environmental structures and processes, (2) the attitudes and perceptions of workers, and (3) the safety-related behaviors of individuals (Cooper, 2000). The No. 1 strategic goal for acute care facilities should be implementation of quality and patient safety initiatives. Nurse leaders must advocate for the organization to place as much emphasis on quality and safety goals as it does on productivity and financial goals (Page, 2004).

Patient safety cultures should include a "no blame" philosophy of managing errors within the environment of care. In that process of no blame, organizations can learn about prevention of errors through identification of systems issues. Reason (1990) describes the work environment and work conditions as the context in which the human error occurs. Error management needs to focus on the environmental elements and generally not the individual as the source of error. Academic medical center hospitals that belong to the University HealthSystem Consortium have the opportunity to participate in electronic tracking of errors and near misses through the use of the Patient Safety Net. Multidisciplinary staff can click on a Patient Safety Net icon on their unit computers and submit errors and near misses. Data are fed back to the manager and the organization, trends are identified, and errors and near misses are compared with other hospitals in the database. Interventions to address errors are shared among hospitals.

The growing national emphasis on patient safety has affected labor expenses associated with the monitoring of safe care. The regulatory requirements for auditing patient care practices and care documentation have placed an additional financial burden on health care organizations. Few organizations have computer technology sophisticated enough to capture the data required for reporting to the regulatory agencies. Therefore nurses and other multidisciplinary staff are expected to participate in manual audits. Projections for personnel and time to complete required audits efficiently for the Centers for Medicare and Medicaid Services, Joint Commission on Accreditation of Healthcare Organizations, Leapfrog, and insurers need to be factored into annual budget projections. Hidden expenses can undermine a nursing budget and can affect patient safety and quality by taking valuable nursing resources away from patient care to do audits.

Health care leaders must influence and unite groups in the organization by articulating values, reinforcing norms, and providing incentives for desired safety behaviors. A comprehensive unit-based safety program was adopted by Johns Hopkins Hospital (Healthcare Advisory Board, 2005). One step of the program includes members of the executive team "adopting a unit." The program is an example of a creative approach in building a culture of patient safety by partnering executives with staff on units to identify and correct safety issues (Pronovost et al., 2004). Patient safety behaviors need to be grounded in the education of all health care professionals, including physicians (Barach & Berwick, 2003; Buerhaus, 2004).

TECHNOLOGY

Nurse leaders of the future need to be more savvy than ever regarding new technology. The implications for technology to improve quality and patient safety need to be assessed and combined with the need to support the effective role of the nurse and expand patient and family involvement in care processes. Some examples of how the growth of technology has supported patient safety initiatives include (1) expanded surveillance capabilities through central cardiac monitoring systems and fetal surveillance systems; (2) safety in medication order transcription and administration through the use of intravenous infusion pump safety systems, bar code readers, and computerized physician order entry systems; and (3) home monitoring devices for chronic disease management that send vital sign assessments electronically via telephone or Internet. Provision of secure access by patients to their medical records is possible through a patient Web portal. Studies indicate better satisfaction with doctor-patient communication and improved adherence to treatment plans with the use of this technology (Earnest, Ross, Moore, Wittevrongel, & Lin, 2004; Ross, Moore, Earnest, Wittevrongel, & Lin, 2004). Nurse leaders will need to evaluate how nursing documentation and education can enhance nurse-patient communication with the use of the patient Web portal. In addition, telenursing, like telemedicine, can be used to connect advanced practice nurses such as a certified wound ostomy continence nurse, in a metropolitan area to nurses in rural hospitals for consultation on wound care. Documentation systems of the future must be designed by vendors to reduce nursing documentation time and to integrate standardized language into their products.

VIEWPOINTS

With the implementation of any new technology comes huge training costs. Nurse leaders must not underestimate these needs.

PATIENT-CENTERED CARE

In *Crossing the Quality Chasm* (2001), the Institute of Medicine proposed an agenda with recommendations, rules, and aims for transforming health care in the twenty-first century that emphasizes the importance of patient-centered care. One of the recommendations for private and public purchasers, health care organizations, clinicians, and patients is that they should work together to redesign health care processes. Rules associated with this redesign are listed in Box 38-1 and represent the increasing emphasis on patient-centered care. Nurse leaders need to be champions for enactment of these rules. The Agency for Healthcare Research and Quality is developing a national standard for assessing and reporting patients' hospital experiences through its Consumer Assessment of Health Plans (CAHPS II) initiative. The initiative represents the combined efforts of the Centers for Medicare and Medicaid Services and other federal agencies to improve patient care. In addition, the National Quality Forum has recommended priorities for research regarding the need to measure patient experiences with inpatient care.

Some current examples of the expansion of patient-centered care include (1) patient and provider attendance at and participation in the Institute of Family-Centered Care conferences and (2) the use of patient decision aids for value-based patient choices regarding health care (O'Connor, Llewellyn-Thomas, & Flood, 2004). Access to Internet health care information has made the patient a more informed consumer of health care services and has heightened expectations of care processes. Patients are demanding a higher level of service, and nurses have a great influence on how patients perceive their service quality. Focus groups have been used to include the consumer perspective during the designing of new hospitals. Patient and family advisory councils deliver valuable information on the consumer perspective related to the patient and family hospital experience (American Hospital Association, 2004). The unique patient/family perspective can be included in strategic planning, allowing patients and families to participate in setting hospital goals and objectives. Nurse leaders of the future need to promote patient and family involvement in advisory councils designed to gain ongoing, valuable patient/family feedback regarding the process of acute care delivery.

BOX 38-1

Rules for Transforming Health Care

Care based on continuous healing relationships
Customization based on patient needs and values
Patient as the source of control
Shared knowledge and the free flow of information
Evidence-based decision making
Safety as a system property
The need for transparency and anticipation of needs
Continuous decrease in waste
Cooperation among clinicians

From Institute of Medicine. (2001). *Crossing the quality chasm: A new health system for the 21st century.* Washington, DC: National Academy Press.

HOSPITAL MARGINS

Hospitals of the future will continue to struggle to meet margins, and access to capital will be one of the highest needs (Healthcare Advisory Board, 2004). Many hospital facilities are getting old and need to be replaced. Nurse leaders must be highly involved in new construction and ensure a focus on patient safety and staff efficiency in the design of new hospitals. In addition, large sums of capital will be needed for technology. Many hospitals cannot get by on operating income alone. Hospitals will rely more on philanthropy, and they will continue to focus relentlessly on cost management (Futurescan, 2004). Having enough nurses to provide care will be critical to hospital financial performance. Fitch, a global rating agency, is interested in hospital registered nurse vacancy rates because these affect future financial performance of hospitals (Fitch Ratings, 2003).

Health care costs continue to rise. A Commonwealth Fund Health Care Opinion Leaders Survey (Commonwealth Fund, 2005) found that one of the priorities for Congress in the next 5 years is to enact reforms to moderate the rising costs of medical care for our nation. With the country facing a huge budget deficit, legislation to provide health care coverage for the uninsured seems unlikely, and hospitals will be faced with providing more uncompensated care. Much of the health care that hospitals deliver is to the elderly and for end-of-life care. New care models are being developed to focus on the needs of these patients. A growing number of Americans have chronic diseases, and experiments are under way to create new models of disease management and care for comorbidities. Hospitals cannot continue merely to decrease expenses; hospitals must look to clinical transformation involving care redesign for these patients (Healthcare Advisory Board, 2004).

WORK ENVIRONMENT

One of the greatest transitions acute care hospitals are focusing on is the need to provide a positive work environment for registered nurses. Hospitals struggled to meet cost reductions in the 1990s because of reduced Medicare reimbursement, reduction in reimbursement from other insurers, and the impact of managed care. Restructuring took place throughout hospitals that affected nursing, and many nurses lost trust in their leaders (Joint Commission on Accreditation of Healthcare Organizations, 2002). Drucker (2004) states that whatever authority one has as a leader comes from the trust the organization has in that person. An Institute of Medicine report (Page, 2004) identified loss of trust in administration by nursing staff and recommended that health care organizations demonstrate trust and promote initiatives to increase trust in nursing staff.

Code Green, a case study of Beth Israel Hospital in Boston (Weinberg, 2003), describes the financial crisis at Beth Israel, the merger with another hospital, the restructuring that took place, and the effect this had on nursing. Beth Israel, a Magnet hospital, went from the gold standard model for professional nursing to a hospital in which nurse vacancies became difficult to fill.

Lack of a positive, healthy work environment is one of the variables contributing to the nursing shortage (American Hospital Association, 2002; NurseWeek/American Organization of Nurse Executives, 2002). Magnet hospitals are known for having work environments that attract and retain nurses (McClure, Poulin, Sovie, & Wandelt, 1983, 2002). All hospitals should set strategic goals to meet the types of standards that Magnet hospitals are required to meet. The American Association of Critical-Care Nurses (2005) has published national standards for establishing and sustaining healthy work environments. The standards represent evidence-based and relationship-centered principles of professional performance (Box 38-2). As hospitals look to the future, they know there will be a shortage of nurses and a shortage of all workers. Hospitals must become employers of choice because there will be fierce competition for this scare resource. One cannot become an employer of choice without providing a positive work environment.

Nurse leaders must keep a pulse on the nursing work environment by measurement of staff nurses' perceptions of the environment. Kramer and Schmalenberg

---

BOX 38-2

American Association of Critical-Care Nurses Standards for Establishing and Sustaining Healthy Work Environments

1. Skilled communication: Nurses must be as proficient in communication skills as they are in clinical skills.
2. True collaboration: Nurses must be relentless in pursuing and fostering true collaboration.
3. Effective decision making: Nurses must be valued and committed partners in making policy, deciding and evaluating clinical care, and leading organizational operations.
4. Appropriate staffing: Staffing must ensure the effective match between patient needs and nurse competencies.
5. Meaningful recognition: Nurses must be recognized and must recognize others for the value each brings to the work of the organization.
6. Authentic leadership: Nurses must fully embrace the imperative of a healthy work environment, authentically live it, and engage others in its achievement.

From American Association of Critical-Care Nurses. (2005). *AACN standards for establishing and sustaining healthy work environments.* Retrieved February 20, 2005, from http://www.aacn.org/aacn/pubpolcy.nsf/Files/HWEStandards/$file/HWEStandards.pdf.

(2002) interviewed 279 staff nurses in 14 Magnet hospitals to determine what essential attributes must be present in the work environment in order for registered nurses to give quality care. Eight essentials were identified and are listed in Box 38-3. The Essentials of Magnetism Tool (Kramer & Schmalenberg, 2004) can be used by nursing leadership to measure staff nurses' perceptions of their work environments. Interventions then can be put into place to address the essentials that have low scores. The data should be shared with top-level leadership in the organization so they have an understanding of issues related to the work environment and the impact on retention and quality of care.

EVIDENCE-BASED PRACTICE

Kitson, Harvey, and McCormack (1998) argue that the successful implementation of research into practice is a function of the interplay of three core elements: the level and nature of the evidence, the context or environment into which the research is to be placed, and the

BOX 38-3

Eight Essential Characteristics of an Exciting and Rewarding Work Environment

Working with clinically competent nurses

Good nurse/physician relationships and communication

Nurse autonomy and accountability

Supportive nurse manager/supervisor

Control over nursing practice

Support for education

Adequate nurse staffing

Culture where concern for the patient is paramount

From Kramer, M., & Schmalenberg, C. E. (2004). Development and evaluation of essentials of magnetism tool. *Journal of Nursing Administration, 34*(7/8), 365-378.

method or way in which the process is facilitated. The diffusion and adoption of evidence-based practice in the 1990s increased significantly and has become part of the language for clinicians, managers, and policy makers (Walshe & Rundall, 2001). One of the drivers for an increase in the use of evidence in nursing practice has been Magnet hospital standards. Magnet hospitals and those applying to become Magnet hospitals must demonstrate how current research appropriate to the practice setting is available, disseminated, and used to change clinical and administrative practice (American Nurses Credentialing Center, 2005). Nurse leaders have been slow to adopt evidence-based management practices. Management decisions often are based on financial decisions or recommendations from consultants and not on evidence. A significant amount of research related to the work environment exists, yet nurse leaders are not using the research to transform their work environments. Evidence-based nursing practice is no longer a "nice thing" for nurse leaders in which to engage, but rather it is an expectation that nurse leaders will facilitate evidence-based clinical practice and, like their clinical staff, they will search for, appraise, and apply empirical evidence from management research (Page, 2004).

NURSING EDUCATION AND COMPETENCY

New studies are beginning to show a relationship between the education of the nurse and the outcomes of the patient. One study examined the effect of education at the baccalaureate level or higher on mortality and failure-to-rescue rates (Aiken, Clarke, Cheung, Sloane, & Silber, 2003). When the hospital had a higher proportion of nurses educated at the bachelor of science in nursing or higher degree, the hospital had lower mortality and failure-to-rescue rates. A 10% increase in the educational level was associated with a 5% decrease in mortality within 30 days of admission and the odds of failure to rescue.

A 2004 benchmarking project conducted by the University HealthSystem Consortium (2004) studied 1592 failure-to-rescue cases in academic medical center hospitals. A higher percentage of failure-to-rescue cases received intervention with presentation of the earliest signs when 50% or more of the registered nurses had a bachelor of science in nursing or higher degree. These studies provide beginning evidence that nurse education has an impact on mortality and failure to rescue. The educational preparation of nurses must be revisited, and the baccalaureate degree must become the entry level for the registered nurse.

Competency of nurses also has been related to quality of patient care. New initiatives to improve competency of practicing nurses must be undertaken. No longer can new graduate nurses be expected to care for hospitalized acute care patients without additional training, knowledge, and skills. Schools of nursing prepare nurses as generalists, and the skills and knowledge needed to care for the complex, acutely ill, hospitalized patient cannot be provided in the 4-year bachelor of science in nursing program. A postbaccalaureate residency program must become the standard (Goode & Williams, 2004). The residency program should be accredited by a national accrediting body, and pass-through dollars should be provided by the Centers for Medicare and Medicaid Services just as they are for medical and pharmacy residents. Transition of the new graduate into practice is rapid, and time for mentoring and training is inadequate (Joint Commission on Accreditation of Healthcare Organizations, 2002). The Joint Commission on Accreditation of Healthcare Organizations president Dennis O'Leary (2003) urged the Centers for Medicare and Medicaid Services to support federal funding for postgraduate nurse residency training programs of at least 1 year in length, and he stated this was a de minimus investment in patient safety. Among the 3000 cases in the sentinel event database of the commission, inadequate orientation or in-service training was a factor in 56% of the cases, and inadequate competency assessment was a factor in 16% of cases (Joint Commission on Accreditation of Healthcare Organizations, 2004).

Research conducted by Kramer and Schmalenberg (2004) found that staff nurses identified the competencies of their peers as the most important factor that must be present in the work environment in order for them to deliver quality patient care. Staff nurses indicated they want to take report from a competent nurse, give report to a competent nurse, and have competent nurses on the unit to help them whenever they have a crisis or untoward event with one of their patients. Staff nurse competency is essential to quality and safety of patient care, and nurse leaders need to implement residency training for new graduates along with in-service training, continuing education programs, and competency testing for senior staff to ensure ongoing competency.

DIVERSITY: PATIENTS AND WORKFORCE

Nurses' patients are becoming more ethnically and culturally diverse. Each immigrant and cultural group has specific health care risks and practices, and there is much for nurses to learn from these diverse patients (Futurescan, 2004). Communication with multicultural groups will become increasingly complex. The demand for oral and written communication will be great, and more resources will be needed for translators and for devices such as translator telephones in order to minimize risk and to improve patient understanding of their illness, treatment, and discharge instructions. Magnet standards are addressing diversity issues, and the standards require hospitals to demonstrate how hospitals address workforce diversity and how they establish a nondiscriminatory climate in which care to patients is delivered in a manner sensitive to diversity (American Nurses Credentialing Center, 2005). Magnet hospitals collect data to determine whether the diversity of the workforce represents the diversity of the patients. Perhaps diversity in health care management can lead to improved quality of care and a better work environment because these leaders may understand better the needs of the diverse patients and staff. Nurse leaders should strive to have a diverse nurse management team representative of the patients for whom they care.

LEARNING ORGANIZATION

Nurse leaders are faced with the demands of keeping abreast with best practices and new knowledge. Garvin (1993) identifies a learning organization as one that is skilled at creating, acquiring, and transferring knowledge and also is skilled at modifying its behavior to implement new knowledge. According to Senge (1990), competency of the learning organization is to master knowledge management and knowledge transfer. That mastery can occur through the use of social networks to share information, knowledge, and resources (Shortell, 2004). Nurse leaders can be experts in networking with other professionals to promote patient safety and quality. The current delays in dissemination of clinical practice innovations can be reduced through technological advances and the expansion of networking. Nurse leaders have a societal responsibility to participate in patient safety initiatives beyond the boundaries of their own organizations. Relationships need to be established with legislators with a purpose to educate and influence local, state, and national health policies. Nursing leaders are accountable for developing and using extensive social networks to influence the process of knowledge transfer regarding patient safety, quality, and patient-centered health care.

SUMMARY

The knowledge and skills needed by nurse leaders continues to grow. Much of the patient experience, the enjoyment of work of the nursing staff, and the quality of care nurses deliver, is influenced by the nurses in leadership positions. As nurses look to the future, they know that patients are more savvy about health care and are paying more attention to health care quality rankings on report cards. Many patients will want to be involved integrally in their care.

Registered nurses are selecting to work in hospitals that provide work environments that allow them to provide high-quality patient care. Nurse leaders must embrace a personal obligation to create a positive, healthy work environment for their staffs. The transitions described in this chapter are stimulating not only to nurse leaders who lead with passion but also to those who continuously seek new knowledge and those who actively manage change through ongoing communication and feedback.

REFERENCES

Aiken, L. H., Clarke, S. P., Cheung, R. G., Sloane, D. M., & Silber, J. H. (2003). Educational levels of hospital nurses and surgical patient mortality. *JAMA: The Journal of the American Medical Association, 290*(12), 1617-1624.

American Association of Critical-Care Nurses. (2005). *AACN standards for establishing and sustaining healthy work environments.*

Retrieved February 20, 2005, from http://www.aacn.org/aacn/pubpolcy.nsf/Files/HWEStandards/$file/HWEStandards.pdf

American Hospital Association. (2004). *Strategies for leadership: Advancing the practice of patient- and family-centered care—A resource guide for hospital senior leaders, medical staff and governing boards.* Retrieved February 20, 2005, from http://www.aha.org/aha/key_issues/patient_safety/contents/resourceguide

American Hospital Association, Commission on Workforce for Hospitals and Health Systems. (2002). *In our hands: How hospital leaders can build a thriving workforce.* Chicago, IL: American Hospital Association.

American Nurses Credentialing Center. (2005). *Application manual.* Silver Spring, MD: Author.

Barach, P., & Berwick, D. (2003). Patient safety and the reliability of health care systems. *Annals of Internal Medicine, 138*(12), 997-998.

Buerhaus, P. (2004). Lucian Leape on patient safety in U.S. hospitals. *Journal of Nursing Scholarship, 36*(4), 366-370.

Commonwealth Fund. (2005). *The Commonwealth Fund health care opinion leaders survey.* Retrieved January 7, 2005, from http://www.cmwf.org/usr_doc/CMWF_OpionLeaders_brief_030805.pdf

Cooper, M. (2000). Towards a model of safety culture. *Safety Science, 36,* 111-136.

Drucker, P. F. (2004). What makes an effective executive? *Harvard Business Review, 6,* 1-8.

Earnest, M., Ross, S., Moore, L., Wittevrongel, L., & Lin, C. (2004). Patients' perceptions on sharing an online accessible electronic medical record. *Journal of American Medical Informatics Association, 11*(5), 410-417.

Fitch Ratings. (2003). *Nursing shortage update.* Retrieved May 13, 2003, from www.fitchratings.com

Futurescan. (2004). *Healthcare trends and implications 2004-2008.* Chicago, IL: Health Administration Press.

Garvin, D. (1993, July-August). Building a learning organization. *Harvard Business Review,* pp. 78-91.

Goode, C. J., & Williams, C. A. (2004). Post-baccalaureate nurse residency program. *Journal of Nursing Administration, 34*(2), 71-77.

Healthcare Advisory Board. (2004). *The new medical enterprise.* Washington, DC: Advisory Board Company.

Healthcare Advisory Board. (2005). *Clinical strategy watch: Patient safety: Hopkins Fosters "Culture of Safety" through six-step initiative tool.* Washington, DC: Advisory Board Company.

Institute of Medicine. (2001). *Crossing the quality chasm: A new health system for the 21st century.* Washington, DC: National Academy Press.

Joint Commission on Accreditation of Healthcare Organizations. (2002). *Health care at the crossroads.* Oakbrook, IL: Author.

Joint Commission on Accreditation of Healthcare Organizations. (2004). *Sentinel event statistics.* Retrieved February 7, 2005, from http://www.jcaho.org/accredited +organizations/sentinel+events/sentinel+event+statistics.htm

Kitson, A., Harvey, G., & McCormack, B. (1998). Enabling the implementation of evidence-based practice: A conceptual framework. *Quality in Health Care, 7,* 149-158.

Kohn, L. T., Corrigan, J. M., & Donaldson, M. S. (Eds.). (2000). *To err is human: Building a safer health system.* Washington, DC: National Academy Press.

Kramer, M., & Schmalenberg, C. E. (2002). Staff nurses identify essentials of magnetism. In M. L. McClure & A. S. Hinshaw (Eds.), *Magnet hospitals revisited: Attraction and retention of professional nurses.* Washington, DC: American Nurses Publishing.

Kramer, M., & Schmalenberg, C. E. (2004). Development and evaluation of Essentials of Magnetism Tool. *Journal of Nursing Administration, 34*(7/8), 365-378.

McClure, M. L., Poulin, M. A., Sovie, M. D., & Wandelt, M. A. (1983). *Magnet hospitals.* Kansas City, MO: American Nurses Association.

McClure, M. L., Poulin, M. A., Sovie, M. D., & Wandelt, M. A. (2002). Magnet hospitals: Attraction and retention of professional nurses. In M. L. McClure & A. S. Hinshaw (Eds.), *Magnet hospitals revisited: Attraction and retention of professional nurses* (pp. 1-24). Washington DC: American Nurses Publishing.

NurseWeek/American Organization of Nurse Executives. (2002). *National survey of registered nurses.* San Jose, CA: NurseWeek Publishing Company.

O'Connor, A., Llewellyn-Thomas, H., & Flood, A. (2004). *Modifying unwarranted variations in health care: Shared decision making using patient decision aids.* Retrieved February 7, 2005, from http://content.healthaffairs.org/cgi/content/full/hlthaff.var.63/DC2

O'Leary, D. (2003, June 11). *Patient safety: Instilling hospitals with a culture of continuous improvement* (Testimony before the Senate Committee on Government Affairs, Washington, D.C.).

Page, A. (Ed.). (2004). *Keeping patients safe: Transforming the work environment of nurses.* Washington, DC: National Academy Press.

Pronovost, P., Weast, B., Bishop, K., Paine, L., Griffith, R., Rosenstein, B., et al. (2004). Patient safety: Senior executive adopt-a-work unit: A model for safety improvement. *Joint Commission Journal on Quality and Safety, 30*(2), 59-68.

Reason, J. (1990). *Human error.* Cambridge, UK: Cambridge University Press.

Ross, S., Moore, L., Earnest, M., Wittevrongel, L., & Lin C. (2004). Providing a Web-based online medical record with electronic communication capabilities to patients with congestive heart failure: Randomized trial. *Journal of Medical Internet Research, 6*(2), e12. Retrieved March 19, 2005, from http://www.jmir.org/2004/2/e12

Senge, P. (1990). *The fifth discipline: The art and practice of the learning organization.* New York: Doubleday.

Shortell, S. M. (2004). Increasing value: A research agenda for addressing the managerial and organizational challenges facing health care delivery in the United States. *Medical Care Research and Review, 61*(3), 12S-30S.

University HealthSystem Consortium. (2004). *Failure to rescue benchmarking.* Chicago, IL: Author.

Walshe, K., & Rundall, T. G. (2001). Evidence-based management: From theory to practice in health care. *The Milbank Quarterly, 79*(3), 429-457.

Weinberg, D. B. (2003). *Code green.* Ithaca, NY: Cornell University Press.

Nursing Employment Issues

Unions, Mandatory Overtime, Patient/Staff Ratios

THOMAS R. CLANCY ◆ CATHERINE H. ABRAMS

Over the past 2 decades, the nursing and health care workforce shortages have brought many challenges. Some of these challenges have moved from individual institutional issues to the legislative agenda and have implications for the profession and industry as a whole. Three of these challenges discussed in this chapter are mandatory overtime, staffing ratios, and unions.

MANDATORY OVERTIME

Definition

Mandatory overtime is defined as involuntary time when the registered nurse (RN) is required to remain for all or part of a subsequent shift or is required to come to work beyond the agreed-upon shift assignment (American Organization of Nurse Executives [AONE], 2003a). The Fair Labor Standards Act defines mandatory overtime as hours worked over 40 hours per week or over 80 hours for a 2-week period. Mandatory overtime does not include those hours for which a staff member has volunteered. The AONE does say that the nurse manager must consider the total number of hours a nurse has worked and the effects of fatigue on human performance when making assignments. Reports of mandatory overtime have been widespread and overblown at times. The AONE views mandatory overtime as the staffing vehicle of last resort.

Patient Safety and Mandatory Overtime

The Michigan Nurses Association (2004) lists the following threats to patient safety and individualized care that result from extensive overtime:

◆ Nurses being less alert to changes in patients' conditions
◆ Nurses having slower reactions
◆ Medication errors: adverse drug events
◆ Errors in clinical judgment

◆ Increase in health care–acquired infections
◆ Increase in decubitus ulcers

The most recent Institute of Medicine report (Page, 2004) spoke strongly for limiting overtime as a means to improve patient safety and reduce the thousands of hospital deaths that are being attributed to overworked and tired nurses.

Status of Mandatory Overtime Legislation in the United States

Currently, 10 states (California, Connecticut, Maine, Maryland, Minnesota, New Jersey, Oregon, Texas, Washington, and West Virginia) have approached mandatory overtime from different perspectives. These approaches range from enacting restrictions on mandatory overtime to prohibiting punitive action against nurses who refuse to work overtime to requiring that health care organizations develop policies and procedures for mandatory overtime. In 2004, 14 other states introduced legislation to prohibit mandatory overtime among nurses (American Nurses Association, 2004). Figure 39-1 graphically illustrates the current environment across the nation.

Mandatory Overtime and Health Care Costs

A review of the literature found few studies that evaluated the relationship of overtime work and health care costs (Stanton & Rutherford, 2004). Though research is limited, what is written suggests that increased fatigue and nurse burnout do carry a significant direct cost and increase the cost of medical liability for the organization. With declining reimbursement on so many fronts, health care facilities are focused on controlling costs. Nurses are especially vulnerable because they compose the greatest proportion of employees in health care organizations (U.S. Department of Labor, "Registered Nurse," 2004). Cost also is added when absenteeism increases or vacancies are created because nurses decide to seek employment

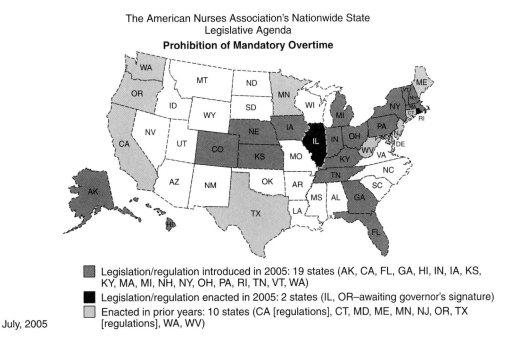

The American Nurses Association's Nationwide State
Legislative Agenda
Prohibition of Mandatory Overtime

July, 2005

■ Legislation/regulation introduced in 2005: 19 states (AK, CA, FL, GA, HI, IN, IA, KS, KY, MA, MI, NH, NY, OH, PA, RI, TN, VT, WA)
■ Legislation/regulation enacted in 2005: 2 states (IL, OR–awaiting governor's signature)
□ Enacted in prior years: 10 states (CA [regulations], CT, MD, ME, MN, NJ, OR, TX [regulations], WA, WV)

FIGURE 39-1 Mandatory overtime legislation among the states, 2004.

in institutions that do not allow forced overtime. The most recent data indicate that recruitment costs to replace an RN on a medical surgical floor are equivalent to the annual salary of the individual being recruited. At current salary levels that could be as much as $50,000 for each medical-surgical nurse and $64,000 for each critical care nurse (Michigan Nurses Association, 2004).

Nursing has always been a profession known for its attention to the care of the sick and vulnerable. With the shortage of appropriately trained and competent workers, it is paramount that the nursing and hospital leaders of today work to support the social contract that nurses have with the community to provide care when it is needed and to do so in a professional, competent, and compassionate manner. Imposing mandatory overtime on an already stressed, fatigued, and aging workforce can only exacerbate the problems faced in health care delivery. The solutions to avoiding mandatory overtime comes from ensuring that nurses are included in decision making and that nurse administrators remain clinically competent and have the ability to assist when the patient acuity and census require it.

The commitment to be available and provide the care needed must be honored by those in positions of leadership. Without this focus, the state of the employee/employer relationship will erode for years to come. Fostering a healthful work environment that

recognizes the value of nursing to the care of patients can avoid mandatory overtime while providing the workforce needed to care for those who require support and intervention daily.

PATIENT STAFF RATIOS

The combined effect of an aging RN workforce coupled with a decline in the number of hospitals nationwide has prompted nurse executives, legislators, physicians, the public, and nurses to focus on nurse-to-patient ratios. In recent years, the movement has been toward mandating the number of patients for which a nurse in a given discipline can care for in a given period. Many believe that mandating nurse-to-patient ratios will improve the quality of care and patient and nurse satisfaction. Others, such as the AONE (2003a), believe that mandating specific staffing ratios during a time of shortage will lead to a reduction in service, increased closures of units and possibly hospitals, and increased expenses as hospitals pay for overtime or temporary staffing.

Legislated Ratios

The first state to pass legislation requiring mandated staffing ratios was California in 2004 (Box 39-1).

One should note that these ratios apply only to RNs and that they do not distinguish between day, evening,

VIEWPOINTS

BOX 39-1

The California Nurses Association Ratios Requirements as of January 1, 2004

- Medical-surgical   1:6
- Emergency department   1:4
- Step-down/telemetry/pediatrics   1:4
- Intensive/critical care   1:2
- Neonatal intensive care   1:2
- Operating room   1:1
- Postanesthesia recovery   1:2
- Labor and delivery   1:2

Data from Ericksen, A. B. (2004). *Nurse-to-patient ratios: Will mandatory guidelines be the wave of the future?* Salisbury, MD: Healthcare Staffing & Management Solutions.

and night shifts. Because most organizations staff fewer RNs per patient on the evening and night shifts because of decreased activities, nurse-to-patient ratios have been difficult to meet.

Factors To Be Considered Before Mandating Ratios

To mandate nurse-to-patient ratios without taking into consideration several other factors is a mistake. These factors include the condition severity of the patient population, the skill and experience of the RN caring for the patients, the design of the facility itself, and the number of support personnel available to perform tasks that do not require RN training or experience. Those who support mandating ratios believe a decrease in patient safety and nurse satisfaction and deterioration of the work environment will occur without this legislation; those who are opposed feel that these same things will happen with mandating the number of nurses per patient (AONE, 2003a).

Each day the number and mix of patients on a unit at the beginning of the shift is not the same as at the end of the shift. Many times a 100% turnover can occur between 7 AM and 3 PM. In most instances, mandating the number of patients per nurse or employing a patient condition severity system cannot replace the professional judgment of the nurse manager or the professional RN who is on duty during this time. Another concern among staff nurses is that if ratios are mandated, the mandate will be viewed as the maximum number of nurses needed, no matter what happens or changes within the patient population. Times definitely arise when more nurses are needed than a mandated ratio may require.

Complexity of the Issue

Again, research is lacking that identifies the appropriate staffing levels, and little has been done to tie evidenced-based and patient care outcomes to staffing guidelines (AONE, 2003a). Patient care on any given unit remains unpredictable. This factor makes it necessary for nurse managers to have the flexibility to determine the appropriate number of staff to meet the needs of the patient population the majority of the time. Other variables include the shift, the availability of hospital resources, the unit volatility (admissions, discharges, and transfers), and the amount of technology on the unit. Only when all of these factors are given the appropriate weight can a sound decision be made as to the number of nurses required to care for the number of patients needing that care.

Several productivity/condition severity systems have been able to predict the number of nursing care hours required per patient per day. Using this as a base, the manager then is able to determine the number of staff and what level of preparation those individuals need. These systems may provide a starting point by which research and ratios could be derived. Removing the ability of the manager and the staff nurse to decide what staff is needed only complicates the issue rather than simplifies it.

Determining the best nurse-to-patient ratios is a complicated issue, and one on which the majority of the members of the nursing profession are not united. The American Nurses Association contends that staffing can best be implemented by identifying nursing quality indicators and mechanisms to determine and assess outcomes. Without solid research, assigning patient care to meet the individual needs of each patient must be determined by the professionals who are living the moment.

UNIONS

The severest test of a nurse administrator's leadership abilities occurs when staff nurses self-organize to form a union. As the term implies, self-organization reflects groundswell support for better representation of nurses' collective interests. The act of nurses self-organizing to negotiate the terms of their employment is the furthermost extension of the employee-employer relationship. However, the seeds of discontent are not planted by unions. Discontent usually results from an underlying atmosphere of mistrust, miscommunication, and feelings of helplessness and creates a unionization climate (Forman & Davis, 2002a). Unions simply take advantage of the discontent.

Why do nurses join unions? Although the literature is exhaustive (New Jersey Hospital Association, 2003), three common themes have emerged: autonomy, patient safety (understaffing), and wages (Forman & Davis, 2002b; Schraeder & Friedman, 2002).

Professional Autonomy

Nurses represent the greatest proportion of staff in virtually any health care setting (hospital, nursing home, physician's office). Of the 12.5 million jobs for wage and salary workers in the health care industry, 2.3 million went to RNs (U.S. Department of Labor, "Registered Nurses," 2004). Historically, nurses have not been afforded a voice in decisions that affect their wages, benefits, and working environment (Forman & Davis, 2002b). Decades of low pay, poor working conditions, and inflexible hospital management have prompted nurses to explore unionization as a means to gain professional autonomy.

The decision to bring health care under protection of the National Labor Relations Act in 1974 dramatically increased RN union organizing activity. Nonsupervisory RNs now were given legal protection through the National Labor Relations Board (NLRB) when seeking a collective bargaining agent (Forman & Davis, 2002b). As a result, the combined efforts of national and state nursing organizations (American Nurses Association and California Nurses Association, for example) and existing labor organizations (Service Employees International Union, The Teamsters, United Auto Workers, American Federation of Teachers) have increased RN union membership to 17.4% of the total RN workforce (Hirsch & Macpherson, 2003).

Although unions provide another avenue for nurses to influence decisions regarding their work environment, controversy exists regarding whether they actually improve professional autonomy (Forman & Powell, 2002). The National Labor Relations Act stipulates that during the collective bargaining process, the parties must confer in good faith with respect to wages, hours, and other terms or conditions of employment (Chatilovicz, Darch, Miller, & Kenwood, 2001). However, health care organizations are not *required* to discuss professional items such as clinical practice, staffing levels, education benefits, clinical ladder programs, or tuition reimbursement as part of the collective bargaining process. In fact, many health care organizations refuse to discuss these issues during contract negotiations.

Patient Safety

Unsafe staffing levels, mandatory overtime, floating, and emotional exhaustion have been cited as major factors influencing recent growth in RN union membership (Aiken, 2002; Schraeder & Friedman, 2002). From 1995 to 1999, RN union membership in the United States grew by 77.66% (American Federation of Teachers Healthcare, 2003). During the same period, American health care organizations began experiencing one of the severest nursing shortages in history (U.S. Department of Health and Human Services, 2002). The effects of cost cutting, reengineering, and downsizing by health care organizations in response to increased managed care and lowered reimbursement over the last decade has affected the work environment of nurses significantly. Understaffing and mandatory overtime issues have contributed to a drop in the proportion of RNs employed by hospitals from 66.5% in 1992 to 59% in 2000 (Buerhaus, Staiger, & Auerbauch, 2000). The typical RN works 8.5 weeks of overtime per year, and mandatory overtime has become a major issue in recent strikes by nurses (Service Employees International Union Nurse Alliance, 2001).

The emotional stress associated with understaffing, floating, and higher patient acuity levels has led to frequent turnover as nurses seek a more stable environment. A study compiled by Aiken (2002) showed that 43% of surveyed nurses reported job burnout and intended to leave their current position within the next 12 months. Peter Hart Research Associates (2001) found that 50% of nurses surveyed had considered leaving the field within the past 2 years for reasons other than retirement. Not surprisingly, in light of these factors, nurses have turned to unions for help.

Wages

Over the last decade, nurses' salaries have fluctuated significantly. From 1992 to 1997 the average weekly wage for RNs declined by 6.2%, whereas wages for the total labor market dropped by only 1.2%. Registered nurse salaries rose by 10.2% between 1997 and 2000 and have leveled off at a 4.1% gain from 2001 to 2002. The net increase in RN weekly wages from 1992 to 2002 was 3.3% compared with a 6.8% gain for the total labor force (U.S. Department of Labor, Bureau of Labor Statistics, 2004). Again, given the dismal net increase in pay, it is not surprising that RNs have turned to unionization as a means to increase compensation. Section 8(d) of the National Labor Relations Act requires an employer to confer in good faith with respect to wages, hours, and other terms of employment. Unionization has paid off for nurses, at least in the area of wages, where the collective bargaining process has resulted in unionized nurses earning 11% more than non-unionized nurses in 2002 (National Labor Relations Board, 1999).

The Union Campaign

The combined effects of the nursing shortage, under-staffing, mandatory overtime, and stagnate pay coupled with a lack of professional autonomy has provided fertile ground for unionization of RNs. A union campaign generally starts with a group of nurses approaching a union representative to seek help. Often a single event such as a layoff or salary freeze acts as a lightning rod to ignite a long-standing period of discontentment among the staff. After assessing the chances of success, unions then assist nurses by providing a structured roadmap for conducting a union campaign.

The foundation of a union campaign is the employee committee that steers the campaign from its inception. Early in the process, union organizers assist nurses to organize their strongest supporters into a formal committee by providing education and direction on how to run a campaign. The initial strategy in a unionization effort consists of rapidly building support among the incumbent nursing staff. Methods include telephone calls from committee members to employees, flyers, and educational meetings held outside of the health care organization, often in a supporter's home or in a local hotel conference room (Forman & Davis, 2002a).

Union campaigns run on emotion, and building momentum quickly and quietly is a key strategy. If successful, administration may be unaware a union effort is even under way until it is too late to stop. Union representatives know this and make every effort to work behind the scenes until they are sure adequate support is present. Once organizing activity is discovered, administration generally reacts quickly to reverse initial campaign momentum.

The National Labor Relations Act specifically outlines how a bargaining representative can be selected. The most common method employees select is through a secret ballot conducted by the NLRB. However, the NLRB cannot conduct such a ballot until a petition is filed requesting one. The NLRB recognizes interest in representation when 30% or more of a "unit of employees" signs a petition or authorization card. A unit of employees is defined as a group of two or more employees who share a community of interest and therefore reasonably may be grouped together for purposes of collective bargaining. Nonsupervisory RNs make up such a group (Chatilovicz et al., 2001).

Conducting a union campaign is expensive. Union representatives often publish extensive education material, rent meeting rooms, provide speakers, and develop video messages and Web sites. That is why most petitions are not filed until at least 65% to 70% of eligible voters have signed a petition or authorizing card. Once a petition is filed, the NLRB will issue it and then set a date for a secret ballet, usually within 42 days (Forman & Davis, 2002a).

Preelection Campaigning

When a petition is filed, employers and employees must adhere to strict rules outlined by the NLRB regarding preelection activities. From an employer's perspective, violation of preelection rules may result in charges of unfair labor practices. If such charges are found to be valid, the NLRB may rerun the election or, in a worse-case scenario, impose a bargaining order. Such an order may require the employer to recognize and bargain with the union even though the union may have lost the election. Examples of prohibited preelection employer activities include the following (Chatilovicz et al., 2001):

- *Threats:* Remarks directly or indirectly threatening the employee with discharge, layoff, loss of pay, loss of benefits, or loss of promotional opportunities if the employee signs a union authorization card, attends union organizational meetings, wears union insignia, and speaks in favor of the union or votes for the union
- *Interrogation:* Supervisors asking employees how many persons attended a union meeting, whether they signed union cards, or how they intend to vote in the election
- *Promises:* Suggestions that an employee will receive better wages, benefits, or working conditions if the employee does not sign a union card, votes against the union, or talks against the union
- *Spying:* Supervisors stationing themselves near union meetings and observing and identifying employees attending the meeting, following union supporters to determine where they go after work, or requesting that employees report on the union activities of co-workers

Before the election the employer will be required to file with the NLRB regional director a voter eligibility list (also known as an Excelsior list). This is a list of all eligible voters and must be filed within 7 days of the NLRB approval of a voluntary election agreement. The Excelsior list outlines the collective bargaining unit and may require a hearing between the NLRB, union representatives, and the employer to build consensus on the final list. Often these hearings can be contentious because the composition of the bargaining unit plays a significant role in the election results.

At the conclusion of the 42-day period, a secret ballot is held at the workplace. Strict instructions are provided by the NLRB regarding who may be present in the polling room and how the ballots are to be handled. Once the polling booths are closed, a representative from the NLRB counts the votes in the presence of the employer and employees. A final count of 50% plus one vote wins the election.

Leadership During a Union Campaign

Prevention is the best strategy for remaining union free. A long-standing atmosphere of helplessness, feeling unappreciated, and poor communication drives nurses to seek union representation. Recognizing the telltale signs of nurse dissatisfaction early and then dealing with them quickly is the key to preventing unionization. Early warning signs include disruptive staff meetings; requests by groups of nurses to meet with the nurse executive or chief executive officer to discuss pay, benefits, and other issues; and signed petitions. Even a change in the atmosphere on nursing units is cause for alarm. The frequent presence of nurses meeting in hallways and then quickly disbanding when a manager approaches or a sudden change in attitude among the staff are telltale signs of a problem.

Often the nurse executive is unaware that union representatives have been contacted until after the steering committee has been formed. By then, a structured drive to contact nurses and gain union support is already under way. That is why it is essential that the nurse executive intervenes and deals with the underlying problem before union representatives are contacted. Interventions include a formal process for identifying what the root problems are. This may include a hospital-wide employee survey or a series of meetings between the nursing staff, nurse executive, and chief executive officer. The use of outside consultants that specialize in labor relations should be considered. The availability of an objective third party may prompt nurses to feel less threatened and may provide an opportunity to solve problems.

The key to preventing RNs from seeking union assistance is open communication and then quick action to solve the problem. Credibility is gained when nurses see that management is serious about addressing issues. One must understand, though, that once a steering committee has been formed and union representatives have become involved, new issues will begin to arise. A union will attempt to drive a wedge between management and employees. Common tactics include discrediting facts presented by the employer or taking credit for any positive changes the employer may implement. The union will try to create a perception that employees are the union and that collectively they can solve all problems (pay, benefits, overtime, staffing, patient care).

Nurse administrators must realize that there is a measured response from unions as the employer reacts to organizing activity. In effect, the harder the employer pushes, the harder the union pushes back. Once organizing activity is acknowledged, it is important that the health care organizations seek legal counseling in labor relations. Union representatives are professional organizers, and attempting to navigate without legal counsel through the unfamiliar rules enforced by the NLRB is dangerous. Unfair labor practices early in the campaign, especially during the union card signing phase, can result in an NLRB-imposed reelection or bargaining order.

The discovery of union activity within a health care organization is a wake-up call. The administrative staff, from the chief executive officer to the shift supervisor, must acknowledge that a serious problem exists in the organization. This means removing as many distractions as possible and concentrating fully on the issues. Once a petition has been issued by the NLRB, only a 42-day window of opportunity exists to reverse momentum. In effect, large projects should be placed on hold to allow managers time to listen and to educate staff regarding unionization.

Tactics used by unions to influence staff are many and varied. As the campaign progresses toward the election, any of the following activities may occur: visits by organizing staff at employee's homes, telephone surveys, regular meetings with speakers from other unionized health care facilities, multiple flyers and brochures including union contracts from other institutions, professionally made videos, and extensive Web site information. Union supporters will begin wearing union buttons and other paraphernalia at the workplace. One should expect staff that have not revealed their voting intentions to be approached constantly by telephone, in their homes, and at the health care organization by union supporters. Some campaigns use the local press as a tactic. Frequent editorials and feature articles by union supporters are not unusual.

Health care organizations should consider many tactics during a union campaign. Taking a position of silence is not one of them. Silence can be interpreted as "not caring" and may lend support to what union organizers have been alleging. The NLRB rules during a campaign are specific regarding employee threats, interrogation, promises, and spying. However, this does not mean managers cannot speak with their staff about unions. In fact, the most important figure in winning employee confidence is the first-line manager. One-to-one communication by the unit manager to answer questions and educate staff is the most effective tactic in preventing unionization.

Although frank discussions between the unit manager and staff are important, they can be contentious. Campaigns run on emotion, and employees will take a strong position on whether to support or oppose a union. Often the nurse manager is caught in the line of fire. A union campaign can drag on for months if there is an extended card signing phase or the NLRB delays the vote because of bargaining unit issues and multiple hearings. Dealing with ongoing conflict on the nursing unit can be exhausting, and nurse executives need to be keenly aware of this. Problems arise when managers start avoiding conflict and stop communicating with their staff. When this happens, the nurse executive must step in and find ways to support the manager. In extreme cases, the nurse executive must make a hard decision and replace the manager midcampaign.

SUMMARY

In the last decade, RN union membership has increased nearly 80% (American Federation of Teachers Healthcare, 2003). Reasons for this dramatic increase are complex but generally follow a common theme. Professional autonomy, patient safety, job security, staffing, mandatory overtime, wages, and benefits have been cited as major factors. Underlying the rise in RN unionization are the economic and demographic variables fueling growth in membership: declining reimbursement, increasing managed care, and an aging RN workforce. Leading in today's health care environment requires an in-depth understanding of the many forces driving nurses to seek unionization.

The key to remaining union-free is prevention. Acknowledging that a problem exists is the first step in winning back the trust and confidence of the RN staff in any organization. Acknowledgment is synonymous with taking action. This means meeting with staff nurses and piecing together the often disparate issues into a unified strategy. Identifying the issues and crafting a strategy must be followed up with quick and decisive action.

In the event union activity is discovered within an organization, legal counsel on labor relations is essential. The rules enforced by the NLRB are specific and require that management be educated on potential violations of the National Labor Relations Act. Nurse administrators also must recognize that union

representatives are professional organizers and that there is a measured response to any actions the organization may take to reverse the momentum gained in a campaign.

The discovery of union activity within an organization is disheartening to nurse administrators. However, how the administrator responds is the key to effective leadership. Reversing the momentum in a union campaign can be the greatest challenge nurse administrators and their management staff will ever face. If successful though, an even stronger, more committed organization can emerge.

REFERENCES

Aiken, L. (2002). Hospital nurse staffing and patient mortality, nurse burnout, and job dissatisfaction. *JAMA: The Journal of the American Medical Association, 288*(16), 1987-1993.

American Federation of Teachers Healthcare. (2003). *The state of the healthcare workforce annual report for 2003.* Washington, DC: Author.

American Nurses Association. (2004). The nationwide state legislative agenda on nurse staffing. In *Legislative trends and analysis.* Silver Spring, MD: Author.

American Organization of Nurse Executives. (2003a). *AONE policy statement on mandated staffing ratios.* Retrieved August 1, 2005, from http://www.hospitalconnect.com/aone/advocacy/ps_ratios.html

American Organization of Nurse Executives. (2003b). *Policy statement on mandatory overtime.* Retrieved August 1, 2005, from http://www.ohanet.org/advocacy/state/issues/position/overtime_AONE.pdf

Buerhaus, P., Staiger, D., & Auerbauch, D. (2000). Implications of an aging registered nurse workforce. *JAMA: The Journal of the American Medical Association, 283*(22), 2948-2954.

Chatilovicz, P., Darch, D. A., Miller, E. B., & Kenwood, Y. C. (2001). Union representation and unfair labor practices. In K. A. Reed & R. J. Mignin (Eds.), *Federal employment laws and regulations: How to comply* (chap. 31). Chicago, IL: American Chamber of Commerce Publishers.

Forman, H., & Davis, G. (2002a). The anatomy of a union campaign. *Journal of Nursing Administration, 32*(9), 444-447.

Forman, H., & Davis, G. (2002b). The rising tide of healthcare labor unions in nursing. *Journal of Nursing Administration, 32*(7/8), 376-378.

Hirsch, B., & Macpherson, D. (2003). *Union membership and earnings data book: Compilations of the current population survey, 2002 and 2003.* Washington, DC: Washington Bureau of National Affairs.

Michigan Nurses Association. (2004). *The costs of mandatory overtime for nurses.* Okemos, MI: Author.

National Labor Relations Board. (1999). *Annual report of the national labor relations board, 1990-1999.* Washington, DC: Author.

New Jersey Hospital Association. (2003). *Labor unions: journal literature, books and Web sites.* Princeton, NJ: Author.

Page, A. (Ed.). (2004). *Keeping patients safe: Transforming the work environment of nurses.* Washington, DC: National Academies Press.

Peter Hart Research Associates. (2001). *The nurse shortage: Perspectives from current direct care nurses and former direct care nurses.* Washington, DC: Author.

Schraeder, M., & Friedman, L. H. (2002). Collective bargaining in the nursing profession: Salient issues and resent developments in healthcare reform. *Hospital Topics: Research and Perspectives in Healthcare, 80*(3), 21-24.

Service Employees International Union Nurse Alliance. (2001). *The shortage of care: A study by SEIU Nurse Alliance.* Retrieved January 20, 2005, from http://www.seiu.org/health/nurses/

Stanton, M., & Rutherford, M. (2004). Hospital nurse staffing the quality of care. In *Research in action* (AHRQ Pub. No.04-0029). Rockville, MD: Agency for Healthcare Research and Quality.

U.S. Department of Health and Human Services. (2002). *Projected supply, demand, and shortages of RNs: 2000-2020.* Washington, DC: Author.

U.S. Department of Labor. (2004). *Registered nurse.* Retrieved January 20, 2005, from www.bls.gov/oco/ocos083.htm

U.S. Department of Labor, Bureau of Labor Statistics. (2004). *Current population survey.* Washington, DC: Author.

CHAPTER

40

Shared Governance Models in Nursing

What Is Shared, Who Governs, and Who Benefits?

JANET P. SPECHT ◆ MERIDEAN L. MAAS

Governance, or self-regulation, has long been recognized as a privilege given to professions that earn the public trust by demonstrating accountability for their specialized practices (Crocker, Kirkpatrick, & Lentenbrink, 1992; Hess, 2004). To ensure that professionals do not misuse autonomy for their own interests, rather than those of their clients, society requires professionals to demonstrate accountability for their actions (Maas & Jacox, 1977). Nursing has developed many self-regulating mechanisms (e.g., codes of ethics, standards, credentialing and accreditation criteria, and guidelines for peer review) that demonstrate the ability to govern its members in the public interest (McCloskey et al., 1994); however, the privilege of governance has been slow in coming. Professional nursing governance in practice settings, where physicians and administrators who benefit from the subordinate employee status of nurses have dominated, has been especially constrained.

Although there are examples of the implementation of professional nurse practice models over several decades and there are current international examples (Anthony, 2004; Caramanica, 2004; Horvath, 1990; Jacoby & Terpste, 1990; Johnson, 1987; Maas & Jacox, 1977; McDonagh, Rhodes, Sharkey, & Goodroe, 1989; O'May & Buchan, 1999; Rose & DiPasquale, 1990; Thompson et al., 2004), recognition of the need for nurse governance became most focused in hospitals in the United States during the nursing shortage of the 1980s. The value of nursing to the delivery of health care in hospitals also became more visible as a result of relentless technological and medical advances and their associated costs. After a period of widespread use of registered nurses (RNs) to provide a variety of services to downsize other departments and workers, hospitals began to reconsider the best use of nursing knowledge and skills. The folly of

using nurses to perform functions for which they are highly overqualified became clearer as the undersupply of nurses compared with demand reached critical proportions. While the demand for nurses grew, increasing numbers of nurses demonstrated dissatisfaction with their jobs and careers by moving to part-time work, leaving nursing for other careers, or moving to other practice settings after a brief period of employment in one hospital (Prescott, 1987). A decreasing number of persons entered the nursing field because of low pay, limited career advancement opportunities, and a greater number of other career options for women (American Nurses Association, 1992). Finally, demands for more accountability for the outcomes of care accompanied the pressures to control costs. The result was that an increasing number of nurse and hospital administrators recognized that the staff nurse, at the point of contact with the patient, is in the critical position to ensure the delivery of quality care (Spitzer-Lehmann, 1989).

These and other factors encouraged nurse executives in hospitals to move to models of nursing practice that increased nurse autonomy for clinical decision making and participation in decision making throughout the organization. Shared governance models were a popular strategy in the 1980s and early 1990s to increase nurse job satisfaction and retention and to achieve cost-effective quality outcomes (Stichler, 1992).

Predictably, however, because of the efforts of nurse educators, the nursing profession, and health care and public policy makers, the supply of nurses increased in the mid-1990s. As concerns about nurse job satisfaction and retention waned with an oversupply of nurses, so did efforts to implement nurse shared governance in practice settings. Further, attention in hospitals shifted to cost reductions to maintain a competitive edge in managed care environments, resulting in downsizing of programs and staff. Shortened hospital stays, increased ambulatory care, and same-day surgeries reallocated health care that previously was provided in hospitals to community settings and families. Downsizing in hospitals was especially brutal in nursing departments. The consequences were another ebb in the number of admissions to nursing programs and many nurses who were "laid off" finding other employment, some in new community nursing opportunities and some in other fields. Again, as predicted, the new millennium dawned with another nurse shortage on the horizon. Combined with the folly of downsizing of organizations by eliminating many nursing positions, the shortage of nurses reached critical proportions. As nurses have come to expect, administrators, encouraged by nurse shortage and concerns about patient safety (Page, 2003), rediscovered their value. Nurses again are concerned about recruitment and retention, and there is a resurgence of interest in nursing shared governance (Anthony, 2004; Hess, 2004).

Many nurse executives and nurses in hospitals have worked to maintain or continue to implement nurse shared governance. Nurse shared governance models also are beginning to appear in community-based settings, such as nursing homes and home health care (Ferguson-Paré, 1996; Melchior et al., 1997; Morrall, 1997). Nurse shared governance also is beginning to appear internationally, especially in the United Kingdom (Gavin, Ash, Wakefield, & Rowe, 1999). Nurses in these settings recognize that the aim of nurse shared governance models to empower nurses within the decision-making system of an organization, particularly regarding increasing nurses' authority and control over nursing practice, not only is important for nurses' job satisfaction but also for outcomes effectiveness. A number of issues, however, need to be addressed as changes are made in organizations to implement shared governance. These issues include the lack of clearly defined criteria for shared governance, mixed motives for the implementation of shared governance, disagreement about how shared governance can and should be implemented, and concerns about the effects of shared governance on different roles within nursing and organization systems. Yet as Porter-O'Grady (2004) notes, the use of shared governance in the United Kingdom with a National Health Service indicates that the model is amenable to different social and cultural circumstances. In the United States the time is opportune to consider and resolve the issues that prevail in advance of increased interest in shared governance models that may accompany the current nursing shortage.

WHAT IS SHARED GOVERNANCE?

Clarification of the concept of shared governance and the structures and processes that must be in place for implementation in employing organizations is necessary if the nursing profession is to honor its contract with society as described in the American Nurses Association *Social Policy Statement* (American Nurses Association, 1980, 1995, 2003). The concept of shared governance comes from the recognition of the need to accommodate two systems of authority when professionals are employed in organizations. In organizations, authority ordinarily is vested in positions arranged in a hierarchy, with positions higher in the hierarchy assigned a greater scope of authority than lower positions. Although professionals employed by organizations occupy positions with corresponding organizational authority, they also have authority as a function of membership in their profession (Minzberg, 1979). For a profession, this authority is based on specialized knowledge. Society gives professionals autonomy to get important work done effectively by experts who also are competent judges of the needed expertise. When professionals are employed by organizations, there is always the danger that the societal needs that are entrusted to the profession will become subordinated to the needs of the organization. This is the critical reason why governance shared by the organization and its employed professionals has evolved. Nurse shared governance is synonymous with professional nursing practice in organizations that employ nurses (Maas & Specht, 1990). In nursing, shared governance means that nurse employees and the organization are partners in meeting the goals of the organization and the mandates of the nursing profession (Porter-O'Grady, 1991a, 1991b). However, descriptions of the requisite structures and processes for claimed shared governance models are often incomplete or unclear. Professional nurse shared governance does not exist unless the authority and accountability of professional nurses is codified in the organization and decision making structures and processes are in place that enable nurses to define and regulate nursing practice and share decisions with administrators regarding the management of resources.

As illustrated in Figure 40-1, specialized knowledge and commitment to a service ideal are the foundation for professional nurse autonomy and accountability (Maas & Specht, 1990). *Professional nurse autonomy* means that professional nurses have the authority to define and decide what services they will provide and what constitutes safe and effective practice.

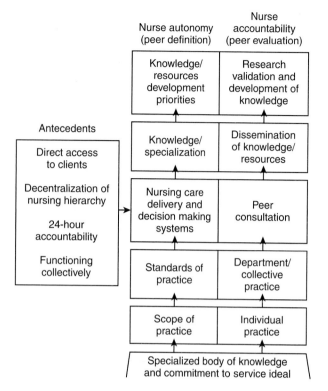

Nurse autonomy (peer definition) | Nurse accountability (peer evaluation)

Knowledge/resources development priorities | Research validation and development of knowledge

Knowledge/specialization | Dissemination of knowledge/resources

Nursing care delivery and decision making systems | Peer consultation

Standards of practice | Department/collective practice

Scope of practice | Individual practice

Specialized body of knowledge and commitment to service ideal

Antecedents

Direct access to clients

Decentralization of nursing hierarchy

24-hour accountability

Functioning collectively

FIGURE 40-1 Iowa Veterans Home model of professional nursing practice.
(From Maas, M. L. [1989]. Professional practice for the extended care environment: Learning from one model and its implication. *Journal of Professional Nursing, 5*[22], 66-76.)

Professional nurse accountability means responsibility and answerability to authority for the services rendered. The profession must take action to ensure that the practice of its members is safe and effective. Thus organizational structures of decision making, coordination, and control set forth in a constitution and bylaws are needed (1) to enable nurse peer definition of the scope of nursing practice, standards of practice, nursing delivery systems, qualifications for the selection of staff, and knowledge and resources required; and (2) to enable peer evaluation of the practice, promotion, and retention of individual nurses, evaluation of the department (collective) practice, peer consultation, dissemination of knowledge, and development of knowledge through research. Contrary to some definitions that describe shared governance as a structure for staff nurse autonomy (Pinkerton, 1988), the structure must enable professional autonomy and accountability of all professional nurses, as individuals and as a collective, if governance is to be shared by the organization and employed

professional nurses (Maas, Jacox, & Specht, 1975). All RNs, regardless of their position in the organization (e.g., staff nurse, clinical nurse specialist, nurse researcher, nurse educator, nurse manager, or nurse administrator) must have professional autonomy and accountability as individuals and as a collective of peers (Maas & Jacox, 1977).

More than 1000 hospitals in the United States implemented shared governance in the 1980s and early 1990s (Porter-O'Grady, 1994); however, many of these shared governance models disappeared as the shortage of nurses abated (Hess, 1998). The correlation of increased adoption of shared governance when nurses are in short supply and its disappearance from many hospitals when there is an ample supply of nurses supports the contention that shared governance may be viewed by administrators as more of a recruitment method than it is a serious recognition of the value of nurses as professionals.

As shared governance models continue to be applied in settings, an important note is that much variation exists in the models implemented under this label. A number of different terms, such as *participation in decision making, participative management, self-governance, empowerment,* and *professional practice* are used at times to be synonymous with share governance and at other times to indicate different organizational models with varying degrees of nurse participation in decision making. The consensus appears to be that shared governance means some amount or type of shared decision making by staff and nursing management. Less clarity and agreement exist regarding what specific decisions are made or are shared by nurses and managers, what staff persons are included in the shared governance, and whether nurses as individuals or as a collective have authority and accountability for certain decisions. Thus models of practice implemented under the label of shared governance range from those with minimal, ad hoc, or informal participation by some or all nursing staff in a limited number of decisions with little or no expectation for nursing staff accountability, to models in which the profession and the organization truly share authority and accountability for the mandates of the profession and the mission of the organization.

Although we contend that nurse shared governance is synonymous with a professional model of nursing practice within an employing organization, other theoretical frameworks have guided shared governance in some settings. For example, Kanter's theory of structural power (1993) emphasizing work empowerment where the emphasis is on management "granting" power to nurses for autonomous actions has guided a number of shared governance initiatives (Erickson, Hamilton, Jones, & Ditomassi, 2003; Laschinger, Almost, & Tuer-Hodes, 2003; Laschinger & Havens, 1996). Self-managing work teams is another theoretical framework described by Anthony (2004). The self-managing work team model posits that work groups jointly responsible for achieving goals lead themselves (Jones, 2004). Organizations that have implemented the self-managing work teams model include those described by Perley and Raab (1994) and Song, Daly, Rudy, Douglas, and Dyer (1997). Empowerment and self-managing work teams, however, beg the question of what is the appropriate model for professionals who are employees of an organization. Professionals empower themselves with their expertise, and it is this expertise that they profess accountably to apply with their clients. Thus professional nurses best serve their employers' objectives if they have control of their practice and are accountable for specific outcomes. Work teams may include persons other than professionals. Although self-managing teams may be more productive and produce higher-quality products, they produce work autonomy not professional autonomy, which includes all aspects of practice, not just the way work is done.

Because all nursing staff do not have the specialized knowledge and socialization to the service ideal that professional nurses do, it should be obvious that democracy in the workplace is not nurse shared governance and vise versa. Nursing staff who assist RNs in the delivery of care clearly are not qualified to govern the profession, although they can and should participate in decision making in the organization.

Discussion of whole-systems shared governance is increasing (Evan, Aubry, Hawkins, Curley, & Porter-O'Grady, 1995; Porter-O'Grady, 1994; Wilson & Porter-O'Grady, 1999). Whole-systems governance is more similar to democracy in the workplace than to professional nurse governance. The basis for sharing in these models is doing the work rather than being a member of the profession. Although whole-systems governance schemes increase participation in decision making for all workers, they do not address control of professional practice by the profession. Whole-systems shared governance reinforces the need for professional nurse shared governance, albeit it complements governance by the profession, but does not supplant it. Both are important for the effectiveness of the organization; however, professional governance enables the application of expert knowledge as the best way to achieve quality outcomes.

The confusion between the concept of participation in decision making and professional governance has contributed to the view advanced by Porter O'Grady (1994) and Wilson and Porter-O'Grady (1999) that whole-systems governance is a progression beyond nurse shared governance. This, however, is not the case. The goals of whole-systems shared governance and professional nurse shared governance are distinctly different. Integration, equity, and communication among disciplines within the organization are fundamental objectives of whole-systems governance, whereas nurse shared governance is a partnership between professional nurses and the organization to meet the mandates of the profession for autonomy and accountability of nurses for client welfare and the goals of the organization. These two approaches to governance come from difference theoretical bases. From an organizational behavior perspective, whole-systems shared governance does not address the societal aegis and function of a profession as does nurse shared governance, which is derived from the sociology of professions literature. The two systems are not mutually exclusive, and both can contribute positively to client outcomes and to effective organizations. The Hartford experience illustrates this (Caramanica, 2004).

Less obvious and still controversial is to assert that not all RNs are qualified to assume autonomy and accountability. All RNs share the mandates of the profession; however, there is great variation in their knowledge, education, and experience. Implementation of shared governance requires that RNs who are expected to assume professional autonomy and accountability are prepared to do so. This means that the first shared decisions of the organization and nursing leadership must be the definition of criteria for admitting RNs to professional decision making privileges and agreement on the programming and resources needed to assist RNs who desire to meet the criteria.

The controversy over what decisions professional nurses and organization management would make mostly focuses on a debate about whether nurses who are not managers can decide matters of resource distribution. This is simply a concern about loss of control on the part of managers and reflects a lack of commitment to professional nurse governance. The importance of this issue is underscored by the results of a survey of 1100 RNs from 10 hospitals that was conducted from June 1993 to April 1994 (Hess, 1995). The study revealed that out of six aspects of governance, including control over professional practice, the nurses rated as most important the influence over organization resources that support practice. Another illustration of the importance of the issue is the recent downsizing of hospitals and elimination of nurse positions with limited participation and essentially no control over the decisions by nurses. In many instances, nurses knew that the cuts were placing patients and nurses in jeopardy. Only after serious effects occurred for some patients and collective action by some nurses is the recklessness of these decisions now being recognized and is beginning to be reversed (Beyea, Killen, & Berlandi, 2002; Clark, 2003; Jackson, Chiarello, Gaynes, & Gerberding, 2002).

Professional shared governance requires that all nurses in the organization develop a consensus about goals and priorities and the expectations that available resources will be allocated accordingly. All nurses are kept aware of the available resources, share the planning of their allocation, and share the responsibility to develop alternatives where there is shortfall. Specific areas of authority and accountability for different roles (e.g., managers, educators, and clinicians) are defined, and control of decisions is placed with those who carry them out (Jenkins, 1991). Disagreements about decisions are resolved through negotiation. Although the development of the consensus, structures, and expectations for shared governance is not easy, resistance to doing it because of concern about who will make the decisions is most often a lack of commitment to professional nursing practice and an unwillingness to relinquish control.

Professional nurse's participation in decision making, empowerment of nurse professionals, participative management, and work redesign are coincident and necessary for professional nurse shared governance, but none is synonymous with it. The goals of work redesign are often to enhance the authority of nurses and rectify organizational problems that contribute to suboptimal use and turnover of professional nurses (Strasen, 1989). Thus the goal of work redesign efforts may be directed toward implementation of shared governance models. The goals of many work redesign efforts, however, also are to increase the participation of nurses in decision making without providing the structures whereby they have professional authority and accountability for all decisions affecting nursing practice. Some work redesign efforts actually obscure the identity of nursing as a professional discipline with obligations of accountability to clients for services rendered. The current emphasis on interdisciplinary efforts and team building, while laudable, often is interpreted as shared authority and accountability without recognizing the necessity of retaining mechanisms for demonstrating

the accountability of disciplines other than medicine. A study of the implementation of nurse shared governance in one hospital described the concurrent implementation of patient-focused care, which resulted in the removal of the term *nursing* from all nurse shared governance documents (Ramler, 1995). Although patient-focused care is approaching the graveyard of other previously ill-conceived models marketed by consultants who play to the desperations and priorities of administrators, it illustrates the lack of clear understanding of professional shared governance and its importance for quality outcomes that tends to prevail.

Many nurse executives have become vice presidents for patient care services (or some similar title), promoting the change in language from "nursing" to "patient care services" and in many instances eliminating departments of nursing (Specht, 1995). Although most nurses applaud the need for a nurse executive to administer all patient services, few seem to analyze the implications critically. They do not appear to note the implications if the nursing department is not a visible and accountable entity. Nor do many appear to discern the need for nursing and each discipline to be autonomous and accountable for the practice of the discipline for interdisciplinary care to be a reality (McCloskey & Maas, 1998). In the circumstances of interpretation of interdisciplinary as negating the identities, unique perspectives, and obligations of individual disciplines it is most critical to have professional nurse shared governance operational, but it is also when it is least likely to be implemented.

Nurses must be astute about the distinction among these concepts so that they are not misled into believing that they are sharing governance with management as professionals, when in fact they are not equal partners in meeting the mandates of the profession or the goals of the organization. If the structures enabling professional autonomy and accountability outlined in Figure 40-1 are not implemented, nurse shared governance is not operational. Figure 40-2 provides one example of decision making, coordination, and control structures defined in a constitution and bylaws that enable nurse shared governance in an organization (Maas & Specht, 1990).

We wondered previously whether there will be a resurgence of interest in nurse shared governance as the current nursing shortage continues. Previously, we noted that clarity about shared governance for nurses is essential if it is to be more than one more "bandwagon" jumped on without being anchored to a clear theoretical base and commitment to enabling professional nursing

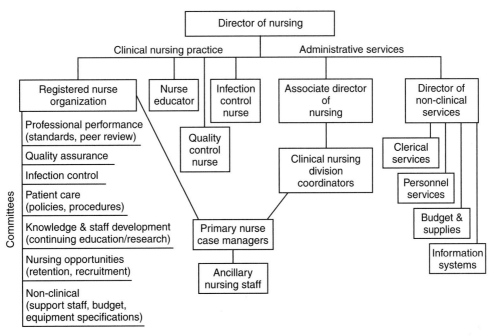

FIGURE 40-2   Iowa Veterans Home department of nursing.
(From Maas, M. L. [1989]. Professional practice for the extended care environment: Learning from one model and its implication. *Journal of Professional Nursing, 5*[22], 66-76.)

practice (Maas, Specht, & Ramler, 1997). Some continue to argue that the knowledge base of nursing is insufficient to support control of practice as professionals and that the majority of nurses do not want professional authority and accountability. Others still complain that shared governance is little more than a philosophy, a fad, or a nursing self-aggrandizement and that there is no evidence that benefits accrue when nurses have more professional autonomy. A few assert that shared governance sounds like a religion when the converted argue its merits. Admittedly, the description of change to shared governance as "transformation" may sound a bit like "being born again," connoting a spiritual experience rather than a functional model of social organization derived from sound theory and validated empirically (Porter O'Grady, 1992; Wilson & Porter-O'Grady, 1999). It is opportune that literature reporting the effects of nurse shared governance is mounting, which we review in a later section of this chapter.

The claim by some (Schwartz, 1990) that nurses are unwilling to exercise self-discipline and act in behalf of the public is unfounded. As a profession, nursing has demonstrated over and over that it is worthy of the public trust and that it is able to govern its members in accord with that trust (Peplau, 1985). Nurse administrators who

observe that staff nurses appear to be unwilling to assume professional authority and accountability too often are noting the behaviors of nurses who have been used and abused to benefit others. These nurses typically have experienced capricious changes, a lack of power and control over a heavy and often dangerously overwhelming workload, and a lack of socialization in the knowledge and skills needed for organizational and interdisciplinary politics. Evidence indicates that professional nurses welcome shared governance if it is implemented with their participation, with ample opportunity to gain the needed knowledge and skills for consensus decision making, and with the appropriate organizational structures for professional authority and control of practice in place (Maas, 1989). Further, evidence indicates that the nursing knowledge base is sufficient to support control of practice and that nurses participate more actively in the development and dissemination of knowledge in a professional model of practice (Brooks, Olsen, Rieger-Kligy, & Mooney 1995; Gulland & Payne, 1997; Maas, 1989; McDonagh et al., 1989; Skubak, Earls, & Botos, 1994; Wilson & Porter-O'Grady, 1999). The increased focus on outcomes effectiveness is an opportunity for nursing to demonstrate its accountability for client outcomes. Regrettably, the structures and processes for the assessment of outcomes effectiveness often are not linked to the structures and processes for professional nurse shared governance.

MOTIVES FOR SHARED GOVERNANCE: IS IT AN OPIATE?

Although the motives for implementing all shared governance models are assumed to enhance the delivery of quality care, these motives are mixed regarding the commitment to enabling the work of the professional nurse. Because shared governance remains an attractive aspect of the work environment for nurses, many hospitals boast shared governance as a desirable feature of their organizations. Yet often minimal structures of shared governance are actually in place (Specht, 1995). In some cases the motive seems to be to increase nurses' perceptions of empowerment for practice without actually divesting power from the organization hierarchy to nurses as professionals (Porter-O'Grady, 1991a, 1991b). Clearly, organization and nurse mangers have been reluctant to relinquish power and control over decisions that influence nursing and the organization. Because of nurse dissatisfaction with the practice environment, collective bargaining and collective action has become more of a threat to nurse and hospital administrators (Kerfoot, 1992). The recent success of California nurses in obtaining legislation to specify minimum safe RN staff-to-patient ratios in hospitals is an example (American Nurses Association, 1999; "California Law Requires Staffing Ratios," 1999; Donaldson, 2001). Administrators' decisions to implement shared governance may be based on a selection of the better of two less than desirable choices; shared governance or a less desirable form of collective nurse influence. When collective bargaining or some other collective threat is perceived, wise nurse administrators seek models that integrate the "threat" with structures of shared governance (Crocker et al., 1992).

Too often, nurses have their hopes raised that they are gaining authority and control over the circumstances of their work and their ability to affect patient care priorities only to have those hopes dashed by the whims of those who hold the real power in the organization. Implementation of shared governance simply may be a strategy to gain what management wants without actual gains in decision making authority for nurses. Nurses initially may not recognize that what is portrayed as shared governance does not provide them with authority to control their practice or to enable nursing

and the organization to meet the professional mandate and the organizational goals as partners with management. Nurses soon recognize the lack of power and become frustrated and disillusioned. This is when nurses are apt to leave employment or withdraw to the safety of the traditional hierarchy, where they seek minimal accountability and investment of time, energy, and risk in their jobs. These circumstances underscore the importance of what shared governance entails in terms of nurses' authority and accountability for decision making and how shared governance is best implemented in organizations. Wilson and Porter-O'Grady (1999) write eloquently about the enlightened leadership that is needed to transform an organization for shared governance.

IMPLEMENTATION OF SHARED GOVERNANCE: IS THERE A BEST WAY?

We have noted that shared governance models are not the same in all settings and that this variation is appropriate because of cultural and system operational differences (Porter-O'Grady, 1987; Wilson, 1989). Debate occurs, however, about whether implementation is best orchestrated from the top down or from the bottom up and whether shared governance can be operationalized as separate unit-based as opposed to organization-wide models. Certainly, there is agreement that the nursing and hospital administrations must be supportive of the changes in any case (Jenkins, 1988; Maas, 1989; Porter-O'Grady, 1991a, 1991b; Wilson & Porter-O'Grady, 1999). Less agreement occurs about how to involve the whole staff in the change process and about which is better—unit-by-unit implementation or simultaneous, phased-in implementation of shared governance throughout an entire nursing department (Caramanica & Rosenbecker, 1991; Fagan, 1991; Porter-O'Grady, 1991a, 1991b). Although unique issues must be addressed with each approach, either is appropriate, depending on the situation and assuming that principles of participative change and socialization are not violated. The important point is that professional nurse shared governance is a developmental process and may require as many as 5 years to implement (Hess, 2004; Maas, 1989; Maas & Jacox, 1977; Thompson et al., 2004).

Leadership from nursing administration and from clinical nurses who have a vision regarding nurse shared governance is essential. These nurses must begin to define the objectives and expectations of nurses and create the organizational circumstances whereby all nurses participate to conceptualize and implement shared governance. Planned change, rather than directed change, is necessary (Hersey, Blanchard, & Johnson, 2000). Paradoxically, bureaucratic methods are used at the outset to reinforce expectations about professional practice, participation, and change. Participation, however, of all nurses to gain an understanding of shared governance and new organizational goals, develop new meanings about the nurse's role and work, and acquire new skills and behaviors needed to enact shared governance soon shifts the predominant decision-making methods to collaboration, negotiation, and consensus. Whether implementation of shared governance is top-down throughout the whole organization or bottom-up unit by unit, nursing administrators and managers become consultants, teachers, coaches, and facilitators.

In either approach, nurses must learn the skills of confrontation, negotiation, collaboration, and consensus decision making (Maas, 1989). They also must understand the requirements of professional practice and what it means to be accountable as professionals (Wilson, 1989). Through consensus decision making combined with the expectation of accountability, nurses must develop shared beliefs and values about standards of practice and the structures and processes that will best ensure their enactment (Maas, 1989). Consensus decision making promotes collegiality and the responsible use of collective action by all nurses, regardless of position.

If the unit-based approach to the implementation of shared governance is chosen, one advantage is that more nurses involved in the change likely will be committed to it from the outset. Implementation is more focused and involves fewer nurses. Following success on one or more units, other units are apt to become interested, choose to implement shared governance, and profit from the experience of the pioneering units. Nursing administration and the nurses on the pioneering units will need to be cognizant of the effects of shared governance in one or a few units on the rest of the department and organization. Different patterns and models of communication and decision making necessarily will exist between the nurses on the units with shared governance and nurses on other units, nurse administrators and managers, persons in other departments, and members of other disciplines. Finally, the scope of shared governance implemented on single units will be constrained at the outset because collective authority and accountability cannot include all nurses in the organization. With unit-based shared governance, the collective, central power and influence of nursing is diluted. Nursing administration will need to retain the prerogative for any decisions that affect the nursing department or organization as a whole until all units implement shared governance and the partnership for decision between all nursing professionals and the organization is defined. For this reason, unit-based implementation may be more appealing to some nurse administrators who wish to dilute the collective power of nurses. Because of the limited scope of unit-based shared governance, progress to a full partnership of nurses and the organization may be slow and may never evolve. Shared governance is not implemented fully until there are structures for all professional nurses to make collective department-wide decisions and to negotiate these decisions with administration (Foster, 1992).

With the organization-wide approach, the issues focus on how to involve large numbers of nurses in the change process so that they learn the skills of consensus decision making, participate in decision making, developed shared meanings, and actualize the behaviors of professional autonomy and accountability. If shared governance is implemented throughout an entire system, individual nurses should be deprived of the choice not to participate and not to be accountable professionals. This can present difficult problems because nurses will have different amounts of understanding and commitment to professional practice. Further, the change process necessarily will occur within an environment that is usually not friendly to the investment of nurses' time in pursuits other than the patient care demands of the day. Nurse staffing most often is not planned to allow nurses much time to think and plan as a group. Nurse administrators therefore must expect all nurses, regardless of position, to plan and implement the changes needed for nurses to share governance with the organization and to provide the circumstances whereby nurses are able to meet these expectations. In this regard, nurse administrators must depend on middle and first-line managers to support the change to shared governance and to alter their roles to become facilitators, teachers, and consultants for staff nurses and each other. If middle managers are not committed to shared governance and resist the needed changes, many problems will ensue. The effects of shared governance on middle and first-line managers—as well as on nursing and organization line and staff roles, staff nurse roles, and the roles of members of other disciplines—must be anticipated with plans carefully made to prepare position occupants for the needed changes and skills (Wilson, 1989).

ROLE AND SYSTEM EFFECTS OF SHARED GOVERNANCE

Reports of data about the effects of nurse shared governance models on the attitudes and roles of staff nurses, managers, and administrators and on the structures and processes or organizational systems are increasing (Wilson, 1989). Discussions focus on the effects of shared governance on the attitudes and roles of the nurse manager and staff nurses with a consistent finding that nurse job satisfaction improves as nurse authority and control over practice is realized (Brodbeck, 1992; Brooks et al., 1995; De Baca, Jones, & Tornabeni, 1993; Edwards et al., 1994; George, Burke, & Rodgers, 1997; Hastings & Waltz, 1995; Kovner, Hendrickson, Knickmin, & Finkler, 1993; Lachinger & Havens, 1996; Ludemann & Brown, 1989; Maas & Jacox, 1977; Porter-O'Grady, 1991a, 1991b; Relf, 1995; Song et al., 1997; Thrasher et al., 1992; Westrope, Vaughn, Bott, & Taunton, 1995). An exception is a finding by Prince (1997) that job satisfaction of staff nurses decreased following implementation of unit-based nurse shared governance. Prince notes that the decrease in job satisfaction likely was due to increased time and workload commitments, increased stress, decreased budget, and reorganization and leadership transition. This finding is consistent with the emphasis on the importance of strong, committed, and skilled leadership to shepherd the change to shared governance and to create the organizational circumstances within which the change can best occur (Hastings & Walz, 1995; Havens, 1994; Maas & Jacox, 1977; Wilson & Porter-O'Grady, 1999).

O'May and Buchan's review of the literature (1999) located 48 studies that described or evaluated implementation of shared governance. The studies reviewed confirm Haven's finding (1994) that confusion exists regarding definition of nurse shared governance, making it difficult to know for certain what is being evaluated. O'May and Buchan (1999) selected and reviewed the studies from organization management and business perspectives, including those that described or evaluated participative management, professional practice, and self-managed work team models. Shared governance models also included whole-system governance models that involved all staff in shared governance. Common inadequacies of research evaluating shared governance implementation are no consistent theoretical framework and assumptions, few longitudinal

studies, a lack of rigor in research designs, many different measurement methods, few studies that address system-level analysis in addition to individual analysis, bias toward documenting positive effects, and a lack of complete evaluation of the redistribution of governance (Anthony, 2004; Gavin et al., 1999; Hess, 1996). Thus the failure to delineate models of nurse professional shared governance clearly using criteria based on the sociology of professions and organizations leaves little remaining research that has evaluated the effects on staff, patient, and organization outcomes. What appears to be evaluated most consistently is the effects of participation in decisions on nurse and other staff attitudes.

Agreement exists that management styles must change along with organizational structures to enable professional nurse shared governance (Maas & Jacox, 1977; Wilson & Porter-O'Grady, 1999). As stated before, the role of management becomes one of consulting, teaching, collaborating, and creating an environment with the structures and resources needed for the practice of nursing and shared decision making between nurses and the organization (Stichler, 1992). This new role is foreign to many managers. Nurse managers must become leaders who change who they are, what they do, and how they do it. To achieve nurse shared governance that is accountable to be responsive to clients and organizations that are increasingly complex and fluid, nurse leaders must be an advocate of staff and model learning and changing (Wilson & Porter-O'Grady, 1999).

Although nurse managers will retain responsibility for specified functions, in a professional model they share accountability with all nurses and should act in accord with the consensus among nurse professionals about goals and priorities. Because rules about sharing decisions between management and professional nurses are ambiguous, managers experience stress and anxiety, especially in the early stages of implementing shared governance (Wilson, 1989). Managers also experience role stress because of the added time and costs required to enable consensus decision making among nurses. If not supported by organization and nursing administration, middle and first-line managers—even though they are committed to shared governance—may not choose to expend the effort or take the risks needed to enable nurses to develop the needed consensus. Nurses need to be able to meet together for consensus decision making, and the manager/leader must lead to facilitate their doing so. Administrators who understand the important gains from unleashing the expertise of professional nurses must lead to prepare managers for the new role and support them throughout the lengthy change process of relinquishing control of the decisions for which all professional nurses are accountable. In other words, nurse leaders must redesign their roles to serve the collective of nurse professionals, enabling professional autonomy and accountability for quality outcomes.

For staff nurses, the critical role changes with shared governance are increased accountability and risk. Problems are no longer blamed on others because all nurses share decisions and are accountable for the outcomes. As noted, new understandings and skills are needed. Perhaps most stressful to nurses is the accountability for knowledge to support the decision-making authority of professionals. Role conflict and ambiguity, however, also are stresses. An important example of role conflict with management is when resources are not considered appropriate for quality care (Porter-O'Grady, 1991a, 1991b). Rather than being avoided or ignored as sources of dissatisfaction, shared governance provides the organizational mechanisms for conflict resolution and role clarification through collaboration and consensus decision making.

Staff nurses should be salaried rather than paid an hourly wage, with salaries commensurate with the added accountability and investment required of a participant in shared governance (Johnson, 1987). Further, salaried staff nurses should have more flexible hours and greater control over their time, with accountability shared among nurses for patient care coverage but held as individuals for the care of specific clients throughout an episode of care. Staff nurses often fear being salaried because they believe administration may take advantage of them and make further inordinate demands on their time without adequate compensation. Administrators often resist paying staff nurses set salaries because they fear they will lose control and be unable to hold nurses accountable for an equitable exchange of investment for productivity. Administrators also resist individual nurses being accountable for specific clients throughout an episode of care. Adherence to the principle of accountability for specific clients is abandoned when an alternative appears to have greater short-run benefits for the organization. Yet accountability is the bedrock of professional practice. Shared governance, with staff nurses salaried, provides the means for the most benefits to accrue to all parties—nurses, the organization, and patients—if nurses are afforded the rights and privileges ordinarily enjoyed by salaried professionals and are held accountable for cost-effective practice as individuals and as a collective.

SUMMARY

Because almost all practicing nurses are employed, nurse shared governance in employing organizations is imperative if the profession is to fulfill its social contract (American Nurses Association, 1980, 1995, 2003). Nurse shared governance also is needed for organizations to perform best in the turbulent, managed care environment. The prediction that future provider contracts will be based on demonstrated quality outcomes should cause greater provider organization interest in nurse shared governance. Magnet hospital status, a recognition sought by many hospitals, also cannot be attained unless there is evidence of nursing control of its own professional activities and its influence over the delivery of patient care. We would agree with Porter O'Grady (2004) that it is difficult to understand why the American Nurses Credentialing Center Magnet Recognition Program has failed to identify this as shared governance. Almost all hospitals that have achieved Magnet status have implemented shared governance to enable professional nursing practice (Kramer & Schmalenberg, 2003). These incentives, combined with the current RN shortage, may produce more efforts to implement professional nursing models of practice in organizations. Implementation of shared governance models that enable professional nursing practice is jeopardized, however, when there is lack of clarity about what shared governance is and when shared governance is confused with other organizational innovations that are similar but not the same. Likewise, it is important that the motives of those who lead the implementation of nurse share governance be consistent with professional authority and control over nursing practice so that the profession can meet its commitments to clients in all practice settings. As Hess (1995) noted, nurses and administrators need to agree on the meaning of shared governance and resolve their different views as to what aspects of authority and accountability are most important for nurses. Shared governance requires that nurses are accountable to define and control nursing practice. Nurses also must be accountable to understand what shared governance is, expect that the necessary structures and processes are present if implementation of shared governance is claimed, be discerning about the motives for implementation, and take the risks and develop the knowledge to support the privilege of professional practice. If the aim of all nurses in an organization is to implement structures and processes that enable the profession to define and control practice, unit-based versus organization-wide implementation does not matter. The critical imperative is that mechanisms for collective nurse decision making are developed for the organization as a whole at some point. Nurses committed to professional nursing practice also must be resolved to complete role adaptations and cope with corresponding stresses that accompany change to shared governance, recognizing the benefits of supportive collegial relationships and consensus decisions among nurses in all roles.

Finally, nurses also must be accountable for the outcomes of their interventions with clients. Research exists that links shared governance to improved job satisfaction and social integration of nurses, but less research links shared governance to improved patient outcomes and least cost to organizations (Anthony, 2004). Although efforts to study shared governance are increasing, more systematic evaluation and publication of the results are needed. As with all organizational innovations, strategies and tools must continue to be developed and tested so that nurse administrators and clinicians conveniently and systematically can evaluate the outcomes of shared governance (Herrin, 2004; McCloskey et al., 1994). Foremost among the needed strategies is a standardized definition of the operations that must be observed for nurse shared governance to be implemented (Hess, 1995). These standardized operations must be agreed upon by managers and staff nurses (Hess, 2004). Nursing clinical information systems containing standardized nursing languages that yield large databases for the evaluation of the effectiveness of nursing organization and clinical interventions also are needed. This will require that the professional nurse collective, including nurse administrators and managers, are accountable for the development of electronic information systems. These systems must include standardized nursing data that are retrievable for data repositories that can be used for analysis of nursing intervention effectiveness. The use of effectiveness data to inform practice and policy decisions will empower nursing. Effectiveness data will prevent the adoption of every "new idea" presented as a panacea and potentially interrupt the destructive cycles of nurse abundance and shortage that often accompany or prompt decisions for change that are made without evidence of the impact on nurse, patient, and organization outcomes.

REFERENCES

American Nurses Association. (1980). *Nursing: A social policy statement.* Kansas City, MO: Author.

American Nurses Association. (1992). Standards of nursing practice. Code for nurses with interpretive statement. The nursing shortage in the 1990's: Realities and remedies. In *Best sellers.* Kansas City, MO: Author.

American Nurses Association. (1995). *Nursing: A social policy statement* (2nd ed.). Kansas City, MO: Author.

American Nurses Association. (1999). *Principles for nurse staffing.* Kansas City, MO: Author.

American Nurses Association. (2003). *Nursing's social policy statement* (2nd ed.). Washington, DC: American Nurses Publishing.

Anthony, M. (2004). Shared governance models: The theory, practice, and evidence. *Online Journal of Issues in Nursing, 9*(1). Retrieved February 11, 2005, from www.nursingworld.org/ojin/topic23

Beyea, S., Killen, A., & Berlandi, J. (2002). Lessons about patient safety from Jean Reeder—Patient safety first. *AORN Journal, 76*(2), 318-321.

Brodbeck, K. (1992). Professional practice actualized through an integrated shared governance and quality assurance model. *Journal of Nursing Care Quality, 6*(2), 20-31.

Brooks, S. B., Olsen, P., Rieger-Kligy, S., & Mooney, L. (1995). Peer review: An approach to performance evaluation in a professional practice model. *Critical Care Nursing Quarterly, 18*(3), 36-47.

California law requires staffing ratios. (1999). *American Nurse, 31*(6), 11.

Caramanica, L. (2004). Shared governance: Hartford hospital's experience. *Online Journal of Issues in Nursing, 9*(1). Retrieved February 11, 2005, from www.nursingworld.org/ojin/topic23

Caramanica, L., & Rosenbecker, S. (1991). A pilot unit approach to shared governance. *Nursing Management, 22*(1), 46-48.

Clark, S. (2003). Patient safety series, part 2 of 2: Balancing staffing and safety. *Nurse Management, 34*(6), 44-48.

Crocker, D. G., Kirkpatrick, R. M., & Lentenbrink, L. (1992). Shared governance and collective bargaining: Integration, not confrontation. In T. Porter-O'Grady (Ed.), *Implementing shared governance: Creating a professional organization.* St. Louis, MO: Mosby.

De Baca, V., Jones, K., & Tornabeni, J. (1993). A cost-benefit analysis of shared governance. *Journal of Nursing Administration, 23*(7-8), 50-57.

Donaldson, N. (2001). Nurse staffing in California hospitals: 1998-2000 findings from the California nursing outcomes collalition database. *Policy, Politics and Nursing Practice 2*(1), 9-28.

Edwards, G. B., Farrough, M., Gardner, M., Harrison, D., Sherman, M., & Simpson, S. (1994). Unit-based shared governance CAN work! *Nursing Management, 25*(4), 74-77.

Erickson, J. I., Hamilton, G. A., Jones, D. E., & Ditomassi, M. (2003). The value of collaborative governance/staff empowerment. *Journal of Nursing Administration, 33*(2), 96-104.

Evan, L., Aubry, K., Hawkins, M., Curley, T. A., & Porter-O'Grady, T. (1995). Whole systems shared governance: A model for the integrated health systems. *Journal of Nursing Administration, 25*(5), 18-27.

Fagan, M. J. (1991). Can unit-based shared governance thrive on its own? *Nursing Management, 22*(7), 104L-149L.

Ferguson-Paré, M. L. (1996). Registered nurses' perception of their autonomy and the factors that influence their autonomy in rehabilitation and long-term care settings. *Canadian Journal of Nursing Administration, 9*(2), 95-108.

Foster, B. E. (1992). Shared governance: Design and implementation. In T. Porter-O'Grady (Ed.), *Implementing shared governance: Creating a professional organization*. St. Louis, MO: Mosby.

Gavin, M., Ash, D., Wakefield, S., & Rowe, C. (1999). Shared governance: Time to consider the cons as well as the pros. *Journal of Nursing Management, 7,* 193-200.

George, V. M., Burke, L. J., & Rodgers, B. L. (1997). Research-based planning for change: Assessing nurses' attitudes toward governance and professional practice autonomy after hospital acquisition. *Journal of Nursing Administration, 27*(5), 53-61.

Gulland, A., & Payne, D. (1997). Daisy chain power. *Nursing Times, 93*(34), 14-15.

Hastings, C., & Waltz, C. (1995). Assessing the outcomes of professional practice redesign: Impact on staff nurse perceptions. *Journal of Nursing Administration, 25*(3), 34-42.

Havens, D. S. (1994). Is governance being shared? *Journal of Nursing Administration, 24*(6), 59-64.

Herrin, D. (2004). Shared governance: A nurse executive response. *Online Journal of Issues in Nursing, 9*(1). Retrieved February 11, 2005, from www.nursingworld.org/ojin/topic23

Hersey, P., Blanchard, K., & Johnson, D. E. (2000). *Management of organization behavior: Utilizing human resources* (8th ed.). Englewood Cliffs, NJ: Prentice Hall.

Hess, R. G. (1995). Shared governance: Nursing's 20th-century Tower of Babel. *Journal of Nursing Administration, 25*(5), 14-17.

Hess, R. (1996). Measuring shared governance outcomes. *Nursing Research, 47*(1), 35-42.

Hess, R. (1998). A breed apart: Real shared governance. *Journal of Shared Governance, 4*(3), 5-6.

Hess, R. G. (2004). From bedside to boardroom-nursing shared governance. *Online Journal of Issues in Nursing, 9*(1). Retrieved February 11, 2005, from www.nursingworld.org/ojin/topic23.

Horvath, K. J. (1990). Professional nursing practice model. In G. G. Mayer, M. J. Madden, & E. Lawrenz (Eds.), *Patient care delivery models*. Rockville, MD: Aspen.

Jackson, M., Chiarello, L., Gaynes, R., & Gerberding, J. (2002). Nurse staffing and healthcare associated infections. *Journal of Nursing Administration, 32*(6), 314-322.

Jacoby, J., & Terpste, M. (1990). Collaborative governance: Model for professional autonomy. *Nursing Management, 21*(2), 42-44.

Jenkins, J. E. (1988). A nursing governance and practice model: What are the costs? *Nursing Economics, 6*(6), 302-311.

Jenkins, J. E. (1991). Professional governance: The missing link. *Nursing Management, 22*(8), 26-30.

Johnson, L. M. (1987). Self-governance: Treatment for an unhealthy nursing culture. *Health Progress, 5,* 41-43.

Jones, G. (2004). *Organizational theory, design, and change* (4th ed.). Upper Saddle River, NJ: Pearson, Prentice Hall.

Kanter, R. (1993). *Men and women of the corporation* (2nd ed.). New York: Basic Books.

Kerfoot, K. (1992, March). *Unit-based shared governance: The federation model*. Paper presented at Shared Governance: Sailing Towards Success, San Diego, CA.

Kramer, M., & Schmalenburg, C. E. (2003). Magnet hospital nurses describe control over nursing practice. *Western Journal of Nursing Research, 25*(4), 424-452.

Kovner, C. T., Hendrickson, G., Knickman, J. R., & Finkler, S. A. (1993). Changing the delivery of nursing care: Implementation issues and qualitative findings. *Journal of Nursing Administration, 23*(11), 24-34.

Laschinger, H. K. S., Almost, J., & Tuer-Hodes, D. (2003). Workplace empowerment and Magnet hospital characteristics. *Journal of Nursing Administration, 33*(7/8), 410-422.

Laschinger, H. K. S., & Havens, D. S. (1996). Staff nurse empowerment and perceived control over nursing practice. *Journal of Nursing Administration, 26*(9), 27-35.

Ludemann, R. S., & Brown, C. (1989). Staff perceptions of shared governance. *Nursing Administration Quarterly, 13*(4), 49-56.

Maas, M. (1989). Professional practice for the extended care environment: Learning from one model and its implementation. *Journal of Professional Nursing, 5*(5), 55-76.

Maas, M., & Jacox, A. (1977). *Guidelines for nurse autonomy/patient welfare*. New York: Appleton-Century-Crofts.

Maas, M., Jacox, A., & Specht, J. (1975). Nurse autonomy: Not rhetoric but for real. *American Journal of Nursing, 20,* 2201-2208.

Maas, M., & Specht, J. P. (1990). Nursing professionalization and self-governance: A model for long term care. In G. G. Mayer, M. J. Madden, & E. Lawrenz (Eds.), *Patient care delivery models* (pp. 151-163). Rockville, MD: Aspen.

Maas, M. L., Specht, J., & Ramler, C. (1997). Shared governance models in nursing: What is shared, who governs and who benefits? In J. C. McCloskey & H. K. Grace (Eds.), *Current issues in nursing* (5th ed., pp. 388-396). St. Louis, MO: Mosby.

McCloskey, J. C., & Maas, M. L. (1998). Interdisciplinary teams. *Nursing Outlook, 46,* 157-163.

McCloskey, J. C., Maas, M., Gardner Huber, D., Kasparek, A., Specht, J., Ramler, C., et al. (1994). Nursing management innovations: A need for systematic evaluation. *Nursing Economic$, 12*(1), 35-45.

McDonagh, K. J., Rhodes, B., Sharkey, K., & Goodroe, J. H. (1989). Shared governance at St. Joseph's Hospital of Atlanta: A mature professional practice model. *Nursing Administration Quarterly, 13*(4), 17-28.

Melchior, M. E. W., Van Den Berg, A. A., Halfens, R., Huyer Abu-Saad, H., Philipsen, H., & Gassman, P. (1997).

Burnout and the work environment of nurses in psychiatric long-stay care settings. *Social Psychiatry and Psychiatric Epidemiology, 32*(3), 158-164.

Minzberg, H. (1979). *The structure of organizations.* Englewood Cliffs, NJ: Prentice Hall.

Morrall, P. A. (1997). Professionalism and community psychiatric nursing: A case study of four mental health teams. *Journal of Advanced Nursing, 25,* 1133-1137.

O'May, F., & Buchan, J. (1999). Shared governance: A literature review. *International Journal of Nursing Studies, 36,* 281-300.

Page, A. (Ed.). (2003). *Keeping patients safe: Transforming the work environment of nurses.* Washington, DC: National Academies Press.

Peplau, H. (1985, February). Is nursing self-regulatory power being eroded? *American Journal of Nursing, 85*(2), 141-143.

Perley, M. J., & Raab, A. (1994). Beyond shared governance: Restructuring care delivery for self-managing work teams. *Nursing Administration Quarterly, 19*(1), 12-20.

Pinkerton, S. E. (1988). An overview of shared governance. In S. E. Pinkerton & P. Schroeder (Eds.), *Commitment to excellence: Developing a professional nursing staff.* Rockville, MD: Aspen.

Porter-O'Grady, T. (1987). Shared governance and new organizational models. *Nursing Economic$, 5*(6), 281-286.

Porter-O'Grady, T. (1991a). Shared governance for nursing. Part I: Creating the new organization. *Association of Operating Room Nurses Journal, 52*(2), 694-703.

Porter-O'Grady, T. (1991b). Shared governance for nursing. Part II: Putting the organization into action. *Association of Operating Room Nurses Journal, 53*(3), 694-703.

Porter-O'Grady, T. (1992). Shared governance: Looking toward the future. In T. Porter-O'Grady (Ed.), *Implementing shared governance: Creating a professional organization.* St. Louis, MO: Mosby.

Porter-O'Grady, T. (1994). Whole systems shared governance: Creating the seamless organization. *Nursing Economic$, 12*(4), 187-195.

Porter-O'Grady, T. (2004). Shared governance: Is it a model for nurses to gain control over their practice? *Online Journal of Issues in Nursing, 9*(1). Retrieved February 11, 2005, from www.nursingworld.org/ojin

Prescott, P. (1987). Another round of nurse shortage. *Image: The Journal of Nursing Scholarship, 19*(4), 204-209.

Prince, S. B. (1997). Shared governance: Sharing power and opportunity. *Journal of Nursing Administration, 27*(3), 28-35.

Ramler, C. L. (1995). *Evaluation of the implementation of a professional nurse shared governance model.* Unpublished doctoral dissertation, University of Iowa, College of Nursing, Iowa City.

Relf, M. (1995). Increasing job satisfaction and motivation while reducing nursing turnover through the implementation of shared governance. *Critical Care Nursing, 18*(3), 7-13.

Rose, M., & DiPasquale, B. (1990). The Johns Hopkins professional practice model. In G. G. Mayer, M. J. Madden, & E. Lawrenz (Eds.), *Patient care delivery models* (pp. 85-96). Rockville, MD: Aspen.

Schwartz, R. H. (1990). Nurse decision-making influence: A discrepancy between the nursing and hospital literatures. *Journal of Nursing Administration, 20*(6), 35-39.

Skubak, K. J., Earls, N. H., & Botos, M. J. (1994). Shared governance: Getting it started. *Nursing Management, 25*(5), 80I-J, 80N, 80P.

Song, R., Daly, B. J., Rudy, E. F., Douglas, S., & Dyer, M. A. (1997). Nurses' job satisfaction, absenteeism, and turnover after implementing a special care unit practice model. *Research in Nursing and Health, 20,* 443-452.

Specht, J. (1995). *Shared governance: Development and features.* Unpublished doctoral dissertation, University of Iowa, College of Nursing, Iowa City.

Spitzer-Lehmann, R. (1989). Middle management consolidation. *Nursing Management, 20*(4), 59-62.

Stichler, J. F. (1992). A conceptual basis for shared governance. In T. Porter-O'Grady (Ed.), *Implementing shared governance: Creating a professional organization* (pp. 1-24). St. Louis, MO: Mosby.

Strasen, L. (1989). Redesigning patient care to empower nurses and increase productivity. *Nursing Economic$, 7*(1), 32-35.

Thompson, B., Hateley, P., Molloy, R., Fernandez, S., Madigan, A., Thrower C., et al. (2004). Journey, not an event: Implementation of shared governance in a NHS Trust. *Online Journal of Issues in Nursing, 9*(1). Retrieved February 11, 2005, from www.nursingworld.org/ojin

Thrasher, T., Bossman, V. M., Carroll, S., Cook, B., Cherry, K., Kopras, S. M., et al. (1992). Empowering the clinical nurse through quality assurance in a shared governance setting. *Journal of Nursing Care Quality, 6*(2), 15-19.

Westrope, R. A., Vaughn, L., Bott, M., & Taunton, R. L. (1995). Shared governance: From vision to reality. *Journal of Nursing Administration, 25*(12), 45-54.

Wilson, C. K. (1989). Develop outcomes. *Journal of Nursing Administration, 26,* 14-19.

Wilson, C. K., & Porter-O'Grady, T. (1999). *Leading the revolution in health care* (2nd ed.). Gaithersburg, MD: Aspen.

HEALTH CARE SYSTEMS

System Reform

Opportunity or Threat?

PERLE SLAVIK COWEN ◆ SUE MOORHEAD

In many ways the only consistency in the U.S. health care system over the last several decades has been the constant presence of change. Much of this change has been focused on trying to reduce the costs of health care, a somewhat elusive goal by any measure available. A key focus on cost-containment efforts and the move toward managed care have been the important strategies of the last decade. These strategies have raised questions about every aspect of the system from where care is delivered, to the best provider of care, to the payer, and even to the status of the patient within the system. Length of stay has been reduced dramatically in hospitals during this time frame, leaving some patients and their families questioning whether the system still works for them. These changes are occurring during a time when patients are better educated about health and have an infinite supply of health information from the electronic world at their fingertips. The current situation is creating a good deal of disturbing turmoil, especially after the downsizing of the 1990s in which jobs were lost and the security of the past was shattered. Even nurses question whether the current system can withstand the many changes needed to ensure quality care for patients. Part of the instability in the system is that nursing as a profession is enduring one of its most severe shortages ever, and most experts state that this shortage will last longer and not respond to the usual stopgap measures. Business models have become the preferred model for change, even in nursing. During times of great change, however, people also look for new solutions to focus on the opportunities rather than the threats. The chapters in this section illustrate the roles of nurses in this changing health care environment. Nurses still are trying to create the elusive health care system that is cost-effective, produces quality patient outcomes, and meets the needs of all Americans.

In the debate chapter for this section, Mooney clearly outlines the dilemma nurses face: Should health care change be systematic and incremental, or should change be radical and systemic? Mooney maintains that the debate is less about whether change is needed and more about the pace, shape, and financing of the changes needed in the current system. As the title of this chapter implies, the assumption today is that Americans have a medical care system that works well for some and that they ought to move toward a comprehensive health care system that will work at some basic level for all. This idea is reinforced by the fact that 100,000 individuals lose their health insurance each month in this country—a truly alarming rate—and that many have to choose between food and medications. Mooney maintains that discussions about change in U.S. health care often surface under the heading of reform and tend to be cyclical and to appear about once each generation. Reform can be framed as improvement and at other times as major repair or amendment to the current system. This chapter raises issues such as should the nation continue to focus on technology and drugs or should the nation focus on increasing individual responsibility and developing caring communities? Are economic factors inappropriate solutions to the individual and social uncertainty generated by trauma and disease? Mooney presents both sides of this issue—incremental systematic change versus radical systemic change. For both viewpoints she discusses the responses to the key components of each. The importance of the role of nursing is stressed throughout this chapter and provides a great opportunity to debate the future that nurses envision and would prefer for the health care system.

In the first viewpoint chapter, Walker, Elberson, and Bibb focus on helping nurses better understand how emerging "business coalitions" within and related to the delivery, financing, and shaping of health care affect nurses individually and collectively in local and global markets. They present examples of coalitions in the market and policy arena and discuss possible new coalitions for the improvement of health care through research. They stress that the bottom line orientation of health care requires that nurses continue to be smart about the business side of the delivery system, the purchasing system (as employees), and how coalitions and partnerships are shaping health care for the future. The chapter includes a definition of coalition and the purposes and reasons to build coalitions and serves as a crash course on organizational structures and coalition building. The authors challenge nurses to become active players in shaping the new health care organizations. Four interesting case studies complete the chapter and illustrate the new wave of coalitions. These case studies focus on a coalition developed to address the need for health care reform in the future; an example of a business coalition built for the purpose of purchasing services/benefits and cost savings; a coalition of groups coming together to address quality of life issues and positive experience in death; and an opportunity related to coalition building that highlights issues in the study and measurement of population health management and improving outcomes in the context of patient safety within the military and federal health system. The authors provide excellent content on coalitions that can be used to build nursing partnerships for the future to improve patient care.

In the next viewpoint chapter, Dodd maintains that professional nursing as it is represented by professional nursing organizations with lobbyists in Washington, D.C., has protected the profession over the last few decades but has not done enough to influence the broader health debates that have occurred as a new health care system has evolved. Only on a few occasions has the profession of nursing demonstrated a commitment to a political ideology. Dodd challenges nurses to develop positions related to how nurses think the U.S. health system should work and to choose a political ideology that matches this belief and work as leaders within professional nursing to make this vision possible. This chapter provides a historical and global perspective on this issue.

The corporatization of health care with a focus on mergers and acquisitions is the subject of the next chapter by Beyers. Mergers and acquisitions use business approaches to achieve service goals. Successful mergers and acquisitions create synergy among the existing and acquired organizations. Although each merger or acquisition is unique and unpredictable, influenced by a number of factors, each produces anxiety and requires good communication and change skills. Success is related to the potential for strategic benefit, integration of the organization to create a new whole, and low employee resistance; and it is important to recognize that the human factor can make or break a merger or acquisition. Beyers discusses the impact of mergers and acquisitions on employees, leadership, sponsors and owners, the community, the organization, the economy, and nursing. Information sharing and having a champion for the change are important. Each of the involved organizations has an established pattern of change so that integrating different change patterns together is critical. The chapter provides four approaches to integration. Research results indicate that there were no significant differences in the outcomes related to one of these four approaches to guide leaders through this process. Beyers believes that the movement from a public service to a business model can be to the advantage of nurses if they are prepared to be involved. Beyers urges nurses to continue to serve as the conscience of health care during the merger process. This chapter provides a good overview of what to anticipate during a time of merger or acquisition.

Rufus Howe provides an insightful viewpoint chapter on the issues of a managed care environment on the role of nurse practitioners. The chapter provides an overview of the key factors in a managed care environment and includes a useful list of terms used in managed care systems that nurses need to know. In addition, Howe discusses some of the important aspects of the role of nurse practitioners in managed care environments. According to Howe, managed care organizations are realizing that nurse practitioners play a vital role in helping to provide careful care through cost-efficient strategies. In the future, federal and state legislators need to take several important steps before significant change occurs, but the prevailing wisdom is that the patients themselves will drive this. Health delivery systems are changing at an incredible pace and so are the expectations of the increasingly aged patients. This is a must-read chapter for anyone interested in working as a nurse practitioner in a managed care environment.

One mechanism for care provision in today's managed health care system is the contract, a legal document that specifies services to be delivered and the payment for these services. In this viewpoint chapter, Zazworsky takes the position that nurses must manage contracts and that the ability to contract directly for nursing services and to receive payment for services delivered is essential for the survival of professional nursing practice. In health care, contracting is tied directly to the recognition nurses' receive for their contributions to health care outcomes, control over practice, and decision making in the allocation of scarce resources. This ability to contract directly for nursing care is the difference between nurses' remaining invisible in health care or shaping the future of the health care delivery system. With contracts, providers assume financial risk when they agree to provide services for a specific price. This chapter provides a good explanation of contracts and the factors that contribute to success or failure. The author argues that being able to price nursing services identifies the value of nursing. Nurses are urged to take an active part in negotiating contracts and to develop expertise in the business side of nursing. This is a chapter that all nurses should read.

In the final viewpoint chapter in this section, Rivers and Pinkerton describe the impact of the Magnet Recognition Program on the ability of hospitals to create a competitive edge in the current U.S. hospital system. A resurgence of interest in this program has occurred as the shortage of nurses grows and intensifies. Becoming a Magnet hospital requires deep-rooted culture change in most cases and creates a more professional model of nursing practice. The authors maintain that an important goal of Magnet status is to improve collaboration and communication among nurses and other health care providers. This is an important focus for quality care. In addition, the authors raise some important questions, such as, Is Magnet designation an achievable goal for all hospitals? Should all hospitals pursue Magnet status?

Can hospitals with this status influence the greater health care environment? Will Magnet hospitals lead the transformation in health care? Will Magnet hospitals be the basis for new reimbursement models? The answers to these questions are important to the future directions of the U.S. health care system. This chapter identifies the potential impact of Magnet status on system reform and represents an important mechanism of change for hospitals in this country.

Although the need for health care reform is obvious, the shape of the reform is not yet clear, and nursing needs to be diligent in providing a well-developed vision of the future. Business practices and decision making have become much more dominant but have not solved many of the issues as expected. What is clear is that there is a definite movement from hospital-based and illness treatment care to community-based and health promotion care. Building coalitions among providers and with consumers is a part of this shift in emphasis and will be a component of any health care reform of the future. The changes nurses are seeing are threatening too many players, and politics continues to be a big part of the success or failure of new efforts. Although the future shape of the health care system is unknown, clearly nurses must take an active role in being part of the solution and advocating for care for public good.

From a Medical Care System for a Few to a Comprehensive Health Care System for All

MARY MARGARET MOONEY

Because the strength of our nation is in its people, their good health
is a proper national concern; healthy Americans live more
rewarding, more productive and happier lives.

Dwight D. Eisenhower (cited in Carter, 1958, p. 31)

A lot can be said about health care delivery in the United States, but not much can be said for it. What can be said for a health care environment in which 100,000 persons lose health insurance coverage each month and segments of the population need to choose between food and medicine? What can be said for an organism that nourishes a thicket of rules and regulations and fuels dissatisfaction in patients and providers?

One thing that can be said for health care in the United States is that it possesses the cutting-edge technology and brain power to do wonderful things that preserve and enhance life. If something physiologically terrible is going to happen to me, I would like to have it strike on the doorstep of one of the nation's leading hospitals. In addition, anyone with a thought to change the way health is interpreted and promoted in this country is ill-advised to ignore the economic significance of the health care enterprise. Although talk tends to be about health care costs, revenue and expense are involved. Estimates vary slightly from expert to expert, but the portion of gross domestic product expended on health care consistently hovers around 13%. These dollars do not just disappear. Somebody's boat is being floated.

> The debate is less about whether change is needed and is more about the pace, shape, and financing of the change.

The title of this chapter is based on an assumption that Americans have a medical care system that works well for some and that Americans *ought* to be moving toward a comprehensive health care system that will work at some basic level for all. The assumption seems well-founded given that politicians (red and blue), physicians, nurses, economists, columnists, and heads of health care systems are calling for change. Nevertheless, no unanimity exists about the type of change that is desired.

Voices are raised in favor of massive systemic change. Equally loud are those speaking for systematic, incremental changes. The debate is less about whether change is needed and is more about the pace, shape, and financing of the change. The side of the debate one chooses is influenced not by the facts, which are common to both sides, but by values—social, technical, and economic. Those who favor miniscule or no change also are oriented to their position by values but are not likely to enter the fray unless threatened because they tend to occupy positions of power that currently control the shape and financing of health care and have little to gain by exposure in the public forum.

Discussions about change in U.S. health care often surface under the heading of reform. These discussions are cyclical and over the past century have appeared about once each generation. Lately, however, such discussions seem to swell about every 10 years. At times the reform conversation is framed as improvement and other times as major repair or amendment. Improvement usually implies acceptance of current American health care practice as the "best system in the world," which of course can be made better. Amendment arguments usually imply censure of the current state of health care in America as "mediocre at best and corrupt at worst" and of course must be radically overhauled.

Recent political events seem to indicate that there is no secure middle ground on which to build a bipartisan consensus to address health care concerns. A nationally recognized business leader has said that he does not see anything—systematic or systemic—happening until a major cataclysmic incident occurs. Are Americans then to be left to wring their hands, avert their eyes, and hope that the fates will permit them and their families to avoid needing significant health care services for the foreseeable future?

> Recent political events seem to indicate that there is no secure middle ground on which to build a bipartisan consensus to address health care concerns.

I do not think so. We are nurses. Neither nurses' professional social contract nor their code of ethics permits them to be uninvolved bystanders to the means and ends manifest in the panorama of health. Nurses need not only to add their voices to the chorus of those asking hard questions but also to listen carefully to those with whom they do not agree. That is the glory and the burden of living in a free and pluralistic society.

This chapter poses opposing arguments for change in health care and its delivery. Should health care change be systematic and incremental, or should change be radical and systemic? Should Americans as a nation continue to focus on technology and drugs, or should they focus on increasing individual responsibility and developing caring communities? Should market forces shape health care, or are economic factors inappropriate solutions to the individual and social uncertainty generated by trauma and disease?

A rationale for incremental systematic change and a rationale for radical systemic change are presented. Following each is a response from the opposing viewpoint. An analytical summary completes the debate segment of this unit. The reader is encouraged to seek more in-depth information about the possibilities for change and to ponder the repercussions of the various courses of action on the health of the nation and on the profession of nursing.

INCREMENTAL SYSTEMATIC CHANGE

The medical care system in the United States is very good, and it has come to its current level of excellence through incremental change powered by the push of entrepreneurship and the pull of beneficence. When mistakes are made along the way, they are corrected by consumer pressure. Mismanagement of managed care, for example, has prompted legislation to ensure things such as minimum length of stay for childbirth and mandated emergency care.

Ability to pay is a powerful predictor of the percentage of gross domestic product allocated to health care. The current medical system honors the quintessential American value of individual freedom. Although it is unfortunate that this often makes the social value of health care a function of the recipient's socioeconomic status, this is preferable to government orchestrating health care services. Government ought to do no more than grease the skids of the marketplace to facilitate good business practices that will reward good medical practice.

> The medical care system in the United States is very good, and it has come to its current level of excellence through incremental change powered by the push of entrepreneurship and the pull of beneficence.

Polls repeatedly indicate that most Americans think that the health care delivery system needs to be changed but are happy with their own doctors and care. What are needed are more avenues for access to and methods of payment for medical care. Health (medical) savings accounts offer an attractive way to set aside money for routine health care expenses. According to this part of the plan for incremental change, an individual or family establishing a health savings account also would have an income tax deduction for high-deductible insurance policies giving protection from financial distress in the event of significant sickness or trauma. Budgeting for health care is as important as budgeting for other needs. Control of one's own resources and responsibility for one's own needs will encourage wise, cost-effective health care choices.

Another aspect of most plans for incremental change is medical liability reform. Dollars now consumed by lawyer's fees, awards, and settlements should be kept in the health care system. Medical liability reform will lower overall health care costs by retaining providers in communities and decreasing malpractice insurance rates. The American Medical Association (2005) suggests that patients are losing access to care because physicians in some areas of the country are forced to retire early, relocate, or give up performing high-risk medical procedures. Twenty states are in "full blown medical liability crisis." These states are Arkansas, Connecticut, Florida, Georgia, Illinois, Kentucky, Massachusetts, Mississippi, Missouri, Nevada, New Jersey, New York, North Carolina, Ohio, Oregon, Pennsylvania, Texas, Washington, and West Virginia. In these crisis states patients continue to lose access to care. Creation of association health plans would give working families greater access to affordable health insurance by allowing small businesses to band together through trade groups and negotiate on behalf of their employees. Refundable tax credits for low-income Americans may make health insurance more affordable for the working poor who constitute a large percentage of the uninsured.

Few issues in health care have as much resonance with Americans as does the freedom to choose one's own physician and point of care. Those in favor of incremental change generally emphasize the loss of this freedom that has been part and parcel of substantive changes such as health maintenance organizations, work to reverse such changes, and decry anything that would jeopardize freedom of choice.

> The great health care institutions were not founded because it was felt that the poor had a right to health care.

A precondition of freedom is the recognition of the individual's capacity to make his or her own decisions. In a free, capitalistic society this capacity resides in the corporation as a legal entity and in the individual citizen. Life enhancement advantages of advances in drug therapy and surgical interventions are the result of decades of research and investment of resources by companies energized by the prospect of profit. If the profit motive is removed, a corporation will not be eager to undertake the risk involved in generating new products.

Health care, including disease prevention and health promotion, is one of many commodities in the free market. Advantages exist to empowering individuals to exert greater control over health care products through increased access and concerted efforts to determine relationships between quality and cost. Nevertheless, the nature of a free society is to advance. Society does not stand still, and it demands the same of its citizens. A free society requires and rewards individuals who are keen to better themselves. The ultimate exercise of freedom is the ability to spend one's money the way one wishes.

American society constitutionally is opposed to any redistribution of wealth (tax and transfer system) that would be required to support the tenuous claim that all citizens have a right to basic health care. The great health care institutions were not founded because it was felt that the poor had a right to health care. These institutions were built by philanthropic or religious impulse and did well in serving the needs of the less fortunate until government intervention forced them to compete on the same playing field as for-profit entities catering to those of means.

In summary, incremental systematic change in health care will occur as it has in the past. Medical science and pharmaceutical discovery will advance best as players in a marketplace with minimum regulatory parameters. Americans of means can continue to enjoy the best health care in the world. Certain segments of the population may need to rely on limited governmental supports and supplemental programs provided by the compassionate volunteerism that is part of the American heritage. The system is not perfect, but no alternative is proved to work better *and* sustain the individual freedom and private property rights that American society values so highly.

RESPONSE TO KEY POINTS OF ARGUMENT FOR INCREMENTAL SYSTEMATIC CHANGE

Incremental changes are too little and too late. Tax subsidies and vouchers are attractive, but the proposed subsides are not enough to purchase adequate insurance. Plans that cap employers' premiums are more likely to shift costs to employees than to diminish growth in overall costs. Health (medical) savings accounts work well for the financially well-off, but if one's income is consumed by day-to-day need for food, clothing, and shelter, health savings accounts (or saving accounts of any kind) are the stuff of fairy tales.

Point-of-care places are not free marketplaces. One simply does not shop for a cholecystectomy the way one shops for a new car. A mother is not going to comparison shop for best urgent care prices when her child spikes a dangerous fever at 8 PM. The conditions of the need to "buy" and the ability to "sell" health care violate underlying parameters of a free market. The unfortunate outcomes of the managed care incentives and mandates of the 1990s offer ample evidence that the power of the market does not work in health care.

Expansion of Medicaid means that fees for services will be so low that even more providers will resist caring for Medicaid patients. Something is distinctly unpalatable about a system that pays a pediatrician $20 for seeing the child of a poor person and $50 for seeing the child of the legislator who supports the legislation that provides for the Medicaid payment for the child of the less-advantaged parent. The problems in health care delivery in the United States are systemic. Incremental changes will exacerbate, not solve, the health care dilemma.

RADICAL, SYSTEMIC CHANGE

Budgets are documents though which those responsible for an enterprise reveal their values. The federal budget for years has been a manifestation of legislative and executive schizophrenia as the growing consensus that there is a "right" to health care confronts the "right" to control one's own income and the "right" to be free of intrusive government regulation. At one point, voluntary managed care insurance products were touted as the way to ensure access to adequate services, to control costs, and to move toward covering nearly all citizens while at the same time avoiding bringing to the table universal health care coverage with its aura of socialized medicine and governmental intrusion. Managed care, as it has come to be synonymous with organized underuse, has shifted from promised child to pariah status.

Although not as great as was hoped, managed care is not as bad *in principle* as the lived experience of many would indicate. The Kaiser Permanente plan enjoyed many years of satisfied patients and providers. Nevertheless, without universal health coverage with uniform benefits, managed care cannot avoid stinting on services in the current environment.

> Budgets are documents though which those responsible for an enterprise reveal their values.

A mixed chorus of individuals and groups has sounded a call for universal health care coverage in the United States. The Institute of Medicine, a quixotic presidential candidate, physician groups, labor unions, county and city health officials, newspaper editorial boards, and the chief executive officer of a national health system are some of the unlikely bedfellows in this chorus. Supporters of universal health care coverage have come to their positions by routes moral and by routes practical.

In addition to increasing solidarity in the belief that all citizens must have access to comprehensive health care, a growing sense is that Americans already are paying as much as universal coverage would cost through pouring a big chunk of every health care dollar into executive salaries and stock options, into drug advertising, and into lobbying by groups that profit from the health care status quo. Furthermore, universal health care coverage is essential to finishing the job of welfare reform.

> A mixed chorus of individuals and groups has sounded a call for universal health care coverage in the United States.

It will cost more to provide comprehensive health care to all citizens—but not that much more. Today almost half of all Americans receive their health insurance from a U.S. government program or have no insurance at all. The other half has, for the most part, insurance through an employer. Various plans that have been proposed differ in total dollars and in rates of increase, but all are within the fiscal ability of the richest nation in the world. Increased direct health care costs will be offset by an increase in individual productivity, the resultant increased competitiveness of American business in the global marketplace, and the recovery of dollars spent on advertising and the paperwork required to support the current bureaucratic system.

The wealthy would pay more in taxes to support the system, but the increase in taxes paid by the non-wealthy would be offset by the elimination of insurance premiums and out-of-pocket expenses. Science and compassion would determine clinical decisions, not insurance status or a voice emanating from the approval department of a faceless corporation.

Several plans for radical systemic change have been proposed. Some are outlines of privately delivered, publicly financed, single-payer systems. Others are less radical and proffer a mix of payers and a mix of public and private financing, so-called play-or-pay schemes. The ideas presented by a group of nursing faculty and the ideas presented by a pair of investigative reporters are two examples of different views on systemic change.

Faculty of the Columbia School of Nursing recently outlined a plan for affordable essential health care that attempts to find a balance between low cost sharing, which often is accompanied by misuse of therapy, and high cost sharing, which often is accompanied by delay of care critical to long-term health and fiscal benefit (Mundinger, Edwidge, Thomas, Smolowitz, & Honig, 2004).

Key elements for success of the Columbia plan include the following:

- Evidence-based clinical decisions
- Mandatory coverage (similar to car insurance protocols)
- Provision of all benefits in the care network
- Privately administered
- A percentage copay/coinsurance for service with an annual cap
- Minimal flat fee for preventive care visits
- Expensive procedures such as transplant would not be covered
- Vision and hearing screening would not be covered
- Cosmetic surgery, podiatry, and alternative therapy would not be covered

Bartlett and Steele (2004) are proponents of universal coverage and of a single-payer mechanism reimbursement for services. They point to the relative efficiency of Medicare as contrasted to the bureaucracy of the private market as support for the single-payer concept. Studies have found the Medicare overhead to be about 10% to 18% less than that of private carriers, notwithstanding that in the current system, Medicare payments usually are administered by private insurance companies with which the government contracts for this service. Similar to the Columbia system, the system envisioned by Bartlett and Steele would be as concerned with preventing disease and trauma as with treating illness and injury. To collect the fees and disburse the payments, a health care council patterned on the Federal Reserve System would be created. Revenue to support the program would come from taxes: a gross receipts levy on businesses and a flat tax on *all* individual income.

In summary, the richest nation in the world can provide for the basic health care needs of all its citizens. The cost-benefit ratio is favorable not only in human terms but also in financial terms. Radical change does not require selection of the most radical of suggested solutions. Single-payer does not imply single plan, nor does universal coverage imply single payer. Dominant social preferences must be respected insofar as they do not sabotage the goal of health care access and affordability for all.

RESPONSE TO KEY POINTS OF ARGUMENT FOR RADICAL SYSTEMIC CHANGE

The debacle of the managed care plans of the 1990s provides sufficient evidence that government financing of medical expenses results in deterioration in the quality of care for everyone—including the aged and the poor.

Nevertheless, the strongest case against radical systemic change is a social-cultural one. A mandated approach is unpalatable to the citizenry because it violates their fundamental value of individual freedom. Nobody has a right to medical care. If a person cannot pay for what he or she needs, that person must depend on voluntary charity. The premise that one gains a moral claim to a good not by earning it but simply by needing it is erroneous.

The argument that universal health coverage will create a fair environment is only partly correct. Universal health coverage will not be fair (and fairness is one of the key elements of an acceptable universal system). Rich persons still will be able to get what they want when they want it. The rest of the population will be treated fairly in that they *all* will have to wait (note the experience in other countries) for the services they want. Furthermore, the distribution of benefits will not coincide with the distribution of costs.

The consensus is that a problem exists in health care. But twenty-first century research models and projections for fixing the problem bear a striking resemblance to those that were found wanting and were rejected in the 1970s and the 1990s. Current problems are due to governmental interference. A solution will not be found in more governmental control. For change to be effective, it must be sustainable. The difficulties being experienced by Social Security and by Medicare demonstrate the inherent difficulty of relying on taxation as a means of financial support for a service.

Universal coverage will not encourage healthful lifestyles. Healthful choices in nutrition, exercise, and recreational practices are not influenced by whether one is eligible for an annual checkup, immunizations, or care for minor and major illnesses. Such choices are the result of character and ultimate goals. Universal coverage will not control costs. Patients will seek more services, and physicians still will provide unnecessary services. The country is too diverse to expect that one health care plan can be satisfactory for all citizens. Racial, ethnic, and geographic barriers to care still will exist.

SUMMARY

Americans, rich and poor, are beginning to feel insecure about their health care coverage. They want something done. This insecurity and the concern that the illness or injury of one member of a family can spell financial doom for the entire family has revived the conversation about change in health care delivery at the micro and macro levels. Americans are not likely to frame this discussion about what should be done as "rationing by class" versus "distributive compassion." Far more likely is that Americans will talk about "market competition" versus "government regulation." Whatever terminology Americans decide to use, these are the questions that must be answered:

◆ Do we want to embrace as policy the de facto practice of endorsing a multitier health system in which a person's health care experience is determined by his or her ability to pay for it?

◆ Do we want to persuade (or force) the upper socioeconomic class of the nation's families to help buy health insurance for the lower socioeconomic class of the nation's families?

> Political feasibility and financial sustainability are essential elements of any change that will have the vigor necessary to weather the test of time.

Although posed as questions to which "yes" or "no" would be an appropriate grammatical response, Americans know the answer is not that simple, not that clear, and not that unambiguous.

Obviously, in the incremental/radical conversation there are few islands of agreement in a surging ocean of points of debate. It appears, however, that both those who favor incremental change and those who favor radical change agree on the following:

◆ Health care spending should be based on appropriate and efficient use of resources.

◆ Continuous improvement of health care services should be promoted.

◆ Patients and their families should have effective participation in decision making.

Perhaps if discussions proceed from these islands of agreement, Americans can navigate the waves of disagreement more safely.

Whichever side of the debate one's philosophical stance favors, a pragmatic approach will be required. Political feasibility and financial sustainability are essential elements of any change that will have the vigor to weather the test of time. Nurses tend to want *the* best scenario, and in individual patient care that scenario is an admirable and necessary goal. In the public policy arena the best *possible* scenario is not usually anyone's individual choice for best scenario. Do Americans lack resources, or do Americans lack the will to use resources differently?

What is the best Americans can do in this county, in this time, to have the best possible health care?

> What nurses may lack as a group is the confidence that they do have something to add to the conversation and that they can affect the outcome of the debate.

Nurses know that effectiveness depends on good clinically managed care, not on hard bargains. Yet how often under the rubric of "effectiveness" are nurses forced to abort clinical decision making because of a hard bargain struck far from the bedside?

By numbers alone, nurses can be a formidable force for change. The pressure required for change is building. Nurses can increase and focus that pressure through thoughtful consideration of what is best for their patients and through participation in their professional organizations. Nurses need to examine their assumptions, their expectations, and their way of doing business so that they expand rather than limit the capacity for change.

By health care expertise nurses have much to add to the debate. Change will not occur until there is a clear, shared vision by a critical mass of citizens. A good idea is no good if the time is not right. Nurses have the moral capital to clarify for the larger public the good, the bad, and the ugly of incremental and radical proposals for change. What nurses may lack as a group is the confidence that they do have something to add to the conversation and that they can affect the outcome of the debate. This confidence is essential for taking an active role in identifying the steps that will be needed to bring about any selected change.

REFERENCES

American Medical Association. (2005). *America's medical liability crisis: A national view.* Retrieved March 13, 2005, from http://www.ama-assn.org/noindex/category/11871.html

Bartlett, D., & Steele, J. (2004). *Critical condition.* New York: Doubleday.

Carter, R. (1958). *The doctor business.* New York: Doubleday & Company.

Mundinger, M., Edwidge, T., Smolowitz, J, & Honig, J. (2004). Essential health care: Affordable for all? *Nursing Economics, 22*(5), 239-244.

Business Coalitions

Defining, Purchasing, and Providing Health Care

PATRICIA HINTON WALKER ◆ KAREN L. ELBERSON ◆ SANDRA C. GARMON BIBB

The U.S. health care industry continues to experience rapid and significant change. Governmental intervention and consolidation throughout the health care system continue to include mergers, alliances, and acquisitions between provider groups (such as hospitals, health maintenance organizations, and preferred provider organizations), insurance carriers, suppliers, distributors, and other related industries. The big have become bigger, and the increase in alliances is growing at all levels of the value chain (Speckman & Isabella, 2000). Managed care is still alive and well in the United States. Many other countries around the globe are managing care in an attempt to achieve the best health outcomes. The international focus (on prevention, primary care, and the health of the public) in many cases has better health statistics than those of the United States, the focus of which is on illness and disease. Balancing cost and quality is still a significant challenge nationally and globally. For consumers and providers, managed care in the United States continues to conjure up negative responses. However, the National Coalition on Health Care, one of the new coalition examples cited in this chapter, is addressing the need for health care reform and calls for changes in the current managed care approaches. Managing care for the improvement of population-based outcomes is here to stay, but the focus should be shifted to include health promotion and prevention, not just disease management. Patient safety issues are also at the front of the current health care delivery agenda, and these issues are here to stay as well. Consequently, nurses need not only to develop and improve business knowledge and literacy in order to be successful but also to learn to define many of the historical issues of nursing in the context of patient safety.

Managed care is still a term used to describe various coalitions, alliances, partnerships, and mergers with the goals of increasing market presence, managing provider practices, and improving patient flow. These organizations still are described as health maintenance organizations, such as Kaiser Permanente; as integrated delivery system that attempts to link hospitals, home health care agencies, and group primary care practices; or as some form of preferred provider organization. Regardless of the particular model or approach, there are generally at least four common goals of any type of managed care organization:

1. To control costs, usually by controlling use of services
2. To use sound business approaches to ensure efficiency, resulting in significant reductions in the health care labor force through work redesign
3. To ensure quality through the measurement of outcomes (clinical indicators, customer satisfaction, and cost)
4. To do all of the foregoing by trying to form coalitions, alliances, or partnerships that will manage care across the wellness-illness continuum for a specified dollar amount (usually negotiated up front in a managed care contract)

Unfortunately, as competition has raged in markets experiencing high managed care penetration, the bottom line is driving many decisions even more than in past years. This has continued to affect negatively the workplace environment, recruitment and retention of nursing staff, and the satisfaction of consumers. However, with patient safety surfacing and receiving the attention of the Institute of Medicine (through reports *To Err Is Human* and *Crossing the Quality Chasm*), issues related to fatigue, staffing, and other workplace problems are the topic of much of the emerging health services research in this new area.

Emerging areas where business coalitions are flourishing and making a difference include development of groups and coalitions to conduct research, particularly health services research; coalitions addressing the need for health care reform; coalitions addressing licensure and mobility of nurses across state lines for practice (Nursing Compact); employer coalitions trying to purchase cost-effective health care; and coalitions for care focused on special issues or populations. As mentioned previously, because of the need to study population health and improve outcomes, to address health disparities, and to improve patient safety, researchers and organizations are participating in partnerships and coalitions in order to address these emerging concerns for the U.S. health care delivery system. Because of the rising costs of health care, health care benefits, and pharmaceuticals, other coalitions and business partnerships are emerging to try to address the future of health care. The National Coalition on Health Care was initiated to address the health care crisis in this country and to describe ways in which the health care system should be reformed.

The challenge of delivering safe, effective, and efficient health care continues to have significant implications for the nursing profession in practice, education, research, and administration. Recent coalition development will have a growing impact on nurses and their families: as consumers of health care, as practitioners in health care systems across the continuum of care, and as employees in the health care delivery system. Emerging concerns related to the high cost of care in the United States; the perceived, critical need for reform in the delivery system of care and the workplace environment; and the crisis presented by the growing shortage of health care workers such as nurses just compound the problem.

This chapter is designed to assist nurses to understand better how these emerging business coalitions within and related to the delivery, financing, and shaping of health care for the coming years affect nurses individually and collectively. We hope that this chapter provides incentives for nurses to be involved in the shaping of the health care system, should reforms suggested by the National Coalition on Health Care be taken seriously. We believe that nurses as providers not only must accept increased responsibility for the delivery of safe and effective care but also must be at the table in increasing numbers as researchers and consumers of research data related to the workplace environment. This chapter presents examples of coalitions in the market and policy arena that are emerging and have an impact on nurses and other health care providers. Additionally, considerations of the expansion and development of new coalitions for the improvement of health care through research will be discussed. We do not have to tell nurses about how the current and impending nursing shortage has unbelievable implications for the patient safety research agenda. Changes in health care delivery continue to provide nurses with the opportunity to affect aspects of care that nurses have valued throughout history: coordinating care across the continuum, attention to prevention of disease and health promotion, attention to the role of the family and community, and empowering the voices of the patients (now clients/consumers/customers) in their own care. The bottom line orientation of health care requires that nurses continue to be smart about the business side of the delivery system, the purchasing system (as employees), and how coalitions and partnerships are shaping health care for the future.

CONTEXT FOR COALITIONS

When health care costs rose significantly in the 1980s, one of the ways that businesses and employers tried to control costs was through the development of coalitions (Rooney, 1992). Usually these coalitions were an attempt to contain costs on a community-wide basis and to control cost shifting from employer to employer. Although this approach met with marginal success, many forms of coalitions continue to grow as one attempt to address some of the problems in the health care delivery system today. These forms of alliances and mergers include entities such as provider groups, hospitals, and buyer-supplier relationships and politically motivated groups addressing many of the financial, ethical, and other related health care issues. New forms of alliances are developing to achieve the outsourcing of nonessential services, which brings unlikely businesses to the health care table; corporate-education contracts to ensure a competent current and future workforce; and technology access (Speckman & Isabella, 2000).

What is a coalition? How does a coalition differ from alliances, partnerships, mergers, and networks? How have technological advances and the advances in access and use of the Internet in health care changed and enhanced the nature of coalitions? What do nurses need to know about emerging new coalitions? And finally, how will this affect nursing, research, and administration? The literature contains many references to coalitions but uses different terms to label them. A thesaurus lists *alliance, network, partnership, affiliation,* and *consortium* in connection with the use of the word *coalition*. *Merriam-Webster's Collegiate Dictionary* (1994) specifically defines a coalition as "a temporary alliance of distinct parties, persons, or states for joint action." Partnership refers to a legal relationship usually involving close cooperation between parties with specified and joint rights and responsibilities; an alliance is an association that furthers common interests of members; and a consortium means an agreement, combination, or group formed to undertake an enterprise beyond the resources of any one member. For the purposes of this chapter, these terms will be used interchangeably, depending on the particular reference.

Is a coalition an organization? How does one study coalitions, learn to work within them, and manage them in the same way as traditional organizations? Can nurses better understand how to work in this newest evolution of organizational change in response to rapid changes in the delivery of health care and in the buying-up, loose-knit, changing organizational relationships in health care? The answers are yes, and it is even more important that nurses and other providers understand what is happening in the evolution of coalition building, particularly in the context of the rapid reshaping of health care. Classic management approaches still apply to the discussion of studying and exploring ways of dealing with emerging coalitions. Tichy (1983) indicates that nurses must understand organizational models to understand how organizations change. He describes a model as a set of assumptions or beliefs that guide managerial action, assist in diagnosing organizational problems, and focus the individuals that work in the organization.

Tichy (1983) described three models—classic or mechanistic, human resource organic, and political—that will sound familiar to most individuals who are experiencing the organizational challenges of emerging new structures for the delivery of care. First, the classic or mechanistic model focuses on structure, span of control, and specialized task functions. This model is similar to a typical bureaucratic organization with detailed job descriptions and a rigid chain of command, where decisions are made along vertical lines with minimum flexibility. Some of the government organizations still are organized in this way. The human resources organic model is more focused on the human perspective, where the model is shared decision making, with lots of interaction vertically and laterally in the organization. Supervisors are usually motivators and facilitators who communicate through expectations rather than strict orders and tasks. Traditional academic organizations and those focused on innovation are more likely to be structured in this way. Each of these two approaches clearly has strengths and weaknesses. The political model is the third approach and can be viewed as an arena in which multiple coalitions vie for control of the organization through ongoing processes of bargaining and negotiation. One best studies this model from the perspective of understanding internal (usually full-time

employees) and external coalitions (partners, alliance members, networked groups) that make up the larger organization (Mintzberg, 1977).

Nurses and other providers need to understand and learn how to influence these types of organizations in which change strategies are based on making political adjustments, understanding where the greatest power and influence is held, and mastering the skills of negotiation, bargaining, and coalition building (Tichy, 1983). The political model, which may be a bit more foreign to providers such as nurses who "just want to provide care," is developing rapidly in the health care field in response to competition for consumers' dollars and market share because it is the most flexible, adaptive, and responsive model. Two weaknesses must be noted in this evolving model, however; sometimes attention to detail and organizational cultural issues are difficult to resolve between different cultures in the different organizations in a coalition (p. 49). Consequently attention to the structure, processes, and outcomes of quality care (production) and the merging of different organizational cultures or values continue to create adjustment problems for providers experiencing the change of emerging coalitions and partnerships in the changing health care delivery structures.

PURPOSES AND REASONS FOR COALITION DEVELOPMENT

Why is the political model or the development of coalitions, alliances, and partnerships continuing to dominate the health care organizational structures at this time? Why do nurses even need to understand this new phenomenon? Again, nurses should look to the business literature for the answers, because if they understand the nature of the organizational change in which they are participating (by choice, chance, or requirement), they can position nursing as a profession and themselves as professionals.

The evolution of alliances, coalitions, mergers, and partnerships is an increasingly global phenomenon. Many companies in a variety of industries are choosing alliances, coalitions, and partnerships as vehicles for change in a tight market economy, and this phenomenon is occurring on a worldwide basis. Competition and rapid positioning continues to be the name of the game, particularly with the rapid expansion of technology and the use of technology to answer some of the patient safety challenges in health care today. Additionally, for the health care consumer and provider, Internet access is changing practice and the business of health care.

Administrators, who are nurses, need to improve their knowledge about business practices, coalition development, and use of technology in order to lead and manage other nurses and interdisciplinary providers in today's organizations. Hamel and Prahalad (1994), in their book *Competing for the Future,* write that "competition for the future is competition to create and dominate emerging opportunities—to stake out new competitive space" (p. 22). Further, the authors say, organizations not only must compete within the boundaries of existing industries (such as hospitals, home health, and insurance industries) but also must shape the structure of industries so that they will be able to compete and dominate the market in the future. This means that "competition will take place within and between coalitions of companies, and not only between individual businesses" (p. 23).

Why is it so important to understand these business trends anyway? Clearly, those nurses and other clinical professionals need to abandon old ways and assist their organization to remain competitive and survive in a changing workforce. New competencies are needed. Meister (1998), in her book *Corporate Universities,* identifies competencies that Fortune 500 companies now are expecting of employees. These include leadership development, collaboration and communication skills, technological literacy, business literacy, learning to learn skills competency, and self-management of one's own career. Because competition is so high at this time in health care, no one organizational structure has evolved to be the solution. Nurses need to understand that many companies are trying to "shape the structures" for managed care through development of different kinds of alliances and coalitions. Subsequently, nurses and other providers then can position themselves to have more influence on quality of care and consumer satisfaction, two of the historic strengths of nursing. Regardless of the type of structure, it is important for nurses to be active players, not only helping to shape future organizations/coalitions but also to contribute meaningfully to innovative ways of getting things accomplished.

One key to assisting health care organizations in developing successful coalitions and alliances is to understand the reasons for coalition development and the process of building coalitions. Coalitions develop for several reasons but most obvious is the reason that no one organization has all the required resources, skills, knowledge, and expertise to produce the product. In health care the product is to provide cost-effective,

quality care across the continuum. A second reason that coalitions are formed is for political advantage. In some cases a coalition is a good way to co-opt potential future competitors or, through partnering, to prevent resources from getting in the hands of a competitor. A political coalition also may provide access to new markets. A third reason for coalition development is to share risks and costs. "Alliances allow participation in high volatile industries, where knowledge spreads rapidly, at substantially lower investment and risk than would be the case for a single organization" (Zuckerman, Kaluzny, & Ricketts, 1995, p. 3).

Because many business coalitions are formed not only for political reasons but also to acquire resources, skills, and knowledge, they may seem to be linkages without logic. Current coalitions that have formed to enhance benefits and provide cost-effective group purchasing are two types of organizations that are dominant in the market place more recently. Coalition building, however, follows no distinctive pattern. According to Bell and Shea (1998), partnerships rapidly are becoming the primary structure of contemporary business as organizations partner with vendors, unions, customers, and even competitors to take advantage of market opportunities, leverage intellectual capital, and create more innovative enterprises.

The literature has evolved from a focus on describing coalitions, alliances, and partnerships to exploration of how to make them last. More alliances fail than succeed today, and this is evident to those who watch their employers change names, ownership, and partnerships frequently. Bell and Shea (1998) liken these evolving partnerships to the level of difficulty of a dance: the highest (most difficult) level of partnership is the tango (with different partners who must move carefully and totally together); the waltz (tamed and simplified interaction); the square dance (with strict rules and protocols but little emotional intensity or closeness—and actions called by outside forces); the twist (moving separately, but somewhat connected); and finally the line dance (partners are completely independent but moving in the same direction without entanglement). Bell and Shea focus on selection of the right partner, the building of trust, evolution of the relationship, and learning from mistakes to improve the dance over time. It would behoove many nurses in health care and education to examine the nature of the partnership and the type of dance in order to prevent unrealistic expectations in the development and growth of the alliances and partnerships they experience in their work settings.

TYPES AND FORMATION OF COALITIONS IN HEALTH CARE

Generally, health care coalitions (as mentioned previously, sometimes referred to as alliances or cooperatives) frequently are established by groups that wish to use collective strength to accomplish that which cannot be accomplished alone. Through the enhancement of bargaining strength, while containing cost and quality through enhanced bargaining strength, and increased competition among insurance plans and medical service providers, health care coalitions share information on the cost and performance of providers and on the terms of contracts. Coalition design varies considerably. Many coalitions tend to be self-governing and organized as not-for-profit membership organizations. Generally, coalitions assess each member group minimal fees to cover operating costs. Only a few have hired staff. The remainder use volunteer management committees made up of representatives from each fund. Some use volunteers to manage through committee, and only a few have managers or employed staff.

Roles of coalitions vary. Some only collect information on clinical quality or sponsor member satisfaction surveys. One example is a coalition of purchasers that uses its collective power to buy the best benefits at the lowest price. Other coalitions may be built through the efforts of multiple employers, single employers, and public or private health plans. Again, economics is the driving force behind these types of coalitions. In the case of health plans, administrative efficiencies and sometimes price discounts can be presented by provider groups to larger purchasers in exchange for increased patient volume. Coalitions of this type can purchase health care services for less money than individual funds could on their own and, at the same time, maximize employee choice (American Federation of State, County, and Municipal Employees, n.d.).

However, many coalitions are formed by employers' groups, but generally speaking, union involvement is limited. Some characteristics include variation in size and geographic coverage, tendency to be self-governing, usually a not-for-profit organization, and usually an assessment of each member group for minimal fees to cover operating costs. The structure of coalitions may vary from "loosely organized," which maximizes autonomy, to "tightly organized" structures that may limit independent activities. For example, in a loosely organized coalition information may be provided on price and quality of health care plans, or endorsement of certain providers with availability of reduced fees or other cost control issues. Individual coalition members have the autonomy to develop independent contracts and negotiate different benefits. Tightly organized coalitions tend to pool their resources and pool their risks in order to contract directly with provider or insurance groups for all of the members of the coalition. The tightly organized coalition would be considered the least flexible but may be the most cost-effective because it offers a common delivery of benefits or services. The bargaining power of individual funds provides an efficient method of purchase through economies of scale and reduction of administrative costs with maximum choices for coalition members (American Federation of State, County, and Municipal Employees, n.d.).

Kaluzny et al. (in Zuckerman et al., 1995) define coalitions and alliances in different language: two general types of coalition—lateral and integrative. As mentioned, similar types of organizations come together to achieve economies of scale by pooling resources, sharing information and human resources, group purchasing, and increasing collective power. When this occurs, a lateral alliance or coalition is formed. Examples of this include hospitals merging or networking together based on type of service, geographic distribution, or religious preferences. Rural hospital networks or consortiums and community hospital partnerships are two specific examples. However, the integrative type is more related to market, strategic positioning, and competitive advantage. Kanter (1989) uses the term *stakeholder alliance* to describe linkages among buyers, suppliers, and customers. This type of alliance usually calls its members stakeholders. In these coalitions, vertical and horizontal integration are evident and include clinical, administrative, financial, educational, and delivery components of the organization.

EXAMPLES OF COALITIONS SERVING A VARIETY OF HEALTH CARE–RELATED FUNCTIONS

We have chosen to highlight four examples of a new wave of coalitions or partnerships in this chapter. These four examples highlight important issues for nursing: a coalition developed to address the need for health care reform in the future; an example of a business coalition built for the purpose of purchasing services/benefits and cost savings; and a coalition of groups on common interest coming together to address quality of life issues and positive experience in death. Finally, an opportunity related to coalition building highlights issues in the study and measurement of population health management and improving outcomes in the context of patient safety within the military and federal health systems. This will be described as an outcome of research conducted by faculty and students in the Graduate School of Nursing at the Uniformed Services University of the Health Sciences in Bethesda, Maryland. These business relationship (coalition) examples also demonstrate the types of dances described by Bell and Shea (1998) in their book *Dance Lessons*.

Example 1: Compassionate Care to Improve Quality of Life

The California Coalition for Compassionate Care (n.d.) is a statewide coalition or alliance of 50 or more regional and statewide organizations that are dedicated to "the advancement of palliative medicine and end-of-life care." The mission statement of this coalition emphasizes the value and promotion of high-quality and compassionate end-of-life care. The focus of the efforts involves the encouragement of increasing advance care planning and palliative services, leadership for the development of these areas of practice, and political involvement attempting to influence systemwide change. The coalition is governed by a steering committee (made up of a member of each of the organizations belonging to the coalition). The roles and functions of the steering committee are periodically to meet and discuss work group accomplishments, new initiatives, and future governance issues. An executive committee manages the coalition and is responsible and accountable for the financial, contractual, and reporting obligations. The work/tasks actually are accomplished and implemented through work groups (supplied from membership within the organizations that belong to the coalition), and these groups have a defined relationship to members of the steering committee. An executive director provides strategic leadership direction and development, along with the programmatic and fiscal responsibilities. Examples of member organizations include organizations serving aging communities, end-of-life groups, the American Cancer Society, religious groups concerned with end-of-life care, home health organizations, hospice and palliative care organizations, home health groups, pharmaceutical groups, and children's service groups concerned about these same issues.

This coalition initially was supported by funds from the Robert Wood Johnson Foundation and subsequently has been supported primarily through the Archstone Foundation. The mission of the Archstone Foundation is to assist society in meeting needs of aging populations. This foundation uses its resources to help all generations plan for the aging process with a focus on healthful aging and independence, and it addresses quality of life and end-of-life issues.

This partnership may be most representative of the square dance described by Bell and Shea (1998) because of the "calls" of outside forces—particularly economic forces and limitations imposed by regulations and financing related to each of the groups/organizations within the coalition. This particular coalition is made up of many different styles and types of partners who are dancing together but somehow in concert through the use of their work groups that work with a steering committee member chairing different work/task dance groups. In square dancing, different groups are dressed differently but belong to that "square" in the dance. Protocols, procedures, and imposed structures and moves are required to manage the different dimensions of this arrangement. The agreements in some cases have been made based on trust that has developed over time. Other partnerships, however, may be based on some economic and political connections that facilitate and support common interests.

Example 2: Business Coalitions Market Overview

As mentioned before, varying forms of business and health care coalitions and alliances have been formed in recent years to purchase health care, pharmacy, and other benefits collectively to reduce costs and increase accessibility to services and products for customers and employees. A key question is how these coalitions obtain the information and data needed to make wise, cost-effective decisions. Business Coalitions Market Overview is essentially a coalition serving coalitions. This market overview coalition provides information, trends affecting the market, and profiles of more than 50 of the leading health care coalitions in the country. Categories of coalitions include food and beverage industry, finance, and health care. Within the health care industry, one can search information regarding market overviews related to biotechnology, medical, and pharmaceutical coalitions. Through the Business Coalitions Market Overview, provider and employer coalitions (for example) can benchmark their services, benefits with other coalitions to ensure market sensitivity, and cost-effectiveness in an every changing market (National Coalition on Health Care, 2005).

This new model for coalitions or alliances and innovative partnerships also is intended to facilitate distribution of information, research, and guidelines for improved, safe, quality care. Nurses and other health care providers need to know of groups such as the Business Coalitions Market Overview to be informed as employees, as providers, and as consumers of health care. According to Bell and Shea (1998), this model would best be described at this time as the twist. Each member of the coalition or alliance is independent and enters the dance based on its own interest and its own "form of dance." All partners have many options, and as long as the options benefit the partnership, these entities will work together in loose-knit ways.

Example 3: The National Coalition on Health Care

A national discussion has been taking place related to the need for health care reform since the great debate(s) in 1993-1994 when a variety of proposals failed to pass legislation. Although this nationwide debate has subsided, at least one coalition, the National Coalition on Health Care, the nation's broadest and largest alliance, has conducted a year of study not only to address the need for change but also to describe some of the specifications for badly needed reform of the U.S. health care delivery system. This coalition is made up of at least 100 organizations such as groups representing patients, consumers, unions, businesses, religious groups, pension and health funds, and health care providers. The coalition was developed purposefully as a nonpartisan organization that was designed truly to represent a cross section of more than 150 million American employees, members, consumers, providers, and congregants (National Coalition on Health Care, 2004).

The U.S. health care system suffers from three large problems: rising costs; a significant, growing number of Americans without health insurance; and substandard care (Business coalitions market overview, 2005). This recent business coalition report examines in detail each of these problem areas, highlighting that despite the significant, escalating costs, the availability, accessibility, quality, and delivery of care is not meeting the needs of the American people. Among their recommendations are (1) that health care reform must be a national priority and is long overdue; (2) that the reform must be systematic and interconnected, not just a list of stand-alone initiatives; (3) and that the reform cannot continue a system for haves and have-nots but must be system-wide, including all payers, patients, and providers. This report makes the case not only for the cost-effectiveness of health care reform but also for the savings to provider groups, employer groups, and the federal government of instituting a health care reform agenda, indicating that the cost of a reformed system would be must less expensive than a reformed system, "saving over 125 billion annually."

The reforms discussed in this report promote four specifics for a future system (Business coalitions market overview, 2005):

> 1) an employer mandate, supplemented by individual mandates; 2) expansion of existing public health insurance programs (such as the State Children's Health Insurance Plan); 3) creation of new targeted public supported programs (for example, a new program modeled on the Federal Employee Health Benefit Plan); and 4) establishment of a universal publicly financed program.

The report from this bipartisan, health care alliance, with so many diverse but critical groups interested in health care reform, could be considered a waltz as described by Bell and Shea (1998). For example, three former U.S. presidents are honorary chairs: former Presidents George Bush, Jimmy Carter, and Gerald Ford. In this case the partnership is built on long-standing relationships and working together in nonpartisan ways to achieve common goals. The challenge for the future is to learn new ways to dance together, practice together, prepare for the performances (when this agenda might appear center stage as a national debate again), and learn from mistakes to improve the dance continually. Health care reform clearly will require new and different kinds of alliances and coalitions such as this National Coalition on Health Care, with unlikely partners if the American public is going to receive safe, cost-effective, comprehensive, quality health care with coverage for all during this century.

Example 4: Exploring Health Outcomes of Federal Sector Coalitions for Care Through Research

The military and federal health systems (including the Veterans Administration) and the U.S. Public Health Service could be described as an unusual structure of alliances and/or coalitions for the purposes of providing care and conducting health care research. The federal business of health care is one of the largest businesses in the United States. This interconnected coalition-like grouping of health care organizations has significant responsibilities for the provision of care; acts as a purchaser of care through the Department of Defense Tricare Management Activity; provides care to military and federal health workers and their beneficiaries; and manages a tremendously large number of providers, including nurses. The National Coalition on Health Care (described previously) identified a health care delivery model such as the Federal Employee Health Benefit Plan as one possible component of a solution for future health care reform. Consequently, research being conducted by faculty and graduate students in the School of Nursing at the Uniformed Services of the Health Sciences is relevant to this discussion on business coalitions.

Nurses (clinicians and researchers) within the Department of Defense Military Health System must be prepared to be clinically competent and clinically relevant to the roles and beneficiary health care requirements of the Department of Defense Military Health System milieu (Bibb et al., 2003; Hinton-Walker, Bibb, & Elberson, in press). Secondary analysis of data contained in existing Department of Defense Military Health System and related clinical databases is an excellent research method for identifying population health status and health needs; measuring outcomes associated with health, quality, costs, and safety; and designing, implementing, and evaluating population health programs (Bibb, 2001; Clarke & Clossette, 2000; Department of Defense, 2005; Department of Defense Tricare Management Activity, 2001; Lincoln, Smith, & Baker, 2000; Proctor & Taylor, 2000; Siegel, Moy, Burstin, 2004; Smaldone & Connor, 2003; Woolf, 2004). However, to date, use of secondary analysis of existing data as a research methodology has been undertaken primarily by health service researchers, and nursing is just beginning to contribute to the body of health care research by means of secondary analysis (Clarke & Clossette, 2000; Smaldone & Connor, 2003). The increased emphasis on population-based health care in the Department of Defense Military Health System and issues associated with the cost and quality outcomes of care delivered in the federal health sector can serve as an effective model for future study and evaluation of care in a reformed health care delivery system—if that happens in the future.

A number of clinical databases have been established and are being used in the Department of Defense Military Health System to conduct research and design programs; however, the nature of these databases varies considerably in relation to completeness and accuracy. In addition, limited published information is available that is related to location and access of these databases, as well as identification of future usefulness of data contained in these databases in conducting population

health research and developing and monitoring population health programs. Various military health care databases currently are influencing quality improvement projects and programs, which in an indirect way has the opportunity to define policy in the federal sector or inform policy in the private health care sector. However, no central depository exists for similar health care data between and among this loosely organized coalition-like structure of the Army, Navy, and Air Force.

The challenge of measuring effectiveness of health programs (health promotion and prevention programs related to fitness and health) and evaluating cost and quality outcomes of health care delivery across the players in this coalition-like federal health system are many, but the potential is great. Questions to ask are whether the Navy Environmental Health Center data is unique to its service, and whether this data also could benefit the Army and Air Force in identifying trends, gaps, and areas for improvement. The Army Health Hazard Assessment database has been in existence since the 1970s and has been a resource for Army managers in the development of medical programs to minimize health hazards associated with military equipment and systems. Again, the question exists of whether this data is unique to the Army, or whether other military services could benefit from this valuable information and perhaps use it to reexamine current policy of that service. Finally, the Air Force recently published an article on its Global Expeditionary Medical System, which provides clinical data on every medical encounter that occurs at U.S. Force medical treatment facilities in theater, boasting high internal validity and reliability for service members deployed in the U.S. Air Force setting. With research projects designed to make use of the data, thorough research can be done to measure effectiveness of health programs and health care delivery across this unique coalition-like organization (Department of Defense Military Health System and the Veterans Health Administration).

The School of Nursing faculty and students at Uniformed Services of the Health Sciences have taken the first step of equipping Department of Defense Military Health System nurses with the skills and expertise required to conduct population health research using existing Department of Defense Military Health System population health data. In addition, a project is being developed and implemented that will assess the completeness and accuracy of the database containing these health data through faculty-directed graduate student research projects. Other student groups (again guided by faculty) are identifying and describing databases used for population health research and program design in the Military Health System that will result in a listing of databases available for population health research and program and policy development and evaluation. The conduct of these studies will develop a method for systematically identifying Department of Defense Military Health System clinical databases across this loosely linked coalition and establish the feasibility of conducting a follow-on studies to evaluate the completeness and accuracy of a sample of Department of Defense Military Health System clinical databases. This research being conducted within the Graduate School of Nursing is the first of its kind and has tremendous value to nursing, the military and federal health system, and to society at large in these contexts: (1) informing policy makers of the value of and effectiveness of the military and federal health care delivery system, which serves a growing diverse population in the United States; (2) measuring similar and differing population health outcomes between and among coalition-like members; and (3) informing the health policy makers in the legislative arena who are interested in addressing the current challenges in the health care delivery system through system-wide reform identified by the National Coalition on Health Care.

IMPLICATIONS FOR NURSES AND NURSING PROFESSION

Rosenstein (1994, p. 53) reports that "newer industry initiatives have begun to focus on the value for the health care dollar where large health care coalitions have begun to selectively contract with those providers who deliver more effective care." Is nursing ready for this challenge? Nurses have a unique opportunity to position themselves for places of influence in the development of new coalitions, alliances, and partnerships. New opportunities are emerging in education and practice, but nurses must accept the challenge of exploring new frontiers, learning new competencies, and responding in entrepreneurial ways. Nurses must accept individual responsibility for mastering and teaching at least six of the competencies identified by Meister (1998) that global corporations will require in the future: (1) learning to learn new skills competence, (2) leadership development, (3) business literacy, (4) collaboration and team building, (5) technology literacy, and (6) management of one's own career. These ideas are not new but are more and more critical to the survival of nurses as individuals and to nursing as a profession in the

twenty-first century. Many roles in managed care exist, but nurses must be willing to take some risk, learn new skills, and work in and with this new market-driven business environment.

Other new roles that are emerging are related to data and research needed to measure cost and quality outcomes of care. Some disease management teams in mature managed care organizations have an expert in data and information analysis on the team as an equal player with the clinician. Primary care practice also will continue to be a challenge to maintain positive health outcomes. In some settings, advanced practice nurses already are managing primary care practices with physicians in a collaborative way. Nurses also must find creative, innovative, and cost-effective ways to facilitate learning across global boundaries. Technology is the answer but will require new ways of teaching, learning, and practicing.

"Many of tomorrow's most intriguing opportunities—interactive television, on-board navigational systems for cars and trucks, cell therapy, remote at-home medical diagnostics, satellite personal communication devices, a national video register of homes for sale, an alternative to the internal combustion engine—will require the integration of skills and capabilities residing in a wide variety of companies" (Hamel & Prahalad, 1994, p. 276). Business coalitions will be increasingly dominant in many global health care markets. How will nurses respond? Which dance will nurses want to perform? How will nurses prepare for the dance? Will nurses join the more complex dances that require significant knowledge and competence in the areas of building and maintaining alliances, coalitions, and partnerships, or will nurses just sit on the sidelines while other professions assume many of the responsibilities that traditionally have belonged to nurses? Nurses can just join the line dance, or nurses can create new dances for local and global challenges of partnership.

REFERENCES

American Federation of State, County, and Municipal Employees. (n.d.). *Health care coalitions*. Retrieved July 23, 2005, from http://www.afscme.org/wrkplace/hcoalfaq.htm

Bell, C. R., & Shea, H. (1998). *Dance lessons*. San Francisco: Berret-Koehler.

Bibb, S. C. (2001). Population-based needs assessment in the design of patient education programs. *Military Medicine, 166*, 297-300.

Bibb, S. C., Malebranche, M., Crowell, D., Altman, C., Lyon, S., Carlson, A., et al. (2003). Professional development needs of registered nurses practicing at a military community hospital. *Journal of Continuing Education in Nursing, 34*(1), 39-45.

California Coalition for Compassionate Care. (n.d.). *About the coalition.* Retrieved July 23, 2005, from http://www.finalchoices.calhealth.org/governance.htm

Clarke, S. P., & Clossette, S. (2000). Secondary analysis: Theoretical, methodological, and practical considerations. *Canadian Journal of Nursing Research, 32,* 109-129.

Department of Defense. (2005). *2005 DoD survey of health related behaviors among military personnel.* Retrieved November 18, 2004, from http://dodwws.rti.org/project.cfm

Department of Defense Tricare Management Activity. (2001). *Population health improvement plan and guide.* Retrieved July 23, 2005, from http://www.tricare.osd.mil/mhsophsc/DoD_PHI_Plan_Guide.pdf

Hamel, G., & Prahalad, C. K. (1994). *Competing for the future: Breakthrough strategies for seizing control of your industry and creating the markets of tomorrow* (p. 23). Boston: Harvard Business Press.

Hinton-Walker, P., Bibb, S. C., Elberson, K. L. (in press). Research issues: Bioterrorism and mass casualty events. *Nursing Clinics in North America.*

Kanter, R. M. (1989, August). Becoming PALs: Pooling, allying, and linking across companies. *Academy of Management Executives, 3,* 183-193.

Lincoln, A. E., Smith, G. S., Baker, S. P. (2000). The use of existing military administrative and health databases for injury surveillance and research. *American Journal of Preventive Medicine, 18*(3S), 8-13.

Meister, J. C. (1998). *Corporate universities.* New York: McGraw-Hill.

Merriam-Webster's Collegiate Dictionary (10th ed., p. 219). (1994). Springfield, MA: Merriam-Webster.

Mintzberg, H. (1977). Policy as a field of management theory. *Academy of Management Review, 2,* 88-103.

National Coalition on Health Care. (2004). Building a better healthcare system: Specifications for reform. Retrieved July 23, 2005, from http://www.nchc.org/

National Coalition on Health Care. (2005). New projections from nation's largest health care coalition show health care reform would produce huge savings. Retrieved July 23, 2005, from http://www.nchc.org/news/press_releases/2005/Press%20Release_final.pdf

Proctor, S. J., & Taylor, P. R. A. (2000). A practical guide to continuous population-based data collection (PACE): A process facilitating uniformity of care and research into practice. *QJM: An International Journal of Medicine, 93,* 67-73.

Rooney, E. (1992). Business coalitions on health care: An evolution from cost containment to quality improvement. *American Association of Occupational Health Nurses, 40,* 342-351.

Rosenstein, A. H. (1994). Cost-effective health care: Tools for improvement. *Health Care Management Review, 19,* 53-61.

Siegel, S., Moy, E., & Burstin, H. (2004). Assessing the nation's progress toward elimination of disparities in health care. *Journal of General Internal Medicine, 19,* 195-200.

Smaldone, A. M., & Connor, J. A. (2003). The use of large administrative data sets in nursing research. *Applied Nursing Research, 16,* 205-207.

Speckman, R. E., & Isabella, L. A. (with MacAvoy, T. C.). (2000). *Alliance competence.* New York: John Wiley & Sons.

Tichy, N. M. (1983). *Managing strategic change: Technical, political and cultural dynamics.* New York: John Wiley & Sons.

Woolf, S. H. (2004). Patient safety is not enough: Targeting quality improvements to optimize the health of the population. *Annals of Internal Medicine, 140*(1), 33-36.

Zuckerman, H. S., Kaluzny, A. D., & Ricketts, T. C., III. (1995). Strategic alliances: A worldwide phenomenon comes to health care. In A. D. Kalzuny, H. S. Zuckerman, & T. C. Ricketts III, *Partners for the dance: Forming strategic alliances in health care* (pp. 1-18). Ann Arbor, MI: Health Administration Press.

WEB REFERENCES

Business coalitions market overview. (2005). Trumbull, CT: Knowledge Source. Retrieved from Mindbranch July 23, 2005, from http://www.mindbranch.com/products/R255-0031.html

Canadian Pharmacists Association
http://www.pharmacists.ca/content/about_cpha/who_we_are/partnerships_coalitions/health_care.cfm

California Coalition for Compassionate Care
http://www.finalchoices.calhealth.org/
http://www.finalchoices.calhealth.org/governance.htm
http://www.finalchoices.calhealth.org/nf_initiative.htm
http://www.finalchoices.calhealth.org/02professional_education.htm
http://www.finalchoices.calhealth.org/03consumer_education.htm
http://www.finalchoices.calhealth.org/04community_coalitions.htm
http://www.finalchoices.calhealth.org/advance_directive.htm
http://www.finalchoices.calhealth.org/pubs_materials.htm
http://www.finalchoices.calhealth.org/public_policy.htm
http://www.finalchoices.calhealth.org/CHIPS.htm
http://www.finalchoices.calhealth.org/links.htm

International Foundation of Employee Benefit Plans. (2005). What are health care coalitions? Retrieved July 23, 2005, from http://www.ifebp.org/knowledge/recohm.asp?coalition

The Challenge

Participate in the Era of Politics—Choose an Ideology and Lead

CATHERINE J. DODD

Since the beginning of the profession, nursing has concerned itself with promoting and protecting the health of those entrusted to the care of nurses. This is the basis on which the profession has long been involved in working to influence the health policy agenda of the United States and international health policy. Much has been published in the last 3 decades about the involvement of nursing in politics, and indeed the profession has achieved higher levels of funding for nursing education and research; advanced practice nurses have been recognized as providers by Medicare and Medicaid; and needle safety legislation has been signed into law. However, this chapter suggests that professional nursing represented by professional nursing organizations with lobbyists in Washington, D.C. has protected the profession but has not done and is not doing enough to influence the broader health debates during key political eras when policies shaping the health care system were being debated. Many individual nurses engage in political advocacy based on their personal political ideology; however, the profession of nursing has only on a few occasions demonstrated a commitment to a political ideology. The objective of the discussion that follows is to challenge nurses to develop positions related to how the U.S. health care system should work, to choose a political ideology that matches their belief, and then to work as leaders within professional nursing organizations to influence the dominant ideologies of the profession. Nursing is one of the most trusted professions. The public values the opinions, beliefs, and ideologies of nurses. The profession of nursing must participate in the debates that will determine the kind of health care system that is created in current and future political eras.

IDEOLOGY, POLITICS, AND POLICY

Policies are developed within political systems: executive-regulative, legislative-statutory, and judicial. Hence policy is linked inextricably to politics. The health policies of the United States are not the "result of a well-thought-out approach to meeting people's health care needs" (Salmon, 2001). They are the result of political ideologies influencing policy development. The policies that have created the U.S. "non-system" of health care are the product of political eras. Political eras are characterized by the political ideologies of the presidents who appoint their cabinets to craft and implement policies that reflect their political ideologies. The political ideology of the majority party in Congress also influences policy. The U.S. "non-system" of health care is the result of dominant political ideologies of several presidents with some influence by opposition from Congress when the majority party in Congress (the House of Representatives or the Senate or both) was different from the president's party.

What Is the Political Ideology of Nursing?

An ideology is a "deeply held system of beliefs that frame the possible and the ethical, orienting us to what is ('reality'), to who we are, and to how we related to the world. Ideologies influence what we conceive of as imaginable and as right and wrong" (Estes, 1994, p. 139). Politicians have ideologies that are reflected in the ideologies of their political parties. Political parties represent systems of beliefs that frame how things should be, what is right, and what is wrong.

During only a few eras in the 110-plus year history of nursing has the *profession* demonstrated a political ideology concerned with how the systems of care are developed, financed, and implemented at national and international levels. Individual nurses have been and are political leaders, and many of them were or are active in professional nursing organizations. However, with the exception of the early 1930s, the 1970s, and the period surrounding the administration of President Clinton (1992-2000), nursing as a profession has not demonstrated an ideology related to health care and the economic systems that influence health at the national level. One should note that some state nurses associations have been and continue to lobby for a broader agenda than the protection and expansion of the nursing profession. This discussion is confined to national political eras and ideologies.

The profession of nursing has been and continues to be involved in electing and lobbying presidents and Congress to protect and enhance the professional status of nursing. The American Nurses Association has lobbied on behalf of nurses since the Spanish-American War and has had a formal presence in Washington, D.C., since World War II. The American Nurses Association Political Action Committee has endorsed candidates in the presidential elections since 1984. Professional nursing advocacy has focused largely on improving the working conditions under which nursing care is provided and on protecting and enhancing the role of nursing in caring for individuals, families, communities, schools, and armies. Nursing has taken positions to establish and support Social Security, to protect Medicare, and to fund preventive care; however, professional organizations devote few resources to working actively to pass policies that will increase access to care, improve quality, and eliminate health care inequities that characterize the health of the nation.

Ideology: Health Care as a Product of the Market

The American dream is to be successful and independent and to make money and purchase everything one's family needs. Individualism and entrepreneurialism are two ideologies that often go hand in hand and that have characterized the development of America. The belief that an unregulated market competition will produce a high-quality product by efficiently using resources and producing a product that consumers demand is at the center of "what makes our country great" and is as "American as apple pie." The American health care system is a "product" shaped by a quasi-regulated market with significant government funding. The regulatory involvement of government (or some might say the intrusion of government) in competitive markets has varied from administration to administration. The government has

the dual charge of preserving a healthy economy and promoting a healthy citizenry to work (and spend) in the economy. In health care the role of government is inconsistent. Policy makers (politicians) say that they want every child to have health care and that they do not want seniors to spend their final years in under-staffed nursing homes, but they continue to enact laws that create a non-system of care. In the previous edition of this book, Salmon (2001, p. 346) said, "our health care 'non-system' is the direct result of such factors as professional self-interest, corporate interest, and political action." These factors represent an ideology, a market ideology that views health care as a commodity (a product to purchase) in a market versus health care as a human right. "Consumer-driven health care," a catch phrase during George W. Bush's first term in office, implies that consumers have responsibility for choosing not only providers but what services they want from those providers and that prudent consumer choices will increase competition and drive down prices while improving quality. If only consumers could choose not to have chronic illnesses.

Political Ideologies and Health Care: A Historical Perspective

In direct contrast is the kind of care promoted by early nursing leaders, in the early 1900s, thousands of immigrants crowded into settlement slums in New York City to work in factories. Lillian Wald, the founder of public health nursing, was active in politics. She successfully lobbied for parks for children and for nurses in public schools, and she brought health care directly to the people in their community at the Henry Street Settlement House (Jewish Women's Archive, 2005). Shortly after the passage of the Nineteenth Amendment granting women suffrage in 1920 during Democratic President Wilson's administration, members of Congress were elected who were concerned about women and children dying in childbirth and of starvation and poverty. Congress passed the Sheppard Towner Act, the first government funding for health care, specifically maternal-child health care. Mary Breckinridge (n.d.), the founder of nurse-midwifery in the United States, sought government funding to bring prenatal care to families in Appalachian Kentucky where the infant and maternal mortality rate was high. The physician in charge of the Children's Bureau, appointed by Republican President Harding (1921-1923), denied Breckinridge funding because of the belief that nurses should not work independently and the money was better spent on private physicians who were beginning to deliver babies in hospitals. Breckinridge was undaunted, and she founded the Frontier Nursing Service in 1925 using her own funds. Her "nurses on horseback" introduced a model rural health care system and provided professional services to neglected people of a thousand-square-mile area in southeastern Kentucky. The system lowered the rate of death in childbirth in Leslie County, Kentucky, from the highest in the nation to substantially below the national average.

Republican President Herbert Hoover's administration (1929-1933) was burdened by the great depression. Hoover was orphaned at a young age and was a self-made man; his ideology exemplified individualism and entrepreneurialism. To address the financial crisis of the country, he created grants to aid states to stimulate business (the market) but said, "while people must not suffer from hunger and cold, caring for them must be primarily a local and voluntary responsibility" (The White House, n.d.).

During this time, poverty plagued every American city. Public health nursing had grown, and the National Organization of Public Health Nurses along with the American Nurses Association (ANA), supported the plan of Democratic President Franklin Delano Roosevelt (1933-1945) for social security (Flanagan, 1976). The President and Democratically controlled Congress (House and Senate) greatly increased government funding for health and social services. Federal aid to the states for health and welfare in the form of funding for "crippled children, the aged, and aid to dependent children" was established (Lee & Benjamin, 1994). In 1935 the Social Security Act passed with 288 Democratic votes, 77 Republican votes, 1 Farm vote, and 6 Progressive votes. The act created a social insurance program for children who had lost a parent, for the disabled who were unable to work, and for the elderly. The program was called the Old Age, Survivors' and Disability Insurance program. Roosevelt appointed the first woman cabinet secretary, Francis Perkins, and she urged him to include health care in the Social Security proposal, but opposition from the American Medical Association and from organized labor (which negotiated health benefits for employees) opposed a national health insurance plan, so Roosevelt decided to wait.

World War II distracted the nation. Democrat Harry Truman completed Roosevelt's term (1945-1953) as the war ended. He then ran for president and won on a platform of adding national health insurance to Social Security. The Democratic majority in the House of Representatives was lost during Truman's midterm election because the American Medical Association funded a campaign to defeat Democratic congressional candidates who supported Truman's national health insurance plan, calling it "socialized medicine" and creating fear that it would put the government in the doctor's office (Denker, 1993). The ideology of personal choice, not having a big government, emerged in this election, and national health insurance never passed. The dominant ideology continues to oppose government intervention health insurance (with the exception of Medicare for the elderly).

During the 1950s and early 1960s under Republican President Eisenhower, the federal government passed the Hill-Burton law and funded the building of hospitals to keep pace with the growth of technology, the cost of medical care increased, and the health "industry" began. Soon there were too many hospitals. Many persons had insurance coverage as a benefit of employment; however, many persons still paid the doctor directly, and payment was costly. Health policy was not on the national agenda again until the presidency of Democrat John F. Kennedy (1961-1963). Many persons could not afford medical care, and the cost of hospitalization drained the savings of many aging persons. During his administration, federal funding to states, counties, cities, and nonprofit organizations for medical care increased. Discussions about creating national programs to fund medical care for the poor and the elderly (Medicaid and Medicare, respectively) began. Under Democratic President Johnson, the largest expansion of government funding for health care was passed: Medicare A, a program to cover hospital costs for the elderly, and Medicaid, a program to pay for health care for the poor, were enacted. The Food and Drug Administration was created to ensure that drugs were safe before marketing. Neighborhood health centers were funded for the first time. The Civil Rights Act passed, removing obstacles to voting for blacks and establishing access to equal health care services (if they could afford them). Many antipoverty programs were put in place. The government began to subsidize private medical care on a large scale, and medical entrepreneurialism blossomed. Private investor-owned hospitals, nursing homes, and clinics sprouted up. The health care industry grew with the influx of public funds. The dominant ideology was to expand access with public funds paid to private business.

ERA OF DEMAND FOR NATIONAL HEALTH INSURANCE

A marked shortage of nurses to staff the many hospital beds newly subsidized by Medicare and Medicaid drew the attention of Congress. Republican President Nixon (1969-1974) reluctantly signed the Nurse Training Act of 1971 in which Congress authorized $885 million for 3 years. Unfortunately, because of the costs of the Vietnam War, President Nixon's budgets were far less than what Congress authorized. Congress added the funding back to the budget in the appropriation process, and Nixon vetoed the appropriation bill. In 1974 the President cut the nursing appropriation from $160 million to $49 million; however, lobbying efforts by the ANA and the National League for Nursing were successful in convincing Congress to reinstate the funding despite President Nixon's cuts (Kalisch & Kalisch, 1982).

During Nixon's administration, the pressure to establish a national health program was great. He proposed national health coverage via an employer mandate to provide coverage, but it failed to garner the support of Republicans and enough Democrats to pass. Democrats opposed linking health coverage to the ability to work, because when persons fell ill and could not work was when they needed coverage the most. Senators Edward Kennedy (D), Russell Long (D), and Abraham Ribicoff (D) and Representative Wilbur Mills (D) introduced national health insurance proposals (Etheredge, 2001) that failed to pass.

Nixon's administration was responsible for the legislation that created health maintenance organizations as a new way of financing health care. Cost would be controlled by consumers choosing a health maintenance organization, creating market competition. Nixon signed legislation initiated by the Democrats in Congress to add the disabled and persons with end-stage renal disease to Medicare.

During this time, nursing began to pay attention to proposals for national health insurance, realizing that Medicare and Medicaid were designed to ensure payment only to hospitals and physicians. In 1974 the ANA adopted a resolution stating that:

> Health, a state of physical, social and mental well-being is a basic human right, government at all levels must act to insure that health care services are provided for all citizens, there is a need for integrated systems to deliver comprehensive health care services that are accessible and acceptable to all people without regard to age, sex, race, social, or economic condition, there is a need for a national program designed to correct serious inadequacies in present health care delivery systems, nursing care is an essential component of health care (Flanagan, 1976, p. 281).

That same year, the ANA formed a political action committee to help elect candidates that represented the ideology of nursing. The ANA also proposed a national health insurance program financed through payroll taxes or payment of premiums by the self-employed and purchase of health insurance coverage for poor and unemployed from general tax revenues. This was an *ideological* position that all persons should have access to care, that nursing should be a part of that care, and that if persons could not pay for care, the government should pay for it out of tax revenues. Beyond just making the statement, the ANA made a commitment to support candidates for federal office who supported this ideology. However, the dominant political ideology was that health care was a product, a commodity to be purchased by consumers within the market created by the health care industry. In 1975 the Supreme Court ruled that antitrust laws applied to professional medical practice, thereby encouraging commercial competition and advertising by physicians. The ruling implied that medical "markets" would serve consumer interests by moderating prices and improving quality. As the cost of care increased, regulatory mechanisms were put in place to limit growth and address the maldistribution of physicians (Folland, Goodman, & Stano, 2004).

In 1975 the ANA established a separate fund to support state ratification of the Equal Rights Amendment, originally introduced in Congress in 1921, and Congress passed the amendment in 1972. The Equal Rights Amendment stated, "Equality of Rights under the law shall not be denied or abridged by the United States or any state on account of sex." The amendment failed to be ratified by 38 states before it died in 1982. The ANA moved its quadrennial convention to participate in the boycott of states that had not passed the Equal Rights Amendment. This action was an example action based on the ideology of nursing, its system of beliefs.

ERA OF MARKET COMPETITION

Republican President Reagan took office in 1981. The Republican ideology was (and continues to be) to decrease the size of government. Reagan greatly downsized the Department of Health and Human Services (Etheredge, 2001). His ideology of a "new Federalism" decreased federal expenditures for domestic social programs and asserted that the role of government is to maintain the national defense and law and order (Estes, 1994). During this era (and subsequent George H. W. Bush and George W. Bush administration eras), the free market was the center of the economy, tax reductions (despite great increases to the national debt) would stimulate the market along with deregulation, and competition would stimulate reform, bringing about cost control. Reagan immediately cut taxes, and in doing so cut the income to pay for government programs. The resulting $200 billion deficit was blamed on increasing costs of Medicaid and Medicare (Etheredge, 2001). Government spending on Medicaid and Medicare became an "economic crisis." To control costs, Reagan implemented diagnosis-related groups, or a lump-sum payment to hospitals based on diagnosis, as an alternative to fee-for-service reimbursement to hospitals. Reagan's ideology also emphasized the cultural image of the traditional family in a time when divorce was becoming more socially accepted. The health care system during the Reagan era became dominated by a powerful medical profession and for-profit medical industries. Not surprisingly, the number of uninsured grew dramatically, and the cost of health care rose at 2 to 3 times the rate of inflation (Lee & Benjamin, 1994).

The ANA, frustrated with the growing cost of health care and with the conditions under which nurses were attempting to care for patients hospitalized for increasingly shorter lengths of stay, took a controversial action and endorsed a candidate in the presidential election, choosing the Democratic nominee in 1984 and 1988. Reagan won reelection in 1984, and George H. W. Bush won in 1988. These bold actions, criticized by many, were the result of nursing standing up for its political ideology of believing that health care is a right, not a product that only the privileged should be able to afford.

Republican President George H. W. Bush (1989-1993) inherited a large debt and continued Reagan's economic ideology, claiming that the economic crisis demanded market intervention for health care cost containment through privatization, competition, and deregulation. His cultural ideology was influenced by the radical religious right, and he placed a "gag rule" on providers at family planning clinics so they could not say the word *abortion,* and he banned fetal tissue research (Estes, 1994). Nursing spoke out against these limits on access to care and research opportunities and withheld campaign support for most candidates who supported Bush's draconian rules. Bush did nothing to stop the investor-owned insurance industry attempts to decrease costs by shortening lengths of stay in hospitals. Consumers and Congress—not the President—insisted on legislation to protect patients from being subjected to "drive-through deliveries" and "drive-by mastectomies." Never before in history was Congress required to intervene to protect patients from insurance companies dictating patient care driven by the need to return a profit to their investors.

During Reagan's and Bush's combined 12 years of market intervention, national health expenditures rose from $25 billion in 1980 to $870 billion in 1992. As insurance premiums increased, many employers eliminated insurance benefits, increasing the number of uninsured. In 12 years, the market had failed to control health costs. A two-tiered system of health care reemerged, and the working poor lacked access to care.

ERA OF HEALTH CARE REFORM

Health care reform, the need to expand access and control costs while preserving quality, was a major issue in the 1992 presidential election. The ANA, along with the National League for Nursing, had developed *Nursing's Agenda for Health Care Reform,* a policy paper that proposed greater use of nurses and advanced practice nurses along with investments in primary care in community-based settings to control costs (ANA, 2001). Nursing had spent the time and money on research to back up the effectiveness of the agenda, and Democratic presidential candidate William Jefferson Clinton's platform for reform paralleled that of nursing. In the 1992 presidential election, nursing demonstrated its ideology and endorsed Clinton for president. After Clinton was elected, the ANA worked with the President to pass his health care reform proposal. Clinton's proposal for "managed competition" was not "national health insurance"; however, it did address quality, access, and cost, and it included nurses as essential providers in all settings. In Clinton's proposal the government played a regulatory role in structuring a market in which employees would choose from several health coverage options (Nichols, Ginsburg, Christianson, & Hurley, 2004) and the government-managed (regulated) premiums, physician reimbursement, and pharmaceutical costs.

In the midterm congressional election (2 years into Clinton's first term), the ANA Political Action Committee withheld support from candidates who did not support the health care reform proposal. Unfortunately, like Truman in his midterm election, Clinton lost the Democratic majority in Congress in 1994. In that election, the American Medical Association and the Health Insurance Association of America targeted swing congressional races where the incumbent supported Clinton's proposal with advertisements suggesting that if Clinton's reform passed with the candidate's support, the government would be in the doctor's office making decisions. Health care reform was stalled, and unregulated health care costs continued to rise. Employers seeking lower health insurance premiums began to limit choices to health maintenance organizations, and many employers dropped health coverage entirely. For-profit health care continued to grow, and investor-owned insurers and health maintenance organizations began to make medical decisions, often denying much-needed care in order to make a profit. Many not-for-profit health care facilities began to resemble their investor-owned competitors, spending money on advertising and atmosphere in order to compete (Relman, 2005).

ERA OF EXPANDING ACCESS

Despite the $490 billion deficit Clinton inherited from George H. W. Bush, Clinton balanced the budget during his term (1993-2001), and when he left office there was a surplus of more than $5.6 trillion over the next 10 years. Clinton proposed and signed into law the largest expansion of government-funded health coverage since the creation of Medicare and Medicaid, the State Children's Health Insurance Plan that provides coverage for children up to 200% over the poverty level by matching state and federal dollars.

ERA OF TAX CUTS AND PRIVATIZATION, MORE MARKET-BASED CONTROL, DEFICITS, AND CUTBACKS

The election (some would call it a selection) of Republican President George W. Bush in 2000 ushered in a new political era of market ideology and privatization of health and social services. Hospital systems were permitted to consolidate to increase market power, but the quality of care did not improve and the cost of care has not gone down because of new efficiencies (Cutler, 2004). Under the guise of adding a prescription drug benefit to Medicare, George W. Bush and the Republican Congress set Medicare policy on the road to privatization. Under the proposal, Medicare covers the cost of prescription drugs under specific circumstances, with no regulation of prescription drug costs that are much more expensive than in other countries occurs, and no mechanism to get lower prices for bulk purchasing is in place. Medicare funds are going to the pharmaceutical industry with no cost regulation.

President Bush's ideology, like that of Republican administrations before him, is to limit government funding for health care. Under the new Medicare law, the government will provide vouchers to Medicare beneficiaries that they can use to purchase health insurance. If the insurance costs more than the voucher, individuals must make up the difference with their own money.

This two-tiered system of health care ensures that the federal government pays a fixed amount for health insurance premiums and that the beneficiary will pay when the premium goes up. The program transfers the cost to the beneficiary, rather than being a public system that treats every beneficiary equally and this voucher system creates a private purchasing program. The other component of the Medicare Prescription Drug plan was the creation of health savings accounts. The market ideology of consumer-driven health care in which consumers (not patients) consume products allows individuals to purchase an inexpensive, high-deductible catastrophic health insurance plan (called a medical savings account, or health savings account [HSA]) with money from their employer that otherwise would be used to pay for insurance coverage. The HSAs allow employers (including the federal government) to pay for a fixed and defined contribution rather than a defined package of benefits. Excess funds in the employee's private HSA account are invested and rolled over each year and can be used to pay only for out-of-pocket medical expenses. Frugal consumers will select inexpensive doctors and hospitals when they need care and theoretically will save money. When the employee turns 65, unspent funds can be spent to augment Medicare coverage.

This proposal does not make financial or quality sense. It discourages routine preventive checkups, and unfortunately, selecting medical expertise is not like buying a car or other product; expecting patients and their families to shop for the best deal on brain surgery will not work. In addition, the HSAs change the risk pool of insurance and will drive up the cost of insurance for persons who do not choose them because young persons without expensive chronic illnesses will choose HSAs. The prescription drug bill had many flaws: one was that the pharmaceutical industry was successful in including a prohibition on bulk purchasing for better prices and on the importation of the same drugs from Canada.

Similarly, Bush's proposal to privatize Social Security promises younger workers a private savings account that they will own. Social Security was designed as a social insurance program with defined benefits for the elderly, the disabled, and children who lose their parents; it was never intended to be a private savings plan. Bush's goal is to decrease the government contribution and increase private investment. The privatization of Social Security will remove millions of dollars from the trust fund and will fail to provide a guaranteed benefit package for future generations, leaving persons just one accident away from poverty. Bush cited an economic crisis as his reason for Social Security reform, yet the Social Security Administration itself states that the fund is solvent until 2042. Removing funds to put in private accounts will shorten the time of solvency and make the problem worse. The real economic crisis was created by the permanent tax cuts enacted by George Bush and the Republican-controlled Congress that are projected to run a deficit of $8.4 trillion by the end of 2010 (not unlike the crises created by the tax cuts of Reagan and George H. W. Bush).

Privatization is the recurring Republican ideology, as is individualism and relying on market competition to keep costs down. Estes (1994) describes dominant power relations as being sustained through ideologies in three ways:

1. Ideologies successfully help create cultural images by policy makers, experts, and the media.
2. Ideologies create an appeal to the necessities of the economic system.
3. Ideologies focus problems and their solutions on familiar organizational structures and professions rather than on the more fundamental issues of class, gender, and race.

The American Nurses Association opposed Republican efforts to privatize public insurance programs and sent letters to Congress; however, these issues were not used as criteria for consideration for campaign contributions and support by the ANA Political Action Committee, and nurses in key districts were not mobilized to lobby their members. In these instances, the ANA did not put "its money where its mouth is" because so few nurse were involved or demanded action by the ANA.

The wealthy will always have access to quality health care; it is the disenfranchised that the profession of nursing must help protect. Women who leave the workforce to care for children and then their aging parents accrue less retirement on lower wages and live longer on their smaller retirement incomes. Privatizing Social Security, privatizing Medicare, and failing to regulate the cost of prescription drugs adversely affects women and persons of lower socioeconomic means. Nurses must be involved in this debate.

ERA OF RISING COSTS AND DECLINING COVERAGE WITHOUT RESPONSIBLE INTERVENTION

Increases in the cost of health care account for the decline in health insurance coverage, as more and more employers eliminate health coverage as a benefit (Gilmer

& Kronick, 2005). Coverage varies from state to state. In Massachusetts, Wisconsin, Ohio, and Minnesota, more than 80% of workers are covered. These states have a higher percentage of non-Hispanics than other states. Only 63% of workers in New Mexico, California, Florida, and Texas have employer-sponsored insurance. When controlling for income, there is a direct correlation between lack of employer-sponsored health coverage and race, ethnicity, and place of birth (Kronick, Gilmer, & Rice, 2004). One in five persons is uninsured at some point in a year. The Institute of Medicine found overwhelming evidence that the uninsured receive poorer care. The uninsured are less likely to receive preventive and screening services, and therefore serious diseases are detected later. The Institute of Medicine estimated that 20,000 persons die each year because they are uninsured (Cutler, 2004). A direct link exists between health insurance as one factor in explaining why people of color rank the lowest on key health status indicators. Three fourths of the 23 million uninsured in communities of color in the United States lived below 200% of the federal poverty level of $37,670 for a family of four in 2003 (Lillie-Blanton & Hoffman, 2005).

It is estimated that 1.9 to 2.2 million American families experience medical bankruptcy caused by medical expenses each year and nearly 76% of them had medical coverage at the onset of their illness (Himmelstein, Warren, Thorne, & Woolhandler, 2005). The Republican Congress passed a bankruptcy bill that makes it easier for the credit card companies to seize assets of families, regardless of health status. After a family declares bankruptcy, the family must rely on Medicaid, the program that provides health coverage for the poor.

Medicaid spending has increased 65% from 2000 to 2005. In an effort to limit federal spending on social programs, President Bush proposed a 20% cut to Medicaid in the 2006 budget. The federal government pays on average 57 cents out of every dollar Medicaid spends, and the state pays the balance. More than 50 million Americans rely on Medicaid for their health care. The greatest number of persons relying on Medicaid are poor families with children; however, the majority of Medicaid dollars are spent on the elderly and disabled, particularly on care provided by for-profit nursing homes. Medicaid pays for two thirds of all nursing home residents in the country (Economist, 2005). The number of persons requiring nursing home care will increase every year, and cutting Medicaid funding will result in less care for the most frail elderly in nursing homes.

Per capita, the United States has the most expensive health care system in the world, yet the United States ranks in the lower one half of health outcome measures internationally, barely higher than Turkey, Mexico, Poland, Hungary, and Korea. The United States also ranks highest in diabetes mortality. Physicians (and nurses) in the United States are paid higher wages than their counterparts internationally, and the average hospital cost per day ranks the highest among the 29 member nations of the Organization for Economic Cooperation and Development. Americans pay 40% more per capita than Germans do for health care and received 15% fewer real health resources with much of the U.S. money spent on high-cost, high-tech solutions to often preventable diseases.

> The cost-benefit of insuring the uninsured is estimated at approximately $33 billion and the savings from reducing mortality alone are estimated at approximately $20 billion (Cutler, 2004).

Now is time for the profession of nursing to be guided and inspired by the ideology asserted over the last several decades. The ideology of nursing must be demonstrated by investing the individual and collective resources of professional organizations to influence the policy makers, to influence campaigns, and to influence the media. Writing letters and wearing buttons is not enough; nurses' actions must speak louder than their words. Nurses need to choose which political party reflects their beliefs about who deserves access to quality, affordable health care. Nurses need to insist that the professional associations that represent them hold elected officials and candidates to the standard that considers health care a right for all persons, not just the privileged.

GLOBAL RESPONSIBILITY OF NURSING

Nursing is a global profession, and beyond influencing domestic policy, the ANA represents the wealthiest country in the world within the International Council of Nursing (ICN), the oldest international health organization. The ICN takes positions on many issues, such as the continued use of land mines, access to safe water, human trafficking, and the marketing of tobacco to children. A central concern for ICN is protecting and enhancing the practice of nursing through regulation and education of nurses and developing mechanisms to meet the global demand for nurses. Throughout the world, wherever nursing is taught in English (the Philippines, South Korea, Australia, the United Kingdom, South Africa, and Canada), U.S. health care recruiting agencies are "stealing nurses." Although the United States voices support for ICN positions, it remains to be seen what the profession of nursing in the United States is doing to stop health care recruiters from stealing nurses who are needed in their own countries. These countries are not as wealthy as the United States, they subsidized the education of their nurses, and the United States recruits them away. Global market forces allow the United States to offer better wages to foreign nurses, yet the United States does nothing to assist in the education and training of nurses in these countries. What does the profession believe about this? What is nursing ideology? What are nurses doing about it? The United States is the largest manufacturer of land mine parts that are sold worldwide. Land mines used during wars can never be removed and render farmland unusable, farm animals dead, and children limbless. The ICN has urged the elimination of land mines. What is nursing in the United States doing to stop the manufacture and sale of these deadly weapons? Does the ANA withhold political support from candidates who support the continued production of land mines? The ANA must take a leadership role on policy issues that the United States dominates and over which it has control.

Nurses have a professional obligation to those entrusted to their care and to society to work individually and collectively to demonstrate that they have political ideologies that serve all of humankind, especially the most vulnerable. Each nurse has an obligation to be involved in politics to shape the policies that govern health care delivery. In the words of former Vice President Hubert Humphrey, "The moral test of government is how that government treats those who are in the dawn of life, the children; those who are in the twilight of life, the elderly; and those who are in the shadows of life, the sick, the needy, and the handicapped." Nurses choose elected officials, and their choice should reflect the ideology of nursing about health care. Nurses must be involved and vocal lest their ideals be silenced and their ideology be invisible.

REFERENCES

American Nurses Association. (2001). *Nursing's agenda for health care reform.* Washington, DC: Author.

Breckinridge, M. Biographical sketch of Mary Breckinridge. Retrieved July 24, 2005, from http://www.lesliecounty.net/history/mary_breckinridge.htm

Cutler, D. M. (2004). *Your money or your life.* Oxford, NY: Oxford University Press.

Denker, P. (1993). Families. In *A.S.A.P. Update.* Washington, DC: Families USA.

Economist. (March 3, 2005). Editorial, *Medicaid Reform: The Next Big Thing.* New York, pp. 29-30.

Estes, C. (1994). Privatization, the welfare state and aging: The Reagan-Bush legacy. In P. R. Lee & C. Estes (Eds.), *The nation's health.* Boston, MA: Jones and Bartlett.

Etheredge, L. (2001). *On the archeology of health care policy: Periods and paradigms.* The Robert Wood Johnson Health Policy Fellowship Program. Washington, DC: National Academies Press.

Flanagan, L. (1976). *One strong voice.* Kansas City, MO: American Nurses Association.

Folland, S., Goodman, A. C., & Stano, M. (2004). *The economics of health and health care* (4th ed.). Upper Saddle River, NJ: Pearson, Prentice Hall.

Gilmer, T., & Kronick, R. (2005, April). It's the premiums, stupid: Projections of the uninsured through 2013. *Health Affairs.* Web Exclusives Volume 24 Supplement 1, Jan-June 2005 Project Hope, Bethesda, MD.

Himmelstein, D. U., Warren, E., Thorne, D., & Woolhandler, S. (2005, February). Market watch: Illness and injury as contributors to bankruptcy. *Health Affairs.* Web Exclusives Volume 24 Supplement 1, Jan-June 2005 Project Hope, Bethesda, MD.

Jewish Women's Archive. (2005). *Lillian Wald: 1867-1940* [See Outdoor Recreation League, New York Immigration Commission, Nursing Insurance Partnership, Federal Children's Bureau, House on Henry Street, Red Scare Resistance]. Available July 24, 2005, from http://www.jwa.org/exhibits/wov/wald/lwbio.html

Kalisch, B., & Kalisch, P. (1982). *Politics of nursing.* Philadelphia, Lippincott.

Kronick, R., Gilmer, T., & Rice, T. (2004, June 2). The kindness of strangers: Community effects on the rate of employer coverage. *Health Affairs.* Retrieved July 24, 2005, from http://content.healthaffairs.org/cgi/content/full/hlthaff.w4.328/DC1

Lee, P. R., & Benjamin, A. E. (1994). Health policy and the politics of health care. In P. R. Lee & C. Estes, *The nation's health.* Boston, MA: Jones and Bartlett.

Lillie-Blanton, M., & Hoffman, C. (2005). The role of health insurance coverage in reducing racial/ethnic disparities in health care. *Health Affairs, 24*(2), 398-408.

Nichols, L. M., Ginsburg, P. B., Christianson, J., & Hurley, R. E. (2004). Are market forces strong enough to deliver efficient health care systems? Confidence is waning. *Health Affairs, 23*(2), 8-24.

Relman, A. (2005). A proposal for universal coverage. *New England Journal of Medicine, 353*(1), 96-97. Retrieved August 1, 2005, from http://content.nejm.org/content/vol353/issue1/index.shtml

Salmon, M. E. (2001). Nursing in a political era. In J. C. McCloskey & H. K. Grace (Eds.), *Current issues in nursing.* St. Louis, MO: Mosby.

The White House. (n.d.). *Herbert Hoover.* Retrieved August 1, 2005, from http://www.whitehouse.gov/history/presidents/hh31.html

The Corporatization of Health Care

Mergers and Acquisitions

MARJORIE BEYERS

Few business approaches illustrate the effects of corporatization on health care as well as mergers and acquisitions do. A common theme in mergers and acquisitions is change. This change reaches every level of the organization from the operations of a health care entity to the corporate structure. Driven by business goals, mergers and acquisitions affect the way health care is financed, organized, managed, and delivered. Terms such as the *health care industry* or *the enterprise* have become commonplace in health care. Increasingly, the capability to provide patient care is recognized as depending on financially healthy organizations. Although the debate about how to preserve patient care in a financially driven market continues, corporatization of health care is now more or less accepted (Beyers, 1999). Mergers and acquisitions not only change ownership and sponsorship but also have the potential to change health care services and the way these services are delivered.

Mergers and acquisitions in the business world have been the subject of many research studies, speculation, and controversy. Recognizing that each merger or acquisition is unique, researchers have identified several factors that appear to influence the success or failure of mergers and acquisitions. Successful mergers and acquisitions create synergy among the existing and acquired organizations (Larsson, Brousseau, Driver, & Sweet, 2004). Success is related to the potential for strategic benefit, integration of the organization to create a new whole, and low employee resistance. The human factor now is recognized to be able to make or break a merger or acquisition. Employee motivation to accept or reject the merger or acquisition is influenced by many factors. One of the most important factors is the reason for the merger or acquisition. When a merger "saves" a community hospital from closing, employee response may be more favorable than when a merger "takes over" the community hospital as part of a strategic plan to increase market share or to achieve corporate growth. The impact of a hostile merger is different from the impact achieved when the involved groups mutually agree on the merger or acquisition from the early stages onward. Yet other factors are the cultures of the organizations, the careers of individuals involved, and the communications before, during, and after the merger. The reasons for change, the degree of support and acceptance by stakeholders, and the leadership significantly affect outcomes of mergers and acquisitions.

Mergers and acquisitions, once rare and anxiety producing in health care, are now more common but no less anxiety producing. The very mention of mergers and acquisitions produces anxiety because they signal significant change that has uncertain outcomes. Mergers and acquisitions have been compared with marriages: some work and some do not. Every situation of merger or acquisition has to be analyzed for its own characteristics, including the organizational cultures, the relationships of the organizations to the community, the financial status of the organizations, and the community perception of service and accessibility. Speculation and real competition for power and control within the organization, anticipation of changes that may be imposed by the new owner or the new executive team, and uncertainty about how the merger or acquisition will affect one's work and career are almost inescapable even in the best planned and executed mergers and acquisitions. Different individuals or groups may respond differently to the merger or acquisition. What some view as a positive move may be perceived by others as negative. Few individuals or groups are untouched by a merger or an acquisition.

THE CHANGING HEALTH CARE ENTERPRISE

The chief reason for mergers and acquisitions is to further the strategic achievement of business goals. Generally, mergers and acquisitions are a way to achieve growth of the corporation. Some common business goals for which mergers and acquisitions are used are to increase the assets of the corporation, to expand product lines, to increase market share, to develop new markets or to strengthen existing ones, to decrease competition, or to attain resources, services, or a presence (Nahass, 2005). In health care, mergers may take place to strengthen the financial and service position of hospitals as in formation of a new system or corporation. Many religious-sponsored hospitals have formed corporations or health care systems to preserve their identity and their capability to continue to serve communities through the combined strength of entities that form the system. Yet another reason for mergers and acquisitions in health care may be to achieve economies of scale and scope by consolidation of resources and services to improve cost and productivity outcomes.

Early on, this consolidation focused on improving cost-effectiveness through increasing the critical mass of users, reducing redundancy, standardizing work processes, and targeting outcomes. However, the expected improvements have not been realized. Unfortunately, a residual outcome of the early mergers and acquisitions is the skepticism among health care workers about their value and the memory of failed organizational restructuring and less than positive change. Much has been learned about the processes of initiating and implementing mergers and acquisitions. They are not always successful. In some cases, the merger is turned around, a sure sign of failure. Some mergers or acquisitions are irrevocable. Today, however, a well-managed strategically positive merger or acquisition may be successful for the community, the corporation, and the employees.

Mergers or acquisitions are a corporate strategy that may be initiated by a given health care entity in a community or by a corporation. The rate of hospital mergers dropped sharply in 2002, reported by the American Hospital Association (2005) as the lowest level in 10 years. A study by Lewin Associates, as reported by the Health Care Advisory Board (2005) however, found that there were 130 mergers in 2004, a 136% increase from 2003; 120 hospital mergers in 2000; 118 in 2001; 98 in 2002; and 55 in 2003. The American Hospital Association publication *Trend Watch* (2005) predicts that the number of mergers and acquisitions will rise in the future. These researchers found that the value of

hospitals rose in this period and that most of the mergers were related to buyouts by for-profit chains. Controversy about the value of mergers continues. On the negative side, mergers are thought to decrease competition and increase the cost of health care. On the positive side, a merger or acquisition may enable a community to retain its health care services.

Mergers, acquisitions, and corporate consolidation are under the purview of the Federal Trade Commission. The Federal Trade Commission can be expected to be more attentive to hospital mergers, acquisitions, and consolidation in the future for several reasons. One is the public interest in mergers and acquisitions in all types of businesses over the past years. Some prevailing reasons related to health care are competition and the cost of health care related to the economic value of health care assets, the impact of health care on communities and businesses, and the concerns about competition and increased costs. The statement of the Federal Trade Commission presented to the Committee on the Judiciary of the U.S. Senate concerning mergers and corporate consolidation in the New Economy emphasized many points relevant to today's market (Pitofsky, 1998). At that time the statement recognized that downsizing and consolidation were forces in hospital mergers, acquisitions, and consolidation. Notable were changes in health care practices, which shifted care to outpatient settings, thereby reducing the hospital capacity needed to serve communities. Acceptable reasons for mergers and acquisitions were improving operations efficiency and meeting public policy goals such as the quality and cost of health care, providing choice, and diversity. Although dated, this statement provides a good understanding of mergers, acquisitions, and corporate consolidation.

Predictions are that the Federal Trade Commission will be scrutinizing health care mergers, acquisitions, and consolidations more closely in the future (Health Care Advisory Board, 2005). The belief that mergers, acquisitions, and consolidation may mean survival for a health care entity continues. In the corporate perspective, growth is an expected strategic goal. Growth in the health care industry may mean development of the continuum of care with ownership or partnerships with nursing homes, home care, clinics, doctor's offices, and community services, or it may mean becoming a larger corporation with more hospitals in more communities. Acquisitions are one way to accomplish "instant" growth, to acquire capital, or to become more competitive by increasing market share. Arnold (2004) presents a thoughtful treatise on growth as a corporate strategy,

VIEWPOINTS

arguing that growth is not always more but can mean strengthening and stabilizing of existing assets. Another important point made in Arnold's work is that although corporations manage globally, they market locally. This point is particularly relevant to health care, which is local. Health care is affected by the local community culture, social and economic environment, and the expectations and needs of customers, whether individuals, families, business health programs, or community services. Reducing competition through acquisitions or mergers may have the effect of decreasing competition and diversity in communities, which are matters of interest to the Federal Trade Commission.

THE PROCESS FOR MERGERS, ACQUISITIONS, AND CONSOLIDATION

Mergers and acquisitions bring about periods of intense change and challenges for individuals. Leadership is needed to help employees navigate the change. Information is key, as is having a champion for the change. Each of the involved organizations can be expected to have an established pattern of change. Bringing different change patterns together in the process of early integration helps one understand how the changes will be made over time. How change is made influences the readiness and willingness of employees to participate (Weaver & Sorrells-Jones, 1999). At the executive level the change is significant. A merger, acquisition, or consolidation almost inevitably means changes in the executive management structure. The acquiring corporation may provide organizational services for areas such as human resources and finance, effectively changing the jobs in those areas. Some individuals may lose their jobs, whereas others find that their work has changed significantly. The management structure may change. Some individuals may leave in anticipation of this change, whereas others may not fit the new corporate culture. Yet others are absorbed into the new structure. At the operations level, employees when learning of change may be concerned about their future, particularly in relation to their jobs, their work, their salaries, and their careers. Most employees providing direct patient care have more job security than others because they provide the core business services and they are also in demand. Recognizing that change affects everyone in the situation, well-managed mergers, acquisitions, and consolidations plan for employee involvement in the change.

The eventual success or failure of a merger, acquisition, or consolidation is affected by every step in the process.

Initially, the idea to pursue a merger, acquisition, or consolidation usually takes place in boardrooms or executive suites as part of strategic plan development. Some corporations strategically plan for mergers and acquisitions to meet objectives for growth, to become more competitive, to become more financially stable, to better serve regions or communities, to improve market share through expanded and more diverse services, or to consolidate services to decrease bed capacity and stabilize facilities. An infinite number of reasons exist for pursuing a merger, acquisition, or consolidation, and each situation is different, depending on the community and the organizations involved. A great variety also exists in the types of business arrangements and agreements that can be crafted to achieve these goals. Buyouts, partnerships, joint ventures, and other arrangements are possibilities. The motivation for the merger, acquisition, or consolidation has much to do with public perception of the value of the change. In some cases the beginning exploration of possibilities is a well-kept secret. In other cases, there may be community knowledge of the potential for change. In all cases, communication about potential or pending changes must be planned carefully to ensure that people understand the reasons for the change, are informed, and when appropriate, are involved in decisions surrounding the change and have a place to voice their concerns, ideas, and preferences.

Once the decision to merge or to acquire an organization is made, the due diligence process begins. During this time, every aspect of the target organization is investigated to determine the feasibility of the merger or acquisition. Finance, market share, services, employees, facilities, and community culture are explored in this due diligence process. How the organization is structured and managed and how it performs are analyzed along with the potential for improvements and increased effectiveness of operations and services. Essentially the value of the organization to the acquiring or merging corporation is analyzed to determine whether the merger or the acquisition is in the best interests of the participating groups. Hospitals experiencing financial pressure may have little choice in pursuing the change, and it is not always easy to put a positive face on the merger or acquisition. A hospital may seek to merge or to be acquired for many reasons. Difficulty attracting and retaining physicians, outdated facilities that would require extensive capital investment to renovate, difficulty maintaining market share, availability of labor, and high insurance costs are some of the reasons cited (Byrd & McCue, 2003). Byrd and McCue cite access to capital as one of the primary reasons that not-for-profit hospital boards seek partnerships with others.

Hospitals have been and continue to be stressed in many ways. Low revenues, low profits, shortages of health care professionals, technological advances in health care, changing demands and expectations of the community and individual patients and families, high insurance premiums, low returns on investments, demands for patient safety and transparent quality, and short life cycle for equipment and supplies are only part of the extensive list of factors that stress hospitals today. These stresses are more or less constant over time and are felt by even the most solvent, well-endowed hospital. Thus Byrd and McCue (2003) raise the question, "Can your hospital remain independent?" Advantages they cite include not only access to capital but also the access to management expertise, the potential to achieve economies of scale through joint purchasing of equipment and supplies, increased access to managed care contracts and negotiating leverage with third-party payers, and improved systems for management information and patient billing. Areas for which employees, physicians, and the community should gain commitment from the acquiring company include continuation of all services provided by the hospital, ensuring employment for a given period, development and implementation of a physician recruitment plan, maintaining a community board, and continuing the existing charity care policies. Byrd and McCue recommend a thorough self-assessment by the hospital before it pursues partnerships or business arrangements with others, assuming that the hospital would prefer to remain independent if possible.

Although mergers and acquisitions achieve similar purposes, they are different. Both are complex, but acquisitions tend to be more straightforward than mergers. Mergers usually involve integration of two or more similar businesses into one organization to secure its future or to support growth. Compared with the processes of acquisitions, the processes of merging are long term and often diffuse. The impact of the merger is colored by the reasons for the merger, conditions of the merger, and negotiated terms such as the percentage of ownership and protections for the community and employees. Acquisitions usually are undertaken to expand a business. The acquired business becomes a component of the parent, and the extent of integration varies. In some cases the acquired business may continue in its present state with no major changes other than reporting relationships. In other cases the financial and management structures may change, but the expertise and work processes of the acquired entity remain much the same, largely because the work is different from that of the new owner. Acquiring existing assets, products, or services allows an organization to expand its products and services to customers. Another reason for acquisitions is to establish new distribution channels or expand customer bases useful to build comprehensive services, as in the patient care continuum.

This viewpoint is focused on the traditional hospital and long-term care and home care sectors of the health care industry. Once dominant in the industry, these sectors now are joined by and sometimes overshadowed by emerging health care sectors including specialty hospitals, producers of technology such as devices and information systems, and pharmaceutical companies. Vince Gallaro (2004), in a *Modern Healthcare* article, noted that what he called the "blizzard of deals" is a sure sign of a robust industry in which companies have gotten into the spirit to merge and to acquire. Looking at the health care industry as a whole, $140 billion was exchanged in 652 deals in 2004 compared with $92.8 billion in the previous year. The major themes in his article affirm that merger and acquisition activity is unpredictable; that there is value in becoming bigger to increase negotiating power in financial markets, with government payers, and others; and that there is real advantage in the economies of scale and size. Gallaro clearly states the difference between acquisition to gain assets and consolidation to improve competition and services. Clearly, the health care industry in the broad sense has changed to encompass not only service providers but also the health-related businesses surrounding health care. This broadened perspective of the health care industry has affected the entire industry just as it has been affected by the growth of the for-profit service sector.

As stated before, much of the merger and acquisition activity is taking place in the for-profit sector of the health care industry. The for-profits have the benefit of buying power stemming from stock offerings and access to credit. Many companies seek opportunities to purchase hospitals to improve profitability. Strategies used to increase profits are well honed and can be applied to newly acquired hospitals. Improving the facility, garnering efficiencies of scale and management approaches, and brand name advertising and customer service design are some of the ways that the for-profit sector approaches mergers and acquisitions. Many communities report satisfaction with the acquisitions, noting that they have expanded services, do not have to travel to receive selected specialty services, enjoy improved financial status, and prove to be an asset to the community economy. In many cases the hospital is the largest single employer in some communities (Kirchheimer, 2001). Attitudes about for-profits have changed over the years. The for-profits are anchored in the industry. Private, not-for-profit hospitals, often reluctantly are selling to or joining with for-profits in various types of partnerships. The broadening of the definition of health care industry and the inclusion of the for-profit sector have changed the perspective of business in health care. It seems inevitable that health care will adapt to other business practices as they emerge.

ONCE THE DECISION IS MADE

The decision to merge, to be acquired or to acquire, or to consolidate is never easy. Once the decision is made to change based on positive due diligence information, self-assessment, and strategic business goals, the development of a strategic approach to making and closing the deal and to beginning the implementation of the decision is critical. In this phase, communication is the key to success. Uncertainty prevails until the deal is closed. Employees and the community continue to experience uncertainty during the implementation of the merger or acquisition. Planning strategically for this phase of mergers and acquisitions requires attention to leadership and communication, the two factors that have the greatest impact on eventual success or failure of the merger or acquisition. Leadership and communication influence employee readiness and willingness to change. As noted before, employee attitude is a key factor in the success or failure of mergers, acquisitions, and consolidation. Employment of firms experienced in mergers and acquisitions to assist with strategic planning and implementation is common practice. Many firms now specialize in health care mergers and acquisitions and have developed approaches to facilitate the implementation process. Seeking this help is often important because the leaders of the organization must deal with the organization, with the change, and with employees, a tall order at best. However, trusted leaders are influential in these processes, which involve complex planning, implementing, and sustaining a merger or an acquisition.

Resources for these leaders include consultation, anecdotal information from peers and colleagues, case studies of other mergers or acquisitions, and business analysis.

The capability to work diligently to achieve an effective merger or acquisition challenges leadership. Positive attitudes toward change and the ability to support others in the change processes are required to lead employees and community members in the changes associated with mergers or acquisitions. Many leaders must come to grips with their own values and beliefs to deal effectively with leading a merger or acquisition. For example, views differ about growth as a corporate goal. Schulman (2004) expresses the notion that a new growth model is needed for corporate America. In his view, mergers and acquisitions are for many executives a fast track to expansion and personal gain. He puts forth the argument that organic growth is preferable to acquired growth. Organic growth from within strengthens the organization. Mass (2005) explores the relative value of growth in terms of chief executive officer performance. Is growth or increased margin the most important? Other authors relate growth to innovation and savvy managing of the growth agenda for businesses (Gulati et al., 2004). Leaders who would prefer to remain independent must come to terms with the meaning of growth, the expectations of performance, and the real situation of the organization when determining the value of some type of merger partnership or of being acquired. Leaders who have made these deliberations thoughtfully are in a better position to help others accept and adapt to changes.

Mergers and acquisitions present a leadership challenge. Charismatic leadership is key in successful mergers and in acquisitions, although difficult in the latter (Waldman, 2004). Waldman presents a model for chief executive officer charismatic leadership. In the premerger phase the chief executive officer is engaged in organizational differentiation, that is describing and accounting for the key features of the assets and due diligence processes, and in differentiation of cultures. The first, organizational differentiation, is used to plan for postmerger integration throughout the organization. The second is used to integrate cultures between and among the merged entities. Organizational and cultural factors are considered and used to plan change strategies, which influence resistance to change and ultimately the success or failure of the merger. This model is not as applicable to acquisitions because leadership may change depending on the approach to the acquisition. In this case, integration is the predominant theme for planning change.

Although leaders are negotiating the terms of mergers and acquisitions over time, they also must be providing clear communication appropriate to the various groups affected by the merger or acquisition. Each group—the board, the community, health care professionals, all employees, colleagues in the industry, the media, and others—has a different interest and agenda and needs information tailored to that agenda. To be effective, a communication plan must carry the core message in terms appropriate for each target group. One should note that during merger or acquisition negotiations, providing appropriate information in a timely way can be complex, particularly if the negotiations are limited to a few individuals behind closed doors because of competition or other issues. The phases of negotiation can be communicated. Usually mergers and acquisitions are negotiated in phases, beginning with the business portfolio, followed by integration of personnel and processes of the organization. Most employees and many community members have difficulty waiting for the business side to be completed because their interests lie in the personnel and processes of the organization.

INTEGRATION

When organizations come together through mergers, acquisitions, or one of the many forms of partnerships, a new organization is formed through integration. A number of different integration approaches may be used. Ellis (2004) conducted a study of approaches to acquisitions to determine their impact on acquisition success. The following are the four approaches selected for in-depth study:

◆ *The preservation approach* results in minimum change for the targeted organization. In this approach the organization continues functioning as it did before being merged or acquired. The staff of the target organization has decision-making autonomy and may consider suggestions or recommendations from the corporate parent. The parent provides organizational resources to improve operations as needed.

◆ *The absorption approach* involves preintegration planning to absorb the target organization into the parent organization and management structures. Key integration issues are identified and negotiated as part of the deal, and employees and other stakeholders receive information throughout the process on a timely basis. A calendar of events with timetables is provided along with information to minimize uncertainty and to speed up the process. The transition is planned to move into the new structure, usually within an aggressive time frame.

◆ *The symbiotic approach* facilitates a period of getting to know one another. The target and parent firm spend time to learn about each other's organization and processes and then use this information to plan organizational changes that are implemented gradually. The goal is to blend both firms to create interdependent organizations through cooperation, shared organizational responsibility, and development of transition paced to the situation.

◆ *The transformational approach* focuses on best practices of each organization and may involve changes in organizational culture and operations. This approach uses transition to move from the existing to the new values, organizational structure, practices, and processes. Usually a plan for transformation is developed as part of the negotiations, and a strategic vision, goals, and plans for the new companies are communicated. Managers of both organizations are involved in establishing and participating in transition activities.

Study results indicated that in many ways, no significant differences were found in the outcomes related to one of these four approaches. The transformational approach was found to result in the more detailed planning, prioritizing, identification of best practices, and collaboration than the other approaches. Better understanding of what approaches work best in specific types of situations will be informed by future research. At this time, the value of strategic planning, leadership, communication, and attending to the human factor in the merger, acquisition, or consolidation appears to be imperatives for success.

The success of mergers or acquisitions often is evaluated on the degree of integration achieved. Some mergers or acquisitions are successful; some are not. When two or more organizations merge or when an organization is acquired, the goals of integration are to improve productivity, cost-effectiveness, quality, and consistency in services in addition to the profitability and growth goals that usually drive the merger initially. For health care professionals, a successful merger, acquisition, or consolidation is marked by improved and expanded services that meet the needs of the community, patients, families, and significant others for health and for care when needed. Health care professionals are drawn to organizations that value accessible, patient-centered care that uses the best technology and that is provided in an environment that values patients and employees.

In some of the early mergers or acquisitions within health care there was an expectation that clinical integration would follow naturally once the financial and organizational leadership issues were resolved. This expectation did not prove to be the case in practice. Clinical integration continues to be difficult. The various cultures and financial aspects of clinical services are often barriers to integration. A key issue is lack of clarity on the meaning of clinical integration (Formella & Balner, 1999), which continues to be defined in various ways. In some situations clinical integration refers to access to linked services in the continuum of care. In others, integration refers to multidisciplinary standardization of care processes, technology, and patient safety/quality processes. Perhaps even more significant than definition is the nature of hospital organizations and the way people who work within them perceive themselves and each other. Peter Drucker (2002) cites hospitals as an example of the splintered organization. He writes that hospitals are "altogether the most complex human organization ever devised" (p. 118). In Drucker's analysis, about half of the hospital workers are knowledge workers, with nurses and specialists in business departments among the largest of the groups. Each type of knowledge worker has a specialty, with its own rules, requirements, and accreditation. Each type needs and wants administrative support and understanding. Because of the specialized knowledge and small numbers of many of the professionals in a given specialty, there are few opportunities to further one's career. At the height of the restructuring movement, these specialties were referred to as "silos." A continuing challenge in hospitals—whether they are independent, merging, or being acquired or acquiring—is collaboration and cooperation among the knowledge workers and all employees to achieve organizational wholeness, which is as good a definition as any for clinical integration.

The variation in cultures and operational processes within health care entities continues to confound the issue of clinical integration. As indicated, one strategy to gain participation and support of employees is to negotiate aspects of integration in the negotiating phase, with continued work on detailed planning and prioritizing in the implementation phases. Key elements important in integration are retaining key employees and maintaining consistency in community services during the change. Incentives are needed to retain talent during times of change. Another compelling reason for retaining employees is that employees throughout the organization have the priceless "organizational memory," a valuable commodity in organizations. This employee memory is aligned closely with employee loyalty, a valuable asset in any organization.

Employees accepting of change can ask the right questions about the logic of the change and about the work processes, which can save time and resources as the merger or acquisition unfolds.

THE HUMAN FACTOR

Influence of the human factor on the outcome of a merger, acquisition, or consolidation now is recognized and valued. This human factor applies to a variety of groups and individuals involved with or affected by the change in some way. For example, the human factor applies to the board, which makes the ultimate decision to merge, to acquire, or to be acquired. Board members are key stakeholders and leaders in determining the vision and strategies for the organization who guide decision making. Board members are responsible to the community and sponsors and thus may be conflicted about change. The future of the board often is negotiated in the premerger or preacquisition discussions. Thus board members are informed and privy to decisions that directly affect them and the organization. Often the board recommends and/or approves not only the terms of the deal but also the preprocesses and postprocesses including communications, naming the new organization, and shaping the new culture for the changed organization. In all of these scenarios, to be the acquiring is easier than to be the acquired. Many health care organizations have deep historical roots that are meaningful in the organization and the community served. One strategy is to retain presence of community leaders in facilities, on committees, and in other ways to exhibit valuing of their contribution and of their importance. The support of these leaders influences responses of others and thus the impact of the change.

The community benefit of a hospital has been a subject of inquiry for the past several years. Not only do hospitals provide a source of employment and economic stability for communities, but also they attract businesses, families, and events that depend on or value access to health care. Health care is local, and people within a community may have strong feelings about their community hospital. Thus community members, organizations, and groups are important to the success or failure of change in that these people are the customer base, the employee pool, and contributors to events and fund-raising activities of hospitals and related social, public welfare groups. The unique interdependence between communities and their health care organizations is grounded in the interdependence. Health care is an essential community service, providing help and support. Most hospitals reach out to the community to provide help and advice on key health issues, to support action on population needs for health care, and to participate in or sponsor projects to improve community health. Because health care is integral to the community life, mergers or acquisitions evoke community response and reactions. Community leaders may block a merger or acquisition or may support the change fully, depending on their perspective. The community accountability is a strong countervailing force in deliberations about mergers and acquisitions.

Mergers and acquisitions affect employees at every level. Job security is a major issue for individuals whose jobs are affected by mergers and acquisitions. Job identity is as strong an issue for many when they perceive that their role or function will be altered significantly in the merger or acquisition. Typically, administrative and management positions are most vulnerable in mergers or acquisitions, but employees in all types of positions usually share feelings of vulnerability about their jobs, relationships, and future employment, even in times of shortages of health care workers in their specialty or profession. Employees are aware that in many situations, the hospital or health care system is a financial driver, and any changes in the hospital or health system are likely to affect other aspects of the community economy and thus the lives and well-being of their families, friends, and neighbors.

Nursing now is recognized as an important asset in hospitals. Nurse executives participate in the teams involved in decision making about mergers, acquisitions, or consolidation and provide invaluable knowledge and resources regarding clinical practices; patient requirements for care; multidisciplinary care requirements and needs; the priorities for technology, equipment, devices, and supplies; and most importantly the valuing and recognition of employees at every level. Nurse leaders contribute to the success of mergers and acquisitions through knowledge transfer and learning processes. Their contacts are developed and enhanced through participation in shared governance multidisciplinary teams, affinity groups, networking groups, professional associations, and interaction with colleagues. Many nurses are engaged in identifying and sharing best practices across organizations and within organizations and multidisciplinary team work, affinity groups, and colleague networking. Many serve as the leaders in development of case management, patient safety, quality, and customer service initiatives that are imperatives in today's health care environment.

Experiences over the past decade have prepared nurses to accept and to shape change. Changes in health care have necessitated development of new models for care delivery and new management structures that more closely resemble the new "boundaryless" organization. In fact, in many situations, nurses' vision has outpaced the rate of change (Ashkenas, Ulrich, Todd, & Kerr, 2002).

Recognition that the human factor is significant in merger or acquisition outcomes has led to study of factors that favorably affect success. Not unexpectedly, intangibles often have been found to be more important than the tangible assets or features of mergers and acquisitions. These intangibles may be highly personal or may be imbedded in culture and are therefore difficult to identify and to study. What is known, however, is that strategic readiness for change involved human capital, information capital, and organization capital (Kaplan & Norton, 2004). Those who have studied quality outcomes and processes have learned never to underestimate the value of or the importance of learning, teamwork, and loyalty to mission and values. Informed integration of organizations that are merging or in the acquiring process builds on this knowledge. Coaching and team development for managers, ongoing education and interactive groups for employees, and focus on assets related to the core business of patient care are part of the integration process. In many ways the integration of organizations in the merger or acquisition processes is similar to the processes many organizations use to create the organization of the future. The positive side of mergers and acquisitions is that they provide opportunities for planned and well-executed change to improve patient care, thereby improving nurse, physician, and employee satisfaction. They also provide the opportunity to examine and revise, discard or renew processes and structures that serve to support individuals who provide and receive the care. Standardization is now part of the move toward patient safety and quality. Standardization now is expected of all and is no longer a threatening factor in mergers and acquisitions.

Change is inevitable in mergers, acquisitions, and consolidation. Nursing leadership is challenged to provide direction, to keep the focus on professional nursing practice, and to ensure that the standards of clinical nursing practice are upheld as the tools, procedures, and supports are assessed and adapted to the new organization. Futuristic leaders recognize the opportunity to analyze the change and to identify or recognize opportunities to strengthen or enhance clinical patient care. The statement that corporatization of health care provides an entrée for nursing to strengthen and expand the clinical care role of nurses (Beyers, 1999) is affirmed by recent challenges to create a new environment for nursing practice that effectively uses new technology, multidisciplinary participation, and resources to provide innovative, quality, and safe care. Nurses are in a good position to design patient care services, to evaluate the quality of patient care services, and to debate the issues of health care rights. Nurses are also well positioned to debate the issues not only of how to finance health care but also of how the resources should be deployed in the evolving health care system. To move toward this future, nursing will be pressed to ensure a strong financial and business base for nursing services. As with any service, the success of the financial and business base depends on the quality of the service. Designing quality patient care services continues to be an essential role for nurse administrators. The business and finance aspects can be viewed as tools to accomplish the goals of the patient service design.

Nurses also are aware of the "human condition" in the communities they serve. In many cases, people in these communities require health services that do not have a cost or price. These services, which may be categorized as public or community service, are just as important as the reimbursed services. Consequently, nurses should consider carefully whether it is prudent fully to buy in to the business approaches that achieve health care corporatization. Some community health care services such as the outreach programs do not fit the corporate business model. Yet these services are important to the health care mission. Nurses have long served as the conscience of health care. Nurses are with patients 24 hours a day, in every setting where health care is delivered. Patients trust nurses. Nurses are perceived to be patient advocates because they put the patient first. Nurses understand what patients experience in their health care complexity. Nurses know that some of the most salient aspects of health care do not have a price, cannot be packaged or branded, and would not be considered useful for leverage or other business purposes. Nurses relate to and speak for the human condition, which transcends corporatization.

REFERENCES

American Hospital Association. (2005). *Trend watch.* Chicago, IL: Author.

Arnold, D. (2004). *The mirage of global markets: How globalizing companies can succeed as markets localize.* Upper Saddle River, NJ: Prentice Hall.

Ashkenas, R., Ulrich, D., Todd, J., & Kerr, S. (2002). *The boundaryless organization.* San Francisco: Jossey-Bass.

Beyers, M. (1999). The future of nursing. In R. W. Gilkey (Ed.), *The 21st century health care leader* (pp. 278-289). San Francisco: Jossey-Bass.

Byrd, C.W., Jr., & McCue, M. J. (2003). Can your hospital remain independent? *Healthcare Financial Management, 57*(9), 40-44.

Drucker, P. F. (2002). *Managing in the next society* (p. 118). New York: St. Martin Press.

Ellis, K. M. (2004). Managing the acquisition process: Do differences actually exist across integration approaches? (pp. 111-132). In A. L. Pablo (Ed.), *Mergers and acquisitions: Creating integrative knowledge.* Malden, MA: Blackwell Publishing.

Formella, N. M., & Balner, J. (1999). Role transitions for patient care vice presidents: From a single entity to a system focus. *Journal of Nursing Administration, 29*(4), 11-17.

Gallaro, V. (2004). Blizzard of deals: In a sure sign of robust industry, companies recently have gotten in the spirit to merge and acquire. *Modern Healthcare, 34*(12), 6.

Gulati, R., Freeman, K. W., Nolen, G., Tyson, J., Lewis, K. D., & Greifeld, R. (2004). How CEOs manage growth agendas. *Harvard Business Review, 82*(7/8), 124-132.

Health Care Advisory Board. (2005). *New report shows hospital mergers, acquisitions up 136% in 2004.* Retrieved February 11, 2004, from http://www.advisory.com/members

Kaplan, R. S., & Norton, D. P. (2004). Measuring the strategic readiness of intangible assets. *Harvard Business Review, 82*(2), 52-63.

Kirchheimer, B. (2001). Acquisition binge: The sequel: Flush with cash, for-profit chains are once again buying and rebuilding hospitals. *Modern Healthcare, 31*(4), 50.

Larsson, R., Brousseau, K. R., Driver, M. M., & Sweet, P. L. (2004). The secrets of merger and acquisition success: A co-competence and motivational approach to synergy realization (pp 7-19). In A. L. Pablo (Ed.), *Mergers and acquisitions: Creating integrative knowledge.* Malden, MA: Blackwell Publishing.

Mass, N. N. (2005). The relative value of growth. *Harvard Business Review, 83*(4), 102-112.

Nahass, G. (2005). *Merger integration in Silicon Valley? Part three, integration management structure.* Retrieved February 16, 2005, from http://www.pwc.com/extweb/execpers.nsf/docid/C67411C724D9CE6B85257019007D1305

Pitofsky, R. (1998). *Statement of the Federal Trade Commission. Presented by Robert Pitofsky, chairman, before the Committee on the Judiciary, United States Senate, concerning mergers and corporate consolidation in the New Economy, June 16, 1998, Washington, D.C.* Retrieved July 28, 2005, from http://www.ftc.gov/os/1998/06/merger98.tes.htm

Schulman, J. M. (2004). *Getting bigger by growing smaller: A new growth model for corporate America.* Upper Saddle River, NJ: Prentice Hall.

Waldman, D. A. (2004). The role of CEO charismatic leadership in effective implementation of mergers and acquisitions (pp. 194-211). In A. L. Pablo (Ed.), *Mergers and acquisitions: Creating integrative knowledge*. Malden, MA: Blackwell Publishing.

Weaver, D., & Sorrells-Jones, J. (1999). Knowledge workers and knowledge-intense organizations, Part 2. *Journal of Nursing Administration, 29*(9), 19-25.

Nurse Practitioners

Issues Within a Managed Care Environment

RUFUS HOWE

Few care settings have been more challenging for the nurse practitioner than the managed care environment. Managed care and nurse practitioners have "grown up" together, and as this chapter shows, there are still significant issues to resolve on both sides. The purpose of this chapter is to give the reader a sense of what managed care is at its roots and how nurse practitioners are fitting in and could fit within the managed care model.

MANAGED CARE EVOLUTION

Although the origins of managed care can be traced back to the establishment of prepaid health plans in the early 1900s, the movement really accelerated with two significant milestones. In the early 1970s, Dr. Paul Elwood coined the term *health maintenance organization*. Dr. Elwood and his Jackson Hole Group recognized that traditional fee-for-service arrangements were causing spiraling health care expenditures without a commensurate increase in health care quality (Ellwood, 2001). In 1973, Congress passed the Health Maintenance Organization Act and supplied start-up funds for health plans to begin offering health insurance products (Uylhara & Thomas, 1975). The intent of this act was to provide incentives to providers to contain costs by reducing unnecessary care and to concentrate on best practices. Over the next decade, managed care and Congress lifted certain limitations on the original legislation that prompted rapid changes resulting in a growth of insured lives from 6.3 million in 1977 to 29.3 million in 1987 (Kongstvedt, 1997). Today, more than 115 million patients are covered by managed care organizations in the United States, and approximately 70% of all physicians work with at least one managed care organization, although

many work with more than 12 at one time (MacLeod, 1994).

MANAGED CARE STRUCTURE

Managed care began with a vision to provide health care to an enrolled population that would satisfy the provider and the patient. This vision was to be accomplished through forming provider cooperatives called networks that would charge discounted rates for their services to the sponsoring managed care organization. The enrollees would benefit through this arrangement by paying less for their health care through the power of being a member of a risk pool. This vision demanded a two-pronged approach to health care financial (transactional) mechanisms that would ensure that fees were fair and equitable and that clinical mechanisms would ensure the highest quality care possible. Over time, other managed care structures emerged as the industry emerged and were formed largely as a market reaction to changes in customer preferences and financial issues. Today, the three main kinds of managed care plans are health maintenance organization, preferred provider organization, and traditional indemnity.

Health Maintenance Organizations

Health maintenance organizations were the first model for managed care. In a health maintenance organization, patients select a primary provider from a prearranged network of providers. This primary care provider functions as the gateway from which all care is delivered, including to which procedures and specialists patients have access. This arrangement otherwise is known as a gatekeeper model. The advantage of this model is price. Health maintenance organization pricing is generally the lowest cost option because the patient trades the choice of providers for a flat-fee, one-provider model.

Preferred Provider Organizations

For a higher premium, preferred provider organizations allow the patient to select within a preferred provider group. In some cases, these providers have been pre-selected because they have the best care quality profile and are willing to accept discounted charges from the health plan. In the preferred provider organization model, there is no gatekeeper. The patient determines which providers to see and when to see them.

Traditional Indemnity Model

In the traditional indemnity model the health plan pays for any provider a patient sees at the rate the provider charges. This model most closely matches how care was delivered before the advent of managed care. Although this model has the most flexibility, the cost to the patient is significantly higher. The current Medicare model is a traditional indemnity model.

It is safe to say that the rise of managed care organizations is related directly to the rapid rise of health care expenditures. For a 20-year span, health care expenditures increased from 10% to 13% a year—far outpacing inflation (Health Care Financing Administration, n.d.). A Wall Street analysis of managed care reveals that profit margins are expanding slowly, premium prices have undergone double-digit increases over the past 5 years, the commercial market is offering more flexible plans to accommodate for changing market preferences, and many are reducing their penetration in the Medicare supplemental market (Healthcare Financial Management, 2003).

MANAGED CARE TAXONOMY

Managed care has its own set of terms that nurse practitioners must understand to work with the system. What follows is a sample of the key managed care terms:

◆ *Capitation:* A fixed amount of money—or allotment—per patient given to the provider per year and regardless of the number of services the patient uses. This is a budgeted amount that depends on there being an average cost across a given provider panel. In a capitated model, the provider receives incentives to limit unnecessary use of tests, specialists, or in some cases medications.

◆ *Coinsurance:* A portion of a health care premium that is paid by the insured.

◆ *Co-payment:* A set amount paid by the insured after the deductible is paid. In most cases the co-payment is based on care setting. Office visit co-payments are generally much less expensive than emergency department co-payments. Co-payments also are applied to medications in a tiered fashion. This is done to encourage the use of generic drugs or lower-cost medications over the newer, more expensive ones that may or may not result in better efficacy.

◆ *Covered lives:* The total number of persons in a health plan or a component of the health plan.

◆ *Deductible:* The amount that must be paid before the insurance plan begins its benefits.

◆ *Employer contribution:* The amount an employer contributes to the health insurance premium.

◆ *Exclusions:* Health conditions not covered by a health plan. Exclusions sometimes are known as preexisting conditions and are meant to not skew the risk pool adversely.

◆ *Fee-for-service:* This is another way to describe the traditional indemnity design. Fee-for-service is best thought of as "pay as you go."

◆ *Maximum out-of-pocket costs:* Health insurance plans place a limit on the total amount of money they will make patients pay for their care for a specified amount of time. This mechanism is meant as a protection for the insured and is covered financially by reinsurance companies that provide insurance to health plans to soften the financial burden of very high-cost patients.

◆ *Network:* A preset group of providers (physicians, hospitals, laboratories, pharmacies, durable medical equipment companies, skilled nursing facilities, rehabilitation facilities) that have agreed to the health plan negotiated rates.

◆ *PHO (physician hospital organization):* This organization is a group or cooperative of physicians who have banded together for the purpose of selling their services to a health plan.

◆ *Precertification:* Most health plans require a provider to seek approval for nonemergent elective procedures, surgeries, and sometimes medications before they are performed. Precertification process usually use established best practice guidelines to ensure the service is indicated and follows the most cost-effective process.

◆ *Preexisting condition:* A condition, such as human immunodeficiency virus infection, renal failure, or diabetes that existed before one applied for health insurance. Although the list of conditions vary, most health plans have such a list and are allowed to deny health plan membership based on the applicant having one of these conditions.

◆ *Premium:* The cost of health insurance to the patient.

◆ *Preventive care:* From a health plan perspective, preventive care includes any service that may prevent a patient from becoming ill. Screening examinations such as prostate tests, mammograms, Pap smears, screening colonoscopies, and well-baby care are examples. Lower-priced health plan products may not cover these services.

◆ *Provider:* Providers are defined broadly as persons (e.g., physicians, nurse practitioners, and physical therapists) and places (e.g., hospitals and skilled nurse facilities). In each case, the health plan has specific contractual agreements.

◆ *TPA (third-party administrator):* A company that administers claims processing and payment on behalf of an employer. In most cases the care management (clinical) aspects of the benefit are an add-on or are covered by another entity.

NURSE PRACTITIONER EVOLUTION

What started 30 years ago at the University of Colorado as training for pediatric nurse practitioners for the rural population is today more than 49,000 nurse practitioners in all manner of settings, specialties, and locations. Nurse practitioners are regarded as advance practice nurses along with nurse anesthetists, clinical nurse specialists, and midwives.

Although nurse practitioners are subject to individual State Boards of Nursing or in some cases boards of medicine, the basic premise of what a nurse practitioner is trained to do remains the same. Nurse practitioners are trained to "assess, counsel, diagnose, prescribe, and manage the primary needs of a caseload of clients in collaboration with other care professionals" (American Nurses Association, 1996, pp. 21-31).

Nurse practitioners have always practiced in primary care roles and have managed simple to complex cases. Over the years the educational preparation and work experience have combined to ensure the highest degree of clinical competence. Nurse practitioners manage health via careful history taking, physical assessment, and interpretation of a wide variety of laboratory and procedural tests. They are expected to synthesize clinical data to come to a reasonable diagnostic conclusion and then to render a plan that is sensitive to individual preferences and situations.

Nurse practitioner credentialing has evolved into four national certification groups:

◆ American Nurses Credentialing Center
◆ National Certifying Board of Pediatric Nurse Practitioners
◆ American Academy of Nurse Practitioners
◆ National Certification Corporation

Each of these certifications requires retesting every 5 to 6 years or regular clinical experience within the nurse's scope of practice.

Nurse practitioner salary data for 2003 indicate that the average annual pay is $69,203, well below a board-certified family practice or internal medicine physician (Advance for Nurse Practitioners, 2005). Even though a gap exists in market value, there appears to be a positive trend toward market recognition of the nurse practitioner's worth. A direct correlation between salary level and practice setting exists. Nurse practitioners who work in acute care facilities or those who own their own business tend to earn more than those who are embedded in a physician-run general practice.

Managed care organizations are often reluctant to contract with a nurse practitioner–owned business without evidence of physician collaboration. In many states, nurse practitioners pay collaboration fees that satisfy this requirement. Under this arrangement a physician charges a fee for whatever the regulation or contract requires. This might mean a monthly chart review procedure and availability for consultation. In practice, nurse practitioner charts are more comprehensive (Lenz, Mundinger, Hopkins, Lin, & Smolowitz, 2002) and rarely will need physician consultation. This arrangement varies with state regulatory boards. Eight states do not have a collaboration clause in their regulations. Oregon is one of the more lenient states in this regard. The Oregon nurse practitioner statutes state, "The nurse practitioner is responsible for recognizing limits of knowledge and experience and for resolving situations beyond his/her NP expertise by consulting with or referring clients to other health care providers" (Oregon Secretary of State, n.d.).

Nurse practitioners also shine in their ability to adhere to published standards of care in their practice. In several studies (Fain & Melkus, 1994; Larne & Pugh, 1998), the overall rate of compliance was shown to be inconsistent in physician and nurse practitioner groups, but in the Lenz et al. studies (2002), the documentation of certain diabetic standards of care was higher for the nurse practitioner group. This and other similar factors should increase the attractiveness of nurse practitioners to managed care because of their reliance on health employer data and information set (HEDIS) scores to gain accreditation. The data set HEDIS is used by the National Committee for Quality Assurance to assess and monitor the quality of health care services provided in managed care arrangements.

It would seem that for the nurse practitioner or, for that matter, any lower cost primary provider, that the environment is ripe for increased exposure and stature. Certainly the literature demonstrates that nurse practitioners are at least on par with, if not better than, their physician counterparts in health care outcomes, cost, and satisfaction (Mason et al., 1999; Mundinger et al., 2000; Perry, 1995; Salkever, 1982). Even when nurse practitioners are studied in acute care settings, the traditional domain of physicians, they fair well. Rudy et al. (1998) showed in their study on care activities and outcomes of patients cared for by acute care nurse practitioners that there were no market differences between the nurse practitioners and physicians.

From a managed care perspective, this should be good news for nurse practitioners. Unfortunately, barriers remain to entry to practice. After all, if the managed care organization is able to reduce the cost of delivering services—that is, charges for office visits without a loss in health care quality—then it is reasonable to believe that a credible provider of primary care services such as a nurse practitioner would be welcomed.

MANAGED CARE ORGANIZATION CONTRACTING

Many health plans reimburse nurse practitioners if they are under the direct supervision of a physician and do not directly contract with them. The following text extracted from Tufts Health Plan (2003) in Boston, Massachusetts, is a typical example of this policy and illustrates the barriers to professional recognition faced by nurse practitioners:

> Tufts Health Plan reimburses medically necessary services performed by a Nurse Practitioner (NP) or a Physician Assistant (PA), when care is provided under the supervision of a participating Tufts Health Plan physician. Tufts Health Plan does not contract directly with NP's or PAs in Massachusetts. It is the responsibility of the supervising physician to educate the NP and PA on all Tufts Health Plan policies, procedures and guidelines. The supervising physician is responsible for maintaining appropriate state licensing information for all NPs and PAs under his or her supervision. The supervising physician must also maintain proof of appropriate professional malpractice liability insurance coverage for all NPs and PAs under his or her supervision.

REIMBURSEMENT

Nurse practitioners and physician assistants are reimbursed according to the Tufts Health Plan contracted rate of the supervising physician that is submitted on the claim, regardless of where the service is rendered. Claims are subject to payment edits that are updated at regular intervals and generally are based on Centers for Medicare and Medicaid Services specialty society guidelines and correct coding initiative.

Despite a wealth of supporting and positive evidence of the efficiency and efficacy of nurse practitioner practice, nurse practitioners continue to experience difficulty blending into the professional practice environment. According to a recent American Academy of Nurse Practitioners survey completed in April 2003, more than 41% of nurse practitioners reported they had problems with recognition as a primary care provider, 25% with recognition for pharmacy distribution, and 17% with receipt of samples. In other words, 83% of nurse practitioners had problems with the things that put them in good standing with a managed care organization.

Reimbursement options for nurse practitioners vary across managed care contracts, but they are all restrictive. On a positive note, the U.S. Balanced Budget Act of 1997 allowed reimbursement of nurse practitioners for all settings, yet fell short by setting the payment rate at only 85% of physicians. All types of managed care organizations pay nurse practitioners less than physicians for the same services (Buppert, 1998). The lower reimbursement rates make it difficult for the nurse practitioners to establish their own business, practice, and caseload.

Nurse practitioners are a revenue/profit provider, not a liability. In many arrangements, nurse practitioners are salaried employees within a physician practice, cloaking the profit impact. The fact is that nurse practitioners typically are giving away their economic value under this arrangement. Buppert and Billing (2002) estimate that given the usual nurse practitioner salary and workload numbers, the practice will make $69,500 per nurse practitioner in profit after accounting for salary and overhead. If the relationship between the nurse practitioner and the "collaborating" physician were different, the profit would go to the nurse practitioner, not the practice.

Because the payer environment is not favorable, the onus is on the nurse practitioner to understand clearly the state licensing agreements, state health regulations, managed care contracting language, upcoming legislation, and finally negotiation strategies.

MEDICARE

Medicare is the government version of a traditional indemnity form of managed care and represents a growing number of high-use beneficiaries over 65 years old. Medicare recognizes nurse practitioners as providers as long as they meet the following requirements:

1. They meet Medicare nurse practitioner qualification requirements. Starting in January 2003, nurse practitioners must have a master's-level preparation and national certification.
2. The practice that hired the nurse practitioner must accept Medicare payments at the 85% rate off the physician's scheduled charges.
3. The claimed services are the same as that for which a physician would bill.
4. There must be a collaborative agreement with a physician.
5. The nurse practitioner must stay within the scope of practice of the state.

The ultimate goal is for the nurse practitioner to be able to bill the payer directly, thus tying the service to the source of the service (McCloskey, Grey, Deshefy-Longhi, & Grey, 2003). A related goal is for the nurse practitioner to have a unique provider number. This number differs from a Drug Enforcement Administration prescribing authority number. The unique provider number is awarded per managed care or payer contract. Physicians typically have many provider numbers, one per payer source.

It is said, "Law leads change." Specifically, nurse practitioner state scope of practice language should be updated or addressed to reflect the current nurse practitioner practice. Nurse practitioners and physicians are captive to a system with 50 separate state codes with differing agendas and needs. Federal legal codes are mired in language that in some cases is more than 30 years old—before the emergence of nurse practitioners. This situation creates confusion, conflict of interest, and loss of health care potential.

NURSE PRACTITIONER MANAGED CARE STRATEGIES

Nurse Practitioner as Independent Contractor

Medicare allows nurse practitioners to be independent contractors if the supervising physician changes the practice type from sole practitioner to group practice. The nurse practitioner then can perform Medicare-authorized services such as nursing home, hospital, or home visits and any other assessment and diagnostic procedures approved by the state scope of practice. For the instances that nurse practitioners are working independently, they can bill under their unique provider number. When the nurse practitioner is working in the office and under physician supervision, the nurse practitioner must use the physician's provider number for billing.

Obtaining Status as a Managed Care Panel or Network Provider

A nurse practitioner should strive to be a unique provider recognized within a managed care provider network. This benefits the entire practice by ensuring that the managed care organization acknowledges the presence and role of the nurse practitioner, thus limiting the liability inherent in an implied provider relationship. Other positives include increasing panel size of the practice, broadening the services of the practice, and creating more clinical value for the insured patients.

According to Buppert and Billing (2002), the following checklist is helpful when one is attempting to change the managed care organization policy to allow nurse practitioners to be network providers:

1. Ascertain whether state law allows nurse practitioners to be managed care providers.
2. Identify the individual or individuals at the managed care organization who can make the decision to change company policy.
3. Ask for a meeting and present the case for empanelment of nurse practitioners.
4. In the meeting, ask what stands in the way of nurse practitioners getting on provider panels.
5. Address the barriers to empanelment with the provider panels.
6. Work with the appropriate individuals or committees to effect policy change. The entity most likely to persuade a managed care organization to change its policy is a large employer that purchases health services through the managed care organization.
7. If policy does not change, follow up with the organization every 6 months asking, "What stands in the way of nurse practitioners getting on provider panels?"

MINUTECLINIC

One of the most promising programs for nurse practitioners is the MinuteClinics in St. Paul, Minnesota, and Baltimore, Maryland. Staffed by nurse practitioners and physician assistants, the clinics are prepared to treat a wide variety of acute minor illnesses and to provide routine testing and vaccines (Box 45-1). Often these

BOX 45-1

Example Treatments, Screenings, and Vaccinations Provided by MinuteClinics

TREATMENTS AND SCREENINGS

Allergy testing
Athlete's foot
Bronchitis
Cold sores
Deer tick bites
Ear infections
Female bladder infections
Flu treatment
Laryngitis
Minor skin infections
Mononucleosis
Pink eye and styes
Poison ivy
Ringworm
Seasonal allergies
Sinus infections
Strep throat, rapid test
Swimmer's ear

VACCINES

Hepatitis B (child and adult)
Pneumonia
Tetanus, diphtheria

clinics are located in consumer-friendly locations such as department stores and employer campuses. Care is delivered through carefully constructed evidence-based guidelines that include standard therapies and indicators for referral when the clinical picture is more complex. The company has invested in a clinical information system that contains the clinical protocols and knows when a patient has a pattern of repeat infections that will trigger a referral to a specialist.

The premise for the clinics is simple enough, and the combination of the right care at the right time and at the right cost is winning over quite a few people. The clinics are strictly walk-in (no appointments). Patients usually are seen quickly, and the appointments last no longer than 15 minutes. Managed care organizations are supporting this clinic model because the cost difference between traditional care settings and MinuteClinics is significant. Consider a weekend visit for a sore throat with fever, for example. If the patient were lucky enough to have a doctor that offers weekend clinic hours, the average cost would be $109, and the more likely emergency department visit would cost $329, whereas a MinuteClinic visit is only $48. This represents a significant savings for

all concerned. The patient saves the more expensive insurance co-payment, and the insurance company saves $61 and $281, respectively. One can see how this care model would be attractive once the benefit is calculated over the number of insured lives. A few health plans are so excited about this concept that they provide incentives for the use of these clinics through lower co-payment arrangements.

MEDICARE CHRONIC CARE IMPROVEMENT PROGRAM

The recent Medicare Chronic Care Improvement Program may provide the much-needed stimulus to move things in a positive direction. The Chronic Care Improvement Program is a remarkable piece of legislation that calls for an intentional effort to apply evidence-based medicine process to the Medicare-enrolled population. The programs will emphasize the kind of care issues that nurse practitioners have been delivering: adherence to standards of care, self-care strategies, and appropriate treatment. The Chronic Care Improvement Program will begin in earnest during the summer of 2005, serve approximately 180,000 chronically ill beneficiaries, and last 2 to 3 $1/2$ years.

The Chronic Care Improvement Program will be a highly visible care management program that will catch the eye of all constituents of the health care industry. Careful attention also will be given to the clinical and financial impact of these efforts, leading to more ammunition in the move to a more equitable distribution of provider sources.

SUMMARY

Despite the issues surrounding the role and professional standing of nurse practitioners in managed care, the future is hopeful. Managed care organizations are realizing that nurse practitioners are playing a vital role in helping to stem their medical losses via careful care and cost-efficient strategies. Federal and state legislators need to take several important steps before a significant movement occurs in this area, and the prevailing wisdom is that the patients themselves will drive this. Health care delivery systems are changing at an incredible pace, and so are the expectations of the increasingly aged patients.

REFERENCES

Advance for Nurse Practitioners. (2005). *2003 national salary survey of nurse practitioners.* Retrieved July 1, 2005, from http://nurse-practitioners.advanceweb.com/Common/editorial/editorial.aspx?CC=27264

American Academy of Nurse Practitioners. (2003). *Results of 2003 AANP membership survey.* Austin, TX: Author.

American Nurses Association. (1996). *Scope and standards of advanced practice nursing.* Washington, DC: American Nurses Publishing.

Buppert, C. (1998). Reimbursement for nurse practitioner services. *Nurse Practitioner, 28*(2), 67, 70, 72-76, 81-82.

Buppert, C., & Billing, J. D. (2002). For nurse practitioner services: Guidelines for NPs, physicians, employers, and insurers. *Medscape Nurses, 4*(1), 2002.

Ellwood, P. (2001). *Does managed care need to be replaced?* Presentation to the Graduate School of Management [Speech], University of California, Irvine, October 2, 2001. Retrieved July 1, 2005, from https://www.medscape.com/viewarticle/408185_print

Fain, J. A., & Melkus, G. D. (1994). Nurse practitioner practice patterns based on standards of medical care for patients with diabetes. *Diabetes Care, 17*(8), 879-881.

Health Care Financing Administration, Office of the Actuary. (n.d.). *National health expenditures aggregate and per capita amounts, percent distribution, and average annual percent growth by source of funds: Selected years 1960-94.* Boston, MA: Author.

Healthcare Financial Management. (2003). Fitch sees negative financial outlook for health care; CMS sees mixed outlook - Industry Watch - Brief Article. From http://www.findarticles.com/p/articles/mi_m3257/is_9_57/ai_108443769#continue

Kongstvedt, P. R. (1997). *Essentials of managed care* (2nd ed.). Gaithersburg, MD: Aspen.

Larne, A. C., & Pugh, J. A. (1998). Attitudes of primary care providers toward diabetes barriers to guideline implementation. *Diabetes Care, 21*, 1391-1396.

Lenz, E. R., Mundinger, M. O., Hopkins, S. C., Lin, S. X., & Smolowitz, H. (2002). Diabetes care processes and outcomes in patients treated by nurse practitioners or physicians. *Diabetes Educator, 28*, 590-598.

MacLeod, G. (1994). Roots of managed care. In P. Kongstvedt (Ed.), *The managed health care handbook* (2nd ed.). Gaithersburg, MD: Aspen.

Mason, D., Alexander, J. M., Huffaker, J., Reilly, P. A., Sigmund, E. C., & Cohen, S. S. (1999). Nurse practitioners' experiences with managed care organizations in New York and Connecticut. *Nursing Outlook, 47*(5), 201-208.

McCloskey, B., Grey, M., Deshefy-Longhi, T., & Grey, L. J. (2003). APRN practice patterns in primary care. *The Nurse Practitioner, 28*(4), 39-44.

Mundinger, M. O., Kane, R. L., Lenz, E. R., Totten, A. M., Tsai, W., Cleary, P., et al. (2000). Primary care outcomes in patients treated by nurse practitioners or physicians: A randomized trial. *JAMA: The Journal of the American Medical Association, 283*(1), 59-68.

Oregon Secretary of State. (n.d.). *Oregon Administrative Rules 851-050-0005.* Retrieved January 11, 2002, from https://arcweb.sos.state.or.us/rules/OARS_800/OAR_851/851_050.html

Perry, K. (1995). Why patients love physician extenders. *Medical Economics, 95,* 58-67.

Roderick, S., Hooker, P. A., Potts, R., & Ray, W. (1996). Patient satisfaction: Comparing physician assistants, nurse practitioners, and physicians. *Permanente Journal.* Retrieved January 5, 2006 from http://xnet.kp.org/permanentejournal/sum97pj/ptsat.html

Rudy, E. B., Davidson, L. J., Daly, B., Clochesy, J. M., Sereika, S., Baldisser, M., et al. (1998). Care activities and outcomes of patients cared for by acute care nurse practitioners, physician assistants, and resident physicians: A comparison. *American Journal of Critical Care, 7*(4), 267-281.

Salkever, D. S. (1982). Episode-based efficiency comparisons for physicians and nurse practitioners. *Medical Care, 20,* 143-153.

Tufts Health Plan. (2003). *Nurse practitioner and physician assistant facility guideline.* Retrieved January 1, 2004, from http://www.tufts-healthplan.com/providers/pdf/billing_guidelines/NP-PA.pdf

Uylhara, E., & Thomas, M. A. (1975). *Health Maintenance Organization and the HMO Act of 1973, RAND Corporation Research White Paper.* Retrieved January 5, 2005 from http://www.rand.org/pubs/papers/P5554/

Contracting for Nursing Services

DONNA ZAZWORSKY

The thought of contracting for nursing care is unsettling for many nurses. Contracts are associated with a business model of health care. They raise images of compromising the nurse-patient relationship for a financial transaction. It is not uncommon to hear, "I became a nurse to serve patients. Money has no place in nursing care." In this view, contracts, which represent the exchange of payment for service, should not be a part of nursing practice nor of concern to nurses. I disagree.

VIEWPOINT. The ability to contract directly for nursing services and to receive payment for services delivered is essential for the survival of professional nursing practice. Contracting is tied directly to recognition of nurses' contributions to health care outcomes, to control over practice, and to decision making over allocation of scarce health care resources. The ability to contract directly for nursing care is the difference between nurses' remaining invisible in health care or shaping the future of the health care delivery system.

WHAT IS A CONTRACT?

Most simply, a contract is a legal document between two or more parties that specifies services to be delivered and the payment for those services. The context for the services usually is defined in great detail, including where the services will be provided, how often they will be provided, how they will be reimbursed, the penalties for nondelivery of services or missing agreed-upon time frames, insurance coverage for liability for adverse outcomes, and processes for dispute resolution and termination.

In health care today, contracts are the major vehicle for health care organizations to provide care to a target population and be paid for it. Hospitals, home care agencies, skilled nursing facilities, and physician groups alike contract with a variety of entities such as government agencies, employers, insurance companies, and health maintenance organizations to provide one or more components of the full continuum of health care services. Without contracts, it is possible to provide health care services, but it is unlikely that the service will be reimbursed.

Individuals and organizations that enter into health care contracts agree to deliver services or to pay for them. Depending on the type of reimbursement, provider and payer of services may take on varying degrees of financial risk. For example, fee-for-service payment is not associated with substantial risk for a hospital or health care organization as long as the agreed-upon payment allows a certain margin of profit. The hospital or health care organization just needs to make sure that it maintains sufficient volume of services to cover costs and make a profit.

In contrast, contracts that use capitated payment are common in managed care arrangements and may be associated with significant financial risk for providers of care. Under capitated payment, providers are reimbursed *in advance* for the delivery of a defined set of services for a certain population. For example, a primary care physician is assigned 1000 patients from a certain health maintenance organization. The health maintenance organization agrees to pay the physician $10 per member per month. Thus the physician receives $10,000 each month to provide primary care services to this group of patients *whether or not the patients use any primary care services.*

It is possible to make or lose substantial sums of money in capitated contracts depending on the extent to which services covered in the contract are used. No matter how much service the population uses, whether more or less than estimated, the contracted provider remains financially responsible for delivering services under the terms of the agreement of the contract. Providers who enter into capitated contracts, also called risk contracts, do so with the premise that they will be able to manage service use and costs and thus have dollars remaining from the prospective capitated payment at the end of the month. Today, health care professionals and organizations can enter into a variety of different types of contracts, each associated with different amounts of financial risk. For profit and nonprofit organizations alike, the goal is to deliver quality services and to make enough money to continue, to expand services, and to pay stockholders investing in the organization.

Contracting is considered art and science. Although many of the financial components of a contract such as costs and expected use of services can be estimated with some degree of accuracy, numerous factors contribute to the success or failure of health care contracts. The mix of contracts held by an organization, the health needs of patients covered by the contract, and service use patterns affect profitability. Not surprisingly, as health care professionals participate more in contract negotiations and share more of the financial risk, their interest in mastering the skills of contracting has grown tremendously. The health care literature contains numerous articles with advice on how to negotiate and manage contracts, especially capitated or risk contracts (Gallagher, 1997; Hodnicki & Doughty, 2005; Knight, 1997; Monarch, 2002; Potter, 1999).

NURSES AND CONTRACTS

In many practice settings, nurses have owned businesses and entered into contracts for decades. In the early 1900s, Lillian Wald, the visionary leader of the Visiting Nurse Service of New York, contracted with several benefit societies on the lower east side of New York City to provide home nursing care to the members (Denker, 1993). In 1909, Wald initiated an experiment with Metropolitan Life Insurance Company that ultimately led to the first national system of insurance coverage for home-based care. She managed not only to convince insurers about the benefits of home nursing care but also to negotiate a successful capitated contract almost a century ago.

Following on the heels of the success of leaders like Lillian Wald, numerous nurses have chosen to become entrepreneurs. Today, nurses own and manage small businesses and large health care companies. In competitive arenas such as home care and case management, nurses provide skilled nursing services for health care organizations and insurers. Their businesses rely on contracts and direct payment for nursing services for income and survival.

Private practice opportunities for advanced practice nurses are becoming more evident. Many hospitals no longer can afford to provide specialty services such as diabetes self-management education or specialized case management services that extend beyond the hospital walls. Advanced practice nurses are establishing subcontracts or "carveouts" with health plans, worker's compensation, employers, physician providers, and lawyers to provide specialized case management services or other specialty services that the advanced practice nurse is certified to do (Mahn-DiNicola & Zazworsky, 2005).

Today, however, there continues to be a number of settings that do not bill directly for nursing care. In hospitals and nursing homes, for example, nursing care typically is included in the price of room and board. In many primary care settings, nurse practitioner services are billed under the physician's payment code.

What difference does it make whether nursing services are paid for directly or indirectly? As long as nurses can provide good nursing care and get paid, why make an issue of nursing being included in contracts or receiving direct payment? When you go into a grocery or department store and pay for an item of food or clothing, do you think about the skill sets or time of different individuals whose work went into the production of that item? Do you distinguish any specific group for their contributions to the quality of the item or demand that their seal of approval come with the purchase?

In settings that do not bill directly for nursing care, the purchasers may be aware that nursing is included in the negotiated price but usually have limited knowledge of the expertise they are buying. Contract discussions usually revolve around the cost of hospital care, not skilled nursing care, even though skilled nursing care is the largest component of hospital expenses. When patients receive their hospital bill or notification of insurance payment, more often than not they do not associate the bill with the quality of the nursing care they received. In effect, nursing is invisible to payers and the public.

In American society the willingness to pay for services is tied directly to the value placed on the service. Consumers do not pay for services they do not value. Conversely, nurses need to ask, do consumers value services they are not aware they are paying for? If payers and the public do not link the hospital or primary care bill to the outstanding nursing care they received, what is the likelihood that they will demand that nurses receive payment commensurate with their expertise? How likely are they to become involved in issues that affect the quality of nursing care? Invisibility has been and continues to be costly to the profession of nursing.

For nursing, the ability to contract (and thus, be paid) directly for nursing services does the following:

◆ Reflects the value placed on nursing care by consumers and payers
◆ Recognizes that nurses offer a distinct service
◆ Provides control over nursing care decisions and resulting dollars
◆ Permits public evaluation of the contribution of nursing to care
◆ Generates dollars to serve vulnerable and underserved groups
◆ Improves the contracting process

Americans' willingness to pay for a service or product is associated with the value they place on it. Individuals and insurers pay for health insurance and services because they want and value health care or their customers demand it. Although there is ongoing debate about the extent to which health care follows typical market principles, the way that health care dollars are allocated still reflects the value placed on varying services. Services that are exchanged for payment at the contract table are those that the payer wants and which the payer is willing to pay for.

Inclusion of nursing care in contracts indicates that nursing is recognized as a distinct and valuable service. Specific identification of nursing as a covered service indicates that the payer wants the service, is willing to pay for it, and holds the organization accountable for the quality of that care. Most other health care professionals, such as physicians or therapists, are named in contracts and thus have the opportunity to negotiate the terms under which their services are delivered. Invisibility at the contract table means not only having nursing services sold for unacceptable rates but also a missed opportunity to educate and reeducate contractors and payers about nursing.

When payment is hidden, included in the room fee, or attributed to another professional, nurses lose a critical opportunity to demonstrate their contribution to health care. In primary care settings that bill services delivered by a nurse practitioner "incident to" physician services and under the physician's name, data about the services included on the billing statement are connected to the physician, not the nurse practitioner. Yet nurse practitioners have to complete the same credentialing process as any physician delivering services to a plan. Mason et al. (1999) note, "Reimbursement under the physician PIN [provider identification number] may generate more profit for the practice but it eliminates recognition of the nurse practitioner as the service provider and clouds accountability" (p. 207).

Medicare does allow nurse practitioners and clinical nurse specialists legally authorized under their state Nurse Practice Act to bill independently once they have received their own provider identification number. However, direct reimbursement is only 85% of the Medicare physician fee schedule for services (Mason, Leavitt, & Chaffee, 2002). Unfortunately, plans that recognize nurse practitioner direct billing usually follow the Medicare reimbursement trends. Even with landmark studies published in *JAMA: the Journal of the American Medical Association* demonstrated no difference in the effectiveness of nurse practitioners and physicians in primary care clinics run by Columbia University in New York City (Mundinger et al., 2000).

The ability to contract and thus generate direct revenue has major implications for participation in decision making and control over allocation of health care resources. Nursing directors in hospitals and nursing homes oversee areas associated with the largest component of hospital budgets. In fact, without nurses, hospitals and nursing homes would not exist. Yet across the country, nursing directors are being moved farther from the seat of power and decision making. Nurses must ask, "Would this be happening if nursing directors controlled all access to nursing resources and were the primary negotiators for nursing care during contracts?" How might this affect the ability of nurses to take control over nursing delivery models?

Clearly, most nurses are not in nursing for money or to make a profit. Nurses have a distinguished record of serving vulnerable and underserved populations. The reality experienced by many nurses who have been involved in caring for these groups, however, is that maintaining funding for even the most essential programs is difficult. Contracting is a vehicle to generate dollars that can be used to pay for services for which there is no reimbursement. Community nursing centers have done an extraordinary job of maintaining services for uninsured and vulnerable populations by increasing income from contracts (Box 46-1). A common saying in health care goes, "No margin, no mission." Nurses in community health centers and other settings have demonstrated that successful contracting prevents this unacceptable cycle.

Finally, nursing involvement in contracts is an important way to improve health care contracts. Individuals who negotiate health care contracts for most large health care institutions and insurance companies are not usually clinicians or practitioners. Although they may be expert at the financing of health care, they often do not understand the operational dynamics of service

BOX 46-1

Contracting for Nursing Services in Today's Community Nursing Centers: Contracting With Peter to Pay Paul

Community nursing centers emerged more than 3 decades ago to serve individuals and populations without access to traditional health care services. Today, more than 300 community nursing centers (CNCs) are estimated to be across the United States in inner-city and rural settings, providing care to individuals of all ages and ethnic groups (Watson, 1996).

Most of the CNCs started in academic health centers and received funding through federal grants. Grants from the Department of Health and Human Services, Division of Nursing, have been instrumental in enabling nursing faculty to set up innovative community care models.

Although grant funding is an excellent vehicle to jump-start much needed community-based health initiatives, eventually grants end and programs are faced with finding the money to continue operations. Community nursing centers are challenged particularly in this regard because they typically serve populations for which there is limited or no reimbursement for services. Much of the current literature on CNCs addresses their economic viability and survival.

Today, many of the mature CNCs—that is, those that have been around for a long time—report an important new step toward long-term financial survival. They have diversified their funding streams to balance expenses associated with reimbursable and nonreimbursable care. Income from Medicare, Medicaid, and state contracts augments grant support, and together they permit successful CNCs to continue to carry out their mission of service for vulnerable populations.

Without a funding menu that includes contracts, CNCs could not continue to provide health care services to the thousands of uninsured and vulnerable individuals and families they see each year. For CNCs, the ability to compete for and win contracts is essential to reaching out and responding to unmet community needs.

---

delivery or the interdependence of health care services. Contracts that appear to be reasonable financially often result in frustration and financial losses because they do not work clinically or overlook essential services or incentives that make the whole package work better. For example, any nurse who works in a hospital knows how critical the services that follow hospitalization are to preventing subsequent admissions and emergency department visits. Yet some contracts create incentives to minimize or delay the use of postacute services. Having skilled nurses at the contract table avoids perverse scenarios that diminish quality of care and ultimately increase expenses.

GETTING TO THE CONTRACTS TABLE

Participation in contracts requires expertise and data. Contract negotiations incorporate the art of bargaining and compromise and the science of finance and economics.

Nurses who engage in contracting come prepared. They are able to do the following:

- Define the services for which they are to be reimbursed
- Specify the costs of the services, for example, cost per visit
- Provide data about the quality of their service

- Assume the responsibility and risk associated with the terms of the contract
- Walk away from the contract when it is unacceptable

In some settings, nurses readily can generate the necessary information to engage in contracts. Financial and information systems are developed sufficiently to capture major outcomes and expenses associated with the delivery of nursing care. In other settings, considerable effort and capital must be infused into developing the infrastructure needed to support this effort.

There is no getting away from the fact that credible data are a requirement for successful contracting. Settings that are unwilling or unable to allocate resources to document nursing outcomes and costs in a systematic and ongoing way must be considered suspect in their commitment to deliver nursing services. Without data and contracts, nursing programs may continue to exist at the whim of the current administrators and may remain extremely vulnerable.

To negotiate successfully with all the knowledge, experience, and data necessary for contracts, nurses must work to put to rest the "nurses should not deal with money" issue and any associated issues related to feelings about competition. Expertise and experience on the business side of health care is a necessary means to a desired end of better health care for the persons nurses serve. The refusal to deal with money or competition is also a refusal to participate at the level that critical decisions about allocation of health care resources are made.

In addition, nurses need to work actively to remove other barriers to participating in contracts and receiving equitable reimbursement for their services. Legislative advances such as the Balanced Budget Act of 1997, which mandated Medicare reimbursement for advanced practice nurses, are essential to level the playing field for nurses. Hopefully, future legislation will rectify issues related to equal pay for equal work for nurses.

SUMMARY

Every nurse must come to terms with the role that money plays in health care today. Whether the nurse works as employee or independent practitioner, someone or some organization is paying directly or indirectly for the services nurses provide. The distance between the payment for services and the paycheck may be short or long, but nurses fool themselves if they ignore the fact that money and financial incentives drive much of their behavior and decisions in health care. Nurses should watch what happens when Congress changes the methods for reimbursing Medicare or Medicaid if they have any lingering doubt.

For a growing number of nurses, this strong message about the importance of reimbursement and contracting is a case of preaching to the converted. All too many, however, still have a long way to go. The need to bring nurses into the twenty-first century of health care represents a critical opportunity for nursing educators and administrators to work together to shape the future of nursing and health care. It would be a national tragedy if professional nursing goes the way of the dinosaur because it refused to learn and master the lesson of integrating business and mission.

REFERENCES

Denker, E. P. (1993). *Healing at home: Visiting Nurse Service of New York.* New York: Visiting Nurse Service.

Gallagher, R. M. (1997). What APRNs need to know about contracting with managed care organizations. *Nursing Trends & Issues, 2*(6), 1-8.

Hodnicki, D. R., & Doughty, S. E. D. (2005). Marketing and contracting considerations. In A. B. Hamric, J. A. Spross, & C. M. Hanson (Eds.), *Advanced practice nursing: An integrative approach* (3rd ed., pp. 749-779). Philadelphia: W.B. Saunders.

Knight, W. (1997). *Managed care contracting: A guide for health care professionals.* Gaithersburg, MD: Aspen.

Mahn-DiNicola, V. A., & Zazworsky, D. J. (2005). The advanced practice nurse case manager. In A. B. Hamric, J. A. Spross, & C. M. Hanson (Eds.), *Advanced practice nursing: An integrative approach* (3rd ed., pp. 617-675). Philadelphia: W.B. Saunders.

Mason, D., Alexander, J. M., Huffaker, J., Reilly, P. A., Sigmund, E. C., & Cohen, S. S. (1999). Nurse practitioners' experiences with managed care organizations in New York and Connecticut. *Nursing Outlook, 47*(5), 201-208.

Mason, D. L., Leavitt, J. K., & Chaffee, M. W. (2002). *Policy and politics in nursing and health care* (p. 257). St. Louis, MO: Saunders.

Monarch, K. (2002). *Nursing & the law* (pp. 149-162). Washington, DC: American Nurses Association.

Mundinger, M. O., Kane, R. L., Lenz, E. R., Totten, A. M., Tsai, W. U., Cleary, P. D., et al. (2000). Primary care outcomes in patients treated by nurse practitioners or physicians: A randomized trial. *JAMA: the Journal of the American Medical Association, 283,* 59-68.

Potter, L. (1999). The managed care contract: Survival or closure? *Nursing Administration Quarterly, 23*(4), 58-62.

Watson, L. J. (1996). A national profile of nursing centers. *Nurse Practitioner, 21*(3), 72-80.

Magnet Designation

Gold Standard for Nursing Excellence

ROSE RIVERS ◆ SUEELLEN PINKERTON

This chapter is about the competitive edge. Magnet recognition through the American Nurses Credentialing Center Magnet Recognition Program (2005) is the gold standard for excellence in nursing care and patient outcomes. In addition, Magnet recognition creates a visible link between nursing and overall hospital success. Being Magnet designated calls for a transformation, and the level of thinking in the organization must change to whole systems thinking in order to change the level of practice.

MAGNET RECOGNITION: A SOLID FOUNDATION

The Magnet Recognition Program provides a road map and blueprint for improving patient care quality, specifically the impact of nursing care on quality. The focus on nurse-sensitive indicators lays the groundwork for nurses to focus on their sphere of influence. The *Scope and Standards for Nurse Administrators* (American Nurses Association, 2004) are the foundation for the program. These standards support the principles for professional practice models including role expectations for the chief nursing officer (CNO). Fourteen Forces of Magnetism (American Nurses Credential Center [ANCC], 2005) provide structure for document submission to the ANCC. These 14 forces form the basis for evaluating nursing leadership and administration, professional practice, and professional development. An important note is that these forces were identified through research on Magnet-designated hospitals as the hallmark for their sustained success.

During a severe nursing shortage in the early 1980s, some hospitals were recognized for their retention of quality nurses. These hospitals were not experiencing nurse vacancy and turnover as were their counterparts. The American Academy of Nursing commissioned a study to determine factors associated with the success of these hospitals. Forty-one hospitals participated in the study that identified and described variables contributing to an environment that supported the recruitment and retention of nurses. These hospitals were assigned the status of "magnet hospitals" because they were able to attract nurses in the midst of a severe shortage. The original study was published in 1983 as *Magnet Hospitals: Attraction and Retention of Professional Nurses* (McClure, Poulin, Sovie, & Wandelt, 1983). Researchers continued to study these Magnet hospitals, building on the work of the original study, which resulted in a compilation of the works that was published by the American Nurses Association (2002) in *Magnet Hospitals Revisited: Attraction and Retention of Professional Nurses.*

Continued shortages of nurses called for long-term sustainable strategies to address the issues affecting the recruitment and retention of qualified nurses. In 1993 the ANCC began a Magnet Hospital Recognition Program. A few years later, this program became the Magnet Nursing Services Recognition Program for Excellence in Nursing Services. The initiative began with a pilot program to identify Magnet hospitals, and in the late 1990s the program was extended to all hospitals and long-term care facilities. Currently, more than 160 hospitals have achieved Magnet status, including a long-term care facility. The Magnet Recognition Program has grown to achieve international status and influence.

The Magnet Recognition Program took the lessons from the first generation of Magnet-designated hospitals to build the current program. Research has built the framework for excellence that is the basis for Magnet designation; the framework is not a set of standards that was "made up." In addition, as noted in a White Paper by the Joint Commission on Accreditation of Healthcare Organizations (2002), *Health Care at the Crossroads: Strategies for Addressing the Evolving Nursing Shortage,* the Magnet Forces and Standards align with the goals of the commission. The goals of the Institute of Medicine regarding patient safety are congruent with the focus of the Magnet program on the nurse work environment. Many of these strategies are noted in the Institute of Medicine report *Keeping Patients Safe: Transforming the Work Environment of Nurses* (Page, 2003).

THE IMPORTANCE OF MAGNET RECOGNITION

Magnet recognition is gaining attention in environments external to the health care system. Havens and Johnston (2004), in focus groups conducted with chief nurse executives and Magnet coordinators, had one CNO report that the chief executive officer and chief operating officer of the hospital were surprised to find out that the bond raters, at their annual bond rating meeting in New York, knew about Magnet hospitals. The bond raters also wanted to know the vacancy rate, turnover, and general health of the nursing staff in the hospital. They recognize the benefit of a strong nursing force to the viability of the hospital. "They said that the financial picture of a hospital is in jeopardy if they do not have a strong nursing department" (p. 581). Magnet recognition also is mentioned as a factor in the placement of hospitals on the *US News & World Report* "Best Hospitals" list and in naming the Best Children's Hospitals. Magnet recognition also has been a factor in the successful negotiation of managed care contracts.

Recent popular magazines and newspaper articles have recommended Magnet designation as a factor consumers should support and consider in selecting a hospital. This assumes consumers have some voice in selecting a hospital. Most recently, recruitment ads for chief nurse executives have mentioned looking for a CNO who will lead the Magnet effort. In a position of influence, the ANCC (2005) has set educational requirements for the hospital CNO, who, if applying for Magnet status, must possess a master's degree by January 1, 2008, and either the master's degree or bachelor's degree must be in nursing. Some schools of nursing also are looking for Magnet facilities only to use as clinical sites for student experiences.

THE PATH TO MAGNET RECOGNITION

Magnet recognition creates a visible link between nursing and overall hospital success. Today's hospitals cannot afford to have nursing be the weak link in the chain. A Magnet culture strengthens the nursing link. To be successful, hospitals must have a great purpose and vision. Magnet status can be the tool to achieving this

purpose and vision. Magnet status is about doing the right things right. Magnet status is about positioning nurses to give better care to patients. Magnet status is about saying "no" to mediocrity and saying "yes" to excellence through application of evidenced-based leadership, management, and clinical practices.

The effect of the nursing shortage has created a momentum for examination of current practices in hospitals. Some of the benefits of achieving Magnet status are high patient and family satisfaction, high quality of nursing care with improved clinical outcomes, strong collaborative relationships, and improved recruitment and retention of nurses.

A healthy, growing phenomenon is to help other hospitals, typically thought of as competitors, to achieve Magnet status. Promoting the "Magnet environment" as the norm presents an opportunity to change the image of nursing from being a difficult, unattractive career choice to becoming a prestigious, enticing profession. A "Magnet culture" encourages innovation regarding professional development. Creating new opportunities that foster growth by making the best use of experienced expert nurses is a win-win-win situation for the hospital, nurse, and patient. With these benefits, the question becomes how to sustain them. Historically, the nursing shortage has generated solutions such as a variety of bonus pay programs. Some popular programs offers 40 hours' pay for 24 hours worked (usually on the weekend) and other variations to attract nurses. These models have not been sustainable in the long run. Costly gimmicks are not the answer. Cultural transformation is required to sustain results.

Becoming a Magnet hospital requires deep rooted culture change. Magnet status is not a cover-up with a pretty headdress. Magnet status requires changing old ways of thinking and doing, including the thinking and doing of senior leadership. Magnet designation infers excellence and sets the expectation for excellence for consumers and providers. Magnet status sets the expectation for continuous learning because excellence is a journey. It has no finish line.

A WHOLE SYSTEM EFFORT

Pursing Magnet designation is creating an environment for all to succeed. Support of nursing is support of overall patient care quality. Positioning nursing leadership leverages staff nurses to improve patient care quality. A significant focus on nurses is required to improve patient outcomes, given their centrality to patient satisfaction and quality of care. Magnet designation as an

VIEWPOINTS

organizational goal becomes a catalyst to align the hospital vision, mission, philosophy, and values. Nursing leadership becomes an anchor. Organizational response to nursing becomes a unifying force in which collaboration is the norm to meet patient demands. Nursing governs nursing practice, including human resource allocation, in this type of environment.

The challenge to achieve Magnet designation is a call to action and for action. The challenge is CNO driven and hospital supported. It helps to build bridges between nurses and the CNO. It opens the door for "crucial conversations" (Patterson, Grenny, McMillian, & Switzler, 2002) that address long-standing issues and concerns, such as professional jealousy and horizontal violence. Magnet designation as a mutual goal serves to improve collaboration and communication. Other departments are major players in the pursuit of Magnet status, often participating to the extent of completing a gap analysis on their own departments. Pursuing Magnet designation is not a solitary struggle. Nursing is not an island unto itself; therefore interdisciplinary partnerships are key to achieving Magnet designation.

FUTURE IMPLICATIONS FOR MAGNET DESIGNATION

As more and more hospitals seek Magnet designation, some not successfully, one question is whether Magnet designation is an achievable goal for all hospitals. Should all hospitals pursue Magnet designation? Can Magnet-designated hospitals influence the greater health care environment? Will Magnet hospitals lead the transformation in health care? Will Magnet hospitals be the basis for new reimbursement models? Will Magnet hospitals have fewer risk management issues? Will compassion fatigue (Figley, 2003) be a factor in Magnet hospitals? Should the ANCC determine standards for hospitals and CNO educational preparation? How can non-Magnet hospitals influence the standards set by the ANCC? What is the balance between the American Nurses Association collective bargaining activities and Magnet designation? What is the role of the American Organization of Nurse Executives in Magnet designation? Will tensions between non-Magnet and Magnet hospitals have an effect on unifying nursing?

CASE STUDY

Maggie Winters was hired recently by the New Light Hospital as the CNO. Part of her hiring goals was to examine Magnet designation for the hospital. She completes a careful gap analysis and finds a large gap between her goals and the goals of the nurse managers regarding Magnet recognition; they are not convinced that the hospital should pursue Magnet designation. What should be her course of action? Should she wait? Should she expect them to follow her lead? What if they try to undermine her goals? Should she gain staff nurse support and hope nurse managers follow? What is the role of education? What resources are available to Maggie to educate the leadership? How does Maggie quantify the cost-benefit of Magnet recognition?

REFERENCES

American Nurses Association. (2002). *Magnet hospitals revisited: Attraction and retention of professional nurses.* Washington, DC: Author.

American Nurses Association. (2004). *Scope and standards for nurse administrators* (2nd ed.). Washington, DC: Author.

American Nurses Credentialing Center. (2005). *ANCC Magnet Program: Recognizing excellence in nursing services application manual 2005.* Silver Spring, MD: Author.

Figley, C. R. (2003). *Treating compassion fatigue.* New York: Brunner-Routledge.

Havens, D. S., & Johnston, M. A. (2004). Achieving Magnet hospital recognition: Chief nurse executives and Magnet coordinators tell their stories. *Journal of Nursing Administration, 34*(12), 579-588.

Joint Commission on Accreditation of Healthcare Organizations. (2002). *Health care at the crossroads: Strategies for addressing the evolving nursing shortage.* Retrieved November 9, 2005, from http://www.jcaho.org/about+us/public+policy+initiatives/health_care_at_the_crossroads.pdf

McClure, M. L., Poulin, M. A., Sovie, M. D., & Wandelt, M. A. (1983). *Magnet hospitals: Attraction and retention of professional nurses.* Kansas City, MO: American Nurses Association.

Page, A. (Ed.). (2003). *Keeping patients safe: Transforming the work environment of nurses.* Washington, DC: National Academies Press.

Patterson, K., Grenny, J., McMillian, R., & Switzler, A. (2002). *Crucial conversations tools for talking when stakes are high.* New York: McGraw-Hill.

HEALTH CARE COSTS

A Concern for Costs

PERLE SLAVIK COWEN   ◆   SUE MOORHEAD

Since the last edition of *Current Issues in Nursing* the debate over costs of health care has become a central concern of most Americans. This focus has come about as discussions of reform of Medicare have intensified and the costs of medications and use of prescription drugs have soared. Americans are concerned about the escalation of out-of-pocket costs associated with health insurance and the increasing issues of medical errors. In spite of this focus on costs, not many nurses have developed programs of research or careers around nursing economics. The concern for costs is determining a number of decisions that affect nurses and the patients for whom they care. This section introduces some of the issues around the costs of nursing and health care in today's health care environment.

In the debate chapter, York and Gibson maintain that spending on health care in the public and private sectors has followed an upward trajectory since the early 1960s and has become one of the most challenging public policy issues facing the United States. This chapter examines how different aspects of the health care market contribute to the high cost of health care and then explores the effectiveness of various strategies to control health care spending in this country. York and Gibson summarize the health care spending drivers as hospital services, prescription drugs, physician services, the link between medical conditions and health spending, technology and medical innovation, and personal disposable income. On the consumer side the implications are increased cost sharing, costs of drugs, availability of health coverage, and the effect of public health care programs on costs. The strength of this chapter is the detailed examination of potential solutions to the problem. In the end the authors conclude that consumers should participate in health care treatment decisions, especially from a financial standpoint. This chapter provides an excellent foundation for the viewpoint chapters that follow.

In the first viewpoint chapter, Maddox examines the evolution of managed care, the financial factors that have created the current health care system, and the impact of the changes on nursing. The chapter contains numerous financial facts and offers the reader an excellent overview of the financial aspects of health care. The author covers the evolution of the third-party payer system and clearly explains the functions of Medicare and Medicaid and prospective payment systems. The chapter gives an overview of different models of managed care and discusses in some detail the preferred provider organization and the health maintenance organization. The last half of the chapter focuses on the impact of managed care and current reimbursement methods on hospitals, ambulatory and outpatient services, long-term care, nurse staffing, and selected nursing roles such as the advanced practice nurse and the nurse manager. Maddox also discusses three use management strategies: prospective, concurrent, and retrospective. The Balanced Budget Act of 1997 brought several changes, including the recognition of nurse practitioners, clinical specialists, and physician assistants as authorized Medicare providers eligible for direct reimbursement. Maddox concludes that with this new role comes increased responsibility for the provider. This is an informative chapter about the history and current issues related to reimbursement trends in the United States and the impact on health care and nursing.

The changes and challenges in home health care is the topic of the next chapter by Anderson, Clark, and Dusio. Home health care is the delivery of continued nursing and therapeutic services provided in a home-based setting. Six Medicare-covered disciplines typically are involved in home health care: skilled nursing, home health aides, physical therapy, occupational therapy, speech therapy, and social services. The focus of these services is on preventing complications and preserving client independence and health. This chapter highlights the funding of home health care in the United States, including the recent establishment of prospective payment. The authors describe current challenges in home health care such as technology and differentiated clinical practice. As care increasingly moves into the home setting, all nurses must be concerned with the funding and quality of care available to consumers in their homes.

Reimbursement for nurses and other nonphysician providers is the subject of the chapter by Lee. The proliferation in consumer use of alternative therapies such as autogenic training, biofeedback, massage, acupuncture, Ayurvedic techniques, and reflexology has resulted in the recognition that there needs to be a way to document the use of such therapies and bill for reimbursement as they become more accepted. Today, consumer demand for alternative therapies is great, and these therapies increasingly are included in mainstream practice and medical and nursing journals. In 1996 the Health Insurance Portability and Accountability Act called for the setting of a national standard to communicate with all providers (not just physicians) electronically in a standardized way. This act, combined with the widespread and growing dissatisfaction with the *Current Procedural Terminology,* opened the door for the development of the *Complete Complementary Alternative Medicine Billing and Coding Reference.* The *Reference,* published for the first time in 1999, includes Alternative Billing Codes (ABCs) developed by a group known as Alternative Link in Las Cruces, New Mexico. In this coding system, *alternative* is defined as any provider other than an allopathic physician and the treatments provided by these providers. Thus nursing is included (although most nurses do not think of themselves as alternative providers). The ABCs include interventions from the Nursing Interventions Classification, the Home Health Care Classification, and the Omaha System. The ABCs have been included in the *American National Standards Implementation Guideline* and the National Library of Medicine Unified Medical Language. The system not only includes language for thousands of alternative therapies but also provides the legal scope of practice for multiple-practitioner groups. This chapter highlights the progress of alternative reimbursement systems and demonstrates its usefulness for nursing. This is a must-read for all advanced practice nurses. Will the growing use of alternative therapies be documented?

The next chapter by Rhodes, a nurse attorney whose practice focuses on compliance with the Health Insurance Portability and Accountability Act (HIPAA), provides an overview of the impact of the act. This act, passed in 1996, is a federal statute that includes several complicated health care provisions, the most well-known being the privacy provisions. The act takes its name from the notion that employees can carry insurance from one job to another ("health insurance portability"). It focuses on three areas: privacy, electronic and computer security, and the processing of medical claims. Rhodes maintains that one of the absurd assumptions is that the enactment of the HIPAA rules would save money and reduce the costs of health care. This is supported by the facts that the HIPAA rules were imposed on a complex system of health care that is already expensive, is distributed unequally, and is increasing in cost every year and that the rules apply to every provider, regardless of size, location, or history of violation of privacy. The chapter provides an excellent overview of HIPAA regulations and important information on the costs of this policy.

In the final viewpoint chapter, Judge-Ellis and Sorofman argue that drugs are too cheap and that health care providers do not acknowledge the dangers of drugs. They support this view with the idea that drugs are toxic if used too much and are debilitating if used in a manner that does not address the physiological needs of the patient. They suggest that not enough focus is put on medication mismanagement. This interesting perspective is an important contribution to this section on costs and includes a case study to illustrate the scenario that drugs are too cheap. This is a timely discussion topic given the ongoing debate of the costs of prescription drugs in this country and is a growing concern of many senior citizens.

The nursing profession continues to face a variety of economic issues in practice. These are important issues for the profession and for the patients for whom nurses care in all settings. Today, nurses and nursing students are gaining critical knowledge about costs of health care, and nursing is playing an increasing role in health care cost-containment efforts. Nurses need to continue to make the costs of health care a nursing concern and take appropriate actions whenever the opportunities arise.

Controlling Health Care Costs

Is There an Answer?

JOSEPH W. YORK ◆ MARY M. GIBSON

S pending on health care in the public and private sector has been on an upward trajectory since the early 1960s and has become one of the most challenging public policy issues facing the United States. Health care spending continues to grow faster than the overall economy and employee compensation, raising concern that greater numbers of Americans, particularly those with lower incomes, may lose access to health care. Factors generally cited as contributing to the dramatic rise in health care spending include growth in pharmaceutical expenses, new medical technologies, increased consumer demand, the cost of health care labor, greater negotiating power on the part of hospitals and providers, and the aging of the population (Heffler et al., 2004; Thorpe & Ginsburg, 2001).

Although many Americans have benefited from this increasing investment in health care, the size and pace of growth has placed strain on the systems used to finance health care, including public programs such as Medicare and Medicaid and private employer-sponsored health care coverage. Efforts to control spending through market forces or government regulation have had little long-term effect. The question of affordability and whether individuals receive a corresponding value in relation to the escalating cost of care has caught the attention of policy makers, legislators, employers, and consumers. These individuals collectively must decide how to balance effective cost-control policies with the increased demand for services that will inevitably come with an aging but prosperous population.

This chapter looks at how the different aspects of the health care market contribute to the high cost of health care and then explores the effectiveness of various strategies to control health care spending in this country.

HEALTH CARE SPENDING DRIVERS

The dominant factors underlying the increase in total health care spending are inpatient and outpatient hospital services, drugs, and physician services.

Hospital Services

Inpatient and outpatient hospital services accounted for more than half of the increase in health care spending per privately insured person during 2003, with spending on outpatient care being the fastest growing category (Strunk & Ginsberg, 2004a). Innovations in medical technologies and continued pressure from payers to provide services in the most cost-effective setting continue to drive services into the outpatient setting. As a cost driver, hospital prices, rather than utilization accounted for much of the overall growth in hospital spending.

The trend in hospital prices has continued to accelerate in recent years as hospitals have consolidated their negotiating power over health plans in many areas of the country. Several additional factors have contributed to the acceleration in hospital prices over this period, including a strong labor market for hospital workers, especially nurses. A shortage of trained personnel has driven up wage rates and the number of hours worked, and many health care facilities have passed the increased wage costs along to payers, including health plans and consumers. Another factor driving up prices may be that with diminishing profit margins for Medicare patients, hospitals are continuing to shift more costs to private payers. In the future, however, the recent Medicare payment rate reduction "give backs" following payment cuts mandated by the Balanced Budget Act of 1997 could put downward pressure on hospital price increases.

In contrast, on the inpatient side, utilization management tools that were relaxed in the late 1990s by managed care plans are being implemented with renewed enthusiasm by health plans and payers in an effort to keep downward pressure on the use of inpatient hospital services. Insurers are reinstating tools such as prior authorization requirements and are enhancing disease and case management programs to target selectively the high-use and high-cost services in an effort to keep hospital costs and premiums under control. In addition, cost sharing for hospital care is becoming more common in plan design. Per-stay and per-day co-payments for inpatient care are being added to plans as an additional incentive to reduce utilization and length of stay.

Prescription Drugs

After becoming a major cost driver in the late 1990s, the trend for drug spending has slowed recently, reflecting changes in the use and price of drugs. However, pharmaceuticals still remain the faster-growing health sector. Decreased spending on the introduction of new drugs and direct-to-consumer advertising also has slowed the rate of growth in this sector.

Many health plans have instituted drug co-payment plan designs that create incentives for patients to use lower-cost generic drugs. Employers also are increasing co-payments for drugs or are instituting a coinsurance plan in which individuals pay a percentage of their drug costs rather than a fixed dollar amount. As a result, individuals are motivated to use less expensive generic drugs rather than brand name or other preferred drugs. Incentives that result in higher out-of-pocket costs also might slow the growth of prescription use as individuals turn to commonly prescribed drugs that are now available over the counter or to brand name prescription drugs that recently have lost their patent protection and now face stiff competition from lower-cost generic drugs.

In the mid-1990s the availability of newer, higher-priced drugs and rising per capita prescription use fueled increases in spending that were several times higher than for hospital care or physician services. Factors often cited as contributing to the double-digit growth rates include spending on research and development; spending on promotion, including heavy direct-to-consumer advertising; and the availability of prescription drug coverage.

More recently, however, prescription drug spending trends have slowed from the high rates of growth in the late 1990s and early part of this decade. Greater use of generic drugs, which tend to be priced lower than name brand equivalents, and tiered pharmacy benefit plans under which individuals pay more for name brand drugs have helped to slow the rate of drug spending. In addition, many employers now are requiring individuals to pay more toward the cost of prescription drugs through higher co-payments or through coinsurance, where an individual pays a percentage of the total cost instead of a fixed-dollar amount. In December 2003, Congress passed the Medicare Prescription Drug, Improvement, and Modernization Act (MMA) of 2003.

Until the passage of the MMA, many seniors purchased supplemental insurance plans to cover prescription drugs that were not part of the original Medicare benefit package. The MMA is expected to reduce the rate of growth in spending in the private sector as individuals who now have supplemental coverage enroll in Medicare. However, whether overall spending on prescriptions will be affected is difficult to predict.

Although the use of increased cost-sharing incentives also may have helped to slow the trend in drug use rates, several other factors have been important. Fewer new drugs have been approved for sale, several blockbuster prescription drugs have been removed abruptly from the market, and other drugs have been reclassified to over-the-counter status. However, spending on prescription drugs is expected to grow and may do so at an increasing rate once the new Medicare prescription drug program is implemented beginning in 2006. As more individuals in the population become eligible for Medicare benefits, the rate of growth may jump again. Moreover, the pursuit and demand for new and better pharmaceuticals is unlikely to abate. Discoveries in science, particularly in the field of genomics, will open the door to new classes of drugs requiring large investments in research and manufacturing.

Physician Services

According to the Strunk and Ginsberg (2004b), the trend in spending on physician services continues to be the slowest-growing component of health care spending for privately insured patients. This is most likely due to the transition to less tightly managed care, with the growth in use and price contributing equally to the increase in spending on physician care.

Medical Conditions and Health Care Spending. Understanding the link between health care spending and specific medical conditions also can shed light on spending growth. A recent study using data compiled by the U.S. Department of Health and Human Services found that 15 medical conditions accounted for half of the growth in spending between 1987 and 2000 (Thorpe, Florence, & Joski, 2004). Of these, heart disease, mental disorders, asthma, cancer, and trauma were responsible for nearly one third of the increase. Researchers also were able to show that spending could be explained as changes in the number of individuals treated, the cost per treated case, or spending because of population growth and that the importance of these factors varied by medical condition.

For some conditions, increased spending could be explained by the rise in the number of individuals treated, reflecting two trends: better recognition and diagnosis of the disease and increased prevalence in the population. For instance, the cost of treating mental disorders nearly doubled as a result of improvements in diagnosis, whereas the increased cost of treating asthma appeared to be related to an increased number of individuals suffering from the disease.

For other conditions the cost to treat each case rose significantly. For instance, in heart disease, the cost to treat each case rose nearly 70% between 1987 and 2000, reflecting the use of new medical technologies and drugs. However, although spending per person went up, death rates associated with heart disease decreased. This observation suggests that some spending increases are warranted when health indicators improve as a result of treatment.

Technology/Medical Innovation. The consensus about the effect of technology on health care spending is not universal. Many believe that advances in medicine—including technological and clinical developments that result in new products, processes or procedures, whether they are diagnostic, therapeutic, preventive, or administrative—are a key driver in the escalating cost of health care. Others support the position that the subtle and complex relationship between technological innovation and health care spending is not well understood and that medical technologies are not inherently cost increasing. Individual technologies can (1) reduce or increase the unit cost of treatment, the risk of complications, clinical incomes, or hospital revenues; (2) require repetitive use or eliminate the need for further treatment; (3) expand or leave constant the population of those at risk for medical treatment; or (4) improve or complicate the patient's quality of life.

Personal Disposable Income. With consumers paying a larger portion of the cost of services, disposable personal income may become an important driver in trends in private spending on medical services, particularly those currently not well covered by many payers such as dental services, medical equipment, and other professional care services. Nursing home services currently also have high out-of-pocket cost sharing, although the relationship to disposable income is less direct, given the contributions of Medicare and the potential eligibility for benefits under Medicaid for longer stays.

IMPLICATIONS FOR CONSUMERS

Implications for consumers focus on several areas such as increased cost sharing, prescription drugs, and availability of coverage.

Increased Cost Sharing

Although the growth in health insurance premiums fell slightly in early 2004 after years of accelerating rate increases, the continuing rise in health care spending will exert upward pressure on premiums into the foreseeable future. Employers have responded to the continuing rise in health insurance premiums by shifting more costs to consumers through various types of cost-sharing arrangements. This premium buy-down in the form of higher deductibles and co-payments is expected to result in an increased share of consumer disposable income going for medical costs. Employees also are paying a greater portion of the premium through higher monthly contributions.

In addition to co-payments for physician services, a growing number of individuals with employer-sponsored coverage now have separate hospital cost-sharing arrangements. In spite of rising costs, employers have been reluctant to reduce covered benefits, preferring instead to implement cost-sharing arrangements. Once rare, these cost-sharing arrangements can include a separate annual deductible and co-payment for hospital services, coinsurance for hospital services, or both.

Prescription Drugs

Prescription drugs account for the largest share of out-of-pocket spending by consumers. To control expenses, employers have redesigned their prescription drug benefit plans to include mail-order discount programs or multitier cost-sharing formulas under which the individual's share varies with the type of drug prescribed and availability of brand or generic options.

Availability of Coverage

Health cost increases threaten to make health care coverage less affordable and more difficult to extend coverage to those currently without it. Although large firms continue to offer health insurance coverage, smaller firms often experience difficulties in finding affordable coverage because of the costs of administering smaller programs. The number of jobs offering health insurance has fallen in this country, although this does not always translate into loss of coverage; some individuals might have access to a second policy through a family member, the individual health insurance market, or a public program.

Individuals Covered Under Public Programs

Implications of increased health care spending to individuals with Medicare and Medicaid differ in some ways from those with private insurance. Medicare has coped with spending increases in much the same way that private insurance does: by increasing premiums and deductibles and co-payments. Medicaid beneficiaries, however, are more likely to lose benefits as states adjust eligibility rules that exclude a portion of the population at the margin. In addition, some states are experimenting with small deductibles for Medicaid recipients to discourage overuse of health care services.

Outlook for Cost Trends

Nothing indicates that the overall growth in health care spending will abate any time in the foreseeable future. Current projections suggest that the overall growth in health care spending will increase at an average annual rate that is 2.1 percentage points greater than the growth of the national economy. As a result, spending on health care is expected to increase from 14.9% in 2002 to 18.4% of the gross domestic product in 2013. If this trend continues, health care premiums will continue to rise and payers likely will push for additional tools to manage the growth in underlying health care costs. The growth in personal health care spending also is expected to continue. Factors converging to influence the rate of growth include use and intensity of services, prices for services, and the state of the economy, including labor markets, health insurance plan designs, and an aging population.

Administrative tools to control costs will include greater financial responsibility for patients in the form of higher deductibles and co-payments and a relatively new tool, health savings accounts. All of these strategies are designed to motivate individuals to consume health care more judiciously.

APPROACHES TO CONTROLLING HEALTH CARE SPENDING

Concern over rising health care costs has led to numerous approaches to control spending. One natural way of distinguishing among the various programs and proposals is to think of them in terms of government regulation versus market forces. For instance, the federal government has attempted with some success to slow the rate of health care costs in its own programs, Medicare and Medicaid. Market-driven strategies, however, arise from individual organizations such as insurance companies and employers who use various methods to reduce health care spending by their policyholders and employees. Some of these strategies include controlling access to health care, bargaining with providers (hospitals and

physicians, for instance), and shifting costs to individuals. Some newer innovations include strategies that combine government and market approaches, such as health care spending accounts and exerting pressure on government to reform medical liability rules. Finally, some organizations have begun looking at ways to compensate health care providers for quality and efficiency. This section will look at several of these current and developing strategies.

Government Regulation

Before World War II, government regulation of health care was largely absent. Proposals to expand insurance availability and to nationalize health care first emerged in the 1930s in response to widespread poverty resulting from the Great Depression. However, opposition by the American Medical Association effectively undermined these efforts (Starr, 1982, pp. 271-275). At the end of the twentieth century, America remained one of the few industrialized countries that had not instituted a nationalized health care plan. However, because of programs such as Medicare and Medicaid, direct federal expenditures on health care totaled 45% of all U.S. spending (Pipes, 2004, p. 1). Government thus has a vested interest in controlling health care expenditures and also has the power of law to enforce regulations intended to hold down health care costs.

Medicare and Medicaid

Although the aim of the Medicare and Medicaid programs was primarily to improve the health of vulnerable populations, early estimates of the costs of these programs proved to be optimistic. In the case of Medicare, reimbursement rates to providers were for "reasonable and customary" charges, based on the fees charged in the same community by similar providers. Little was done to control the rise in health care services during the high-inflation years of the 1970s and early 1980s. Finally, in 1983, Congress passed the Medicare Prospective Payment Plan, which established diagnostic-related groups. Rather than pay for each service or supply provided in the course of a patient's care, the diagnostic-related group established a set fee that would be paid to a hospital for treating a patient with a particular disease. The system included adjustments for case severity, teaching hospitals, and disproportionate share of uncompensated care related to a particular hospital, but even with adjustments, the program put the responsibility for controlling the cost of care directly on the provider.

Despite constant adjustments to the prospective payment plan program, Medicare spending continued to grow disproportionately through the next decade. In 1997 the Balanced Budget Act was passed. The act included provisions to reduce payments to providers further while maintaining benefits for Medicare enrollees. The natural reaction of physicians and hospitals has been to raise their prices to other patient populations, especially commercial insurance and self-pay patients, a practice termed *cost shifting*. Thus even when the federal government has been able to regulate its own expenditures, the overall health care spending of the nation has been affected little by the various adjustments to Medicare.

Spending on Medicaid programs also has increased dramatically over time, but for different reasons. From the outset, Medicaid has set reimbursement rates for providers so that government could regulate the growth in fees charged by hospitals and physicians. However, the number of eligible individuals tends to grow during economic downturns, resulting in increases in overall spending. In the first years of the millennium, overall rates for Medicaid spending grew by upwards of 9.5% annually, even as state and federal tax revenues fell while the country suffered through a recession. Medicaid also is distinguished from other programs in that it is administered by individual states with differing rules for coverage. The states receive varying amounts from the federal government, which allots anywhere from 50% to 83% of the Medicaid budget of a state, depending on the overall economic strength of the state.

Efforts to manage Medicaid spending growth focus on a few key strategies. First, eligibility requirements can be modified. Most states place family eligibility in terms of the family's earning power compared with the national definition for the poverty level. Typically, a state may rule a family eligible for Medicaid benefits if its income is no greater than 1.5 to 2 times the national poverty level. States can sweep large numbers of eligible individuals and families into and out of their programs by modifying the means test. Second, states can tighten reimbursement rates to providers. This tactic works well in regions where the Medicaid-eligible population is small and cost shifting can cover the revenue shortfall for hospitals and physicians. However, providers who care primarily for Medicaid populations often cannot handle reductions in revenue and may shut down or, in the case of individual physicians, move elsewhere. In these cases, states often must provide additional grants and funding to certain providers to ensure that they can continue to care for these needy populations. A third approach has been to require small deductibles and co-payments by Medicaid patients. However, because of the severely limited financial resources of most Medicaid patients, how great an impact this action will have is not clear. Finally, most states have adopted managed care plans for their Medicaid populations to better regulate use of services. The managed care plans usually consist of states contracting with existing health providers to furnish care for Medicaid patients, often at a capitated rate (meaning that the state will prepay a set amount per individual enrolled without regard to how much service the patient consumes). The incentives for developing a managed care mechanism include controlling costs for the state, which negotiates an overall lower rate with the managed care company than it currently spends on fee-for-service, and at the same time encouraging more rational use of health care by Medicaid populations via the managed care plan. The performance of managed care plans for Medicaid populations has been successful where the rates paid were sufficient to cover costs. However, over time, significant numbers of plans have folded or refused to accept further enrollments because of the low capitation rates offered by some states. Thus although managed care has promise for controlling Medicaid spending, it often is hampered when managed care plans decide the rates being offered are not attractive.

Single Payer/National Health Insurance Plan

Dissatisfaction with many aspects of the United States health care system has led to proposals for a *single-payer system*, often referred to as *national health insurance*. A single-payer plan would ensure coverage for every person for any medically necessary service, regardless of age, employment, or economic status. Such plans exist in the United States at present in the form of the Medicare and Medicaid programs. Both of these plans are seen by many as templates for offering comprehensive health care to all citizens and legal residents of the United States.

Proponents of single-payer plans see many advantages to these proposals over the current mix of plans now in operation in the United States. These advantages include the following:

◆ The cost of administering multiple public and private plans (Medicare and Medicaid, along with insurance companies and health maintenance organizations, to name a few) would be reduced to one administrative unit.

◆ Hospitals and doctors would spend less on maintaining complex billing and collection systems because they would have to bill only to one entity.

- Charges by providers (hospitals, clinics, physicians, and other health care professionals) could be controlled through prospective rate setting. Rates would be decided through negotiation between the national plan and providers, such as now is the case with Medicare. Because all patients would be covered by the plan, costs could not be shifted to self-paying or insurance-covered patients.
- Pharmaceutical costs, the fastest-rising segment of health care at present, could be controlled by a national formulary that specified approved drugs and supplies. Pharmaceutical companies and retailers also would be subject to rate setting that ensured a reasonable cost for each product.
- Better access to health care, including coverage for drugs and supplies, may reduce the incidence of patients deferring treatment only to be admitted later for more serious problems, with resulting large hospital charges.

In 1994 a national panel convened by former First Lady Hillary Clinton developed a proposal for a national health care plan that was intended to guarantee universal health care coverage regardless of an individual's employment status, income, or other factor (*The President's Health Security Plan,* 1993). Titled the Health Security Act, this plan proposed to reduce the overall health care expense burden of the nation by creating one simplified administration system. Regions and individual states would administer health boards that reviewed use and approved referrals to specialists much as managed care systems do. Funding would be provided by a tax on employers, regardless of the size of the company, or 7.9% on wages. All Americans would be covered automatically and would receive comprehensive care from the physician of their choice. The proposal differed from many national health care plans in that it preserved individual choice and had a decentralized orientation through the state and regional administrations. Unfortunately for the Clinton administration, the public debate quickly grew acrimonious with questions about funding and the actual freedom of consumers to choose medical treatments, and the proposal ultimately was dropped.

The success of a single-payer plan in the United States can be analyzed only in the abstract because no one has been successful in implementing it in this country. However, critics have focused on two bodies of evidence to argue against development of such a plan. The first body of evidence comes from experience with Medicare. Because all health care administered to citizens over age 65 is paid through Medicare, one can look at the financial performance of this plan to see how a restrictive payer plan might function. For instance, an important feature of Medicare is its deductibles and co-payments for many services. These patient payment features have risen at rates of 5% and up in recent years as Medicare attempted to close the gap between spending and income from payroll deduction.

The other perspective on single-payer plans comes from comparisons with other countries that have adopted a national health insurance plan. In this respect, the evidence is not promising. The most direct comparisons can be made with the systems in Canada and Britain. These two countries are most like the United States in terms of culture and especially in regard to diverse populations as measured by ethnic background, economic status, and dispersion between urban and rural populations. The major difference between Canada and Britain and the United States is that Canada and Britain provide national health plans that cover all citizens in those countries, whereas the majority of U.S. citizens must receive coverage through an employer or purchase individual private health insurance plans. Nonetheless, when comparisons were drawn between the two systems, although health care costs as a proportion of gross domestic product are highest in the United States, lower in Britain, and lowest in Canada, the following were found (Goodman, Musgrave, & Herrick, 2004):

- Average length of hospital stay is 5.9 days in the United States, 6.2 days in Britain, and 7.1 days in Canada.
- Mortality rates for breast cancer (percent of patients diagnosed with the disease who die from it) are 25% in the United States, 28% in Canada, and 46% in Britain. For prostate cancer, the U.S. rate is 19%; Canada, 25%; and Britain, 57%.
- Infant mortality rates are higher in the United States (7.2 deaths per 1000 deliveries) than in Canada (6.1 per 1000) or Britain (6.9 per 1000). However, when geographic and ethnic differences are examined within a single country, the mortality rates for the United States are substantially the same for similar populations in the other two countries. For instance, the infant mortality rate in New Hampshire is 4.4, compared with 4.6 for Prince Edward Island in Canada, a relatively prosperous province. The rate in Saskatchewan is 9.1, reflecting its largely rural and poorer population. Similar comparisons can be drawn for United Kingdom regions.

These findings suggest that health care delivery is neither more efficient nor more effective for national plans versus the private system of the United States.

The United States tends to have shorter lengths of stay and better outcomes for serious diseases. Countries with national plans tend to provide better screening and routine care because individuals are more likely to see a doctor when they do not have to pay a large amount for the visit. These observations may reflect the decision on the part of national plans to focus on routine care and screening of their populations while restricting access to more complex care for the smaller segment of the population with serious illness. Economists often discuss the trade-off between time and money; in this case the national health plan requires patients to wait longer for certain procedures, saving money in the process because it hires fewer specialists and purchases smaller numbers of specialized equipment. For instance, a comparison of the numbers of patients having to wait more than 4 months for elective surgeries indicated that for Britain the proportion was 36%; for Canada, 27%; and for the United States, only 5%. This may correlate with the cited mortality rates for breast and prostate cancer (Goodman, Musgrave, & Herrick, 2004, p. 23).

In summary, although national health care plans are less expensive than private plans on a nationwide basis and demonstrate better overall health standards, the savings may be at the cost of the seriously ill populations in those countries. Regulating spending on more expensive procedures may equate with longer waiting times and potentially higher mortality rates. Whether this is a trade-off that citizens are willing to make is a question that requires serious public debate.

MARKET-DRIVEN STRATEGIES FOR CONTROLLING HEALTH CARE SPENDING

Although many countries around the world encourage private enterprise, the United States may stand apart in terms of its constitutional restrictions on government function and its emphasis on market-driven philosophy. Not surprisingly then, the 75% of Americans who are not in government health care programs (i.e., Medicare and Medicaid) rely in large part on the private sector for financing their health care. For most of this country's history, health care has been provided on a fee-for-service basis, with patients paying for services as they were provided, directly or through a third-party such as private insurance. Even Medicare for much of its early existence paid for services using a menu of reasonable and customary fees that reflected a community standard to determine an acceptable level of payment.

However, during the 1980s, rapidly accelerating health care spending led government and private insurers to search for ways to contain this growth. Not only was it a component of a high overall inflation rate, but also it was making it difficult for American companies to compete with international counterparts that did not have to absorb high costs for employee health services. The response from the commercial marketplace has been managed care, along with sharper bargaining on the purchase of health care services and attempts to manage utilization better.

Managed Care

The term *managed care* actually encompasses a variety of systems designed to control individual access to the health care system by restricting the available providers and participating in the decision of what care should be delivered. It is hard today to imagine that only 25 or 30 years ago, persons with an insurance card could make an appointment to see any doctor they chose, including specialists, and that the physician could decide with little oversight from the insurance company where the patient might be hospitalized, for how long, and what procedures might be performed. Today, even the simplest health insurance plans require choice of a primary care doctor who acts as a gatekeeper for access to the health care system, coupled with approval by the plan for most procedures, and justification for any hospitalization of the patient.

Managed care organizations did not have a large presence in the United States until passage by Congress in 1973 of the Health Maintenance Organization Act. This law sought to promote health maintenance organization (HMO) growth by requiring employers to offer an HMO choice in their employee health care plans and also provided start-up funding for HMOs. The impetus for the act came from the observation that fee-for-service plans encourage health care providers to offer more, rather than fewer, services and procedures, whereas a prepaid plan would be more efficient and careful in what services it provided to members (referred to as utilization) (Kongstvedt, 2002, p. 10). In exchange, the managed care plan could offer lower premiums to employers.

Over the following years, HMOs grew in size and numbers. However, concerns over the restrictions placed on patients who could see only the doctors employed by their particular HMO and could be hospitalized only in the institution specified by the HMO led to different arrangements such as preferred provider organizations. These organizations differ from HMOs in that they allow patients to seek care outside the system, but with a reduced reimbursement rate, such as 60% to 70% of allowed charges. Preferred provider organizations still require certification for hospitalization and other mechanisms for managing use.

Estimating the impact of managed care organizations on health care spending in the past 2 decades is difficult. Perhaps most telling is that these organizations have replaced traditional health insurance plans almost completely with company-sponsored benefits. However, the growth in health care spending appears to have risen with few exceptions at a rate well over inflation in the period in which managed care plans dominated the private sector of health care funding. Why has managed care not lived up to its promises? One possible reason is that employers, who purchase health care benefits for employees, have been caught in the middle when managed care organizations refuse to provide services that employees demand but may not be justified. To placate certain classes of workers, employers have sought more liberal plans (Nichols, Ginsburg, Berenson, Christianson, & Hurley, 2004). Secondly, competition among managed care organizations has not been as strong as expected. Within cities and regions, dominant managed care organizations hold near-monopoly positions and do not feel threatened about losing patients to other systems. Thus, for instance, although a city such as Chicago (population of 4 million plus might have five or six large provider systems, towns with populations of 250,000 may have only one large private system that is not motivated to negotiate lower prices.

Managed Competition

Managed competition describes a concept in which, unlike managed care, the consumer (employer or individual) joins groups that have the market power to negotiate lower costs from providers. One way this might work is for employers to set a fixed price for health care services, with employees making up any additional charge. This would lead to competition among providers to become more efficient or to distinguish themselves by some value-added component such as quality or cutting-edge technology. Public agencies, employer groups, or government would establish the base price for coverage.

The forces needed to drive managed competition have not emerged in the past decade. As noted in the previous section on managed care, employers are often reluctant to force their workers into making tough decisions about health care. Because health care quality is traditionally difficult for the layman to assess, providers have not been eager to promote themselves based on relative health outcomes for their patients. Finally, the competition concept is only operative where competing organizations exist, and as noted previously, many communities do not have multiple health care organizations competing in the same niche. Thus although managed competition has much to merit as a concept, it has yet to play out in the marketplace.

Disease Management

A recent concept is of *disease management,* which occurs when providers focus their management on a few chronic diseases prevalent among their patient population. Problems such as diabetes, asthma, hypertension, and coronary artery disease consume a disproportionate share of health care spending as a reflection of their prevalence and difficulty in management. By establishing standards of care and protocols based on best evidence, the hypothesis is that costs will go down as efficiency and effectiveness of treatment rises. This is similar in concept to quality improvement programs in industry, where focusing on the most expensive steps in production can improve quality and lower cost by addressing human error, inefficient processes, and redundancy.

Many providers use disease management concepts as an approach to working with populations with common chronic diseases. The growing popularity of evidence-based medicine as a means of analyzing the literature to determine what treatments work best with particular populations is a starting point for the development of standard treatment plans. When standard plans are in place, health care workers at lower levels can be trained to work with patients, a potential cost savings. By providing better care to patients, spending also is expected to drop as a result of fewer emergency room visits and hospital stays. Finally, quality of life should improve for the patients, a real and positive consideration for developing disease management protocols.

Unfortunately, demonstration of actual savings through the implementation of disease management has not materialized. A report by a group practice that provides care to Kaiser Permanente members in California (Fireman, Bartlett, & Selby, 2004) looked at treatment for approximately 3000 patients with coronary heart disease, heart failure, diabetes, and asthma over a 6-year period in which disease management procedures (e.g., clinical guidelines, patient self-management education, frequent testing, control of risk factors, and performance feedback to health care workers) were implemented. What Fireman et al. discovered was a number of improvements in disease indicators, such as reduction in blood pressure, fasting glucose levels, and cholesterol, and better compliance in taking medications. Another important finding was that for patients with diabetes or asthma, hospitalizations decreased (although total inpatient days did not), as did emergency room visits for asthmatics. However, despite very good quality measures, the authors could not demonstrate a reduction or even stabilization of costs associated with the four diseases selected. Even when costs were adjusted for increases in the Consumer Price Index, real increases of 19% to 27% were reported. What this study may demonstrate is that the cost of effectively managing certain chronic diseases will lead to higher health care consumption as patients receive more frequent screenings and seek more care when warning signs occur. Because disease management leads to better health outcomes, it is a compelling approach to treating patients. However, disease management cannot be advanced as a cost-reduction technique without additional study.

Consumer-Directed Health Care

In the sixth edition of *Current Issues in Nursing,* Seefeldt, Garg, and Grace (2001, p. 385), note that in the discussion of health care costs, "the biggest stakeholder of all, the consumer of health care services, is rarely mentioned as part of the debate." Yet the trend has been to reduce consumer choice at the point of service and to encourage use of services provided within a network. One problem with encouraging patient choice is what economists term a *moral hazard.* When employees are handed an insurance card that is accepted by most providers, they have no incentive to shop for health care based on price or efficiency. In fact, they may not have enough information to search out quality, relying instead on advertisements and recommendations from friends and family. The moral hazard occurs because health care then becomes a "free good" for these consumers; they tend to overuse the available services because someone else is paying the bill.

A simple solution to the moral hazard issue is to require patients to pay a portion of their bills. This can be in the form of deductibles (patient pays the initial portion and only then does the coverage begin) or co-payments (patient pays a percentage of the total bill). However, cost sharing by patients has not had a noticeable effect on the rise of health care spending, and in many cases, employers have found it difficult to persuade employees to accept insurance plans that require significant out-of-pocket expenditures.

Shifting health care costs to employees and individuals is a practice that has real limits and one that places the greatest burden on individuals who need care the most, for themselves or for members of their families. Health savings accounts (HSAs) recently have emerged as a solution that combines cost sharing with protection from the expense of chronic or catastrophic disease or injury. Briefly, HSAs are accounts into which employees deposit pretax funds (in other words, they do not pay income tax on the money put into the account). The employees can withdraw funds to reimburse deductibles, coinsurance, prescriptions, eyeglasses, hearing aids, and many over-the-counter health care items. As long as the withdrawal pays for an allowed service or supply, the amount is not taxed. Health savings accounts have been in existence for a number of years, but until the December 2003 Medicare revision, they had significant disadvantages, chief of which was that money not spent in an account by the end of a calendar year was forfeited. This required careful planning on the part of the employee, and many avoided investing funds that might be lost because of changes in health needs. The forfeiture provision was eliminated in the 2004 law, and the move from "use it or lose it" to "keep it and save it" has resulted in large numbers of companies offering HSAs to employees; and some estimates indicate by 2006 that more than 80% of companies will include this benefit.

Health savings accounts can be attractive benefits to employees and employers. The employer can offer lower-cost health insurance policies that have higher deductibles and co-payments, and even can pass along the savings to employees to encourage them to start up their funds. Employees can use the funds for a variety of health care needs, including out-of-system care that otherwise would be too expensive. If employees move to a different company, the funds can accompany them. Some programs even issue a debit card that the employee can use to pay for goods and services, eliminating virtually all paperwork. From a larger, national perspective, it is hoped that HSAs will motivate individuals to make more careful decisions on how to spend their health care funds and encourage them to seek out lower-cost services.

Early evidence that HSAs can have an economic impact is encouraging. In 2003, Aetna launched its Healthfund (Aetna, 2004), a patient directed account with many of the features of HSAs. In the first 12 months of operation with 13,500 subscribers, Aetna found the following:

◆ Employers experienced a 3.7% medical cost increase, compared with double-digit increases for a similar population.
◆ For the one full replacement plan sponsor in the study, medical costs decreased by 11%.
◆ The low medical cost increases for all members in the study were driven by two major factors: a reduction

in certain physician visits, including a 115 reduction in primary care office visits, and a modest 3% increase in specialist visits; and a reduction in use of facility services, including a 3% decrease in emergency room visits, a 14% decrease in outpatient cases, and a 5% decrease in inpatient admissions.

◆ Members experienced a 5.5% decrease in pharmacy costs driven by a 13% decline in overall prescriptions and a 7% increase in overall generic drug use.

These are dramatic results, and further experience is needed to confirm whether HSAs can sustain decreased health care spending. However, because HSAs address some of the fastest growing health cost drivers such as pharmacy and outpatient procedures, they may have an overall effect on health care spending.

THE EMERGING ISSUE OF QUALITY

Interest in reimbursing health care providers based on performance has risen in recent years, in part related to concerns over quality of care, error, and outcomes. Sometimes referred to as "pay for performance" (Rosenthal, Fernandopulle, Song, & Landon, 2004), the aim of these financial incentives is to motivate providers to demonstrate high quality in terms of "structural" indicators, referring to the presence of appropriate staff, equipment, and procedures that are associated with high-quality care and good outcomes, or in the treatment of specific diseases or even patients. Incentives can range from HMOs paying a small incentive per month per subscriber to bonuses of hundreds of dollars to physicians for maintaining good health indicators in patients with chronic disease to large annual payments to providers for maintaining overall quality measures.

Another approach to quality is the development of patient safety programs. Concern over the number of medical errors occurring in health care settings has led to federally funded research into improvements in patient safety and protection for institutions that develop and use error-reporting mechanisms. Reducing error can lead to lower health care spending by mechanisms such as decreasing inpatient length of stay, eliminating extra procedures and services needed to reverse the injury caused by the initial error, and ultimately to reducing professional liability premiums.

It is too early to tell whether these programs will lead to better efficiency and lower spending in the treatment of patients. However, a number of problems will have to be solved to ensure the viability of quality programs. In terms of reducing spending, examination of the Kaiser Permanente program by Fireman et al. (2004) suggests that costs do not decrease where quality is the focus. Health care providers also may object to this level of scrutiny of their operations, claiming that the measures are not valid indicators of quality. This most likely might occur for those providers who are of marginal quality and would most benefit by the improvements. Financial incentives also will have to be significant enough to fund operational changes by providers. If payments are too small, physicians and hospitals may decide to ignore them. However, very large payments may divert funds from other uses and result in overall spending increases. Finally, "what gets measured gets done." Providers may become focused on those services and indicators that are part of the quality program and may neglect others because the financial incentives do not exist to improve them. This could lead to paradoxical decreases in quality in other areas of the practice or institution.

PROFESSIONAL LIABILITY INSURANCE REFORM

Professional liability insurance to individual health professionals and to institutions often has been cited as a major driver of health care expense. Many physicians face malpractice premiums in the range of $150,000 to $250,000 annually (Albert, 2004), and some have retired or moved in response to these heavy expenses. Providers also pass along increased insurance premium costs to their patients, contributing to rising spending rates. Another indirect consequence of high liability costs is the practice of "defensive medicine," which refers to physicians ordering tests and procedures not directly related to the patient's well-being but that could protect the physician from accusations that they missed a condition or problem that was not obvious or suspected. No one has reliable figures on the cost of defensive medicine because physicians often rationalize the additional services in terms of better care for the patient.

Faced with the unpleasant prospect of losing physicians who move to areas where their malpractice insurance premiums might be lower, many states have sought to reduce increases in insurance premiums by setting maximum awards for pain and suffering. From time to time the U.S. Congress considers national professional liability reform. Approaches include setting national caps on noneconomic awards (pain and suffering, for example) and punitive damages, reducing joint and several liability (where any one party can be made to pay the entire award if other parties to the suit cannot), and even limited the fees that an attorney can charge for bringing a malpractice suit to court. Evidence that these could be effective provisions comes from California, where increases in professional liability insurance premiums have been lower than in other states in part because California was one of the first states to set award caps.

SUMMARY

What works? Despite the best combined efforts of government and the private sector, no strategy has emerged that leads to stability in health care spending. Advocates for government administration ("Medicare for all") see economies in a single-payer plan that can control prices and access, whereas promoters of market-based plans focus on economic incentives that combine aspects of choice, quality, and competition. Unlike other consumer goods and services, however, health care often is "purchased" under stress and without adequate information for the consumer. Coupled with that is the sentiment that no expense be spared (especially if it involves a third-party payer) to maintain health and well-being. The conclusion of the authors of the previous edition of this chapter was that consumers should participate in health care treatment decisions, especially from a financial standpoint. That sentiment continues to resonate through this chapter, and it may turn out that the best solution to rising spending will be to return the control of spending to the consumer. Whether mechanisms such as HSAs will have a significant impact on health care spending is yet to be seen. However, the failure of every other strategy so far is a compelling argument to consider new perspectives and fresh ideas in how to manage the cost of health care while maintaining quality.

REFERENCES

Aetna HealthFund® First-Year Results Validate Positive Impact of Health Care Consumerism (2004). Retrieved on October 23, 2005 from http://www.aetna.com/news/2004/pr_20040622.htm

Albert, T. (2004, November 15). Liability premium increases slowing, yet rates remain at record highs. *AMNews, 47*(43), 1-2.

Fireman, B., Bartlett, J., & Selby, J. (2004). Can disease management reduce health are costs by improving quality? *Health Affairs, 23*(6), 63-75.

Goodman, J. C., Musgrave, G. L., & Herrick, D. M. (2004). *Lives at risk: Single-payer national health insurance around the world.* New York: Rowman & Littlefield.

Heffler, S., Smith, S., Keehan, S. L, Clemens, M. K., & Zezza, M. (2004). Health spending projections through 2013. *Health Affairs* retrieved October 23, 2005, from http://content.healthaffairs.org/cgi/content/abstract/hlthaff.w4.79v1

Kongstvedt, P. R. (2002). *Managed care: What it is and how it works.* Gaithersburg, MD: Aspen.

Nichols, L. M., Ginsburg, P. B., Berenson, R. A., Christianson, J., & Hurley, R. E. (2004). Are market forces strong enough to deliver efficient health care systems? Confidence is waning. *Health Affairs, 23*(2), 8-21.

Pipes, S. C. (2004). *Miracle cure: How to solve America's health care crisis and why Canada isn't the answer.* Vancouver, BC: The Fraser Institute.

The President's Health Security Plan. (1993). New York: Time Books.

Rosenthal, M. B., Fernandopulle, R., Song, H. R., & Landon, B. (2004). Paying for quality: Providers' incentives for quality improvement. *Health Affairs, 23*(2), 127-141.

Seefeldt, F. M., Garg, M., and Grace, H. K. (2001). Controlling health care costs: Regulation versus competition. In J. M. Dochterman & H. K. Grace (Eds.), *Current issues in nursing* (6th ed., pp. 337-386). St. Louis, MO: Mosby.

Starr, P. (1982). *The social transformation of American medicine.* New York, NY: Basic Books.

Strunk, B. C., & Ginsberg, P. B. (2004a, June 9). Tracking health care costs: Trends turn downward in 2003. *Health Affairs.* Retrieved April 2, 2005, from http://content.healthaffairs.org/cgi/content/full/hlthaff.w4.354/DC1

Strunk, B. C., & Ginsburg, P. B. (2004b). Tracking health care costs: Spending growth slowdown stalls in first half of 2004. *EBRI Notes, 25*(12), 1-7.

Thorpe, K. E., Florence, C. S., & Joski, P. (2004, August 25). Which medical conditions account for the rise in health care spending? *Health Affairs.* Retrieved April 2, 2005, from http://content.healthaffairs.org/cgi/content/full/hlthaff.w4.437/DC1

Thorpe, K. E. & Ginsburg, P. B. (2001). Factors driving cost increases. *AHRQ's User Liaison Program* Retrieved October 23, 2005 from http://www.ahrq.gov/news/ulp/costs/ulpcosts1.htm

Managed Care, Prospective Payment, and Reimbursement Trends

Impact and Implications for Nursing

P. J. MADDOX

In the 1980s the rising cost of health care prompted policy makers to consider serious structural reform of the U.S. health care system. State and local governments have faced poor economic conditions, budget constraints, and growing public demands for health and social services (especially Medicaid and Medicare). This has occurred as the aged and low-income populations have grown and employer-subsidized health insurance coverage has declined (Henry J. Kaiser Family Foundation, 2005). Through the 1990s, these approaches were the cornerstone of health care cost containment, followed by efforts to "right-size" care delivery systems and improve service quality.

Struggling to cover rising health care costs, policy makers have adopted a myriad of strategies (i.e., reducing coverage and limiting access) to try to control or at least limit rising costs. Employers also have become concerned about the rising cost of health care. As a result, they have demanded that insurers be more aggressive in their efforts to reduce the rate of premium increases while changing their approaches to coverage for employees (i.e., passing on premium costs to employees and offering insurance plans that require co-payments and deductibles). Among the many strategies used to curb rising costs is adoption of prospective payment and managed care (financing strategies designed to provide incentives to health care providers to use health services/resources efficiently). These strategies and their impact are the focus of this chapter.

System expectations of nurses as health service providers, managers, and resource stewards are affected profoundly by the economics of health care delivery and changing reimbursement/financing schemes (Dranove, 2000). As noted, economic pressures have created the momentum for changes in the delivery and financing of health care that have affected nursing practice. System changes brought about by patient care process redesign,

the prospective payment system (PPS), and rising concerns about health care system safety, regulatory avoidance, and the rise of consumerism are continuing to challenge the status quo (Christiansen & Bender, 1994; Dranove, Shanley, & White, 1993; Sovie, 1995; Wilson & Porter-O'Grady, 1999; Wunderlich, Sloan, & Davis, 1996). To cope with rising health costs, health care service organizations have responded by eliminating excess capacity, improving economies of scale by integrating services, merging and/or consolidating, and focusing on operational efficiency (Agency for Healthcare Research and Quality, 2001; Buerhaus & Needleman, 2000; Stanton & Rutherford, 2004). The focus of this chapter is twofold: to examine the evolution of managed care and the demographic, economic, and financial factors that have served as the motivation for changing the U.S. health care system and to examine selected effects that managed care and economic pressures have exerted on nursing roles and practice in recent years.

ECONOMIC TRENDS AND THE U.S. HEALTH CARE SYSTEM

The U.S. health care system is a diverse collection of subindustries that are involved directly or indirectly in the provision of health care services. The major "players" in the industry are health professionals who provide health care services, pharmaceutical and equipment suppliers, insurers (public/government and private), employers and other stakeholder entities such as educational institutions, consulting and research firms, professional associations, and trade unions. Today, the health care industry is large and pervasive, with characteristics and operational differences that vary widely between geographic region and type of community (rural or urban).

The infrastructure of the U.S. health care system has evolved rapidly since the 1950s, producing unprecedented increases in the overall cost of health care and shifting the responsibility for payment. From 1950 to 1980, growth in national health care expenditures were attributable to the rise of first dollar private health insurance coverage (no deductible, or amount that you have to pay, for a covered medical expense) and the advent of government-financed health insurance programs (Medicare and Medicaid). Today, even without universal access to health insurance, the United States spends more on health care than any nation in the world, averaging more than $3659 per person (Dranove, 2000; Mechanic, 2004).

The increase in health care expenditures during the 1980s in particular led to widespread adoption of managed care by employer-sponsored health plans. To a lesser degree, public programs followed. By the 1990s, Medicare reimbursement changes and the proliferation of managed care slowed the rate of growth in health care expenditures (Fronstein, 1994). In 1980, U.S. health care expenditures totaled $245.8 billion and accounted for 8.8% of the national gross domestic product. By 2003, per capita expenditures had increased to $1678.90 and accounted for a rise in gross domestic product to 15.3%. Table 49-1 depicts the growth of total U.S. expenditures and changes in public/private expenditures over time.

Analysis of health care expenditures by service category points to some with higher rates of spending increases over others (hospitals, physicians, and pharmaceuticals). These particular sources have attracted the interest of public policy makers and have been the focus of more rigorous regulatory oversight and more restrictive reimbursement policy in recent years. Table 49-2 summarizes category-specific expenditures from 1980 to 2003.

TABLE 49-1

National Health Care Expenditures 1980-2003: Total per Capita (Private and Public) and Percent Gross Domestic Product

Year	Total National Health Expenditures (in billions)	Per Capita Expenditures: Private Sources (in billions)	Per Capita Expenditures: Public Sources (in billions)	Percent Gross Domestic Product	U.S. Population (in millions)
1980	$245.8	$140.9	$104.8	8.8	230
1990	$696.0	$413.5	$282.5	12.0	254
1995	$990.2	$533.4	$456.8	13.4	271
2000	$1309.9	$717.5	$592.4	13.3	287
2003	$1678.9	$913.2	$765.7	15.3	296

From Centers for Medicare and Medicaid Services. (2005). *National health expenditures tables.* Retrieved June 1, 2005, from http://www.cms.hhs.gov/statistics/nhe/historical/.

TABLE 49-2

National Health Expenditures by Selected Service Category, 1980-2003

Spending Category	Expenditures by Year (in billions of dollars)				
	1980	1990	1995	2000	2003
National expenditures	245.8	696.0	990.2	1309.9	1678.9
Hospitals	101.5	253.9	343.6	413.1	515.9
Physicians	47.1	157.5	220.5	290.2	369.7
Home health	2.4	12.6	30.5	36.5	40.0
Nursing home	17.7	52.7	74.6	95.3	110.5
Prescriptions	12.0	40.3	60.8	121.5	179.2
Administration	12.1	40.0	60.5	81.9	119.0
Research	5.5	12.7	17.1	29.1	40.2

From Centers for Medicare and Medicaid Services. (2005). *National health expenditures tables.* Retrieved June 1, 2005, from http://www.cms.hhs.gov/statistics/nhe/historical/.

Expenditures for hospitals, physicians, and prescription drugs account for the majority of cost increases, with prescription drug spending outpacing all other categories in recent years. Figure 49-1 depicts current expenditures (2003) for all categories.

Left unchecked, expenditures for care and services (all categories) are expected to continue rising because of demographic changes such as aging of the population and chronic illness trends. Factors driving health care expenditures are explained in the sections that follow.

DEMOGRAPHICS AFFECTING HEALTH CARE COSTS

Demographic changes are under way in the United States, including the aging of the population and "epidemic" health problems such as asthma, diabetes, hypertension, obesity, and chemical dependency. Changes in population demographics and health status have

tremendous implications for health service providers and affect the overall cost of health care. Because the majority of the aged and other special populations receive services though publicly funded programs, increasing health needs among these populations has considerable impact on public insurance programs, especially Medicaid and Medicare (Heller, 2005). Figure 49-2 illustrates the distribution of resources by payer source in 2003. In the future, payer shifts are expected to continue from private to public sources, along with other approaches such as shifting some of the cost of premiums and access to services to consumers (Fronstein, 1994; Mechanic, 2004).

IMPACT OF AN AGING POPULATION

Population aging is expected to affect health services more than any other demographic factor, putting

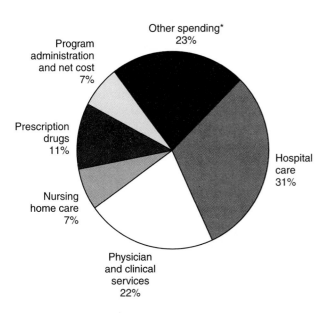

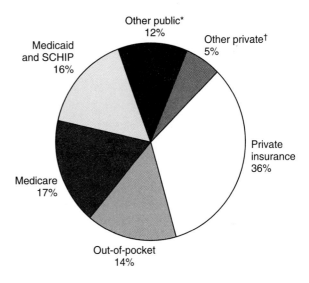

* "Other spending" includes dental services, other professional services, home health care, durable medical products, over-the-counter medicines and sundries, public health activities, research and construction.

FIGURE 49-1 National health care expenditures by category, 2003. "Other Spending" includes dental services, other professional services, home health care, durable medical products, over-the-counter medicines and sundries, public health activities, research, and construction. (From Centers for Medicare and Medicaid Services. [2005]. *The nation's health dollar: 2003.* Retrieved June 1, 2005, from http://www.cms.hhs.gov/ statistics/nhe/historical/chart.asp.)

* "Other public" includes programs such as workers compensation, public health activity, Department of Defense, Department of Veterans Affairs, Indian Health Service, and state and local hospital subsidies and school health.
† "Other private" includes industrial in-plant, privately funded construction, and non-patient revenues, including philanthropy.

FIGURE 49-2 Health service payer distributions, 2004. "Other Public" includes programs such as workers compensation, public health activity, Department of Defense, Department of Veterans Affairs, Indian Health Service, and state and local hospital subsidies and school health. "Other Private" includes industrial in-plant, privately funded construction, and non-patient revenues, including philanthropy. (From Centers for Medicare and Medicaid Services. [2005]. *The nation's health dollar: 2003.* Retrieved June 1, 2005, from http://www.cms.hhs.gov/ statistics/nhe/historical/chart.asp.)

increasing pressure and importance on Medicare cost containment (Hurley, Grossman, & Strunk, 2003). By 2030 the baby boomer generation will compose up to 21% of the population aged 65 and older, and the number of frail elderly (older than age 85) will double. Table 49-3 depicts age cohort growth projections.

Even as life expectancy and functional health status have been increasing, the elderly continue to consume a disproportionate share of financial resources in the last years of life. Although the new "young" elderly (independent and active 60 year olds) are expected to live longer, they also are expected to acquire multiple chronic conditions that become disabling with advanced age. The aged are admitted to hospitals 3 times more often than the general population, and their average length of stay is more than 3 days longer. The elderly also visit physicians more often and constitute a larger percentage of nursing home residents (Andersen & Hussey, 2000). Table 49-4 illustrates the economic impact of funding health services for those over age 65.

The rising number of aged also spurs concerns about funding health care in the future because of shifts in the ratio of individuals working to those retired. Working adults (through income and Social Security payroll taxes) are the primary source of funds for the Medicare; as the population ages and retirement rates increase, the Medicare funding base decreases.

Macrodemographic indicators termed *dependency ratios* inform policy makers about economic and physical support requirements for servicing the elderly. The elderly support ratio (number of persons 65 years and over divided by the number of individuals age 20 to 64 multiplied by 100) is an indicator of requirements necessary for economic and physical support. As Table 49-5 indicates, the elderly support ratio is projected to increase sharply over time. As a result, some policy makers believe that system reforms are needed to ensure adequate financing and infrastructure for delivery of health care and "daily living" services to an aging population.

Policy-related reform options under consideration include increased age limits for Medicare eligibility, means testing for Medicare eligibility, increased availability and coverage for long-term care insurance, incentives for prevention, and less expensive and more efficient delivery arrangements and care settings such as managed care (Gold, 2003; Heller, 2005; Hurley et al., 2003). Meanwhile, the debate continues as to how best to handle future funding for Medicare as public demands for coverage enhancements (especially pharmaceuticals) and provider choice continue (Blegen & Vaughn, 1998; Holohan, Weil, & Weiner, 2003; Lesser, Ginsburg, & Devers, 2003).

EVOLUTION OF U.S. HEALTH CARE SYSTEM FUNDING

Since the 1960s, total spending by all private and public (federal, state, and local government) programs has increased, with the percentage of expenditures attributable to private sources decreasing in relation to public

TABLE 49-3

	Percent Increase in Population Estimates by Age Cohort, 1995-2030		
Age and Period	Lowest Estimate (%)	Middle Estimate (%)	Highest Estimate (%)
65+			
1995-2010	10.8	17.5	24.2
1995-2030	75.6	106.8	136.4
75+			
1995-2010	14.5	24.1	35
1995-2030	71.8	116.2	164
85+			
1995-2010	37.9	56	79.1
1995-2030	59.1	132.7	235.1

From U.S. Bureau of the Census, National Aging Information Center, 1999.

TABLE 49-4

U.S. Health Spending for the Elderly, 1995				
Percent Total Health Spending on Elderly, 1995	Ratio of Health Spending for Persons >65 and <64	Estimated Percent GDP Spent on Health Care for the Elderly	Percent GDP Spent on Health Care	Health Care Spending per Capita, 1997
38	3.8	5.0	13.6	$12,090

From Organization for Economic Cooperation and Development, 1999 Health Data, from Andersen, G. F., & Hussey, P. S. (2000). Population aging: a comparison among industrialized countries. *Health Affairs, 19*(3), 195.

expenditure increases. Among public sources, the percentage paid by the federal government is increasing most rapidly. From 2000 to 2003, the rate of national health care expenditures for publicly funded programs stabilized compared with prior decades. This stabilization is largely attributable to the impact of the PPS and efficiency gains from managed care financing arrangements (which are discussed later in this chapter).

In 1980, national health care expenditures totaled $246 billion; by 2003, they had risen to almost $1679 billion. Of this, public expenditures accounted for nearly $766 billion (46% of all expenditures), with federal programs accounting for the largest component of public expenditures ($542 billion). Table 49-6 depicts changes in national health care expenditures from 1970 to 2003.

FINANCING TRENDS IN THE U.S. HEALTH CARE SYSTEM

National health care expenditures are projected to grow at an average annual rate of 6.5%, reaching $2.2 trillion by 2009. If this projection is on course, national health care expenditures will compose 16.2% of the gross domestic product. Over time, the United States has developed a dependence on private source funding through employer-subsidized health insurance. Although public funding has been and continues to increase, it is important to understand changes unfolding in the private sector regarding the development and growth of third-party payers (Fronstein, 1994; Lesser et al., 2003). This development is occurring as third-party payment programs determine the external threats and opportunities health care organizations and providers inevitably must manage.

EVOLUTION OF THE THIRD-PARTY PAYER SYSTEM

Scientific and technical advances in the U.S. health industry have occurred rapidly since the 1950s, with hospitals becoming the dominant locus for the diagnosis and treatment of disease. The 1930s (a period in which the United States experienced rising health care costs and the economic depression), however, explain

TABLE 49-5

Elderly Support Ratio by Age, 1990-2050		
	Ratio by Age-Group	
Year	**65-74 Years**	**75+ Years**
1990	12.4	8.9
2050	16.5	21.7

From Hobbs, F. B., & Damon, B. L. (1996). *Current population reports special studies, 65+ in the United States.* Washington, DC: U.S. Bureau of the Census.

TABLE 49-6

National Health Expenditures by Source of Funds, Selected Years 1970-2003							
	Expenditures by Selected Year (in billions of dollars)						
Source of Funds	**1970***	**1980†**	**1993***	**1997†**	**1999†**	**2001†**	**2003**
National health expenditures	73.1	245.83	888.1	1093.1	1222.2	1426.4	1678.9
Private funds total	45.4	140.95	497.7	589.8	671.9	771.8	913.2
Private insurance	25.1	58.2	146.9	162.0	184.7	202.0	230.5
Out-of-pocket	15.5	68.2	360.7	360.7	413.7	496.6	600.6
Public funds total	27.6	104.8	390.4	503.2	550.3	654.6	765.7
Federal total	17.6	71.3	274.4	360.0	386.2	463.8	541.7
Medicare	7.7	37.4	148.3	209.4	213.0	248.8	283.1
Medicaid	2.8	14.5	76.8	94.8	108.4	131.8	158.7
Other	7.1	19.4	49.3	55.8	64.7	83.2	99.8
State/local total	10.0	33.5	116.0	143.3	164.1	190.8	224.0
Medicaid	2.4	11.5	44.8	64.7	78.4	91.9	109.9
Other	7.6	22.0	71.1	78.6	85.7	99.0	114.1

From Centers for Medicare and Medicaid Services, Office of the Actuary, National Health Statistics Group.
*Average annual growth, 1960-1970.
†Average annual growth from prior year shown.

the motivation for the third-party insurance dependence. During the Depression, physicians and hospitals (through the American Hospital Association) encouraged the development of insurance plans, primarily Blue Cross and Blue Shield, to stabilize funding streams for their services. As a result, employee benefit health insurance developed and grew rapidly, especially following World War II. In 1966, Medicare and Medicaid programs were established as government-sponsored "insurance" programs for the elderly and the poor because these populations were not covered under employer-dependent plans. These government-sponsored programs have been the primary focus of action for health care cost containment and health care access reform efforts since the 1970s. A closer examination of publicly financed health care programs follows.

MEDICARE AND MEDICAID

Medicare is a federal health insurance program designed selectively to cover the cost of health care services for the following: citizens aged 65 years and older and those less than 65 with qualified disabilities or end-stage renal failure. In 2003, almost 35 million aged and 6 million disabled persons were enrolled in Medicare (Centers for Medicare and Medicaid Services, 2004).

The growth of Medicare eligibles and rising health care costs (the rate of annual cost increases continues to outpace the rate of inflation) has led some to predict the bankruptcy of the Medicare system by 2015 unless substantial changes are made (Smith, Cowan, Sensenig, Catlin, & the Health Accounts Team, 2005; Smith, Heffler, & Freeland, 1999). This concern and increasing dissatisfaction with cost-containment efforts have led to recent proposals for Medicare reform (MedPAC, 2004).

Medicare Program Coverage

Medicare has four parts, each with its own federal trust fund designed theoretically to ensure that adequate funds are available. The health insurance portion (Part A) pays for inpatient hospital care, posthospital skilled nursing care, home health services, and hospice care. Supplemental medical insurance (Part B) covers physician services, hospital outpatient services, and selected other services. Part C refers to the Medicare Advantage program (formerly known as Medicare +Choice) under which private health maintenance organization (HMO) plans provide services to enrollees. Part D is the new voluntary outpatient prescription drug benefit that was passed in 2003 (scheduled for implementation in 2006). Part A is funded primarily through payroll taxes; Part B, by charges to enrollees. Table 49-7 outlines selected

TABLE 49-7

Medicare Program Milestones and Costs, 1965-2005

Year/Selected Changes/Milestones	Medicare Part A Deductible	Medicare Part B Deductible	Beneficiaries Covered
1965 Medicare established (amendment to Social Security legislation)	$40/year	$2/month	
1966 Medicare began	$52/year	$4/month	20.4 million
1975 First system amendment establishing disability coverage for disabled under age 65, HMOs, and PSROs	$92/year	$6.70/month	24.9 million
1980	$180/year	$8.70/month	28.4 million
1982 Tax Equity and Fiscal Responsibility Act established prospective payment, replaced PSROs with PROs, and required federal employees to pay health insurance payroll tax			
1983 Diagnosis-related groups (DRGs) were adopted as the hospital prospective payment mechanism			

TABLE 49-7

Medicare Program Milestones and Costs, 1965-2005—cont'd

Year/Selected Changes/Milestones	Medicare Part A Deductible	Medicare Part B Deductible	Beneficiaries Covered
1984 The Deficit Reduction Act froze doctor fees and established "participating" physicians program and fee schedules			
1985	$400/year	$15.50/month	31.1 million
1986, 1987 Omnibus Budget Reconciliation Acts (OBRA) revised payment procedures, imposed quality standards for nursing homes, and froze payments			
1988 Largest Medicare expansion included outpatient prescription drug benefit, and expanded hospital and skilled nursing facility benefits; Medicaid began coverage of Medicare premiums and cost sharing for low-income eligibles (<100% federal poverty level); 1989 Medicare Catastrophic Coverage Act repealed some 1988 benefits			
1990 OBRA established low-income Medicare beneficiary group, requiring state Medicaid programs to cover premiums for those between 100% and 120% of federal poverty level	$592/year	$28.60/month	34.3 million
1995	$716/year	$46.10/month	37.6 million
1997 Balanced Budget Amendment Act included broad changes in provider payments to slow Medicare spending; established Medicare +Choice HMO and the Medicare Payment Advisory Commission			
2000 Medicare, Medicaid, and SCHIP Benefit Improvement and Protection Act; increased Medicare payments to providers and Medicare +Choice plans	$776/year	$54.40/month	39.7 million
2003 Medicare Prescription Drug, Improvement and Modernization Act provides for outpatient drug benefits beginning in 2006, established income-related Part B deductible, and created financial incentives for private health plans to contract with Medicare			
2005 Established "Welcome to Medicare" physical, preventative services, and screening tests	$912/year	$78.20/month	42.3 million

From Henry J. Kaiser Family Foundation. (2005). *Medicare: A timeline of key developments* [1965-2005]. Retrieved June 1, 2005, from http://www.kff.org/medicare/medicaretimeline.cfm.
HMO, Health maintenance organization; *PSRO,* professional standards review organization; *PRO,* professional review organization; *SCHIP,* State Children's Health Insurance Program.

Medicare program policy changes (milestones) since its inception, along with premium rate growth and beneficiaries covered.

In 2003, Medicare spent more than $280 billion on benefits and administration: 45% on inpatient or outpatient hospital services, 17% for physicians' fees, and 9% for home health and skilled nursing facility expenses (Caplan & AARP Public Policy Institute, 2005).

Medicaid Program Coverage

Medicaid is a federal- and state-funded health and long-term care insurance program for approximately 52 million low-income citizens. Medicaid covers three groups: low-income children and parents, the elderly (65 and older), and individuals (age 65 and less) with disabilities. Federal and state governments jointly fund Medicaid, although the federal government establishes the minimum requirements for Medicaid eligibility and defines essential services that must be covered. States design the scope of their own programs, using federal requirements as a minimum and receive roughly $1 in matching federal funds for each state dollar of coverage. States also may receive federal matching funds for covering other populations such as the elderly poor who are not eligible for supplemental security income. Complex regulations determine core mandatory and optional coverage, and states have considerable flexibility in designing optional eligibilities/population groups (Table 49-8).

Because states bear only about half of the costs of Medicaid programs, some policy makers believe the federal contribution has created incentives for states to expand Medicaid coverage beyond the original intent of the program. Currently, discussion is under way about ways to overhaul (reform) federal Medicaid contributions and systems requirements.

Prospective Payment Systems

As part of the Tax Equity and Fiscal Responsibility Act of 1982, Congress established a new hospital payment based on a predetermined cost-per-case basis. In 1983 amendments to the Social Security Act defined the case payment system of reimbursement to hospitals based on diagnosis-related groups (DRGs). The PPS applied to hospitals in fiscal years beginning on or after October 1, 1993. Under the PPS, hospital payments were to be phased in through 1991 to this preestablished amount per case treated with a payment rates adjustment mechanism for some case variation. Initially, DRGs classified patients into 23 major diagnostic categories, with 490 subcategories. Specialty hospitals, such as children's long-term care, rehabilitation, and psychiatric hospitals initially were exempt from PPSs. States with approved alternative payment systems (New Jersey and Maryland) were also exempt.

The Medicare DRG payment system originally applied only to a portion of the cost of treating hospital patients (inpatient operating costs). Later, incremental

TABLE 49-8

Medicaid Beneficiary Populations, 2005	
Mandatory Populations	**Optional Populations**
Children age 6 or older, below 100% FPL ($15,670/year for family of three)	Low-income children above 100% FPL (no age mandate)
Children age 6 or less, below 133% FPL ($20,841/year for family of three)	Low-income parents with income above state AFDC level (1996 base)
Parents below state AFDC cutoffs (~42% FPL)	Pregnant women above 133% FPL
Pregnant women, 133% FPL	Disabled and elderly below 100% FPL, less than SSI level ($9310/year per individual)
Elderly and disabled SSI beneficiaries with income, 74% FPL ($6768/year per individual)	Nursing home residents above SSI levels, below 300% of SSI ($1692/month)
Certain working disabled	Individuals at risk of needing a nursing facility (under HCBS waiver)
Medicare buy-in groups (QMB, SLMB, QI)	Certain working disabled (greater than SSI levels)
	Medically needy

From Kaiser Commission on Medicaid and the Uninsured. (2005). *Medicaid: An overview of spending on "mandatory" vs. "optional" populations and services* (p. 2). Retrieved June 1, 2005, from http://www.kff.org/medicaid/7331.cfm.
AFCD, Aid to Families with Dependent Children; *FPL,* federal poverty level; *HCBS,* Home and Community Based Services; *QI,* Qualified individual; *QMB,* qualified Medicare beneficiary; *SLIMB,* specified low-income Medicare beneficiary; *SSI,* supplemental security income.

payments were added under the PPS for indirect medical education costs and for outlier cases (cases involving atypical costs). Payment rates also were established for each of nine geographic regions, and adjustments were added to account for national, urban, and rural differences. Payments for direct medical expenses, capital, and hospital outpatient expenses originally were not included in the DRG PPS. Until October 1991, capital and related costs were paid on a "reasonable cost" basis. Now, covered PPS capital payments use a standard federal rate for reimbursement based on average (national) 1992 Medicare cost per discharge. Updated annually, federal DRG payment rates are published in June and are finalized in September (November or December if there is delayed congressional action).

In 1999, skilled nursing facilities providing subacute cares for Medicaid patients were subject to yet a different PPS. The Medicare skilled nursing facility PPS (established by the Balanced Budget Act of 1997) mandates a per diem payment system modified by case adjustments. These provisions were implemented over a 3-year phase-in period, applied to all facilities paid on or before October 1, 1995. Reimbursements cover all routine, therapy, and capital costs except approved education, and adjustments are made for urban and rural areas and geographic differences in labor costs (Knapp, 1999).

More specifically, the skilled nursing facility PPS system uses resource utilization groups, which measure resident characteristics and staff care time for various categories of patients. Originally, the resource utilization groups system had seven categories of patient condition severity that were established from classifications derived from assessments recorded in the minimum data set at specified intervals of 5-, 14-, 30-, 60-, and 90-day Part A stays. Rates were based on average 1995 costs (national) and were adjusted for area wage differences and case mix, without exceptions or exemptions. Coverage included drugs and therapies under Part B and necessary laboratory tests, radiographs, and ambulance services provided during the skilled nursing care stay.

MANAGED CARE

Managed care plans reflect the current movement to control health care spending by combining providers and insurers into a related entity. This is an approach to managing the quality and costs of providing health care by integrating the financial risks and rewards for service delivery by making reimbursement sensitive to provider decisions. The rewards are oriented toward optimizing efficiency and care outcomes (using the fewest resources to achieve the best result). Measuring the effects of managed care and other delivery system changes on the costs and quality of health care has been difficult, resulting in disagreement as to whether costs have been affected (Fronstein, 1994; Lesser et al., 2003).

No definition of managed health care is commonly recognized. Among the varieties of managed care arrangements are two common characteristics: an authorization system and provider restrictions (limitations on choice of provider). From least to most restrictive the different models of managed care include the following:

- Indemnity insurance with precertification, mandatory second opinion, and large case management
- Service plan with precertification, mandatory second opinion, and large case management
- Preferred provider organization (PPO)
- Point-of-service plan
- "Open access" HMO
- Traditional HMO
    - Open panel HMO
        - Individual practice association
        - Direct contract with provider
    - Network model HMO
    - Closed panel HMO
        - Group model
        - Staff model

The two most prevalent types of formal managed care arrangements are HMOs and PPOs.

Preferred Provider Arrangements

The PPO evolved during the early 1980s and is considered a hybrid of an HMO and traditional health care insurance. The PPOs use many of the same cost-savings strategies as traditional HMOs (such as utilization review and discounted reimbursement by volume service contracting). Typically, however, PPOs do not require beneficiaries to use providers with which the PPO has discounted fee contracts. Unlike HMOs, PPOs do not require beneficiaries to use preselected gatekeeper physicians who serve as the initial contact and authorize all services. The PPOs are less likely than HMOs to provide preventive services and typically do not assume responsibility for system quality control because individual enrollees have a choice among PPO providers.

Health Maintenance Organization Arrangements

The HMO is organized on the premise that a fee-for-service system creates perverse incentives that reward providers for treating patients' illnesses inefficiently and ineffectively and offers few incentives for prevention and rehabilitation services. Full-risk HMOs combine the financing and the delivery of comprehensive health care services into a single system and at least theoretically produce incentives that focus on the prevention of illness over treatment. In recent years, HMO financial incentives and provider decisions have come under attack amid allegations of withholding treatment to curb costs or increase operating margins at the expense of quality care (Blendon et al., 1998; Gold, 2003; Lesser et al., 2003).

The many different types of HMO structures have varying arrangements for ownership and financial incentives (risk). Health maintenance organizations use a variety of methods to control costs, including limiting patients to particular providers, gatekeeper physicians who must authorize specialized services, utilization review to ensure that services rendered are appropriate, discounted rate schedules from providers, and payment methods that transfer some risk to providers. In general, services are not covered if beneficiaries bypass their primary care (gatekeeper) physician/provider or use non-HMO providers. The cost of providing services and the quality of service provided also varies among HMOs nationwide.

Managed Care Trends

Managed care arrangements have proliferated, and enrollment in them has grown rapidly since the 1980s. During this time, HMO plans experienced somewhat greater success in curbing the rate of cost growth with the cost of HMO product premiums (relative to indemnity insurance plans for equivalent coverage) being offered at lower rates. About one third of all insured are estimated to be enrolled in some form of managed care. Among price-conscious large firms, enrollment in managed care plans grew from 5% to 50% from 1984 to 1993 (Gabel, Ginsburg, & Hunt, 1997). Between 1993 and 1997, HMOs and PPOs dominated employer plan offerings and enrollment in small and large organizations. Table 49-9 presents an analysis of enrollment by type of managed care offering and size of organization.

Between 1987 and 1994, total enrollment in HMOs increased from 28.6 million to 39.8 million (4% of the U.S. population). During this period, new forms of managed care began to proliferate: enrollment in PPOs increased from 12.2 million to 58 million; enrollment in point-of-service plans increased from almost none to 2.3 million. In addition, the percentage of managed care organizations using various forms of utilization review increased from 1987 (41%) to 1990 (95%) (Fronstein,

TABLE 49-9

Utilization of Managed Care Arrangements by Organizational Size, 1993-1997

Employer Size	Managed Care Arrangement and Percent Use					
	HMO Only	POS Only	PPO Only	Indemnity Only	Managed Care and Indemnity	Other Combinations
<50 EMPLOYEES						
1993	15	3	23	49	7	3
1997	34	6	34	17	3	6
50-499 EMPLOYEES						
1993	13	3	23	34	16	11
1997	29	6	29	11	10	15
>500 EMPLOYEES						
1993	6	3	13	29	37	12
1997	8	12	19	12	22	27
ALL EMPLOYERS						
1993	10	3	18	34	25	10
1997	19	9	25	12	15	20

From National Employer Health Insurance Survey & 1997 Robert Wood Johnson Foundation Employer Health Insurance Survey, from Marquis, S. M., & Long, S. H. (1999, November/December). Trends in managed care and managed competition, 1993-1997. *Health Affairs*, p. 83.
HMO, Health maintenance organization; *POS*, point of service; *PPO*, preferred provider organization.

1994; Guterman, Eggers, Riley, Greene, & Terrell, 1988; Hurley et al., 2003).

In an effort to achieve the cost savings demonstrated by HMOs and PPOs, in the late 1990s, conventional insurance companies started to apply some of their plan management strategies. Called managed fee-for-service plans, these plans typically use preadmission certification, utilization review, case management, and second opinions to control inappropriate use and limit individual physician options for diagnosis and treatment. Today, enrollment in hybrid HMO and PPO plans that use exclusive provider organization/networks and point-of-service arrangements continues, even as enrollment in traditional managed care programs decreases (Blendon et al., 1998; Lesser et al., 2003).

Although the differences between HMOs, PPOs, and conventional plans were once distinct, considerable overlap now exists in the strategies and incentives they use while striving to offer a choice of providers that the public continues to demand. Thus managed care should be thought of as a continuum of care management and provider practice oversight that varies in the approach to providing integrated insurance and health care service delivery programs.

SERVICE DELIVERY TRENDS AFFECTED BY MANAGED CARE

Before the 1980s, most health care service organizations were freestanding and not formally linked with insurers, providers, or other health care service organizations. The earliest integrated health care systems were those that sought horizontal (service continuum) integration (i.e., home health and skilled nursing service organizations with hospitals). During the 1990s, health care systems and health care providers began adopting more diversified and vertically integrated arrangements. Vertical integration brought the continuum of horizontal services together (often multiinstitutional hospital, ambulatory, and long-term care) and created business and support services efficiencies. Some of the obvious benefits included keeping patients in the corporate network of services, acquiring access to managerial and functional specialists (i.e., marketing specialists), use of information systems (especially administrative) and creation of greater access to capital, and an enhanced ability to recruit and retain management and professional staff. Although delivery settings are discussed as separate entities, vertical corporate integration is recognized as key to system/community stability by establishing more powerful provider collectives, strengthening

patient referrals, and increasing profitability. Vertical integration for a full continuum of health care services taken to the maximum (rarely seen) also integrates payer and service provider functions for insured populations. Trends specific to care delivery setting/sector are discussed in the sections that follow.

Hospitals

Hospitals provide diagnostic and therapeutic services to persons who require more than several hours of care, although most hospitals also provide ambulatory services as well. Hospitals differ in function, length of patient stay, size, and ownership. These factors affect the type and quantity of fixed assets, programs, and management requirements, and the type and level of reimbursement available.

Recent environmental and operational changes have created significant challenges affecting the management of hospitals. According to Medicare Payment Commission (MedPAC, 2003) analyses of Medicare cost data (third quarter 2003), total hospital margins for all payers (Medicare, Medicaid, and private sources) reflected the relationship of all hospital revenues to costs (including inpatient, outpatient, and postacute, and nonpatient services). From 1991 to 1993, total hospital margins increased from 4.4% to 6.3% before declining to 3.5% in 2001. In 2001, 68% of hospitals had positive total margins and accounted for 72% of Medicare inpatient PPS discharges. The Medicare inpatient margin increased from a low of −2.4% (1991) to a record high of 16.7% (1997). After implementation of the Balanced Budget Act of 1997, inpatient margins fell to 4.7% (2002). During the same period, length of stay for all hospital inpatient admissions fell by 22% to 5.1 days. For Medicare, inpatient lengths of stay fell by 32% to 6.0 days from 1991 to 2002.

For varying reasons, urban and rural hospitals have found it particularly difficult to achieve retained earnings after paying for operating expenses because Medicare payments have tightened. Decreasing margins were seen across all types of hospitals, and the payment-to-cost ratio was down for Medicare and private payers. This trend is widely believed to be due in large part to the impact of managed care as a function of changes in hospital length of stay and reductions in the negotiated rate payments. Table 49-10 illustrates (MedPAC) data on U.S. hospital operating margins.

Whether one interprets these changes as good or necessary, there is no doubt that tightening operating revenue and expense ratios are related to the proliferation of managed care (Fronstein, 1994; Mechanic, 2004).

TABLE 49-10

Hospital Operating Margins and Change in Length of Stay, 1991-2001			
Year	Hospital Total Margin	Medicare PPS Margin	Cumulative Change in Total Hospital Length of Stay
1991	4.4	−2.4	0.0
1992	4.4	−0.9	−1.7
1993	4.4	1.3	−4.0
1994	5.0	5.6	−8.1
1995	5.8	11.1	−12.5
1996	6.1	16.3	−16.1
1997	6.2	16.7	−18.4
1998	4.3	14.5	−18.9
1999	3.8	12.3	−20.1
2000	3.8	10.7	−21.0
2001	3.5	8.1	−21.4
2002	NA	4.7	−21.6

From MedPAC analysis of Medicare cost report data (third quarter 2003), Centers for Medicare and Medicaid Services; MedPAC analysis of American Hospital Association annual hospital survey data, Centers for Medicare and Medicaid Services, 2003.
NA, Not available; *PPS,* prospective payment system.

Unfortunately, hospital operating expenses are at an all-time high. In addition to financing expensive new technology, staff payroll and benefit expenses are the largest recurring operating expenses hospitals incur. Of these, nursing service personnel (registered nurses [RNs] and others) usually compose the largest cost object. Thus interest has evolved in recent years in reducing nursing service costs as one method of improving the short-term economic performance of hospitals. Changes in hospital staffing ratios and skill mix reflect this dilemma.

Ambulatory and Outpatient Services

Ambulatory and outpatient care services encompass services including medical practices, hospital outpatient departments, and emergency rooms. In the 1980s, substantial growth in new ambulatory care settings was observed, such as in home health care, ambulatory surgical centers, urgent care centers, diagnostic imaging centers, rehabilitation/sports medicine centers, and clinical laboratories. In general, these new settings offer patients increased convenience compared with hospital-based services, and in many situations, the new centers provide services at lower costs than do hospitals. The Medicare PPS for hospital outpatient services has been the source of controversy and challenges since it was implemented in 2000. According to the American Hospital Association, the negative impact of new outpatient PPS rules resulting under the Balanced Budget Act of 1997 are expected to reduce outpatient service margins under Medicare to between −20.3% and −28.8%.

Although many factors account for the expansion of ambulatory services, technology and cost containment are the leading contributors. Patients who once required hospitalizations because of the complexity, intensity, invasiveness, or risk associated with certain procedures now can be treated in outpatient settings. In addition, third-party payers have encouraged providers to expand their outpatient services through mandatory authorization for inpatient services and by payment mechanisms that provide incentives to perform services on an outpatient basis. Finally, fewer regulatory requirements are associated with building and managing outpatient services compared with establishing new programs and services.

Significant reductions in Medicare reimbursement were targeted for the home health industry by the Balance Budget Act of 1997. Provisions were projected to produce an estimated savings of $40 billion in Medicare payments alone. Additionally, reimbursement for home health services was to be severely curtailed as the Centers for Medicare and Medicaid Services adopted a new PPS to replace the interim payment system.

Long-Term Care

Long-term care entails health and personal services provided to individuals who lack some degree of functional capacity. Long-term care usually covers an extended period, and it may include inpatient and outpatient services (most of which focus on mental health, rehabilitation, and nursing home care). Long-term care services are differentiated by levels of independent functioning with activities of daily living and mobility. Individuals become candidates for long-term care when they become too mentally or physically incapacitated to perform the tasks necessary to live independently, and when their family members are unable to provide the services needed.

Long-term care is typically a hybrid of health and social services. Three levels of nursing home care exist: skilled nursing facilities, intermediate care, and residential care facilities. Medicaid dominates the list of payers for nursing home care, followed by private pay and then Medicare. As the percentage of the U.S. population ages, demand for long-term care is expected to grow (Gold, 2003). The elderly are disproportionately high users of health services and major users of long-term care.

Assisted living is a newer alternative to residential home and long-term care services, focused on support and services to maximize mobility and independence, rather than health care services in the activities of daily living.

Medicare cost savings are expected to come from skilled nursing facilities through implementation of a new Medicare prospective payment. Ironically, as skilled nursing facilities have received patients with higher condition severity from early hospital discharges and have offered higher levels of care, they now are caught between new Medicare payment rules and new skilled nursing facility PPS rates (based on average industry costs for different types of care). In addition to these reimbursement changes, the Balanced Budget Act of 1997 closed loopholes that allowed nursing homes to clear 30% profit margins on respiratory, physical, and occupational therapy.

UTILIZATION MANAGEMENT STRATEGIES

Because health care costs vary by price and volume, utilization management has become a particularly important goal directly or indirectly related to the expansion of managed care. The management of health services and their use in this regard is divided into three types of efforts: prospective, concurrent, and retrospective.

Prospective utilization management involves efforts such as health risk appraisals, demand management, referral services, and institutional services. Demand management involves managing the demand for medical services before use. The most common approaches involve providing home care manuals, increasing access to preventive services, and nurse advice lines. Prospective institutional service management involves authorization or approval before accessing services in inpatient or outpatient settings (e.g., preadmission authorization). Clinical criteria for authorizations are commercially available, or plans develop their own.

Concurrent utilization review typically is applied to inpatient care and large case management. Interventions include inpatient care and continued stay review, large case management, and disease management. Large/population case management refers to the management of catastrophic or chronic disease populations/cases that exceed routine costs and for which active intervention in the timing and nature of service delivery is known to reduce costs and improve outcomes. Cases such as acquired immunodeficiency syndrome, transplants, diabetes, and psychiatric disorders often benefit from case management. Ironically, nurses have been used with greater frequency as case managers to coordinate many

aspects of care planning and client follow-up and management in order to improve the quality of care and outcomes and ultimately reduce costs. Disease management is a special form of large case management. It typically involves selected clinical conditions and works proactively with the patient to control the course of the disease. Disease management differs from preventive care activities in that the diagnosis is clear, and cost savings occur by improving individual outcomes.

Retrospective management typically involves managing use after services have been provided. Two categories of activity are common: case review and pattern analysis. In case review, individual cases are examined for appropriateness of care, billing errors, or other problems. Pattern analysis involves the review of large amounts of use data to determine whether patterns exist. Medical practice/practitioner profiling is one such example.

Although none of these falls into the exclusive domain of managed care, all are potentially useful methods of reducing unnecessary variation in practice. As a result, managed care arrangements typically provide the environment that is most receptive to the oversight and accountability embedded in these efforts. New roles for nurses in implementing institutional service and disease management programs have emerged in recent years, along with roles that involve the coordination of care and use of standardized treatment pathways to improve outcomes.

DIRECT REIMBURSEMENT FOR NURSING SERVICES

Among the diverse provisions of the Balanced Budget Act of 1997, a number are associated with the provision and reimbursement of nonphysician practitioners. The act extends to nonphysician providers (including advanced practice nurses [APNs]) new opportunities and responsibilities. First, nurse practitioners, clinical nurse specialists, and physician assistants were recognized as authorized Medicare providers eligible for direct reimbursement. A Centers for Medicare and Medicaid Services ruling associated with this provision subsequently defined only APNs and clinical nurse specialists with master's degrees in nursing to be qualified to receive payments from Medicare Part B services. The revision also provided for a grace period until 2003 when the minimum education rule was to be enforced (Buppert, 1999, 2005). Less clear and more controversial are provisions for reimbursement of nurses as first surgical assistants, even as MedPAC has expressed concerns about lack of consensus on educational qualifications and the potential for billing duplication.

The Balanced Budget Act of 1997 standardized nurse practitioner reimbursement at 85% of the physician's Medicare fee schedule, regardless of where services are provided. This represents up to a 20% increase in reimbursement for providing services such as those rendered as a first surgical assistant. Advanced practice nurse enrollment in the Medicare program carries with it increased personal responsibility. Medicare has the most aggressive fraud and abuse guidelines of any insurance plans. As such, it is essential the APNs become familiar with billing for services (ICD-9 and CPT codes) and be knowledgeable about using evaluation and management (E and M) codes (Buppert, 1999, 2005). These codes are the only method that the payer can use to substantiate that the level of service provided was equal to the severity and complexity of the presenting problem (Towers, 1999).

Additionally, the Balanced Budget Act of 1997 cedes supervision and legislative scope of practice back to the individual states. This provision effectively removes the requirement for a physician to see a Medicare patient first or to be in the office when services are billed under the APN's provider number. However, APNs must be familiar with state supervision requirements (Buppert, 2005).

Medicare regulations also permit APNs to develop independent contractor arrangements with medical practices and provider entities (called 1099 arrangements). This provides considerable employment flexibility but shifts the income tax responsibility from the practice or organization to the independent contractor (Mazzoco, 2000). To this end, APNs also must be familiar with tax and employment contract responsibilities.

Although these provisions of the Balanced Budget Act of 1997 have done more to influence the course of advanced practice nursing than any other single piece of legislation in the 1990s, the ramifications are many and far reaching. Note, however, that federal provision for the reimbursement of APNs has no effect on private insurance carriers; it only permits APNs to enroll as Medicare providers. Each private insurance plan has its own policies and authorized list of providers. When plans do not recognize APNs to be eligible for direct reimbursement, some practice situations may fall back on "incident to" billing techniques. "Incident to" is an old billing method that permits practices to bill for APN services under the supervising physician's billing number at 100% of the physician's fee schedule, as long as the physician is present in the office at the time services are rendered. Opportunities for APN reimbursement for hospital-based services are more complex.

Recent business and legal rulings have changed the hospital billing landscape, affecting those who bill for hospital-based services (Buppert, 2005). The importance of sorting out the "one bill per patient, per service day" requirement (particularly when there is no shared billing) and ensuring that APNs work within the basic and advanced scopes of nursing practice relevant to each state (not just allowable services under Medicare) cannot be overemphasized. Individual medical directors have the ability to exercise a wide degree of flexibility in interpreting Centers for Medicare and Medicaid Services billing regulations (including down-coding of services provided by APNs) (Zuzelo et al., 2004).

IMPACT OF MANAGED CARE AND SYSTEM COST-CONTAINMENT EFFORTS

Chief among the reasons accounting for the early growth and popularity of managed care with health insurance purchasers (including employers and public sector programs) was the emphasis on cost containment. Research on this topic has indicated that compared with fee-for-service plans, HMO enrollees have lower hospital admission rates, shorter lengths of stay, and reduced numbers of diagnostic tests and procedures (Draper, Hurley, & Short, 2004; Weinick & Cohen, 2000). Many PPOs and point-of-service plans now use the same types of utilization controls as HMOs (i.e., requiring precertification for an approved length of stay and plan review to determine medical necessity), yet they are preferred by consumers because they offer cost savings while retaining consumer choice of provider.

Growth in managed care plan enrollment and increased managed care plan options have produced changes in the types of persons enrolling in managed care plans over time. On average, managed care populations have become less healthy, and the early observations about managed care advantages with respect to lowering hospital use and expenses have been attenuated (Blendon et al., 1998; Lesser et al., 2003).

Additionally, local health care service markets have been affected by managed care expansion. Competitive pressure to reduce expenses by decreasing hospital use has been extended to fee-for-service plans. Weinick and Cohen (2000) examined existing national survey data for managed care enrollment and hospital use in 1987 and 1996. In 1987, statistically significant hospital use differences were found between managed care and nonmanaged care enrollees, with managed care rates being lower. By 1996, the differences were no longer statistically significant because overall changes in hospital costs were attributable to decreased hospital use by nonmanaged care enrollees. This study and others also have observed shifts in the characteristics of managed care enrolled populations, with publicly insured populations more likely to be enrolled in managed care, and managed care organizations thus have attracted a larger number of enrollees in fair or poor health. Many have observed decreased hospital use by managed care and nonmanaged care plans, and practice pattern changes adopted by providers and plans from case management also were identified as a possible influencing factor (Draper et al., 2004; Weinick & Cohen, 2000).

Regardless of whether the changes observed are attributable to shifts in the composition of managed care populations or changes in plans or providers behavior, findings suggest that the competitive advantage of managed care organizations with respect to inpatient hospital use had peaked by 1996 (Draper et al., 2004; Lesser et al., 2003). In the future the ability to generate further cost savings in hospital care by increasing managed care enrollment may be limited as similar patterns of use occur for all payers and types of plans (especially managed care and nonmanaged care plans).

Medicaid Managed Care

Over the last decade, state Medicaid programs have expanded Medicaid managed care programs in order to deliver services to basic and expanded populations. Between 1990 and 2002, Medicaid enrollment increased by 60% (40 million). Of these, almost 23 million Medicaid beneficiaries were enrolled in some form of Medicaid managed care, including HMO and primary care case management (Draper et al., 2004; Gold, 2003). This occurred at the same time that commercial insurers began moving away from traditional managed care programs. According to the Community Tracking Study of 12 U.S. communities, commercial managed care programs decreased by 30% from 1996 to 2002, even as Medicaid-focused managed care increased by 4% in the same period (Centers for Medicare and Medicaid Services, 2004; Draper & Hurley, 2002).

Managed care selective contracting and legislation mandating the PPS has led to many changes in hospital care: fewer inpatient admissions, lower average lengths of hospital stay, higher patient condition severity (Dranove et al., 1993; Guterman et al., 1988). It remains to be seen whether similar effects will be observed in the future in skilled nursing facilities as in hospitals.

As the U.S. health care system continues to undergo considerable change, whether these changes will be attributable to legislative initiatives designed to reduce costs or to the strategies brought to the health care system by managed care remains to be seen. However, considerable consensus exists about cost-reduction strategies continuing to be necessary while increasing the quality and accountability for health care outcomes. In general, two approaches are advocated: the shift of services away from hospital-based delivery systems to ambulatory, home health, and long-term care systems and sector-specific interventions related to improving cost containment and the quality of health and health care service outcomes (Buerhaus & Staiger, 1996; Institute of Medicine, 2001; Shortell, 1993; Sovie, 1995; Weinick & Cohen, 2000). This shift is occurring even as a backlash to manage care is recognized.

According to Mechanic (2004), the managed care backlash is a collective behavioral response galvanized by professional, provider, and special interest communities. The push point for this backlash has been the negative reaction to limiting services (rationing) at the point of service. Americans have become accustomed to choice and autonomy in accessing health care and have reacted negatively to restrictions. High-visibility attacks on health care quality and access under managed care and regulatory initiatives have succeeded in diluting strong utilization management controls once thought possible and desirable under managed care.

MANAGED CARE AND NURSE STAFFING

The effect of managed care on the staffing of nursing personnel and hospitals has been a source of growing concern. Recent newspaper articles report that hospitals have been reducing their use of RNs by replacing them with unlicensed assistive personnel in response to cost-cutting pressures caused by the growth of HMOs (Hall, 1998). Patient advocates, nursing unions, and other observers have argued that staffing changes are reducing the quality of care provided by hospitals, and some states have rushed to provide public policy solutions to a elusive problem (O'Neal & Seago, 2002).

Little research is published on staffing, staffing ratios, and the cost and quality of care. Of the reported research, findings are mixed. Some researchers have reported finding a reduction of full-time equivalent employment of hospital nurses per patient day (Aiken, Clarke, Cheung, Sloane, & Silber, 2003; Aiken, Clarke, & Douglas, 2002; Aiken, Clarke, Sloane, Sochalski, Busse, et al., 2001; Aiken, Clarke, Sloane, Sochalski, & Silber, 2002; Hancock, Pollock, & Kim, 1987); others report increased hours worked in hospitals (Spetz, 1998, 1999). Buerhaus and Staiger (1996) conducted a cross state comparison of RN employment and HMO penetration, identifying slower rates of RN employment growth in states with higher HMO penetration.

Spetz (1999) examined the effects of managed care and the PPS on hospital employment of RNs, licensed practical nurses, and unlicensed assistive personnel in California from 1994 to 1997. She reported that HMOs used fewer licensed practical nurses and unlicensed assistive personnel and that HMOs did not reduce RN demand. Although she concluded that the PPS had a smaller effect on RN staffing in medical-surgical units than on hospital units overall and was not linked to nurse staffing changes, she expressed concern that organizational responses to the PPS might affect care delivery systems and quality of care adversely (Seago, Spetz, Coffman, Rosenoff, & O'Neil, 2003; Spetz, 1999).

In considering the impact of skill mix and staffing (nursing personnel use), impact on quality of care often is questioned. The Institute of Medicine examined the adequacy of nursing personnel staffing and found little research that systematically examined the relationship between skill mix and quality of care (Wunderlich et al., 1996). More recently, contradictory findings were reported in two different studies examining the association between nurse staffing and patient outcomes (Aiken, Clarke, & Douglas, 2002; Blegen & Vaughn, 1998; Mitchell & Shortell, 1997; Seago et al., 2003). Various research groups have reported on the effects of selected organizational characteristics as they affect quality of care, finding that some nurse characteristics may be more important than staffing levels alone (Aiken, Clarke, Cheung, et al., 2003; Blegen & Vaughn, 1998; Clarke & Aiken, 2003). Buerhaus and Needleman (2000) conducted a review of federally funded nursing workforce studies and research efforts that investigated the relationship between hospital nurse staffing and patient outcomes sensitive to nursing. They found an insufficient body of empirical evidence to link changes in hospital nurse staffing to adverse effects on patient care and questioned the utility of mandated minimum staffing levels. These finding come even as claims of reduced nurse staffing and poor quality of care are motivating selected state legislatures to consider regulation of hospital nursing personnel (Hall, 1998; Seago et al., 2003). Legislation has been introduced in several states including Massachusetts, Nevada, California, and Florida to establish minimum hospital staffing levels for the nurses and other staff.

Unions and hospitals have engaged in heated debate about whether nurse staffing levels have been reduced and whether such reductions adversely affect the quality of care. Union contract disputes have drawn additional public attention to nurse staffing changes and nurses' assertion that the quality of care in hospitals has been affected adversely in recent years (Hall, 1998; Hercher, 1997; O'Neil & Seago, 2002).

Because patient care personnel wages (especially RNs) are the largest single item in hospital operating budgets, financial incentives exist to change nurse staffing in order to reduce costs. Although this may be a shortsighted strategy that backfires at times when adverse effects on quality care may be observed, it is nonetheless one strategy used by health care facilities to reduce operating expenditures quickly (O'Neal & Seago, 2002). What is needed now is research to understand nursing contributions to patient outcomes (Blegen & Vaughn, 1998; Buerhaus & Needleman, 2000; Clarke & Aiken, 2003).

MANAGED CARE AND NURSE ROLES

The direct and indirect impact of managed care and PPSs on nursing roles is considerable. Although an extensive discussion about the impact on advanced practice roles (clinical and administrative) and changing RN roles in acute care and other settings is beyond the scope of this chapter, an overview of such trends follows.

Nonphysician clinicians are becoming increasingly prominent as health care providers (Spetz, 1999). A study conducted by Cooper, Prakash, and Dietrich (1998) examined nonphysician clinicians including nurse practitioners, physician assistants, and certified nurse-midwives. The aggregate number of nonphysician clinicians graduating annually in 10 nonphysician clinician disciplines doubled between 1992 and 1997 and was expected to increase by 20% through 2001. The demand was estimated to be highest for physician assistants and APNs (nurse practitioners, clinical nurse specialists, and certified nurse-midwives) who could provide primary care services, as well as certified registered nurse anesthetists. Recently, the demand for hospital-based practitioners ("hospitalist" doctors of medicine and nonphysician clinicians) has increased, especially for highly specialized service areas such as critical care, gerontology, and pediatrics (Cooper, Prakash, et al., 1998; Cooper, Henderson, & Dietrich, 1998).

Until 1977 the reimbursement of APNs (nurse practitioners, certified nurse-midwives, clinical nurse specialists) and physician assistants by Medicare was governed by the "incident to" physician services provision. This allowed nonphysician clinicians employed by physicians to be reimbursed by payment to the employer.

In 1977 the Rural Health Clinic Act permitted Medicare and Medicaid directly to reimburse physician assistants and nurse practitioners working in freestanding, physician-directed rural clinics located in health professions shortage areas. This provision subsequently was expanded to cover care provided in other locations, waiving on-site physician supervision unless it was required by the state. The Balanced Budget Act of 1977 further expanded direct Medicare reimbursement for physician assistants, nurse practitioners, and clinical nurse specialists to include all nonhospital sites and removed the on-site physician requirement. Although nonphysician clinicians are authorized to provide a range of physician services (independent from physicians) and to be reimbursed for providing those services, marked variation has been identified in their scopes of practice, practice arrangements concerning physician independence, and reimbursement (Schaffner, Ludwig-Beymer, & Wiggins, 1995) (Table 49-11).

Although the number of practicing nonphysician clinicians varies from state to state, the number is expected to grow in anticipation of care efficiencies in systems brought about by managed care. Provider organizations such as clinics, physician group practices, and HMOs have reported increased use of nonphysician clinicians in their practices or are offering independent practice agreements (Cooper, Henderson, et al., 1998).

Among the most significant changes associated with managed care have been changes in the use of RNs in a wide variety of organizations and health sectors in order to manage and improve clinical outcomes. Numerous reports of nursing contributions in the management of patient outcomes is found in the literature for nursing roles that are associated with RNs and advanced practice nurses (Long, 2004; Madden & Reid Ponte, 1994; Maddox, 1999; O'Neil & Seago, 2002).

The use of APNs to support case management and population/disease management interventions (including clinical pathways) is increasingly common. Critical pathways and disease management protocols are predetermined courses of progress that patients should be making while undergoing diagnosis and treatment for specific health-related problems with oversight and evaluation of clinical response/progress from ongoing monitoring and evaluation. Analysis of clinician's interventions and patient progress is conducted to identify cost-effectiveness and optimize clinical outcomes.

More recently, the American Association of Colleges of Nursing is leading a multi-stakeholder–endorsed pilot study for implementing a new basic nurse role called the clinical nurse leader. The role and pilot project were developed acknowledging changes in the health care system and recognizing the value of using knowledge, skills, and abilities of clinical nurses in the coordination and oversight of system processes to improve patient outcomes (American Association of Colleges of Nursing, 2005; Long, 2004).

IMPACT OF MANAGED CARE AND NURSE MANAGER PRACTICE

A lengthy discussion of the impact of managed care on nurse manager practice is beyond the scope of this chapter. However, the challenges managed care and PPO payment systems pose to managers in acute and postacute care sectors are tremendous. Since the 1980s, nursing and other health care system managers have been implored to learn how to prepare their facilities and staff for prospective payment and more importantly how to provide the leadership to carry out a strategic plan for survival. Longest (1998) and others have identified a variety of competencies required for senior managers in the rapidly changing health care system.

TABLE 49-11

Number of States Reimbursing Advanced Practice Nurses			
	Medicaid Reimbursement	Private Insurance Mandates	Medicare Reimbursement
Nurse practitioners	48	29	Yes
Certified nurse-midwives	49	37	Yes
Physician assistants	49	3	Yes
Certified registered nurse anesthetists	36	22	Yes
Clinical nurse specialists	36	0	Yes

From Cooper, R. A., Henderson, T., & Dietrich, C. L. (1998). Roles of nonphysician clinicians as autonomous providers of patient care. *JAMA: The Journal of the American Medical Association, 280*(9), 799.

These competencies include conceptual, technical, managerial, clinical, interpersonal, collaborative, political, commercial, and governance skills that are different from those espoused before the 1970s. Initially, the focus of efforts was motivated by a need to reduce operating expenses. More recently, efforts have focused on improving customer service and satisfaction, along with overall quality of care, while operating efficiently (Hancock et al., 1987; Long, 2004; O'Neil & Seago, 2002). New leadership sensitivities and skills associated with managing competing stakeholder relations, allocating scarce resources, and changing organizational culture have been called for (Maddox, 1999; Sovie, 1995; Stahl, 1998). The era of managed care has had a considerable effect on nursing and has demanded considerable change in the management and leadership that nurses provide to organizations and the direct provision of services in all sectors of the U.S. health care system (O'Neil & Seago, 2002; Spetz, 1999; Stahl, 1998).

As outpatient care consumes an increasing portion of the health care dollar and efforts to control outpatient spending are enhanced, the traditional operations role of the ambulatory care manager is changing. In the past, ambulatory care managers typically have met the needs of physician owners by ensuring adequate billing, collections, staffing, scheduling, and patient relations, whereas physicians have tended to make the long-term business decisions. However, changes in reimbursement systems, including managed care contracts, now require a higher level of management expertise. In the future, increasing competitions, as well as the increasing complexity of the health care environment, will force managers of ambulatory care facilities to become more sophisticated in making business decisions, including financial management decisions.

SUMMARY

The "graying of America" is resulting from increased longevity coupled with the aging of post–World War II baby boomers. The trend is of major concern to policy makers because the elderly use a disproportionately high share of health care services, a majority of which is funded through public sources.

Managing the financial viability of the health care organization involves a collection of processes for subsystems to obtain funds for the organization and to make optimal use of those funds once obtained. Most hospitals receive a substantial amount of the revenue from public payers such as Medicare and state Medicaid programs.

Managed care continues to evolve, as does the U.S. health care system. Economic and regulatory forces as described in this chapter also will influence practice patterns among managed care and nonmanaged care providers. Nevertheless the desire to provide access to high-quality, affordable health care will continue to motivate the use of cost-containment and cost-reduction strategies that have been the cornerstone of managed care.

Nurses have played a pivotal role in implementing care management strategies (first used in managed care and now widely used across all reimbursement programs), and nurse managers are considered a critical resource in health care organizations in balancing competing demands for access to efficient, safe health care services juxtaposed with continuing interest in reducing unnecessary expenditures. Whether it be the use of APNs as primary care providers, the case management intervention of nurses, or the intervention of nurse managers in resource allocation decisions, nurses must possess the knowledge, skills, and abilities to participate in a health care system that demands greater accountability and the delivery of high-quality, safe, and efficient health services.

REFERENCES

Agency for Healthcare Research and Quality. (2001). *Making health care safer: A critical analysis of patient safety practices.* Evidence report/technology assessment: No. 43. Rockville, MD: Author.

Aiken, L. H., Clarke, S. P., Cheung, R. B., Sloane, D. M., & Silber, J. H. (2003). Educational levels of hospital nurses and surgical patient mortality. *JAMA: The Journal of the American Medical Association, 290*(13), 1617-1623.

Aiken, L. H., Clarke, S. P., & Douglas, M. S. (2002). Hospital staffing, organization, and quality of care: Cross-national findings. *International Journal for Quality in Health Care, 14*(1), 5-13.

Aiken, L. H., Clarke, S. P., Sloane, D. M., Sochalski, J. A., Busse, R., Clarke, H., et al. (2001). Nurses' reports on hospital care in five countries. *Health Affairs, 20*(3), 43-53.

Aiken, L. H., Clarke, S. P., Sloane, D. M., Sochalski, J., & Silber, J. H. (2002). Hospital nurse staffing and patient mortality, nurse burnout, and job dissatisfaction. *JAMA: The Journal of the American Medical Association, 288*(16), 1987-1993.

American Association of Colleges of Nursing. (2005). *Fact sheet: The clinical nurse leader.* Retrieved June 1, 2005, from http://www.aacn.nche.edu/CNL/pdf/CNLFactSheet.pdf

Andersen, G. F., & Hussey, P. S. (2000). Population aging: A comparison among industrialized countries. *Health Affairs, 19*(3), 191-203.

Blegen, M. A., & Vaughn, T. (1998). A multisite study of nurse staffing and patient occurrences. *Nursing Economics, 16,* 196-203.

Blendon, R. J., Brodie, M., Benson, J. M., Altman, D. E., Levitt, L., Hoff, T., et al. (1998). Understanding the managed care backlash. *Health Affairs, 17*(4), 80-94.

Buerhaus, P., & Needleman, J. (2000). Policy implications of research on nurse staffing and quality of patient care. *Policy, Politics, & Nursing Practice, 1*(1), 5-15.

Buerhaus, P., & Staiger, D. O. (1996). Managed care and the nurse workforce. *JAMA: The Journal of the American Medical Association, 276*(18), 1487-1497.

Buppert, C. (1999). HCFA revises criteria NP Medicare billing. *Clinician News, 3*(8), 29-30.

Buppert, C. (2005). Capturing reimbursement for advanced practice nurse services in acute and critical care. *AACN Clinical Issues, 16*(1), 23-25.

Caplan, C., & AARP Public Policy Institute. (2005). *The Medicare program: A brief overview.* Retrieved June 1, 2005, from http://www.aarp.org/research/medicare/coverage/Articles/the_medicare_program_a_brief_overview.html

Centers for Medicare and Medicaid Services. (2004). *CMS statistics: Medicare enrollment.* Retrieved June 1, 2005, from http://www.cms.hhs.gov/statistics/enrollment/default.asp

Christiansen, P., & Bender, L. H. (1994). Models of nursing care in a changing environment: current challenges and future directions. *Orthopaedic Nursing, 13*(7), 64-70.

Clarke, S. P., & Aiken, L. H. (2003). Failure to rescue. *American Journal of Nursing, 3*(1), 42-47.

Cooper, R. A., Henderson, T., & Dietrich, C. (1998). Roles of nonphysician clinicians as autonomous providers of patient care. *JAMA: The Journal of the American Medical Association, 280*(9), 795-801.

Cooper, R. A., Prakash, L., & Dietrich, C. L. (1998). Current and projected workforce of nonphysician clinicians. *JAMA: The Journal of the American Medical Association, 280*(9), 788-794.

Dranove, D. (2000). *The economic evolution of American health care.* Princeton, NJ: Princeton University Press.

Dranove, D., Shanley, M., & White, W. D. (1993). Price and concentration in hospital markets: The switch from patient-driven to payer-driven competition. *Journal of Law and Economics, 36,* 179-204.

Draper, D. A., & Hurley, R. A. (2002). The changing face of managed care. *Health Affairs, 21*(1), 11-23.

Draper, D. A., Hurley, R. E., & Short, A. C. (2004). Medicaid managed care: The last bastion of the HMO. *Health Affairs, 23*(2), 155-167.

Fronstein, P. (1994). *The effectiveness of health care cost management strategies: A review of the evidence.* Retrieved June 1, 2005, from Employee Benefits Research Institute Web site: http://www.ebri.org/publications/ib/index.cfm?fa=ibDisp&content_id=61

Gabel, J. R., Ginsburg, P. B., & Hunt, K. A. (1997, September/October). Small employers and their health benefits, 1988-1996: An awkward adolescence. *Health Affairs,* pp. 103-110.

Gold, M. (2003, April 2). Can managed care and competition control Medicare costs? *Health Affairs.* Retrieved June 1, 2005, from http://content.healthaffairs.org/cgi/reprint/hlthaff.w3.176v1

Guterman, S. P., Eggers, P. W., Riley, G., Greene, T. F., & Terrell, S. A. (1988). The first 3 years of Medicare prospective payment: An overview. *Health Care Financing Review, 9*(3), 67-77.

Hall, C. (1998, February 5). Evidence doesn't back Kaiser nurse's claims. *San Francisco Chronicle,* p. A1.

Hancock, W. M., Pollock, S. M., & Kim, M. (1987). A model to determine staff levels, cost, and productivity of hospital units, *Journal of Medical Systems, 11*(5), 319-330.

Heller, A. (2005). Social and economic determinants of Medicare managed care participation. *Health Care Financing Review, 26*(3), 1-4.

Henry J. Kaiser Family Foundation. (2005). *Medicare: A timeline of key developments* [1965-2005]. Retrieved June 1, 2005, from http://www.kff.org/medicare/medicaretimeline.cfm

Hercher, E. (1997, August 21). Nurse talks focus on staff levels, *San Francisco Chronicle,* p. A17.

Holohan, J., Weil, A., & Weiner, J. M. (2003). Which way for federalism and health policy? *Health Affairs, W3,* 317-333.

Hurley, R. E., Grossman, J. M., & Strunk, B. C. (2003). Medicare contracting risk/Medicare risk contracting: A life-cycle view from twelve markets, Part 2. *Health Services Research, 38*(1), 375-392.

Institute of Medicine. (2001). *Crossing the quality chasm: A new health care system for the 21st century.* Washington, DC: National Academy Press.

Knapp, M. T. (1999). Nurses basic guide to understanding the Medicare PPS. *Nursing Management, 30*(5), 14-15.

Lesser, C. S., Ginsburg, P. B., & Devers, K. (2003). The end of an era: What became of the "managed care revolution" in 2001? *Health Services Research, 38*(1), 337-355.

Long, K. A. (2004). Preparing nurses for the 21st century: Re-envisioning nursing education and practice. *Journal of Professional Nursing, 20*(2), 82-88.

Longest, B. (1998). Managerial competence at senior levels of integrated delivery systems. *Journal of Health Care Management, 43*(2), 115-133.

Madden, M. J., & Reid Ponte, P. (1994). Advance practice roles in the managed care environment. *Journal of Nursing Administration, 24*(1), 56-62.

Maddox, P. J. (1999). Management skills. In J. Lancaster (Ed.), *Nursing issues in leading and managing change* (pp. 415-431). St. Louis, MO: Mosby.

Mazzoco, W. J. (2000). *The Balanced Budget Act of 1997: Reimbursement for the advanced practice nurse.* Available June 1, 2005, from http://www.medscape.com

Mechanic, D. (2004). The rise and fall of managed care. *Journal of Health and Social Behavior, 45*(Suppl.), 76-86.

MedPAC. (2003, March). *Report to Congress: Medicare payment policy.* Available June 1, 2005, from http://www.medpac.gov/publications/generic_report_display.cfm?report_type_id=1&sid=2&subid=0

MedPAC. (2004). *MedPac data book: Healthcare spending and the Medicare program.* Available June 1, 2005, from http://www.medpac.gov/publications/congressional_reports/Jun04databook.pdf

Mitchell, P., & Shortell, S. (1997). Adverse outcomes and variation in the organization of care delivery. *Medical Care, 35*(11), 19-32.

O'Neil, E., & Seago, J. A. (2002). Meeting the challenge of nursing and the nation's health. *JAMA: The Journal of the American Medical Association, 288*(16), 2030-2031.

Schaffner, J. W., Ludwig-Beymer, P., & Wiggins, J. (1995). Utilization of advanced practice nurses in health of the care systems and multispecialty group practice. *Journal of Nursing Administration, 25*(12), 37-43.

Seago, J., Spetz, J., Coffman, J., Rosenoff, E., & O'Neil, E. (2003). Minimum staffing ratios: The California workforce initiative survey. *Nursing Economics, 21*(2), 65-71.

Shortell, S. M. (1993). Creating organized delivery systems: The barriers and facilitators. *Hospital & Health Services Administration, 38*(4), 447-456.

Smith, C., Cowan, C., Sensenig, A., Catlin, A., & the Health Accounts Team. (2005). Health spending growth slows in 2003, *Health Affairs, 24*(1), 185-194.

Smith, S., Heffler, S., & Freeland, M. (1999). The next decade of health spending: A new outlook. *Health Affairs, 18*(4), 86-95.

Sovie, M. D. (1995). Tailoring hospitals for managed care and integrated systems. *Nursing Economics, 13*(2), 72-83.

Spetz, J. (1998). The effects of managed care and prospective payment on the demand for hospital nurses: Evidence from California. *Health Services Research, 34*(5), 993-1007.

Spetz, J. (1999). Victor Fuchs on health care, ethics and the role of nurses. *Image: The Journal of Nursing Scholarship, 31*(3), 255.

Stahl, D. A. (1998). PPS challenges and post-acute care. *Nursing Management, 29*(8), 10-14.

Stanton, M. W., & Rutherford, M. K. (2004). *Hospital nurse staffing and quality of care. Research in Action.* Rockville, MD: Agency for Healthcare Research and Quality.

Towers, J. (1999). Corner in issues. Medicare reimbursement for nurse practitioners. *Journal of American Academy of Nurse Practitioners, 11*(8), 343-348.

Weinick, R. M., & Cohen, J. W. (2000). Leveling the playing field: Managed care enrollment and hospital use, 1987-1996. *Health Affairs, 19*(3), 179-184.

Wilson, C. K., & Porter-O'Grady, T. (1999). *Leading the revolution in healthcare: Advancing systems, igniting performance.* Gaithersburg, MD: Aspen.

Wunderlich, G. S., Sloan, F. S., & Davis, C. K. (Eds.). (1996). *Nursing staff in hospitals and nursing homes: Is it adequate?* (pp. 173-175). Washington, DC: National Academy Press.

Zuzelo, P. R., Fallon, R., Lang, C., McGovern K., Mount L., & Cummings, B. (2004). Clinical nurse specialists' knowledge specific to Medicare structures and processes. *Clinical Nurse Specialist, 18*(4), 207-217.

WEB SITES

http://www.bls.gov/
U.S. Department of Labor, Bureau of Labor Statistics

http://www.cms.hhs.gov/statistics/nhe/historical/
Centers for Medicare and Medicaid Services, National health expenditures tables

http://www.medpac.gov/
Medicare Payment Advisory Commission

http://www.census.gov/
U.S. Census Bureau

http://www.bea.doc.gov/
U.S. Department of Commerce, Bureau of Economic Analysis

The Cost of Home Health Care

Changes and Challenges

MARY ANN ANDERSON ◆ MARA CLARKE ◆ MARIE E. DUSIO

ome health care is the delivery of continued nursing and therapeutic services provided in a home-based setting (Hood, 2001). Skilled nursing, home health aides, physical therapy, occupational therapy, speech therapy, and social services are the six Medicare-covered disciplines typically involved in home health care (Grimaldi, 2000). Overall, home health care services help to prevent complications and preserve client independence and health (Hood, 2001; Marrelli, 2001).

Home health care has been and continues to be a vital part of the continuum of care. Health care services based outside of the hospital setting have nearly 100-year-old roots. Care in the early 1900s often was provided by volunteer organizations and paid for by charitable contributions, life insurance policies (Portillo & Schumacher, 1998), or the clients themselves. With the advent of Medicare in 1965, selected home care services were a part of the coverage for those aged 65 and older (Saucier-Lundy, Utterback, Lance, & Stainton, 2001).

Home care agencies receive client referrals from a variety of sources, including physician offices, skilled nursing facilities, and the family of the client, but the majority of referrals are from acute care hospitals (Anderson & Helms, 1998). Thus by default, market forces that influence hospitals will affect the home health care industry. When hospitals were reimbursed on a fee-for-service basis, increased costs could be passed on to third-party payers. In the early 1980s a prospective payment system was implemented for hospitalized elderly clients. Payments now are derived from the client's diagnostic-related group and from expected costs, rather than from the individualized care given. Hospitals discharged elderly clients "sicker" and "quicker." Referrals to continuing care agencies, including home health care, grew significantly. Newly discharged clients still were in need of services, such as skilled nursing and therapy, to promote continued rehabilitation. Home health care was considered to be more cost-effective than continued hospital care (Hughes et al., 1997), and eliminated many of the problems associated with hospital stays (i.e., nosocomial infections) (Marrelli, 2001). The home care industry was well situated to fill in the gap created by shortened hospital stays.

The use of home health care services by Medicare-insured elderly clients more than doubled from 1990 to 1997 (Alexy, Benjamin-Coleman, & Brown, 2001; Langa, Chernew, Kabeto, & Katz, 2001; National Association of Home Care, 2001; St. Pierre & Dombi, 2000). Medicare is the largest payer source of medical care, and clients using Medicare are the most frequent clients of home health care services (Hood, 2001; Marrelli, 2001). The growth in the home health care industry resulted not only from the prospective payment system in hospitals but also from the increased number of elderly clients who live longer (Hughes et al., 1997) with increasingly complex, multiple chronic conditions (Anderson & Helms, 2001). Inevitably, such clients require and use more health resources, and health care costs rise. Third-party payers are looking constantly for ways to provide quality care at a more efficient cost.

HOME CARE FUNDING

Traditionally, home care services were reimbursed on a fee-for-service basis. Each service or discipline that provided care to the homebound client billed for services individually. Home care agencies were paid on a per-visit basis according to the Medicare schedule in place at the time that service was delivered (Grimaldi, 2000). Guidelines for payment were in place, and oversight of the reimbursement system relied on what the provider reported and justified as necessary for service delivery (St. Pierre & Dombi, 2000). Home care providers billed third-party payers for the actual costs incurred in delivering care to the client; billing was not based on the hospital diagnostic-related groups.

Services performed by each discipline, within reason, were reimbursed.

In addition, the federal government provided financial incentives for the development of new home care agencies in order to meet the growing number of elderly referred for home care. To recover start-up costs, newly established home care agencies were reimbursed by Medicare at a higher per-visit rate than existing agencies for a limited number of years. The number of for-profit home health care agencies grew dramatically (Portillo & Schumacher, 1998). For-profit home care agencies tended to control their referrals carefully, accepting clients with less complex care needs, better personal economic resources, and better overall insurance. Not-for-profit home care agencies with open mission statements often were left with more complex, less well-insured clients. Client case mix was not regulated (Anderson & Helms, 2001).

The situation continued until 1997 when the largest payer, the federal government through Medicare, began the cost-containment process (Eaton, 2002; Grimaldi, 2000; St. Pierre & Dombi, 2000) beginning with the interim payment system. This system brought about three major changes in reimbursement for home care services. The first was to decrease the aggregate cost limits per agency and the second to take the per beneficiary payment amount into consideration of those amounts. These two combined lead to overall decreased reimbursement rates for visits (Grimaldi, 2000; St. Pierre & Dombi, 2000). Finally, consolidated billing was instituted; all services and supplies provided to a client, regardless if by an outside entity, would be billed to the original agency that initiated care. This change was believed to help prevent service shifting when clients were getting close to meeting their cost limits (Grimaldi, 2000). The interim payment system was a transition to a more permanent payment system. With the interim payment system, beneficiary allotment decreased, and home care agencies were more accountable for services charged. The system, however, did not take into account assessment of outcomes for services rendered (St. Pierre & Dombi, 2000).

Development of an objective system to measure the effectiveness of home care services began in the late 1980s under the direction of the Health Care Financing Administration. The data collected in this system provided the basis for what now is called the Outcome and Assessment Information Set (OASIS) (Shaughnessy, Crisler, & Schlenker, 1998). In 2000, OASIS became the foundation for prospective payment system funding in home care.

Prospective Payment in Home Health Care

The prospective payment system in home health care was initiated by Medicare and began with the first visit following September 30, 2000. The goals of these changes were to improve integration of necessary services and to reduce unnecessary services by setting limits and guidelines. The significant changes that the prospective payment system initiated were billing for episodes of care rather than per visit and the fixed predetermined rates for service (Grimaldi, 2001; Hood, 2001; Shaughnessy et al., 1998). An episode of care is a period of 60 days and begins on the first billable day. A new episode begins on the sixty-first day (Grimaldi, 2001). Also, the rates were based not only on the diagnosis but also on the type and level of services predicted to be required. All of the home care prospective payment system is predicated on the OASIS assessment and the resulting score, completed upon home care admission.

Outcome and Assessment Information Set

A nurse or therapist using OASIS at the first visit assesses clients admitted into home care. The OASIS is a comprehensive evaluative tool that predicts the type and level of care that is to be needed and serves as a means of evaluating treatment outcomes (Grimaldi, 2000; Marrelli, 2001). The OASIS contains three assessment criteria: clinical (C), functional (F), and services utilization (S). The assessment criteria take into consideration elements such as the primary diagnosis, other medical conditions, activities of daily living, the type and location of care before admission, and the number of expected therapy visits. Each component is rated on a scale and is awarded as points (n). The equation then reads CnFnSn (Grimaldi, 2000).

Various combinations of the assessment criteria (CnFnSn) place clients into groups called home health resource groups (HHRGs) according to the severity of their condition. Payment is based on the HHRG. Each HHRG is cost weighted, indicating expected resource use. Discrepancies are monitored closely by payer sources, and inaccurate ratings may lead to increased audits or inadequate reimbursement (Grimaldi, 2000; Marrelli, 2001).

The HHRG may be altered with changes in the client's condition and may be reflected in the reimbursement. This is important because payment is received twice; 60% at the start of care, and 40% after the episode of care is complete. Adjustments in the final payment result from changes in the client's HHRG and may be less or more than the anticipated cost (Grimaldi, 2000).

CHALLENGES AND CHANGES

The prospective payment system in home care undoubtedly has affected the availability and delivery of services (Anderson & Helms, 2001; Marrelli, 2001). Nurses report that the time required for data collection and OASIS form completion has created increased workload stress (Flynn & Deatrick, 2003). Agencies must employ personnel with the requisite skills for electronic data collection and reporting. Continuing education of agency staff now tends to focus on topics related to prospective payment system requirements, not clinical practice (Humphrey, 2002a). Since the advent of prospective payment systems, it is even more critical that home care resources be used efficiently. For example, the importance of consultation with specialists to predict more accurately the resources necessary to meet client needs during an episode of care actually may decrease costs (Humphrey, 2002b). Nurses, as the largest group of health care providers in the United States, definitely affect the quality and costs of care and potentially can identify and implement solutions (Tonges, 1998). Nursing practices are vital to organizational survival (Hood, 2001).

The usefulness of data generated by OASIS is not yet fully understood. Client-level outcomes of care are not well defined, and client improvement or client decline is not well demonstrated by the OASIS instrument. One suggestion is that the relative performance of agencies might be evaluated through comparison of select OASIS factors (Keepnews, Capitman, & Rosati, 2004). Surveyors may look for information related to "zero tolerance" factors, including deterioration of skin integrity and falls in the home (Zuber, 2003).

These changes have not gone unobserved. The U.S. Department of Health and Human Services created an advisory committee on regulatory reform to streamline Medicare reimbursement processes (Utterback, 2002). The use of OASIS data to influence reimbursement rates is considered "hijacking" by some (Zuber, 2003), although the widespread use of prospective payment systems signals the likelihood of permanence or at least long tenure. The goal of the Department of Health and Human Services committee is to identify changes that simultaneously will maintain standards of care, reduce burdens, and streamline the OASIS process. Numerous stakeholders were consulted and hundreds of issues were explored toward this end (Utterback, 2002).

The OASIS admission data may be useful in predicting which older clients are at risk for deterioration of skin integrity (Bergquist, 2003). However, the psychometric dimensions of the OASIS need to be considered carefully when one is extracting data for use in outcomes-based quality improvement (Madigan, 2002). Further studies of data related to specific OASIS factors may demonstrate the risk predictability of those factors. This could provide an opportunity for identification of prevention strategies that may be instituted (Bergquist, 2003).

The sweeping changes in home health care funding have created challenges for the industry. Like the overall health care system, there will continue to be varied attempts to control costs. Evidence of such strategies is exemplified in the areas of technology application and the increasing differentiation of nursing practice in home care.

Technology

Point of care technology and other ways to automate information and clinicians are trends for improved use of scarce resources (Humphrey, 2002a). Home-based telemonitoring is a less expensive care approach that allows nurses to assess client status with fewer, more costly in-person home visits (Cherry, Dryden, Kobb, Hilsen, & Nedd, 2003; Tweed, 2003). A wide range of clients may be served by telehealth modalities (Chetney, 2003; Dansky, Bowles, & Palmer, 1999). Clients generally are satisfied with and perceive the benefits of technology applications in health care (Dansky & Bowles, 2002; Ryan, Kobb, & Hilsen, 2003). Nurse-hours are a precious commodity, even more so under prospective payment. Any tools that enhance nursing care without adding nurse-hours provide a mechanism to assist agencies in maintaining financial solvency.

Another application of technology in the home care realm involves professional education. Rapid and continuous changes in the art and science of nursing care require that nurses become lifelong learners if they are to continue to practice competently. The around-the-clock nature of nursing practice combined with the distances between nurses' homes, work sites, and educational institutions can present barriers to nurses attempting to meet their continuing education needs (Atack & Rankin, 2002). The use of technology is growing in professional education for home care. Technology may prove especially beneficial in agencies that serve vast geographic areas. Web-based instruction is increasing in popularity as a means to assist nurses in overcoming issues of geography and scheduling that can limit educational choices (Atack & Rankin, 2002; Cragg, Humbert, & Doucette, 2004; Kiehl, 2004). Small groups or even individuals now can access professional education; such instruction would have been cost prohibitive before the advent of technology (Cragg et al., 2004). Asynchronous instruction is especially useful when scheduling issues predominate (Kiehl, 2004). Videoconferencing use has expanded since the mid-1990s in education and in client care (Sackett, Campbell-Heider, & Blyth, 2004). Teleconferences are a cost-effective staff development delivery method (Humphrey, 2002a). A shift from telemedicine to telehealth was instrumental in shifting the application of videoconferencing from medicine to nursing and home care (Sackett et al., 2004). Further advances in technology may improve the already developing distance technology face of nursing.

Differentiated Clinical Practice

Clients are released from acute care institutions earlier, with greater condition severity, and in need of costly skilled care (Bradford, Sutton, & Byrd, 2003). Concurrent with the changes associated with implementation of prospective payment systems, the practice of home health care nursing also has changed. Advances in technology, pharmacology, and the evidence base are making the generalist role in home care nursing obsolete. The traditional pattern of nursing care delivery was that of fairly autonomous primary care nursing. Clients also often received care from therapists and home care aides, but usually on visits independent from those of the primary nurse. Counter to past home care practice, teams of nurses with areas of specialization may be necessary to improve outcomes and best use agency resources in the most cost-efficient manner (Humphrey, 2002a).

Nurse case managers can serve as a vital link between the client, agency, and physicians. The importance of effective case management likely only will increase in an environment of managed care with capitation (Tonges, 1998). Intake clinicians can decrease costs and maximize appropriate delivery of care by screening potential clients before the lengthy admission and OASIS completion processes. A retention coordinator can assist with readmission to the home care agency after discharge or subsequent hospitalizations (Humphrey, 2002b). Additionally, the large number of clients with skin integrity issues will necessitate that wound care competency is or will become a standard for home care nurses (Humphrey, 2002a, 2002b).

Most individuals want their accomplishments to be recognized (Kravutske & Fox, 1996), and nurses are not immune to this desire. Attempting to use output measures of nursing care, which encompass only quantities of tasks completed, or the element of time necessary for task completion presents an inaccurate measure of the work of home care nurses. Nursing is a complex science

with tasks that encompass a range and depth of knowledge, skills, and attitudes. Productivity measures in nursing should take into consideration the effectiveness and efficiency of the care delivered (Benefield, 1996). Despite this, the lack of a meaningful productivity standard for home care nurses existed before the implementation of prospective payment systems and has not yet been remedied adequately (Humphrey, 2002b).

Salary compression often serves as a disincentive to nurses with long tenure (Hamric, Whitworth, & Greenfield, 1993) and can have a negative impact on nurse morale, possibly contributing to cyclical nursing shortages (DeGroote, Burke, & George, 1998). The existence of nurses' negative perceptions of their workplaces can negatively affect productivity, client satisfaction, and client compliance with treatment regimens (Tonges, 1998). Although nurse case managers enjoy increased autonomy, influence, and improved collaboration with other disciplines—including physicians (Tonges, 1998)—compensation must reflect the requisite education and expertise required of these positions if it is to be perceived as equitable (DeGroote et al., 1998).

Clinical ladders originally were introduced into nursing in the 1970s (Goodloe et al., 1996; Nuccio et al., 1996). They were developed as an alternative method of promotion for nurses who preferred direct client care to administrative roles (Hamric et al., 1993; Krugman, Smith, & Goode, 2000). Clinical ladders reward and recognize excellence in practice (Goodloe et al., 1996) and help retain nurses who provide direct client care (Krugman et al., 2000; Nuccio et al., 1996). Clinical ladders also assist in shaping and defining a workforce inclusive of varied educational and skill levels (Krugman et al., 2000). Clinical ladders provide a mechanism for delivery of quality care and job satisfaction in environments where nurses possess a variety of abilities, educational levels, and interests (Goodloe et al., 1996; Nuccio, et al., 1996) and may enhance professional development (Nuccio et al., 1996). Nurses exhibit different levels of clinical practice, leadership, professional development, and research ability. These differences should be reflected in the structure of the clinical ladder (Kravutske & Fox, 1996).

Many clinical ladders embody Benner's novice to expert theoretical framework, a five-level model (Benner, 1984; Goodloe et al., 1996; Hamric et al., 1993; Kravutske & Fox, 1996; Krugman et al., 2000; Nuccio et al., 1996). This formative model distinguishes between ability levels in nurses (Benner, 1984; Goodloe et al., 1996). Clinical ladders based on Benner's work can provide a defining framework for assessment of achievement of practice expectations (Goodloe et al., 1996). Nurses compare themselves to a standard, not each other. Clinical ladders provide a mechanism to evaluate and document nursing practice levels and should be progressive, including different roles at different levels (Hamric et al., 1993; Krugman et al., 2000).

Implementation of a clinical ladder can produce major changes in the culture and practices of an organization (Hamric et al., 1993). Positive and negative reactions are anticipated to arise during transitions (Hamric et al., 1993; Nuccio et al., 1996). Nurse leaders strongly influence the reactions to and outcomes of change processes. Managers should strive to be supportive of staff and facilitate individuals in achievement of their goals (Nuccio et al., 1996). Nurse managers can assist nurses with developing comfort with transitions by reminding them of the need for change and rationale for appropriateness of the selected approach (Bradford et al., 2003).

Orientation programs are essential, even for nurses with home care experience in other agencies, because each organization likely develops its own strategies and nuances (Humphrey, 2002a). Mindful of the different educational levels of the nurses, level-appropriate educational offerings should be available (Nuccio et al., 1996). Formal and informal educational offerings may help with transition (Hamric et al., 1993), and mentorship should be encouraged (Hamric et al., 1993; Nuccio et al., 1996). Nurse managers and supervisors should serve as mentors to ensure adequate role model cohorts at all levels (Krugman et al., 2000). The common mission of the nurses in each agency should be supported through the ladder and processes, and the implementation of change should be incremental (Bruhn, 2004).

Two attributes identified as important to home care staff nurses were the ability to discuss client care with a supervisory nurse and availability of real-time telephone support from nurses with expertise and authority. Development of care teams will identify nurses with the clinical and system expertise, familiarity with clients and service area, and team and peer support attractive to home health care nurses. Incorporation of these roles can help achieve realistic workloads and adequate staffing (Flynn & Deatrick, 2003) because staffing mixes can be altered to provide continuous, quality, and individualized care.

SUMMARY

As the usefulness and meaning of the generated OASIS data become better understood, the allocation of resources may reflect the findings of nursing intervention research more appropriately. This also may provide a framework to identify high-risk clients on admission with increased precision and allow for identification of other factors not previously noted. The OASIS data one day may be used to identify interventions that are evidence-based and cost-effective.

Home health care practice is likely to continue to evolve to embrace the ever-advancing technological applications. Supplementing nurses with user-friendly technology may produce improved outcome measures and cost efficiencies so vital in a capitated payment environment. As the client pool ages and the comfort level with technologically assisted care grows, the inclusion of some form of technology likely will become an expectation for clients in the future.

Differentiated practice may serve to address quality and quantity of care issues. Through rational assignment of care to the most appropriate provider, the scarce resources for American home health care may be distributed best to meet client needs. The continued aging of the population, especially the large number of baby boomers, and outcomes of attempts to remedy the current nursing shortage also will present new challenges and contribute to changes in the American health care system. Changes in third-party payer practices, Medicare, and Social Security cannot be accurately predicted yet, but also may influence the future of home health care.

REFERENCES

Alexy, B., Benjamin-Coleman, R., & Brown, S. (2001). Home healthcare and client outcomes. *Home Healthcare Nurse, 19*(4), 233-239.

Anderson, M. A., & Helms, L. B. (1998). A comparison of continuing care communication. *Image: the Journal of Nursing Scholarship, 30*(3), 261-266.

Anderson, M. A., & Helms, L. B. (2001). Outliers in home care. *Home Care Provider, 6*(3), 81-82.

Atack, L., & Rankin, J. (2002). A descriptive study of registered nurses' experiences with Web-based learning. *Journal of Advanced Nursing, 40*(4), 457-465.

Benefield, L. E. (1996). Component analysis of productivity in home care RNs. *Public Health Nursing, 13*(4), 233-243.

Benner, P. (1984). *From novice to expert: Excellence and power in clinical nursing practice.* Menlo Park, CA: Addison-Wesley.

Bergquist, S. (2003). Pressure ulcer prediction in older adults receiving home health care: Implications for use with the OASIS. *Advances in Skin and Wound Care, 16*(3), 132-139.

Bradford, R. J., Sutton, M. M., & Byrd, N. K. (2003). From survival to success: It takes more than theory. *Nursing Administration Quarterly, 27*(2), 106-119.

Bruhn, J. G. (2004). Leaders who create change and those who manage it. *The Health Care Manager, 23*(2), 132-140.

Cherry, J. C., Dryden, K., Kobb, R., Hilsen, P., & Nedd, N. (2003). Opening a window of opportunity through technology and coordination: A multisite case study. *Telemedicine Journal and e-Health, 9*(3), 265-271.

Chetney, R. (2003). The Cardiac Connection Program: Home care that doesn't miss a beat. *Home Healthcare Nurse, 21*(10), 680-686.

Cragg, C. E., Humbert, J., & Doucette, S. (2004). A toolbox of technical supports for nurses new to Web learning. *Computers, Informatics, Nursing, 22*(1), 19-25.

Dansky, K. H., & Bowles, K. H. (2002). Lessons learned from a telehomecare project. *Caring, 4,* 18-22.

Dansky, K. H., Bowles, K. H., & Palmer, L. (1999). How telemedicine affects patients. *Caring, 8,* 10-14.

DeGroot, H. A., Burke, L. J., & George, V. M. (1998). Implementing the differentiated pay structure model: Process and outcomes. *The Journal of Nursing Administration, 28*(5), 28-38.

Eaton, M. K. (2002). Home health access dilemma. *Journal of Nursing Administration, 32*(1), 9-11.

Flynn, L., & Deatrick, J. A. (2003). Home care nurses' descriptions of important agency attributes. *Journal of Nursing Scholarship, 35*(4), 385-390.

Goodloe, L. R., Sampson, R. C., Munjas, B., Whitworth, T. R., Lantz, C. D., Tangley, E., et al. (1996). Clinical ladder to professional advancement program: An evolutionary process. *Journal of Nursing Administration, 26*(6), 58-64.

Grimaldi, P. L. (2000). Medicare's new home health prospective payment system explained. *Healthcare Financial Management, 54*(11), 47-55.

Hamric, A. B., Whitworth, T. R., & Greenfield, A. S. (1993). Implementing a clinically focused advancement system: One institution's experience. *Journal of Nursing Administration, 23*(9), 20-28.

Hood, F. J. (2001). Medicare's home health prospective payment system. *Southern Medical Journal, 94*(10), 986-989.

Hughes, S. L., Ulasevich, A., Weaver, F. M., Henderson, W., Manheim, L., Kubal, J. D., et al. (1997). Impact of home care on hospital days: A meta analysis. *Health Services Research, 32*(4), 415-432.

Humphrey, C. J. (2002a). The current status of home care nursing practice. *Home Healthcare Nurse, 20*(10), 677-684.

Humphrey, C. J. (2002b). The current status of home care nursing practice. Part 2: Operational trends and future challenges. *Home Healthcare Nurse, 20*(11), 741-747.

Keepnews, D., Capitman, J. A., & Rosati, R. J. (2004). Measuring patient-level clinical outcomes of home health care. *Journal of Nursing Scholarship, 36*(1), 79-85.

Kiehl, E. M. (2004). The traveling classroom. *Nurse Educator, 29*(2), 49-51.

Kravutske, M. E., & Fox, D. H. (1996). Creating a registered nurse advancement program that works. *Journal of Nursing Administration, 26*(11), 17-22.

Krugman, M., Smith, K., & Goode, C. J. (2000). A clinical advancement program: Evaluating 10 years of progressive change. *Journal of Nursing Administration, 30*(5), 215-225.

Langa, K. M., Chernew, M. E., Kabeto, M. U., & Katz, S. J. (2001). The explosion in paid home health care in the 1990's: Who received the additional services? *Medical Care, 39*(2), 147-157.

Madigan, E. A. (2002). The scientific dimensions of OASIS for home care outcome measurement. *Home Healthcare Nurse 20*(9), 579-583.

Marrelli, T. M. (2001). Prospective payment in home care: An overview. *Geriatric Nursing, 22*(4), 217-218.

National Association of Home Care. (2001, November). *Basic statistics about home care.* Retrieved February 14, 2003, from http://www.nahc.org/Consumer/hcstats.html

Nuccio, S. A., Lingen, D., Burke, L. J., Kramer, A., Ladewig, N., Raaum, J., et al. (1996). The clinical practice developmental model: The transition process. *Journal of Nursing Administration, 26*(12), 29-37.

Portillo, C. J., & Schumacher, K. L. (1998). Graduate program: Advanced practice nurses in the home. *AACN Clinical Issues: Advanced Practice in Acute and Critical Care, 9*(3), 355-361.

Ryan, P., Kobb, R., & Hilsen, P. (2003). Making the right connection: Matching patients to technology. *Telemedicine Journal and e-Health, 9*(1), 81-88.

Sackett, K. M., Campbell-Heider, N., & Blyth, J. B. (2004). The evolution and evaluation of videoconferencing technology for graduate nursing education. *Computers, Informatics, Nursing, 22*(2), 101-106.

Saucier-Lundy, K., Utterback, K. B., Lance, D. K., & Stainton, M. E. (2001). Home visiting, home health and hospice nursing. In K. Saucier-Lundy & S. Janes, (Eds.), *Community health nursing: Caring for the public's health* (p. 893). Sudbury, MA: Jones and Bartlett.

Shaughnessy, P. W., Crisler, K. S., & Schlenker, R. E. (1998). Outcome-based quality improvement in home health care: The OASIS indicators. *Topics in Health Information Management, 18*(4), 56-69.

St. Pierre, M., & Dombi, W. A. (2000). Home health PPS: New payment system; new hope. *Caring, 19*(1), 6-11.

Tonges, M. C. (1998). Job design for nurse case management: Intended and unintended effects on satisfaction and well-being. *Nursing Case Management, 3*(1), 11-23.

Tweed, S. C. (2003). Seven performance-accelerating technologies that will shape the future of home care. *Home Healthcare Nurse, 21*(10), 647-650.

Utterback. K. (2002). CMS regulatory reform advisory committee update. *Home Healthcare Nurse, 20*(9), 552.

Zuber, R. F. (2003). Medicare survey shifts focus to outcomes. *Home Healthcare Nurse, 21*(3), 187-191.

Reimbursement for Alternative Providers

JUDY LEE

An examination of the fairly recent history of consumers' demands for complementary and alternative medicine (CAM) calls for the inclusion of developing data on the positive contributions of professional nursing to patient outcomes and costs. In the history of nursing, there was never a mechanism that allowed for development of this information. Historically, nursing charges have been lumped into untrackable "day charges" or vague time-based "visit" charges, without documentation of what actually was being done for the patient.

DOCUMENTING THE CONTRIBUTIONS OF NURSING

Nursing interventions, recorded in actuarial data as part of a "package of services," do not allow for validation of the actual value of the nursing contribution to patient outcomes. Having this hard data made available for the first time in the history of nursing makes a major, positive impact on the nursing profession as a whole by (1) giving the profession the measurable credibility it has long deserved; (2) developing actuarial data that will allow insurance companies to underwrite independent nursing services as plan benefits; (3) increasing the potential for development of independent, entrepreneurial nursing practices; (4) leveling the playing field for reimbursement for those services; (5) increasing consumers' access to independent nursing services; and (6) expanding services to medically underserved areas of the nation.

OVERVIEW OF THE HISTORY OF COMPLEMENTARY AND ALTERNATIVE MEDICINE

Healing approaches that incorporate emotional and spiritual elements have been around for years in one form or another, but the mainstream providers of health care have treated them like poor stepchildren and have relegated them to the fringes of alternative medicine (Pert, 1997). Nurses are actually on the forefront of incorporating CAM techniques into traditional allopathic models. Early on, many nurses received education in therapeutic touch and inaugurated it into their practices. The American Holistic Nurses Association was already founded by 1980. As far back as 1996 the *Nursing Interventions Classification* (McCloskey & Bulechek, 1996), which reflected advanced practice nursing, for many years had included "alternative therapies" such as autogenic training, biofeedback, calming techniques, hypnosis, meditation, simple guided imagery, and simple relaxation therapy. In the 2000 edition, the *Nursing Interventions Classification* included forgiveness facilitation, spiritual growth facilitation, religious addiction prevention, and others as alternative therapies (McCloskey & Bulechek, 2000). By the 2004 edition, nursing interventions for timely issues such as obesity reduction in individual and group settings were included in the *Nursing Interventions Classification* (Dochterman & Bulechek, 2004).

Naturopathy, osteopathy, and chiropractic practitioners, who once had a large following, effectively were squelched in the United States by serious, concerted efforts of the American Medical Association (Coulter, 1995). Strong consumers' demand for these and other CAM services became even more widespread during the 1970s and 1980s. Complementary and alternative medicine became a virtual health care buzzword by the early 1990s, so much so that consumers choosing nonallopathic options could not be ignored. Over these 3 decades, increasing numbers of consumers realized that wellness-oriented systems were more beneficial and cost-effective than illness-oriented models. Consumers began to vote with their pocketbooks, seeking out these services without the blessing or support of traditional third-party reimbursement models. They paid for most of the services primarily out of their own pockets. In 1990 alone, 44% of Americans used CAM providers, and the resulting 425 million visits translated into more than $12 billion spent (Eisenberg, Kessler, et al., 1993). Data from the 2002 National Health Interview Survey (NHIS), conducted by the Centers for Disease Control and Prevention and the National Center for Health Statistics, reported, "Given the breadth of CAM therapies queried in the NHIS, it is not surprising that NHIS estimates of CAM use (62.1%) are greater than previously reported in the literature" (Barnes et al., 2004, p. 6).

A resurgence of the classic models of chiropractic and acupuncture benefited many Americans and were being expanded creatively. An innovative combination of chiropractic and acupuncture techniques was pioneered in the West by Dr. George Goodheart, founder and developer of applied kinesiology. Significant contributions were seen with the development of network spinal analysis (Association for Network Care, n.d.). Dr. Devi Nambudripad's NAET (Nambudripad allergy elimination technique) also drew significant international attention to professions with effective, nonimmunization allergy desensitization in large populations (Nambudripad, 1999b). Widespread international success of NAET grew into the establishment of the Nambudripad Allergy Research Foundation, and in 2005 the first edition of the *Journal of NAET Energetics and Complementary Medicine* was unveiled. This journal details data supporting the amazing improvement of allergy-related autism, which warranted further study (Nambudripad, 1999a).

Another example is demonstrated by statistics collected nationally for many years by the Midwives Alliance of North America. These data documented the dramatically reduced cesarean section rates—3.4% average—for planned out-of-hospital births with midwife attendants (Davis & Johnson, 1999). This significant reduction occurred while cesarean section rates were spiraling upward of 28% throughout the nation. The modalities of chiropractic, naturopathy, midwifery, homeopathy, and Western and Asian herbs regularly were being bantered about in social discourse and discussed in great depth in the popular press. The dramatically changing view of the consumer concerning "health and healing" in all areas of life is well reflected in Dr. Donald Epstein's Social Myths chart (Table 51-1) in *Healing Myths, Healing Magic* (2000).

CONSUMER DEMANDS

Consumer demands have been so dramatic, even mainstream medical journals such as the *Journal of the*

American Medical Association dedicated an entire issue to alternative medicine in December 1998. *Advance for Nurse Practitioners* regularly carries articles such as "Alternative Health Trends" (Cozic, 2000). Even massage therapy services have become mainstream, creating a strong demand for books such as *The Medical Massage Office Manual* (Callahan & Luther, 1999), which provides effective instruction on properly filing insurance claim forms. In the second edition (1999) of the textbook *Massage during Pregnancy,* certified nurse-midwife Bette L. Waters added a full three-page addendum instructing massage therapists on how to become preferred providers on managed care networks. The information still is included in the third edition of this high demand textbook (Waters, 2004). The face of health care delivery in the United States has changed rapidly and is continuing to do so.

PHYSICIANS' RESPONSES

"In recent years, holistic providers have faced hostile medical boards and organized opposition from segments of the biomedical community," stated internationally renowned attorney Michael H. Cohen (1998) in *Complementary and Alternative Medicine: Legal Boundaries and Regulatory Perspectives.* Pioneering physicians such as Ted Rozema and many others, integrating CAM techniques into their own allopathic practices, often have been subjected to personal and professional attack by peers, perhaps even more cruelly than other providers. For example, despite formal physician protocols, rules of conduct, and positive outcome studies, EDTA chelation therapy providers came under peer attack. "Like all pioneering ventures in virtually any field, turf battles have to be fought, sometimes for years before acceptance comes" (Lonsdale, 1997, p. 3). This delicate phrasing was used by the American College for Advancement in Medicine when referring to some of the ongoing attacks. Legal and illegal attacks on the practice of midwifery and the introduction of national precedent setting "any willing provider" legislation is outlined in a book titled *Vaginal politics: A midwife story* (Lee & Waters, 2004).

In 1997 a conservative estimate of out-of-pocket expenses of *$34.4 billion* for CAM was comparable to total out-of-pocket monies spent for *all physician services in the United States* (Eisenberg et al., 1998). Following the money, if not the many years of consumers' demands, medical doctors all over the country gradually are beginning to implement some of these alternative modalities into their own practices. By the late 1990s, chelation therapy, acupuncture, homeopathy, Ayurvedic techniques, and referrals to massage therapists, reflexologists, and

TABLE 51-1

Social Myths

The Tree of Knowledge	The Tree of Life
THE SUPREME AGENCY	
The conscious mind through the gaining of knowledge. The intellect can be used to solve every problem or challenge that might ever occur.	Life itself, through a fuller, richer experience of life. Life contains all the miracles and wisdom of the universe and all solutions to every challenge that might ever occur.
HOW SUCCESS IS ACHIEVED	
By manipulation of the environment and others. Insulation of the individual from unwanted events, circumstances, and situations is vital.	By being sensitive to the timing and rhythms of nature, as well as the rhythms, pulsations, and vibrations of our body. Every step in life then becomes obvious and requires little work other than to be awake and aware.
RELATIONSHIPS	
Valued for what they can offer us in achieving personal advancement or success.	Valued for expanding our participation in the world and for nurturing, and being nurtured by, the people and opportunities that come into our life.
PHYSICAL SYMPTOMS	
Viewed as annoyances or interruptions in life, to be eliminated, controlled, or avoided.	Viewed as gifts that have an important message to give us and that guide us toward healing and a deeper experience of life.
HEALTH	
The state in which the individual is not deterred from living a normal life. Achieving our personal goals without physical limitations or discomfort.	The state of optimal physical, emotional, mental, social, and spiritual well-being. Health is associated with gaining a deeper connection with the vibrations, pulsations, and rhythms of life through our body-mind.
SOLUTIONS CHOSEN	
Exclusive, competitive, and logical. More is better. The more complicated, the higher the educational degree, the more difficult to master, or the more sacrifice, money, or risk is involved, the greater the dividend or benefit. A greater result requires greater intellect or force.	Inclusive, noncompetitive, and illogical. Those that magically appear or become self-evident at the time of need. Internal biological and spiritual forces guide the process, which may not always be logical. Solutions often include unexpected gifts that life presents us.
AVOIDANCE	
Avoid the unexpected, chaotic, emotional, or spiritual unless prior planning allows it to be controlled.	Avoid ideas, practices, and situations that do not seem to work in our life, including attitudes and actions that separate us from other people, or our body-mind and its feelings, rhythms, and sensations. Avoid whatever detracts from our experience of wonder and awe for the power of life.

From Epstein, D. M. (2000). *Healing myths, healing magic: Breaking the spell of old illusions, reclaiming our power to heal*. San Rafael, CA: Amber-Allen Publishing.

herbalists became more common. By the turn of the century, the most popular classes in many medical schools were those newly introduced, teaching integrated medicine. The lack of a standardized language describing this myriad of CAM and "integrative" services was a major problem. Providers, even within the same profession, often were not using the same words to describe the same procedures. The problem was compounded significantly by cross-profession conversations and documentation efforts.

NEED FOR STANDARDIZATION

In establishing the National Center for Complementary and Alternative Medicine (NCCAM) in October 1998, Public Law 105-277 mandated the director to "study the integration of alternative treatment, diagnostic and prevention systems, modalities, and disciplines with the practice of conventional medicine as a complement to such medicine and into health care delivery systems in the United States" (Public Health Service Act, 1998).

On December 13, 1999, in a program announcement, NCCAM announced a new Complementary and Alternative Medicine Education Project Grant (R25). The NCCAM Education Project Grant was designed to enhance the integration of CAM and conventional medicine. According to the announcement (PA No. PAR-00-027), "A significant percentage of patients being treated by conventional medical practitioners are also employing CAM practices; yet communication between CAM and conventional practitioners is low. Without appropriate integration of treatments and attitudes between the two healing systems, there exists the possibility of suboptimal, contraindicated or even deleterious treatment" (NCCAM, 1999).

Further nightmares were created daily as insurance companies and providers incorporated CAM and tried to communicate in the existing vague and nonstandardized vocabularies. They were faced with an urgent need to track efficacy and costs because insurers cannot take the financial risk of fully underwriting a plan benefit until actuarial data are accumulated. Early attempts to address this problem further complicated the intent. Local (in-house) billing code sets and dummy billing systems proliferated across the country as managed care organizations rushed to provide these alternative services. Because one system could not talk with the other, claims processing was all but impossible, and no nationally valid data could be developed. Imagine trying to use an automated teller machine card if each bank in the world spoke in its own native "dialect" and was unable to interpret the electronic data "language" of another bank to do business. Also imperative was the need for any new electronic messaging format adopted for CAM to be incorporated easily into the existing health care model. The Centers for Medicare and Medicaid Services (CMS) 1500 Universal Claim Form, formerly known as Health Care Financing Authority HCFA 1500, is the Medicare-Medicaid industry standard insurance billing claims form. Any revision would make the forms electronically unreadable and likely would cost the industry and all stakeholders hundreds of billions of dollars. Yet standardization would save all stakeholders money in the long run according to a *Wall Street Journal* article (Gentry, 2000). A lack of comparative information hinders the advancement of CAM. According to a study by Pelletier and Astin published in the *Journal of Alternative Therapies in Health and Medicine* in 2002, lack of research on clinical or cost effectiveness and ignorance about the exact nature of CAM services were cited by managed care organizations and insurers as common obstacles to incorporating CAM into mainstream of health care.

THE GOVERNMENT RESPONSE

The Health Insurance Portability and Accountability Act of 1996 (HIPAA) was the response by the U.S. Congress to contain costs and address many varied health-related issues (104th Congress of the United States, 1996). The act implicitly called for setting a national standard to communicate effectively with *all providers* electronically in a common "language." In an attempt to eliminate the proliferation of local code sets, HIPAA required the secretary of the Department of Health and Human Services to "name" a national electronic standard no later than August 2000. Work on implementation of the many mandates in HIPAA proceeded slowly with regular and ongoing delays. The urgency to continue was highlighted by many surveys in 1998 and 1999 that reported 70% to 86% of the nation's largest health maintenance organizations were covering or stated their intention to incorporate and pay for some type of alternative modalities by 2000 (Goodwin, 1999). Not all CAM groups were convinced this government intervention was the answer. D.H. Leavitt, CEO/founder of the ChiroCode Institute, publisher of the *ChiroCode Deskbook,* had this comment regarding HIPAA: "Doctors and Providers can be assured of two HIPAA realities: (1) It is a benign little "hatchling" today which only requires a 'good faith' effort towards compliance in its infancy. (2) It will surely grow into another monolithic bureaucracy" (ChiroCode Institute, 2005).

THE AMERICAN MEDICAL ASSOCIATION

Throughout this period the American Medical Association (AMA) apparently had good financial reasons basically to ignore nursing and CAM/integrative models of practice. The association had issued only four chiropractic and two acupuncture billing codes, and this did not occur until the mid-1990s. By then, much work had been done by several nursing organizations to classify and create a taxonomy for nursing procedures and to gain national licensing. National licensing efforts remained in the embryonic stage into the new millennium. This put nursing in the same boat as all other "alternative" providers, who had differing scopes of practice and licensing requirements in every state. Despite traditional allopathic provider status and ongoing efforts to secure them, nurses had not been blessed with any Current Procedural Terminology (CPT) billing codes, which are developed and owned by the AMA. By one estimate, HIPAA-compliant health-related data standards do not exist for more than 80% of licensed health care providers. The gaps in the nation's HIPAA code sets result in missing or substandard data on care delivered by 84.7% of the nation's caregivers, including more than 2,700,000 advanced practice and registered nurses (Figure 51-1).

The AMA membership roles dropped significantly over the last 2 decades of the twentieth century, and the membership that remains frequently has engaged in ongoing challenges of leadership and policies. When questioned in 1999 by its own members about "using brute force and domination," Board Chair D. Ted Lewers said, "we recognize the fact that we have acted like an 800-pound gorilla" (Boothe, 1999). Even the role of the AMA in controlling the CPT Standard for Electronic Transaction and Codes Sets was being challenged publicly by its own members and the Association of American Physicians and Surgeons. During the 1998 public comment period to HIPAA and the Health Care Financing Administration proposed response (Proposed Rule HCFA-0149-P), the president of the Association of American Physicians and Surgeons made several significant points:

> Even most members of the AMA—who constitute a small fraction of physicians—have no meaningful rights to participate in the decision making of the leadership. The Proposed Rule allows the AMA to revise the CPT coding system at its discretion without any procedural safeguards. The AMA has a financial incentive to perpetuate ambiguities and complications so that physicians will be required to purchase from the AMA and its licensees publications [contributing] $100 million per year in CPT-related revenue. Indeed physicians are not even allowed to attend the meetings, at which revisions are considered, and the AMA decision makers are neither elected by nor accountable to the vast majority of physicians affected (Association of American Physicians and Surgeons, 1998).

Although physicians all over the country were attacking the perceived arrogance and lack of inclusiveness of the AMA to their own medical doctors, alternative providers were voicing concerns that a conflict of interest existed by having the AMA develop billing codes for non–medical doctor providers' models of care. The AMA never bothered to request from the Department of Health and Human Services the right to do so by the formal 1998 deadline. Yet once a solution to this multifaceted problem was developed by an autonomous entity, the AMA, again with possible vested financial interests, began implementation of a brand new series of billing codes. These Category III "temporary" codes totally bypassed the long-time internal review criteria and processes of the AMA that require that payable coding be subjected to "technology assessment" standards established by conventional Western physicians. Many of these temporary codes duplicated those in the code set of the other entity and began being released not just once a year, like their other codes, but biannually. This appeared to industry experts to be a desperate attempt by a monolithic trade association to usurp control and continue limiting direct reimbursement to non–medical doctor providers. Apparently, this was also in direct contravention of the intent of HIPAA objectives disallowing the proliferation of duplications in code sets.

THE MISSING LINK IS FINALLY FOUND

As fate would have it, inside a small, nondescript building in Las Cruces, New Mexico, a curious mixture of

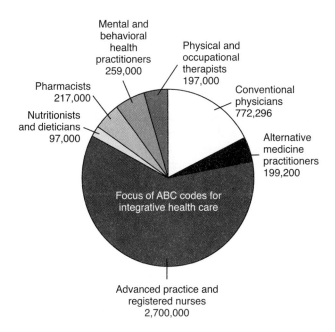

FIGURE 51-1   Nursing pie chart ABC.

insurance specialists, lawyers, health care administrators, midwives, massage therapists, accountants, acupuncturists, marketing executives, physicians, and computer geeks had been laboring doggedly to put the finishing touches on this exact "missing link" for CAM reimbursement. Melinna Giannini, a licensed and credentialed third-party health administrator, and Marion Stone, a self-described "grandmother/entrepreneur," had first begun assembling the strange mix of experts in 1996, well before HIPAA was published. With input from their "experts" and state and national provider associations and credentialing bodies, by late 1998, Alternative Link Systems, Inc., was able to birth the Alternative Billing Concepts (ABC) codes for billing. These 4000 totally new billing codes, equal to approximately half of those developed by the AMA, meet the intent and criteria of HIPAA to contain costs while accurately reflecting the actual patient encounter with all providers. In the 1996 edition of the *Nursing Interventions Classification,* editors McCloskey and Bulechek (p. 8) stated, "Indeed, reimbursement to nurses is a key issue in the reduction of health care costs." In 1998, as director of research for Alternative Link Systems, Inc., I was able to incorporate most of the Nursing Interventions Classification interventions into the system. In addition, Home Health Care Classification, the OMAHA System, and Sexual Assault Nursing Examinations also were integrated into the billing system by the year 2000. Contractual commitments to continue doing so also were implemented.

In February 2002, Synthia Laura Molina, BS, MBA, joined Alternative Link Systems, Inc., as chief executive officer, contributing her expertise of 2 decades of helping health care pioneers lead emerging markets. Before joining Alternative Link Systems, Molina specialized in industry transformation, market leadership, and quality systems. She was the founder and chief executive officer of Mission: Accomplished, an industry analysis, strategic planning, and business development consulting firm, and director of the Drucker master of business administration degree program at the Claremont Colleges.

BECOMING A NATIONAL STANDARD

Alternative Link Systems, Inc. cleared numerous hurdles and met the Department of Health and Human Services 1998 deadline for submitting this billing code set for consideration as a national standard. This was the only code set submitted that included alternative medicine providers and procedures and met all the criteria outlined by the department. As mentioned previously, the secretary of the Department of Health and Human Services already had been required by HIPAA to "name" an electronic billing coding set that would cover the activities of all providers by August 2000. A U.S. patent was awarded in 1998 for the Alternative Billing Concepts (ABC codes) coding system, "A Coding System for the Billing and Reimbursement of Alternative Medicine Services." Patent pending filings also had been obtained in 90 other countries. While awaiting adoption of the codes as a national standard, in 1999 the American National Standards Institute (ANSI-X12N) voted the ABC codes into their implementation guide. An official optional code set can be used immediately by any payer. Unique coding information on nursing and alternative interventions was included in the Unified Medical Language System of the National Library of Medicine, where the CPT codes of the AMA for allopathic medicine also reside.

The original ABC coding manual, *The Complete Complementary Alternative Medicine Billing and Coding Reference* (Hall, 1999), was prepared for use, with related patented information, to expand the existing capabilities of current allopathic coding systems. This was accomplished by uniquely addressing (the complex and changing clinical and legal) varying state-specific requirements governing providers and payers in the area of CAM and nursing. The ABC codes are paired with terminology and definitions that accurately describe what is said, done, ordered, prescribed, or distributed by 17 practitioner types (Box 51-1). The system was planned specifically as a living document and was designed purposely for easy expandability to include more treatments and more licensed providers.

More than 11 million code combinations are possible within the structure to support emerging services, and more than 1200 modifiers can be added to support future licensed providers *without any costly additions to the health care industry or any stakeholders.* The system was built on the belief that the codes will greatly improve entrance of nursing and CAM/integrative procedures into mainstream health care. The codes provide the infrastructure needed for payers of all types to measure the effectiveness and costs of CAM services side by side with conventional medicine, thus facilitating responsible patient access to integrated health care. The codes support comparisons of the economic and health outcomes of conventional, complementary, and alternative approaches to care, as well as medical doctor and non–medical doctor caregivers. The codes help give employers and public payers a way to reduce health benefit costs and generate greater employee and beneficiary accountability for

BOX 51-1

Reimbursement for Integrative Health Care Practitioner Types in the 2005, Seventh Edition of the *ABC Coding Manual for Integrative Healthcare*

CODE IDENTIFIERS*

1H = Advanced nurse practitioner
1F = Clinical nurse specialist
1A = Doctor of chiropractic
1L = Doctor of osteopathy
1M= Holistic medical doctor
1B = Licensed massage therapist
1E = Naturopathic doctor/physician
1G = Certified nurse-midwife
1C = Doctor of Oriental medicine/acupuncturist
1N = Physicians assistant
1J = Licensed practical nurse or licensed vocational nurse
1D = Direct-entry midwife
1K = Registered nurse
1S = Christian Science practitioner
1T = Spiritual care nurse
1U = Reflexologist
1V = Naprapath

*Other licensed practitioners can be added to the system. Please call Alternative Link Systems, Inc., for more information at 505-875-0001 and ask for the research department.
© Alternative Link Systems, Inc., 2005, Albuquerque, New Mexico.

---

health-related choices. They help give health care policy makers a more complete, accurate, and precise picture of the financing, administration, and delivery of care. This results in the identification of best practices across settings, caregivers, and care philosophies to support cost-effective, evidence-based care that ensures that more Americans gain access to the right care in the right place and time at a rational cost.

According to Leavitt and Lehtinen (2003), "If it allows a head-to-head comparison of conventional, complementary, and alternative methodologies of care, ABC has the potential to identify and advance the most health-promoting and cost effective health care practices and to make clear what works and what does not ... (it) could be one of the most positive events in health care since surgeons started boiling their instruments."

Anyone can use ABC codes when submitting paper claims. In 2003, then-Secretary Tommy Thompson, Department of Health and Human Services, allowed electronic use of ABC codes under HIPAA for those who "registered" during a limited time period. More than

10,000 individuals and organizations secured the rights to use the codes in electronic commerce. Since a ruling by the department in 2004 extends this right to their "trading partners," virtually every participant in U.S. health care can use the codes.

In a 2004 report to the secretary of the Department of Health and Human Services, CEO Molina and others from Alternative Link Systems precisely recapped the steps that were taken between 1996 and 2003 to secure timely, objective, and transparent evaluation of the ABC codes as a HIPAA standard. The report also mentioned that before the development of ABC codes, a health practitioner trade association was the primary coding authority for health interventions, whether delivered by medical doctors or independent health care practitioners. Many of the codes this organization developed for independent health care providers were not sufficiently granular to support direct billing. Independent health care providers could bill directly if they had access to the ABC codes. Although not mentioning the AMA by name, this was a thinly veiled reference to the vested self-interest of the AMA in maintaining the status quo. *The Commercial Use and Cost-Benefit of ABC Codes in HIPAA Transactions and the NHII* was submitted for review on October 11, 2004, to the Office of the Secretary of U.S. Department of Health and Human Services by Alternative Link Systems, Inc. (Giannini & Molina, 2004).

Alternative Link Systems sought the opportunity to respond to any concerns or questions that might have been raised by CMS reviewers. Despite being completed well before, over nine months passed before reviewers finding were finally released to Alternative Link Systems. This release occurred only after direct intervention by Sen. Pete Domenici (Republican from New Mexico) and other members of congress. Alternative Link Systems took issue with many of the statements in the review and has since provided proof that certain statement made by reviewers (such as ABC codes are not supported by participants in the health care industry) were not true. As many of you are aware, the American Nurses Association, representing over 2.6 million nurses, has supported inclusion of ABC codes as a HIPAA standard. This is along with strong support from national insurance companies, a national PPO network alliance, Alaska Medicaid, a New Mexico Medicare Advantage Plan and over 12,000 entities that registered to use ABC codes in HIPAA transactions. The Alaska Medicaid program alone successfully processed over 540,000 HIPAA transactions using ABC codes by January of 2005.

The National Foundation for Women Legislators, representing over 1,500 elected women legislators in the

U.S. passed a resolution calling for the adoption of ABC codes under HIPAA. Congress appropriated funds for Alternative Link Systems to help develop codes for care provided by the military and to measure the effect of this care on force readiness, rehabilitation, retention, and reintegration. A beta site in the Department of Defense has requested assistance in integrating ABC codes into their system stating, "We want to be poised when alternative reimbursement for nurses becomes available."

ABC codes were expected to be named a mandatory national standard under HIPAA by the end of 2005, according to Molina (2004a). HHS set precedence for adding health care codes to its national coding system without requiring National Proposed Rule Making, a HIPAA exception or a cost-benefit analysis. Examples are vision, home infusion, and limited mental healthcare service codes. Yet, by the end of October 2005, Secretary Leavitt still had not enacted ABC codes.

Melinna Giannini, founder and board chair of Alternative Link Systems, Inc., in this same 2004 report to the Department of Health and Human Services, showed data supporting the claim that ABC codes and other gap-filling health-related data elements to improve health care are projected to save more than $51 billion a year through administrative simplification and elimination of coding-related anomalies that generate systemic inefficiencies in U.S. health care. Over time, they will support even greater annual savings through improvements in (1) health benefit plan design, (2) managed care and provider contracting, (3) utilization and clinical practice management, (4) billing and claims management, (5) outcomes research, and (6) a variety of actuarial analyses.

BENEFITS FOR NURSING PRACTICE

Until the advent of the ABC codes system, no standardized coded data for CAM existed that allowed cost and outcome data to emerge. Non-ABC code sets focus on the practices of less than 15.3% of the health practitioners in the U.S. health care system, leaving some 84.7% of practitioners, including more than 2,700,000 nurses, without adequate billing codes to reflect their practices. Although not all nursing services automatically will be covered by third-party reimbursement at some point in the future just because a billing code exists, *not* having a billing code to describe each of them is an absolute guarantee that they will never be covered. By ensuring that every health care intervention can be represented through standardized and digitized information, ABC codes ensure the health industry can realize the same

efficiencies and good management practices that the retail industry achieved by adopting universal product codes. Used with older coding systems, ABC codes provide an essential solution to the health care crisis: complete, accurate, and precise documentation of patient encounters and a common language for comparing the economic and health outcomes of competing approaches to care. As nurses have suspected for many years but have not had hard documentation to prove, ABC data should validate that those patients who receive appropriate levels of nursing care in a timely manner do better, get well faster, and save the health care system untold billions of dollars in the long run. Add to that the data supporting the vast positive impact of advanced practice nurses working independently in medically underserved areas of the nation.

With this ABC coding system, the insurance industry immediately can secure legal scope of practice information electronically and can incorporate independent health care nurses and other providers into plan benefits. This will broaden availability of desperately needed services to the public. Equally important, underwriters now can compare all credentialed nurses by coded treatment patterns to assess the costs and benefits associated with the addition of these services. It becomes more and more apparent why the AMA might not wish for this data to develop.

Other data elements available through Alternative Link Systems, Inc., include the following:

1. Provide the backbone for insurance underwriting.
2. Improve health care research, management, and commerce. These data elements include the following:
   a. Expanded definitions that correspond to ABC codes to reduce the need for lengthy explanations of care and claims attachments
   b. Relative value units for thousands of independent health care interventions to support pricing and payment determinations
   c. Two-character independent health care practitioner identifiers that are used as code modifiers to establish the type of caregiver who provided a particular health care service or supply item
   d. Legal practice guidelines based on statutes, administrative regulations, and case law that can be accessed on a per intervention, per practitioner, and per state-specific basis to determine the legality of delivered care
   e. Independent health care practitioner training and licensing standards to support credentialing and other mechanisms for establishing caregiver qualifications. The strategic allies of Alternative Link

provide corresponding independent health care clinical efficacy and cost-effectiveness guidelines.

Beta site testing of the Alternative Link Systems to make it user-friendly was accomplished in 1998 and 1999. The coding system began to be introduced gradually on a state-by-state basis into other payer systems, starting in early 2000. When looking closely at how the system works, one can see the inherently elegant solution for the providers and the payers. Figure 51-2 shows the life of an electronic claim and tasks supported by Alternative Link Systems products and services. As any billing clerk knows, "kickbacks or pending of claims" (not paying for a service while asking the provider for more information) occurs at many junctures in this process. Requests for more information such as narrative reports and SOAP (subjective, objective, assessment, plan) notes takes place regularly with all current allopathic coding systems. Because of design oversights that have not been corrected, by the AMA or CMS, to date no in-depth allopathic information is able to be transmitted electronically on a code-by-code basis.

Payment or cash flow to providers is stopped at each point at which more information is requested. Because of the ease of playing these "pending games" in their favor, payers have long collected enormous sums of interest by holding monies owed to providers. Writing and reading nonstandardized reports is also costly to all parties in staff time and money. Even into early twenty-first century, with Nurse Practice Acts still vary significantly state by state, it is most important to payer and nurse to have a claim that is processable electronically, ensuring legality of treatment and payment, as well as prompt reimbursement. In 2005, Robert Honigsfeld, DC, a past president of the American Board of Chiropractic Consultants and nationally known expert witness, reported to the Ohio State Chiropractic Association that a "clean" electronic claim costs approximately 10 cents to process. Although a paper claim costs about $2, a nurse-reviewed claim costs more than $5, and a peer review costs a minimum of $50 but often ranges upward of $200.

The designers of the ABC codes were aware of the many problems in the existing arcane allopathic models used for health care billing. They purposely circumvented old design flaws with the inclusion of solutions. In electronic format an "expanded definition" was attached to each billing code and explains, in a formalized set manner, to providers and payers exactly what transpired or is being billed for (Table 51-2). This is of great value to the provider because it (1) eliminates claim "pending" by a payer (who will not pay for a service that has been rendered already until receiving more information from the provider), (2) reduces the possibility of inadvertently "unbundling" global fee types of services (some services must be billed as a package only) or "upcoding" (charging for a similar but not identical procedure that pays a higher price), (3) reduces the possibility of CMS-levied fines of up to $10,000 per claim for "not reflecting the actual patient encounter" appropriately, and (4) speeds up reimbursement, thereby improving provider cash flow and profit margins of the practice. This method of transferring accurate billing data allows for electronic direct deposit of insurance monies into the provider's account, further speeding up the influx of monies to practices. Having to write reports continually to get paid appropriately is also in direct conflict with the HIPAA mandate to reduce paperwork.

In a piecemeal effort, in 2000 the CMS began introducing provider-specific code modifiers into its own Healthcare Common Procedure Coding set. Again, there were outcries that this was potentially a surreptitious attempt to do an end run around acceptance of the ABC codes as a mandatory national standard. However, without legal scope of practice information, CMS "modifiers" are really just taxonomy codes. So far, the industry is not widely using provider taxonomy codes because they still do not yet meet industry needs on the level of a procedural claim. However, Alternative Link Systems, the developers of ABC codes, has the capability simply to map the modifiers to the CMS and nursing taxonomy codes. This mapping would preserve the legal logic that is currently tied to ABC modifiers, giving the industry substantial necessary data on the level of a procedural claim.

In the above-mentioned report to the Department of Health and Human Services and CMS, Giannini and Molina (2004) also specifically reported on how the timely introduction of ABC codes as a mandatory standard directly affects more than 2,700,000 nurses and saves all stakeholders substantial amounts of time and money.

This report projects a $51 billion net benefit from ABC codes within 1 year of deployment by using the following:

- *Quantitative evidence* of the cost-benefit of ABC codes in HIPAA transactions, supporting administrative simplification and generating greater business and industry efficiencies
- *Qualitative evidence* of the value of ABC codes to individual and public health, the U.S. health care system, and the nation's socioeconomic development

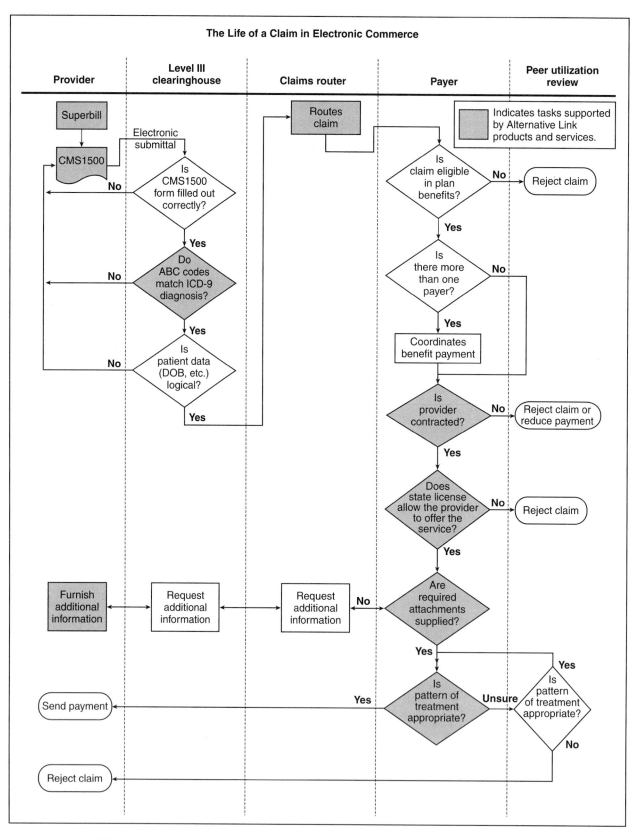

FIGURE 51-2 The life of a claim: electronic commerce (averages 14 days). (© Alternative Link Systems Inc., 2005, Albuquerque, New Mexico.)

TABLE 51-2

An Expanded Definition

1. Supports submission of electronic claims with attachments the payer needs to "pass" on claims.
2. Builds precise communication between the provider and payer, thus saving time and money for both.

ABC Code	Description	Expanded Definition
CCAAA	Block technique, general, chiropractic services, practice specialties	The application of wedge blocks to specific anatomical sites before, after, or as manipulation.
CCAAB	Educational kinesiology, 15 minutes, general, chiropractic, practice specialties	Fifteen-minute period of applying specific exercises, ranges of motions, and/or strengthening procedures to rehabilitate a compromised joint.

© Alternative Link, LLC, 1999, Las Cruces, New Mexico.

BOX 51-2

Training Standards*

ABC CODE CEEAC[†]: CERTIFIED NURSE-MIDWIFE TRAINING STANDARD IN ARIZONA

Registered nurse practitioners (RNP) in Arizona, including nurse midwives, must be certified by the State Board of Nursing, complete a nurse practitioner education program approved and recognized by the board, and hold current certification from the American College of Nurse Midwives. After 2001, an RNP must also have a master of science degree.

ABC CODE CEEAC: REGISTERED MIDWIFE TRAINING STANDARD IN ARIZONA

A midwife in Arizona must be a high school graduate; have current certification in CPR and neonatal resuscitation; and submit one written recommendation from a physician, certified nurse midwife or licensed midwife, and one written recommendation from a mother who has received the midwife's services. A midwife must also pass each of the required core subjects from accredited college-level courses, or through self-study and demonstration of competences, receive an above average or excellent assessment in essential skills from a preceptor, and pass a qualifying examination administered by the Department of Health Services. If licensed to practice midwifery in another state, a midwife must complete a midwifery apprenticeship program or state-licensed and professionally approved midwifery school.

ABC CODE CEEAQ: NATUROPATHIC DOCTOR TRAINING STANDARD IN ARIZONA

A naturopathic physician in Arizona must be a graduate of an approved school of naturopathic medicine, have completed an approved internship, preceptorship or clinical training program in naturopathic medicine and pass the examination conducted by the North American Board of Naturopathic Examiners.

*Training standards for different practitioner types are contained in machine-readable format by code.
[†]Note the five-digit, all alpha format of the ABC codes. Training standards vary on a state-by-state basis for each provider type for legal use of the *same* code.
© Alternative Link Systems, Inc., 2005, Albuquerque, New Mexico.

♦ *A legal analysis* that establishes the addition of ABC codes to the Healthcare Common Procedure Coding System as a HIPAA code set maintenance step rather than a modification step, making its use mandatory under HIPAA.

Not only does the ABC code system describe the actual patient encounter accurately, more importantly, it explains to all payers that the service being billed is, or is not, within the legal scope of practice of that provider. Training standards also are attached electronically to each code, indicating legal scope of practice details (Box 51-2).

This information is state-by-state specific for all provider types covered by the system. The amount of ongoing research that is required to keep up with this rapidly changing area of health care delivery in all 51 regions of the United States is impossible to describe here. Expansion to include other providers is an integral part of the system design. By 2000 the system included the legal state-specific scope of practice information for 13 provider types. Included were those for practical nurses, registered nurses, nurse-midwives, advanced practice nurses, and clinical nurse specialists. Led by

Connie Koshewa, current director of research, the legal research team developed the 2005 version (*ABC Coding Manual for Integrative Healthcare,* seventh edition) and added 4 additional provider types to the original 13. The system now contains more than 4327 ABC codes and 53 new assessment codes using nursing diagnoses.

By ensuring that every health care intervention can be represented through standardized and digitized information, ABC codes ensure the health industry can realize the same efficiencies and good management practices that the retail industry achieved by adopting universal product codes.

HOW IT ALL WORKS

Alternative Link Systems code books, databases, and support tools are designed for providers, payers, claims adjusters, medical managers, provider network developers, third-party payers, and software producers throughout the health care industry. The products support paper and electronic claims. The system was created to save health care entities time, money, and the risk of potential legal liability. A "technical" summary indicates that providers and payers, connected by the Alternative Link Systems, gain the following benefits (Giannini & Koshewa, 2000):

◆ Providers file accurate descriptions of the patient encounter on standard claim forms.
◆ Payers use the same information as the provider filing the claim, thus enhancing communication.
◆ Claims adjusters have references for each claim filed to ensure compliance with state laws.
◆ Payers develop cost and outcome data (without needing to purchase new software system).
◆ Payers underwrite insured benefits for CAM and nursing based on the cost and outcome data.
◆ Providers and payers save time and money by not having to create or interpret written reports.
◆ Providers and payers reduce the risk of liability of claims falling outside the scope of practice laws.
◆ Provider networks negotiate fees with payers in any locale using existing business models.

NUTS AND BOLTS

In plain English, all of this is much simpler. Do you believe that a physician trade organization is the most suitable group to develop national billing codes for nurses and other potentially competing practitioners? For the first time in the history of U.S. health care, with the use of the ABC codes, payers can compare apples

to apples when it comes to patients' costs and outcomes. Information develops stemming from the identical source of warehoused allopathic data, the *International Classification of Diseases, Ninth Revision* (ICD-9), and diagnosis code. (The United States is the only developed nation that has still not yet implemented the ICD-10CM version.) If thousands of patients have an identical diagnosis and one group is treated using typical allopathic methods and the other is treated using nursing and/or alternative medicine, costs and outcomes develop and can be compared. Reliable information quickly tells payers which providers contain costs while helping patients stay well longer or get well more quickly. Managed care organizations in particular are looking for ways to enhance their bottom line. The historical emphasis of nursing and CAM/integrative medicine has been on preventive activities that are designed to keep people well and to avoid costly crisis intervention-type health care as much as possible. The savings on visits to emergency departments and inpatient services alone could be astronomical. Documenting the monies that are saved by using chelation therapy to avoid bypass surgery also should prove to be interesting. Anecdotal evidence has shown most CAM procedures to be significantly less costly in general than much of allopathic medicine. An analysis of data from malpractice insurers from 1990 to 1996 stated, "claims against (CAM) practitioners occurred less frequently and typically involved injury that was less severe than claims against physicians during the same period" (Studdert et al., 1998). Now a way exists to demonstrate which providers and which modalities contain costs while providing excellent outcomes. This task was simple, but not easy, until the Alternative Link Systems was established.

Access and inclusiveness to the system have been guaranteed by Alternative Link Systems, Inc., policy. Provider associations easily can request additional codes or inclusion of additional provider types simply by submitting a form to Alternative Link Systems (*www.alternativelink.com*). Typically, there is no charge for this service, and expansions can be implemented in a timely manner. A nonprofit organization, the Foundation for Integrative Health Care, was created in 1999 to identify and advocate cost-effective and evidence-based integrative health care practices. This helps to level the playing field for third-party reimbursement for all providers. For example, a study on the use of ice massage on specific acupoints to reduce the pain of labor was conducted over a 3-year period by Waters and Raisler. After the results were published in the *Journal of Midwifery and Women's Health* (and later also summarized for online inclusion in the Medscape library), the introduction of a billing code for ice massage was addressed by Alternative Link Systems, and in 2004 an ABC billing code (BAAAE) was created.

CHALLENGES

Consumers are now much more well-educated and well-armed than ever before. Use of pretax monies in high-deductible consumer-driven health care plans also is giving them more choices than ever before. Patients *will* be showing up in your office with a proliferation of articles and "studies" pulled from widespread press and off the World Wide Web. Between 2003 and 2005, enormous numbers of trade and popular press magazines carried articles about CAM/integrative procedures and the use of ABC codes. An example is an article by Molina (2004a), "ABC Codes: an Essential Tool for Health Benefit Cost Management and Consumer-Driven Health Plans" in *Compensation Benefits Review* published by Sage Publications. This will only become more commonplace.

Be prepared to discuss the pros and cons of all treatment options in depth. Now is an appropriate time to educate yourself and perhaps decide which of these alternative modalities might be appropriate and interesting to incorporate into your own practice. Nurses, particularly nurse practitioners who are trained in alternative therapies, are in a unique position to enhance patients' well-being and help them take realistic charge of their own health and future.

Using this system, nurses quickly will be designing incredibly creative studies that will play a major role in a healthier and happier population. Other nonpharmaceutical pain relief such as the "ice massage study" mentioned before, the use of meditation, family planning and genetic counseling, spiritual care, obesity counseling in group settings, parenting education and skills training, and outcomes associated with including massage as part of routine prenatal care are only some interesting areas worthy of exploration. Molina (2004b) stated that there is a new opportunity to capture clinical nurse specialist's contributions to U.S. health care. Because of the active involvement of the National Association of Clinical Nurse Specialists, the codes will improve and expand over time, so that data collection, analysis, and communication will more and more reflect real-world practices and provide a basis for advancement of the profession and U.S. health care.

REFERENCES

Association of American Physicians and Surgeons. (1998). *Proposed rule HCFA-0149-P. Comments on standards for electronic transactions and code sets (070198)-64 of 184.* Baltimore: Author.

Association for Network Care. (n.d.). *Network spinal analysis.* Retrieved August 1, 2005, from http://www.associationfornetworkcare.com/whatisnsa.shtml

Barnes, P. M., Powel-Griner, E., Division of Health Interview Statistics, McFann, K., Nahin, R. L., & National Center for Complementary and Alternative Medicine, National Institutes of Health. (2004). Complementary and alternative medicine use among adults: United States, 2002. *Advance Data from Vital and Health Statistics, 343,* 1-20.

Boothe, B. (1999, September 6). AMA leaders promise more collaboration with specialties. *American Medical News. 42*(33), 5-6.

Callahan, M. M., & Luther, D. W. (1999). *The medical massage office manual* (2nd ed.). Steamboat Springs, CO: Callahan/Luther Partnership.

ChiroCode Institute. (2005). *2005 ChiroCode deskbook.* Phoenix, AZ: Author.

Cohen, M. H. (1998). Complementary and alternative medicine: Legal boundaries and regulatory perspectives. Baltimore: Johns Hopkins University Press.

Coulter, H. (1995). *Use divided legacy* (Vol. 4). Washington, DC: The Center for Empirical Medicine.

Cozic, A. (2000). Complementary health care, alternative therapies, tools for the new millennium. *Advance for Nurse Practitioners, 8*(1), 64-66.

Davis, B., & Johnson, K. (1999). Hospital procedures for 9,966 intended home and birth center births—MANA 1999. *Midwives' Alliance of North America Newsletter, 17,* 6-14.

Dochterman, J. C., & Bulechek, G. (2004). *Nursing interventions classification (NIC)* (4th ed.). St. Louis, MO: Mosby.

Eisenberg, D. M., Davis, R. B., Ettner, S. L., Appel, S., Wilkey, S., Rompay, M. V., et al. (1998). Trends in alternative medicine: Use in the United States, 1990-1997. *JAMA: The Journal of the American Medical Association, 280,* 1569-1575.

Eisenberg, D. M., Kessler, R. C., Foster, C., Norlock, F. E., Calkins, D., & Delbanco, T. (1993). Unconventional medicine in the United States. Prevalence, costs, and pattern of use. *New England Journal of Medicine, 328,* 246-252.

Epstein, D. M. (2000). Healing myths, healing magic: Breaking the spell of old illusions, reclaiming our power to heal. San Rafael, CA: Amber-Allen Publishing.

Gentry, C. (2000, January 3). Health-care firms face costly change. *Wall Street Journal,* pp. 3A-4A.

Giannini, M., & Koshewa, C. (Eds.). (2000). *The complete complementary alternative medicine billing and coding reference* (2nd ed.). Newton, MA: Integrative Medicine.

Giannini, M., & Molina, S. (2004). *The commercial use and cost-benefit of ABC codes in HIPAA transactions and the NHII.* Submitted on October 11, 2004, by Alternative Link

Systems, Inc., to the Office of the Secretary, U.S. Department of Health and Human Services.

Goodwin, J. (1999). A health insurance revolution. *New Age Journal, 6*(1), 66-69.

Hall, D. (Ed.). (1999). The complete complementary alternative medicine billing and coding reference. Newton, MA: Integrative Medicine.

Honigsfeld, R. (2005). Paper presented at the Ohio State Chiropractic Association Meeting, Bellville, OH.

Koshewa, C. (2005). *ABC coding manual for integrative healthcare* (7th ed.). Albuquerque, NM: Alternative Link Systems.

Leavitt, D. H., & Lehtinen, R. (2003). As simple as ABC: New coding system spells good news for chiropractic. *Chiropractics Economics Magazine, 49*(12). Retrieved August 1, 2005, from http://www.chiroeco.com/article/2003/issue12/mgmt2.html

Lee, J., & Waters, B. L. (2004). *Vaginal politics: A midwife story.* Deming, NM: Bluwaters Press.

Lonsdale, D. (1997). Special issue protocols for chelation therapy. *Journal of Advancement in Medicine, 10*(1), 3.

McCloskey, J. C., & Bulechek, G. M. (Eds.). (1996). *Nursing interventions classification (NIC)* (2nd ed.). St. Louis, MO: Mosby-Year Book.

McCloskey, J. C., & Bulechek, G. M. (Eds.). (2000). *Nursing interventions classification (NIC)* (3rd ed.). St. Louis, MO: Mosby.

Molina, S. L. (2004a). ABC codes: An essential tool for health benefit cost management and consumer-driven health plans. *Compensation Benefits Review, 36*(5), 71-77.

Molina, S. (2004b). ABC codes. A new opportunity to capture CNS contributions to U.S. healthcare. *Clinical Nurse Specialist, 18*(5), 238-247.

Nambudripad, D. S. (1999a). *Say goodbye to allergy-related autism.* Buena Park, CA: Delta Publishing.

Nambudripad, D. S. (1999b). *Say goodbye to illness.* Buena Park, CA: Delta Publishing.

National Center for Complementary and Alternative Medicine. (1999). *Complementary and alternative medicine (CAM) education project grant.* Retrieved August 1, 2005, from http://grants.nih.gov/grants/guide/pa-files/PAR-00-027.html

104th Congress of the United States. (1996). Health Insurance Portability and Accountability Act, Public Law 104-191. *Congressional Record, 142,* 1-180.

Pert, C. B. (1997). *Molecules of emotion.* New York: Scribner.

Public Health Service Act. (1998). 42 U.S.C. 287c-21

Studdert, D. M., Eisenberg, D. M., Miller, F. H., Curto, D. A., Kaptchuk, T. J., & Brennan, T. A. (1998). Medical malpractice implications of alternative medicine. *JAMA: The Journal of the American Medical Association, 280,* 1610-1615.

Waters, B. L. & Raisler, J. (2003). Ice massage for the reduction of labor pain. *Journal of Midwifery and Women's Health, 48*(5), 317-321.

Waters, B. W. (1999). *Massage during pregnancy* (2nd ed.). Deming, NM: Bluwaters Press.

Waters, B.W. (2004). *Massage during pregnancy* (3rd ed.). Deming, NM: Bluwaters Press.

Impact of the Health Insurance Portability and Accountability Act

ANN M. RHODES

Perhaps one of the most absurd assertions about health care costs made in recent years (an economic arena in which absurd assumptions and assertions are all but routine) is that the enactment of the Health Insurance Portability and Accountability Act rules would save money and reduce the costs of health care, particularly the costs of processing health insurance claims. The Health Insurance Accountability and Portability Act of 1996 (HIPAA)[1] is a federal statute that includes several complicated health care provisions, the most well-known being the privacy provisions. The original intent of the legislation was to address "job lock": the problem of employees who have health conditions and change jobs to find that they are "locked out" of employee health insurance coverage because of a preexisting condition clause in the health plan at the new job.

The Health Insurance Portability and Accountability Act takes its name from the notion that employees can carry insurance from one job to another ("health insurance portability"). The statute authorized administrative rules (which have the force of law) in three areas. All of these areas affect health care costs. The first is *privacy*. The statute created the authority for extensive regulations for a national standard for health care privacy, applying to all health care providers that transmit information electronically. The second area is *electronic and computer security*. Rules were developed that create consistent standards for physical, technical, and administrative safeguards for all computers that contain information that is identifiable and relates to a person's health or medical treatment. The third area relates to the *processing of medical claims* and requires the use of a uniform set of identifiers and transaction codes for all providers and health insurers in processing claims for reimbursement. This is intended to achieve greater efficiency and cost-effectiveness in the processing of health care claims.

Briefly, the HIPAA statute and rules were put into place without any realistic or systematic assessment of the actual cost of implementation and compliance. Because the Department of Health and Human Services believes that the HIPAA standards ultimately will result in savings to the provider community, the costs of implementation and compliance were not factored into the base year calculations for the prospective payment system (the federal prospective payment fees for service are the benchmark for many private insurers). This means that the HIPAA regulatory mandates come at the expense of patient care: the money required to meet the standards for privacy and computer security by the federal rules must be reallocated from existing budgets. This generally means cuts in areas that have a direct impact on patient care.

The first part of the HIPAA rules to be implemented, and the area in which institutions have the most experience, is the Privacy Rule. Most institutions assumed enormous costs in hiring individuals to serve as privacy officers (a requirement of the federal rules), paying for consultants to assist in compliance efforts, and in time spent developing policies and procedures that specifically are required by the Privacy Rule. In addition, the unquantifiable costs of the diminished quality of patient care are a consequence of poorer communication between and among caretakers because of questions about what communications are appropriate under the Privacy Rule.

During the development of the legislation, extensive congressional hearings were held and a significant number of constituent comments were made to members of Congress on the subject of privacy of patient care information. In the hearings, individuals testified about problems they had experienced when information about their health status or medical treatment was shared without their authorization. Particular concern was focused on electronic transmission of health information and the use of fax, cellular telephones, e-mail, Internet communication, and database management. This led Congress to address through statute the preventable, improper disclosure of information and improper access to information.

The statue authorized the Department of Health and Human Services to enact, through its rule-making authority, detailed standards to protect privacy. The Privacy Rule[2] went into effect on April 14, 2003. This created a minimal national threshold for privacy standards aimed at protecting and avoiding improper dissemination of protected health information. The stated objectives of the privacy standards include streamlining and promoting efficiency in the electronic information-sharing process, establishing parameters and limitations on health information sharing, and reducing costs in health care and billing functions.[3]

This chapter addresses the impact of HIPAA on health care costs and specifically whether the stated goal of reducing costs has been, or is likely to be, achieved. To put this issue in context, it is important to discuss (1) the scope of HIPAA and (2) the nature of health care costs in the United States.

THE SCOPE OF HIPAA

First, HIPAA and the subsequent administrative rules established standards and requirements in areas besides privacy. A set of rules on computer security[4] went into effect in April 2005, and additional rules requiring uniform identifiers for health care entities and establishing consistent standards for electronic transactions are still to come. The most visible rule, however, is the Privacy Rule.

Privacy Rule

The Privacy Rule applies to three types of entities: health care providers, health plans (insurers), and health care clearinghouses (such as billing services) if they meet the following criteria: they must transmit protected health information in electronic form.[5] *Health care provider* is defined further in one section of the law by place of service such as a hospital, skilled care facility, outpatient clinic, home health agency, or hospice.[6] In another section, *health care provider* is defined by the services provided and the nature of the provider. This specifically includes nurses and nurse practitioners.[7]

Institutions must comply with the Privacy Rule, and institutions have a number of responsibilities to perform and document to show compliance. If the provisions of the Privacy Rule are violated, the institution

can be subject to civil and criminal penalties (fines and money damages). A recent (June 1, 2005) opinion from the U.S. Department of Justice stated that the institution (rather than individuals, supervisors, or board members) will be liable for damages resulting from an unlawful disclosure in most circumstances.[8]

The Privacy and Security Rules are specific and prescriptive, affecting medical records, billing records, enrollment, case management, and claims records of an individual. This includes any record in any format or medium that is used to make any health care decision. *Protected health information* is defined broadly to include any information that relates to the past, present, or future physical or mental health or condition of an individual, the provision of health care to an individual, or the payment for health care provided to the individual that identifies the person or could be combined with other information to identify the person. Protected health information be disclosed only if it is authorized, permissible, or compelled.[9]

The Privacy Rule requires the following: a privacy officer to oversee implementation and compliance; the use of a privacy notice that is distributed to each patient and describes the patients' rights under the Privacy Rule; and a substantial body of policies and procedures with an institutional structure to monitor compliance, conduct audits, and investigate concerns. All consent forms and patient information materials must be HIPAA compliant, which means that the materials must contain the required notices to advise patients of their rights, and they must not disclose protected health information inadvertently. The Privacy Rule also mandates that every staff member receive training in the rule.

Compliance with HIPAA is expensive. Compliance requires experienced, skilled staff; the production of thousands of pages of documents; and the time and energy of all employees. Some costs can be quantified: the salary of the privacy officer, for example, and the cost of printing privacy notices. More significant is the time and expense required to train staff to maintain a high level of awareness of these complex rules. The Privacy Rule requires that every patient receive a "Notice of Privacy Practices," the content of which is dictated by rule. The health care entity needs to document that the patient received this notice. Patients receive this notice on their first encounter with a hospital or a clinic. Although a great deal of useful information is contained in the document about the patient's rights regarding health care information and its use and protection, it is reasonable to assume that many patients and family members are unable to comprehend much of the contents because of the stress of being in the health care system and the complexity of the information. In addition, patients from diverse backgrounds may find the information in the privacy notice difficult to absorb. Concern about the effectiveness of communication with diverse groups has been raised by a number of consumer groups and was summarized in a report by the General Accounting Office of the first year's experience with the HIPAA Privacy Rule.[10]

Under the Privacy Rule, every patient has a number of rights that can be exercised by the patient or on the patient's behalf by a personal representative. These include the right to be assured that the personal health information will be treated in a respectful manner and disclosed only when necessary; to request a restriction on the uses and disclosures (*use* generally refers to revealing information within an institution among health care professionals, and *disclosure* refers to making information available to an entity outside the institution or for a purpose unrelated to care; consequently, use and disclosure are two different things, although the information may be the same); to request confidential communications; to access protected health information; to amend the record if an error has been made; and to receive an accounting of the disclosures made of the information in the record.[11]

Patients have the opportunity to object to some uses of protected health information: inclusion in the directory of the institution and release of information for marketing purposes.[12] In these instances, patient requests to be excluded must be respected. One note, however, is that one of the costly but unquantifiable consequences of the Privacy Rule is the staff time involved in complying with the patient requests in these areas, communicating the patient requests, and following up to ensure the requests are handled appropriately.

Some uses of protected health information can occur without patient authorization, and these categories are broad in some cases, much broader that most patients know. These uses include the following: uses and disclosures required by law; uses and disclosures for public health activities; uses and disclosures to monitor communicable diseases; uses and disclosures to monitor workplace injuries; disclosures about victims of abuse, neglect, or domestic violence; uses and disclosures for health oversight activities (audit, licensure, accreditation, inspections, or other activities); disclosures for judicial and administrative proceedings; disclosures for law enforcement purposes; uses and

disclosures for specialized government functions; uses and disclosures to avert threats to the public health; uses and disclosures for research purposes; and uses and disclosures to determine cause of death or for organ transplantation.[13] Some of these provisions could be used by law enforcement to obtain a great deal of information about patients, and in this area the Privacy Rule in fact may have reduced patients' privacy protection.

Security Rules

The second major area of action under HIPAA was the enactment of Security Rules that require physical, technical, and administrative safeguards of electronic data. Institutions are required to designate a security officer to oversee compliance efforts and to conduct an extensive audit of current systems. Based on the audit that covers everything from password protection to disaster recovery plans, the institution determines what needs to be done to bring the systems into compliance. For many institutions, compliance means significant investment in new equipment or additional programming costs. Many institutions are required to purchase new systems and software, conduct extensive training, employ consultants and additional staff, send staff to training sessions, and assume substantial costs for consultants to conduct audits and advise them on compliance. All of the actions have to be documented, and as with the Privacy Rule, dozens of policies and procedures have to be developed.

In the commentary that accompanied a draft of the Privacy Rules, the Department of Health and Human Services estimated that the regulations would cost $17.6 billion initially but would lead to cost savings over time. In the commentary that preceded the Security Rules, the Department of Health and Human Services acknowledged the "seeming disconnect" between two statements: in Section A of the Security Standards the comments state, "no individual small entity is expected to experience direct costs that exceed benefits as a result of this rule," and in Section E (factors in establishing the Security Standards) the comment is "we cannot estimate the per-entity cost of implementation because there is no information available regarding the extent to which providers', plans' and clearinghouses' current security practices are deficient."[14]

This comment is significant for two reasons: first, it makes clear that the rules are being enacted with no idea what the fiscal impact is on the entities affected by them, and second, and perhaps more problematic, is the statement that there is no evidence that there are any known deficiencies in the systems that the rules are intended to address. Is it any surprise, then, that a contributing factor in the increase in health care costs is the unfunded mandate of federal legislation by rule?

Since the 1960s, health care costs have risen steadily, generally at a rate far exceeding the overall inflation rate. In 1999 the cost of health care was $1.2 trillion a year, and health care consistently absorbs 14% of the annual gross national product. Many theories are advanced to account for this: the cost of medication (12% to 14% per year), with demand for specific medications encouraged by massive, high-cost advertising; high technology and expensive equipment that are widely available despite early efforts to control costs by limiting the proliferation of expensive services; an aging population; more treatments available to extend life in formerly fatal illnesses; public health problems such as smoking and obesity that result in medical problems. In addition, consolidation of hospitals and insurers that exercise substantial market power and the conversion from nonprofit to for-profit of hospitals (with the resulting concentration of uninsured and underinsured in public hospitals) have contributed to rising costs of care and of health insurance premiums.

Employer health costs have been increasing by 12% to 13% per year nationally for the past 4 years, and projections are that increases will be 10% to 11% annually for the next 4 years. To put this in perspective, if one buys an average midsize car, $1400 of the purchase price is attributable to employee health care costs.

The HIPAA rules were imposed on a complex system of health care that is already expensive, is distributed unequally, and is increasing in cost every year. The rules apply to every provider, regardless of size, location, or history of violation of privacy. The HIPAA rules are a classic unfunded mandate: a legal requirement with penalties for noncompliance but no funds provided to meet the requirement. The health care entities identified for the application of the HIPAA rules are required to comply with the rules and to absorb the cost of compliance, which means increasing rates for services (which may not be recovered by payments) or reducing other things in the budget to cover the costs associated with meeting the requirements of the rules. Both of these alternatives have an impact on costs and care.

COSTS OF HIPAA

How much do the HIPAA rules cost? The cost to each institution can only be estimated, and it is virtually impossible to determine an accurate aggregate figure.

The estimates from the Department of Health and Human Services (the entity writing the rules) and the estimates from the representatives of provider groups are vastly different. The Department of Health and Human Services has asserted that the use of electronic transaction and code set standards will result in a savings of $29.9 billion over 10 years.[15] The rationale is that the regulations related to uniform transaction and code sets (the third part of the HIPAA rules) streamline the processing of health care claims, reduce the volume of paperwork, and provide better service. This component of the rules establishes standard data elements, codes, and formats for submitting electronic claims. All health care providers will be able to use the standard transaction to bill for services.

The American Hospital Association estimated that the cost of implementing only the Privacy Rules (keep in mind that HIPAA encompasses the Privacy Rule, Security Rules, and uniform transaction and code sets) was $22 billion.[15] This number includes only hospitals represented by association. Other organizations (clinics, academic units) have spent billions more on compliance, including consultants, computer systems integration assistance, printing of privacy notices, and staff training.

Have costs gone down as predicted by the Department of Health and Human Services? No. Has efficiency and greater accuracy been achieved through the use of the standard transaction and code sets? It is too soon to tell, in part because the effective implementation date of those rules was moved many times because so many institutions did not have the computers and software to comply.

Has the protection of patient privacy improved? This is not likely. Because these rules have been in effect for 2 years, it is possible only to assess the financial and the substantive effect of the rules.

Regarding cost, no one ever suggested that the Privacy Rule would save money. Implementation and compliance are costly in staff time and direct expense. The question becomes, Is this substantial investment paying off in better protection of patient privacy?

I would suggest that the answer to that is "no." The protection of confidentiality, no doubt, is an essential obligation to a patient. The expectation of privacy is the foundation of the patient-provider relationship. Violation of a patient confidence is prohibited by law in most states (located in the rules that define and regulate professional practice, generally), and protection of the patient's privacy is an element of professional codes of ethics. Most institutions have policies that require all staff members to maintain confidentiality. There are (and always have been) exceptions: disclosures that are required by law in the case of child abuse, for example.

In addition, violation of privacy is recognized as a compensable injury in tort law in most jurisdictions. If a patient can demonstrate that confidential health information was disclosed and that the disclosure caused harm, a lawsuit can be filed and money damages recovered. This means that before the Privacy Rule promulgated under HIPAA, health professionals already were required by law and by professional ethical standards to maintain patient confidentiality. Violating confidentiality, except under the legally permissible disclosure requirements (such as child abuse), subjects a professional to possible licensing sanctions and civil liability, as well as discipline in the workplace. Violations also may undermine patient care by violating the trust of a patient and diminishing the patient's confidence in the system and reducing the likelihood that the patient will be candid and forthcoming in future communications with health professionals.

Thus substantial incentives to maintaining the integrity of health information were in place before HIPAA. During the congressional testimony that preceded the enactment of HIPAA, the focus of violations of patient confidentiality was twofold: anecdotal evidence of breaches of confidentiality caused by unusual circumstances (such as a truck containing patient records overturning, causing the records to be blown across fields) and misuse of health data for discriminatory purposes by employers, insurers, and lending agencies. During the hearings, members of Congress did not hear that there was widespread violation of privacy by health providers, but the burden of complying with the Privacy Rules has affected every practicing professional.

Hospitals and other health care providers have incurred enormous costs to comply with the security standards. Interestingly, the department that wrote the standards admits that the costs of compliance cannot be determined: "We are unable to estimate, of the nation's two million-plus health plans and one million-plus providers that conduct electronic transactions, the number of entities that would require new or modified security safeguards and procedures beyond what they currently have in place. Nor are we able to estimate the number of entities that neither conduct electronic transactions nor maintain individually identifiable electronic health information but may become covered entities at some future time. As we are unable to estimate the number of entities and what measures are or are not already in place, or what specific implementation will be chosen to meet the requirements of the regulation, we are also unable to estimate the cost to those entities."[17]

Thus the rules have been expensive (and not quantifiable) to implement in response to a problem that may not have existed and for which protections and remedies at law were in place already for individuals who suffered violations of privacy. The predicted savings and efficiencies have not yet occurred and consequently cannot be measured.

An additional area in the HIPAA Privacy Rule has had a demonstrably negative effect: research. A recent article suggests that the Privacy Rule may create a substantial burden and prohibit the development of valuable research.[18] Cardiovascular researchers at the University of Michigan evaluated their ability to obtain patient consent to participate in a patient registry during two 6-month periods. The first period was before the implementation of the Privacy Rule, and the second was after the Privacy Rule was in effect. One should note that the Common Rule,[19] which contains strict safeguards and consent requirements when research of any type is done on human subjects, was applicable during both study periods. The researchers found that a strict interpretation of the Privacy Rule resulted in a decreased ability to obtain consent from patient subjects to participate in research and in different rates of response and possible selection bias.[20] The authors of this study conclude that the strict interpretation of the Privacy Rule in research will result in less representative registries of patient populations, potentially biased populations, and increased costs.[21]

SUMMARY

The rising cost of health care, commonly called a crisis, has been the subject of debate, commentary, and politicization since the 1970s. To date, costs keep rising, the percentage of the gross national product devoted to health care keeps going up, the number of uninsured is increasing, and a gap in the quality of care between the insured and the uninsured and underinsured is growing. In the complex world of health care and undesired medical inflation, does the federal government have any business dictating privacy and security standards to health care entities by law when this action will surely drive up medical costs? The federal government, as the nation's largest purchaser of care, is in a unique position to tell all providers how the business of providing care will be run, even if this results in increased costs and only marginal benefits to patients. The agency that funds care can impose rules on the providers that deliver the care, even if the rules are expensive and ineffective.

The Health Insurance Portability and Accountability Act as a "prescription" for cost control is not delivering as promised, at least so far. And the act has some unpleasant side effects: cost increases, substantial staff time invested in documenting compliance, patient confusion, and potential damage to research. Nonetheless, the rules are here to stay.

REFERENCES

1. Health Insurance Portability and Accountability Act, Pub. L. No. 98-457, codified at title 1 §101; 42 U.S.C. Chapter 67, subchapter 1, §5101 (1996).
2. Privacy Rule, 45 CFR §160, 164 (2003).
3. 42 U.S.C. §1320 d-7 (2000).
4. 45 CFR §160, 162, 164.
5. 45 CFR §164.104, §160.102.5.
6. 42 U.S.C. §1395x(u).
7. 42 U.S.C. §1385x (5)(2)(K) and (L)(2).
8. U.S. Department of Justice. (2005, June 1). *Scope of criminal enforcement under 42 U.S.C. §1320d-6* [memorandum]. Washington, DC: Author.
9. 45 CFR §164.501.
10. GAO-04-965: *Health information: First-year experiences under the federal Privacy Rule*, at 19 (September 2004).
11. 42 CFR §164.522(a)(1).
12. 45 CFR §510.
13. 45 CFR §512 (a), et seq.
14. 68 Fed. Reg. 34, at 8364 (February 20, 2003).
15. Armstrong, D., Kline-Rogers, E., Jani, S. M., Goldman, E. B., Fang, J., Mukherjee, D., et al. (2005). Potential impact of the HIPAA Privacy Rule on data collection in a registry of patients with acute coronary syndrome. *Archives of Internal Medicine, 165*(10), 1125-1129.
16. 45 CFR 46.
17. Armstrong et al. (p. 1128).
18. Armstrong et al. (p. 1129).

Drugs Are Too Cheap

TESS JUDGE-ELLIS   ◆   BERNARD SOROFMAN

The debate rages over access and affordability of medications. Most argue that medications should be financially attainable; some argue that high prices are the unavoidable outcome of new product development for new miracle cures. Regardless of the opinion, there is controversy. This chapter focuses on the use of medications: the costs and implications of their use for patients, the health care system, and society.

A different perspective is that medications, the wonders that they are, are inherently dangerous: toxic if used too much and debilitating if used in a manner that does not address the physiological need. Individuals do not comprehend the power and problems of medication mismanagement. The easy accessibility of medication yields little respect for their power. Inattention to the knowledge required to maintain health results in further mismanagement and harm. So consider for a moment a radical notion: Drugs are too cheap; raise prices to improve health.

Dorothy Hanson is a 78-year-old woman. She was admitted to the hospital after falling and breaking her wrist. She underwent an open reduction internal fixation of her left wrist yesterday. Mrs. Hanson lives in a city of approximately 250,000 people. She has two children and six grandchildren. Her husband, Don, died 4 years ago of lung cancer, and she lives alone. She is a retired school teacher and spends most of her free time with her bridge club and traveling to visit family. Mrs. Hanson is comfortable financially with her teacher's retirement and she has little, if any, debt. Her insurance is Medicare, and she has a supplement that covers 60% of the cost of her medications. Her medical history is significant for hypertension and hypothyroidism for which she takes hydrochlorothiazide, lisinopril, and levothyroxine.

THE CLINICAL SITUATION

Medications are toxic substances that heal and harm (Manasse, 1989a, 1989b); a dynamic clinical dance occurs between the miracle of pharmacotherapy and the dramatic problems that medications can cause. In 2003, medication use in the United States exceeded $182 billion

("Almost Half," 2004). In the last week, 81% of the adults in the United States used a medication; more than 50% used a prescription drug (Kaufman, Kelly, Rosenberg, Anderson, & Mitchell, 2002). With such high use rates, problems abound no matter whether the medication use is appropriate or a drug misadventure. Such easy and poorly controlled access to medications is a health hazard. The best way to manage this situation is to put a greater value on prescription drugs: raise the prices. Drugs are too cheap and that results in continued problems.

In fact, drug-induced disease is common. The latest estimates on drug-related morbidity and mortality are pushing $200 billion (Ernst & Grizzle, 2001). An estimate of the incidence of drug-related illness in older citizens ranges from 5% to 25% (Gandhi et al., 2003). Hospitalization and medical visits resulting from medication use are a daily phenomenon. Although the data are difficult to pin down, about 15% of all hospitalizations (Lazarou, Pomeranz, & Covey, 1998), with an estimated range of 2% to 25% (Einarson, 1993), are due to drug-induced disease; estimates of drug-related emergency room visits range from nearly zero to more than 10% (Wintersetin, Sauer, Hepler, & Poole, 2002). One report indicated that posthospitalization admissions resulting from drugs have been estimated at 19% (Foster, Murff, Peterson, Gandhi, & Bates, 2003).

Awareness of the incidence of drug-induced disease is important for nurses. This knowledge informs clinical reasoning and guides how nurses ask and illicit information from patients. Not only may this help avoid a needless hospitalization in the future, but also it affects patient teaching and may provide useful information to other members of the health care team.

Mrs. Hanson says, "Yes, they just added that lisinopril to my blood pressure medication about five weeks ago." You note that her blood pressures have been running 105/68 to 110/74 since she has been hospitalized. She says, "I took my blood pressure at the drug store, and it ran about one ten over seventy. I thought that was pretty good." Upon further questioning, Mrs. Hanson says that she is definitely more dizzy and unsteady when she first gets up from being seated. "I'm so used to just popping up and going! I guess I am a little impatient with having to make changes because of a little light-headedness." She denies light-headedness currently. You review the importance of rising slowing, especially after being placed on new blood pressure medication. You also make a note to talk to the doctor and the home health nurse about your concerns about her light-headedness since she began taking the lisinopril. This very well could have contributed to her fall.

One reason why medications are problems in the health care world is the concept of patient adherence—the use of pharmaceuticals in a manner consistent with patient-provider communication. Nonadherence is common and ranges between 20% and 80%, depending on the patient, the clinical condition, and the pharmaceutical situation. The reasons for adherence or nonadherence vary. Provider-patient communication is complex and is made more difficult by provider insensitivity or ignorance of patient literacy, hearing problems, complex instructions that the patient cannot understand in a rushed visit, language barriers, and inconsistent health/illness belief model, for example. Regardless of the reason, it follows that with improved adherence to the prescribed regimen, disease states would be easier to manage. Nonadherence because of expensive medications is low, less than 6% (Kennedy, Coyne, & Sclar, 2004). Patients place a higher value on medications that cost more; expensive medication means valuable therapy, and treatment adherence is improved. More expensive medication often is in a once per day dosing (versus 3 times daily or 4 times daily dosing on less expensive or generic medication), which improves adherence.

Nurses must be aware of the wide variety of adherence issues and keep those in mind as they apply a nonjudgmental attitude when asking and receiving sensitive patient information. Patients need to know that the nurse is open and is willing to listen to their information.

Mrs. Hanson has been discharged from the hospital to home health care. You admitted her yesterday to your agency and established a plan. At the end of your visit the following week you again say, "What other concerns do you have today, Mrs. Hanson?" After several seconds she says, "Well, I guess I need to tell you that I have not filled that Fosamax prescription." You ask, "What kept you from filling that?" Mrs. Hanson says, "Well, the cost is really high, but that isn't it entirely! What really is the problem is that I am scared to take it! My sister had medication coverage—her copay was nine dollars—and she went on this medication. She thought she was doing the right thing, but I don't know. Now she has all sorts of stomach troubles. Did you know that she can't even have a cup of coffee without having to take a handful of antacids!" Mrs. Hanson looks visibly upset and crosses her arms in front of her.

THE REALITY: EASY AND INEXPENSIVE ACCESS FOR CONSUMERS, PATIENTS, AND PROVIDERS

As drug prices go down, access increases (Kennedy & Erb, 2002), more persons purchase the medications, consumption increases, and drug-related morbidity expands. More medications in the environment mean more can be taken inappropriately, and this establishes the necessary situation to create drug-related harm. Drugs are cheap and are easily replaceable. This means they have little value and are not protected as a valuable resource.

Patients are insulated from the high cost of pharmaceuticals. Insurance pays; as one patient put it, "All my drugs cost ten dollars." Most Americans have health insurance (Henry J. Kaiser Family Foundation, 2004). Insurance plans pay the primary costs of the medications, and in many cases patients are not aware of the medication costs. Billing is direct to the insurer, and the patient only sees a copayment; the "distance" reduces responsibility and value for the medications. The low cost of drugs makes them easy to obtain and provides few incentives to decrease access to the pharmaceuticals.

To be taking a medication is a choice. Yet who makes that choice, and what are the driving forces for the choice? Providers also are influenced by a variety of cost-related issues such as choosing the least expensive medication and the availability of sample medications. Prescribing often is dictated by whether patients have insurance coverage for prescription medications and whether an insurance company formulary restricts certain medications (Kolchinsky, 2003). Although these factors are important ones to consider, the patient often can be left out of the discussion, and equivocal decision making on a clinical condition might well be determined by the extent of one's insurance coverage.

Sample medications are often given out. More than 50% of elderly in one study of more than 24,000 patients received free samples from their physicians. In fact, the more often that elderly visit the physician, the greater likelihood that they will receive samples. Overall, the study reported that 9% of Medicare recipients receive drug samples. Compliance was an issue with those patients who received drug samples. Of the 14% of patients who reported skipping medications or taking fewer medications than prescribed, 73% of these reported taking medication samples versus 53% who had no financial difficulties (Taira, Iwane, & Chung, 2003). The reason most often cited by physicians for dispensing sample medications is patient inability to afford a prescription. However, it is acknowledged that drug samples are provided by drug companies that desire to introduce new medications to the physician and consumer. One concern is that although drug samples initially may cost the patient nothing, eventually having to purchase this medication from a pharmacy actually may be costly.

More and more medications are being sold over the counter (e.g., loratadine [Claritin] and famotidine [Pepcid AC]). Patients are able to diagnose and treat many medical conditions without having to seek professional opinion. Patients may not recognize over-the-counter medications as medication and may fail to report these drugs when they are asked to give a medication history.

> You are a little taken aback by Mrs. Hanson's strong reaction to her sister-in-law's stomach trouble. It seemed a little out of character. You offer to get her a glass of water, and when you return you ask, "Mrs. Hanson, how is your stomach doing for you? Do you have any trouble there?" Mrs. Hanson states that she does have some stomach trouble, but it isn't really a problem as long as she takes that "stomach medicine" she buys at the pharmacy, at which point she shows you the package for the over-the-counter lansoprazole (Prevacid). "Nancy can't even enjoy her chocolate anymore! That would be just horrible for me!"

Patients share medications. Although there is not much published on this, a recent study of medication sharing among teenagers provides a window into this situation. Students shared and borrowed medications (Daniel, Honein, & Moore, 2003). This becomes an interesting phenomenon; medications are given away. Now medications are free of cost, and because it is outside the health professional sector, they may lose the knowledge that must travel with them to create healing and avoid harm. An expensive and valued commodity would not be given away as freely and may retain more of its clinical knowledge properties.

Medications are available 24 hours a day on the Internet, and the convenience of home shopping cannot be ignored. One can sit at one's computer, and not only can one request that inexpensive medications be sent directly to one's home, but also some consumers can find online physicians to diagnose a condition and prescribe the medications. Regulatory control is weak for Internet medication shopping (Gallager & Colaizzi, 2000) and consumer interest is high (Picard, Nau, McKercher, & Schumock, 2004). The Internet opens up a whole new level of economic consideration.

One can buy medications from many manufacturers from all over the globe, often avoiding the expensive costs of patent protection. Medications can be imported from many international sources. The current debate focuses on Canadian imports but cannot be so limited. The importation of medicines allows the public to purchase their medications at discounted prices. Internet supply sources compete on a global scale, leading to reductions in price and increase in availability. Inexpensive sources of drugs create a concern about counterfeit medications from international sources (U.S. Department of Health and Human Services, 2004). Drugs can be fabricated easily. The consumer does not have the ability to analyze the product for quality. In the United States, quality assurance is provided by a series of federal and state regulations. International sources often are not monitored, and one cannot assume that the medications received are safe and effective.

Generic drugs make medications more affordable (Anonymous, 2002). A generic drug is by Food and Drug Administration definition one that is the same chemical entity as the brand name and patented drug. In general, generic drugs are sold at lower prices because they were developed without most of the research and development costs inherent in the development of new pharmaceuticals. In addition, generic drugs can be sold through contract agreements while a drug is still on patent or after patent restrictions are removed. However, in international settings some patent exclusivity is not respected, and the drugs are manufactured. Consumers do not realize that generic drugs in the United States are generally cheaper than brand drugs from Canada (Bren, 2004). Nor do they realize that the Internet market is changing and evolving rapidly. Many times the purchase is the same brand as the United States, and many times the medications are the same generic versions available in the United States. Access is too easy. The patient gets ready access to medications at a reduced price.

Patients shop around for the best deal. Medications are a product in today's society, and patients are savvy consumers. More than 3 billion prescriptions were filled at pharmacies in 2003 (National Association of Chain Drug Stores, 2005). These stores entice consumers by price-matching and discount prescriptions. Value-added aspects range from the convenience of having one's prescription on a national data bank to being able to get all of one's grocery shopping done while one waits for the prescription. One should consider the value of the long-term relationship with one's family pharmacist when one considers the price of medications.

SOLUTION

An old adage is "the most expensive medication is the one that is not used appropriately." The costs of medications are an enormous burden on health care in the United States. Cost savings compete with health outcomes. A choice between medications and food or other basic needs is not uncommon. For Americans, travel to Canada or Mexico for prescription medications is now commonplace. Ordering discounted prescriptions from online pharmacies is commonplace. Medication expenses made up 14.1% of the gross domestic product in the United States in 2002 ("Almost Half," 2004). The federal government has passed legislation to reduce the cost of prescription medication for American seniors through the Medicare prescription drug program. This legislation was passed in the spring of 2004, and its implementation and impact are still pending.

NURSING IMPLICATIONS

Nurses are sophisticated problem solvers. Nurses must continue to fine tune their curiosity and clinical reasoning skills, however, and direct consumers toward the area of medications and medication management. Medications must be viewed as potential or current problems. Nurses must achieve a respect for the clinical problems that arise from medication use, keep medications on their clinical "radar screen," and learn to ask the right questions. A medication history that simply is a copy of the patient's medication list is not enough. Questions should be detailed enough to explore a patient's clinical puzzle thoroughly; for example, "When was the medication started?" "Have you recently had a dosage change, or is this the way that you have always taken your medications?" "How do you pay for your medications?" "What do you do when you miss a dose?" "How often does this occur?" and finally "Any concerns about your medication?" These questions and others like them transmit a respect for medications and their affect on patients.

Nurses are champion patient advocates. Nurses must view this as a role that extends into the medication arena. For example, a patient may feel torn between the desire to not "go against" a doctor's order and yet feel extremely uncomfortable taking a medication. The nurse in the foregoing case example was able to validate the patient's concerns and give her space to talk about her medication and the choices that she is making. When nurses display sensitivity to the complexity of concerns surrounding medications, patients may feel more comfortable disclosing their concerns or medication misadventures. Nurses are then in a wonderful position to assist the patient.

Nurses are model team members. Drawing other members of the health care team, such as the pharmacist, into the clinical discussion is another wonderful way to empower the patient. Pharmacists can offer suggestions for different dosing strategies; other medications that might be appropriate; different formulations that may not cause discomfort; and many other helpful solutions. Increased knowledge in pharmacology will better inform the nurse and the patient.

Do medications cost too little? Should prices be increased? What safeguards for individuals and society should be put in place? Whatever one's position, one can be assured that the issue is complex; the principles are heavily woven into the fabric of society, and solutions are debatable from more than two perspectives. Nursing is at the forefront of the battle to ensure that medications heal.

ENDNOTE

This case study is written with a focused perspective to create thought, discussion, and, we hope, debate. Our personal positions on this topic diverge from this manuscript in many ways.

REFERENCES

Almost half of all Americans on prescriptions. (2004, December 3). *Medical News Today*. Retrieved April 1, 2005, from http://www.medicalnewstoday.com/medicalnews.php?newsid=17269

Anonymous. (2002). Generic drugs. *Medical Letter on Drugs & Therapeutics, 44*(1141), 89-90.

Bren, L. (2004). Study: U.S. generic drugs cost less than Canadian drugs. *FDA Consumer, 38*(4), 9.

Daniel, K. L., Honein, M. A., & Moore, C. A. (2003). Sharing prescription medication among teenage girls: Potential danger to unplanned/undiagnosed pregnancies. *Pediatrics, 111*(5), 1167-1170.

Einarson, T. R. (1993). Drug-related hospital admissions. *Annals of Pharmacotherapy, 27,* 832-840.

Ernst, F. R., & Grizzle, A. J. (2001). Drug related morbidity and mortality: Updating the cost of illness model. *Journal of American Pharmaceutical Association, 41*(2), 192-199.

Foster, I., Murff, H. J., Peterson, J. F., Gandhi, T. K., & Bates, D. W. (2003). The incidence and severity of adverse effects affecting patients after discharge from the hospital. *Annals of Internal Medicine, 138*(3), 161-167.

Gallager, J. C., & Colaizzi, J. L. (2000). Issues in Internet pharmacy. *Annals of Pharmacotherapy, 34,* 1483-1485.

Gandhi, T. K, Weingart, S. N., Borus J., Seger, A. C., Peterson, J., Burdick, E., et al. (2003). Adverse events in ambulatory care. *New England Journal of Medicine, 348*(16), 1556-1564.

Henry J. Kaiser Family Foundation. (2004, August 27). *Daily health policy report.* Retrieved February 21, 2005, from http://www.kaisernetwork.org/daily_reports/rep_index.cfm?DR_ID=25474

Kaufman, D. W., Kelly, J. P., Rosenberg, L., Anderson, T. E., & Mitchell, A. A. (2002). Recent patterns of medication use in the ambulatory adult population of the United States. *JAMA: The Journal of American Medical Association, 287*(3), 337-344.

Kennedy, J., Coyne, J., & Sclar, D. (2004). Drug affordability and prescription noncompliance in the United States: 1997-2002. *Clinical Therapeutics, 26*(4), 607-614.

Kennedy, J., & Erb, C. (2002). Prescription noncompliance due to cost among adults with disabilities in the United States. *American Journal of Public Health, 92*(7), 1120-1124.

Kolchinsky, P. (2003, September). Drug pricing principles. *BioProcess International.* Retrieved April 1, 2005, from Pharmalicensing.com: http://pharmalicensing.com/features/disp/1066849957_3f96d6a52730a

Lazarou, J., Pomeranz, B. H., & Covey, P. H. (1998). Incidence of adverse drug reactions in hospitalized patients. *JAMA: The Journal of American Medical Association, 279,* 1200-1205.

Manasse, H. R. (1989a). Medication use in an imperfect world: Drug misadventuring as an issue of public policy. Part 1. *American Journal of Hospital Pharmacy, 46,* 929-944.

Manasse, H. R. (1989b). Medication use in an imperfect world: Drug misadventuring as an issue of public policy. Part 2. *American Journal of Hospital Pharmacy, 46,* 1141-1152.

Picard, A. S., Nau, D. P., McKercher, P. C., & Schumock, G. T. (2004). Importation of prescription medications: Experiences, opinions, and intended behaviors of U.S. Community Pharmacists. *Journal of American Pharmacists Association, 44,* 666-672.

Taira, D. A., Iwane, K. A., & Chung, R. S. (2003). Prescription drugs: Elderly enrollee reports of financial access of free samples, and discussion of generic equivalents related to type of coverage. *American Journal of Managed Care, 9,* 305-312.

U.S. Department of Health and Human Services, Task Force on Drug Importation. (2004). *Report on prescription drug importation.* Washington, DC: Author.

Wintersetin, A. G., Sauer, B. C., Hepler, C. D., & Poole, C. (2002). Preventable drug-related hospital admissions. *Annals Pharmacotherapy, 35,* 1238-1245.

ROLE CHALLENGES, COLLABORATION, AND CONFLICT

Colleagues and Conflict

PERLE SLAVIK COWEN ◆ SUE MOORHEAD

Health care is undergoing many changes, some welcome and some unwelcome, as demonstrated in the other sections of the book. A combination of increasing demands for resources and decreased time for communication can create a situation that leads to difficult and at times fractious interactions among colleagues. The 2004 Institute of Medicine report on transforming the work environment of nurses pays particular attention to collaboration among health professionals, listing conflict management as one of the key characteristics of such collaboration. The report also encourages health care organizations to institute human resource policies that include conflict management skills. In the health care environment, change has become a constant state of affairs in which old roles are evolving and new roles are emerging. These roles involve collaboration and conflict, two topics that the chapters in this section explore in some detail.

The debate chapter for this section is about collaboration between nurses and physicians. Nurse leaders have long desired more collaborative roles and relationships with physicians. Keenan and Tschannen build on previous work by Baggs and examine and summarize 22 recent research studies that were identified as having evaluated changes in the state of the science on nurse/physician collaboration. The critical attributes used to define collaboration included sharing in planning, decision making, problem solving, goal setting, and responsibility; working together cooperatively; and coordinating and communicating openly. In their findings, Keenan and Tschannen identify antecedent environmental and professional factors that clearly foster or impede nurse/physician collaboration and note that "higher levels of perceptions of nurse/physician collaboration are associated with important patient and professional outcomes." Obstacles to collaborative practice include traditional communication patterns, decision-making prerogatives of physicians, and reluctance on the part of nurses to accept greater responsibility for decision making. The authors provide a graphic model of the characteristics proposed as necessary for effective collaboration to occur.

The authors identify and encourage changes in educational programs to promote collaborative learning and changes within practice settings to facilitate collaborative problem solving. This chapter contains an excellent and comprehensive review of the literature on nurse/physician collaboration.

The changing roles of nurses reflect the changing roles of women in society. In the first viewpoint chapter, Chinn explains that because most nurses are women and because nurses' role of caring for the sick has been assigned to women worldwide, feminism and nursing are connected inextricably. Chinn structures her chapter around a statement by Florence Nightingale: "Passion, intellect, moral activity—these three have never been satisfied in woman." Chinn discusses these three values historically and in modern times. She relates passion to feminism as a culture grounded in women's experience and a political stance to right injustices against women; intellect to feminism as a discipline seeking to give voice to women's experience; and moral activity to feminism as an ethic of valuing women and women's experience. Feminism, she says, is not an ideology but a perspective that values diversity. She concludes her chapter with a set of suggested readings and questions to explore further some of the ideas that she has raised. Chinn's chapter is highly recommended as a classic for all women and men in nursing who value the contributions of both sexes.

The unique perspective and contribution that nurses bring to the patient is labeled by Pike and Maas in the next chapter as "nurses voice." They urge nurses to choose colleagueship over silence and note that nurses' voices have been silenced by external and internal forces. Among the new external constraints is the restructuring of health care in the United States. These constraints, according to the authors, have inflicted wounds on nurses' professional self-esteem. Pike and Maas urge nurses to speak out, to define themselves as colleagues, rather than acting out the appealing victim role and remaining silent and blaming physicians. The taking up of the conflict requires an understanding of the uniqueness of nursing, a breadth of clinical experience, a language to communicate to others the nature of nursing, and an understanding of the constraints imposed on nurses. Using two case studies, the authors illustrate that nurses' silences have significant implications for patient care and for nurses' role and satisfaction. All nurses should read and act on this thought-provoking and important chapter.

Edwards, Grover, and Woods address collaboration between nursing and medicine in the delivery of services to the community. Community-based care requires a shift in power from the hospital and expert professionals to community members. A new collaborative approach to the education of medical and nursing students is necessary in order to embrace the new philosophy. Edwards, Grover, and Woods identify the key collaboration factors as empowerment, emotional intelligence, principled negotiation, and teamwork. The chapter includes the societal, professional, and economic forces that work against collaboration between physicians and nurses. A few successes of effective collaboration are beginning to be documented. The chapter describes in details the 15-year successful collaborative education model at East Tennessee State University designed to provide health care to the Blue Ridge mountain community. A large community need and a series of grants from the W.K. Kellogg Foundation have enabled community leaders and health professionals in the colleges of medicine, nursing, and public and allied health to work together to establish a successful multidisciplinary education and practice model. Although the setting and driving forces may not be the same as other parts of the country, the accomplishments of this group are clearly visionary and admirable. In this day of rapid change in health care and recognized need to refocus nursing education and services to the community, everyone should read this chapter.

Conflict and its resolution is also the subject of the last chapter by Kritek. She opens with a story of a typical conflict that nurses confront daily and describes how "conflicts shape the day-to-day work experiences of health care providers and their perception that much of that conflict arrives 'out of the blue' and implicitly sends a message that no recourse is possible." Kritek introduces us to alternative dispute resolution, a new approach focused on the exploration and implementation of policies and practices that address conflict by seeking alternatives to mutual harm to the participants. Conflict is costly, and Kritek provides a table one can use to estimate the cost of conflict in a given unit or department. Her chapter is a personal philosophical reflection on the nature of conflict in nursing and ways that nurses handle conflict. Her constructive and creative discourse on "lessons from the trenches" covers three premises: (1) nurses already have many conflict resolutions skills mastered, (2) nurses avoid conflicts where they feel disadvantaged, and (3) nurses can enhance their alternative dispute resolution competencies. Following her summary, Kritek provides a list of good reading materials and Web sites. Kritek wants nurses to think of themselves as persons who can assist in the resolution of conflicts creatively and constructively. The first step, she says, is to recognize that the nursing profession is at an "uneven table" and that the approach being used is harmful. Kritek says that conflict in health care will increase, and she wants nurses to transform their current behavior to that which is beyond mere manipulation. This is a thoughtful, challenging chapter, one that many of us should read several times.

Collaborative practice for nurses is closer to reality than in the past because of the changes in society and in health care delivery. Collaboration requires certain skills, however, and a risk-taking attitude. In a sense, the opportunity for collaboration creates conflict. When nurses choose collaboration, they choose conflict. This realization and knowledge of strategies to deal with conflict may move us closer to a preferred future.

Collaboration Issues Between Nurses and Physicians

GAIL KEENAN ◆ DANA TSCHANNEN*

A comprehensive review of the state of the science on nurse/physician collaboration was presented in the sixth edition of *Current Issues in Nursing* (Baggs, 2001). The critical attributes used to define collaboration included sharing in planning, decision making, problem solving, goal setting, and responsibility; working together cooperatively; and coordinating and communicating openly (Baggs & Schmitt, 1988). The current chapter builds on the previous review and examines subsequent changes in knowledge about this area. In addition, we discuss the implications of the changes to practice and directions for future research.

HISTORICAL PERSPECTIVE

In the previous synthesis of nurse/physician collaboration, Baggs (2001) addressed the following questions: What is it? Does it exist? and Why does it matter? To answer the first question, Baggs reviewed the literature and presented a model of the factors associated with nurse/physician collaboration. The model was composed of the precursors or antecedents of nurse/physician collaboration and the outcomes of it. The antecedents included professional and organizational factors; time, availability, receptivity, assertiveness, and problem-solving skills of the nurse and physician; and supportive work group norms. The outcomes influenced by nurse/physician collaboration included patient and professional factors, quality of care, mortality rates and cost of care, patient satisfaction, and nurse job satisfaction and retention.

In answering the question "Does it exist?" Baggs asserted that evidence indicates that the two professions are moving toward stronger levels of collaboration between nurses and physicians. Nonetheless, the major challenge identified was that nurses and physicians do not agree on the meaning of interdisciplinary collaboration. Nurse writers and researchers typically describe it as a balanced or equal sharing of professional knowledge, decision making, and responsibility for patient care. Physicians, conversely, rarely write about it and tend to describe nurse/physician collaboration as excellent communication with nurse members of a health care team headed by the physician leader and primary decision maker. Moreover, when questioned, physicians consistently report significantly higher levels of collaboration with nurses than their nurse colleagues.

Baggs (2001) interpreted the disciplinary discrepancies in the definitions of nurse/physician collaboration mainly to occur because of the different educational requirements of the two professions. Stereotypical thinking about education fosters automatic reinforcement of the assumption that the ideas of the more educated are superior to those of the less educated. Baggs asserted, however, that as nurses continue to achieve higher and higher levels of education, the two disciplines will engage correspondingly in more collaborative communication. In conclusion, Baggs explained why collaboration between the professions matters. Specifically, she argued that recognizing and equitably weighting the unique contributions of nurses and physicians in care decisions ultimately accrues to the patient benefit in multiple ways while simultaneously supporting positive professional outcomes.

RECENT NURSE/PHYSICIAN COLLABORATION RESEARCH

Through a variety of means, 22 related research studies were identified to evaluate changes in the state of the science on nurse/physician collaboration following the Baggs (2001) review. All studies reviewed, with the exception of 3, were reported in 2000 or later. Nine are interventions studies, and the remaining 13 are cross-sectional or longitudinal. Seventeen of the studies were

*We wish to express our gratitude to Milisa Manojlovich, PhD, RN, for her review and thoughtful input on this manuscript.

conducted in three or fewer hospitals: one hospital ($n = 11$), two hospitals, ($n = 3$), and three hospitals ($n = 3$). One study was conducted with graduate student nurses, and the remaining 4 were conducted in multiple (17, 84, 64, and 65) hospitals. Physicians (n range, 3 to 269) were the subjects in 7 of the studies, patients (n range, 124 to 1326) were subjects in 8 studies, and nurses (n range, 3 to 1973) were subjects in 17. Convenience sampling was used as the primary mode of accessing subjects in 18 of the studies. In 3 of the studies a randomized experimental control group design was used, and in 1 study administrative data from a large database were examined randomly. Surveys were the primary source of data, with a few studies reporting the use of data from observations, administrative and other large databases, and chart audits. The key study characteristics are presented in tables organized into research predominantly focused on the antecedents of nurse/physician collaboration (Table 54-1) or the outcomes of collaboration (Table 54-2). In general, most of the studies provided additional evidence to support previous findings. Several new factors, however, were examined and found to be significantly associated with nurse/physician collaboration.

As is noted in Table 54-1, the antecedents "effective communication styles" and "supportive environmental conditions" again were found to be associated significantly with higher levels of nurse/physician collaboration (Chaboyer, Najman, & Dunn, 2001; Coeling & Cukr, 2000; Doran, Sidani, Keating, & Doidge, 2002; Foley, Kee, Minick, Harvey, & Jennings, 2002; Keenan, Tschannen, Aebersold, & Kocan, 2005; Tschannen, 2004, 2005). New and more specific environmental factors found to be significant included job autonomy, job control, and the extent of the nurse manager's participation in clinical and administrative decisions (Chaboyer et al., 2001; Doran et al., 2002; Foley et al., 2002; Krairiksh & Anthony, 2001; Tschannen, 2004). New professional factors examined included staffing levels, nurse experience, and nurse education. Foley et al. (2002) found a significant positive relationship between nurse/physician collaboration and expertise, a measure of the amount of formal and informal education, whereas Tschannen (2005) found a significant positive association between staffing levels and experience and no relationship to education level.

The more recent research also indicates that nurses and physicians continue to disagree significantly on the levels of nurse/physician collaboration in their work environments (Copnell et al., 2004; Hojat et al., 2001; Keenan et al., 2005; Rosenstein, 2002; Tschannen, 2005). As found previously, physicians perceive higher levels of collaboration and respect in their relations with nurses than their nurse colleagues indicate. Nurses, however, rate the importance of nurse/physician collaboration to be higher than physicians.

In an interesting intervention study, Keenan et al. (2005) identified a pattern of nurse deference in observations of the communication of two collaborative task groups each composed of two physicians, two nurses, and a professional facilitator. In the analysis of the four 2-hour sessions for each task group, nurses had significantly less talk time and verbalized significantly more support agreement statements than their physician counterparts. This discrepancy was considered to be particularly significant given the problem focus of each group, and solutions to be derived were of equal concern to the physicians and nurses. Moreover, the discrepancy occurred under conditions in which it was the sole job of the facilitator to ensure balance in the communication and in which team members (nurses and physicians) had been selected based on being identified as informal leaders. Though balance in communication was achieved in both groups by sessions three and four, the findings suggest that norms of nurse deference remain strong and unconscious in the nurse/physician dyad and that eliminating such norms will require powerful efforts. In another study by Copnell et al. (2004) designed to improve nurse-physician collaboration through implementing a nurse practitioner case management model, no significant changes in collaboration were found between the preintervention and postintervention valuation periods. It must be noted, however, that the absence of significant findings likely was due, in part, to insensitive measures and a small sample. An interesting finding reported by Tschannen (2005) was that nurses' daily reports of the levels of nurse/physician collaboration had no association to their general perceptions of nurse/physician collaboration on their units. The finding suggests that general reports of collaboration may be of little value in evaluating whether nurse/physician collaboration takes place when it is most needed.

The list of professional outcome variables (see Table 54-2) significantly influenced by nurse/physician collaboration was expanded to include job stress, group cohesion, and nurse satisfaction with decision-making processes (Adams & Bond, 2000; Boyle & Kochinda, 2004; Bratt, Broome, Kelber, & Lostocco, 2000; Dechairo-Marino, Jordan-Marsh, Traiger, & Saulo, 2001) and error rates (Donchin et al., 1995). Several studies reconfirmed the positive relationship between nurse/physician collaboration and nurse satisfaction, turnover (Adams & Bond, 2000; Bratt et al., 2000; Coeling & Cukr, 2000; Mark,

Text continued on p. 494

DEBATE

TABLE 54-1

Studies of Antecedents to Nurse and Physician Collaboration (1998-2005)

Study	Design	Sample	Selected Variables	Methods/ Measures	Selected Findings
(Chaboyer et al., 2001)	Descriptive Random Australia	3 Hospitals 189 RNs CC = 57% RR RNs Non-CC = 55% RR	Job valuation Autonomy Collaboration with MDs Independent action	Mailed survey Comparison of means	Non-CC RNs reported significantly higher levels of autonomy than CC RNs ($p < .05$); CC RNs reported significantly higher levels of RN/MD collaboration, job valuation, and independent action ($p < .05$).
(Copnell et al., 2004)	Intervention (I) Pretest and posttest	1 Hospital 2 ICUs Pretest 47 RNs Pretest 15 MDs = 41% RR Posttest 59 RNs Posttest 16 MDs = 37% RR	I = Neonatal nurse practitioner model— advance clinical management of newborn RN/MD perceptions of RN/MD relationship and communication	Survey Comparison of means pretest and posttest	No significant differences between pretest and posttest RN/MD perceptions of the RN/MD relationships and communication; significant differences found between RN/MD groups' perceptions.
(Doran et al., 2002)	Descriptive, cross-sectional survey design	1 Hospital 26 Med-surg units 254 RNs = 35% RR 372 Patients = 73% RR	Patient = demographics, medical diagnosis, functional health status, therapeutic self-care, mood disturbance RN = demographics, autonomy, role tension, time for care, care quality, RN/MD communication and coordination	RN and patient surveys Chart audits Structural equation modeling	Significant findings: Job autonomy ($p = .29$) and education of RNs ($p = .27$) had a positive effect on communication; length of experience ($p = -.24$) and role tension ($p = -.34$) had a negative effect; communication had a positive effect on therapeutic self-care ($p = .20$).

	Design	Sample	Variables	Methods	Findings
(Foley et al., 2002)	Descriptive	2 Military hospitals 8 Units 103 RNs = 56% RR	Autonomy Control over practice RN/MD collaboration Nursing expertise	Survey Correlations	RN/MD collaboration significantly and positively related to autonomy ($p = .01$), control over practice ($p = .01$), and nursing expertise ($p = .05$); no significant differences were found for military ($n = 59$)/civilian ($n = 41$) on perceptions of RN/MD collaboration. Military group was significantly younger ($p \leq .01$), with more educated ($p \leq .01$), more males ($p \leq .01$), and more certifications ($p \leq .05$), and indicated greater autonomy ($p \leq .05$) than civilian counterparts.
(Hojat et al., 2001)	Cross section Descriptive Convenience Anonymous 2 Countries	3 Hospitals 1 U.S. hospital: 84 RNs, 118 MDs 2 Mexican hospitals: 279 RNs, 149 MDs (no RR)	Attitudes toward RN and MD collaboration	Survey Comparison of means	U.S. RNs and MDs expressed significantly more positive attitudes toward RN/MD collaboration ($p < .01$) than Mexican MDs and RNs; U.S. RNs had significantly more positive attitudes toward collaboration than U.S. MDs and Mexican MDs and RNs ($p < .01$).
(Keenan et al., 2005)	Intervention (I) Pretest and posttest Longitudinal	1 Hospital 2 Units pre-post RNs: 47 = RR 66%; 38 = 55% MDs: 18 = RR 53%; 16 = 46% 2 (I) Units A, B RNs: 2, 2 MDs: 2, 2	Perceptions work group MDs and RNs collaboration Intervention (I) 4 2-hour facilitated group sessions for problem identification, solution, implementation, and evaluation plans Quality of RN and DR collaborative communication	Repeated survey to work group pretest and 6 months posttest Videotaped I sessions MD and RN comparisons of talk time and message types	MDs from unit B posttest collaboration scores were significantly higher than pretest scores ($p = .031$); MDs' talk time was significantly greater than RNs' ($p = .043$), balanced by sessions 3 and 4; MDs had significantly more "gives opinion responses" than RNs ($p = .003$); RNs had significantly more "support/agreement" responses than MDs ($p = .011$).

Continued

TABLE 54-1

Studies of Antecedents to Nurse and Physician Collaboration (1998-2005)—cont'd

Study	Design	Sample	Selected Variables	Methods/ Measures	Selected Findings
Krairiksh & Anthony, 2001)	Cross section Descriptive	3 Hospitals 28 Units 279 RNs = 43% RR	Participation in phases of clinical and administrative decisions; problem identification, evaluation of alternatives, and selection of solution, perceptions RN/MD collaboration, extent that manager takes lead in decisions	Survey Correlations	Perceptions of RN/MD collaboration significantly correlated with RN participation in all phases of administrative ($p < .01$) and clinical ($p < .01$) decisions and perceived extent that manager takes lead in administrative ($p < .05$) and clinical ($p < .05$) decisions.
(Rosenstein, 2002)	Descriptive	84 Hospitals 720 RNs 173 MDs 26 administrators 281 (title unknown)	Collaboration Respect Disruptive behavior	Survey Comparison of means	MDs perceived respect for RN input in collaboration, MD level of support for RNs in RN/MD conflict, and overall atmosphere of RN/MD relations in one's setting to be significantly more positive than RNs perceived ($p < .01$). RNs rated the overall significance of RN/MD relationships and importance to RN satisfaction significantly higher than MDs' ratings ($p < .01$).
(Tschannen, 2004)	Nonexperimental	1 Hospital 2 Units 71 RNs = 65%-71% RR 34 MDs = 50%-56% RR	RN/MD collaboration Teamwork Organizational commitment	Secondary analysis of survey data Regression	Strong perceptions of teamwork and organizational commitment were related to strong perceptions of collaboration for RNs and MDs ($p < .05$); perceptions of teamwork and organizational commitment explained 55.1% of the variance in collaboration levels for MDs ($p=.06$) and 14.7% for RNs ($p = .045$).

| (Tschannen, 2005) | Nonexperimental Longitudinal | 2 Hospitals 4 Units 135 RNs = 75% RR 310 Patients | Nurse staffing (expertise, education, hours per patient day, skill mix, experience) RN/MD collaboration Length of stay | Survey Administrative data Correlations Regressions Analysis of variance | Stronger perceptions of RN/MD collaboration was associated with higher staff levels ($p = .00$), higher experience levels ($p = .03$), and a more positive perception of the environment ($p = .00$). RNs' daily reports of RN/MD collaboration did not significantly correlate with RNs' general reports of RN/MD collaboration. |

CC, Critical care; *DR,* distribution ratio; *ICU,* intensive care unit; *MD,* medical doctor; *RN,* registered nurse; *RR,* response ratio.

TABLE 54-2

Studies of Outcomes of Nurse and Physician Collaboration (1998-2005)

Study	Design	Sample	Selected Variables	Methods/Measures	Selected Findings
(Adams & Bond, 2000)	Descriptive Predictive Prospective	17 Hospitals 117 Units 834 RNs	Collaboration with MD staff Collaboration with other staff Cohesion among nurses Job satisfaction	Survey Correlations Regressions ANOVA	Job satisfaction was significantly correlated with collaboration MD staff ($p < .001$), collaboration with other professionals ($p < .001$), and cohesion among nurses ($p < .001$); the most important predictors of job satisfaction included cohesion among nurses, staff organization, and collaboration with MD staff.
(Boyle & Kochinda, 2004)	Intervention (I) Pretest and posttest Convenience	2 Hospitals 2 Units (A and B) Unit B: 24 RNs and MDs Intervention group (I) 7 RNs 3 MDs	Collaborative intervention (I) = 6 educational modules (leadership, communication, conflict resolution, change adaptation, teams, trust) Unit performance, job stress, job satisfaction, intent to stay	Survey Comparison of means pretest and posttest non-I staff and I staff	Non-I staff RNs' and MDs' (Unit B, $n = 21$) perceptions of problem solving between groups and RN leadership increased significantly ($p = .013$); non-I staff RNs ($n = 15$) reported lower job stress (p = .001); paired t-tests of the I staff revealed significant increases ($p < .05$) in satisfaction with leadership and communication.
(Bratt et al., 2000)	Cross-sectional United States and Canada	65 institutions 1973 staff RNs	Group cohesion Job stress RN/MD collaboration RN leadership Organizational work satisfaction	Survey Correlations Regressions	Significant correlations were found between job stress and group cohesion (−), professional job satisfaction, RN/MD collaboration, RN leadership behaviors, and organizational work satisfaction; (−) job stress, group cohesion, job satisfaction, collaboration, and RN leadership behaviors explained 52% of the variance in organizational work satisfaction.

Study	Design	Sample	Variables	Methods	Findings
(Coeling & Cukr, 2000)	Posttest Nonequivalent groups	Group 1 38 RN students 208 Interactions Group 2 27 RN students 131 Interactions	Communication pattern Quality of care to target patient RN/MD collaboration Nurse satisfaction	RN students' evaluations of descriptions of personal real-time encounters with MDs	Usage of an attentive style and nonusage of a contentious or dominant style resulted in significantly greater perceptions of collaboration, improved quality of care, and increased nurse satisfaction ($p = .000$).
(Curley et al., 1998)	Intervention (I) Randomized control trial	1 Hospital 3 Intervention units 535 Patients 3 Control units 567 Patients	I = Interdisciplinary rounds C = Traditional MD rounds	Patients matched on age, insurance, and case mix Comparison of means	Significantly lower LOS ($p = .002$) for patients receiving interdisciplinary rounds for period 11-9-1993 to 5-31-1994.
(Dechairo-Marino et al., 2001)	Intervention (I) Pretest and posttest quasi-experimental	1 Hospital 2.5 Units Pretest: 87 RNs Posttest: 65 RNs	I = Integrated a multidisciplinary component into the education, communication, documentation, and team structure for RN/MDs Collaboration = ability to reach agreement among divergent opinions to accomplish mutual goals	Surveys Convenience Sample	Strong correlation between collaboration reported by the nurses and the nurses' satisfaction with decision-making process ($r = .76$, $p < .01$). T-tests revealed no change in terms of the relationship between collaboration and nurse satisfaction with decision making postintervention.

Continued

TABLE 54-2

Studies of Outcomes of Nurse and Physician Collaboration (1998-2005)—cont'd

Study	Design	Sample	Selected Variables	Methods/Measures	Selected Findings
(Donchin et al., 1995)	Observational study, concurrent incident Random patient sampling	1 ICU 46 Patients 8178 Activities	Planned activities, initiated activities, reactive activities of all personnel in contact with patients (including visitors and family members), errors observed and recorded during those activities, verbal communication among staff members	24-hour continuous observations of activities and errors recorded on a specially developed form (pre-pilot tested).	Verbal communication was observed in only 9% of activities. Most communications were exclusively among physicians or exclusively among nurses. In only 2% of activities did physicians communicate with nurses, but in 37% of errors, verbal exchanges between RNs and MDs were involved.
(Henneman et al., 2001)	Intervention (I) Pretest and posttest quasi-experimental Power analysis	1 Hospital 1 Unit 124 (experimental) patients 77 (control) patients	I = Interdisciplinary weaning protocol involving daily plans, assessments, and communication Length of stay, weaning, cost	Administrative data Comparison of means and cost	Weaning time ($p = .06$) and LOS ($p = .03$) were significantly less for I patients; average cost per stay was lower for I patients ($43,213) versus control ($52,789) patients ($p = .16$).
(Jitapunkul et al., 1995)	Intervention (I) Experimental and control	1 Hospital Control unit = 199 Patients I (Experimental) unit = 218 Patients	Interdisciplinary (MDs and RNs) rounds and conferences 4 times/week Length of stay	Patients matched on case mix, age (3-month period) Compare means	No significant difference was found in LOS between the control and intervention unit study patients.

Citation	Design	Sample	Variables	Method	Findings
(Mark et al., 2003)	Random Test of causal model Longitudinal	64 Hospitals 124 Med-surg units 1682 RNs = 74% RR 1326 Patients ≥ 80% RR (for 99/124 units)	Hospital characteristics Nursing unit characteristics Professional practice model (PPM) = autonomy, decentralization, and collaboration Outcomes; RN and patient satisfaction	Survey Time 1: context and PPM variables 6 Months after outcome	Availability of services (positive, $p < .05$) and unit size (negative, $p < .05$) significantly related to PPM; PPM significantly related to RN job satisfaction (positive, $p < .01$) and turnover (negative, $p < .05$); higher RN skill mix related to higher levels of patient satisfaction ($p < .10$).
(Mosimaneotsile et al., 2000)	Intervention (I) Longitudinal	1 Rehabilitation hospital 1239 Stroke patients	Integrative care delivery model = multidisciplinary team, care maps, documentation, and cross-training	Retrospective review of patient data 1994-1997	Significant decrease was found in LOS from 18 days (1994) to 15.6 (1997) ($p < .05$).
(Pronovost et al., 2003)	Intervention (I) Pretest and posttest cohort study	1 ICU (16-bed surgical oncology) 3 RNs 6 MDs (residents)	Implementation of a daily goals form used during rounds, ICU length of stay, MD residents and RNs understanding of daily goals	Presurvey and postsurvey of RNs and MD residents	Less than 10% of MDs and RNs understood the goals of care at baseline. Postsurvey: >95% of MD residents and RNs understood goals of care; ICU LOS decreased from presurvey 2.2 to postsurvey 1.1 mean days.
(Rosenstein, 2002)	Descriptive	84 Hospitals 720 RNs 173 MDs 26 Administrators 281 (title unknown)	Collaboration Respect Disruptive behavior	Survey Comparison of means	RNs rated the overall significance of RN/MD relationships and importance to RN satisfaction significantly higher than MDs' ratings ($p < .01$).
(Tschannen, 2005)	Nonexperimental Longitudinal	2 Hospitals 4 Units 135 RNs = 75% RR 310 Patients	Nurse staffing (expertise, education, hours per patient day, skill mix, experience) RN/MD collaboration Length of stay	Survey Administrative data Correlations Regressions ANOVA	RN/MD collaboration was associated with higher number of days than expected on the unit ($p = .059$).

ANOVA, Analysis of variance; *ICU*, intensive care unit; *LOS*, length of stay; *MD*, medical doctor; *RN*, registered nurse; *RR*, response ratio.

Salyer, & Wan, 2003; Tschannen, 2005), and patient satisfaction (Mark et al., 2003). A relationship between nurse/physician collaboration and length of stay was found in a number of studies (Curley, McEachern, & Speroff, 1998; Henneman, Dracup, Ganz, Molayeme, & Cooper, 2001; Jitapunkul et al., 1995; Mosimaneotsile, Braun, & Tokishi, 2000; Pronovost et al., 2003; Tschannen, 2005), though the relationship was not always in the same direction. For example, Tschannen (2005) found that higher levels of collaboration were associated with increased length of stay; whereas Curley et al. (1998) found a significant inverse relationship, and Jitapunkul et al. (1995) found no difference in length of stay.

In seven studies (see Table 54-2) a collaborative intervention was implemented and outcomes were evaluated by contrasting pretests and posttests. Five of these studies involved the implementation of a specified rounding process (Curley et al., 1998; Henneman et al., 2001; Jitapunkul et al., 1995; Mosimaneotsile et al., 2000; Pronovost et al., 2003). With the exception of Jitapunkul et al. (1995) previously noted, all studies of nurse/physician rounding reported significant positive outcomes. The remaining two intervention studies focused on providing educational support to improve the collaboration skills that in turn were expected to improve satisfaction with decision making (Boyle & Kochinda, 2004; Dechairo-Marino et al., 2001). In the former study there was a significant positive change in satisfaction preintervention and postintervention; in the latter there was no significant change.

SYNTHESIS

In summary, the more recent studies discussed generally support findings of previous research conducted on nurse/physician collaboration; that is, antecedent environmental and professional factors clearly foster or impede nurse/physician collaboration, and higher levels of perceptions of nurse/physician collaboration are associated with important patient and professional outcomes. Nonetheless, the more recent review underscores the previously identified problems and limitations of research in the area of nurse/physician collaboration that make it difficult to interpret and apply findings to clinical practice. We believe the major limitations are (1) nurses and physicians do not share a common meaning for nurse/physician collaboration, (2) nurse/physician collaboration has been conceptualized differently across studies, and (3) the differences between groups versus one-on-one nurse/physician collaboration have not been specified.

Baggs (2001) in the earlier review also noted the fact that nurses and physicians define nurse/physician collaboration in different ways. The seriousness of this problem has become more apparent in recent research, given that virtually no studies conducted to date have addressed this problem. In fact, without the support of physicians for equitably weighting nurse input into patient care decisions, collaboration as defined by Baggs and Schmitt (1988) cannot exist. Unless both parties are willing to consider each other's positions, collaboration cannot occur. Moreover, although nurses indicate perceiving less collaboration than physicians, nurses also seem to attribute a slightly different meaning than the Baggs definition to nurse/physician collaboration. In several studies, nurses indicated perceiving stronger levels of collaboration than did outside observers (Keenan et al., 2005; Lamb & Napadano, 1984), and in one study, nurses' general reports of nurse-physician collaboration did not correlate with daily reports of collaboration (Tschannen, 2005). The Keenan et al. (2005) study also suggests the power of traditional norms to limit the nurses' ability to engage in true collaboration with physicians.

Compounding the discrepancy in the disciplinary meanings of nurse/physician collaboration was the wide variation in how collaboration was measured in these studies. For example, rounding was used as a proxy for nurse/physician collaboration in several studies without specifying the type, amount, and format of what constituted collaboration in the study. Given that not all forms of rounding produce positive outcomes, it would be useful to describe and measure more specifically the extent that nurse/physician collaboration actually takes place, if at all, in rounds and the specific impact on desirable outcomes. Designing a successful rounding process requires an understanding of the key features that produce the positive outcomes. Nurse/physician collaboration also has been conceptualized as a conflict management strategy, whereas others describe it as a form of open communication. Lack of consistent meaning of the concept across the disciplines and the inconsistencies in measurement of nurse/physician collaboration continue to make it difficult to know just what the findings mean for clinical practice and how to apply them. Moreover, though it appears that researchers are evaluating some form of positive communication between the nurse and physician, the communication mode does not seem to be what Baggs (1988) and others have agreed constitutes "true collaboration."

Finally, no studies to date have contrasted the characteristics of group versus individual level nurse/physician collaboration, nor have the conditions when collaborative problem solving is not appropriate been described. It would be most helpful to understand the nuances of when to use group versus individual nurse/physician collaboration and when not to use collaboration at all. Clearly, collaborative communication is not always the most effective form of communication between two parties. For example, the physician may have no expertise in "the promotion of patient self-care" and thus is not in a position to collaborate with the nurse on this issue. Instead the physician may be interested in seeking information in his or her communication with the nurse. So too, if a physician orders routine vital signs, with rare exception, it is probably a waste of time for the nurse to insist on collaborating about the times of measurement. In line with this, we suggest that future research be focused on developing a typology of the different modes or types of communication applicable to multidisciplinary issues and the creation of specific measures for each mode. Once developed, the typology and measures could be used in subsequent research to isolate the best match between an interdisciplinary issue and the most effective communication mode. Data from this research then could be used to improve the efficiency of nurse/physician communication and correspondingly the satisfaction of each discipline with it.

IMPLICATIONS FOR PRACTICE

Though our review suggests there are a number of gaps in our knowledge of effective nurse/physician communication, this section is dedicated to suggesting ways one might apply what has been learned from this research. In spite of the gaps, the more recent studies provide further evidence of the importance of nurse/physician communication. Moreover, a variety of factors have been linked to the quality of nurse/physician communication (collaboration being one mode) at any given point in time. With the current recognition that many medical errors are caused by communication failures, there is great interest in redesigning health systems to limit communication failures (Institute of Medicine, 2003; Kohn, Corrigan, & Donaldson, 2003; Page, 2004).

At a minimum, it seems that most authors consider collaboration to involve a form of communication in which at least two parties engage in a problem-solving discussion with the intention of identifying a solution for a problem not well understood (Baggs & Schmitt, 1988; Keenan, Cooke, & Hillis, 1998; Keenan et al., 2005; Tschannen, 2005). Therefore problems that do not have ready solutions are good candidates for collaboration. It is recommended that nurse and physician managers

attempt to identify the types of problems amenable to collaboration and how and when these manifest in day-to-day practice. Having this information in hand, the managers then can design conditions to support desired levels of collaboration more effectively in day-to-day practice. As has been noted (Baggs, 2001; Keenan et al., 2005; Tschannen, 2005), collaboration requires that the nurse and physician have sufficient time, relevant expertise, receptivity to each other, availability, and appropriate communication skills. If any of the factors are missing, the quality of the communication and outcomes achieved will be influenced adversely. Thus two critical considerations include ensuring the adequacy of staffing numbers and the appropriate staff mix. The Tschannen (2005) and Foley et al. (2002) findings suggest that experienced nurses are more likely to engage in problem-solving communication with a physician than their novice counterparts. It makes sense to conjecture that problem-solving skills most likely are developed and refined through experiences across time. It therefore seems prudent to encourage the nurse managers to consider the potential impact of expertise on interdisciplinary communication and factor for it when designing their unit staffing plan and policies. For example, experienced staff might be teamed with the less experienced staff to ensure the availability of nurses who can and will engage in effective problem solving with physicians as needed. In turn the experienced nurses would be serving as role models to the novices. Figure 54-1 provides a graphic model of the characteristics proposed as necessary for collaboration to occur.

In certain cases, issues requiring mutual problem solving may be solved best in formal task groups. In particular, when problems are of concern to the broader community of unit nurses and physicians, the problem solving should be assigned to a representative subgroup of the community for mutual resolution. Again, attention must be given to meeting the conditions supportive of effective mutual problem-solving communication. The nurses and physicians selected for this group must have sufficient time, relevant expertise, receptivity to each other, availability, and appropriate communication skills. When assigning groups to engage in mutual problem solving, we recommend balancing the number of physicians and nurses and assigning a professional facilitator who is responsible for ensuring the balanced input of group members in the problem-solving process. As Keenan et al. (2005) found, nurses tended to demonstrate automatic physician deference until it was clear to the nurses that their input was desired and valued. Assuming true group collaboration will take place,

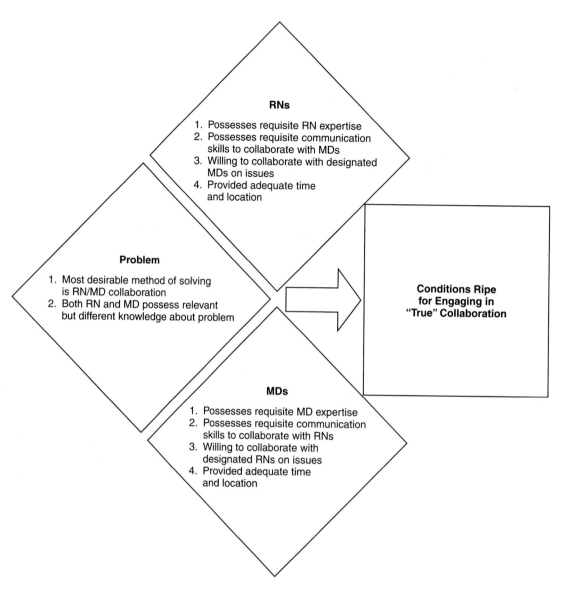

FIGURE 54-1 Requisite components for successful registered nurse (RN) and medical doctor (MD) collaboration in groups and one-on-one.

without taking positive actions to ensure it does, will lead to physician-dominated teams that create solutions conducive to physicians' and not nurses' interests. The potential and costly backlash of one-sided solutions is a reduction in nurse job satisfaction, which in turn is related to increased turnover (Adams & Bond, 2000; Bratt et al., 2000). Therefore it is in the best interest of all parties to make certain that nursing provides adequate input into decisions that have an impact on the day-to-day practice of nursing.

In addition, nurse managers might consider offering educational programs to assist novices and experts to be aware of their own communication skills and to strengthen those skills. This knowledge then can be used to help the novice and expert work together to select nurse/physician communication strategies in line with the skills and knowledge of the involved nurses and physicians. Figure 54-2 provides an example of the mental steps the individual nurse can exercise routinely when deciding the mode of communication to be taken

RN/MD Communication Sequence

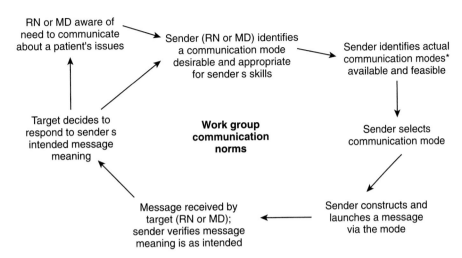

*Modes of communication may include (but are not limited to) collaboration, information sharing, expert advice, and order requests.

FIGURE 54-2 Registered nurse (RN) and medical doctor (MD) communication sequence.

to address a nurse/physician/patient issue. A step in this model not previously discussed is one in which the "sender" ensures that the message sent is received and understood by the "target" as intended. This step is included because a main source of error is the tendency to assume that the target of the message has received and understood the message as intended without verification (Sutcliffe, Lewton, & Rosenthal, 2004).

Finally, to engage in true collaboration, parties must possess expertise and be able to articulate this expertise when communicating with each other. Nurses and physicians must be aware of their own domain knowledge and must be able to articulate this effectively to members of the health care team. Before recent times, nursing knowledge has not been represented in ways that support clear articulation of the nursing component of health care. Consequently, this has fostered the belief by others that nursing has no unique body of knowledge and has limited the nurse's ability to articulate confidently the value and worth of nursing work. To address this problem, researchers have been developing and refining standardized terminologies as a means of enhancing nursing communication by providing the language to clarify and make nursing practice more visible. Keenan et al. (2005) have been involved in this effort and specifically focus on integrating standardized nursing terminologies into practice. As part of their mission, the Hands-on Automated Nursing Data System research

team is dedicated to refining a technology-supported care planning methodology that will facilitate the continuous and accurate communication of nursing care information to nurses and other members of the health care team. In conclusion, we encourage nurses to get involved in learning and integrating standardized terminologies into practice as a means of enhancing the effectiveness of disciplinary and interdisciplinary communication.

REFERENCES

Adams, A., & Bond, S. (2000). Hospital nurses' job satisfaction, individual and organizational characteristics. *Journal of Advanced Nursing, 32*(3), 536-543.

Baggs, J. G. (2001). Collaboration between nurses and physicians in the 21st century. In J. C. McCloskey & H. K. Grace (Eds.), *Current issues in nursing* (6th ed., Chap. 57). St. Louis, MO: Mosby.

Baggs, J. G., & Schmitt, M. H. (1988). Collaboration between nurses and physicians. *Image: The Journal of Nursing Scholarship, 20,* 145-149.

Boyle, D. K., & Kochinda, C. (2004). Enhancing collaborative communication of nurse and physician leadership in two intensive care units. *Journal of Nursing Administration, 34*(2), 60-70.

Bratt, M. M., Broome, M., Kelber, S., & Lostocco, L. (2000). Influence of stress and nursing leadership on job satisfaction of pediatric intensive care unit nurses. *American Journal of Critical Care, 9*(5), 307-317.

Chaboyer, W., Najman, J., & Dunn, S. (2001). Factors influencing job valuation: A comparative study of critical care and non-critical care nurses. *International Journal of Nursing Studies, 38*(2), 153-161.

Coeling, H. V., & Cukr, P. L. (2000). Communication styles that promote perceptions of collaboration, quality, and nurse satisfaction. *Journal of Nursing Care Quality, 14*(2), 63-74.

Copnell, B., Johnston, L., Harrison, D., Wilson, A., Robson, A., Mulcahy, C., et al. (2004). Doctors' and nurses' perceptions of interdisciplinary collaboration in the NICU, and the impact of a neonatal nurse practitioner model of practice. *Journal of Clinical Nursing, 13,* 105-113.

Curley, C., McEachern, J. E., & Speroff, T. (1998). A firm trial of interdisciplinary rounds on the inpatient medical wards: An intervention designed using continuous quality improvement. *Medical Care, 36*(8 Suppl.), AS4-AS12.

Dechairo-Marino, A. E., Jordan-Marsh, M., Traiger, G., & Saulo, M. (2001). Nurse/physician collaboration: Action research and the lessons learned. *Journal of Nursing Administration, 31*(5), 223-232.

Donchin, Y., Gopher, D., Olin, M., Badihi, Y., Biesky, M., Sprung, C. L., et al. (1995). A look at the nature and causes of human errors in the intensive care unit. *Critical Care Medicine, 23*(2), 294-300.

Doran, D., Sidani, S., Keating, M., & Doidge, D. (2002). An empirical test of the nursing role effectiveness model. *Journal of Advanced Nursing, 38*(1), 29-39.

Foley, B. J., Kee, C. C., Minick, P., Harvey, S. S., & Jennings, B. M. (2002). Characteristics of nurses and hospital work environments that foster satisfaction and clinical expertise. *Journal of Nursing Administration, 32*(5), 273-282.

Henneman, E., Dracup, K., Ganz, T., Molayeme, O., & Cooper, C. (2001). Effect of a collaborative weaning plan on patient outcome in the critical care setting. *Critical Care Medicine, 29*(2), 297-303.

Hojat, M., Nasca, T. J., Cohen, M. J. M., Fields, S. K., Rattner, S. L., Griffiths, M., et al. (2001). Attitudes toward physician-nurse collaboration: A cross-cultural study of male and female physicians and nurses in the United States and Mexico. *Nursing Research, 50*(2), 123-128.

Institute of Medicine. (2003). *Crossing the quality chasm: A new health system for the 21st century.* Washington, DC: National Academy Press.

Jitapunkul, S., Nuchprayoon, C., Aksaranugraha, S., Chalwanichsiri, D., Leenawat, B., & Kotepong, W. (1995). A controlled clinical trial of multidisciplinary team approach in the general wards of Chulalongkorn Hospital. *Journal of the Medical Association of Thailand, 78*(11), 618-623.

Keenan, G., Cooke, R., & Hillis, S. L. (1998). Norms and nurse management of conflicts: Keys to understanding nurse-physician collaboration. *Research in Nursing and Health, 21*(1), 59-72.

Keenan, G., Tschannen, D., Aebersold, M., & Kocan, M. (2005). *Pilot of the collaborative communication process intervention.* Unpublished study.

Kohn, L. T., Corrigan, J. M., & Donaldson, M. S. (Eds.). (2003). *To err is human: Building a safer health system.* Washington, DC: National Academy Press.

Krairiksh, M., & Anthony, M. K. (2001). Benefits and outcomes of staff nurses' participation in decision making. *Journal of Nursing Administration, 31*(1), 16-23.

Lamb, G. S., & Napadano, R. J. (1984). Physician-nurse practitioner interaction patterns in primary care practices. *American Journal of Public Health, 74,* 26-29.

Mark, B. A., Salyer, J., & Wan, T. (2003). Professional nursing practice: Impact on organizational and patient outcomes. *Journal of Nursing Administration, 33*(4), 224-234.

Mosimaneotsile, B., Braun, K. L., & Tokishi, C. (2000). Stroke patient outcomes: Does an integrated delivery model of care make a difference? *Physical & Occupational Therapy in Geriatrics, 17*(2), 67-82.

Page, A. (Ed.). (2004). *Keeping patients safe: Transforming the work environment of nurses.* Washington, DC: National Academies Press.

Pronovost, P., Berenholtz, S., Dorman, T., Lipsett, P. A., Simmonds, T., & Haradan, C. (2003). Improving communication in ICU using daily goals. *Journal of Critical Care, 18*(2), 71-75.

Rosenstein, A. H. (2002). Nurse-physician relationships: Impact on nurse satisfaction and retention. *American Journal of Nursing, 102*(6), 26-34.

Sutcliffe, K., Lewton, E., & Rosenthal, M. (2004). Communication failures: An insidious contributor to medical mishaps. *Academic Medicine, 79*(2), 186-194.

Tschannen, D. J. (2004). The effect of individual characteristics on perceptions of collaboration in the work environment. *MedSurg Nursing, 13*(5), 312-318.

Tschannen, D. J. (2005). *Organizational structure, process, and outcome: The effects of nurse staffing and nurse-physician-collaboration on patient length of stay.* Unpublished dissertation, University of Michigan, Ann Arbor.

Feminism and Nursing

Reclaiming Nightingale's Vision

PEGGY L. CHINN

Passion, intellect, moral activity—these three have never been satisfied in woman. In this cold and oppressive conventional atmosphere, they cannot be satisfied. To say more on this subject would be to enter into the whole history of society, of the present state of civilization.

Florence Nightingale (1979, p. 29)

These words were written by Florence Nightingale in 1852, just after she pursued her nursing training at Kaiserswerth. They appear in an essay titled *Cassandra*. For years in her young adulthood, Nightingale yearned to pursue a social calling to serve people, but as a Victorian woman her options were severely restricted. Her essay *Cassandra* is an outcry against the plight of Victorian women like herself and reflects her strong conviction that women had many lost talents and abilities that could be developed.

Nightingale's quote illustrates several aspects of feminism that are equally important today. Even though much has changed for women in many parts of the world since Nightingale's time, "passion, intellect, and moral activity" are three key aspects of women's experience that still are being addressed by feminists today. Nightingale's observation that these three "have never been satisfied in woman" is a fundamental premise of feminist activism. Today, some women in the world can exercise these capacities, but many more remain constrained by the same kinds of social forces that existed in Nightingale's day. Feminist activists seek to right the wrongs and injustices that persist against women, not only through equal opportunity but also through seeking to understand women's experience in the world and to break down the barriers to valuing that experience. Finally, Nightingale's observation that "to say more on this subject would be to enter into the whole history of society, of the present state of civilization" summarizes precisely what feminist authors have set about to accomplish in the past several decades. In other words, feminism is not the singular, polemical, or fanatical fad that is portrayed in the media. Rather, feminism encompasses many perspectives that have entered the whole history of society and the present state of civilization (Young, 1997).

Feminist thought and action is grounded in women's experience and takes stances that assume that women's experience is real and valuable. Feminist thought and action is inherently political. Feminist thought and action challenges the prevailing attitudes that tend to devalue and discount women. The actions and writings that come from feminist thinking are motivated by a desire to benefit women, with the underlying conviction that if it is not good for women, it is not good. Because what affects women affects the world, and what affects the world affects women, feminist concerns are as broad as the world, even the universe.

Nursing and feminism, regardless of definitions of either concept, are inescapably connected because of the presence of women. Not only are most nurses women, but the social role—to care for the sick—of nursing is one that historically has been assigned to women worldwide. Therefore many of the actions and concerns that nurses assume in their day-to-day work are those that are associated with being female in gender. The *American Heritage Talking Dictionary* (1994) gives the following as one of the definitions of *nurse*: "One that serves as a nurturing or fostering influence or means." Generally, those who nurture are women, and when men provide formal nurturing roles in society, they usually enter social realms where women predominate. What usually are not associated with nurturing roles are precisely the three concerns that Nightingale addresses: passion, intellect, and moral activity. Caring for others and fostering their growth generally is viewed as ordinary—something that anyone can do—and certainly not requiring intellectual interest or ability.

Furthermore, caring for others generally is prescribed to women by the dominant culture; therefore exercising independent moral activity is not presumed to be required (Reverby, 1987). Although the world has changed remarkably for women in the Western world since Nightingale's time, women remain tied to their socially accepted female roles, and the roles associated with women are devalued. Even more striking is the fact that worldwide, not much has changed for women since the time of Nightingale.

I will explore feminist perspectives on Nightingale's three concerns—passion, intellect, and moral activity—and will show how these perspectives can assist nurses to move toward changes that are consistent with what is good for nurses, for women, and for all people. These concerns are interrelated. They have distinct aspects, but when one turns to the suggested readings listed at the end of this chapter, one will find that they weave together to form a whole, a global concern.

PASSION

When shall we see a life full of steady enthusiasm, walking straight to its aim, flying home, as that bird is now, against the wind–with … calmness and … confidence? (Nightingale, 1979, p. 36)

For Nightingale, the idea of passion included powerful emotion, even sexual desire—all of which were severely restricted for women in her time. Her primary interest, however, was what she termed "high sympathies," which in her view need to be fed and nurtured in order to serve society well. She said,

If, together, man and woman approach any of the high questions of social, political, or religious life, they are said (and justly—under our present disqualifications) to be going "too far." That such things can be! (Nightingale, 1979, p. 28)

Activists and theorists of the feminist movement of the second half of the twentieth century began to recognize the oppressive dynamic of being ridiculed with accusations of going too far (Morgan, 1968), when in fact they could see clearly that women had not gone far enough. And so women began, with an intensity and seriousness never before seen in human history, to approach the high questions of social, political, and religious life.

In speaking of passion, Nightingale (1979) stated that "poetry and imagination begin life" (p. 30). Nightingale believed that women begin life with vivid and rich imaginations and that their dreams and imaginations hold a key to developing the intellect and moral activity that is required for meaningful social action. She speculated, however, that women learn early to subdue their imaginations because it is so dangerous. Young girls and women receive messages early that society does not want, and that she cannot want, to fulfill her imaginations and dreams.

Nightingale identified the daily circumstances of women's lives that restrict them from developing the seeds of social action that lie dormant in their imagination: lack of time, time consumed by service to the home, time constantly interrupted. Speaking of the constant demands made on women's time by anyone and everyone, Nightingale stated,

Yet time is the most valuable of all things. If they had come every morning and afternoon and robbed us of half-a-crown we should have had redress from the police. But it is laid down, that our time is of no value. (p. 35)

Indeed, when the feminist movement of the second half of the twentieth century began, women realized that they must gain control over their own time in order to begin to change social and political structures that held control over their lives. They began to meet together in small groups to form the art and imagination that is necessary for social activism. The method of feminism—consciousness-raising—was developed in small group processes. In sharing stories of their lives, women began to discover patterns in their lives and among their lives. They began to see individual circumstances of a woman's life in the context of the social and political patterns that sustain women's oppression. And thus was born the idea that the personal is political.

The insight that "the personal is political" represents recognition of the interrelatedness of all things. The insight is expressed in many forms, calling for the joining together of what has been torn apart by centuries of patriarchal dominance. Passion, which is presumed to reside in the personal realm, is actually in all aspects of life. Passion is the necessary fire that gives energy to sustain action in the public world when all seems futile. Through passion the life of thought and the life of action can be brought together.

The enterprise of bringing together that which has been torn apart is a cultural and political enterprise. Culture teaches and reinforces the values that are thought by its members to be good and right. Politics is the ability to enact those values in a social arena. Take, for example, the cultural norm that sustains different moral codes for the personal life from those of the public life. Undertaking to bring together a single moral code for all of life is a project of huge proportions, requiring enormous energy, vivid imagination, and commitment to action.

In nursing, the splits are many: mind-body splits, practice-theory splits, real-ideal splits, public-private splits, work-home splits. Feminist ideas and historical models provide a framework from which to begin to understand the origins of these splits, to understand how they are sustained, and to begin to form action to bring them together into one (Chinn, 1989).

INTELLECT

What wonder if, wearied out, sick at heart with hope deferred, the springs of will broken, not seeing clearly where her duty lies, she abandons intellect as a vocation and takes it only, as we use the moon, by glimpses through her tight-closed window-shutters? (Nightingale, 1979, p. 37)

Nightingale (1979) reasoned that the sphere in which women were required to remain—the private sphere of home and family—was much too narrow a field for development of the mind. Speaking of the systematic ways in which women's lives and interests were curtailed, she said, "This system dooms some minds to incurable infancy, others to silent misery" (p. 37).

Nightingale had a strong conviction that women have the mental abilities to achieve whatever they wish to achieve: compose music, solve scientific problems, create social projects of great importance. But the material limitations on women's lives robbed them not only of the time to devote to such activities but also of the development of the mental and physical skills required to achieve socially meaningful actions. Out of this conviction came her resolve and action to establish nursing as a profession whereby women could develop the intellectual abilities to contribute meaningful service to society.

More than a century later, as feminist thought and action developed, nursing began to be seen in different contexts. Feminists began to recognize the hazards of sustained sex-segregation in occupations and ways in which this social and cultural pattern sustained women's oppression (Greenleaf, 1980). Feminists also challenged the unquestioning acceptance by women of their nurturing and caring roles in society and often saw nurses as sustaining this unquestioning acceptance (Chinn & Wheeler, 1985). However, out of a commitment to value women and women's experience, feminist insights also began to give new meaning to the nature of nurturing and caring and to recognize the essential value of the attitudes, skills, and knowledge that are required to be in relation with others in a caring and nurturing way (Gilligan, 1982; Larrabee, 1993; Noddings, 1984, 1999).

Nursing as a profession did accomplish what Nightingale envisioned: it provided an avenue for nurses to leave the relatively restricted environment of home and family and to enter a broader world of social service. Nursing has provided, worldwide, an avenue for women's education. For many women, becoming a nurse has been the only way to obtain an education, to develop the intellect. But has this been enough? What has been the nature of this education, and has it served women well?

Jo Ann Ashley (1976, 1980), feminist nurse historian, studied the history of nursing education in hospitals. She concluded not only that were nurses not served well by apprenticeship education but also that all nurses continue to suffer the remnants of attitudes and beliefs that continue to influence the content and the processes of nursing education and of nursing.

Consider, for example, the persistent language that sustains nursing's subservience to medicine. The phrase "physician's orders," which nurses are still legally responsible to follow, has not been changed or replaced since the earliest days of nursing as a profession. Alternatives have been suggested (e.g., physician prescription and medical treatments). The alternatives suggest the nature of physician work and relationship with the patient compared with the implications of the physician-nurse relationship in the phrase "physician orders." But nurses still are being educated in many parts of the world in ways that differ little from the earliest days of nursing to follow physician orders and, more importantly, not to question the terminology, practices, or orders themselves.

MORAL ACTIVITY

Women dream of a great sphere of steady, not sketchy benevolence, of moral activity, for which they would fain be trained and fitted, instead of working in the dark, neither knowing nor registering whither their steps lead, whether farther from or nearer to the aim. (Nightingale, 1979, p. 38)

Nightingale has been criticized for her insistence on the moral character requirements that she imposed on the earliest nurses and the heritage of emphasis on character that the profession inherited from her early views. Many of these criticisms are well founded from the perspective of more recent contexts; moral and ethical necessities change over time. However, it is now possible also to consider sustained values in her views on moral activity. Her essential concern in the essay *Cassandra* was that women's perspectives are not valued. She believed that when women's values are not realized, society suffers. She decried the waste of human resources when women are denied the circumstances in which they can develop and know their own moral sense of what is good and what is right.

For Nightingale, two circumstances are required to develop moral activity: time for learning and reflection (bringing together passion and intellect) and sustained experience in applying or acting on what is reflected upon, or experience. She states,

> Women … long for experience, not patch-work experience, but experience followed up and systematized, to enable them to know what they are about and where they are "casting their bread" and whether it is "bread" or a stone. (Nightingale, 1979, p. 39)

She speculated how any profession or occupation could be developed at odd times, which is what women generally are required to do in developing anything. She wonders how an art can be developed if it is viewed only as an amusement, which is how women's arts typically are viewed. She likened the situation of women's sketchy opportunities for development of the intellect and moral activity to starvation and saw it as serious a situation as if women were starved physically of food for the body. She viewed women's unquestioning acceptance of prescribed social roles as a moral problem:

> With what labour women have toiled to break down all individual and independent life, in order to fit themselves for this social and domestic existence, thinking it right! And when they have killed themselves to do it, they have awakened (too late) to think it wrong. (Nightingale, 1979, p. 42)

Nightingale's criticism about women's unquestioning acceptance of their social and domestic existence in her day is a serious issue that deserves consideration today. Consider how her words would read if revised to apply to nursing today:

> With what labor nurses have toiled to break down all individual and independent life, in order to fit themselves for this social and professional existence, thinking it right! And when they have killed themselves to do it, they have awakened (too late) to think it wrong.

Today, nurses do have models and frameworks with which to begin to judge what is right and what is wrong in their nursing practice (Fry, 1992). However, much of what is practiced in nursing is not questioned, and if it is questioned, it feels much too dangerous to act on

the insight. So now we turn to the question, What is a nurse to do?

FEMINIST PERSPECTIVES ON BEING, KNOWING, AND DOING

> Nothing can well be imagined more painful than the present position of woman, unless, on the one hand, she renounces all outward activity and keeps herself within the magic sphere, the bubble of her dreams; or, on the other, surrendering all aspiration, she gives herself to her real life, soul and body. For those to whom it is possible, the latter is best; for out of activity may come thought, out of mere aspiration can come nothing. (Nightingale, 1979, p. 50)

Today, the choice of action does not require women also to surrender all aspiration. A multitude of possibilities for action have emerged out of the dreams and imaginations of feminist activists and theorists of the past few decades. In fact, feminists directly have opposed the disjunction between thought and action, and healing that disjunction is a major enterprise of feminist activists and theorists. Feminist activists in the second half of the last century struggled with the choice of whether to develop theory or to take social and political action. Not everyone did both, but the prevailing practice that emerged was to be sure that theory (thoughtful reflection) and action always characterized feminist enterprises (Redstockings, 1975).

Table 55-1 summarizes definitions of feminism and the concerns—in aspiration and in action—that feminism has developed in the last century. The Suggested Readings at the end of this chapter provide classic and recent resources where one can find additional information on each of these concerns. The following sections describe the various definitions linked with Nightingale's ideas of passion, intellect, and moral activity and provide a sketch of ways in which women actually have claimed places in society to exercise these three.

Passion: Feminism as a Culture Grounded in Women's Experience

Feminist writers, scholars, and activists indeed have entered the whole history of society and the present state of civilization. They have developed extensive cultural resources from which to change women's experience and from which to change the patriarchal tendencies of the dominant culture. Consistent with other social movements, a major concern has been to reclaim women's heritage in history, religion, the arts, and the emergence

TABLE 55-1

Definitions and Characteristics of Feminism

Definitions	Characteristics
A culture grounded in women's experience	• Reclaims women's heritage in history, religion, and culture • Reclaims women's personal and social power • Reclaims women's wisdom • Celebrates women as healers, artists, creators, and statespersons
A political stance to right injustices against women and the earth	• Acts on the premise that the personal is political • Connects gender socialization and women's roles with larger political issues, including restoring the ecology of the earth • Critiques the institutionalization of patriarchal norms • Seeks an end to private and public violence • Seeks balance of power in economic and political terms
A discipline seeking to give voice to women's experience	• Critiques patriarchal norms, practices, and theories • Relates the diverse experiences of women to social, political, philosophical, and scientific interests • Explores the dynamics by which women are silenced and ways to end the silence and invisibility of women • Explores women's health and development • Revises criteria of worth for scholarship and for what counts as knowledge about women
An ethic of valuing women and women's experience	• Critiques "malestream" morality and ethics • Develops ethics of caring and relationship • Reunites as one the public/private ethic • Redefines meanings of responsibility, truth, right, justice, good, and beauty

of civilization. Feminists have been persistent in asking, "Where were the women, and what were they doing?" in every period of known human history. Out of this question has come new appreciation of women as healers, artists, statespersons, creators, and inventors.

From knowledge of women's heritage, women have reclaimed women's personal power to create, to shape the values of the culture, and to bring women's wisdom to bear on the higher questions of society.

Passion: Feminism as a Political Stance to Right Injustices

No other perspective has remained so persistent and broad-based in its concern for righting injustices. Although women's well-being is a central focus, feminist insights link the rights and well-being of women with children, all people (particularly other oppressed groups), and the earth. Women's historical and current situation in the family and society are linked with far-reaching issues such as economics, agricultural, industrial production, war and other forms of social violence, ecological health, and prevailing patterns of

political violence. Feminist writers have shown how women's roles in the family and society are sustained by the larger political patterns and in turn sustain the nature of local, national, and global political patterns.

Feminist examination of political issues and creation of new theories of politics have given rise to new meanings for political concepts such as equality, justice, rights, peace, and diversity. For example, rather than merely accepting the prevailing notion that "equality" means "equal to white middle-class males," feminists seek carefully to construct meanings, criteria, and standards for "equality" that examines what is "good" for all. Out of these insights and commitment to bringing together the personal and the political, feminist activists have taken significant local, regional, national, and international stands.

Nurses and nursing have benefited particularly from feminist political activism that demanded equitable pay for women's work. For example, the landmark case of nurses in Denver who fought to be paid more than tree trimmers established the idea that work should be paid in accord with its educational and skill requirements, not in accord with the gender of the person who typically performs it.

Intellect: Feminism as a Discipline Seeking to Give Voice to Women's Experience

Feminism has developed as a discipline that seeks to give voice and understanding to women's experience. One focus is the plight of women in the patriarchy and the search to find ways for women to change their existence in the patriarchy, as well as ways to change the patriarchy or to create a different world order based on women's aspirations. Another aspect of feminism as a discipline is consideration of the biology-culture debate, addressing questions concerning the extent to which women's experience is shaped by biology and to what extent it is shaped by culture or experience.

Women's health and development is a large area of concern for feminist scholars. Feminists pose questions such as how women's health and development, particularly mental health and development, have been defined, distorted, created, or shaped by the patriarchy. Redefining what health is and what healthful development is for women is a major feminist enterprise. Redefinition does not occur in an ivory tower vacuum; rather, it happens in conjunction with experience, with practice, with action. An example of the redefinition of women's health and development is the work of the Boston Women's Health Book Collective, producers of many books for women about women's health.

Another important area of study for feminist scholars has been discovery of the ways in which women have been silenced, their work rendered invisible in society, and exploring of ways to change women's experience so that they know what it is to be valued, to be heard, to be strong and courageous, to act in the world. Related to explorations of women's silence has been work that is directed toward revising the criteria by which something is judged to be worthy of scholarly attention or worthy to count as knowledge. Feminist scholars have insisted that what concerns women cannot any longer be excluded as worthy of scholarly attention.

Moral Activity: Feminism as an Ethic of Valuing Women and Women's Experience

Feminist ethics is thought and action directed toward values that sustain life, well-being, peace, nurturing, and growth for all. Feminist ethics includes critique of "malestream" morality and ethics, particularly the prevailing patriarchal morality that differentiates standards of ethical behavior at home and in the workplace. Feminist ethics seeks to reunite as one the public and private ethic.

Explorations of the relationship between gender and moral development has led to a better understanding and valuing of women's experience, as well as valuing of the perspectives that tend to emerge when women's values are taken into account. Women tend to value relationships and perceive personal and social obligations in terms of relationships and the well-being of significant others. This perspective redefines what it means to be responsible, to act justly, or to know what is good or right.

Much of the tension that nurses experience in their work lives involves difficult ethical dilemmas for which there are no resolutions if only the traditional patriarchal perspectives of justice and worth are considered. This is largely because patriarchal ethics does not take into account that which most concerns nurses—the quality of relationships and the meaning of caring. As nurses embrace more fully perspectives of feminist ethics, it will be possible to embrace ethical sensibilities that more closely align with the fundamental values of nursing.

SUMMARY

Contrary to popular perception, feminism is not an ideology. Feminism embraces many ways of viewing the world that bring women, women's experiences and perspectives, into focus. Feminism embraces perspectives that value seeing clearly the diversity that exists among all women, not an attempt to define "woman." As you think about what I have presented and as you explore some of the suggested readings, ask yourself the following questions:

- In what ways do I value women? Who am I in relation to women?
- Do my views and values benefit women and in turn all people?
- What do I know about women and nurses in history? Are my assumptions about women and nurses in history accurate and well conceived?
- What do I know about the experience of women who are not like myself in economic status, culture, ethnic background, or belief?

REFERENCES

American heritage talking dictionary (Windows, Mac). (1994). Cambridge, MA: Softkey International.

Ashley, J. (1976). *Hospitals, paternalism, and the role of the nurse.* New York: Teachers College Press.

Ashley, J. (1980). Power in structured misogyny: Implications for the politics of care. *Advances in Nursing Science, 2*(3), 3-22.

Chinn, P. L. (1989). Nursing patterns of knowing and feminist thought. *Nursing Outlook, 10*(2), 71-75.

Chinn, P. L., & Wheeler, C. E. (1985). Feminism and nursing. *Nursing Outlook, 33*(2), 74-77.

Fry, S. T. (1992). The role of caring in a theory of nursing ethics. In H. B. Holmes & L. M. Purdy (Eds.), *Feminist perspectives in medical ethics.* Bloomington: Indiana University Press.

Gilligan, C. (1982). *In a different voice: Psychological theory and women's development.* Boston: Harvard University Press.

Greenleaf, N. P. (1980). Sex-segregated occupations: Relevance for nursing. *Advances in Nursing Science, 2*(3), 23-37.

Larrabee, M. J. (1993). *An ethic of care: Feminist and interdisciplinary perspectives.* New York: Routledge.

Morgan, R. (1968). *Going too far: The personal chronicle of a feminist.* New York: Vintage Books.

Nightingale, F. (1979). *Cassandra.* New York: The Feminist Press.

Noddings, N. (1984). *Caring: A feminine approach to ethics and moral education.* Berkeley: University of California Press.

Noddings, N. (1999). Care, justice, and equity. In M. S. Katz, N. Noddings, & K. A. Strike (Eds.), *Justice and caring: The search for common ground in education* (pp. 7-20). New York: Teachers College Press.

Redstockings, of the Women's Liberation Movement. (1975). *Feminist revolution: An abridged edition with additional writings.* New York: Random House.

Reverby, S. M. (1987). *Ordered to care: The dilemma of American nursing, 1850-1945.* New York: Cambridge University Press.

Young, S. (1997). *Changing the wor(l)d: Discourse, politics, and the feminist movement.* New York: Routledge.

SUGGESTED READINGS

Achterberg, J. (1991). *Woman as healer.* Boston: Shambhala.

Alcoff, L., & Potter, E. (1993). *Feminist epistemologies.* New York: Routledge.

Bunch, C. (1987). *Passionate politics: Feminist theory in action.* New York: St. Martin's Press.

Chinn, P. L. (2004). *Peace & power: Creative leadership for building communities* (6th ed.). Boston: Jones and Bartlett.

Daly, M., & Caputi, J. (1987). *Websters' first new intergalactic wickedary of the English language.* Boston: Beacon Press.

Edwalds, L., & Stocker, M. (Eds.). (1995). *The woman-centered economy: Ideals, reality, and the space in between.* Chicago: Third Side Press.

Freeman, J. (1995). *Women: A feminist perspective* (5th ed.). Mountain View, CA: Mayfield Publishing Co.

Freeman, S. J. M., Bourque, S. C., & Shelton, C. M. (Eds.). (2001). *Women on power: Leadership redefined.* Boston: Northeastern University Press.

Frye, M. (1983). *The politics of reality: Essays in feminist theory.* Freedom, CA: Crossing Press.

Hine, D. C. (1989). *Black women in white: Racial conflict and cooperation in the nursing profession, 1890-1950.* Bloomington: Indiana University Press.

Hooks, B. (2000). *Feminism is for everybody: Passionate politics.* Boston: South End Press.

Humm, M. (1995). *The dictionary of feminist theory* (2nd ed.). Columbus: Ohio State University Press.

Johnstone, M.-J. (1994). *Nursing and the injustices of the law.* Sydney: Harcourt Brace.

McCann, C. R., & Kim, S.-K. (2002). *Feminist theory reader: Local and global perspectives.* London: Routledge.

Mohanty, C. T. (2003). *Feminism without borders: Decolonizing theory, practicing solidarity.* Durham, NC: Duke University Press.

Noddings, N. (1989). *Women and evil.* Berkeley, CA: University of California Press.

O'Reilly, A. (2004). *From motherhood to mothering: The legacy of Adrienne Rich's Of woman born.* New York: State University of New York Press.

Rich, A. (1986). *Of woman born: motherhood as experience and institution* (10th anniversary ed.). New York: W.W. Norton.

Roberts, J. I., & Group, T. M. (1995). *Feminism and nursing: An historical perspective on power, status, and political activism in the nursing profession.* Westport, CT: Praeger.

Rowe-Finkbeiner, K. (2004). *The F-Word: Feminism in jeopardy—Women, politics and the future.* Emeryville, CA: Seal Press.

Spender, D. (1982). *Women of ideas and what men have done to them: From Aphra Behn to Adrienne Rich.* Boston: Routledge & Kegan Paul.

Tong, R. (1998). *Feminist thought: A more comprehensive introduction* (2nd ed.). Boulder, CO: Westview Press.

CHAPTER 56

Entering Collegial Relationships

The Demise of Nurse as Victim

ADELE W. PIKE • MERIDEAN L. MAAS

Scholars of women's development have observed uniqueness in women's ways of thinking, of knowing, of relating to others, and of being (Belensky, Clinchy, Goldberger, & Tarule, 1996; Gilligan, 1993; Miller, 1987). They refer to this uniqueness as "women's voice." Their metaphor of voice is borrowed here and applied to nurses. "Nurses' voice" thus refers to the unique perspectives and contributions that nurses bring to patient care. Disturbingly, this voice is often silent, and that silence is seriously demoralizing to nurses. For patients the consequences are more grievous because the silence denies them the integration of the nursing perspective into the care they receive.

The factors involved in silencing—in censoring—nurses affect the way nurses define their professional self-concept, often leading them to perceive themselves as helpless victims. Most of the factors are rooted in cultural and social mores that, despite being outdated and no longer applicable in present-day health care, are deeply etched in memory. Despite the persistence of their legend, the power of these traditions to silence nurses should be rendered invalid.

For this to occur, nurses must appreciate that they are presented with opportunities for choice: the choice to remain silent or to become essential colleagues in the health care team. This chapter presents an analysis of the factors that suppress nurses' voice and of the significance of the choice nurses make with regard to making their voices heard. In discussing the implications of this choice, critical incidents (Benner, 2001) depicting patients and families facing ethical dilemmas are used to contrast two divergent outcomes that result from the different ways in which nurses choose to exercise their voice.*

---

*The critical incidents published in this paper initially appeared in Pike (1991). The incidents were adapted and used with permission.

SILENCING OF VOICE

Numerous forces affect nurses' voice. Many of these forces are external, such as the historical role of nurse as handmaiden, the hierarchical structure of health care organizations, the perceived authority and directives of physicians, hospital policy, and the threat of disciplinary or legal action. Alarmingly, the restructuring of health care in this country has imposed additional and powerful constraints on nurses' voice. Changes in health care financing and reimbursement have led to reductions in staff and consequent work speedups, leaving nurses little time for reflection and discourse. Likewise, the current nurse shortage with nurses who care for large numbers of patients over long periods, often working extra shifts, results in feelings of job dissatisfaction, powerlessness, and apathy. Repeated health care "reform," mostly in hospitals, has led to the closing of nursing units, displacements of nurses, and layoffs (Aiken, Clarke, & Sloane, 2002; Pike & Alpert, 1994). The real threat of job loss, combined with the turmoil that accompanies downsizing of health care systems and institutions, quickly and insidiously can lure articulate professionals into the perceived safety of being but a cog in a bureaucratic wheel.

Equally ominous and plentiful are the internal forces that constrain nurses' voice. Characteristics such as role confusion, lack of professional confidence, timidity, fear, insecurity, or sense of inferiority lead nurses to *choose* silence as often as external forces impose silence on them (DeMarco, 2002; Pike, 1991; Yarling, & McElmurry, 1986).

These internal and external constraints inflict wounds on nurses' professional self-esteem. The wounds deepen and expand the innate capacity for self-doubt that nurses, like all individuals, have. Having been wounded, nurses experience great difficulty believing in their own capacity, ability, and right to contribute to patient care as vital and essential professionals. Their ambitions and aspirations are stifled. Their vision grows myopic, and they fail to recognize their opportunities and their obligation for self-advancement. Such an inclination establishes a pattern in which nurses perceive themselves as inferior and unable to change their lot (Belensky et al., 1996; Steele, 1991).

This poor professional self-concept sabotages any possibility of collaboration between nurses and other care providers because it identifies nurses as embattled victims and customarily marks physicians as their antagonists. Such a relationship urges an adversarial stance in which the victims place the onus of responsibility for the problematic relationship on their perceived aggressors rather than accepting responsibility and accountability for who they are and what they want to be (Steele, 1991).

The stance of victimization is seductive; and there are many incentives for maintaining this role. Victims are perceived as innocent, and by assigning the locus of their control to external forces, they avoid responsibility and accountability. Victims are spared the stress of change, because in the matrix of victimization, it is the oppressor who must change in order for the victim's condition to improve (Cooper, 1991; Steele, 1991).

There can be no argument that in the past nurses were the victims of oppression and were made to suffer the subjugation of physicians and hospital administrators. They had little choice but to be exploited as conveniences, as loyal and obedient servants. Today, nurses must grapple with the memory of this exploitation but also with the real threat that continues in the current crisis in health care economics to drive back the gains, yet insufficient, that have been made in countering role subservience. It will take tremendous courage and strength of professional character for nurses to maintain and further the success that advances in nursing practice, education, research, and administration have made toward unraveling the traditional socialization of health care providers and culture of health care organizations. Nurses are thus faced with a critical choice: to consider themselves helpless victims of past injustice and present-day economic threats or to define themselves as full-fledged and essential members of the health care team (McCloskey & Maas, 1998; Pike & Alpert, 1994).

The choice is not easy, given the unconscious incentives to remain victims (Cooper, 1991; Haggerty & Goodman, 2003). Defining oneself as an equal professional means being responsible and accountable, which are stressful, difficult, and frightening burdens. The definition obligates nurses to exercise their voice; to articulate their unique knowledge of patients and their responses to illness; and to participate with other health care professionals as colleagues rather than as subordinates (McCloskey & Maas, 1998). It means overcoming self-doubt and timidity and resisting the forces that threaten to corrupt nurses' obligations to patients. Overcoming the internal and external constraints that inhibit the voice, the aspirations, and talents of nurses requires relentless effort. Although the choice to exercise nurses' voice is risky, the choice to remain silent is an unacceptable alternative (Pike & Alpert, 1994).

BEING A COLLEAGUE

Part of the difficulty for nurses in defining themselves as colleagues of other health care professionals is that so little is known about how best to operationalize the role (Alpert, Goldman, Kilroy, & Pike, 1992; Petro, 1992; Prescott & Bowen, 1985; Stein, 1967; Stein, Watts, & Howell, 1990). Colleagueship involves entering into a collaborative relationship that is characterized by mutual trust and respect and an understanding of the perspective each partner contributes (McCloskey & Maas, 1998). Collaboration involves a bond, a union, a depth of caring about one another and about the relationship. The colleagueship this bond breeds obliges individuals to put aside their feelings of interprofessional competition and antagonism that are rooted in history so that the work and expertise of all participants may be integrated and patient care maximized (Alpert et al., 1992; Aradine & Pridham, 1973; Pike, 1991; Pontius, 2002; Weiss & Davis, 1985).

Colleagues openly acknowledge that they share a common goal—the health and comfort of patients in their care. They recognize their interdependence and, accordingly, share responsibility and accountability for patient outcomes. Collegial relationships are safe. Each participant accepts the other as someone who is well-intentioned and trying to do his or her best. When conflict arises, colleagues address it at its source and do not push it up a hierarchical chain of authority (Alpert et al., 1992; Mangiardi & Pellegrino, 1992; Pike, et al., 1993).

Colleagueship has many characteristics of a caring relationship, as defined by the ethic of care. It dispenses with hierarchical habits of relating, replacing dominance and rank with mutual respect and shared decision making. As colleagues, individuals attend to each other's growth and development, protect each other from belittlement, and enhance each other's professional dignity

VIEWPOINTS

(Daiski, 2004; Gadow, 2004; Mayeroff, 1990; Noddings, 2003; Watson, 1999).

Incorporating the concept of colleague into one's professional identity is a developmental process that requires critical self-reflection. To collaborate with others, a nurse must understand and value the unique perspective that nursing offers. Being a colleague requires a breadth of clinical experience that solidifies professional confidence. Nurses who define themselves as colleagues must develop a language that allows them to articulate their unique perspective to nonnurses so that they will be understood (Maas & Delaney, 2004; McCloskey & Maas, 1998). This definition of professional self also requires the maturity to recognize the incentives to remain victimized and to reflect on how one might be seduced by these incentives. Additionally, one must understand the historical and cultural roots to the internal and external constraints imposed on nurses and appreciate that their influence quickly can subjugate nurses at a time when patients can ill afford a silencing of nurses' unique perspectives. Nurses who choose to define themselves as colleagues must overcome these constraints and learn to manage their backward pull.

Operationalizing the concept of professional self as equal colleague frees nurses from the internal constraints that contribute to the silencing of their voice. Once the influence of these internal forces is curtailed, nurses can question, challenge, and overcome external constraints. Colleagueship is difficult work fraught with anxiety, confusion, and frustration; but it is also a fruitful enterprise offering tremendous promise and benefits to nurses and patients (Pike, 1991).

CONSEQUENCES OF CHOICE

The way in which nurses choose to construe their professional selves has significant implications for patient care and nurses' role and satisfaction. The consequences of their choice are particularly dramatic in the care of patients and families in the throes of ethical uncertainty. Consider the following critical incident involving Mr. S. This incident describes a dilemma not unfamiliar to nurses, and it leaves powerful images of morally unacceptable care.

Mr. S. was a 72-year-old man admitted to the hospital from a nursing home as a result of his failure to thrive and a severe infection. On admission he was frail, cachectic, and minimally responsive. He had a temperature of 101.8° F, heart rate 160 beats per minute in atrial fibrillation, respiratory rate of 28 breaths per minute, and an unstable blood pressure. His blood tests suggested severe dehydration.

Mr. S.'s peripheral veins were small and fragile, and repeated attempts to start an intravenous line in his arms were unsuccessful. A line was finally established in his foot, and intravenous fluids and antibiotics were administered.

Long before his admission, Mr. S. had made it known that he did not want "heroic measures" taken to prolong his life in the event of a grave illness. It was documented and well known that "do not resuscitate" applied in his case.

Physicians were unable to determine the source of his infection. Even gentle attempts to provide hydration exacerbated his congestive heart failure and atrial fibrillation. His kidneys failed, and his lungs, damaged by years of smoking, were barely able to meet the increased demands of his illness. It seemed clear that Mr. S. was dying. His nurses worked to minimize any pain or distress he might suffer during his terminal illness.

On his fourth hospital day, Mr. S.'s intravenous line infiltrated and another peripheral line could not be placed. On the following day, the physicians involved in Mr. S.'s care felt obliged to establish a central intravenous line, since in the absence of peripheral access, Mr. S. was not receiving any fluid or antibiotics. At the time, no one openly questioned this decision, despite the fact that his nurses considered such an invasive, aggressive intervention to be wrong in the context of Mr. S.'s illness and wishes.

During the central line insertion, Mr. S. suffered a pneumothorax, and an emergency chest tube was inserted. At this point, he exhibited notable signs of pain and discomfort, which had been absent during the earlier days of his admission.

Mr. S.'s family was called, and they were distressed that invasive interventions had been carried out. They requested that no further aggressive treatment be used in his care.

Mr. S. was given oxygen and morphine for comfort. He died less than 2 days later but continued to show signs of respiratory distress throughout this period.

The nursing staff agonized over the pain and suffering he experienced. They began to place blame and among themselves, spoke of the callousness, aggressiveness, and insensitivity of physicians … of their ability "only to cure, not to care." The nurses felt anger, frustration, pain, remorse, and guilt.

The story of Mr. S. is one of moral failure and moral outrage that resulted in large measure from the silencing of nurses' voice. Mr. S.'s nurses encountered a moral dilemma while they cared for him about whether to place a central venous access line and continue hydration or forgo the line and allow him to die. Faced with this dilemma, the nurses reasoned that Mr. S. was at the end of his life and wanted to prevent his pain and suffering.

Mr. S.'s physicians, faced with the same dilemma, reached a different decision. Tragically, there was no discourse, and the authority and directives of the physicians took precedence over the nurses' plan. The physicians' actions were seen as unquestionable, and this perception served as a constraint to the nurses who had legitimate concerns about Mr. S.'s suffering. The physicians' response—and the nurses' willingness to subjugate their own moral reasoning—effectively censored the nursing perspective.

It is true that the physicians acted in an authoritative manner and never solicited nursing advice, but they had accomplices in this censorship. The nurses caring for Mr. S. chose to be silent: "No one openly questioned this decision." The words used by the nurse reporting this incident suggest that she and her peers were disturbed, even horrified, by the physicians' decision. Yet no nurse spoke up.

The nurses responded to their silencing with moral outrage. An emotional response to the inability to carry out moral choices or decisions, moral outrage is characterized by demoralizing frustration, anger, disgust, and a sense of powerlessness (Noddings, 2003; Pike, 1991). The nurses were furious about the moral failure of Mr. S.'s care, yet they only blamed the physicians, failing to recognize their own contribution to this tragedy. Had any one of Mr. S.'s nurses defined herself as a colleague, instead of a helpless victim, a nurse's voice would have been heard, moral outrage would have been averted, and moral discourse would have ensued. In the end, Mr. S. most likely would have received more morally appropriate care.

In contrast, the following case illustrates the morally acceptable care that resulted from a nurse's choice to see herself as an integral and full-fledged colleague of physicians.

Mrs. H. had been a healthy, active 65-year-old woman until she suffered massive intracranial bleeding. She showed severe neurological impairment, with only occasional and minimal responses to noxious stimuli. The prognosis for neurological recovery was grim. Mrs. H. had prepared a handwritten statement 2 years earlier, at the time of her husband's death from cancer. It was a request that her life not be sustained in the event of an irreversible illness or injury. A photocopy of this statement was placed in her chart and all physician and nurse staff were informed of the statement.

Mrs. H.'s children, however, expressed their desire to pursue every treatment possible. They were adamant that they wanted their mother resuscitated in the event of a cardiac arrest. Mrs. H.'s physician felt obliged to comply with her children's wishes. The nurse understood and respected his feeling of obligation but found it morally conflicting, as most likely the physician did also.

Mrs. H. was deteriorating daily. Aggressive, invasive care continued. The nurse had to leave the room more than once during invasive procedures due to the assaultive nature of the treatments. She saw them [as being] clearly in opposition to Mrs. H.'s wishes.

The nurse spoke with her children and her physician each day. Although she could see and appreciate the agony they were experiencing in light of the massive ethical issues facing them, it

was as if they were all speaking in different dialects of the same language. A three-way conversation to help all parties understand the perspectives of each person was needed.

The nurse arranged a conference during which she, the patient's family, and [the] physician reviewed Mrs. H.'s condition and prognosis, and elaborated care plan options. Her family spoke of their grief and their feelings that they would be abandoning their mother if invasive treatments were discontinued. The physician and nurse explained that their mother would never be abandoned. We discussed how we could provide care for her in accordance with her wishes, and what the specifics of that care would be. In the end, Mrs. H.'s family decided to change the aim of care and keep her comfortable until she died.

This is a difficult and poignant story. There was clearly a dilemma and clearly conflict. At an earlier point in her professional development, Mrs. H.'s nurse might have taken on the role of helpless victim and remained silent. The conflict would have simmered and bred moral outrage. Instead this nurse chose to see herself as a colleague who had the right, the duty, and the ability to facilitate discourse among all involved parties. In doing so, she not only avoided her own moral distress but also transformed the meaning of the situation from conflict to miscommunication. Her actions prompted a discussion that allowed all perspectives to be integrated into Mrs. H.'s care. Her exercise of nurses' voice changed the nature of the care for this patient, making it more consistent with the patient's wishes and more comfortable for her family.

SUMMARY

These critical incidents strongly suggest that the choice a nurse makes about how she defines her professional self affects not only her moral nature but also the nature of care her patients receive. When a nurse identifies herself as the victim of deeply rooted social and economic constraints, she increases the probability that her voice will be silenced. The stance of victimization can lead to feelings of moral outrage and denies patients the benefits of the nursing perspective. However, when a nurse makes the choice to define herself as a professional and a colleague, participating in patient care as an integral member of the health care team, she seizes opportunities for professional fulfillment while affording patients the benefits of integrated care.

The responsibility and accountability for defining oneself as a professional colleague resides in individual nurses. Perhaps it does not seem fair that nurses, because they have inherited internal and external constraints to their professional identity, autonomy, and aspirations, now have to rescue themselves from subjugation. Perhaps it would seem fairer if those whose predecessors exploited nurses made concessions. Fairness aside, history shows that members of dominant groups generally do not offer restitution to those whom they have exploited (Steele, 1991). Although growing numbers of physicians are to be commended for enlightened attitudes and behaviors, nurses will only grow increasingly frustrated waiting for past injustices to be repaid.

Although the issue of fairness will always linger, it is, ironically, fortunate that compensation is not forthcoming. For the possibility of compensation keeps the responsibility for collegiality with physicians and leads to the familiar slogan among nurses, "We're ready to be colleagues just as soon as the doctors change." Making colleagueship depend on changes among physicians maintains nurses as victims; it asks nonnurses to exercise nurses' voice. The only one who can declare herself or himself an essential colleague is the individual nurse, and to do so the nurse must emancipate herself or himself from internal and external constraints.

Nurses' choice to define themselves as colleagues, as full-fledged vital members of the health care team, holds great moral significance for nursing and for patient care. In making this choice, nurses take the opportunity to overcome subjugation and to assume a stance of empowerment. By defining themselves as colleagues, nurses initiate a move on their own behalf and on behalf of their patients to make their voice heard (Cooper, 1991; Falk-Rafael, 2001). Such a professional self-concept is a prerequisite for and a driving force in the development of collaborative relationships with physicians, health care administrators, and in this era of managed care, even third-party payers. Collaboration unifies the contributions of all involved in patient care, making that care more efficient, effective, and comprehensive (Aiken, 1990; Knaus, Draper, Wagner, & Zimmerman, 1986; Pike, 1991; Prescott & Bowen, 1985; Zwarenstein & Reeves, 2002). By choosing to make their voice heard, nurses afford patients not only the advantage of the nursing perspective but also the full benefit of integrated care (Bishop, 2002). The promise this holds for advancing the care delivered to patients and families cannot be underestimated.

REFERENCES

Aiken, L. H. (1990). Charting the future of hospital nursing. *Image: The Journal of Nursing Scholarship, 22*(2), 72-78.

Aiken, L. H., Clarke, S. P., & Sloane, D. M. (2002). Hospital staffing, organization, and quality of care: Cross-national findings. *Nursing Outlook, 50,* 187-194.

Alpert, H. B., Goldman, L. D., Kilroy, C. M., & Pike, A. W. (1992). 7 Gryzmish: Toward an understanding of collaboration. *Nursing Clinics of North America, 27*(1), 47-59.

Aradine, C. R., & Pridham, K. F. (1973). Model for collaboration. *Nursing Outlook, 21*(10), 655-657.

Belensky, M. F., Clinchy, B. M., Goldberger, N. R., & Tarule, J. M. (1996). *Women's ways of knowing: The development of self, voice, and mind.* New York: Basic Books.

Benner, P. (2001). *From novice to expert: Excellence and power in clinical nursing practice.* Menlo Park, CA: Addison-Wesley.

Bishop, V. (2002). Editorial. *NT Research, 7*(6), 400.

Cooper, M. C. (1991). Response to moral outrage and moral discourse in nurse-physician collaboration. *Journal of Professional Nursing, 7*(6), 362-363.

Daiski, I. (2004). Changing nurses' dis-empowering relationship patterns. *Journal of Advanced Nursing, 48*(1), 43-50.

DeMarco, R. (2002). Two theories/a sharper lens: The staff nurse voice in the workplace. *Journal of Advanced Nursing, 38*(6), 549-554.

Falk-Rafael, A. (2001). Empowerment as a process of evolving consciousness: A model of empowered caring. *Advances in Nursing Science, 24*(1), 1-16.

Gadow, S. A. (2004). Nurse and patient: The caring relationship. In A. H. Bishop & J. R. Scudder (Eds.), *Caring, curing, coping: Nurse-physician-patient relationships* (pp. 31-43). Tuscaloosa: University of Alabama Press.

Gilligan, C. (1993). *In a different voice.* Cambridge, MA: Harvard University Press.

Haggerty, L. A., & Goodman, L. A. (2003). Stages of change-based nursing interventions for victims of interpersonal violence. *Journal of Obstetric, Gynecologic, and Neonatal Nursing, 32,* 68-75.

Knaus, W. A., Draper, E. A., Wagner, D. P., & Zimmerman, J. E. (1986). An evaluation of outcome from intensive care in major medical centers. *Annals of Internal Medicine, 104*(3), 410-418.

Maas, M., & Delaney, C. (2004). Nursing process outcome linkages: An assessment of literature and issues. *Medical Care, 42*(2), II-40–II-48.

Mangiardi, J. R., & Pellegrino, E. D. (1992). Collegiality: What is it? *Bulletin of the New York Academy of Medicine, 68*(2), 292-296.

Mayeroff, M. (1990). *On caring.* New York: Harper Collins.

McCloskey, J. C., & Maas, M. (1998). Interdisciplinary team: The nursing perspective is essential. *Nursing Outlook, 46*(4), 157-163.

Miller, J. B. (1987). *Toward a new psychology for women.* Boston, MA: Beacon Press.

Noddings, N. (2003). *Caring: A feminine approach to ethics and moral education* (2nd ed.). Los Angeles: University of California Press.

Petro, J. A. (1992). Collegiality in history. *Bulletin of the New York Academy of Medicine, 68*(2), 292-296.

Pike, A. W. (1991). Moral outrage and moral discourse in nurse-physician collaboration. *Journal of Professional Nursing, 7*(6), 351-363.

Pike, A. W., & Alpert, H. B. (1994). Pioneering the future: The 7 North model of nurse-physician collaboration. *Nursing Administration Quarterly, 18*(4), 11-18.

Pike, A. W., McHugh, M., Canney, K., Miller, N., Reilly, P., & Seibert, C. P. (1993). A new architecture for quality assurance: Nurse-physician collaboration. *Journal of Nursing Care Quality, 7*(3), 1-8.

Pontius, J. M. (2002). On being a colleague. *Journal of the Oklahoma State Medical Association, 95*(4), 239.

Prescott, P. A., & Bowen, S. A. (1985). Physician-nurse relationships. *Annals of Internal Medicine, 103*(127), 127-133.

Steele, S. (1991). *The content of our character.* New York: St. Martin's Press.

Stein, L. I. (1967). The doctor-nurse game. *Archives of General Psychiatry, 16*(6), 699-703.

Stein, L. I., Watts, D. T., & Howell, T. (1990). The doctor-nurse game revisited. *New England Journal of Medicine, 322*(8), 546-549.

Watson, J. (1999). *Nursing: Human science and human care.* New York: National League for Nursing.

Weiss, S. J., & Davis, H. P. (1985). Validity and reliability of the collaborative practice scales. *Nursing Research, 34*(5), 99-305.

Yarling, R. R., & McElmurry, B. J. (1986). The moral foundation of nursing. *Advances in Nursing Science, 8*(2), 63-73.

Zwarenstein, M., & Reeves, S. (2002). Working together but apart: Barriers and routes to nurse physician collaboration. *Journal of Quality Improvement, 28*(5), 233-234.

Health Professions Education in Community-Based Settings

A Collaborative Journey

JOELLEN B. EDWARDS • SUSAN GROVER • JOY E. WACHS

The delivery of health care in the United States has undergone unprecedented change in recent years. Increasingly, the U.S. "system" of health care delivery is recognized as not being a system at all; rather, uncoordinated sectors of care delivery operate within narrow spans of interest and expertise. Little communication occurs among professional disciplines caring for the same clients or among professionals practicing in various levels of care delivery such as acute care, home care, primary care, and long-term care (Greiner & Knebel, 2003). Systematized interdisciplinary care is not readily available to persons coping with chronic illness in community settings. Even in acute care hospitals where health professionals from many disciplines practice daily, lack of interdisciplinary communication can lead to mistakes that can inconvenience or harm clients (Kohn, Corrigan, & Donaldson, 2000). An unacceptably high number of medical errors and the resultant dire consequences to individuals are a call to health professionals to improve quality, accountability, and effectiveness in health care processes. A key factor in the nation's potential for success in transforming health care delivery processes into a safer, more cohesive and seamless system is the ability of health care professionals to collaborate in interdisciplinary teams and across health care delivery settings (Institute of Medicine, 2001). This concept, so simple in vision yet so difficult to achieve, is one that must be operationalized if safe, effective care is to be achieved.

The purposes of this chapter are to explore collaboration within the context of health professions education and to describe the evolution of long-term collaborative relationships at East Tennessee State University among health professions faculty and students and with regional communities. East Tennessee State University

is a doctoral/research-intensive regional institution with a specific mission to educate health professionals. East Tennessee State University is one institution that has attempted to improve collaborative skills through the education of its health professions students in community-based settings and in interdisciplinary learning activities.

NURSING AND MEDICAL EDUCATION

The evolution of education in nursing and medicine—the health professions disciplines that contribute most directly to client care—has a profound impact on the ability of all health professionals to collaborate effectively. Nursing and medicine arose from the tradition of caring for the health and illness needs of people, but as the disciplines became formally recognized, distinct differences in their educational patterns and patient care roles became institutionalized. Early in the twentieth century, the medical profession organized schools at the graduate level in university settings, creating a single path to the legal right to practice medicine. Nursing remained closely aligned with service and gender-based subservience in hospital training schools. Thus autonomy and societal acceptance of medicine as a profession was established readily, whereas recognition of nursing as a profession was stifled. As medical schools developed, they fostered the professional autonomy and the idea that the physician was the sole decision maker and ultimate authority in all client care, an idea that continues to compromise client safety and the multidisciplinary practice environment today. Nursing schools, however, fostered subservience to physicians that paralleled women's gender role expectations, a historical occurrence that still shadows the profession (Group & Roberts, 2004).

Nursing and medicine maintain different philosophical approaches to the education of students and to their professional practice. Although changes are beginning to occur, medicine has been found to value content, rationality, data, and assimilation of scientific information in the educational strategy over attention to the social and relational aspects of health care (Bloom, 1988; Greenlick, 1992). Nursing, however, has been shown to value and teach a more holistic and relational approach to care for well and ill persons (Linderman, 1995). These values are transmitted to and reinforced continually in students through educational processes.

One similarity between nursing and medical education is that for many years the focus of educational experiences for groups has been centered in hospitals. Hospital care has made significant contributions to the preservation of human life and offers unparalleled opportunity for health professions students to care for acutely ill patients with highly complex conditions. Yet today's students also must gain the competencies needed to prevent illness, promote health, provide primary care, address environmental issues, and help individuals and families cope with the effects of chronic illness in their own life setting. Health professions students need the opportunity to find their place outside hospital walls as participants and leaders in improving the health of the community. Community-based interdisciplinary approaches to learning can make a significant difference in graduates' expectations for practice.

COMMUNITY-BASED EDUCATION AND PRACTICE

Community-based education and practice tends to be perceived and defined differently by medicine and nursing, with each perception consistent with the implicit and explicit values of the profession. Nurses tend to view "community-based" as the incorporation of the entire community—homes, schools, homeless shelters, stores, day care centers, public housing units, primary care practices and others—into the education of nursing students and as sites for professional practice (Edwards & Alley, 2002). Medicine, outside the community-oriented primary care movement (Nutting, Wood, & Conner, 1985) more often views "community-based" as the incorporation of precepted primary care experiences into the medical school or residency curriculum, and community-based practice as a physician enterprise outside the acute care setting.

However, if the voice of national health care policy leaders is heard, community-based education and practice will become more than the site of clinical learning. Community-based education will become a method for shifting power from institutions and professionals to a shared relationship with communities and clients that will create a system of safe, effective, and culturally appropriate health care. People in communities, in partnership with health care professionals, will define the health needs to be met and maintain control of the strategies for meeting those needs. This hoped-for pattern is in direct opposition to the current system of education and practice, in which health care organizations and expert professionals decide what the community needs and maintain control of the services offered.

If students are to emerge from health professions education programs ready to participate fully in a delivery system that meets the health needs of the populations, significant changes in the approach to medical, nursing, and allied health education need to be made. True collaboration among the disciplines and health professionals with their communities will be the key to success.

COLLABORATION

To meet the diverse and complex health care needs of communities, the entire health care team must work in concert with clients, families, and community groups to identify appropriate processes to reach the health-related goals set by all the participants. No one profession can dictate the priority need and essential intervention or ignore the input of the individual or community receiving care. Rather, respectful, trusting relationships among health care professionals and clients must be established to generate the multifaceted, effective solutions to health problems that challenge communities today. Effective collaboration is essential to meet the health needs of the community. Sullivan (1998) describes collaboration as "a dynamic, transforming process of creating a power sharing partnership for pervasive application in health care practice, education, research and organizational settings for the purposeful attention to needs and problems in order to achieve likely successful outcomes" (p. 6).

Collaboration can involve two individuals, an individual and a group of people, or two groups of people. In health care a collaborative relationship might evolve between a nurse and a physical therapist in a home health care agency, a public health nurse and the members of the hospital medical staff, or the emergency department staff and the community rescue squad. The key to collaboration is the flat, rather than hierarchical, structure of mutual respect and shared power needed to take a bird's-eye view of situations, identify priority needs, and develop a comprehensive response.

Collaboration Between Medicine and Nursing

The diverse perspectives of medicine and nursing exemplify the opportunities and challenges of collaboration in today's health care settings. Modern medicine has been male-dominated and focused on cure, treatment, and technology. Modern nursing has been female-dominated and focused on care, comfort, and relationships. It would seem that these two disciplines would fit together perfectly, and yet the professional dyad has experienced conflict that is not overcome easily.

Power relationships between the two disciplines have proved a significant barrier to true collaboration because the clear balance of traditional societal, economic, and professional power lies with the physician (Group & Roberts, 2004). These historical patterns of interaction must be replaced with collaborative and team-oriented approaches so that the expertise and knowledge of all professions are equally available to patients and so that coordination of care for the improvement of patient safety can occur effectively (Greiner & Knebel, 2003). Health professions educators and practitioners increasingly recognize that collaboration between medicine and nursing is not only advisable but critical to the quality and safety of health care in the nation.

Collaboration Among Health Professionals and the Community

Relationships between community members and health professionals also can be challenging. Health professionals maintain their own language that sometimes excludes those who do not understand the terminology. Professional jargon or conversely, colloquial terminology, can lead to misinterpretation among potential collaborators. The perceived power of health professionals over community members is real and can disrupt the opportunity for true collaboration. Health professionals and community members often have differing values, beliefs, and priorities. Difficulty in valuing and appreciating the contributions of community members and professionals can arise. Collaboration with community, like collaboration among professionals, is a shared process.

Health professionals can begin the collaborative sharing process by becoming part of the community process rather than being in control of community health–related decisions. Through the experience of interdisciplinary community-based teaching and learning in rural Appalachian communities, Wachs, Goodrow, and Olive (1998) retrospectively identified four stages of the collaborative process.

When the program started, university representatives began meeting with community members and deciding on community interventions. Faculty and students, at their best, worked "for" the community and, at their worst, "did to" the community. This stage was analogous to the parallel play of toddlers; the community and the university worked on similar goals, sometimes in the same space, but not together as one entity. Health fairs planned by students and presented "to" the community are an example of this stage.

As the program matured, faculty and students began to work "with" community members. In this stage, university personnel began to see the strengths of the community members and their ability to take care of themselves, given the resources. When students realized the desires and needs of the community, they were able to use their creativity to develop innovative approaches to meet community needs. For instance, health programs were presented in schools based on topics requested by teachers and administrators.

After several years and a constant commitment to the community, faculty and students "became part of" the community, volunteering, assuming leadership positions, and becoming a focal point for social justice and community change. Slowly, the university voices became integrated with and were overshadowed by community voices. Community members began to realize their own power. Collaborations emerged that strengthened the relationships among community members, students, and faculty and yielded positive results that could not have occurred otherwise. For example, primary care and behavioral health services were integrated in a rural health clinic owned by the College of Nursing, and a community member was hired by the university to improve the behavioral health care system through grassroots organizing.

Actions such as these moved the collaborative process to the stage of "empowerment," where the community now takes steps to meet its own needs in ways that reach far beyond what was ever conceived by the health professions faculty and students. The community believes that anything worthwhile can be accomplished, given commitment, time, resources, and collaborative partners. For instance, the community has partnered with the Tennessee National Guard to establish a local organization aimed at reducing the impact of drugs and alcohol on this rural county; and a few committed citizens were able to open and maintain a halfway house for paroled women and a drop-in center for residents with chronic behavioral health concerns.

STRATEGIES TO ENHANCE COLLABORATION

Collaboration takes time, energy, and commitment. Collaboration is best when the parties involved come from a variety of diverse perspectives. However, the strength of diversity also creates challenges. Diverse individuals and groups see the world from a variety of perspectives and may have difficulty setting aside their own views to appreciate the perspectives of others. To improve the potential for successful collaboration to occur, health professionals must develop new and more complex skills including collaborative problem solving and decision making, conflict management, and teamwork.

Collaborative Problem Solving and Decision Making

One foundational approach to improving collaborative problem-solving and decision-making skills is the concept of emotional intelligence. *Emotional intelligence* is understood best as how individuals "handle themselves and their relationships" (Goleman, Boyatzis, & McKee, 2002, p. 6). Individuals with high levels of emotional intelligence effectively manage themselves and their emotions. They know their strengths and limitations, are positive about their own abilities, and can identify how they are feeling and the impact of those emotions on themselves and others. Because they know themselves so well, they can control the impact of their emotions and be transparent, adaptable, and optimistic. They are the persons who take the initiative to move a project forward and reach the agreed-upon goal and are able to form teams and manage conflict (Goleman et al., 2002). Emotionally intelligent individuals also possess social competence and are able to display empathy in terms of individuals and organizations. They are the servant leaders first described by Greenleaf (1996). Emotional intelligence fosters collaboration through positive communication and expression of mutual concern.

The concept of emotional intelligence as a basis for problem solving and decision making has been used in interdisciplinary faculty development within the community-based learning initiatives and as new groups of students struggle to establish productive and respectful relationships with each other and with community members. The concept of emotional intelligence is used by some faculty as a guide to the self-awareness and other awareness that increases the potential for collaboration.

Conflict Management

Conflicts are inevitable among groups of people. Effective collaboration requires that conflicts be managed in a positive, productive way. *Principled negotiation,* as described by Fisher and Ury (1981), is a method to manage conflict by deciding issues on their merits rather than through bargaining over positions. Negotiators look for mutual gains, but when interests conflict, negotiators insist on basing the outcome on fair standards rather than the will of either side. Principled negotiation should be efficient, produce a wise agreement, and improve the relationship between the two sides. For the process to be effective, negotiators must "separate the people from the problem, focus on issues rather than positions, invent options for mutual gain, and insist on using objective criteria" (p. 15). If an agreement cannot be reached, negotiators select the best alternative, which is usually better for one side than the other and may result in another negotiation effort to move the group further toward a mutual goal.

Conflict at the beginning of the East Tennessee State University community-based interdisciplinary efforts was high and required much trial and error in learning to manage disagreements. As in every academic endeavor, conflicts continue to arise over course content, schedules, projects, and personalities. As faculty, students, and community members enter and exit the program, the collaborators strive to stay focused on their vision of community-based interdisciplinary education and to remain principled in their negotiation of conflict.

Teamwork

Teamwork is another part of the collaborative process that assists participants in understanding different perspectives and strengthens relationships. A successful team requires a shared vision of the future with resulting performance goals, committed team members, wise leadership, adequate resources, effective communication, and a motivating environment (Wachs, in press; LaFasto & Larson, 2001; Mattessich, Murray-Close, & Monsey, 2001). A successful team cannot be created in one meeting but rather takes time to evolve. During this time, team members must understand fully their purpose and the team goal, as well as learn to trust each other and the team leader.

In the East Tennessee State University collaborative health professions education initiatives, team building has been fostered consciously. Faculty development, planning retreats, external facilitators, student orientation to the communities, and classroom activities have been used to strengthen team relationships. An interdisciplinary curriculum committee brings team members together regularly to monitor courses and student outcomes, plan future initiatives, and connect the interdisciplinary activities directly to established curriculum structures within the university. Team-building experiences such as problem solving, fine arts, and adventure leadership activities have been used in various parts of the program. Numerous resources include books, equipment, and vendors to assist in the work of team building that ultimately will affect the effectiveness of collaboration (Wachs, in press). Like management of conflict, team building must receive continuous attention as faculty, students, and community members change.

LONG-TERM COLLABORATION AMONG HEALTH PROFESSIONS FACULTY, STUDENTS, AND COMMUNITIES: AN EVOLUTION

The East Tennessee State University collaborative journey began in 1990 when the Colleges of Nursing and Medicine were approached by business and governmental leaders from a rural county for assistance in rebuilding their shattered health care system. This beginning partnership led to the award of three W.K. Kellogg Foundation grants between 1991 and 1998, all aimed at integrating university and community and improving the lives and health of people of the region. These early efforts provided the basis for a 15-year interdisciplinary community-based health professions education effort that has evolved constantly over the years and is guided by a governance structure that includes representatives from all involved disciplines and from partner communities (Behringer, Bishop, Edwards, & Franks, 1999).

In this continuing educational effort, selected medical, nursing, and public health students share specific learning experiences carried out in long- or short-term partnerships with communities in the region. Faculty members teach and practice in partner communities and are deeply involved in activities that contribute to the community and create learning opportunities for students. Community members identify health-related issues and participate in the curricular process.

Together, the collaborators have made a significant impact on two rural Appalachian communities, the health professions colleges, and the university itself. Box 57-1 provides a time line of the activities of the interdisciplinary community-based effort.

Undergraduate Health Professions Education

In 1991 the goal of the effort was to educate multidisciplinary health professions students in rural primary care settings and communities. The goal was founded in the belief that students who studied and practiced together in communities would be more likely to value the contributions of all professions to patient care and would choose to locate their practices in underserved communities. Undergraduate medical, nursing, and public and allied health students entered the program and stayed together as a cohort for six semesters. As they studied and practiced in partner communities over time, they were expected to collaborate with each other and with community members. As a result of this working relationship, students have helped promote health in partner communities (Goodrow et al., 2001).

A recent study of the outcomes of early graduates confirmed the value of this collaborative educational program. The findings of the 10-year cohort follow-up study demonstrated that graduates of the program had significantly greater interest in rural practice, primary care, community health, providing care for the underserved, and interdisciplinary group collaboration compared with traditional students. In a comparison of "partnership" students' and traditional students' employment location, there was a statistically significant difference ($x2 = 4.397$; $p < .05$) with more partnership students currently working in a rural setting. Work in primary care or community health was significantly more important ($x2 = 10.459$; $p < .01$) to community partnership students compared with traditional students (Florence, Goodrow, Wachs, Grover, & Olive, 2004). These outcomes reflect the successful achievement of objectives in the original iteration of the interdisciplinary community-based health professions program.

These successes spurred the development and approval of an interdisciplinary collaborative course in health communication. Beginning medical and bachelor's-level nursing and public health students are required to take a course together in small interactive groups in which they practice communication skills among the disciplines and with standardized clients. Communication is approached as a skill, and an emphasis is placed on developing quality relationships

BOX 57-1

Major Events in Collaboration, 1990-2005

1990	• Community requests collaboration
	• Primary care clinics established in rural community
1991	• Community-university formal governance structure established
	• W.K. Kellogg Foundation grant, "Community Partnerships for Health Professions Education," awarded to undergraduate health professions students
1992	• Community input into interdisciplinary curriculum
	• Rural partnership cohort of nursing, medicine, and public health students enters first site
1993	• Primary care clinic establishes second rural community rural partnership
1996	• Undergraduate interdisciplinary curriculum revised
	• "Graduate Health Professions Education" grant awarded for graduate health profession students
1998	• Two additional communities added
	• "Expanding Community Partnerships" grant awarded for all disciplines on campus
1999	• Interdisciplinary health communication course required for all health professions undergraduate students
2000	• University mission statement revised to focus on community-based, interdisciplinary collaboration
	• Undergraduate interdisciplinary curriculum revised
2001	• Graduate interdisciplinary experience revised
2003	• Additional interdisciplinary, community-based grants received (Centers for Disease Control and Prevention, National Institutes of Health, BHP)
	• Interdisciplinary health care ethics course and course on collaboration included in the doctor of science in nursing program
2004	• Undergraduate interdisciplinary curriculum revised to include applied community-based research and project
2005	• Revised interdisciplinary undergraduate curriculum implemented

whether between client and clinician or between student nurse and student doctor. The concepts of emotional intelligence and principled negotiation are foundational to this interdisciplinary learning experience. This continuing course sets the expectation for collaboration, allows interdisciplinary professors to role-model expected patterns of behavior, and breaks down traditional professional stereotypes that often can be barriers to effective working relationships and can compromise client safety.

Curriculum is never static, and the program initiated in 1991 has evolved with the ever-changing health care and educational environment. The community-based approach to education begun in the partnership program gradually was integrated into medical and nursing curricula for all students. To maintain its role in curricular innovation and to meet the current needs of students and communities, the program continues to evolve. The newest iteration, begun in January 2005, is a planned series of three collaborative interdisciplinary

courses for senior nursing, first-year medical, and graduate public health students in three partner communities. The first course is an orientation to rural community health that occurs in the community with faculty and community members serving as leaders and facilitators. Participation in team-building skills and immersion in the culture, social, political, and economic status of the community provides an introduction to the community. This course is followed by a rural health research and practice course in which students participate in experiential, community-based, participatory research. The focus on research methodology and process culminates in a plan for a community-guided interdisciplinary research and service project that is implemented in a subsequent semester. This version of interdisciplinary community-based education fits with an increased emphasis on applied research within the university and coincides with rising community awareness of the importance of research. The effectiveness of this newest undergraduate initiative will be monitored for effectiveness over time.

Graduate Health Professions Education

Graduate students have been included in the community-based collaborative education efforts as well. In 1996, again funded by the W.K. Kellogg Foundation, a plan to bring together family medical residents, graduate family nurse practitioner students, and graduate public health students was implemented (Edwards & Smith, 1998). The focus of this iteration was on joint seminars, student-faculty groups that studied specific topics and carried out projects in partnership with community groups, and clinical assignment in sites that modeled exemplary interdisciplinary care. After graduate-level funding was completed, interdisciplinary seminars continued to be offered and assignments were made to interdisciplinary clinical sites by medical and nursing program faculty. Graduate experiences evolved to include doctor of science in nursing students when that program was initiated in 2003. These collaborative ventures have opened the door for other joint projects in teaching, service, and research.

Collaborative Education Across the University

The success of these collaborative and interdisciplinary community-based efforts affected the entire university. In 1998 an additional project, the Expanding Community Partnership Program, was funded by the W.K. Kellogg Foundation. This project brought the potential for every academic unit on campus to participate in community-based, interdisciplinary education (Behringer et al., 2004). The governance structure of the health professions initiative was widened to incorporate all East Tennessee State University colleges, and two more rural counties joined the partnership.

In this effort, community members partnered with faculty and students to implement a wide array of projects that would benefit all participants. Examples of partnership projects included the development of a leadership program for rural youth, the production of an award-winning original historical drama about a rural Tennessee town, the initiation and continuation of a Hispanic newspaper, widespread participation in collecting the memories of World War II veterans, and fitness activities and nutrition education for rural school children. These accomplishments laid the foundation for widespread service-learning experiences integrated into curriculum across the university and continuing community partnerships across the region.

SUMMARY

The task of transitioning from a traditional model of health professions education to a collaborative, interdisciplinary, community-based one entails changes in the organizational culture that encompass faculty expectations and knowledge (Reece, Mawn, & Scollin, 2003). Although this transition can be daunting, the challenge and synergy that result from collaboration positively affects students, faculty members, communities, and the fabric of institutions. As a direct result of these projects, interdisciplinary faculty members have taught together, conducted research and practice projects, published and presented collaboratively, and become personally acquainted as human beings. Interpersonal conflict still occurs, and turf battles still occasionally arise. However, when a conflict occurs, it is most often about individual differences rather than a professional stereotype or bias and usually is negotiated in a principled manner.

The impact of the institutional change cannot be overstated. The university mission statement was revised to focus on community-based, interdisciplinary collaboration. Curricula within the health professions colleges have undergone significant changes that now include community-based service, education, and projects across the curriculum. The number of spontaneous interdisciplinary projects within the university and with community partners has grown, crossing lines that were not imagined in the past. The challenge of interdisciplinary work entails sustained, committed effort and hard work (Long, 2000). The journey toward collaboration described in this chapter has been arduous, but the positive outcomes for students, faculty members, and communities have been well worth the effort.

REFERENCES

Behringer, B., Bach, B., Daudsitel, H., Fraser, J., Kriesky, J., & Lang, G. (2004). *Pursuing opportunities through partnerships: Higher education and communities.* Morgantown: West Virginia University Press.

Behringer, B., Bishop, W., Edwards, J., & Franks, R. (1999). A model for partnerships among communities, disciplines, and institutions. In D. Holmes & M. Osterweis (Eds), *Catalysts in interdisciplinary education* (pp. 43-58). Washington, DC: Association of Academic Health Centers.

Bloom, S. (1988). Structure and ideology in medical education: An analysis of resistance to change. *Journal of Health and Social Behavior, 29,* 294-306.

Edwards, J., & Alley, N. (2002). Transition to community-based nursing curriculum: Process and outcomes. *Journal of Professional Nursing, 18*(2), 78-84.

Edwards, J., & Smith, P. (1998). Impact of interdisciplinary education in underserved areas: Health professions collaboration in rural Tennessee. *Journal of Professional Nursing, 14*(3), 144-149.

Fisher, R., & Ury, W. (1981). *Getting to yes.* New York: Penguin Books.

Florence, B., Goodrow, B. A., Wachs, J. E., Grover, S., & Olive, K. (2004). *Community partnership: A ten year outcome analysis of rural health professions education at ETSU.* Unpublished manuscript, East Tennessee State University, Johnson City.

Goleman, D., Boyatzis, R., & McKee, A. (2002). *Primal leadership. Realizing the power of emotional intelligence.* Boston: Harvard Business School Press.

Goodrow, B., Olive, K., Behringer, B., Kelley, M., Bennard, B., Grover, S., et al. (2001). The community partnerships experience: A report of institutional transition at East Tennessee State University. *Academic Medicine, 76*(2), 134-141.

Greenleaf, R. K. (1996). *On becoming a servant leader.* San Francisco: Jossey-Bass.

Greenlick, M. (1992). Educating physicians for population based clinical practice. *JAMA: The Journal of the American Medical Association, 267*(12), 1645-1648.

Greiner, A. C., & Knebel, E. (Eds.) (2003). *Health professions education: A bridge to quality.* Washington, DC: National Academies Press.

Group, T., & Roberts, J. (2004). *Nursing, physician control, and the medical monopoly.* Bloomington: Indiana University Press.

Institute of Medicine. (2001). *Crossing the quality chasm.* Washington, DC: National Academies Press.

Kohn, L., Corrigan, J., Donaldson, M. (Eds.). (2000). *To err is human: Building a safe health system.* Washington, DC: National Academies Press.

LaFasto, F., & Larson, C. (2001). *When teams work best: 6,000 team members and leaders tell what it takes to succeed.* Thousand Oaks, CA: Sage Publications.

Linderman, C. (1995). *Refocusing undergraduate nursing education.* Atlanta, GA: Southern Council on Collegiate Education in Nursing with the Southern Regional Education Board.

Long, J. (2000). Using the OJKSN as a teaching tool with RN/BSN Students. *Online Journal of Knowledge Synthesis in Nursing, 22*(7), 2E.

Mattessich, P. W., Murray-Close, M., & Monsey, B. R. (2001). *Collaboration: What makes it work.* St. Paul, MN: Amherst H. Wilder Foundation.

Nutting, P., Wood, M., & Conner, E. (1985). Community oriented primary care. *Journal of the American Medical Association, 253*(12), 1763-1766.

Reece, S., Mawn, B., & Scollin, P. (2003). Evaluation of faculty transition into a community-based curriculum. *Journal of Nursing Education, 42*(1), 43-47.

Sullivan, T. J. (1998). *Collaboration: A health care imperative.* New York: McGraw-Hill.

Wachs, J. E., Goodrow, B. A., & Olive, K. E. (1998). *Community partnerships: Education of health science students, service to the community.* Battle Creek, MI: W.K. Kellogg Foundation.

Wachs, J. E. (in press). Building the occupational health team. *AAOHN Journal.*

Some Reflections on Conflict Resolution in Nursing

The Implications of Negotiating at an Uneven Table

PHYLLIS BECK KRITEK

Peggy, the charge nurse of a thriving, busy, and respected orthopedic unit, on a hectic Monday morning full of interns, residents, rounding, and two patients who believe their pain medications are inadequate, gets a call from Betsy in admissions. "We'll be sending up two admits this morning; they'll be covered by the Internal Medicine Department." Peggy is at first a bit disoriented by the message. "Medicine's patients? This is an ortho unit!"

Betsy tries to sound calm, though she does not feel all that calm. "Maybe you didn't hear: we closed a medicine unit because of low admissions in the service, so we are dispersing medical patients throughout the house. You have the beds, so you get the patients." Peggy is getting steamed now. "We can't cover medicine; this is an ortho unit. Why wasn't I in on this decision?"

Betsy tries to sound even calmer. "I don't know, but the admissions will be coming." Peggy cannot find a reasonable retort, so slams down the receiver. Betsy goes to her boss and confides, "Peggy, on Ortho, just went ballistic about the admissions. She hung up on me, slammed down the phone!"

Anyone working in health care today recognizes this story. Not only is it a tale about cost savings and organizational choices, but also it is a story about how conflicts shape the day-to-day work experiences of health care providers and their perception that much of that conflict arrives "out of the blue" and implicitly sends a message that no recourse is possible. The story also creates the conditions for Betsy and Peggy to begin to dislike, distrust, and even verbally discount one another. Over time, this conflict can begin to shape decisions in the organization, and most involved will not remember how the story started.

We do have options. We may not know what they are, or we may believe that pursuing them is too time consuming or dangerous, but the options exist. Peggy and Betsy can make choices that can alter their exchange and bring back to the organization a set of new choices to change such situations in the future. We can manage conflict differently than we are now. We do have options.

ALTERNATIVE DISPUTE RESOLUTION

Alternative dispute resolution (ADR) is a relatively young but thriving field focused on the exploration and implementation of policies and practices that address conflict by seeking alternatives to mutual harm to the participants. Alternative dispute resolution sometimes has been dubbed "appropriate dispute resolution" to highlight this departure from destructive responses to conflict, including all forms of interpersonal violence. Although ADR is a global movement, much of the richest and most expansive work was birthed in the United States, a country that continues to provide leadership in this field of endeavor.

Alternative dispute resolution has an array of sites of practice. Labor/management negotiation and international diplomacy are examples of early investments in the policies and practices. The term *alternative* actually infers an alternative to adjudication and emerges from the discipline of law, another major site of practice. In the last few decades, work in a variety of ADR applications has expanded, with an array of theoretical approaches and arenas, including diverse emphases such as divorce mediation and environmental protection negotiation. The names of these arenas point to some of the modalities of ADR, which range from simple dialog through negotiation, mediation, and complex formal arbitration. Each is a modality designed to assist parties to a conflict in finding a constructive and mutually satisfying resolution to that shared conflict.

More recently, corporations have discovered ADR and have initiated efforts to incorporate the competencies and values of ADR into their organizational practices. Health care has been slow to follow suit, despite the fact that the focus of health care is arguably a more compelling arena for finding constructive outcomes to conflict. Unresolved conflict in health care not only harms the parties involved but also can harm those health care professionals purport to place in their protection and care.

Why Bother With Alternative Dispute Resolution?

Many industries have begun to embrace ADR, not primarily because of some altruistic concern for employees and consumers but simply because it is good business. A particularly compelling dimension of ADR is its potential to reduce cost substantively in a variety of ways. Table 58-1 provides an overview of some of the

TABLE 58-1

Health Care Organization Conflict Cost Factors

Factors Associated With Conflict That Consume the Resources of a Health Care Organization	Estimated Annual Cost
Wasted time for employees	
Bad decisions made during conflicts	
Lost/resigned employees	
Unnecessary restructuring	
Sabotage	
Theft	
Strained cross-professional communication	
Disruptive behavior of personnel	
Damage to property	
Lowered job motivation	
Lowered job morale	
Lost work time	
Verbal abuse and its sequelae	
Employee replacement	
New employee orientation	
Health costs associated with job stress	
Staffing disruptions	
Scheduling dilemmas	
Absenteeism	
Tardiness	
Work not completed before shift ends	
Errors	
Failure to rescue	
Falls and injuries	
Patient safety neglect	
Endless, pointless meetings	
Meetings focused on power distribution	
Repetitive policy manifestos	
Provider career changes	

© Phyllis Beck Kritek, RN, PhD, FAAN

ways unresolved conflict is costly and can be used to estimate the cost of conflict in a given unit or department. The table thereby can document the ways ineffectively resolved conflict erodes the capacity of an organization to flourish.

The virtual obsession in the United States with cost containment in health care has focused on a variety of cost centers, many that nurses find disturbing. Certainly the wholesale and formulaic elimination of much of the nursing enterprise in the 1990s is an excellent case in point. This process involved unreflective implementation of three interacting forces: decreased length of stay, attendant increased patient condition severity, and downsizing of nursing departments. This simplistic solution since has demonstrated its capacity for harm, and the efforts to reverse the damages are incomplete. An analog can be crafted comparing this process to implementation of ADR. Finding out how "the way we do business" in patterns that create conflict has been embraced less readily, perhaps because of our country's culture of preference for the quick fix and the easy solution.

Alternative dispute resolution is not that, of course. Alternative dispute resolution does take time and energy and asks a great deal of individuals. Alternative dispute resolution deals not only with the conflict but also the systems, values, practices, and interests of all involved parties, and that is complex. Nonetheless, ADR can save money and it can improve work environments. In the end, computing the cost of conflict and comparing that to the cost of effective conflict resolution readily demonstrates that in the comparative absorption of organizational resources, ADR is a cost-effective alternative.

The positive impact of conflict transformation practices, however, goes well beyond the considerations of cost management. As the national push to improve the work environments of nurses is examined as a nursing shortage factor, this tool for enhanced work environments is a worthy focal point. The recent report from the Institute of Medicine (Page, 2004) on transforming the work environment of nurses pays particular attention to collaboration among health professionals, listing conflict management as one of the key characteristics of such collaboration (p. 214). Further, the report encourages health care organizations to institute human resource policies that include conflict management skills in performance evaluations (p. 217). As is perhaps obvious, evaluation of a worker on skills neither taught nor rewarded is inappropriate.

Gardner (2005) notes that collaboration in health care environments is encouraged repeatedly and practiced rarely in part because little has been done to explain the actual process of collaboration clearly. To address this void, using her own extensive experience base, she lists "ten lessons in collaboration" (p. 1), the third of which is "develop constructive conflict resolution skills" (p. 5). As she observes, "conflict resolution is the cornerstone of collaborative success" (p. 6). Our collective caution in mastering conflict resolution skills serves as harbinger to the realization that we continue to struggle with the challenge of collaboration.

If It's So Great, Why Aren't Nurses Doing It?

The presence of conflict in health care is hardly news, and for several decades nursing has incorporated "stories" of conflict as part of its folklore in its oral and written traditions. Although many nursing publications discuss conflict and its management, most of this literature is anecdotal or prescriptive. The integration of the fields of nursing and ADR is a work in progress, with a limited number of workers engaged in the task.

Perhaps one of the most useful reports on ADR in nursing is one published by Valentine (2001). In effect, Valentine provided nursing with a meta-analysis of work done to date on nurses' preferred conflict management styles, using the most accepted tool for this appraisal, the Thomas-Kilmann Conflict Mode Index (Thomas & Kilmann, 1974, 2002). Her outcomes are revealing and compelling.

What Valentine was able to document—admittedly with a limited number of studies, albeit more than many where strong conclusions are argued—was that nurses are conflict aversive. In addition, if nurses cannot avoid conflict successfully, we tend to opt for conflict management behaviors that disadvantage us, using either accommodation where we forego our interests to accommodate the other participant in the conflict or compromise where neither party tends to be satisfied with the outcomes, the quintessential "quick fix" that ensures the conflict will reemerge.

The ideal of course is collaboration; a mode nurses purport to value but appear ill equipped to understand. No wonder nurses are wary of exploring conflict resolution. We have learned over time, albeit in part through our own behaviors, that trying to deal with conflict is dangerous, costly, and unsatisfying.

Then Why Bother?

My own introduction to the field of ADR emerged from a Kellogg Leadership Fellowship (1986-1989) where I studied with leaders in the field throughout the United States, accompanied by 13 colleagues, two of whom were also in health care. We learned early on that health care and ADR had not yet connected significantly. We also learned that "selling" ADR to health care communities was a sizable challenge.

These extraordinary opportunities for learning also revealed to me that the ADR community, largely constructed by the "dominant culture," was framed, much as health care is, to reflect and address the world-view of the dominant culture. Having raised questions about this concern repeatedly, one of the leaders of the field observed to me that of course I was correct in my assessment, and if I wished to hear other voices in the dialog, I should raise my voice, or as he said, "write the book"—so I did.

My interest was focused on the uneven table, a place where the assurance of justice and fairness in outcomes is unlikely. Although I was encouraged, as a mediator, to "set an even table," I noted that I personally felt I had never been at one. Over time I have become convinced that in their purest sense, such tables simply do not exist. If indeed there are no even tables, then what does one do when one finds oneself seated at an uneven table, particularly as the disadvantaged party?

The most spontaneous response is to try to "get even," often carrying with it a flavor of revenge. Revenge is a form of violence, and all violence begets further violence. Hence the first response may not be the most constructive or the most creative. If one wishes to be constructive and creative, what is the alternative? My answer to this question became the focus of my book, *Negotiating at an Uneven Table: Developing Moral Courage in Resolving Our Conflicts* (Kritek, 2002).

I describe all of this to unveil the personal journey that got me to the point of writing this chapter in this book. Why did I bother? Because what nurses were doing with conflict seemed destructive and self-defeating, and alternatives were attractive to me. Because it made more sense to me to try to find an alternative than to concede defeat to processes I knew harmed nurses and others. And finally, because over time I learned that conflict need not simply be bad news. Embedded in the process of effective conflict resolution is also the opportunity for growth, self-discovery, and personal and organizational transformation. Not a lot of options are out there that can deliver such a promise. Of course, it is difficult, but then being torn apart by daily conflict on the job looks difficult too.

So in addition to cost savings, running a better shop, creating an improved work environment, and using tools well documented for their potential to enhance outcomes, I learned that ADR can be one pathway to self-actualization and self-fulfillment; hence my interest in conflict transformation. The pathway is not easy (as if there were some), yet it delivers an enormous gift. So I do this work full time after more than 35 years in nursing education.

LESSONS FROM THE TRENCHES

Over the last 15-plus years, I have been training people in conflict resolution and more importantly, conflict transformation, the latter emphasizing the positive opportunities embedded in conflict situations. Most of this work has been done in the United States and most of it with nurses. I concurrently have "done the work" myself, working with groups in conflict, serving as a mediator and facilitator. Although much of my early work focused on the lessons embedded in the book on negotiation, more recently I have been exploring with groups the findings that have emerged from my experiences. This chapter identifies some of those findings and their implications. The discussion focuses on nurses but can be generalized to several comparable groups.

Lesson 1: Nurses Already Have Many Alternative Dispute Resolution Skills Mastered

Even a cursory scan of the health care environment reveals that nurses are confronted with conflict daily and resolve much of it effectively. This is particularly true with patients and their families, with whom nurses often function as effective mediators. Over time, observing these skills led me to create a list of observable competencies nurses demonstrate in a role that I have called "The Health Care Diplomat." Table 58-2 lists these competencies, subdivided into categories of values, responsibilities, and skills. This starter set of ADR abilities positions nurses as ideal mediators in the health care environment.

Hence nurses already have numerous ADR competencies and are called upon daily to use them. However, although nurses do have many formal roles that call forth mediation, much of their work as mediators is essentially informal and unacknowledged. In addition, the role of mediator has not yet been normalized as a central nursing role. Finally, because nurses are conflict aversive, they may be effective in resolving some conflicts and more inclined to avoid others.

The take home lesson is simple: if we already have several competencies and are going to be called upon daily to use them, why not get good at this? When do we avoid conflict and why? What do we want to do about it?

TABLE 58-2

Existing Alternative Dispute Resolution Nurse Competencies	
Checklist	**Nurse Competencies**
	VALUES
	Belief in the worth and value of each human person
	Commitment to quality of services provided
	Advocacy for patients and families
	Sensitivity to patients and families and their needs
	Fairness in treatment of patients and families
	Compassion
	Care and concern for others
	Commitment to constructive work environments
	RESPONSIBILITIES
	Surveillance
	Physiological therapies
	Helping patients compensate for loss
	Providing emotional support
	Educating patients and families
	Integrating care
	Documentation of activities and outcomes
	Seeking information needed
	Supervision
	SKILLS
	Communication with diverse individuals
	Relationship competencies
	Knowledge of system and its processes
	Listening ability
	Monitoring and anticipation of adversity
	Systems-based conceptual thinking
	Connectivity with the entire organization
	Intuition
	Critical thinking
	Differential diagnosing
	Awareness of the importance of timing
	Sense of humor

© Phyllis Beck Kritek, RN, PhD, FAAN

Lesson 2: Nurses Avoid Conflicts Where They Feel Disadvantaged

To posit nurses as diplomats is all well and good, and a second scan of the health care environment readily demonstrates that this is not always the case. Certainly, expert nurses use mediation skills as part of effective patient care, negotiating with patients and their families to ensure a desired outcome. Nurses also negotiate with co-workers and colleagues. They also can find themselves deeply conflicted with these same co-workers and colleagues.

No matter how many mediation skills a nurse has, if he or she feels disadvantaged, it often may seem unwise to take on the conflict and try to resolve it. It seems to be a losing proposition, and the solution too often is avoidance, unattractive compromises, accommodation, or manipulation. Having been taught all of these behaviors as a student nurse and even rewarded for them, I understand the behavior. The behavior is the basis for my book. Nonetheless, we can do more.

An interesting contextual factor shaping nurses' mediator role is the impact of public trust. The Gallup organization has polled U.S. citizens for decades asking them to identify the most trusted professions. Nursing was added only 6 years ago and every year since its addition has scored as the most trusted profession, with the exception of the poll immediately after the 9/11 tragedy, in which firefighters warranted "most trusted" status. In the most recent poll (Moore, 2004) published in December 2004, 79% of respondents indicated that the honesty and ethics of nurses were viewed by the public as "very high" or "high." In 2003 the ranking was 83% (Carroll, 2003). Other health disciplines tend to rank high, but not as high as nurses. Apparently, patients and their families invest substantive trust in nurses. They are the persons to whom Americans want to address their conflictual care situations.

The summary lesson is again simple. Although nurses cannot modify the behavior of others and may view nurses' sociopolitical relationships in health care settings as remarkably resistant to change, nurses certainly can expand their skill base and master new areas of ADR. Indeed, the public trusts nurses to do so. These added abilities better equip nurses to expand the scope of their mediation abilities and promise to ensure more frequent desired outcomes.

Lesson 3: Nurses Can Enhance Their Alternative Dispute Resolution Competencies

Uneven tables are frustrating, and I, like many nurses, would like to banish them. They persist however, so it makes more sense to develop an expanded skill base in dealing with these troublesome situations. Nurses do have choices, and the choices do have consequences.

After about 10 years of training diverse nurse groups about ADR, I noticed that the areas of difficulty for groups were consistent, and hence I began to record these. Over time, I have isolated those areas where nurses appear persistently to manifest less robust skill levels. These are the places where nurses can learn, practice, study, and indeed transform their environments and themselves. These areas are presented in the following section of this chapter; suffice it to say here that identifying learning needs and goals is the first step in expanding knowledge.

The summary lesson is once more simple. If I want to become better at managing conflict, I can decide to do so. Having made this decision, I then set out to develop the competencies that are essential to that end.

Some Noteworthy Disclaimers, Precautions, and Suggestions

Before sketching out the options in competency building, some disclaimers, precautions, and suggestions are useful. The realistic addition of skills to one's bag of tricks takes time and energy, something a lot of nurses find in short supply. Hence a decision to make the investment is important, embedded in the limits of time and possibility. Hence one is wiser to become a student of ADR than to anticipate one will learn some recipes and be done with the task once and for all. I am convinced that I still will be learning new competencies as I die, and I think this keeps me open to possibility.

When attempting to enhance competencies, it is wise to focus, taking one specific conflict and focusing on that rather than trying to fix all of them as they emerge. As with any other skill, a gradual building of ability occurs. Though many suggestions are presented in this chapter, I encourage you to select only two or three to start and to add on as you go. Make the goals realistic so they can be met.

Finally, beware of tackling the hardest conflict first; start with the easiest one. You want to experience early success, not frustration and defeat. Health care professionals, in the main, are trained to set priorities: nurses respond to the fracture or the respiratory distress before they worry about the bruise or the sore wrist. Hence picking the easiest conflict from which to learn may seem counterintuitive. Again, you are seeking success. If you have a history of avoiding certain kinds of conflict, show compassion for yourself and proceed at a realistic rate. This work is complex and it takes time; there are no quick fixes.

A SELF-DEVELOPMENT ROAD MAP

If you have made a decision to expand your competencies, then information helps. As noted, in addition to identifying the starter set nurses already have in place, I have collected specific examples of areas of challenge for most nurses. These too fall in the categories found in Table 58-2: values, responsibilities, and skills. Each is presented as checklists so that the reader can identify the one or two attractive ones that might serve as a point of departure in altering current conflict behaviors.

Value Cultivation

Table 58-3 presents a list of values that are useful in the effort to reconceptualize one's responses to conflict and to imagine ADR as a useful resource. This list identifies the value clarification activities that can move the willing student toward enhanced effectiveness with conflict transformation. As is evident from the list, none of these are easy, and all are inherently attractive and congruent with the traditions and values of the profession.

These values are also ones that expert nurses apply to patient care situations daily. The interesting challenge embedded in this dimension of self-development is the commitment to expand this application to include colleagues and co-workers. What is noteworthy is that the values indeed may be familiar and that the application of these values to selected groups may have been avoided in the past.

Manifesting these values will alter the work environment significantly simply because someone in the environment is "taking a stand" and all other participants will be challenged to adapt. Hence, although the values apply specifically to one person's commitments, they touch the lives of all who encounter that person, changing everyone's experience of a given environment. This actually can be adventuresome and fun.

Responsibility Integration

Table 58-4 provides a checklist of responsibilities to be integrated into one's work role. The challenge embedded

TABLE 58-3

Alternative Dispute Resolution Value Cultivation Checklist for Nurses	
Commitments	**Professional Values to Be Cultivated**
	Courage to face and transform conflict
	Compassion with those with whom I differ
	Embracing diversity as an opportunity and an advantage
	Forgiveness
	Pursuing mission congruence as a challenge
	Inclusiveness in my relationships
	Justice as a complex but worthy goal
	Manifesting "do no harm" as a lifestyle
	Peace building

© Phyllis Beck Kritek, RN, PhD, FAAN

TABLE 58-4

Alternative Dispute Resolution Responsibilities Checklist for Nurses	
Commitments	**Professional Responsibilities To Be Integrated Into Work Role**
	Differentiating between critical thinking and judging others
	Differentiating between humor and ridicule
	Differentiating between problems and essential polarities
	Differentiating between accommodation and collaboration
	Becoming willing overtly to own my own power
	Publicly committing to my professional code of ethics
	Acknowledging and owning my role in conflicts on the job
	Anticipating that the "other side" can teach me something
	Understanding the manifestations of oppression
	Confronting and mastering my fear of retribution
	Detaching from the need for the "right answer"
	Detaching from mindsets of powerlessness
	Detaching from "victim-think"
	Detaching from deprivation expectation
	Imagining that conflict can even be fun
	Learning from conflicts I experience

© Phyllis Beck Kritek, RN, PhD, FAAN

in these responsibilities involves no longer opting for behaviors that may have become habitual, most in response to the frustration of uneven tables and the cost they exact on others who feel disadvantaged. Once an individual forgos the option of vengeance or self-pity, then the unevenness is merely true, not a cause for ranting and raving or, alternatively, whining. It just is.

That being the case, it becomes important to realize that I continue to have the power of my personal moral agency, my integrity and honesty, and my commitment to the constructive resolution of conflict. Starting on the "high ground" enhances my degrees of freedom and the clarity with which I can present my viewpoint. As is apparent, much of this list requires detachment from counterproductive behaviors. Such detachment is a choice, and it does have consequences. Clinging to resentment has thus far resolved little.

Perhaps noteworthy here is that the recent revision of the American Nurses Association *Code of Ethics for Nurses* (2001) includes clear prescriptions for constructive conflict resolution. "The nurse maintains compassionate and caring relationships with colleagues and others with a commitment to the fair treatment of individuals, to integrity-preserving compromise, and to resolving conflicts" (p. 9). The code elsewhere discusses the frequent exposure to conflict inherent in patient care and observes, "Nurses strive to resolve conflicts in ways that ensure patient safety, guard the patient's best interests and preserve the professional integrity of the nurse" (p. 10).

This discipline-specific stance about ethical conduct implies mastery of conflict resolution, an implication not reflected in the preparation or continued professional development opportunities for nursing. Perhaps of greater concern is a lack of direction about the nature of such work.

The field of conflict resolution, or ADR, mushroomed in the 1960s and saw its coming of age in the 1990s (Dukes, 1996), the latter characterized by substantive knowledge generation. This knowledge generation included diversification of theories about ADR. For some, negotiations are distributive, where the goal is to get the most of what I want in the process, with little emphasis on the outcomes for others (Mayer, 2002, p. 148). For others, negotiations are integrative, where I am seeking outcomes that meet all parties' essential needs, which maximize benefits for everyone (p. 151). This latter approach is interest-based but focuses on all participants as partners and emphasizes relationship, communication, education, and the use of a principled process.

This distinction is noteworthy because courses and literature on ADR do not always make this distinction, so that many propose negotiations that are essentially distributive and can intensify further a participant's sense of getting even or inadvertently disadvantaging other parties to the conflict. Seeking to improve one's ADR skills without attention to the type of negotiation being used is important.

A third approach to ADR was developed by Bush and Folger (1994) and gained visibility in the 1990s: transformative mediation, which focused on the transformative potential of conflict for all parties, including the mediator, and emphasized strength instead of weakness and compassion instead of selfishness. This approach has enjoyed a growing following and has built a substantive body of literature; for example, Folger and Bush (2001). Transformative mediation is noteworthy for its congruence with nursing values and practices. Thus beginning to take accountability for conflict resolution may be better served by a transformative approach than one seeking "integrity-preserving compromise" (American Nurses Association, 2001, p. 10; see the foregoing discussion).

To begin to focus on this process of integrating ADR into one's work role is not enough. Study and training are needed, and the first step involves a careful assessment of the varied approaches to ADR. Picking the one that best fits nursing is part of the challenge. Certainly the work of Mayer on integrative negotiation or Bush and Folger on transformative mediation shows greater potential for ethical outcomes than the many authors, particularly those focused on business negotiations, which encourage "getting what you want" and "out-negotiating everyone." Choices have to be made here.

As is perhaps apparent, the list provided in Table 58-4 rejects the potentially opportunistic approaches advocated in distributive negotiation. Nonetheless, many actively market this approach, for example, in labor-management negotiations. Important choices have to be made in the simple act of beginning to learn more about ADR.

Skill Expansion

Table 58-5 provides a list of useful skills that might reasonably be enhanced. As is perhaps self-evident, none of these are simple skills, and all can be enriched continuously with practice and experience. The list is provided largely to encourage reflective consideration of some skill areas of emphasis. Some skills warrant focused attention.

In my experience, nurses often make quick judgments about the nature of a conflict without taking the

TABLE 58-5

Alternative Dispute Resolution Skills Checklist for Nurses

Commitments	Negotiation/Mediation Skills To Be Added or Enhanced
	Picking my tables deliberately
	Conducting a careful and complete conflict analysis
	Identifying when the conflict is actually a system problem, not a person problem
	Discovering the interests of everyone participating in the conflict
	Asking questions often and well
	Asking others how I might help in the conflict
	Acknowledging the strengths of others in a conflict
	Doing my homework before trying to deal with the conflict
	Learning to observe myself objectively during a negotiation
	Reframing all aspects of a conflict before trying to deal with it
	Generating numerous options before selecting one
	Creating the unimagined option
	Clarifying all possible choices and their consequences
	Knowing my boundaries and maintaining them
	Using integrative and constructive humor
	Following up on a process to see it through to its conclusion
	Creating closure
	Affirming my outcomes

© Phyllis Beck Kritek, RN, PhD, FAAN

time for careful analysis, including not just the conflict itself, but the identification of all parties involved (which can be expansive), interests of all parties (which sometimes take exploration to identify), range of potential outcomes (which evokes imagination), and costs of ignoring the conflict (which can be motivating). Identifying parties' interests presumes seeking information, and the habit of assuming one knows another's interests can be a serious deterrent to a careful assessment. Attempting to craft a reasonable resolution with

misinformation is a serious threat to successful mediation and negotiation.

Another important point of emphasis is the need to take the time to assess one's own role in the conflict. The culture of blame that has pervaded health care makes this a difficult challenge, yet can be productive in increasing options and deterring unreflective reactions. As is perhaps apparent from the list, if one can overcome a tendency to fear and avoid conflict and begin to reframe it as an opportunity, in time it can be seen as constructive and educational and sometimes even fun.

COMING FULL CIRCLE

This chapter opened with a story of a typical conflict that nurses confront daily. Imagine alternatives. If Peggy and Betsy had the opportunity to learn about ADR, they first might have approached the entire exchange differently, with openness toward the challenges faced by each person. Peggy might have asked questions about the decision process rather than react, attempting to find out whether the system had a communication glitch that could be addressed. Betsy might have provided information on that glitch and acknowledged that some alternative model needed to be created.

Both women might have watched themselves in the exchange and learned a good deal about what their personal interests were. Betsy might have approached Peggy later and rebuilt a bridge and discussed the situation after the heat of the moment had eased. She may have elected to say nothing to her supervisor, knowing that Peggy's response was reactive and temporary. Peggy might have called Betsy back and apologized. They even might have had a discussion about how to avoid this kind of exchange in the future.

If none of this had happened, the system itself might have noted the problem and, using the in-house conflict management system, conducted an evaluation of what had happened. They might have created a meeting for Betsy and Peggy to talk out the situation and to heal that breach. They might have explored the lack of involvement in and communication about the decision process further and explored ways to correct the situation in the future. They might even have imagined a better solution to the problem than the one used.

This scenario does not exhaust possibilities, but it begins to demonstrate that they exist. What is clear is that blaming, feelings of powerlessness, desire for retribution, and persistent hopelessness are patterns that will not alter or improve the situation. The situation as described was unpleasant for everyone; imagining competencies that could alter that situation, even make it transformative, is a worthy point of departure for reflection.

SUMMARY

This chapter provides an array of observations about ADR in health care. The chapter is intended as an invitation to the reader to pursue further opportunities and invest in ethical commitments to enhanced competency in conflict resolution and hopefully, conflict transformation. To further support this intent, some useful Web sites are provided to introduce the reader to online options in this endeavor. In addition, a list of useful books is provided. My hope is that this array of options will provide guidance and impetus to move forward in nurses' collective commitment to enhanced conflict resolution in health care.

REFERENCES

American Nurses Association. (2001). *Code of ethics for nurses with interpretive statements.* Washington, DC: Author.

Bush, R. A. B., & Folger, J. P. (1994). *The promise of mediation: Responding to conflict through empowerment and recognition.* San Francisco: Jossey-Bass.

Carroll, J. (2003, December 1). *Public rates nursing as most honest and ethical profession.* Retrieved February 1, 2005, from http://www.gallup.com/poll/

Dukes, E. F. (1996). *Resolving public conflict: Transforming community and governance.* Manchester, UK: Manchester University Press.

Folger, J. P., & Bush, R. A. B. (Eds.). (2001). *Designing mediation: Approaches to training and practice within a transformative framework.* New York: Institute for the Study of Conflict Transformation.

Gardner, D. (2005, January 31). Ten lessons in collaboration. *Online Journal in Nursing, 10*(1). Retrieved February 1, 2005, from http://www.nursingworld.org/ojin/topic26/tpc26_1.htm

Kritek, P. B. (2002). *Negotiating at an uneven table: Developing moral courage in resolving our conflicts* (2nd ed.). San Francisco: Jossey-Bass.

Mayer, B. (2002). *The dynamics of conflict resolution: A practitioner's guide.* San Francisco: Jossey-Bass.

Moore, D. W. (2004, December 7). *Nurses top list in honesty and ethics poll.* Retrieved February 1, 2005, from http://www.gallup.com/poll/

Page, A. (Ed.). (2004). *Keeping patients safe: Transforming the work environment of nurses.* Washington, DC: The National Academies Press.

Thomas, K. W., & Kilmann, R. H. (1974, 2002). *Thomas-Kilmann conflict mode index.* Palo Alto, CA: CPP.

Valentine, P. E. B. (2001). Gender perspective on conflict management strategies of nurses. *Journal of Nursing Scholarship, 33*(1), 69-74.

WEB SITES

www.ACRnet.org
The Association for Conflict Resolution is the major professional organization for ADR scholars and practitioners in the United States and provides information on membership, specialization groups, emerging certification programs, educational offerings, ethical codes, and related information.

www.crnetwork.ca
This site provides an overview of some of the rich work being done in Canada in the field of ADR, including educational and training programs, reading resources, and news in the field.

v4.crinfo.org
This site is an information resource managed by the Conflict Resolution Consortium at the University of Colorado. The site is a free online clearinghouse indexing more 25,000 Web pages, books, articles, audiovisual materials, events, and news articles.

www.healthcaremediations.com
This site provides information on a successful conflict management company headed by a nurse, Debra Gerardi. The site demonstrates the impact a nurse such as Deb can have in changing work environments.

www.mediate.org
This is the site of one of the most well-established and respected ADR companies, with 35 years of experience in the training and practice of ADR. Their course offerings are a particularly useful resource.

www.opm.gov/er/adrguide
This is part of the official site of the federal governments human resource agency, the Office of Personnel Management. It provides a resource guide for ADR techniques and practices in federal agencies along with bibliographies, Web sites, and information of the Administrative Dispute Resolution Act of 1996 that mandated the use of ADR processes for all agencies.

www.peacemakers.ca
This Canadian charitable organization is dedicated to research and education on conflict transformation and peace building; hence their site provides extensive bibliographies, case studies, and related resources.

www.transformativemediation.org
This site provides an array of options for persons interested in the work of Bush and Folger on transformative mediation, including educational and organizational resources.

www.usip.org
This is the site of the United States Institute of Peace, an independent, nonpartisan federal institution created by Congress to promote the prevention, management, and peaceful resolution of international conflicts.

SUGGESTED READINGS

Babcock, L., & Laschever, S. (2003). *Women don't ask: Negotiation and the gender divide.* Princeton, NJ: Princeton University Press.

Cloke, K., & Goldsmith, J. (2000). *Resolving conflicts at work: A complete guide for everyone on the job.* San Francisco: Jossey-Bass.

Diamond, L. (2000). *The courage for peace: Daring to create harmony in ourselves and the world.* Berkeley, CA: Conari Press.

Johnson, B. (1992, 1996). *Polarity management: Identifying and managing unsolvable problems.* Amherst, MA: HRD Press.

Kolb, D. M., & Williams, J. (2000). *The shadow negotiation: How women can master the hidden agendas that determine bargaining success.* New York: Simon & Schuster.

Kolb, D. M., & Williams, J. (2003). *Everyday negotiation: Navigating the hidden agendas in bargaining.* San Francisco: Jossey-Bass.

Kritek, P. B. (2002). *Negotiating at an uneven table: Developing moral courage in resolving our conflicts.* San Francisco: Jossey-Bass.

Lederach, J. P. (1997). *Building peace: Sustainable reconciliation in divided societies.* Washington, DC: United States Institute of Peace.

Mayer, B. (2000). *The dynamics of conflict resolution: A practitioner's guide.* San Francisco: Jossey-Bass.

Mayer, R. J. (1995). *Conflict management: The courage to confront.* Columbus, OH: Battelle Press.

Moore, C. W. (1986). *The mediation process: Practical strategies for resolving conflict.* San Francisco: Jossey-Bass.

Rosenberg, M. B. (2003). *Nonviolent communication: A language of life.* Encinitas, CA: PuddleDancer Press.

Slaikeu, K. A., & Hasson, R. H. (1998). *Controlling the costs of conflict: How to design a system for your organization.* San Francisco: Jossey-Bass.

Ury, W. (1999). *Getting to peace: Transforming conflict at home, at work, and in the world.* New York: Penguin.

Yarbrough, E., & Wilmot, W. (1995). *Artful mediation: Constructive conflict at work.* Boulder, CO: Cairns Publishing.

CULTURAL DIVERSITY

Diversity in Nursing

A Challenge for the United States

PERLE SLAVIK COWEN ◆ SUE MOORHEAD

Diversity has always been a key component of American society. Although the United States remains a nation built primarily through immigration, factors such as socioeconomic status and discrimination have influenced the benefits that a diversified population can bring to society. In reality the "melting pot" did not happen. Cultural diversity has become a major goal of many universities in the last few years as a way of enriching the community of scholars and providing experiences for students that are not part of a less diverse environment. International experiences during collegiate programs are also on the rise to enhance these types of experiences for students. Technology has made it possible to communicate easily worldwide, increasing the opportunities for students to learn from students from around the world. In spite of these goals of enhancing diversity in educational experiences, nursing continues to struggle with attracting potential students from diverse cultural groups. This remains a tough challenge for nursing.

Throughout history, nursing has been a pathway for social mobility, especially for women. With relatively few career options outside of the home, acceptable career choices for women were in the fields of teaching, nursing, and secretarial work. White women, first from rural backgrounds, found nursing an acceptable and safe field in which they might advance economically. Ironically, this has not been the case for women from minority groups. Women from underrepresented groups have been relegated primarily to roles of servitude within the health care system as nursing aides or as practical nurses. Entrance into the system in these roles has limited severely the ability to advance within the mainstream of nursing.

Since the 1960s, considerable advances have been made in the ability of women in previously underrepresented groups to participate in all levels of society. But in nursing the situation has remained static, with little advancement on the part of nurses of color. For a profession that prides itself on being an advocate for the rights of patients of all creeds, colors, or national origins, the lack of diversification of the nursing workforce has received only minimal attention. As nurses move into the twenty-first century, the diversity of the population of the United States is increasing significantly. Although the percentage of minorities within the general population continues to increase, nursing continues to lag substantially behind with only about 10% minority representation within the profession. This problem is compounded by the fact that the largest number of minorities entering the profession are educated through associate degree programs. Advancement to higher education, particularly to the doctoral level, is difficult to achieve for minorities, and this creates a lack of diversity among nurses prepared at the doctoral level.

Why does this situation remain unchanged? All of the usual reasons can be offered, and they are the focus of this section: the image of nursing; difficulty in recruiting students into the profession; difficulty in retaining them through the educational programs; and once into practice, difficulty in encouraging their career development. Although these are all valid observations, why is there not more of a concern for the future of the profession if this situation is not reversed dramatically? How can nurses continue to be advocates for patients, when the majority of nurses are white and middle class and the populations they serve are increasingly people of color? Diversity in nursing is not just an ideal but a necessity for the profession to flourish.

In the opening debate chapter, Warda addresses the question of racism and genderism in nursing. This chapter highlights the historical background of diversity in the United States. Warda believes that the image of nursing is a barrier to the recruitment of minorities. This chapter provides an overview of the statistics that show the nursing profession falling far behind in diversity to match that of the general population and addresses the implications of these data related to the appropriateness of care for patients. Warda then outlines some of the factors that serve as barriers for entrance to the field and the ways in which these might be addressed. One of the major persistent problems is that most students from underrepresented groups enter nursing at the lowest end of the career hierarchy, as practical nurses or through associate's degree programs. Educational progression then becomes more difficult, and the percentage of nurses from underrepresented groups becomes even sparser in leadership roles within the profession. The few faculty members and nurses in visible leadership positions do not offer enough role models for potential students wanting to advance in the profession. Without a concerted effort on the part of the nursing profession as a whole, the prospects for change are limited. The factors affecting diversity are many and involve complex personal, academic, and environmental/cultural factors. The continued lack of diversity in nursing requires the immediate attention of many groups: educators, researchers, practitioners, and students of all races and ethnic groups.

In the first viewpoint chapter, Castiglia focuses on the issues of racial diversity in academic programs and stresses the importance of including content on cultural competence in the preparation of nurses. She argues that the delivery of culturally competent care requires that the nurse understand the culture of the patient. If there are no nurses representative of the culture of the patient, this understanding is severely limited. Castiglia addresses issues related to the recruitment, retention, and progression of minority students, particularly Hispanics, and makes suggestions about the support systems necessary to address these inequities. Castiglia suggests that multiple strategies are required, along with financial assistance. Pressure is increasing for all systems to be accountable to achieve diversity and cultural competence. Strategic planning for minority recruitment and retention is essential because students and faculty need formal and informal support services to be successful.

Bullough discusses the issues associated with attracting men into nursing and feels that nursing in the United States will need to change considerably before it can become an attractive career for many men. This chapter notes the increased percentage of males enrolled in nursing educational programs (10%) and traces the historical roots of genderism in nursing. Bullough believes that women will remain the dominant force in nursing for the foreseeable future and that men will have to be aware of the anxieties and fears that women have about men. The author advises nursing and nurses to recruit more men through conscious and deliberate campaigns.

The future for men in nursing is promising, and the percentage of men choosing nursing as a career will increase. This chapter provides food for thought for all nurses, male or female.

In another viewpoint chapter, Dennis addresses issues related to blacks in nursing. The history of blacks in America parallels the history of black nurses in America. Both histories influenced the course of black health within a cultural context that often has clashed with the dominant white culture. Inclusion of the worldview of the black patient and tailoring nursing actions appropriately are essential in good care. Dennis describes particular cultural beliefs and values of blacks and presents health disparities between blacks and whites. Dennis notes that 70% to 90% of recognized illnesses in blacks are managed outside the formal health care system. Because of the history of exploitation and experimentation, blacks understandably are suspicious of health care providers. If health care for blacks is to improve and if the patterns of disease and mortality are to be ameliorated, increased numbers of black nurses providing culturally competent care are an important part of the solution.

Asians and Pacific Islanders represent 4.2% of the total U.S. population or 11.9 million people and are considered the fastest-growing group, increasing about 70% between 1990 and 2000. The five largest groups within this population, in descending order, are the Chinese, Filipino, Asian Indian, Vietnamese, and Korean. These five groups make up about 80% of the Asian/Pacific Islander population. Noting that this categorization masks wide differences between groups, Inouye details the differences in incidence of disease of particular groups. In general, Asian distrust of Western medical care stems from their long history of herbalist or shamanistic healing. Nurses providing care to Asians and Pacific Islanders need to be sensitive to the other cultural values, such as the importance of the family and the reverence for elders. The chapter highlights the 10 leading causes of death in this population. The author uses proverbs and sayings to illustrate health beliefs in an effective way.

Torres and Castillo address the challenge of the growing demographic changes occurring within this country, what they call the "browning" of America. The largest numbers of Hispanics/Latinos in the United States are Mexican Americans, followed by Central or South Americans, Puerto Ricans, and Cubans. When combined, California and Texas are home to more than half of the nation's Hispanics. Because of the economic plight of this population, most Hispanic nurses in the profession enter largely through the associate degree programs. Many more are needed to address the health care issues of this population. The number of nurses that advance to graduate education and to doctoral preparation in particular are even fewer, and they have no ethnic role models. A comprehensive program of recruitment, support systems, and mentoring are recommended as a way to begin to redress the complex problems of increasing the numbers of Hispanics/Latinos in the nursing profession. This is an important challenge for nursing to meet.

In the final chapter in this section, Keltner, Smith, and Slim address the issue of bridging of cultures with Native-American communities and nursing. American Indians face lower life expectancy and higher age-adjusted mortality rates. These realities define many aspects associated with individual, family, and social life. History validates that American Indians have been isolated by poverty, inadequate services, and lack of coordination through interdisciplinary approaches to complex problems. The communities themselves have been exploited, and a general disregard of traditions essential to health behavior and health service use

has occurred. The authors caution nurses to build a framework for building bridges rather than a blueprint and believe that cultural competence has three key components: sensitivity, specificity, and synergy. The natural characteristics of American Indians include their strength and resilience as a people, strong family bonds, and religion as a key foundation of life. When the nurse provides care, the authors suggest that the nurse reinforce these values rather than undermine them. Any treatment needs to focus on the whole person. An increase in the numbers of American-Indian nurses would do much to bridge cultures and produce culturally relevant care. To work well, the bridging of cultures requires true partnerships rather than the more traditional paternalistic approach of health care professionals, including nurses.

This section highlights the slow process of building diversity in nursing. Much remains to be done to reach this goal. The chapters in this section highlight the accomplishments to date, but nursing must be committed to diversity for the future. Diversity can increase the professional status of nursing and lead to better patient outcomes.

Why Isn't Nursing More Diversified?

MARIA R. WARDA

Diversity has always been a major strength of American society. Although the United States remains "a nation of immigrants," socioeconomic stratification and discrimination have limited the benefits that a diversified population can bring to society. In the United States, incongruity exists between the increasing number of racial and ethnic groups and their power to influence and access health care. Recent immigrants, members of ethnic minority groups, and the poor are affected adversely because disparities in income and education levels are associated with differences in the occurrence of illness and death. Higher incomes result in enhanced access to health care, better housing, and safer neighborhoods and increase the opportunity to engage in health-promoting behaviors. Health disparities experienced by members of ethnic minority groups are hypothesized to be the outcome of a set of complex interactions among genetic variations, environmental factors, and specific health behaviors (U.S. Department of Health and Human Services, 2000). Ensuring the cultural competence of all health care workers and increasing the diversity among health care professionals are key strategies that could address some of these inequalities.

Diversity includes consideration of numerous characteristics, such as gender, race, ethnicity, social class, religion, and sexual orientation (The Sullivan Commission, 2004, p. 48). From its beginnings the United States has struggled with the ways that values and value conflicts relate to diversity. The U.S. health care delivery system was conceived within a Eurocentric model that originally excluded nonwhite patients and providers. The civil rights movement of the 1960s eventually ended the more visible racial and ethnic barriers, but it did not eliminate entrenched patterns of inequality in health care. Historically, racial and ethnic minorities have always been underrepresented in the health professions in America (Byrd & Clayton, 2002). The current shift in U.S. demographics has proved more effective in promoting a multicultural society than the institutional summons for cultural equity. The realities of the demographics of the future mandate greater attention to embracing and celebrating diversity in American communities.

As this nation debates issues of equal access, opportunity, and representation, the chosen course of action takes on a more serious urgency in the twenty-first century. The growth in the number of ethnic minority groups is reshaping the composition of future student pools and the labor force in the United States. In this new millennium, ethnic minorities are expected to compose an estimated 28.2% of the U.S. population and to increase to 37% in the year 2025 (U.S. Census Bureau, 1999). The increasing numbers of ethnic minorities will continue to create social and political changes throughout society, particularly in health care, where demands on the financing and delivery systems will increase to equalize the health status between minorities and the majority population.

Nursing schools have the highest proportion of underrepresented minority students of any health professions except for public health (Grumbach, Coffman, Rosenoff, & Munoz, 2001). Between 1991 and 2003 the number of students from underrepresented minority populations enrolled in baccalaureate nursing programs rose 44%. This increase may be attributed to many factors, including targeted recruitment efforts of nursing schools, strong advocacy from minority nursing organizations, and increased federal funding for programs aimed at diversifying the nursing workforce (The Sullivan Commission, 2004, p. 58).

The representation of American Indians in the nursing student population has changed little over the past 10 years with an increase of only 0.1% in baccalaureate, master's, and doctoral programs. In 2003, African Americans accounted for 10.7% of nursing graduates, whereas Hispanic (5.3%), Asian (4.6%), and American Indian (0.9%) nurses accounted for almost 11% of all baccalaureate nursing graduates (American Association of Colleges of Nursing, 2001). Approximately 2.2 million nurses are employed in the U.S. health care system. Although African Americans, Hispanics, Asian Americans, and American Indians represent more than 30% of the U.S. population, their total representation in the nursing profession is slightly more than 12% (Institute of Medicine, 2004). Data from the Health Resources and Services Administration (2001) show that in 2000, African-American registered nurses composed 4.9% of all registered nurses; Hispanics, 2.0%; Asian/Pacific Islanders, 3.7%; and American Indian/Alaskan Natives, 0.5%. Thus the proportion of ethnic minorities in the nursing profession and those entering the profession still falls short of the proportion of minorities in the total U.S. population. Continued efforts need to focus on identifying obstacles to nursing careers and to enhance access to nursing education for underrepresented ethnic minority students.

To address the question of why nursing is not more diversified, this chapter examines the complexity of racism in American social history and the educational environment in which nursing professionals learn and develop. The point being debated is whether nursing will take action to bring about systemic change that will address the scarcity of minorities in the profession or whether it will remain a passive witness to the demographic changes taking place in social and academic systems.

HISTORICAL AND SOCIAL CONTEXT

American society is characterized by a delicate interplay between equity and inequity. Evidence of a national policy based on supremacist ideologies and practices can be identified from the time of establishment of the Thirteen Colonies. From its beginnings the United States enlisted its educational institutions as tools for shaping and preserving cultural homogeneity or the Anglo-Saxon conception of righteousness (Bessent, 1997).

The support of legalized discrimination remained until the mid-twentieth century with laws that kept people of color from equal access and participation in education and employment. As with early medical and dental professions, African Americans also faced overt racial barriers to entry into the nursing profession. Nursing schools in the northern United States maintained quota limits for "colored" students, and Southern schools barred them completely. When national registration for nurses was established in 1903, Southern states routinely banned black nurses from licensing examinations. Black nurses routinely were paid lower salaries than their white counterparts, and as a group

they did not enter hospital duty in any significant numbers until the 1960s (Hine, 1989).

In 1916 the American Nurses Association instituted a formal policy of only accepting nurses through their state associations. Consequently, in states with associations that excluded blacks, as they did in 16 Southern states and the District of Columbia, blacks could not become members of the national association. As a result, black nurses began organizing their own societies. African-American health care professionals, including nurses, shared the common problem of exclusion from the health care system well into the second half of the twentieth century (Hine, 1989).

The 1964 Civil Rights Act led to legislative, executive, and judicial influences that placed pressure on corporations and universities to increase the participation rates of underrepresented minority groups. The policy of affirmative action directed federal contractors to take measures designed to achieve nondiscrimination. Affirmative action aims to encourage aggressive means to overcome the negative effects of past discrimination in employment and college admission practices. Affirmative action is a controversial measure that continues to be challenged to this day. The main debate regarding affirmative action efforts is that they unduly may burden other groups or have the potential for "reverse discrimination." Opponents of affirmative action assert that preferential treatment and other remedies result in the selection of unqualified individuals.

In addition to the few studies that have provided credible and convincing evidence that affirmative action is beneficial to students, higher education institutions, and society, the 2003 Supreme Court ruling on the affirmative action policies of the University of Michigan is the strongest legal decision in support of affirmative action measures. This landmark Michigan decision upheld the practice of using race and ethnicity-conscious admissions and lifted the legal cloud over affirmative action. Of critical importance was how the business community came together in unprecedented support of the affirmative action policies of the university. In the court briefs the companies and corporations emphasized that workforce diversity is imperative for business success in the increasingly diverse and interconnected global markets. In particular, diversity in higher education was identified as critical for the development of skills necessary to participate and compete in the global economy. The ability to work with and build consensus with diverse individuals is an outcome of learning environments that bring together different points of views and foster new models of creative thinking and problem solving.

For the health professions the main benefits of a diverse workforce is the consumers' enhanced access to health care providers of their own racial or ethnic background, a privilege enjoyed disproportionately by white Americans. Several studies show strong evidence that minority practitioners are significantly more likely than their white counterparts to serve in minority and medically underserved communities (Solomon, Williams, & Sinkford, 2001; Stinson & Thurston, 2002).

At its core the discussion of diversity in the formulation of social policy calls upon us to revisit questions about sensitivity, knowledge, and skills needed for constructive relations among people who are different, and the principles that underlie a just and democratic society. The gift that diversity gives is the insistent invitation to ask hard questions about what nurses mean by access and opportunities for education, how nurses teach, which persons should be included as students and teachers, and what nurses are accomplishing in schools and universities. The next section offers a focused discussion of the image of nursing and the misunderstanding of the practice of nursing.

THE IMAGE OF NURSING

Minority populations, as well as the population at large, are poorly informed about careers in nursing. They have inaccurate perceptions about the contributions and roles of nurses in the health care delivery system. The findings of a study that explored young adult perceptions of nursing indicate that their impressions bear little resemblance to the actual responsibilities of nurses and career opportunities that the nursing profession offers. Study participants indicated that nursing continues to be associated with activities such as "bedpans and making beds" and that most choose other professions instead (Dower, McRee, Briggance, & O'Neil, 2001). Many aspects of nursing such as a commitment to helping others, working with cutting-edge technology, relative professional autonomy and flexibility, and a wide variety of career options within the field could be used effectively to attract potential nurses into the profession.

The concept that minority parents hold negative views of nursing has received limited attention in the nursing literature. The University of California Center for the Health Professions is one of the few organizations that has included this variable in its investigations of barriers to minority representation in nursing. Dower et al. (2001) tested the theory that parents of Hispanic and Asian/Pacific Islander ancestry discourage their daughters from entering nursing because of the poor reputation this career has in their countries. The study findings offered only limited support for this assumption. Family circumstances, including acculturation to U.S. norms, family knowledge about career options and educational pathways, and socioeconomic status mediate this notion. For families within these minority groups who are "close" to their home cultures (less acculturated), perceptions of nursing as a career are influenced by the status and work conditions of nursing in their countries. Families who are familiar with the stability, benefits, and respect associated with nursing and other skilled health professions in the United States do not discourage their daughters from pursuing this career. Level of acculturation and knowledge about career options, therefore, may outweigh any cultural bias among these ethnic minority communities.

More attention is being paid in the literature to the need to familiarize students early on in their school years with opportunities to get to know health professionals personally in order to understand better what it is like to be a nurse, a doctor, or a dentist, and what it takes to get there. Evans (2003) reported on a project that used qualitative research methodology to produce a recruitment film to attract Indian and Hispanic students into baccalaureate nursing programs. The main aim of the film was to empower minority individuals and communities by demonstrating that American Indians and Hispanics can become successful nurses. The film also attempts to enhance the cultural competence and appreciation for diversity of other nursing students and nurse educators.

An approach to disseminating accurate and up-to-date information on nursing careers to young adults is for schools of nursing to develop and participate in summer intern programs. These programs can provide young adults direct contact with nursing environments, thus improving the knowledge of college-bound junior high and high school students about the nursing profession. The opportunity to interact personally with practicing nurses, faculty, and nursing students has the potential to influence more favorable opinions about nursing. Such interaction demonstrates to the participants and other minority and underrepresented students that come in contact with nurses that nurses do important work, are respected by other health professionals and patients, use scientific information, and receive competitive salaries. The participation of minority alumni and current students in these early academic recruitment strategies provides needed role models, in addition to access to program information. The critically important benefit to the use of minority nursing student recruiters is that many potential applicants would like to know "what it is like to be a student at your institution," and this is particularly important to minority applicants. Adequate financial and personnel resources are required to ensure the implementation and evaluation of innovative recruitment approaches. Stipends should be provided for students who participate in summer programs to replace lost summer earnings and to encourage students to enroll.

The diversity of career opportunities available to women is affecting enrollment in nursing schools negatively. How can nurses view this as a negative outcome? Diversity of opportunities brings an end to years of oppression and inequality for women. The feminists' profession of nursing needs to support the progress of women while directing efforts to improve the image of nursing. The design of nursing programs that are creative and flexible and that reflect the needs of nontraditional and emerging majority students will bring more diverse individuals into the nursing profession. The infrastructure necessary for the recruitment and retention of the changing pool of candidates is addressed next.

BARRIERS TO RECRUITMENT

Studies point to multiple reasons why underrepresented minority group members do not pursue nursing, including role stereotypes, economic barriers, inadequate primary and secondary school preparation and counseling, a lack of mentors, gender bias, lack of direction from early authority figures, misunderstanding about the practice of nursing, and increased opportunities in other fields (American Association of College of Nursing, 2001). The barriers specific to the nursing education system include high costs, lack of articulation between allied/auxiliary training and nursing education, overreliance on standardized testing in the admission process, unsupportive institutional cultures, and limited adult education options (Dower et al., 2001; The Sullivan Commission, 2004). Box 59-1 provides a comprehensive list of barriers to college education for minorities. Thus the questions to be considered, knowing as much as nurses do, are Why is there such little sustained progress in increasing the number of minorities in nursing? and Why isn't nursing more diversified?

Recruitment Approaches

Increasing the ethnic diversity in the health care workforce has been identified by government, professional nursing, and community groups as a means of enabling

---

BOX 59-1

Barriers to College Education for Minorities

Negative perceptions of nursing
Inadequate secondary school preparation and counseling
Cultural/environmental barriers
Fewer successful role models
Cost of higher education
Limited access to higher education information
Lack of familiarity with the college admission process
Restrictive admission criteria
Perceived and actual racial biases

---

access to culturally appropriate health care (American Association of Colleges of Nursing, 2001; The Sullivan Commission, 2004). Current nursing literature offers little help in identifying effective approaches to recruitment and retention of minority students, and few studies have focused on assessing the effectiveness of such programs (Health Resources and Services Administration, 2000). Many schools are relying exclusively on traditional recruitment efforts such as open houses, personal contacts with faculty and alumni, and distribution of brochures at career fairs and conferences.

The changing economic, social, and demographic conditions in the United States are reshaping the composition of student pools. Research indicates a serious disconnect between the attributes, values, goals, and orientation of students and the nursing profession. Ernst (2000) found that tomorrow's workers hold the following values and orientation: (1) immediacy (managing and moving multiple pieces of information quickly using high technology); (2) independence (autonomy and latitude to feel productive and fulfilled); (3) work-life balance; (4) social responsibility (at the community and individual levels); (5) flexibility (regarding time at work translating to job sharing and telecommuting); and (6) diversity. The incompatibility with nursing in its present form is clear. Increasingly across the nation the potential pools for health professions schools are ethnically diverse and nontraditional students (older, studying part-time, working and supporting families). What are their goals and values? What are educators and employers doing to understand and meet these goals and values? Why are some members of these pools choosing, or being directed into, one career over another?

The Sullivan Report *Missing Persons: Minorities in the Health Professions* (2004) examined the causes of minority underrepresentation in the health professions and offered detailed recommendations based on three principles: (1) to increase diversity in the health professions, the culture of health professions schools must change; (2) new and nontraditional paths to the health professions should be explored; and (3) commitments must be at the highest levels of government and in the private sector. The commission addressed the need to review and enhance health professions schools admission policies to enable a more holistic, individualized screening process. The use of attributes that help determine an applicant's suitability for health professions education was recommended; among them are motivation/goals, maturity/perseverance, social support structure, experience with diverse populations, leadership experience, and letters of recommendation.

Reports from various governmental and private agencies are calling for reform of professional nursing education that could have a significant impact in fostering a larger and more diverse nursing workforce (Dower et al., 2001; The Sullivan Commission, 2004). The most often cited recommendation is for baccalaureate colleges and health professions schools to provide and support "bridging programs" that enable graduates of 2-year colleges to succeed in the transition to 4-year colleges. Graduates of 2-year community college nursing programs should be encouraged (and supported) to enroll in baccalaureate degree-granting nursing programs. The percentage of individuals who enter nursing with an associate's degree in nursing may be as high as 60%, and only 17% of these graduates go on to complete baccalaureate or higher degrees (The Sullivan Commission, 2004, p. 77). The Sullivan Commission supports the belief that community colleges represent a valuable resource for recruiting minority students to 4-year colleges and health professions schools.

Another promising source of future nurses that has been identified in the literature is allied and auxiliary health care workers and other types of second-career individuals. The advanced practice beyond the level of registered nurse has developed well, but considerable work needs to be done in developing the career pathways that can capture and track new employees from care assistant types of roles into professional nursing practice. These career paths should consider the need to incorporate education components at the work site. In addition, nursing schools should facilitate distance learning opportunities to enrollment and completion of educational programs. In the past few years the number of schools that are implementing accelerated bachelor of science in nursing and master's entry programs for college graduates with nonnursing degrees has increased dramatically. The controversy that surrounded the development and implementation of these programs when they were first established has been resolved by reports of their success in enrolling and graduating diverse, highly qualified nurses (Boylston, Peters, & Lacey, 2004; Rodgers & Healy, 2002; Shiber, 2003).

The high costs of health profession education pose a formidable barrier for students of underrepresented minorities, who are more likely to come from low-income groups. Data on costs and debts related to nursing education are not gathered routinely. However, preliminary data from the National League for Nursing indicate that for 1990-1991 and 2000-2001, the tuition for public and private registered nurse programs nearly doubled (Smedley, Butler, & Bristow, 2004). Evidence is increasing that the type of financial aid available may influence enrollment in college for low-income students. Grants were shown to influence enrollment greatly; however, loans were not linked with increased rates of enrollment for this group (Grumbach et al., 2002). The Sullivan Commission (2004) reached the consensus that unattached scholarships—not loans—should be a major mechanism for financing education for ethnic minority students and a major strategy to increasing diversity among the health professions. Federal and state loan forgiveness programs should be implemented widely, with priority for low-income students who are dedicated to caring for underrepresented minorities.

Organizational commitment to achieve diversity in the health professions must include the highest leadership levels of chancellor, university president, and deans. Their leadership is required in developing and implementing new policies and procedures that can change the cultures and attitudes that have promoted and sustained homogeneity in the health professions. Minimal attention has been given to considering educational system changes or adjustments required to develop culturally based recruitment and retention strategies. Health professions schools should have senior program managers who oversee recruitment and retention strategies to (1) enhance diversity, (2) assess the institutional environment for diversity, and (3) provide diversity training to students, faculty, and staff. Effective recruitment efforts need to respond to changes in American society and the nursing profession by enhancing access for an increasingly broader range students and by developing academic structures, policies, and practices that can accommodate differences in cultural values. Leadership beyond the institutional level is also essential. Professional organizations and federal and state agencies need to promulgate guidelines, set standards and regulations, and develop other strategies for promoting cultural competency and diversity within the health professions.

Barriers to Retention

Successful recruitment is ultimately a failure if the applicants do not gain admission, are not provided with enriching academic and personal experiences, and fall short of graduation. Most of the factors related to low retention rates among minorities enrolled in schools of nursing can be grouped under three categories: personal, environmental/cultural, and academic/system. Box 59-2 lists the major factors related to retention as reported in the literature.

Personal Factors. A theme that has emerged as an obstacle to retention involves the lack of academic preparation. Many minority students are first-generation college students, and they and their families are unprepared to understand the challenges and rigors of higher education. They are unprepared for the amount of study required in college courses, and lack good study habits (Abriam-Yago, 2002). Heller (2002) described an aggressive precollege education project launched by the

BOX 59-2

Major Factors Related to Retention Among Minority Students in Schools of Nursing

PERSONAL
Self-efficacy
Determination
Study skills
Grade point average
Language proficiency
Precollege education

ACADEMIC
Lack of faculty support
Unavailability of mentors
Lack of program flexibility
Inadequate academic services
Lack of financial aid
Devalued cultural perspectives
Lack of peer support
Pressures to conform

CULTURAL/ENVIRONMENTAL
Family support
Family responsibilities
Hours of employment
Disconnect between attributes, values, and
    orientation of students and nursing profession

University of Maryland School of Nursing. The program is a partnership with middle schools, high schools, and community colleges to encourage enrollment in professional nursing education. The School of Nursing provides mentorship, training, leadership development, and college preparatory opportunities for ethnic minority students in underserved areas of Baltimore. This innovative, community-based initiative is designed specifically to provide college-bound youth with the tools and resources they need for academic success in 4-year university nursing programs. Informational sessions with high school guidance counselors focused on educational and career aspects of nursing are another integral part of the program.

Other personal factors that should be investigated further are perseverance and self-determination. A study that identified the barriers and bridges to educational mobility of Hispanics in nursing described the participants who succeeded in obtaining nursing education as having inner strength, power, and determination (Villarruel, Canales, & Torres, 2001). A qualitative study of minority nurses' experiences in nursing education resulted in many recollections of painful experiences of discrimination and racism. The themes and patterns that emerged are illustrative of concepts such as determination, endurance, and self-efficacy (Evans, 2003). These attributes of resilience are necessary for the minority student to gain access and successfully cope in majority white institutions.

The literature on the lack of diversity within nursing is limited, and a classic article by Barbee (1993), though dated, is worth considering. Barbee stated that minority nursing students and nurses are acutely and chronically aware of racism in the profession and in health care generally. Minority individuals in nursing spend much time and energy combating institutional discrimination and racism, whereas a segment of European-American nurses spend as much time and energy denying that racism exists. Until nursing schools are transformed into educational systems that welcome and celebrate diversity, minority students may need to rely on characteristics of personal strengths almost exclusively.

Environmental/Cultural Factors. Increasingly, the family environment has been addressed as an important factor influencing academic achievement and retention. Environmental barriers may include family members who discourage aspirations for college education, family responsibilities such as child care, and the need to negotiate day-to-day transactions for relatives with limited English proficiency. Paradoxically, family environment also has been described as a facilitator to educational mobility. Minority students have described the importance of having the encouragement and support of parents, siblings, husbands, and friends (Villarruel et al., 2001). The stress of having to balance full- or part-time employment with school and home responsibilities also has been identified as a major barrier to success in nursing school (Furr & Elling, 2002; Hurd, 2000; Villarruel et al., 2001).

Academic System Factors. The campus climate/ environment embraces the culture, habits, decisions, practices, and policies of the educational institution. Academic and social adjustment to the college environment has been identified as a central theme in the attrition rate among ethnic minority students (Childs, Jones, Nugent, & Cook, 2004; Hurd, 2000). The most often cited barriers to retention are faculty attitudes and inadequacies in meeting minority students' needs, lack of minority faculty to serve as role models and mentors, lack of financial aid, and a failure of nursing education programs to integrate diverse cultural values, attributes, and orientations in their curricula. Dower et al. (2001) report difficulty in the ability of nursing students to reconcile their cultural values and beliefs with those of the nursing profession. European-American values of individualism, self-confidence, and straightforwardness are powerful influences in the development of nursing school curricula and grading criteria. Ethnically diverse students are likely to espouse values related to mutual interdependence and a group versus individual focus, along with a preference for smooth interpersonal relations, cooperation, tolerance, and accommodation of others. A curriculum that pointedly ignores the contributions and the lifestyle of a significant part of its population contributes to the belief that anything nurses know about diverse groups is knowledge about a subculture or deviant nonnorm behavior. This disconnect in the embedded structure of beliefs, values, attitudes, and symbols points out the degree of institutionalized racism in nursing education. The reason why white nursing faculty and students likely would deny that racism exists in nursing education is their belief that racism is an individual attribute rather than a deeply imbedded attitude in the profession and in American society (Barbee & Gibson, 2001).

Retention Strategies

Few institutions establish programs that meet the needs of minority students, and those that do are poorly funded and receive low priority. Most minority recruitment and retention programs are viewed as temporary, time-limited

obligations or as the concerns of specific, committed individuals and as such are not an institutional obligation (Andrews, 2003; Barbee & Gibson, 2001). The lack of a critical mass of minority students, a lack of academic support services, a lack of mentor programs, and the lack of a culture of diversity perpetuate the status quo of nursing education, and the homogeneity of the nursing profession.

A critical aspect of changing institutional climate and culture is increasing the number of minority faculty and administrators. Their presence enhances the minority students' bonds with the institution and demonstrates to all students that minorities can serve in leadership roles, thus providing a basis for future acceptance and expectation. Therefore the examination of campus culture also must include an evaluation of its hiring and recruitment policies.

The literature has identified that effective retention programs must provide peer and faculty mentoring, advising, academic support, and cultural awareness in an environment that celebrates diversity (Childs et al., 2004; Heller, 2002). However, few nursing studies have addressed the issue of retention of disadvantaged minority students, and there has been little effort to document the outcomes of retention approaches. This inertia, or at best lip service to diversity, without deep-rooted commitment to developing and evaluating a plan of action to enhance diversity in nursing education, practice, and leadership will prove catastrophic in view of the rapid demographic changes occurring in American society.

SUMMARY

The complex personal, academic, and environmental/ cultural factors related to the lack of diversity in nursing deserve the immediate collaboration of educators, researchers, practitioners, and students of all races and ethnic groups. The significant discrepancies between the racial and ethnic profile of the general population and that of the nursing profession easily lead one to focus on the question "Why isn't nursing more diversified?" However, this perspective may produce no more than the sugar coating of traditional recruitment and retention approaches. These types of marketing approaches do not include a critical analysis of key cultural concepts and their value to nursing education or their impact on potential minority applicants. A more valuable perspective for serious reform is to ask "How can we directly and intentionally deal with institutional racism in nursing?" "How can we integrate the diverse values, beliefs, and attributes of the potential pool of minority nursing students into nursing curricula?" and "How do we increase diversity in nursing?"

REFERENCES

Abriam-Yago, K. (2002). Mentoring to empower. Retrieved January 5, 2005 from http://www.minoritynurse.com/features/undergraduate/05-29-02a.html

American Association of Colleges of Nursing. (2001). *Effective strategies for increasing diversity in nursing programs* [Issue bulletin]. Washington, DC: Author.

Andrews, D. R. (2003). Lessons from the past: Confronting past discriminatory practices to alleviate the nursing shortage through increased professional diversity. *Journal of Professional Nursing, 19*(5), 289-294.

Barbee, E. L. (1993). Racism in nursing. *Medical Anthropology Quarterly, 7*(4), 346-362.

Barbee, E. L., & Gibson, S. E. (2001). Our dismal progress: The recruitment of non-whites into nursing. *Journal of Nursing Education, 40*(6), 243-244.

Bessent, H. (1997). Closing the gap: Generating opportunities for minority nurses in American health care. In H. Bessent (Ed.), *Strategies for recruitment, retention, and graduation of minority nurses in colleges of nursing*. Washington, DC: American Nurses Publishing.

Boylston, M. T., Peters, M. A., & Lacey, M. (2004). Adult student satisfaction in traditional and accelerated RN-to-BSN programs. *Journal of Professional Nursing, 20*(6), 23-32.

Byrd, W. M., & Clayton, L. (2002). *An American health dilemma* (Vol. 2). New York: Routledge.

Childs, G., Jones, R., Nugent, K. E., & Cook, P. (2004). Retention of African-American students in baccalaureate nursing programs: Are we doing enough? *Journal of Professional Nursing, 20*(2), 129-133.

Dower, C., McRee, T., Briggance, B., & O'Neil, E. (2001). *Diversifying the nursing workforce: A California imperative*. San Francisco: California Workforce Initiative at the University of California—San Francisco, Center for the Health Professions.

Ernst, C. T. (2000, Summer). Continuity through conversation: A voice for generation X. *Human Issues in Management,* pp. 20-25.

Evans, B. C. (2003). The spirit, that thing inside: Using qualitative research techniques to produce a recruitment film for Hispanic/Latino and American Indian students. *Nursing Education Perspectives, 24*(5), 230-237.

Furr, S. R., & Elling, T. W. (2002). African American students in a predominantly white university: Factors associated with retention. *College Student Journal, 36,* 188-202.

Grumbach, K., Coffman, J., Munoz, C., Rosenoff, E., Gandara, P., & Sepulveda, E. (2002). *Strategies for improving the diversity of the health professions*. San Francisco: University of California—San Francisco, Center for California Health Workforce Studies.

Grumbach, K., Coffman, J., Rosenoff, E., & Munoz, C. (2001). Trends in underrepresented minority participation in health professions schools. In Institute of Medicine, *The right thing to do, the smart thing to do: Enhancing diversity in health professions. Summary of the symposium on diversity in health professions in honor of Herbert W. Nickens, M.D.* (pp. 185-207). Washington, DC: National Academy Press.

Health Resources and Services Administration. (2000). *A national agenda for nursing workforce: Racial/ethnic diversity*. Rockville, MD: National Advisory Council on Nurse Education and Practice.

Health Resources and Services Administration. (2001). The registered nurse population: National sample survey of registered nurses—March 2000. Cited in *Changing demographics: And the implications for physicians, nurses, and other health workers*. Spring 2003. Retrieved January, 4, 2005, from http://www.bhpr.hrsa.gov/healthworkforce/reports/changedemo/Content.htm#3.3

Heller, B. R. (2002). Strategies for increasing student diversity in schools of nursing: Lessons learned. *Hispanic Health Care International, 1*(2), 68-70.

Hine, D. (1989). *Black women in white: Racial conflict and cooperation in the nursing profession 1890-1950*. Bloomington: Indiana University Press.

Hurd, H. (2000). Staying power: Colleges work to improve retention rates. *Black Issues in Higher Education, 17*(18), 42-46.

Institute of Medicine. (2004). *In the nation's compelling interest: Ensuring diversity in the health-care workforce* (B. D. Smedley, A. S. Butler, & L. R. Bristow, Eds.). Washington, DC: The National Academies Press.

Rodgers, M. W., & Healy, P. F. (2002). Integrating master's-level entry education into an established BS and MS program. *Journal of Professional Nursing, 18*(4), 190-195.

Shiber, S. M. (2003). A nursing education model for second-degree students. *Nursing Education Perspectives, 24*(3), 135-138.

Smedley, B. D., Butler, A. S., Bristow, L. R. (Eds.). (2004). *In the nation's compelling interest: Ensuring diversity in the health care workforce*. Retrieved November 22, 2004, from http://www.nap.edu/books/030909125X.html/

Solomon, E. S., Williams, C. M., & Sinkford, J. C. (2001). Practice location characteristics of black dentists in Texas. *Journal of Dental Education, 65*(6), 571-574.

Stinson, M. H., & Thurston, N. K. (2002). Racial matching among African American and Hispanic patients and physicians. *Journal of Human Resources, 38*(2), 411-428.

The Sullivan Commission. (2004). *Missing persons: Minorities in the health professions. A report of the Sullivan Commission on diversity in the healthcare workforce*. Retrieved December 12, 2004, from http://admissions.duhs.duke.edu/sullivan-commission/documents/Sullivan_Final_Report_000.pdf

U.S. Census Bureau. (1999). *Tables: Resident population of the United States: Estimates by sex, race, and Hispanic origin with median age; resident population of the United States: Middle Series Projections*

2015-2030, by sex, race, and Hispanic origin, with median age. Retrieved October 1, 2004, from http://www.census.gov

U.S. Department of Health and Human Services. (2000). *Healthy People 2010: With understanding and improving health and objectives for improving health* (2nd ed., 2 vols.). Washington, DC: U.S. Government Printing Office.

Villarruel, A. M., Canales, M., & Torres, S. (2001). Bridges and barriers: Educational mobility of Hispanic nurses. *Journal of Nursing Education, 40*(6), 245-251.

Minority Representation in Nursing

*Is Cultural Competency in Nursing
Achievable and When?*

PATRICIA T. CASTIGLIA

Questions concerning the achievability of cultural competency in nursing persist as nurses enter the twenty-first century. How do nurses not only encourage cultural diversity but also actually achieve it in a profession that continues to exhibit homogeneity? In all the health care professions, but especially in nursing, the demographics do not reflect the demographics of the general population of the United States. Should they reflect this? Is this a real and necessary attainment? If so, how do nurses encourage and retain minority people in nursing? Would a more accurate interpretation of minority representation be based on local and regional population statistics? For example, is it more reasonable to expect a greater number of Hispanic nurses in the Southwest than in the Midwest? Might there be other minority groups in those regions who are not being represented and who are the real minority? In other words, if a minority group becomes the majority group, who then becomes the minority, and how do nurses address their needs?

Where minority representation is small, can educated, culturally competent nurses be successful in administering holistic health care by virtue of their knowledge regardless of their individual culture, race, or ethnicity? If one geographical area has a small minority representation, will nurses in this area be able to give culturally competent nursing care when they do encounter persons of minority status? These same questions have been asked and addressed in the literature since the 1980s. Many individual nursing programs have instituted measures to try to address the recruitment of minorities, the retention of those students, and the education of all students in developing competency in nursing. Competency must include the constructs of culture and diversity. The Sullivan Commission (2004) identified three characteristics for racial and ethnic diversity in

the workforce. First, all racial and ethnic groups from the community must be represented. Second, incorporation of varied skills, talent, and ideas from those groups must be systemwide. Third, at all levels of an organization (institution) a sharing of professional development opportunities, resources, responsibilities, and power must occur (pp. 13-14).

Clearly, some improvements have been made over the last 40 years, but not enough. A review of the literature indicates few recent publications dealing with cultural diversity in nursing but many addressing the nursing shortage. Is the nursing shortage the only reason one should consider minority representation in nursing? Definitely not, but the shortage at least has made nursing administrators in practice and academia recognize the importance of diversity if nurses are to maintain quality nursing care. That minorities are better represented in nursing today than they were 10 years ago is true. True also is that representation is not at the level it should be.

Nursing education programs are challenged by these facts as they strive to prepare graduates for a comprehensive health care system. Graduates must master core competencies for practice, including developing effective interpersonal relationships. Language and cultural barriers are well recognized as able to create misunderstandings that may result in ineffective health care practice and treatment. Despite this recognition, the impact of culture has not always been incorporated into practice by nursing education programs as reflected in recruitment and retention strategies. Since 1990, affirmative action programs, many of which began in the 1960s, have been a subject of considerable continuous and escalating debate. Civil rights protests, including marches on Washington, D.C., in the 1960s, did much to formulate more proactive policies to assist members of minority groups into schools and positions formerly closed to them. Once again nurses are addressing these issues with the optimistic belief that things will change in relation to the representation of persons of minority status in nursing. Why is this important? In writing this chapter, now for the fourth consecutive edition of this book, I find minority representation in nursing to be important. Not only must nurses address this issue, but also nurses must find workable solutions so that future nurses can provide quality, competent nursing care designed to consider and meet the needs of the diverse population. "We hold these truths to be self-evident, that all men are created equal"—the Declaration of Independence recognizes diversity and it is the nurses' responsibility to ensure that diversity is valued.

DIVERSITY IN THE GENERAL POPULATION

The U.S. Census 2000 report indicates a total U.S. population of 281.4 million. Of that number, 77.1% reported themselves to be white; 13%, black; 13.3%, Hispanic; 4.4%, Asians and Pacific Islanders; 1.5%, American Indian and Alaska Native; and 0.43%, Arab (de la Cruz & Brittingham, 2003; Greico, 2001; McKinnon, 2003; Ogunwole, 2002; Ramirez & de la Cruz, 2003; Reeves & Bennett, 2003). Although data on race have been collected since 1790, the 2000 census was the first to offer the ability for persons to identify themselves as belonging to more than one race if they desired to do so.

The 2000 census is also the first time that the U.S Census Bureau has reported on the Arab population. This is also historically important because it legitimizes the people of Arab descent as a recognized minority group. The designation of Arab includes persons with ancestries originating from Arabic-speaking countries or areas of the world usually categorized as Arab. Data on ancestry was collected first in the decennial census in 1980 but not disseminated in a special report. The U.S. Arab population increased from 0.27% in 1980 to 0.42% in 2000. Of those persons reporting, the greatest increase was in the number of individuals of Egyptian ancestry (de la Cruz & Brittingham, 2003, p. 1).

Other interesting factors emerged from the 2000 census. Persons found to be under 18 years of age were identified as follows: 34.4% Hispanic, 33% black, 26% Asian and Pacific Islander, and 23% non-Hispanic white. Approximately one third of the major minority groups are under 18 years of age compared with almost one fourth of the non-Hispanic white population. In addition, the white population has increased more slowly than the minority populations from 1990 to 2000.

The minimum-maximum range for whites (race alone–race combined) of 5.9% to 8.6% is in contrast to a total population growth of 13.2%. Clearly, this has an effect now and will have an escalating effect on the educational systems, the professions, health care, and political governance in the future.

DIVERSITY ISSUES AND LEGISLATION

The original purpose of affirmative action was to attempt to remedy wrongs done to black/African-American people. The fiftieth anniversary of the Supreme Court decision *Brown v. Board of Education* was marked in 2004. This decision ruled that segregation in public schools was illegal. For the last 10 years, major debate in academia, as in the workplace, has centered on the concept of reverse discrimination; that is, that qualified whites are being denied access to academic programs because they do not have a recognized minority status. The Bakke decision in 1978 (*Regents of the University of California v. Bakke*) endorsed the use of race as one factor in admissions decisions. In the case of Podberesky, a Hispanic student, the U.S. Court of Appeals for the Fourth District ruled that the University of Maryland at College Park had failed to meet the legal tests for offering a minority scholarship. This suit challenged a scholarship for black students at the university, and that decision is the only one at the appellate level that deals with a minority challenge. The ruling stated that past discrimination was not sufficient cause for a race-based remedy and that such discrimination must exert some present effect (Jaschik, 1993). The Adarand decision in June 1995 held that race could be used only for preferential treatment if it can withstand "strict scrutiny" by the federal courts (Michaelson, 1995). As it is interpreted, this decision affects higher education because all colleges and universities are to some extent governed by state and federal civil rights laws in order to receive federal and state money. Therefore strict scrutiny would have a far-reaching effect. In 1996 the Adarand decision was used when the federal Fifth Circuit Court ruled on a suit brought by law students at the University of Texas at Austin regarding preferential treatment given to minority applicants. The ruling on the case, *Hopwood v. U.T. Austin Law School*, stipulated that universities in the Fifth Circuit jurisdiction could not use race or ethnicity as factors in determining admission to the university, to special programs, or for scholarships or financial aid (Kauffman, 1996). Admissions could be made, for example, based on economic disadvantage, bilingual ability, or regional or geographical needs. This legislation meant

VIEWPOINTS

that educational institutions in Texas had to find new or additional ways to continue to improve diversity in their student bodies.

In the case of *Smith v. University of Washington Law School* (2000), the Supreme Court in the process of review discussed five hallmarks of a narrowly tailored affirmative action plan. These hallmarks are (1) the absence of quotas; (2) individualized consideration of applicants; (3) serious, good-faith consideration of race-neutral alternatives to the affirmative action program; (4) that no member of any racial group was unduly harmed; and (5) that the program had a sunset provision or some other end point. Two important recent cases involving the University of Michigan were decided in 2003. In *Grutter v. Bollinger* (2003) the decision was made that the University of Michigan law school did not violate the equal protection clause of the Fourteenth Amendment to the Constitution and that student body diversity justified the use of race in university admissions. The use of race by the law school was not the only criterion used, and the admissions policy of the law school was in accord with the stated goal of the school. Applicants were evaluated individually in relation to stated criteria for admission. These criteria included looking beyond grades and scores to "soft variables." Bonilla-Silva (2003) maintains that Justice O'Connor's opinion in *Grutter v. Bollinger* uses color blindness to perpetuate racial inequality without sounding racist. Color-blind racism is founded on the belief that race no longer matters. Only the most limited use of race in admissions will withstand legal close scrutiny. A review of Bonilla-Silva's book by Walsh (2004, p. 3) concludes that "adherence to color-blind racism in America's highest court may already be stunting the growth of racial progress in the U.S. at a time when racial equality is still an unrealized dream."

The second case, often called that companion case to *Grutter v. Bollinger,* is that of *Gratz v. Bollinger* (2003). This case was filed by an applicant denied admission to the University of Michigan, College of Literature, Science, and the Arts. In this case the policy of the college of admitting by a point system that automatically awarded 20 points to African Americans, Hispanics, and Native Americans was challenged. The court found that this policy violated the equal protection clause of the Fourteenth Amendment because the policy was not tailored narrowly to achieve educational diversity. The decision also stated that the admissions policy did not provide individualized assessment of each characteristic of applicants.

Alexander and Schwarzchild (2004) state that the two racial preference admission policies of the University of Michigan were the perfect basis for Justice O'Connor's decision that rejected transparent racial goals—that is, quotas—and endorsed disingenuous ones. The remaining question was whether affirmative action is a "good" thing. Alexander and Schwarzchild believe it is not. One reason given is that race and ethnicity are arbitrary terms. They further stress that racialism is not the same as racism. Racialism means paying close attention to race and to thinking in racial terms. Racism means thinking some people are less worthy; that is, they deserve less concern or respect solely on the basis of race. These authors state that this presents a danger by diluting admissions, which results in grade inflation and the creation of bogus departments and majors in universities (p. 4). In their opinion, universities are interested in race but not in a diversity of views or backgrounds (p. 6). Their recommendation is that Americans should seek to promote people's common humanity, not their superficial differences (p. 7).

Another case of interest is that of *Smith v. University of Washington Law School* (2004). This case was submitted by the same plaintiffs as in 2000 to appeal the previous judgment of the district court. Three white plaintiffs claimed that they were denied admission to the University of Washington Law School because of the unconstitutional consideration of race and ethnicity for admissions to the law school. Under consideration at this same time was a voter initiative, Initiative 200, which was approved by Washington voters in 1998. Initiative 200 prohibited race-based affirmative action plans; however, the plaintiffs were filing on actions taken in 1994, 1995, and 1996 before the passage of the initiative in 1998. The judgment of the district court in favor of the Law School was upheld. No racial quotas, targets, or goals for admission or enrollment had been established. No damages were awarded.

In California, Proposition 209 was passed and prohibits race-conscious admissions. As a result, black student enrollment at the University of California in 2000 and 2001 was about 20% below the level before this legislation (Walsh, 2004). This differs from the Texas experience after the Hopwood case in which the percentage of minority student was almost the same after 3 years as it had been when the state ended affirmative action programs in 1996. This was purported to be attributable to stronger recruiting efforts and new financial aid programs (Carnevale, 1999). The admission of minority students in Texas was addressed through legislation that offered admission to students in the top 10% of their high school graduating class regardless of their grade point average or results of standardized tests.

This resulted in minority and disadvantaged students in the state having guaranteed admission if in their school they were in the top 10% of the graduating class. An important note is that the University of Texas System currently is considering the development of legislation that would permit the use of race for admissions to health professions schools. Preliminary discussions focused on medical and dental schools, but current discussions have expanded to include other health professions disciplines including nursing.

CULTURAL COMPETENCY IN A RACIST SOCIETY

Many terms have evolved in attempts to recognize and deal with members of a divergent American society. Recognition of these terms as evidence of the struggle to come to grips with "how to manage minorities" is important. This phrasing is deliberate because it almost has seemed that simply by naming it, one can put parameters around it and devise ways to manage it. Terms used over the past 20 years have evolved from *cultural awareness* to *cultural sensitivity* to *cultural competence*. The Sullivan Commission (2004) stated that it was understood for their deliberations that cultural competence is the set of behaviors, attitudes, customs, policies, and resources that come together among professionals that enable them "to work effectively in cross-cultural situations" (p. 16). Other terms that interplay with attempts include *diversity, racial equality, multiculturism, transculturism* (Leininger, 1994), and *racial pluralism*. All of these terms are meant to conjure up an awareness of the experiences of minorities and to decide and act on measures to rectify inequalities. Leininger has been among the most prolific authors in nursing, urging culturally congruent care as one of the highest priorities in nursing. One positive result is seen in Medicare contracts that mandate the ability to offer linguistically and culturally appropriate care as a condition of awards made to managed care institutions (Salimbene, 1999).

The construct of cultural competence has developed because awareness, sensitivity, and cultural knowledge have proved to be insufficient. One must ask why. Of course the task is fraught with many issues that people do not like to discuss or even acknowledge exist. Most "enlightened" Americans blanch at the words *discrimination, prejudice,* and *racism*. Yet members of minority groups frequently use these terms when relating to life experiences. Hence an understanding of the meaning of each term is important. Discrimination occurs when there is unfair treatment of an individual because of some class or categorization without considering the individual's merits. Discrimination often is based on prejudice, which is formed by thoughts, attitudes, insensitivity, and ignorance. A negative form of prejudice is called racism (American Nurses Association, 1998). In an earlier white paper the American Nurses Association (1991, p. 2) established the impact of culture on "perceptions, interpretations, and behaviors of persons in a specific cultural group." Terhune (2004) stated that perceptions, minds, and attitudes must change if diversity is to exist at the sociocultural level. Increased diversity offers increased opportunities to reach this goal and to expand changing realities in the real world to academic settings. Salimbene (1999) made an important distinction when she emphasized that equal care does not mean the same care in a multicultural society. Salimbene further emphasized that providers need to acquire enough cultural information that they will be able to anticipate possible barriers that would affect access to health care and compliance. She identified 10 competencies as essential for cultural competence, including awareness, sensitivity, tolerance, understanding, knowledge, and skills that are culturally relevant. The final criterion is "confidence in one's ability to offer care to patients of other cultures" (p. 31). The 10 competencies developed by Salimbene apply to nursing education and practice. The final criterion for faculty would be "confidence in one's ability to teach nursing students of various cultures the knowledge and skills necessary for nursing competence."

Does racism exist in nursing? Barbee and Gibson (2001) state that a culture of racism indeed exists in nursing education. By this they mean that an embedded structure of beliefs, values, attitudes, and symbols about non-whites is passed on to future generations. Most white people would think this is not true and that any racism is an individual characteristic, not a collective attitude. Overt racism has disappeared, if not completely. Signs prohibiting people of color from places and hangings of blacks are no longer common occurrences. Racism today is indeed more subtle but nonetheless effective. Racism is masked in words, references, and the perpetuation of myths. Yet nursing calls itself the caring profession, which makes it all the more difficult to acknowledge the racism. Dreher and MacNaughton (2002) emphasize that the clinical setting is where the expectation of cultural competency is most crucial. They further maintain that cultural competency is really nursing competency.

Projections of population growth illustrate the growth of minorities in the general population. In fact, many futurists postulate a reversal in minority-majority status for at least certain areas of the country. With this growth in mind, development of an infrastructure for the future that builds upon minority strengths and develops well-educated minority members of communities is important. Nowhere is this more true than in the health care professions.

MINORITY REPRESENTATION IN NURSING AND NURSING EDUCATION

Positions in nursing are increasing at a rate that cannot be met unless some changes occur. The changes necessary include many factors related to professionalism, status, education, and diversity. Interwoven with the issues related to minorities in nursing are a number of issues that reflect societal views toward women, toward subcultures in society, and toward demographic changes that have occurred over time. Nursing can no longer sustain itself without incorporating, to a greater extent, diverse minority groups into the profession. Although the number of men in nursing has increased, the profession remains predominantly female, approximately 94.6% (Spratley, Johnson, Sochalski, Fritz, & Spencer, 2000, p. 8). Therefore gender socialization across cultures has played and continues to play a major role in the continuation and the development of nursing. Stereotypes related to gender and ethnicity cannot be separated artificially when examining the past, present, and future considerations of minorities in nursing.

Basic influences when selecting a career relate to one's beliefs about oneself. Where do I belong or fit? What is an acceptable career from the viewpoint of my family and my social group? Where can I find personal fulfillment? Financial reward? Advancement? Security? Ability to be mobile, yet permanence in a career?

In 2000 there were 2,694,540 registered nurses in the United States (Spratley et al., 2000, p. 8). The number of nurses identifying themselves as belonging to one or more racial minority groups or to the Hispanic/Latino group was 333,318; nearly triple the number in 1980. Minority nurses increased from 7% in 1980 to 12% in 2000 (pp. 8-10). American Indians/Alaska Natives and Asians/Native Hawaiians/Pacific Islanders had the greatest increase in this 20-year period, 197% and 207%, respectively. The number of Hispanic/Latino nurses increased by 164%, and the number of African-American/black nurses increased 119%. These growth rates may be deceiving because the actual numbers remain small. Hispanic nurses, for example, remain the most underrepresented group in relation to the number of Hispanics in the population. Only 2% of the registered

nurse population is Hispanic although Hispanics compose 12.5% of the general population (pp. 10-11).

The National Sample Survey in 2000 disclosed some interesting statistics related to the nursing workforce (Spratley et al., 2000). Minority nurses were more likely to be employed in nursing and to work full-time than white nurses. The majority of registered nurses of Asian/Native Hawaiian/Pacific Islander descent (54.3%) received their basic nursing education in baccalaureate programs. The highest percentages of master's or doctoral degrees were achieved by Native Hawaiians and other Pacific Islanders (16.4%), whereas other groups had the following representation: African American/ black (11.1%) and white (10.4%). The smallest group achieving graduate education was Asian nurses, although they had the largest number of nurses educated at the baccalaureate level (p. 18). In terms of advanced practice, nearly 10% of advanced practice nurses were from minority backgrounds. Of these, most of the respondents were nurse practitioners (11%); 8% to 10% were in other advanced practice roles (p. 22).

The National League for Nursing (2003) survey of registered nurse programs identified the total number of basic registered nurse preparation programs in 2003 as 1444. Of these, 529 were baccalaureate programs; 846, associate's degree programs; and 69, diploma programs. The racial composition in baccalaureate programs was as follows: black, 12.9%; Hispanic, 4.7%; Asian, 4.9%; and American Indian, 0.2%. The racial composition in associate degree programs was almost the same: black, 12.6%; Hispanic, 5.9%; Asian, 4.2%; and American Indian, 1.1%. Diploma programs had fewer minorities in all categories: black, 11.6%; Hispanic, 3.7%; Asian, 4.0%; and American Indian, 0.2%. This may have some relationship to the location of diploma schools or may indicate that potential minority students interested in nursing prefer associate's degree or baccalaureate programs for entrance into the profession. Actually, the figures reported by the National League for Nursing for blacks and Hispanics do mirror closely the figures reported for the general population. For all types of nursing programs, minorities, with the exception of Asians and Pacific Islanders, are represented less than in the general population.

The *2003-2004 Enrollment and Graduations Programs in Baccalaureate and Graduate Programs in Nursing* report (Berlin, Stennett, & Bednash, 2004a) revealed the following data in relation to race/ethnicity: 75.3% of baccalaureate students enrolled are white, 10.4% are black/African American, 4.2% are Hispanic/Latino, 0.6% are American Indian/Alaskan Native, and 4.6% are

Asian/Native Hawaiian/Other Pacific Islander. Whites are the majority in all types of doctoral programs, but a large number of black/African-American nurses are enrolled in clinical-focused doctoral programs. Enrollments for all minority groups increased for the 10-year period of 1993 to 2003 with a total minority increase of 7.2% in baccalaureate programs and 10.4% for master's programs. At the doctoral level the increase for that 10-year period was 6.4% (p. 22). Faculty and academic administrative positions in schools of nursing do not reflect the general population: 91.3% of all deans are white, 5.4% are black, 2.0% are Hispanic, 0.2% are Asian, and 1.2% are Native Hawaiian/Other Pacific Islander. Faculty racial configuration is almost the same: 91.1% white, 5.4% black, 1.8% Hispanic, 0.4% American Indian, 1.6% Asian, and 0.3% Native Hawaiian/Other Pacific Islander (p. 3).

In this chapter in the previous edition, the following questions were posed, and three have been answered. "Are members of minority groups attracted to nursing?" It would appear that the numbers are rising. "Do they successfully complete programs of study?" American Association of Colleges of Nursing data suggest a high completion rate. "Do they remain in the profession?" Yes, they compose the largest number of full-time nurses. The last two questions posed, "Why should we be concerned about the representation, or rather the lack of representation, of significant numbers of minorities in nursing?" and "What directions should we pursue?" remain to be explored further.

Shireman (2003) suggests that the following questions be asked when evaluating recruitment and retention strategies for minorities:

1. Is race alone a factor in nonsuccess, or is it really race combined with another factor such as socioeconomic status, or is socioeconomic status the real factor across all student groups?
2. When concentrating on recruitment strategies, do we concentrate on the high schools with the racial, economic, and cultural profiles where we want to recruit in order to promote diversity? Are we recruiting in the best arenas to achieve our goals?
3. When we analyze our graduates, how many go on to graduate school? Are racial minorities concentrated in certain types of work specialties? Why?
4. What does the curriculum include in relation to diversity, and how explicit is that content? Does the curriculum help students to examine and incorporate their own heritage and traditions into the learning experience? How are students treated? Are they treated in accord with what is taught? Do students indicate that the atmosphere in the classroom is culturally sensitive?
5. Does the faculty complement reflect diversity? Does it reflect the student population? The student population could be different from the community population. What efforts are being made for faculty recruitment of qualified individuals from minority backgrounds?
6. What is the relationship of the school of nursing with the university community, the professional community, and the general community concerning creating a diverse student body? Do minority residents of the community feel welcome to enroll in the school? Do the faculty members visit the local schools, act as resources for them, and work on projects with them?

A final question to add to Shireman's list is, "How is mentoring used?" Is mentoring being confused with advisement programs or, in the case of faculty, with orientation programs? How are mentors selected, and how long do most mentors serve in that capacity?

FACTORS AFFECTING CHANGE IN MINORITY REPRESENTATION

A persistent decline in the number of young persons eligible for college admission has been documented nationwide. Concurrently, the number of older students (those over 25 years of age) who are interested in pursuing college careers, including nursing, has increased. It is imperative that nursing schools strengthen efforts to attract more minority students, including men. "Considering the fact that females comprise about 51 per cent of the population and minority group representation is rapidly approaching 33 percent, today's nursing students do not mirror the nation's population" (American Association of Colleges of Nursing, 2001, p. 1).

Applications to nursing programs recovered from the slump of the 1980s as a result of the compounded impact of the nursing shortage; a lack of access to health care for many Americans; an aging population; a shift in emphasis to primary community health care; cost-containment efforts by hospitals, including the use of diagnostic-related groups; and a movement to break down barriers between the health professions through expanded reimbursement by Medicaid, Medicare, and third-party insurers for specifically prepared nurses. These factors have forced the health care system to upgrade salaries and benefits for nurses. When adequate financial reimbursement occurs in a profession, members of that profession develop an increased sense of self-esteem, and colleagues in other professions develop an increased respect.

As health care moved to a managed care system, downsizing of the number of beds and nursing staff occurred in hospitals. Unfortunately, adequate remuneration has not extended to areas of need beyond hospital settings. Public health nurse salaries, school nurse salaries, and salaries of nurses in extended care facilities still lag. This is a serious manifestation of the blatant lack of provision for quality health care to the poor, to rural and urban underserved and underinsured citizens, and to minority populations and particularly a diminished commitment to health promotion and disease prevention activities.

The question of quality in nursing practice continues to be a factor that must be considered carefully. In the past, nursing schools were tempted to make exceptions to admissions requirements to maintain programs through sustained enrollments. Now the pendulum may swing toward admitting only the most highly qualified applicants in relation to quantitative measures such as American College Test (ACT) scores, Scholastic Aptitude Test (SAT) scores, or grade point average. Because of the increased applicant pool, admissions committees may be tempted to fill classes with only the best students as measured by traditional criteria. If efforts are not made on elementary, middle, and high school levels to prepare minority students better, nurses may find that equal opportunity access has been thwarted and that minority students may suffer because they will not be afforded the opportunity to attempt to succeed.

The recruitment of minorities is being enhanced by a variety of strategies. Professional nursing organizations have developed media campaigns to stimulate interest in nursing. Johnson & Johnson Company has supported a television spot on nursing as a profession. Cues including race and gender are integrated into most of these efforts. Individual nursing schools have developed projects, many of which have been funded. One such project is the Wisconsin Youth in Nursing program designed to introduce middle and high school students of color to college and nursing opportunities. This program is one of the University of Wisconsin–Oshkosh precollege programs. Students are brought to the campus for a 2-week campus experience. Parents visit to see the facility, and students have the opportunity to participate in general education classes and special interest nursing classes (Stewart & Cleveland, 2003).

Traditionally, minority students have been classified as high-risk students because they often experience higher attrition rates than white students. The most frequently used criteria on which admission to nursing is based include grade point average, high school rank, interviews, health data, college grade point average, ACT scores, SAT scores, and autobiographical essays. A number of conflicting studies have been done regarding the usefulness of these criteria for the prediction of success in a nursing program. Those studies were from the 1970s and 1980s and varied in their recommendations but generally favored some quantifiable measure, be it high ACT scores, high SAT scores, or high final high school grade point average. An interesting note, however, is that almost 30 years ago, Schwirian (1977) maintained that less that 50% of attrition really is related to academic difficulty and that attrition rather may be due to greater social and economic disadvantages.

Women have been attracted in increasing numbers to professions other than the traditional occupations of nursing and teaching. The attractiveness of the nursing profession has been enhanced during the past 40 years, however, by the development of new and expanded roles in nursing. These new roles are characterized by increased autonomy and by increased appreciation and recognition from the public and from professional colleagues. Efforts have increased by Sigma Theta Tau International Honor Society and the National Student Nurses' Association to raise the consciousness of the general public and particularly junior high school students to nursing as a profession (Fitzgerald, 2000). Many of these expanded roles require advanced education, often at the master's level. Because many of these roles (nurse practitioner, nurse-midwife, nurse anesthetist, and nurse administrator) do require a graduate degree, many nursing schools have developed "fast track" and "second degree" programs. The intent of these programs is to assist the student in achieving her or his personal goal in as efficacious a manner as possible.

Other strategies nursing schools use include more visibility of men in advertisements, especially in settings perceived as macho (the University of Texas Health Science Center at Houston); marketing diverse opportunities in nursing as represented by ethnically diverse nurses (University of Maryland); reaching potential minority students in areas where they live, such as geographical marketing (Intercollegiate College of Nursing/Washington State University); and providing incentives for bilingual students to pursue nursing and to stay in their own communities (Washington State University). Other efforts center on recruitment beginning at the elementary and middle school levels. Mentoring has proved useful in recruitment and retention. Some schools include sensitivity training for faculty as an integral part of efforts to provide prepared mentors. As always, however, the one-on-one interface determines success. Specialized individualized learning programs such as the Success in Learning: Individualized Pathways Program (SLIPP) at Loma Linda University in Southern California has been successful in recruitment and retention.

The Sullivan Commission report (2004), conducted by the Institute of Medicine of the National Academies and funded by the Kellogg Foundation, suggests that medical lobbies and universities actually are discouraging minority enrollment in many health care fields. Medical, nursing, dental, and other health professions schools were reported as being "chilly" toward minority students and disinterested in diversity. This report focuses on institutional strategies by which students are trained and on policy arenas after they are trained. Schools are directed to look beyond standardized testing for admission and to consider commitment to service, community orientation, leadership, and experience with diverse populations among their criteria for admission. A second commission recommendation is to provide more funding to poorer students and suggests that private funds be used to increase the number of health care professionals in underserved, disadvantaged areas. The third recommendation is an admonition to use more individualized approaches to admissions, and the fourth is to provide money to Latino nursing students in the form of scholarships, loans, and payback programs. The remainder of the report recommendations are (5) focus on retention; (6) use community benefit (the legal term applied to nonprofit hospitals) by actually giving something tangible back to the community; (7) involve accreditation organizations by taking diversity into consideration for accreditation; and (8) aim to produce better doctors not tractable students; that is, students who are easy to teach. The Sullivan Commission report does not ask for new legislation; rather it appeals to the health care professions to apply strategies to further cultural diversity (Stern, 2004).

HISPANIC REPRESENTATION IN HIGHER EDUCATION AND NURSING

In 2002, persons of Hispanic origin could report their origin for the U.S. Census as Mexican, Puerto Rican, Cuban, Central and South American, or some other Latino origin. Hispanics, of course, may be of any race. In 2002, 37.4 million Latinos were in the U.S., representing 33% of the total population. Of these, 66.9% indicated that they were of Mexican heritage, 14.3% were Central and South American, 8.6% were Cuban, and 6.5% were of other Hispanic origin (Ramirez & de la Cruz, 2002).

As might be expected, Hispanics were found to live in the West (44.2%) and in the South (34.8%). Nearly half of all Hispanics live within a metropolitan area (45.6%) (Ramirez & de la Cruz, 2002). Mexicans accounted for the smallest number (23.6%) of those workers employed year-round earning $35,000 annually. Hispanics are more likely to live in poverty and to have larger families and are less likely to graduate from high school. In fact, Hispanics represented 17.7% of all children in the United States but represented 30.4% of all children living at the poverty level (p. 6). Those Hispanics achieving a bachelor's degree were found to be 18.6% Cuban, 17.3% Central and South American, 19.7% other Hispanics, and 7.6% Mexican (p. 5).

Why are Mexican Americans highest in poverty and least well-educated of all Hispanic groups while having the greatest numbers? The answers are compound but not complex: immigration status, discrimination, lack of social and financial support, and an inability to access available resources. Culture certainly may be a factor, especially for women. Family cohesion is an important characteristic of Mexicans. Women (Chicanas) in Mexican society are encouraged to marry and have children. This presents a conflict for Chicanas, many of whom view education as a means to socioeconomic mobility and independence. Dissonance occurs for many of these young women in terms of their expected role in Mexican society as wife, mother, and subservient mate to the man. All of these factors exert an influence to diminish professional career expectations. In addition, Mexican American students often are steered into taking noncollege preparatory courses in high school. This may be promulgated by the family as a means of keeping women in less demanding work, which in turn is perceived as having a less negative impact on the woman's traditional role. Such advice from family members may be reinforced by educators who often stereotype Mexican-American students as unable to prepare for more challenging careers. Most of these students need financial assistance and generally rely heavily on scholarships and work-study programs and, to a lesser extent, on loans. Because of the difference in cultures and the difficulty in acculturation, many of these minority students feel more comfortable in smaller colleges or community colleges. Support systems such as associations and organizations that can recognize, promote, and reinforce cultural values are important for student adjustment regardless of the size of the educational setting. Because emotional support is as important as financial support, it is important to get the parents involved and supportive of the student's college experience. Parents need to view college not as a way to "tear apart" the family but as a way to maintain the family for the future. Supporting the student's academic goals and including the student in family and community activities are ways to strengthen and maintain family bonds. Few schools adequately address this aspect of support.

In 2000, 22% of all 18- to 24-year-old Hispanics were enrolled in colleges and universities; up from 16% in 1980. They composed 10% of total college/university enrollment in contrast to 4% in 1980. Fourteen percent were enrolled in 2-year colleges, and 7% in 4-year colleges/universities (U.S. Department of Education, 2005).

Hispanic Serving Institutions are degree-granting public or private institutions of higher education eligible for Title IV funding because they have a documented Hispanic enrollment of 25% or more full-time undergraduate students. In 1999, one half of all Hispanic student college enrollments (45%) were at Hispanic Serving Institutions compared with 29% in 1990 (U.S. Department of Education, 2005). It would appear that Hispanic Serving Institutions have established infrastructures that positively influence the enrollment and graduation of Hispanic students.

In relation to nursing students in colleges and universities, the American Association of Colleges of Nursing reported a Hispanic enrollment of 5.4% in 552 registered nurse programs in fall 2003 and a 4.6% graduation rate for 552 undergraduate programs from August 1, 2002, to July 31, 2003, with an increase in Hispanic enrollment of 3.1% from 1993 to 2003 (Berlin et al., 2004a, p. 21). At the master's level a modest increase in Hispanic enrollment occurred from 2002 to 2003, 3.7% to 4.2%, but doctoral enrollment remained almost the same in research-focused doctoral programs (2.1% to 2.7%), and a drop occurred in clinically focused doctoral enrollment from 2.9% to 0 (pp. 34-35). A small graduate enrollment for Hispanics may result because when the graduates begin earning money, they have familial expectations for that money or because the graduates "fall back" into the traditional female role once they have completed the baccalaureate.

It would appear self-evident that Hispanic students, like other students, would tend to persist in their education when their parents have higher educations and when parental occupations result in higher incomes. Low family income, for many students, results in dropping out of school. Because Mexican-American families generally have lower incomes and larger or extended family to absorb those incomes, their children are at risk for attrition. Efforts must persist, therefore, to obtain scholarships and grants to attempt to alleviate some of this financial pressure. Perhaps a program similar to that of the U.S. Public Health Service by which the graduate pays back through service could be initiated on a federal or state level. A number of hospitals already have instituted such programs for all nurses, not just Hispanic nurses. In 1991 the Department of Health and Human Services instituted a scholarship program called Scholarships for Disadvantaged Students. These scholarships recognize that the concept of being disadvantaged is not necessarily tied to ethnicity alone but rather is tied to socioeconomic factors including deficits in the ability of a particular school district to offer enriched programs for students.

BLACK REPRESENTATION IN HIGHER EDUCATION AND NURSING

The term *black* has been selected for this edition rather than *African American* because it is the term used more often in current literature. In 2002, 13% (36 million) persons in the United States identified themselves as black, with most of those reporting living in the South (33%). More than half of all blacks (52%) lived in a central city within a metropolitan area (McKinnon, 2003, pp. 1-2). More blacks are under 18 years old than the other designated population groups, and most of these are females (30%). At the other end of the age spectrum, however, only 7% of black males and 9% of black females were found to be 65 years of age or older (p. 2). Clearly, the black population is a young group with a shorter life expectancy than non-Hispanic whites. Contrary to a commonly held belief that blacks do not marry, the 2002 Population Survey indicated that nearly half (48%) of all black families were married couple families (p. 3). The poverty rate for the nation was 12% overall, but 23% of those in poverty were black (p. 6).

In 2000, 31% of 18- to 24-year-old blacks were enrolled in colleges and universities. This was an increase from 19% in 1980. Blacks account for 12% of the student enrollment in 2-year institutions and two thirds of the black enrollment is female (Hoffman, Llagas, & Snyder, 2003). Only 17% of blacks earned at least a bachelor's degree, with black females earning more than black males. In terms of nursing at the baccalaureate level, the American Association of Colleges of Nursing (Berlin et al., 2004a) reported that

12.2% of the total enrollment of 552 nursing programs was black in fall 2003, a 3.1% increase from 1993 to 2003.

From August 1, 2002, to July 31, 2003, 10.7% of the graduates of 555 nursing programs were black. At the master's level, black enrollment almost doubled from 1992 to 2003, from 5.8% to 10.5%. The graduation rate for 2002 to 2003 was 9.1% (Berlin et al., 2004a, p. 21-22). This increased enrollment and graduation is significant because blacks, in terms of general health, tend to be sicker than the general population, and the low number of black nurses presents a barrier to treatment because of the lack of integration of their cultural beliefs, values, and practices. Compliance to treatment has been shown to be affected by cultural values, and there are few black nurses to positively affect the integration of black cultural values.

Nursing education historically has provided one of the few avenues for black women to acquire a respected profession. For many years, however, that education primarily was obtained in black hospitals and colleges. New graduates worked only with black patients. As the nursing profession evolved, an elitist system developed in which most white schools had racial quotas. An early effort to recruit black nursing students was stimulated during World War II by the Cadet Nurse Corps program. Today the emphasis is on attracting black and other minority students, not to fill quotas but to develop a cohort of professional nurses who better represent the general population. Historically, problems with the admission and retention of black nurses have occurred. Between 1976 and 1982 the National Advisory Committee on Black Higher Education and Black Colleges and Universities studied the policies and practices at seven predominantly white universities. Although this committee no longer exists, the problems persist.

Black students, like other minority students, often receive a poor secondary education. Their self-esteem has been low and the university setting generally has been perceived as hostile to them. Not only have high school counselors failed in encouraging black students to pursue higher education, but university counselors have not been able effectively to thwart the feelings of loneliness and alienation that black students frequently experience. As with Hispanic students, the lack of financial resources has proved to be a barrier to a large number of potential black nurses. In addition, blacks are still less likely to complete college than whites but are more likely to graduate than Hispanics (Hoffman et al., 2003, p. 106).

GRADUATE NURSING EDUCATION AND THE MINORITY STUDENT

Minority enrollment in graduate nursing programs consistently has been a small segment of the total enrollment regardless of geographical or population-specific considerations. In 1980 the highest educational level for most nurses was the diploma. Enrollment in diploma programs has declined steadily over the last 20 years. In 2000, 34.3% of all nurses reported that the associate's degree was their highest level of education, and 32.7% indicated that the bachelor's degree was the highest level. Bachelor's degrees for nurses increased at a higher rate than associate's degrees. This was the complete reverse of the pattern in the previous 20 years. The impact of increased numbers of nurses with bachelor's degrees has resulted in the increase of nurses with master's or doctoral degrees. In 1980, 5% of the registered nurse population had graduate degrees; in 2000 that percentage rose to 10% (Spratley et al., 2000, p. 7).

Minority enrollment in graduate nursing programs remains a small segment of the total enrollment. Gains have occurred from 1993 to 2003. Blacks continue to be the largest majority-minority group in nursing. Black enrollment rose from 5.8% to 10.5% in that 10-year period. Hispanic enrollment more than doubled from 1.8% to 4.3%, as did Asian/Native Hawaiian/Other Pacific Islander enrollment (3.1% to 6.2%). American Indian/Alaska Native enrollment remained the same at 0.5%. As these figures indicate, the total minority enrollment from 1993 to 2003 rose from 11.2% to 21.6% (Berlin et al., 2004a, p. 22).

Doctoral education also witnessed increases in minority representation in the same time period from a 10.8% enrollment in 1993 to 17.2% enrollment in 2003. Blacks increased from 6.1% to 9.7%, Hispanics from 1.6% to 3.0%, Asians/Native Hawaiians/Other Pacific Islanders from 2.6% to 3.8%, and American Indians/Alaska Natives from 0.6% to 0.7%, remaining almost the same (Berlin et al., 2004a, p. 22). An interesting note is that within the types of doctoral programs available in nursing (research-focused, clinical-focused, or doctor of nursing professional degree), most blacks selected clinical-focused doctoral programs (7.1% in 2002 and 12.9% in 2003). American Indians/Alaska Natives enrolled only in research-focused doctoral programs in 2002 and 2003 (p. 35). Interpretation of program choice must be approached cautiously because the selection of programs is influenced by many factors, including geographical location, financial aid available, program flexibility, and personal goals. From 2002 to 2003, graduation rates for master's programs indicate an increase in black graduations (7.7% to 9.0%) and a decrease in white graduations (81.8% to 70.6%). Increased graduation rates occurred for blacks and Asians in research-focused doctoral programs; decreased for clinical-focused programs; and increased for blacks and whites in doctor of nursing programs (p. 37). Because actual numbers are small, interpretation is limited. Variations in time for doctoral degree completion are common, so data for any 1- or 2-year period may be an artifact of delayed program completion.

The expansion of advanced educational preparation in nursing is related to increased specialization in the practice arena, necessitating increased preparation in terms of the complexity and competency required to administer quality nursing care and to pursue relevant research. Funding for students to attend graduate programs is always subject to the legislators' awareness of the importance of and need for such funding. Federal monies distributed as a result of the Nursing Education Act primarily are allocated for nurses pursuing advanced preparation as nurse practitioners, nurse-midwives, nurse anesthetists, and advanced clinical nurse specialists. Students seeking preparation as nurse administrators had been barred in the past but were included again in recent years.

Universities and colleges have struggled to find ways to increase diversity in the graduate and professional programs and at the baccalaureate level. One such effort was that of the Bethune-Cookman College (a historic black college) and the University of Florida. The goal of this program was to initiate a collaborative relationship that would result in improving access to graduate education for Bethune-Cookman College graduates and increasing graduate student diversity at the University of Florida. The collaboration included career planning, financial planning, mentoring, program flexibility, and continued support in the graduate program. A 3% increase in the enrollment of minority students resulted, and all the initial participants (10) graduated (McWhirter, Courage, & Yearwood-Dixon, 2003). Obviously the numbers of minority students seeking higher education in nursing are not representative of the general population, especially in the case of Hispanics. Therefore these nurses are not able to move within the profession to positions of leadership and power. Why does this happen? Once again a variety of factors interact. The following interpretation is a premise for those of Hispanic origin. Because of the low economic status of most Mexican-American families, when the student completes the basic nursing program, she or he is expected to go to work immediately, often the day after graduation, to contribute to the family's finances. In more than one instance, the graduate is expected to put the next child through college. In addition, at this stage in their lives, marriage and child rearing become a focus. The Mexican-American family culture frowns on leaving children at day care centers or in the care of nonfamily caregivers. In addition, the basic cultural value of the dominant male figure often overrides a career drive. In other words, the nurse resumes life in a culture that generally does not encourage advanced preparation. Survival of the family unit is the primary motivator. This is not to judge that value but rather to acknowledge that it exists and that it may be a factor that discourages minority nurses from pursuing graduate education.

STRATEGIES TO IMPROVE THE ETHNIC MIX IN NURSING

Racial discrimination is a persistent problem in America. The civil rights legislation in the 1960s helped with overt discrimination, but the legacy remains (Brown et al., 2003, p. 227). Forty years later, Americans still are struggling with the effects of generations of discrimination. People of color have not been able to accumulate wealth in the same ways that whites have. Even after World War II, blacks did not have the same opportunities to further their education that whites had. Although many white middle-class people were able to take advantage of the educational opportunity afforded by the GI bill and raise their socioeconomic status by obtaining managerial and professional positions, black veterans were not able to progress and build as deep an economic foundation. That is not to say that blacks did not prosper in many ways after the war. There were more jobs, but those open to them were low-paying jobs with few opportunities to advance. Discrimination in jobs and housing have contributed to keeping minorities in settings that foster poverty, crowding with resultant high crime rates, and the erosion of the family as a unit. Racism persists although there is a facade of a nonracist American society.

Bonilla-Silva (2003) has coined the phrase "color-blind racism." This type of racism ostracizes blacks in more subtle ways through speech, writings, and casual everyday references. For example, interracial marriage is viewed in terms of a concern for problems that the children of such unions may have in the future, or minorities do not achieve because they are lazy, not because of their race. Whites purport that Americans are all equal and yet know full well the economic and educational disadvantages that minorities suffer because of their living situations, the ghettos of urban America. Everyone acknowledges that a college degree becomes a path to wealth and subsequently to power. Considering race in admissions is necessary to achieve diversity, not through quotas but through the recognition of other factors that may ensure the desirability of admission and the probability of success. It must be understood that diversity benefits not only minority students and minority communities but also the white majority by challenging them to identify and consider their values and beliefs. This is especially important in nursing, where quality care and competency must extend to all in need.

As minority populations grow, there will be an increased need for nurses who can relate to, understand, and be accepted by the community. Two important roles in health care have evolved: (1) assisting persons who have been deprived of access to health care to participate in the existing health care system and (2) molding the future health care system to be responsive to their needs. To accomplish these goals, federal, state, and local financial support must be available. Inequities in public education must be addressed. Local public school boards must direct resources toward the goal of quality educational opportunities for all children. Poor school tax districts must receive assistance from the state. At the postsecondary level, institutions must provide counseling and tutorial services and financial aid. Retention of minority students may be affected negatively by "stereotype vulnerability." In this situation, minority students disengage themselves from the anxiety of performance; that is, they accept the view that they lack the ability to succeed (Davidhizar, Dowd, & Giger, 1998).

Factors inhibiting minority members from attaining a career in nursing include feelings of powerlessness and inadequate academic preparation, especially in the sciences; financial costs and the actual and projected decrease in financial aid; inadequate career counseling; and more and better recruitment strategies by other disciplines. In 2003 the U.S. Health and Human Services Department awarded 16 grants totaling nearly $3.5 million to support opportunities for persons from disadvantaged backgrounds to enter nursing (U.S. Newswire, 2003). The grants funded scholarships, stipends, and/or preparatory and retention activities for disadvantaged students including those from racial and ethnic minority groups. The schools receiving the grants had a minority enrollment of 38%, which was double the national average of 19%. In 2005 the University of Massachusetts—Amherst received almost a million dollars in a grant for Nursing Workforce Diversity from the Department of Health and Human Services to connect students interested in nursing at the middle and high school levels to four nursing programs in the area. The program will focus on mentoring and tutoring in math and science, nursing clubs for middle school students, and social and information sessions for high schoolers (University of Massachusetts, 2005).

A major problem in nursing education is the few members of minority nursing faculty. The American Association of Colleges of Nursing report *2003-2004 Salaries of Instructional and Administrative Nursing Faculty in Baccalaureate and Graduate Programs in Nursing* (Berlin, Stennett, & Bednash, 2004c) indicated that 9% of the faculty members of 554 schools reporting were minorities. In another American Association of Colleges of Nursing report (Berlin, Stennett, & Bednash, 2004b), 5.4% of the faculty members were black; 1.8%, Hispanic; 0.4%, American Indian/Alaska Native; 1.6%, Asian; and 0.3%, Native Hawaiian/Other Pacific Islander. Figures for deans of nursing programs were almost the same: 5.4% black; 2.0% Hispanic; 2.0% American Indian/Alaska Native; 0.2% Asian; and 1.2% Native Hawaiian/Other Pacific Islander. The composition of nursing faculties must reflect an ethnic and racial mix, not token representations or the reflection of a specific community. Nursing faculties should strive to become a living model of diversity in collaboration that stresses competence, academic ability, caring, and true equality. Potential minority faculty members must be identified as early as possible in their academic careers and must be supported in their efforts to obtain graduate degrees. In one possible scenario, the graduates could pay back the financial support of the institution through a committed service period. These young faculty members, like all junior faculty, must be nurtured through a mentoring program. They have the potential to serve as role models for minority students and in time can serve as mentors themselves. Unfortunately, research by minority faculty members often not only is unappreciated but also is denigrated. For example, colleagues in nursing may look disparagingly upon research concerning American Indian rites related to health or black nutritional practices. If culturally based research is not valued, minority faculty members may not be tenured. No tenure usually means no career advancement or limited opportunities to contribute to the academic nursing profession.

Philosophical discussions about whether there should be organizations for minorities in nursing, such as the National Association of Hispanic Nurses or the

National Black Nurses Association continue. It would appear that these organizations provide support and networking for minority nurses who may not be able to take advantage of opportunities in the major nursing organizations because of their small numbers. Therefore until the minority nurses themselves feel that a need no longer exists, local chapters of these organizations should be encouraged. Professional nursing success that is necessary to advance in the profession can be interpreted as psychological success whereby an internalized goal includes ego involvement. Psychological success increases self-esteem and strengthens a commitment (Hall, 1976). A supportive social network is a means of minimizing the threat to one's sense of self-worth and fostering career enhancement.

SUMMARY

Nursing education has a direct responsibility to educate practitioners for the future. The demographics of the United States are evolving as they have since its founding. Spanish has become a second language in many parts of the country, and nurses must educate their own to meet these changes.

Health care reform issues mandate minority representation in all health professions. Will the United States move toward universal health care coverage? Surely nurses are almost there with the Children's Health Insurance Program and Medicare and Medicaid for older and disabled adults. The evolving U.S. health care system must reflect our communities, because as health care increasingly moves into the community, health care provider–community partnerships must be formed. Ethnically and racially diverse minority health care providers have been found to be more likely than nonethnic minority health care providers to practice in culturally diverse settings after graduation. "Despite their small numbers, minority nurses are significant contributors to the provision of health care services in this country and leaders in the development of models of care that address the unique needs of minority populations" (American Association of Colleges of Nursing, 2001, p. 1).

The literature on recruiting and maintaining minority representation in nursing is considerable, although much of it is becoming "old" and new contributions in the literature are needed. Some educational institutions recruit heavily from minority institutions. They offer excellent financial assistance to students and woo faculty members with high salaries. The fact that many of these programs experience difficulty in retaining minority

students and faculty members should send a message to everyone. Although acknowledging linguistic and cultural differences, nurses have failed dismally in attempts to meet the needs of minorities adequately. Bosher (2003) analyzed multiple-choice nursing course examinations for linguistic and cultural bias. She found 28 types of flaws occurred at least 10 times. Item bias occurs at two levels: linguistic (overly complex items), structural (long, unclear, or awkward phrases), and cultural (content not equally available to all culture groups).

Multiple strategies are required, and financial assistance, although important, is not solely sufficient. All systems must hold themselves accountable and are held accountable to achieve diversity and cultural competence (The Sullivan Commission, 2004, p. 102). Unless strategic planning for minority recruitment and retention is implemented, all efforts will be doomed. For example, hiring minority faculty members, without mentoring and assistance in the assumption of leadership roles, will not be successful as a long-term strategy. For students and faculty, formal and informal support services can assist in resolving cultural dissonance. Such strategies must be incorporated throughout the curriculum. Content areas such as interpersonal skills, communication skills, leadership ability, and professionalism must be blended. Leadership in forwarding diversity and true accountability are essential if nurses are to make progress. Finally, nurses must admit to racial color blindness and seek to open their eyes to subtle and covert discrimination and bias so that in the next 50 years they will not be asking the same questions about diversity in nursing that they have been asking for the last 40 years.

REFERENCES

Alexander, L., & Swarzschild, M. (2004). From Brown to Grutter: Affirmative action and higher education in the South, constitutionalizing and defining racial equality: Grutter or otherwise. Racial preferences and higher education. *Tulane Law Review, 78,* 1767. Retrieved December 31, 2004, from http://web.lexis-nexis.com/universe/printdoc/

American Association of Colleges of Nursing. (2001). *Effective strategies for increasing diversity in nursing programs.* Washington, DC: Author. Retrieved January 10, 2005, from http://www.aacn.nche.edu/Publications/issues/dec01.htm

American Nurses Association. (1991). *Ethics and human rights position statements: Cultural diversity in nursing practice.* Retrieved January 18, 2005, from http://nursing world.org/readroom/position/ethics/etcldv.htm

American Nurses Association. (1998). *Ethics and human rights position statements: Discrimination and racism in health care.* Retrieved January 18, 2005, from http://nursing world.org/readroom/position/ethics/etdisrac.htm

Barbee, E., & Gibson, S. E. (2001). Our dismal progress: The recruitment of non-whites into nursing. *Journal of Nursing Education, 40*(6), 243-244. Retrieved January 18, 2005, from http://vnweb.hwwilsonweb.com

Berlin, L., Stennett, J., & Bednash, G. D. (2004a). *2003-2004 Enrollment in baccalaureate and graduate programs in nursing* (pp. 21-22, 34-37, 64). Washington, DC: American Association of Colleges of Nursing.

Berlin, L., Stennett, J., & Bednash, G. D. (2004b). *2003-2004 Salaries of deans in baccalaureate and graduate programs in nursing* (p. 3). Washington, DC: American Association of Colleges of Nursing.

Berlin, L., Stennett, J., & Bednash, G. D. (2004c). *2003-2004 Salaries of instructional and administrative nursing faculty in baccalaureate and graduate programs in nursing* (pp. 7-8, 54, 69). Washington, DC: American Association of Colleges of Nursing.

Bonilla-Silva, E. (2003). *Racism without racists.* Lanham, MD: Rowman & Littlefield.

Bosher, S. (2003). Barriers to creating a more culturally diverse nursing profession: Linguistic bias in multiple-choice nursing exams. *Nursing Education Perspectives, 24*(1), 25-34.

Brown, M. K., Carnoy, M., Currie, E., Duster, T., Oppenheimer, D. B., Shultz, M. M., et al. (2003). *White-washing race: The myth of a color-blind society.* Berkeley: University of California Press.

Carnevale, D. (1999, September 3). Enrollment of minority freshmen nears pre-Hopwood levels at University of Texas at Austin. *The Chronicle of Higher Education,* pp. A71.

Davidhizar, R., Dowd, S. B., & Giger, J. N. (1998). Educating the culturally diverse healthcare student. *Nurse Educator 23*(2), 38-41.

de la Cruz, G. P., & Brittingham, A. (2003). *The Arab population: 2000. Census 2000 brief* (Pub. No. C2KBR-23). Washington, DC: U.S. Department of Commerce, U.S. Census Bureau.

Dreher, M., & MacNaughton, N. (2002). Cultural competence in nursing: Foundation or fallacy? *Nursing Outlook, 50*(5), 181-186.

Fitzgerald, T. (2000, January 10). Nurse appeal: Profession tries new tactics to woo next generation of nurses. *Health Week,* p. 15.

Gratz v. Bollinger, 539 U.S. l244. (2003). Copr. 2004 West. No Claim to Orig. U.S. Govt. Works. Second source retrieved on December 31, 2004, from http://lexis-nexis.com/ universe/printdoc/

Greico, E. M. (2001). *The white population: 2000.* Washington, DC: U.S. Department of Commerce, U.S. Census Bureau.

Grutter v. Bollinger, 539 U.S. 306. (2003). Copr. 2004 West. No Claim to Orig. U.S. Govt. Works. Second source retrieved on December 31, 2004, from http://lexis-nexis.com/ universe/printdoc/

Hall, D. T. (1976). *Careers in organizations.* Pacific Palisades, CA: Goodyear.

Hoffman, K., Llagas, C., & Snyder, T. D. (2003). *Status and trends in the education of blacks.* Jesssup, MD: U.S. Department of Education.

Jaschik, S. (1993, February 10). Supporters say threat to minority scholarship outlasts the Bush years. *The Chronicle of Higher Education,* p. A25.

Kauffman, A. H. (1996, August). The Hopwood Case: What it says, what it doesn't say, the future of the caser and the rest of the story. *Intercultural Development Research Association (IDRA) Newsletter,* pp. 7-8.

Leininger, M. (1994). Transcultural nursing education: A world-wide imperative. *Nursing and Health Care, 15*(5), 254-257.

McKinnon, J. (2003). *The black population in the United States: March 2002.* Washington, DC: U.S. Department of Commerce, U.S. Census Bureau.

McWhirter, G., Courage, M., & Yearwood-Dixon, A. (2003). Diversity in graduate nursing education: An experience in collaboration. *Journal of Professional Nursing, 19*(3), 134-144.

Michaelson, M. (1995, July 28). Building a comprehensive defense of affirmative action programs. *The Chronicle of Higher Education,* p. A56.

National League for Nursing. (2003). *NLN 2002-2003 survey of RN nursing programs indicates positive upward trends in the nursing workforce supply.* Retrieved July 19, 2005, from http://www.nln.org/newsreleases/prelimdata12.16.03.pdf

National League for Nursing. (2004). *Nursing data review academic year 2003: Vol. 1. Contemporary RN education.* New York: Author.

Ogunwole, S. U. (2002, February). *The American Indian and Alaska Native population: 2000.* Washington, DC: U.S. Department of Commerce, U.S. Census Bureau.

Ramirez, R. R., & de la Cruz, G. P. (2002). *The Hispanic population in the United States.* Washington, DC: U.S. Department of Commerce, U.S. Census Bureau.

Reeves, T., & Bennett, C. (2003). *The Asian and Pacific Islander population in the United States: March 2002.* Washington, DC: U.S. Department of Commerce, U.S. Census Bureau.

Salimbene, S. (1999). Cultural competence: A priority for performance improvement action. *Journal of Nursing Care Quality, 13*(3), 23-25.

Schwirian, P. (1977). *Prediction of successful nursing performance: Part 2. Admission practices, evaluation strategies and performance prediction among schools of nursing* (HEW Pub. No. HRA 77-27). Washington, DC: U.S. Government Printing Office.

Shireman, R. (2003, August 15). 10 Questions college officials should ask about diversity. *The Chronicle of Higher Education,* pp. B10, B12.

Smith v. University of Washington Law School. (2000). Retrieved January 5, 2005 from http://lib.law.washington.edu/ research/smith_v_lawschool.html

Smith, K. E., Rock, A., Pife, M., v. University of Washington Law School. (2004). U.S. Court of Appeals for Ninth Circuit, 2004 U.S. App. Lexis 26429.

Spratley, E., Johnson, A., Sochalski, J., Fritz, M., & Spencer, W. (2000). *The registered nurse population: Findings from the National Sample Survey of Registered Nurses.* Washington, DC: U.S. Department of Health and Human Resources, Division of Nursing.

Stern, G. M. (2004). Bias at work in training health care workers: Report offers criticism and recommendations. *Ethnic News, 14*(17), 33-35.

Stewart, S., & Cleveland, R. (2003). A pre-college program for culturally diverse high school students. *Nurse Educator, 28*(3), 107-110.

The Sullivan Commission. (2004). *Missing persons: Minorities in the health professions.* Retrieved on January 10, 2004, from http://admissions.duhs.duke.edu/sullivancommission/documents/Sullivan_Final_Report

Terhune, C. (2004). From desegregation to diversity: How far have we really come? *Journal of Nursing Education, 43*(5), 195-196.

University of Massachusetts: Minority recruitment plan could ease nursing shortage. (2005, January 22). *Law & Health Weekly* via LawRx.com via NewsRx.com and NewsRx.net. Retrieved January 17, 2005, from http://web.lexis-nexis.com.lib.buffalo.edu/universe/document?_m=d37679f72671f540

U.S. Department of Education. (2005, January 13). *Highlights from the status and trends in the education of Hispanics: Enrollment in colleges and universities (NCES 2003-008). National Center for Education Statistics.* Retrieved on January 13, 2005 from http://www.ed.gov/index/htm

U.S. Newswire. (2003, June 2). *HHS awards nearly $3.5 million to promote diversity in the nursing workforce.* Retrieved on January 17, 2005, from http://web.lexis-nexis.com.gate.lib.buffalo.edu/Universe/document?_m=d37679f72671f540/

Walsh, K. R. (2004). Color blind racism in Grutter and Gratz. (Reviewing E. Bonilla-Silva, *Racism without racists: Color-blind racism and the persistence of racial inequality in the United States.*) 24 B.C. Third World L.J. 443-467. *College Third World Law Journal.* L.J.443, 22. Retrieved December 31, 2004, from http://web.lexis-nexis.com/universe/

Nursing at the Crossroads

CHAPTER

Men in Nursing

61

VERN L. BULLOUGH

Statistics about men in nursing are difficult to come by. In 1997 it was estimated that 6.5% of the 2 million registered nurses in the United States were men, but other statistics for the same period indicated that only 5.4% were, and still another gave slightly more than 6%. Despite the contradictions, the numbers are increasing slowly, and in recent years more than 10% of the students receiving degrees in nursing in the baccalaureate programs and associate of arts programs were men, and these percentages have been rising. Visibly also, male nurses are playing an increasingly important role in nursing, particularly in fields such as anesthesia (American Nurses Association, 1946, 1994; *Hospital and Health Network*, 1994; National Center for Education Statistics, 1999; National Center for Health Workforce, 2000). In this age of growing gender equality, however, women still dominate in nursing, and this is more due to historical circumstances than any other factor. Worth noting is that in nursing, men are facing many of the same obstacles that women in the past had to face when they tried to be physicians, accountants, scientists, managers, professors, college administrators, or even professional athletes. Undoubtedly, there are still barriers for women in many areas, but they are well on the way to being overcome, and the same holds true for men in nursing. Part of the difficulty is simply that the history and image of nursing since Florence Nightingale has been a feminine one. And the "girly man" in Arnold Schwarzenegger's terms is still a put down of men willing to challenge past stereotypes. As gender stereotypes change, the labeling decreases.

Interestingly, male nurses in some countries where they are more plentiful proportionately than they are in the United States had to face even more rigid stereotypes but somehow managed to overcome them at a more rapid pace than they did in the United States. In Cyprus, for example, where many men went into nursing, as late as the 1960s they were called "sisters" (which also was used in England but much more restrictively). In my interviews of some of the male nurses in Cyprus, one in particular stands out. He was married and the father of several children and told me that he was willing to put up with the term *sister* because the pay was so good. Many other men in Cyprus felt the same way, and compared with the United States, there was a disproportionate number of male nurses. Their willingness to become a nurse emphasizes that there are other factors involved in men choosing nursing despite the feminine image it often had, namely pay and working conditions, or as in Cyprus, the lack of suitable alternative jobs. For much of American history, the economic aspects of nursing were not particularly attractive compared with alternative jobs available. Salaries were low, working hours were long, and attempts to control the personal life of the nurse were deeply ingrained. Many women who went into nursing might well have been unhappy with these same problems, but fewer alternatives were open to them.

Nursing in the United States had to change considerably before it could seem attractive to any but the most dedicated men. Even if men did decide to enter nursing, employment opportunities were limited and often not attractive. Before World War II in the United States, most nurses who continued to practice were employed as private duty nurses. Such an assignment often entailed family care and nursing duties and in many cases required the nurses to live in the home of the patient. Even if the men had been willing, the nursing registries often were controlled by the local nursing associations, and the American Nurses Association for much of its early history did not admit men. Jobs in hospitals were limited because most of the nursing care actually was done by students, who often held jobs even as head nurses in their senior year. In short, pay was poor, hours were long, and employment opportunities for men were limited.

For the nature of nursing to change, it was necessary for medicine to change, and it gradually began to do so as standards for medical schools were raised and subpar medical schools were closed. Instead of being isolated from the universities with which a minority was affiliated, most of the surviving schools established or became closer to their existing university affiliation. At the same time, hospitals grew larger and became more important as more and more patients were moved from their homes to the hospitals for treatment. Nurses were employed increasingly in the hospitals, and the role of nursing itself began to be redefined, but usually men were not included in these new definitions.

A major problem in the United States was the difficulty men had in becoming a nurse. Nursing education took place mainly in the hospital schools, and almost no hospital school would admit men. Interestingly, one of the major reasons for this refusal was the question of how to house male students. Nursing schools required their students to live in nursing homes where their lives were rigidly controlled, and in these sex-segregated institutions there was no place for a male student. Occasionally, a small minority of hospitals did take a male student who usually was given a special room in a janitorial quarter or in the larger hospital with the medical interns, but few men entered nursing because they did not feel welcome. Most of those who did become nurses came through programs specially established for men or in monastic orders such as the Alexian Brothers. Even if a man managed to become a nurse, there was discrimination. In the Second World War, for example, nurses who were women entered the services as officers, but the military refused to commission any male nurse, although he might end up as an enlisted man in the medical corps. In short, sex discrimination was rampant, and in nursing it was men who suffered from it, although in the workforce at large, women in general were discriminated against.

Undoubtedly also many female nurses were reluctant to encourage men to be nurses, fearful that nursing itself might end with men becoming as dominant as they were in other occupations. Some went so far as to argue that nursing by its nature was feminine. If nursing was in the first half of the twentieth century, it had not always been.

BACKGROUND

Through much of history, men, as they had done traditionally in most jobs outside the home, dominated (Bullough & Bullough, 1993a), although within the home itself women were more likely to care for the sick and injured than men. The military, at least since Greek and Roman times, had their own attendants to care for the sick, although when on the march, they often turned to camp followers (i.e., women who were wives or girlfriends or even mothers of the soldiers) who usually settled down near the military camps and often followed the troops in battle doing laundry, sometimes cooking, and doing other tasks. In battles, where it was important every able-bodied man fight, men undoubtedly helped take care of the wounded. Special religious orders for men such as the Knights Hospitaller took care of the sick in the military. Some religious orders for women also took up nursing, notably the Sisters of Charity. The number of hospitals was limited, and these were mainly for the poor and homeless or travelers away from home. Only in the last decades of the nineteenth century, particularly in urban areas where the family support systems that existed in villages and small towns was not available in the large and growing cities, did hospitals begin to grow in numbers. Great disparities in wealth existed, and the vast number of people lived from hand to mouth. If illness struck in such situations, there was no place to go. If the poor were aged and infirm and if family was not nearby, they also needed institutions such as hospitals to care for them.

Hospitals were seen as a growing necessity in a community but were seen primarily as charitable institutions run by religious groups or local government (in the United States it was the county). But who was to staff these institutions? Often the least well patients in most of these so-called hospitals were cared for by other patients who were not as ill or infirm. Sometimes there were paid employees, but any expertise they had was acquired on the job. As the situation worsened, recognition was growing that simply housing such people was not enough. They needed caretakers. In Catholic countries, the caretakers were often nuns, and many of the Protestant groups in the nineteenth century began establishing similar orders, most of which were known as deaconesses. The women who joined these orders did not take the lifetime vows of celibacy and service that the nuns did. Note that the emphasis in Catholic and Protestant areas was on women, although as indicated previously, male religious orders still were dedicated to the care of the sick.

Gender stereotypes were supported by law and custom. As a general rule until well into the twentieth century, women were under the legal control of their husbands, fathers, brothers, or even sons. For modern Americans to realize just how dominant the male role was in the past is sometimes difficult. In fact, much of modern history can be interpreted as a story of women's efforts to break free of the limitations and restrictions put on them by a male-dominated society and to be recognized as important persons in their own right. The world essentially was defined by men who simply assumed they were the high-status sex and women were supposed to be subordinate to them. Although women had special abilities such as childbearing that made them indispensable, this was seen as justification of the necessity for males to protect them. To put it simply, biology was regarded as destiny, and being female slotted a woman into a special category with all kinds of restrictions imposed on her to "protect her."

Economic and social status did have some effect on what was or was not permissible for a woman, but regardless of class, women usually had severe restrictions on their ability to act independently. Being a mother and nursing children, however rewarding this may be, does not in itself mean that women cannot do other things as well. Many women aspired to have more diverse opportunities, and some, often with the encouragement of the men in their lives, were successful. Not infrequently the women who broke the male-only barriers often were described, by themselves and by others, as having a manly mind, manly courage, or manly ability; that is, their biology was slightly different from that of normal women. Many also claimed to be inspired by God to claim a special mission. Regardless of the restrictions, a handful of women still managed to gain special recognition by society for their achievements, and they and their male allies campaigned for changes.

Helping to undermine these traditional assumptions about women were basic changes in society. The industrial revolution of the eighteenth and nineteenth centuries challenged traditional ways of life, and the intellectual movement known as the Enlightenment similarly challenged long-held ideas. Although the emerging factories, first in England, and then elsewhere, employed the village women in greater numbers than before, this only accentuated the problems of the middle class women who lacked opportunities to make themselves useful or somewhat independent. Even women who worked in the growing number of factories ultimately were seen as taking jobs away from men, and so employment increasingly became limited to unmarried women or widows. Their jobs were not regarded as "careers" but a temporary phase in their life until they married. Most of the women who worked long term did so as domestics or washerwomen or in similar tasks

regarded as belonging to the female world. Such positions were not available to middle class women, because as one woman wrote in the middle of the nineteenth century,

> . . . a "proper" woman could not work for profit, or engage in any occupation that money can command, lest she invade the rights of the working classes. . . . Men in want of employment have pressed their way into nearly all the shopping and retail businesses that in my early years were managed in whole, or in part, by women. The conventional barrier that pronounced it ungenteel to be behind a counter, or serving the public in any mercantile capacity is greatly extended. The same in household economy. Servants must be up to their offices, which is very well, but ladies, dismissed from the dairy, the confectionary, the store room, the still room, the poultry yard, the kitchen garden, and the orchard have hardly yet found themselves a sphere equally useful and important to the pursuit of trade and arts to which to apply their too abundant leisure (Greg, 1969, pp. 315-316).

Many of the more well-to-do women tried to participate in the intellectual ferment by becoming hostesses coordinating and participating in intellectual discussions. The term *blue stocking* often was used to describe such women because they tended to dress more informally at such literary events. The problem that middle-class women faced was how to break through the barriers yet retain the proper feminine image. An obvious solution was to busy oneself with traditional women's activities and somehow make these activities into a profession. Such activities included care for the sick, raising and educating small children, visiting and helping neighbors, raising the cultural consciousness of the men in their lives, assisting their husbands in their work or profession, and managing the household. From these "wifely" tasks nurses, elementary school teachers, friendly visitors (who eventually came to be called social workers), librarians, and secretaries emerged, although the last case depended on the invention and widespread use of the typewriter (Bullough & Bullough, 1978, 1984).

The first efforts of women in all these fields were essentially charitable enterprises, and only gradually did these tasks become paying jobs. Whether consciously or unconsciously, women who wanted to challenge tradition seized on the nineteenth-century notion that they constituted a special class; the very biology that made them different and unable to compete with men gave them a weapon they could use. This was the belief that they were made of finer and more delicate material than men. This was interpreted by men to mean that women had to be protected because life in the real world could destroy or weaken them more easily compared with the hardy, more rugged men, and if this happened, they might end up as prostitutes or other types of "bad" women. It also meant that women were set aside to be guardians of culture and tradition, even though few fit the stereotype of wan, ethereal, spiritualized creatures that some of the literature of the time tried to make them. In fact, such portrayals bore little resemblance to the real world of lower-class women who operated machines, worked the fields, washed clothes by hand and took care of large households. Nonetheless, these portraits were endorsed by the science and religion of the time at least for middle- and upper-class women. Some male physicians even went so far as to claim that the female biology prevented a woman from cultivating her intellect too seriously since so much of her bodily resources had to be expended on developing her reproductive organs (Bullough & Bullough, 1978, 1984).

Florence Nightingale was in a full-scale, ladylike rebellion against such an image. She did not want to marry and turn her fate over to some man; rather she wanted to be her own woman and still be socially useful. Money was of no concern to her because she was independently wealthy, and this gave her considerable freedom in making decisions. Nursing came to be her answer because it allowed her to fit the image of the proper woman yet still be on her own. She had the family connections to open up doors that were locked to others. One of her friends was Sidney Herbert, the minister of defense during the Crimean War, which began in 1851. The British, who were allies of Turkey in a war against Russia, were ill prepared for the casualties they suffered, and news about the dreadful care of the sick and wounded threatened the ability of the government to survive. Herbert wanted to show that the government cared about the soldiers and with the prompting from his wife, a friend of Florence Nightingale, and from Nightingale herself, conceived of a public relations coupe by sending a contingent of women to nurse the troops (Bullough & Bullough, 1978, 1984). Nightingale and her nurses became what in today's terms would be called a media sensation and continued to be one because the female nurses proved to be extremely effective. The American poet Henry Wadsworth Longfellow made her a mythical heroine in his poem that included the following lines:

> A lady with a lamp shall stand
> In the great history of the land,
> A noble type of good
> Heroic womanhood.

THE AMERICAN EXPERIENCE

Inevitably, Nightingale became a heroine for all young women, and her life became standard reading material (somewhat highly embroidered) for generations of girls who wanted to make something of themselves (Vicinus, 1990). When Nightingale came back with money donated to her by the grateful troops, she established a nursing school for women that soon, at least in name, became widely imitated. With Nightingale as an example, many women sought to emulate her experience during the American Civil War and many did so. In the years following the war, some women hoped to build on this nursing experiment and follow Nightingale's lead by establishing a nursing school. In 1873, groups of women in New York City; New Haven, Connecticut; and Boston, acting independently, organized schools for women to become nurses using the model that Nightingale had established at St. Thomas Hospital in London. Their action came at a crucial time because hospital building soon increased rapidly in the United States following the development of aseptic techniques and the growing need for institutional care of the poor and homeless in America's growing urban centers.

Medicine also was changing. Procedures formerly reserved for the home, including childbirth, began to move into the hospital setting as physicians took over tasks previously performed by midwives and other nonprofessional healers. Nursing made the growth of the hospitals possible and was seized upon by the medical establishment, especially when it became clear that students were cheap labor. They could staff the hospitals in return for room and board and a modicum of education. Because the hospital administrators (mostly physicians) wanted the nurses available on short notice, hospitals established homes for them, a concept that also fit in the perceived need to protect women. The nursing schools in a sense became a sex-segregated ghetto, with nursing students segregated not only from males but also from other students and from mainstream developments in education. The hospital became the defining educational experience for nurses as it was for medicine. But medicine itself, as indicated, was changing.

As late as the 1950s it was possible to get into medical school in one's junior year in college and receive a doctor of medicine degree after 3 years. Medicine when it became part of the new research-oriented university, however, moved into the university on its own terms. Medicine had a separate and clearly defined expertise and a strong power base. Nursing, however, did not fit into the traditional college and university subject matter, and it was not strong enough or independent enough to establish itself in the university. When nursing first entered the university, it was through schools of education within a university setting that were not highly ranked. The pattern was to combine a traditional hospital nursing program with a specialty in nursing education for a college degree. This affiliation had one major benefit; namely, that students received university credits for their nursing courses in the hospital and that these were transferable. Credits from hospital schools in their own right simply were not accepted by most colleges or universities, and nurses who wanted to continue their education often had to take an undergraduate degree in a different subject to get into a graduate program.

Even in the best of the institutions, such as Teachers College, Columbia University (the dominant graduate school for nurses until the 1950s), the subject matter taught in the universities did not emphasize nursing research but educational research, and the two are not the same thing. Public health nurses, the one nursing specialty for which a bachelor's degree often was required, were regarded primarily as teachers of public health, although they carried out the regular nursing duties as well. So oriented to education were public health nurses that there was a debate for a time whether regular teachers should be given more health training instead of giving nurses the educational background essential for them to become school nurses or to work in public and community health agencies. Still the entrance of nursing education into the university raised the level of nursing even for those schools that had no university affiliation. Anyone who has read the basic texts ranging from history to principles and practices of nursing for many of the courses in the hospital training school, in the first few decades of the twentieth century, comes away distressed by the simplified texts in nonnursing subjects. Courses such as nursing history, often taught in the hospital schools, were full of simplistic if not erroneous information. In most if not all schools, the nonclinical courses that furnished the basis of nursing—such as anatomy, physiology, or pharmacology—generally were taught by physicians on the assumptions that nurse teachers would not have adequate background to teach theses subjects, whereas the actual clinical experience was acquired in what can only be called an apprenticeship mode (Bullough & Bullough, 1978, 1984).

THE PLACE OF MEN

This description of the struggle nurses had to mount to overcome the obstacles put in their path, largely because they were women, is not to put down nursing but to emphasize why so few men went into it. Nurse training in many ways was similar to that of apprenticeship in many of the male occupations such as those of machinists, mechanic, carpenter, and electrician, but far more confining. There was just no room for men because the whole system was viewed as a woman's field, and whole structure was designed to discourage men.

The major exception was in the mental hospitals, where it was believed nurses needed greater strength. This led to schools for men only, such as that established by the Department of Mental and Nervous Diseases at Pennsylvania Hospital or the Mills School of Nursing for Men at Bellevue. Although no real evidence indicates that women in nursing took a strong stand against men in their ranks, clearly nursing was conceived by most of them as a women's profession. In fact, not until the 1930s were the membership bylaws of the American Nurses Association revised to include properly qualified male nurses (Nash, 1936). Male nurses where they existed were not in the mainstream of nursing (Bullough & Bullough, 1978, 1984).

Men who might have wanted to be nurses were ambivalent about their place in the field. Although it was permissible for a woman to strive to be more manlike, for a man to enter a woman's world such as nursing was perceived to mean that he might be labeled as somehow "not quite a man." The anxiety and fear of the public over homosexuality meant that the men who did go into nursing had to be willing to take a lot of "guff" about their manliness, and it was not until the feminist movement and the gay liberation movement of the 1960s that attitudes began to change. As indicated previously, male nurses also faced discrimination by military authorities who accepted them as pharmacist's mates in the navy or as orderlies or assistants in hospitals, but the commissions went to the female nurses.

The first real effort of nurses to help out the men in their midst came from the initiative of Leroy Craig, director of the School of Nursing for Men at Pennsylvania Hospital. He and his allies (men and women) persuaded the American Nurses Association at its 1940 convention to set up a section for "men nurses." Although the section focused its attention on many issues, including upgrading patient care and raising salaries for nurses, its members were not successful in changing the treatment of male nurses in the military. Luther Christman, the real barrier breaker for male nursing, was a 1939 graduate of the Pennsylvania Hospital Nursing School for Men. He tried to enlist in the Army Nurse Corps but was refused. He found, much to his dismay, that male nurses were not even given priority enrollment in the medical corpsmen school, perhaps, because as some have argued, their knowledge often intimidated their less well-educated military instructors. Christman tried to bypass the issue by joining the merchant marines as a medical corpsman and then petitioning for appointment to the Army Nurse Corps and for assignment to the front lines (where female nurses then were not assigned). He was unsuccessful. Enrollments of men in nursing schools during this period dropped drastically from 725 in 1939 to 169 in 1945 (American Nurses Association, 1946, 1994), and most nursing schools affiliated with mental hospitals simply closed.

Conditions for men in nursing began to change following the end of World War II when male enrollments in nursing school slowly started to build. Men did not climb very high until there were alternatives to the segregated diploma hospital schools. The big change came with the establishment of the associate's degree programs in community colleges and expansion of university-based nursing schools, which were not so numerous. The new university schools for the most part were not affiliated with education, but nursing itself was recognized as a subject deserving of university study, which marked a breakthrough for nursing.

What might be called psychological barriers still existed, and men had to overcome them. One of the difficulties that nurses faced in a male-dominated medical world was how to be recognized by physicians as having knowledge and ability of their own. Many did so by playing what came to be called the "doctor-nurse game," in which a nurse in order to get the treatment she felt the patient needed, carefully had to feed the physician the information she felt he needed to make the decision she wanted. To do so too directly seemed to threaten a large number of physicians, who then would put the nurse down and ignore her suggestions. Male nurses did not play this well, and until the pathological behavior was challenged publicly, as it eventually was, the male nurse remained at a disadvantage. Recognition and description of the game was the first step to changing this feminine coping pattern in nursing and removing a barrier for men. Perhaps more important was the rise of the nursing clinical specialties such as nurse anesthetists. Nurse anesthetists had existed since the end of the nineteenth century, but they had been more

or less excluded from mainstream nursing organizations. The rise in their numbers came after World War II, pushed by, among other groups, the U.S. Army. The development of the nurse practitioner and physician's assistants also forced a redirection in nursing (I bear some of the scars of that battle with the ambivalence of organized nursing toward this change). I know the success of the movement shook nursing to its roots and emphasized something that people like Luther Christman had long been agitating for; namely, the importance of clinical expertise.

As the collegiate nursing schools began to give their own master's degrees and ultimately their own doctorates, research became a major element in nursing, and it was now research on subjects of importance to clinical nursing, not on how to develop a curriculum. The explosion of nursing journals is indicative of the rapid increase in research. For a time in the 1950s there were basically only two national nursing journals after the *Trained Nurse* had discontinued publication; namely, the *American Journal of Nursing* and *Nursing Outlook*. A public health nursing journal, the one specialty journal in nursing, had been published, but it too was discontinued. Only in the late 1950s did other nursing journals enter the field so that nurses could claim an increasingly large section of health care as their own and where their expertise was greater than that of the physicians (Bullough & Bullough, 1978, 1984).

As nursing changed, so did the role of men in nursing. A major indicator of change was the granting of military commissions to male nurses through legislation initiated by Rep. Frances Bolton of Ohio, a longtime supporter of nursing. This legislation led to Edward Lyon becoming the first male registered nurse to be commissioned as a reserve officer in the U.S. Army Corps on October 6, 1955. The change in the military status of male nursing was rapid, and by 1990 approximately 30% of the registered nurses in the various military nurse corps were men, more than 4 or 5 times their ratio in civilian nursing. During the Vietnam War, more than 500 male nurses were drafted and were given commissions in the various military nurse corps.

In the long run, however, the most important factor in attracting men to nursing was the improvement in salaries and working conditions during the 1950s and 1960s. Men initially benefited more from this than women. Census data indicates that in the 1970s male nurses generally were paid more than female nurses (Bullough & Bullough, 1975), a fact that made it look like even in a "women's profession," wagewise women were second class. A major reason for the disparity was due to the fact that a disproportionate number of men were nurse anesthetists or nurse administrators or held other high-paying nursing jobs. Still, pay was a sore point with the female colleagues who had encouraged men to enter nursing. Only as the new wave of feminism occurring at the same time began to demand equal pay for equal work was the salary gap between men and women lessened in and out of nursing.

Tensions came from other directions as well, and these became more noticeable as the number of men entering nursing grew. Nursing educators who had taught only women found that men behaved somewhat differently. They reported that the men were not as submissive as the female students traditionally had been, and they often used different problem-solving methods. Most of these alleged problems with male students required simple adjustments that most teachers soon made (Bush, 1976; Schoenmaker, 1976), but a few influential members of the nursing community simply did not want to adjust and opposed the growing number of men in nursing.

Many of those in opposition turned to newly developing field of nursing theory to justify their opposition (Bullough, 1994). As nursing entered the mainstream of academia, nurses in academic positions became convinced that a nursing theory was necessary to provide a bridge between practice and research and that theory-based research was the key to broadening nursing knowledge (Dickoff, James, & Wiedeback, 1968). The result was the development of a number of grand theories.

Among the most troublesome of such theories to men are the caring theories, particularly those that emphasize caring as a particularly feminine trait. Although rooted in the work of Dorothy Johnson (1959), who distinguished between curing and caring, many others also contributed. Kreuter (1957, p. 303) defined caring as the special task of the nurse clinician: "Care is expressed in tending to another, being with him, assisting, protecting … providing his needs and wants with compassion-tenderness." Caring became a part of Watson's theory (1979, 1985) and led her to establish an early caring center. The concept of caring was given special sanction by the American Nurses Association in its 1965 position paper, *Educational Preparation for Nurse Practitioners and Assistants to Nurses,* in which the professional role of the nurse was defined as social psychological support, teaching, and sustaining care.

From a male point of view, there is nothing inherently wrong with emphasizing caring because caring obviously is one of the basic fundamentals of nursing. The problem, however, is the way some theorists implemented it.

One faction of nursing of which Chin is representative feels that caring is a unique feminine quality. In Chin's words (2001), nursing and feminism, regardless of the definitions of either concept, are inescapably connected. By implication, caring was something that men (as males) were not especially qualified to do. This essential necessity for nurses, which so depends on what she calls the feminine values, will be changed if male nurses grow in numbers. This to some extent is true, but many of the so-called feminine qualities also exist in men. The problem is to blend them together to make better nurses. Still the emphasis by some on the uniqueness of caring to women contributes to male uneasiness. One male graduate student in the mid-1990s, in a letter he wrote to a magazine, reported some of his experience in a graduate course (Ross, 1995, pp. 58-60):

> There was a cohort of vehement feminists in the program. It became rapidly apparent to me that not only did these women have strong opinions about traditional science, but they also felt that men had no place in nursing.

These feminists were critical of empirical methodologies and proposed that nursing science should be much more qualitative and based on intuitive knowledge. It was the feminists' contention that traditional science was paternalistic and male-oriented and thus suspect at all levels. They stated that men's and women's minds operated in dramatically different ways. "Men's science" dissected an event and attempted to empiricize it and in the process lost the gestalt that was essential to understanding the event. It was the feminists' contention that only women could understand a holistic viewpoint (Ross, 1995, pp. 58-60).

The next stage of the feminist's arguments was that nursing is an eclectic and holistic science that requires an understanding of each individual's gestalt. Because nursing practice required a holistic view of patients and men could not comprehend this view, nursing research and the knowledge base of nursing should be developed by women. Their next conclusion was that caring requires specific mental function that men are not able to accomplish. Therefore men are incapable of "caring" (Ross, 1995, pp. 58-60).

To the extent that such an attitude exists, and Ross was careful to state that the caring views he criticized were not held by the majority of nurses, many strongly hold these views and make male nurses uncomfortable. In my own experience, I have met a few female nurses who would not recognize me as a nurse because I am a man. The sad part is that most current gender research would indicate that caring is not particularly confined to women. As one who has specialized in gender research, I can state that it is true that men statistically tend to be more aggressive than women and seemingly have special mathematical skills, but these statistical differences show up at the skewed end of the spectrum. The most interesting finding in gender research is the tremendous overlap in talents between most men and women (Bullough & Bullough, 1993b; Hyde, 1986). Moreover, some of the most obvious differences are as much or more cultural than biological.

NURSING IN THE TWENTY-FIRST CENTURY

Nursing changed radically in the twentieth century and will continue to change in the twenty-first. Women will remain the dominant force in nursing in the foreseeable future, and if men in nursing are to become a greater force, they have to recognize some of the anxieties and fears that many women have about men. This was emphasized by a study of men in nursing in the United Kingdom, which has a higher percentage of men in the field than in the United States. A study done in the 1980s found that half of the top posts in nursing within the British National Health Service were held by men (Nuttal, 1983). Men also were found to hold disproportionate strength in the Royal College of Nursing, where 15 of the 31 elected members were men. One female nurse felt that once male power was established, it would tend to be self-perpetuating, making it difficult for women to regain leadership (London, 1987). These fears have carried over into American nursing (Ryan & Porter, 1993). Unique factors in the British system have encouraged what might be called the "disproportionate" power of men. These factors are not present in the United States, but they still trigger a real fear for women in nursing. Even though I feel that with the changing power relationships between men and women in American society, such fears are greatly exaggerated, they still need to be confronted openly. As an academician for more than 50 years, I have observed the rapid change in the role of women, not only in American higher education but also in the business and professional worlds. There might still be a few isolated campuses where the dean of nursing is the only woman in the higher ranks of administration, but this is now rare, and female administrators now are found everywhere, many of them serving as presidents or chancellors.

It might be, as one theory holds, that the problems faced by gender minorities tend to increase as their numbers in a particular occupation grow, until they reach a critical mass, when the barriers more or less disappear.

If this is the case, then it is important to determine this critical mass where the barriers collapse. Kanter (1977) estimated that this percentage in any group ranges between 20% and 40%. Testing this theory in nursing was a study comparing women in law enforcement and men in nursing (Ott, 1989). Ott's study supports the theory in law enforcement, where women tended to see increasing resistance to their presence, but not in nursing, where men found greater acceptance in their increasing numbers. This tends to illustrate that women, or at least those in nursing, are more willing to share their domain with men than men in typically male occupations and professions such as law enforcement have been with women. In spite of Kanter's theory, nursing already has reached a critical mass, which obviously is much lower than 20%. It also would indicate that those uncomfortable with men in the nursing profession constitute only a small minority and that men are more easily accepted in nursing than many would think.

In fact, as women seek jobs in other than the traditional women's professions, the major source of potential new recruits in the future clearly will be men. Those women who do enter nursing will be far more committed to it than those who once entered merely because there seemed to be no alternative. Now women can become engineers, physicians, dentists, automobile mechanics, drivers of 18-wheel trucks, Supreme Court justices, or secretary of state, and almost no occupational position automatically is closed to them. This commitment to nursing as a profession, common among the new female students, undoubtedly will be true of the men who enter as well. It is important, however, that every nurse who is a man should be made conscious of the tremendous contribution that women have made to the profession.

Interestingly, although much of the empowerment of women in the marketplace has come through Title IX of the Civil Rights Act, no similar provision exists for men. This only emphasizes that nursing is helping to change itself by recruiting men, an act which is a credit to the profession because it was not forced to change by the law. Like any minority, men in nursing need occasionally to meet with some of their own, and for this reason the National Male Nurse Association was organized in 1971. The objectives of the organization, as defined in 1981 when it was renamed the American Assembly of Men in Nursing, are as follows:

1. Men and boys in the United States are to be encouraged to become nurses and join together with all nurses in strengthening and humanizing health care for all Americans.

2. Men who are now nurses are encouraged to grow professionally and to demonstrate to each other and to society the increasing contribution made by men within the nursing profession.

3. The American Assembly for Men in Nursing intends that its members be full participants in the nursing profession and its organizations and uses their association to achieve these goals.

The association holds that every professional nurse position and every nursing educational opportunity shall be equally available to those meeting the entry qualifications, regardless of gender. These are not particularly revolutionary goals, nor should they be. Men today go into nursing because they want to be nurses, and that is the way nursing should be and hopefully will be in the twenty-first century as it continues to emphasize the caring potential in both genders. Nursing has become a different profession from the one Nightingale first visualized, but the caring element remains its foundation.

As the twenty-first century progresses, the profession is ridding itself of the handicaps that existed throughout much of the twentieth century because it was regarded as a woman's profession (a good example being the ghetto of the diploma school), and yet the profession has managed to keep the benefits that the female predecessors have brought to nursing. Men undoubtedly will help change nursing, but it will be joining with the women to do so. Nursing is radically different at the beginnings of the twenty-first century than it was at the beginning of the twentieth, and men finally have arrived at a position where they help shape its future. Of the 210 active National Institute for Nursing Research grants, 183 recipients are women, 18 are men, and for 9 the gender could not be determined, indicative that men are contributing (Grant Doctor, 2004) at least in proportion to their membership. What the future will hold for men in nursing is that their percentage will increase and that nursing itself will continue to change, hopefully preserving the best of the past but growing with the future.

My advice to nursing and nurses is to recruit more men through conscious and deliberate campaigns. Few special programs now exist, and they are badly needed to deal with the percentage decline of women entering nursing. Yet in spite of the American Nurses Association recognition of the need to recruit men, there is a need to do more. In a survey of scholarships specifically directed to men, there is only one, the Deloras Jones RN Scholarship available through Kaiser Permanente in California. Even the nursing scholarships specifically directed to "minorities" in nursing are reserved for ethnic and racial minorities, and men are not a particular focus (Grant Doctor, 2004). In this changing world where many traditional jobs for men have disappeared or are disappearing, nursing offers men a great future, but a special effort needs to be made to make them aware of it.

REFERENCES

American Nurses Association. (1946). *Facts about nursing.* Kansas City, MO: Author.

American Nurses Association. (1965). *Educational preparation for nurse practitioners and assistants to nurses.* Kansas City, MO: Author.

American Nurses Association. (1994). *Facts about nursing.* Kansas City, MO: Author.

Bullough, B. (1994). Nursing theory and critique. In B. Bullough & V. L. Bullough (Eds.), *Nursing issues for the nineties and beyond* (pp. 64-82). New York: Springer.

Bullough, B., & Bullough, V. L. (1975). Sex segregation in health care. *Nursing Outlook, 23,* 40-45.

Bullough, V. L., & Bullough, B. (1978). *The care of the sick.* New York: Neale Watson, Prodist Science History.

Bullough, V. L., & Bullough, B. (1984). *History, trends, and politics of nursing.* Norwalk, CT: Appleton-Century-Crofts.

Bullough, V. L., & Bullough, B. (1993a). Medieval nursing. *Nursing History Review, 1,* 217-226.

Bullough, V. L., & Bullough, B. (1993b). *Cross dressing, sex, and gender.* Philadelphia: University of Pennsylvania Press.

Bush, P. J. (1976). The male nurse: A challenge to traditional role identities. *Nursing Forum, 15,* 390-405.

Chin, P. L. (2001). Feminism and nursing: Reclaiming Nightingale's vision. In J. M. Dochterman & H. K. Grace, *Current issues in nursing* (pp. 441-447). St. Louis, MO: Mosby.

Dickoff, J., James, P., & Wiedenback, P. (1968). Theory in practice discipline. *Nursing Research, 17,* 415-435, 545-554.

Grant Doctor. (2004). Men in nursing. *Science.* Retrieved from http://nextwave.sciencemag.org/cgi/content/full/2002/01/24/4

Greg, M. (1969). *Women workers and the Industrial Revolution 1750-1850* (pp. 315-316). London: Frank Case.

Hospital and health network (Computer database). (1994, October 5). 68(19), 78.

Hyde, J. S. (1986). Gender differences in aggression. In J. S. Hyde & M. C. Linn (Eds.), *The psychology of gender* (pp. 51-60). Baltimore: Johns Hopkins University Press.

Johnson, D. (1959). A philosophy of nursing. *Nursing Outlook, 7,* 198-200.

Kanter, R. M. (1977). *Men and women of the corporation.* New York: Basic Books.

Kreuter, E. R. (1957). What is good nursing care? *Nursing Outlook, 5,* 302-305.

London, F. (1987). Should men be actively recruited in nursing? *Nursing Administration Quarterly, 12*(1), 75-81.

Nash, H. J. (1936, August). Men nurses in New York State. *Trained Nurse and Hospital Review,* p. 123.

National Center for Education Statistics, U.S. Office of Education. (1999). *Digest of education statistics, 1998.* Washington, DC: U.S. Government Printing Office.

National Center for Health Workforce. (2000). *Registered nursing workforce, 7th survey.* Washington, DC: U.S. Government Printing Office.

Nuttal, P. (1983). British nursing: Beginning of a power struggle. *Nursing Outlook, 31*(3), 184.

Ott, E. M. (1989). Effect of the male-female ratio at work: Police-women and male nurses. *Psychology of Women Quarterly, 13*(1), 41-57.

Ross, D. (1995, July-August). Letter. *Skeptical Inquirer, 10,* 58-60.

Ryan, S., & Porter, S. (1993). Men in nursing: A cautionary comparative critique. *Nursing Outlook, 41*(6), 262-267.

Schoenmaker, A. (1976). Nursing's dilemma: Male versus female admissions choice. *Nursing Forum, 15,* 406-412.

Statistical Abstract of the United States. (1998). Washington, DC: U.S. Government Printing Office.

Vicinus, M. (1990). What makes a heroine? Girls' biographies of Florence Nightingale. In V. L. Bullough, B. Bullough, & M. P. Stanton (Eds.), *Florence Nightingale and her era: A collection of new scholarship* (pp. 96-107). New York: Garland.

Watson, J. (1979). *The philosophy and science of caring.* Boston: Little, Brown.

Watson, J. (1985). *Nursing, human science and human care: A theory of nursing research.* Norwalk, CT: Appleton-Century-Crofts.

Bridging Cultures

Blacks and Nursing

BETTY PIERCE DENNIS

Blacks compose 12.1% of the U.S. population. Socioeconomically, this group is dichotomous, with both a growing middle class and more than 50% in the "poor" or "near poor" income categories (Kaiser Commission on Medicaid and the Uninsured, 2002). For all income levels, blacks are more likely than whites to rate their health as "poor" (National Center for Health Statistics, 2004). More than 300 years after arriving in America, there are outstanding examples of extraordinary achievement and equally outstanding examples of failure to achieve among blacks. The net effect of this is a vastly marginalized population that despite underrepresentation in important political, social, and economic spheres of society demonstrates an impressive chronology of achievements.

Mortality among blacks is higher at each stage of the life span than for American Indians, whites, Latinos, and Asians/Pacific Islanders. Major causes of death at all ages are cancer, heart disease, and diabetes; and human immunodeficiency virus/acquired immunodeficiency syndrome among blacks leads mortality causes for the 25- to 44-year-old age group (National Center for Health Statistics, 2004). To understand how blacks arrived at this juncture requires consideration of a complex set of factors; important among these is the intersection of black history, health, and culture.

The history of blacks in America parallels the history of black nurses in America. Both histories influenced the course of black health within a cultural context that often clashed with white culture. Although American nursing history has been recorded extensively and well documented, most accounts are not complete. The history of black nurses is missing. In omitting black nurses, American nursing history signifies that their role is not significant. Therefore, reconceptualization of that history to recognize the struggles, perspectives, and contributions of black nurses as integral to the history of all nursing is essential.

> *Each generation, says noted historian John Hope Franklin (1986) has the opportunity to write its own history and indeed is obligated to do so. Only in that way can it provide its contemporaries with the materials vital to understanding the present and to planning strategies for coping with the future. Only in that way can it fulfill its obligation to pass on to posterity the accumulated knowledge and wisdom of the past, which after all, gives substance and direction for the continuity of civilization.*

Little attention has been given to (1) how black nurses came to be and what that means to health care; (2) the imprint on black culture by black nurses; and (3) the role of both phenomena in the state of black health. Historical commentaries of nursing rarely examine the role of race and racism. These factors were strong determinants of past events, and they continue to effect events today. Race and racism are not examined with intent to vilify anyone. However, scrutinizing their role can reveal some of the causes and consequences of conflict that overtly characterized past relations and typifies them today in a more nuanced and subtle way.

After the end of the Civil War in 1865, a 10-year period of reconstruction followed. During this brief span, blacks started schools, opened clinics, and established churches. They also entered politics and purchased land. This surge of progress was ended abruptly with the passing of laws that legalized racial subordination through a separate and unequal system, popularly referred to as "Jim Crow" laws. Health care, also governed by these Jim Crow laws, showed the ill effects. Black patients were refused admission to many hospitals. Those that did accept black patients housed them in "colored" wards, outbuildings, basements, or attics and limited the number admitted. Often the linen, gowns, thermometers, and the like were marked "colored" so as not to be mixed with those used by white patients (Sullivan Commission Report, 2004). The mistreatment of black patients as health care consumers in this and countless other instances has resulted in a mistrust of the health care system that persists as an unresolved and problematic issue in research and health care delivery.

Under the Jim Crow laws, potential black health care personnel effectively were prevented from receiving education as practitioners in nursing, medicine, or dentistry. In the South, blacks simply could not enter these training schools, and the North achieved similar results through the use of quotas (Hine, 1989). Segregation laws also were used to exclude blacks from membership in professional nursing organizations and societies.

BLACK HOSPITALS, BLACK NURSES

The answer of the black community to the reimposition of inequitable health care through segregation laws was to establish their own hospitals to care for black patients and to serve as the training ground for nurses, doctors, and dentists. Beginning in the 1890s, blacks established about 200 hospitals. The nurse training schools in many of the hospitals produced black nurses to care for black patients. Without these hospitals, black nurses would not exist. More than 90 hospital schools for black nurse training were established. Few black nurse graduates were hired by white hospitals, and those who were received a lower salary than white nurses (Hine, 1989). In black hospitals, black doctors had admitting privileges and opportunities for internships and residencies. Each hospital had to generate its own fiscal support. Although the role of white philanthropic groups and philanthropists was important, the commitment and determination of black community groups made these institutions happen and bore the responsibility of their ongoing support to develop and improve them as health care resources.

For example, in 1896 the Phillis Wheatley Club, a women's group, established the Phillis Wheatley Sanitarium and Nursing Training School in New Orleans. The institution was a precursor to the Flint-Goodridge Hospital and Nurse Training School. Once established, the schools and their parent hospitals waged a relentless struggle to survive. Student nurse labor was used extensively in this regard. Some white hospitals hired out students, but all black hospitals did.

Student nurses were hired out to black and white families, and the hospital collected fees for their labor. The hired-out student was on the frontline of attack on illnesses growing out of unsanitary food, water, or living conditions. In addition to work outside of the hospital and caring for patients in the hospital, the student nurse also cooked, cleaned, and washed to maintain the patient care environment. The student nurse also might have a vegetable garden or poultry farm to tend (Hine, 1989). Although wanting, these hospitals and nursing schools were the creators of a health care culture that became the bedrock for the growth of black health care professionals.

By the middle of the twentieth century, black hospitals and their nurse training schools began to close. The thrust of nursing education moved to the university. Baccalaureate nursing programs in historically black colleges and universities were begun in 1936 and now number more than 25. The fact that other programs eventually opened their doors to black nurses is less important than the fact that the nursing programs in historically black colleges and universities continue to exist and offer a baccalaureate to black nurses. In 1970, 40% of black women who held college degrees were in traditional fields such as teaching and nursing. By 2000, that number had declined by more than 50% (Mullings & Wali, 2001). However, education among blacks is prized as a major way to achieve success in the face of inequity. Data show that black nurses are more likely to hold baccalaureate and graduate degrees in nursing. Although 41.8% of whites have degrees, 48.1% of black nurses have degrees in nursing (Spratley, Johnson, Sochalski, & Fritz, 2001).

As history documents the entry of the black nurse, it also shows the impact of her presence. The black nurse has health care and cultural significance, perhaps because the two are so close as to be inseparable. Before the Civil War, nursing was considered a low-status job fit for laboring-class women. By the turn of the century, white nurse leaders heralded nursing as ideal work for middle-class women (James, 1979). This change was not reflected in the black community because from the outset, black nurses were held in high regard in the community and their work was well respected. Poverty and marginal and seasonal jobs for black men required black women to work in and out of the home. The option of staying at home was not a choice for black women as it was for whites. White nurses waged their protests of unequal treatment based on gender. Black nurses, however, emerged from a tradition of ministering to blacks and whites and had first to fight for acceptance as a black person and secondly as a woman. Many examples of black nurses with unusual capacity and great courage have come down through history, and their lives illustrate the complex nature of the problems they faced.

Florence Nightingale was not alone in recognizing the role for nurses in the Crimean War. Mary Grant Seacole traveled from Jamaica to England at her own expense to care for British soldiers and other casualties of the war. Although she brought letters of support from British army doctors, Florence Nightingale twice refused to offer her a position as an army nurse. Seacole decided to build and operate a lodging house that provided the troops a restaurant on the first floor and a health care ward on the second floor. Concocting many of her own medicines, she saved countless soldiers from conditions such as cholera, yellow fever, malaria, and diarrhea and is considered by many to be the first nurse practitioner (Messmer & Parchment, 1998). Although never formally enlisted, each evening after working all day in her canteen-cum-clinic, she volunteered at the hospital that cared for the sick and wounded of the Crimean War along with Nightingale (Carnegie, 1995). Posthumous awards to Seacole have been numerous. In February 2004 a poll conducted by the British Broadcasting Company named her the "Greatest Black Briton."

Sojourner Truth, best known as an abolitionist and women's rights advocate, used her talents in other ways as well. She was a nurse to the wounded during the Civil War. As a counselor for the Freedman's Relief Association during Reconstruction in the Washington, D.C., area, she organized a corps of women to clean Freedman's Hospital because "the sick can never be made well in dirty surroundings." She visited Congress to urge that funds be provided to train nurses and doctors. Many of her actions were known to and admired by President Lincoln, whom she met in 1864 (Carnegie, 1995).

Harriett Tubman is regarded widely for her role as an exemplary and fearless humanitarian who led more than 300 enslaved blacks to freedom on the Underground Railroad. Only 5 feet tall and unable to read or write, she again supported the cause of freedom by becoming a spy and a scout for the Union Army during the Civil War and is reported to have led troops into battle. Her work as a tireless and compassionate nurse for Union soldiers and others off the Sea Islands of South Carolina was outstanding. When she retired to her home in Auburn, New York, she took in other elderly persons and cared for them, a precursor to the nursing homes of today. In 1990 the U.S. House of Representatives passed S.J. Resolution 257 recognizing her inspired achievements (Carnegie, 1995).

The legacy of women like these and thousands more permeate American history and culture and the health care system. Mabel Staupers' story illustrates the commitment and tenacity that opened professional opportunities to black nurses. Staupers was one of the early members of the National Association of Colored Graduate Nurses (NACGN), which was founded in 1908. The NACGN gave black nurses their first opportunities for professional development and peer interaction. Staupers was the leader of a successful campaign to include black nurses in the military. Her opponents were powerful and resourceful. She was resolute and skillful. She also fought to include black nurses in the American Nurses Association (ANA). She began petitioning the ANA House of Delegates in 1934, and in 1948 the ANA approved individual membership. This circumvented the requirement to join ANA through the state associations, which still denied membership to black nurses (Staupers, 1961). Having fought successfully to bring black nurses into the mainstream of nursing organizations, Staupers and other colleagues believed that the NACGN was no longer necessary and voted to dissolve it in 1951. The validity of that decision soon came into question, because less than 20 years after the NACGN was dissolved, the National Black Nurses Association was formed to "insure continuity and flow of our common heritage" (National Black Nurses Association, n.d.). This was soon followed by the formation of the Association of Black Nursing Faculty. Chi Eta Phi, a nursing sorority, was begun in 1936 to provide opportunities in leadership development for black nurses and has grown to be an international and interracial organization (Miller, 1968). These organizations continue to play important roles.

What this brief discussion illustrates is how experiences and historical events in the same society hone and shape individuals and groups differently. At present, black and white nurses may find themselves at similar places, but they have arrived by traveling different roads, and as the poet Robert Frost says, "that has made all the difference" (Frost, 1971).

CULTURE AND HEALTH

At its most basic level, culture is an expression of the lifeways of individuals in a group or community. Black and white nurses practice not only from a defined knowledge base but also from their respective lifeways, experiences, and perspectives. Culture is an intergenerational phenomenon enmeshed in a social system, which allows human beings to meet their most basic needs. Through a consideration of history and culture, it is possible to identify the generative layer responsible for the attitudes, beliefs, and values about health held by blacks. The case of Arnella L. shows how the conflict of cultures operative in health care affects health outcomes.

> Arnella L., age 64, woke up one morning unable to see or use her right arm. An ambulance was called and she was taken to the emergency room. Her problem was diagnosed as a "light stroke," and, as the hospital was overcrowded, she was sent home in the care of relatives. The attending clinician gave her a bottle of pills, medication, she was told, that she would have to take for the rest of her life. She, however, felt that "that don't make sense," and discarded the medication. She believed that her blood had "boiled up" in her brains—her own fault for eating too much rich food. She then embarked on her own combination of healing strategies. The first of these was to sleep propped up on pillows, as postural change to allow some of the excess blood to drain back into the body. She then began a course of vinegar and honey in hot water (taken daily for nine days) to bring the excess blood down to a safe level. Finally, she brought in her minister to pray for her; she later reported that she "felt the stroke leave" her body when he laid his hand on her head. In any case, a niece stated bitterly, "The doctors didn't do nothin' for her and that's for sure." (Snow, 1980)

In this case, the patient's health beliefs are presented within their cultural context. Their effects on treatment and patient outcomes are clear. The example also demonstrates the historical reliance of some blacks on self-care or folk medicine (Bushy, 1992; Wilson-Ford, 1992). Seventy percent to 90% of recognized illnesses in blacks are estimated to be managed outside the formal health care system (Kleinman, Eisenberg, & Good, 1978; Phillips, Mayer, & Aday, 2000). Caregivers could have begun a dialogue with Arnella L. by asking a few brief, open-ended questions to begin to learn about her and her illness. This information then would have been used to collaborate with her in devising a mutually satisfactory plan of care that she would follow.

Several cultural assessment tools have been proposed to capture relevant patient data. To date, most of these tools are comprehensive but too lengthy and time consuming for clinical use (Giger & Davidhizar, 1999; Purnell & Paulanka, 2003). More importantly, most tools do not capture the heterogeneity within the group.

Many blacks can identify with Arnella L.; many others cannot. Between those two extremes are a multitude of variations, all subscribed to by blacks at varying levels of income, education, social position, and experience. A promising approach to establishing a cross-cultural interaction is the use of the client's own explanatory system. Included as a fundamental part of the nursing process, the client's cultural parameters can be assessed quickly through the use of open-ended questions, such as those suggested by Kleinman, Eisenberg, and Good (1978, p. 256):

◆ What do you think caused this illness?
◆ What concerns you most about this illness?
◆ Why do you think it started when it did?
◆ How do you feel about it?
◆ What did you do about treating it before coming to the clinic/hospital?
◆ What do you think your sickness does to you?
◆ How serious is this illness?
◆ What kind of treatment do you think you should receive?

These questions are amenable to time and circumstance. One may ask these questions early or late in a client's contact with the health care system. One easily may postpone asking the questions until after the acute phase of an illness.

The case of Arnella L. also raises another issue. Do clients feel that their self-care approaches will be considered seriously or respected? Does the health care system acknowledge that there are nontraditional ways of care and healing? Many blacks are reticent about sharing culturally derived treatment methods. Instead, they may use a technique called "impression management" to project conforming behavior as was played out in the Arnella L. scenario. Using impression management, the client responds as expected and avoids appearing self-destructive or unconcerned. Until the health care system is able to be inclusive and open, patients may resort to techniques like impression management to move through the health care system.

Health is a nonlinear, developmental process usually described in broad and general terms. This makes it difficult to see the prismatic patterns of experience in which health is one of those elements interacting within the larger cultural and historical context. Even after working closely with black clients, many nurses fail to recognize how history has shaped the perceptions of health and the behaviors that relate to health. What is accepted and acknowledged by health care providers is the role played by lifestyle choices such as smoking, exercise, and diet. Clearly, for blacks these lifestyle choices are inseparable from the parallel system of racism, discrimination, poverty, substandard education, and the day-to-day tensions created by racism. The suggestion that cultural consonance and dissonance are primary explanations of ill health in blacks explains only part of the issue. The structural constraints of society in the form of institutional racism have left their mark on the bodies of blacks and have shortened their lives. The continuing disparate health status of blacks attests to this fact.

RACE AND HEALTH

Black health in America has never been good health. For example, over the years the number of black and white infant deaths has declined, but the ratio of black to white infant deaths is almost identical to that recorded in the early part of the twentieth century (Hine, 1989; Centers for Disease Control and Prevention, 2002). Diabetes is 70% higher among blacks (Centers for Disease Control and Prevention, 2002). Asthma is now the most common chronic disease among American children. Age-adjusted deaths from asthma are 3 times higher for blacks than for whites (U.S. Department of Health and Human Services, 2000). Deaths from asthma exceed 70,000 annually. A recent study of mortality data by Woolf, Johnson, Fryer, Rust, and Satcher (2004) suggests that reducing the mortality rate of blacks to that of whites could save 5 times more lives than could be saved by improvements in medical technology. The authors estimate that 886,202 deaths from 1991 to 2000 could have been averted. They also calculated that medical advances averted only 176,633 deaths during that period. These findings have health and economic significance.

The sense of self of all blacks begins as an intragroup attitude but is finely and finally shaped by how the world sees them. The term *African American* is a cognitive construct with uncertain scientific merit. In other words, African Americans are African Americans because they are recognized and treated as such. Variation characterizes all racial and ethnic groups and is thought to move on a continuum; therefore it cannot be captured in neat racial boxes ("Biological Anthropologist," 1995). However, the nature-nurture or genetics-environment concept of disease causation persists as an explanatory model (Anonymous, 1983; Cooper & David, 1986; Langford, 1981; Thomas, 1992).

Race is heavily weighted in perceived meanings of African American. Race is almost always an antecedent of diseases that are defined by genetics or environmental

factors (Freeman, 2004). Variations such as income and education are combined with health measures to form comparative relationships. On the face of it, blacks do exhibit differences in some morbid conditions. They have a low incidence of multiple sclerosis, cystic fibrosis, and skin cancer ("Biological Anthropologist," 1995) and a high incidence of hypertension, diabetes, and cancer (Centers for Disease Control and Prevention, 2002). However, validation of genetic variation requires more than counting of cases. When the aperture is widened to include nontraditional measures, a more complete picture appears. Genes, environment, and culture must be synergized to see how they affect health.

More than one third of black families have incomes below the poverty level, but blacks with higher incomes may have similar health problems. In other words, income is not a protective factor for blacks. Thomas et al. (1985) and Thomas, Semenya, Neser, Thomas, and Gillum (1990) studied precursors of hypertension in a cohort of black physicians for more than 25 years. The mortality of these physicians matched the mortality of low-income blacks rather than that of their white peers. Similarly, hypertension in men in low occupational classes increased when they remained in that status. Although blacks and whites experienced elevated blood pressures, increases in hypertension were greatest for blacks (Waitzman & Smith, 1994). Among blacks, hypertension develops earlier and with greater severity. Sixty-six percent of all cases of end-stage renal disease caused by hypertension occur among blacks (Epstein et al., 2000). Heurtin-Roberts and Reisin (1992) found that among hypertensive black, the patient's cultural beliefs about hypertension influenced their acceptance of treatment and in turn the control of their blood pressure.

Further, when health data are partitioned according to factors such as urban density, outcomes change. Used as a surrogate measure of socioeconomic status, urban density reduces differences in cancer risks between blacks and whites. High-population areas have higher incidences of cancer regardless of race. This may begin to explain why some conditions that have the highest prevalence in blacks are not correlated with income or education (Kressin & Petersen, 2001).

The periodic appearance of reports that indicate a strong association between the race of the patient and the quality of the care received feeds a deep sense of mistrust and skepticism. Examples include reports such as "Mississippi appendectomies" or eugenic hysterectomies performed on black women (Chase, 1980), testing of women for sickle cell anemia without consent

(Farfel & Holtzman, 1986), court-ordered surgical interventions (Kolder, Gallagher, & Parsons, 1987), and the Tuskegee Syphilis Study. Racial differences in drug response were recorded as early as 1929. However, recent studies show that although blacks differ in drug response and disposition, they continue to be underrepresented in clinical trials of new drugs (Shavers, Lynch, & Burmeister, 2002). In 1994, Congress passed the National Institutes of Health Revitalization Act mandating greater representation of minorities and women in research. Gilbert (2004) found that today, these groups continue to be underrepresented in clinical trials. This mistrust is in part the legacy of unethical treatment of the poor, racial, and ethnic minorities by research and medicine (Corbie-Smith, Thomas, & St. George, 2002; Dennis, 1999).

Heart disease is the number one cause of death in blacks, but whites use significantly more of the available treatments for heart disease, such as coronary angioplasty and coronary artery bypass grafting (Wenneker & Epstein, 1989). The Wenneker and Epstein study along with 99 others were examined in an investigation by the Institute of Medicine (2003) that left little doubt about the inequities of the health care system for the black patient. The committee was "struck by the consistency" of the research studies. The following is a summary of the conclusions of this seminal study:

◆ Racial and ethnic disparities in health care exist and, because they are associated with worse outcomes in most cases, are unacceptable.
◆ Racial and ethnic disparities in health care occur in the context of broader historical and contemporary social and economic inequality, and there is evidence of persistent racial and ethnic discrimination in many sectors of American life.
◆ Many sources—including health systems, health care providers, patients, and utilization managers—may contribute to racial and ethnic disparities in health care.
◆ Bias, stereotyping, prejudice, and clinical uncertainty on the part of health care providers may contribute to racial and ethnic disparities in health care. Although indirect evidence from several lines of research supports this statement, a greater understanding of the prevalence and influence of these processes is needed and should be sought through research. A small number of studies suggest that racial and ethnic minority patients are more likely than white patients to refuse treatment. These studies find that differences in refusal rates are generally small and that minority patient refusal does not fully explain health care disparities (p. 19).

These findings on health disparities are rooted in history, as is the underrepresentation of blacks in the health care professions, especially nursing. Today, black nurses are only 4.9% of the registered nurse population, whereas blacks compose more than 12% of the U.S. population. An additional 20,000 nurses would be needed to raise the figure by 1 percentage point (Spratley et al., 2001). The Sullivan Commission Report (2004) found that overarching themes of history, systemic exclusion, and inequality continue to work against the realization of diversity in the health care professions.

NURSING MATTERS

Nurses are positioned uniquely to offer culturally competent care to black patients. Blacks have high incidences of diseases that are preventable. Therefore making a significant difference in the health of this group is highly probable. Since the 1960s the nursing profession has encouraged the incorporation of culture into care. Achieving this, however, has been a slow process. In 1992 the American Academy of Nursing Expert Panel on Culturally Competent Nursing Care concluded that, "there are no excuses for continuing to provide care that is insensitive and [culturally] incompetent" (p. 277). The Eurocentric model of nursing care is used continuously to devise nursing care for all who enter the health care system, but it has never been adequate. The limitation of the North American Nursing Diagnosis Association (NANDA) nursing diagnoses is a case in point. Two hundred and forty-five nurses from eight countries rated the usefulness of the defining characteristics listed by NANDA for three nursing diagnoses. In each instance, the diagnosis had to be expanded and rewritten, a significant number of its diagnostic characteristics deleted and others added (Geissler, 1991). From a cultural viewpoint, many NANDA terms have multiple meanings. Social dysfunction and social isolation are two of those labels that must be defined within their cultural context. Across cultures, their meanings change (Kelley & Frisch, 1992). Nursing diagnoses are a mainstay of the nursing process, but blacks and other culturally diverse groups may not be well served by their use until they are customized.

Data from the recent report of the Institute of Medicine (2004) strongly suggest that beliefs may not be modified by the types of health promotion campaigns that are currently prevalent. Beliefs can be affected, however, when the message is delivered in a culturally sensitive format. The well-intentioned but culturally inappropriate message is apparent in the following two examples. First, black women in abusive relationships, states Campbell (1993), have concepts of independence and female strength that run counter to accepted ways of help seeking and resource use. These women are more likely to remain in their relationships and prefer assistance in working through the abuse problem. This is at odds with the Eurocentric model, which places emphasis on leaving the relationship. The deliberate capture of cultural content must precede real changes in nursing approaches (Camphina-Bacote, 2002). Second, cultural and historical influences are basic to nurse-client relationships, and whether acknowledged or ignored, they frame the interaction. Blacks respond positively to culturally sensitive therapeutics. A pilot project in which music therapists used black music to open avenues of expression for psychiatric clients was remarkably successful when compared with programs using Eurocentric music (Camphina-Bacote & Allbright, 1992).

I believe that as nursing appreciates the impact of culture on practice, the need for greater expertise will advance. As nurses are encouraged to acknowledge cultural patterns, the relevance of history and social context to care will become more apparent. Culture must be allowed to move up in the curricular hierarchy when nursing students are being transformed into professional nurses. Culture also must be integrated as part of the nursing process with a permanent, prominent venue. Given the opportunity to identify their own attitudes, beliefs, and values, nurses can begin to explore ways in which their heritage affects their own behavior.

Nurses are pivotal members of the health care team. They personify one culture (their own), convey another (nursing and health care), and arbitrate a third (the client's). They can lead the way to cultural plurality. Cultural sensitivity is a brave new world—similar to the old and familiar, yet remarkably diverse and different. We may argue as to whether health care is a right or a privilege, but there is no disagreement that it is a choice. Blacks make that choice based on their perceptions of what the health care system offers. Health behaviors are retained because they are functional, but they do not stand alone. Health behaviors are embedded in cultural and historical realities (Dennis & Small, 2003). When black clients are validated by the health care system in all their sociocultural dimensions, a reciprocal, productive relationship can develop that is built on mutual understanding and respect with the ability finally to eliminate health disparities.

REFERENCES

American Academy of Nursing Expert Panel on Culturally Competent Nursing. (1992). AAN Expert Panel report: Culturally competent nursing care. *Nursing Outlook, 40*(6), 277-283.

Anonymous. (1983). Genetics, environment, and hypertension. *Lancet, 1,* 681-682.

Biological anthropologist traces black's genetic heritage. (1995, July 28). *The Chronicle of Higher Education*, pp. A11, A16.

Bushy, A. (1992). Cultural considerations for primary health care: Where do self care and folk medicine fit? *Holistic Nursing Practice, 6*(3), 10-18.

Campbell, D. W. (1993). Nursing care of African American battered women. *AWHONN's Clinical Issues in Perinatal and Women's Health Nursing, 4*(33), 407-414.

Camphina-Bacote, J. (2002). The process of cultural competence in the delivery of healthcare services: A model of care. *Journal of Transcultural Nursing, 13*(3), 181-184.

Camphina-Bacote, J., & Allbright, R. (1992). Ethnomusic therapy and the dual-diagnosed African American client. *Holistic Nursing Practice, 6*(3), 59-63.

Carnegie, M. E., (1995). *The path we tread: Blacks in nursing worldwide, 1854-1994* (3rd ed). New York: National League for Nursing Press.

Centers for Disease Control and Prevention. (2002). *National vital statistics report.* Hyattsville, MD: National Center for Health Statistics.

Chase, A. (1980). *The legacy of Malthus: The social costs of the new scientific racism.* New York: Alfred A. Knopf.

Cooper, R., & David, R. (1986). The biological concept of race and its application to public health epidemiology. *Journal of Health Politics and Law, 11*(1), 97-116.

Corbie-Smith, G., Thomas, S. B., & St. George, D. M. (2002). Distrust, race, and research. *Archives of Internal Medicine, 162*(21), 2458-2463.

Dennis, B. P. (1999). The origin and nature of informed consent: Experiences among vulnerable groups. *Journal of Professional Nursing, 15*(5), 281-287.

Dennis, B. P., & Small, E. B. (2003). Incorporating cultural diversity in nursing care: An action plan. *Journal of the Association of Black Nursing Faculty in Higher Education, 14*(1), 17-26.

Epstein, A. M., Ayanian, J. Z., Keogh, J. H., Noonan, S. J., Armistead, N., Cleary, P. D., et al. (2000). Racial disparities in access to renal transplantation. *New England Journal of Medicine, 343*(21), 1537-1544.

Farfel, M. R., & Holtzman, N. A. (1986). Education, consent, and counseling in sickle cell anemia screening programs. *American Journal of Public Health, 74*(4), 373-375.

Franklin, J. H. (1986). On the evolution of scholarship in Afro-American history. In D. C. Hine (Ed.), *The state of*

Afro-American history: Past, present, and future. Baton Rouge: Louisiana State University Press.

Freeman, H. P. (2004). Poverty, culture, and social injustice determinants of cancer disparities. *Cancer Journal for Clinicians, 54*(2), 72-78.

Frost, R. (1971). *The road not taken: A selection of Robert Frost poems.* New York: Henry Holt.

Geissler, E. M. (1991). Nursing diagnoses of culturally diverse patients. *International Nursing Review, 38*(5), 150-152.

Giger, J., & Davidhizar, R. (1999). *Transcultural nursing: Assessment and intervention* (3rd ed.). St. Louis, MO: Mosby-Year Book.

Gilbert, C. (2004). Fewer minorities than ever in cancer trials. *JAMA: The Journal of the American Medical Association, 291,* 2720-2726.

Heurtin-Roberts, S., & Reisin, E. (1992). The relation of culturally influenced lay models of hypertension to compliance with treatment. *American Journal of Hypertension, 5,* 787-792.

Hine, D. C. (1989). *Black women in white: Racial conflict and cooperation in the nursing profession 1890-1950.* Bloomington: Indiana University Press.

Institute of Medicine. (2003). *Unequal treatment: Confronting racial and ethnic disparities in health care.* Washington, DC: Author.

Institute of Medicine. (2004). *Health literacy: A prescription to end confusion.* Washington, DC: Author.

James, J. W. (1979). Isabel Hampton and the professionalization of nursing in the 1890s. In M. J. Vogel & C. E. Rosenburg (Eds.), *The therapeutic revolution: Essays in the social history of American medicine* (pp. 201-244). Philadelphia: University of Pennsylvania Press.

Kaiser Commission on Medicaid and the Uninsured. (2002). *Analysis of March 2002 Current Population Survey.* Washington, DC: Author.

Kelley, J. H., & Frisch, N. C. (1992). A transcultural concept analysis of social isolation. In R. M. Carroll-Johnson & M. Paquette (Eds.), *Classification of nursing diagnosis: Proceedings of the tenth conference* (pp. 232-233). Philadelphia: Lippincott.

Kleinman, A., Eisenburg, L., & Good, B. (1978). Culture, illness and care. Clinical lessons from anthropologic and cross-cultural research. *Annals of Internal Medicine, 88,* 251-258.

Kolder, V., Gallagher, J., & Parsons, M. T. (1987). Court-ordered obstetrical interventions. *New England Journal of Medicine, 316*(19), 1192-1196.

Kressin, N. R., & Petersen, L. A. (2001). Racial differences in the use of invasive cardiovascular procedures: Review of the literature and prescription for future research. *Annals of Internal Medicine, 135*(5), 352-366.

Langford, H. G. (1981). Is blood pressure different in black people? *Postgraduate Medical Journal, 57,* 749-754.

Messmer, P. R., & Parchment, Y. (1998). Mary Seacole: The first nurse practitioner. *Clinical Excellence for Nurse Practitioners, 2*(1), 47-51.

Miller, H. S. (1968). *The history of Chi Eta Phi Sorority.* Washington, DC: The Association for the Study of Negro Life and History.

Mullings, L., & Wali, A. (2001). *Stress and resilience: The social context of reproduction in Harlem.* New York: Kluwer Academic/Plenum.

National Black Nurses Association. (n.d.). *About NBNA: The beginning years.* Retrieved December 12, 2004, from http://www.nbna.org./beginning.htm

National Center for Health Statistics. (2004). *Health, United States, 2004 with chartbook on trends in the health of Americans.* Hyattsville, MD: Author.

Phillips, K. A., Mayer, M. I., & Aday, L. A. (2000). Barriers to care among racial/ethnic groups under managed care. *Health Affairs, 19,* 65-75.

Purnell, L. D., & Paulanka, B. J. (2003). *Transcultural health care: A culturally competent approach* (2nd ed.). Philadelphia: F.A. Davis.

Shavers, V. L., Lynch, C. F., & Burmeister, L. F. (2002). Racial differences in factors that influence the willing to participate in medical research studies. *Annuals of Epidemiology, 12*(4), 248-256.

Snow, L. F. (1980). Ethnicity and clinical care: American blacks. *Physician Assistant & Health Practitioner, 4*(7), 50-54, 58.

Spratley, E., Johnson, A., Sochalski, J., & Fritz, M. (2001). *The registered nurse population. March 2000: Findings from the National Sample Survey of Registered Nurses.* Rockville, MD: Health Resources Services Administration.

Staupers, M. K. (1961). *No time for prejudice: A story of the integration of Negroes in nursing in the United States.* New York: Macmillan.

Sullivan Commission Report. (2004). *Missing persons: Minorities in the health professions.* Battle Creek: W.K. Kellogg Foundation.

Thomas, J., Semenya, K., Neser, W. B., Thomas, J., & Gillum, R. F. (1990). Parental hypertension as a predictor of hypertension in black physicians: The Meharry cohort study. *Journal of the National Medical Association, 82*(6), 409-412.

Thomas, J., Semenya, K., Neser, W. B., Thomas, J., Green, D. R., & Gillum, R. F. (1985). Risk factors and the incidence of hypertension in black physicians: The Meharry cohort study. *American Heart Journal, 110*(3), 637-645.

Thomas, V. G. (1992). Explaining health disparities between African American and white populations. Where do we go from here? *Journal of the National Medical Association, 84*(10), 837-840.

U.S. Department of Health and Human Services & Centers for Disease Control and Prevention. (2000). *Asthma prevalence, health care use and mortality, 2000-2001.* Hyattsville, MD: National Center for Health Statistics.

Waitzman, N. J., & Epstein, A. M. (1994). The effects of occupational class transitions on hypertension: Racial disparities among working-age men. *American Journal of Public Health, 84*(6), 945-950.

Waitzman, N. J., & Smith, K. R. (1994). The effects of occupational class transitions on hypertension: Racial disparities among working-age men. *American Journal of Public Health 84*(6): 945-950.

Wenneker, M. B., & Epstein, A. M. (1989). Racial inequalities in the use of procedures for patients with ischemic heart disease in Massachusetts. *JAMA: The Journal of the American Medical Association, 261*(2), 253-257.

Wilson-Ford, V. (1992). Health-protective behaviors of rural black elderly women. *Health and Social Work, 17*(1), 28-36.

Woolf, S. H., Johnson, R. E., Fryer, G. E., Rust, G., & Satcher, D. (2004). The health impact of resolving racial disparities: An analysis of US mortality data. *American Journal of Public Health, 94*(12), 2078-2081.

Narrowing the Health Disparities Gap

Asians and Pacific Islanders and Nursing

JILLIAN INOUYE

The Asian-American population, like the Hispanic and Native American populations, now generally are understood to be a heterogeneous group with different languages, cultures, and residency in the United States. They represent 4.2% of the total population, or 11.9 million persons, and are the fastest-growing group, increasing about 70% between 1990 and 2000. The five largest groups in descending order are the Chinese, Filipinos, Asian Indians, Vietnamese, and Koreans, which together make up about 80% of the Asian-American population (U.S. Census Bureau, 2004).

Contrary to the popular belief of longevity in Asians, they have a lower median age than the total U.S. population; 8% of Asians were aged 65 and over compared with 12% of the total population. More than 60% are married compared with 53% of the total population, with an average household of three members (U.S. Census Bureau, 2004).

Sixty-nine percent of all Asian Americans are foreign born, except for the Japanese, of whom 40% are foreign born compared with about 75% each for Asian Indians, Vietnamese, Koreans, Pakistanis, and Thai. Most of the foreign born population (75%) came to the United States over the past 2 decades. This may explain why almost 79% of Asian Americans over 5 years of age speak a language other than English at home, and about 40% speak English less than "very well." The Japanese was the only group with more than 50% who speak only English at home (U.S. Census Bureau, 2004).

Although the percent of those holding a high school education is roughly the same for Asian Americans and all other people, a higher proportion of Asian Americans (44%) versus the total population (24%) earned at least a bachelor's degree. Asian Indians have the highest percentage with a bachelor's degree.

Filipino women have the highest labor force participation rate at approximately 65%, which is more than 2% higher than the next highest rate (Thai); whereas Pakistani women followed by the Hmong and Japanese have the lowest percent in the labor force. For men, Asian Indian and Pakistani men have the highest labor force participation rates (79% and 77%, respectively).

Although a higher percent (45%) of Asian Americans are employed in management, professional, and related occupations compared with the total population (34%), these varied greatly from highest (Asian Indian at 59%) to the lowest (Laotian at 13.4%). Asian Indian, Japanese, and Chinese men had the three top median earnings, and the Japanese, Asian Indian, and Chinese women have the highest median earnings. The median annual income is higher than the median for all families. However, poverty rates for the Asian-American population and the total population were similar despite higher median earnings for Asian Americans. Home ownership is lower for Asian Americans than for the total population (U.S. Census Bureau, 2004).

The 2002 U.S. Census refers to Native Hawaiian and Other Pacific Islanders as those with origins in any of the original peoples of Hawaii, Guam, Samoa, or other Pacific islands. Of the total U.S. population, 399,000 persons or 0.1%, reported themselves as Pacific Islander, whereas 476,000 reported Pacific Islander and other for a total of 0.3% combined. More than half of the Pacific Islander population lives in two states, Hawaii and California (U.S. Census Bureau, 2001). Native Hawaiians, at 401,000, were the largest group, followed by Samoans and Guamanians at 91,000 and 42,000, respectively.

ASIAN AMERICAN/PACIFIC ISLANDER NURSING WORKFORCE

Although underrepresented minorities compose 25% of the nation's population, they compose only 10% of all health care professionals (Ricketts & Gaul, 2004). Asian Americans/Pacific Islanders compose 5.7% of the registered nurse workforce compared with 9.2% for black, 3% Hispanic, and 0.4% Indian/Eskimo Aleutian. The white rate of 81.7% remains relatively stable (U.S. Census Bureau, 2001). Although these figures reflect an "overrepresentation" of Asians/Pacific Islanders among health care professions, because of the heterogeneous nature of each Asian and Pacific Islander subgroup, they do not truly represent the disparities in the workforce.

The data for Asian Americans/Pacific Islanders illustrate the disparities in demographics and cultural variants. How do health care providers address these issues and avoid the tendency to aggregate, stereotype, and stigmatize? This chapter briefly discusses the major identified health disparities, possible reasons for its continuation, and suggested approaches to narrow the gap.

Health Disparities of Asians/Pacific Islanders

The Institute of Medicine report (2002) documents widespread disparities in health and use of health care services among racial and ethnic minority groups in the United States. The report points to causes that are multifactorial and include patient-, physician-, and system-level factors such as trust, cultural competency and bias, health insurance coverage, and knowledge. The Commonwealth Fund 2001 Health Care Quality Survey, sampling 669 Asian Americans, found that they reported poorer quality of health care than the overall population. Specifically, they had greater communication difficulties with their physicians, fewer preventive services, less chronic disease care, and less satisfaction with the quality of their health care (Collins et al., 2002).

Asian Americans represent both extremes of socioeconomic and health indexes: although more than a million Asian Americans live at or below the federal poverty level. Asian American women have the highest life expectancy of any other group. For the total U.S. population, the age-adjusted death rate for Native Hawaiians is 901 per 100,000 compared with 524 per 100,000 for the general population (President's Advisory Commission on Asian Americans and Pacific Islanders, 2001). Asian Americans suffer disproportionately from certain types of cancer, tuberculosis, and hepatitis B (U.S. Census, 2000).

According to the National Center for Health Statistics (2003), the 12 leading causes of death in the United States in 2001 for Asian Americans/Pacific Islanders were malignant neoplasms, heart disease, cerebrovascular disease, unintentional injuries, diabetes mellitus, chronic lower respiratory diseases, influenza, pneumonia, suicide, nephritis, nephrotic syndrome, neoplasms, and homicide. Native Hawaiians and Other Pacific Islanders have a disproportionately high prevalence of the following conditions and risk factors: hepatitis B, human immunodeficiency virus/acquired immunodeficiency syndrome, and tuberculosis. Furthermore, Asian Americans have a disproportionately high prevalence of the following conditions and risk factors: chronic obstructive pulmonary diseases, hepatitis B, human immunodeficiency virus/acquired immunodeficiency syndrome, tobacco smoke, and tuberculosis.

According to the 2000 U.S. Census, about 21% of Asian Americans/Pacific Islanders lack health insurance compared with about 16% of the general population. For cancer, from 1988 to 1992 the highest age-adjusted incidence rate of cervical cancer occurred among Vietnamese-American women (43 per 100,000), almost 5 times higher than the rate among non-Hispanic white women (7.5 per 100,000). From 1988 to 1992 the highest incidence rate of liver and intrahepatic bile duct cancer was seen in Vietnamese-American men (41.8 per 100,000), more than 10 times higher than the rate among non-Hispanic white men (3.3 per 100,000). Asian Americans/Pacific Islanders had the highest tuberculosis case rates (33 per 100,000) of any racial and ethnic population in 2001 (14 per 100,000 for non-Hispanic blacks, 12 per 100,000 for Hispanics/Latinos, 11 per 100,000 for American Indians/Alaska Natives, and 2 per 100,000 for non-Hispanic whites). Although the rate of acute hepatitis B among Asian Americans/Pacific Islanders has been decreasing, the reported rate in 2001 was more than twice as high among Asian Americans/Pacific Islanders (2.95 per 100,000) as among white Americans (1.31 per 100,000). From 1996 to 2000, Native Hawaiians were 2.5 times more likely to be diagnosed with diabetes than non-Hispanic white residents of Hawaii of similar age. In 2000, infant mortality among Native Hawaiians was 9.1 per 1,000, almost 60% higher than among whites (5.7 per 1,000). Native Hawaiians in Hawaii had an asthma rate of 139.5 per 1,000 in 2000, almost twice the rate for all other races in Hawaii (71.5 per 1,000). In 2000, 30.9% of Native Hawaiians in Hawaii reported smoking cigarettes, compared with 19.7% of Hawaii residents overall.

VIEWPOINTS

Factors potentially contributing to prolonging these disparities for Asian Americans include lack of adequate data and research, language and cultural barriers, lack of mentoring for health care professionals, stigma associated with certain conditions, and beginning efforts on the part of federal agencies to develop strategic plans to address the needs.

Barriers to Narrowing the Health Disparities Gap

LACK OF DATA. The 2000 Census recently provided needed information in disaggregating the Asian Americans and the Pacific Islanders as two distinct groups. This allows distinguishing of disparities for Asian Americans/Pacific Islanders and Pacific Islanders as separate groups. However, little research and data exist on specific health problems in the different ethnic groups. For example, little research has been done with Filipino Americans across the social strata, across generations, and across genders, despite the large numbers in the population and in the workforce. Because of this, explanations or causes for the disparities and measures to address them are difficult to identify. Nor can the relationships between health disparities and demographics be explained. Because data drive almost all programs and services, without research and the resulting data, many Asian Americans/Pacific Islanders may be excluded from participation in federal programs (President's Advisory Commission on Asian Americans and Pacific Islanders, 2001) and having culturally tailored interventions as a result of evidence-based research.

COMMUNICATION BARRIERS. The Asian American/Pacific Islander subgroups speak more than 100 different dialects and languages. A thorough review by Yeo (2004) examined how language barriers may contribute to health disparities. She found consequences of language barriers ranging from miscommunication to inefficient use of health care services such as understanding the side effects of medication, satisfaction with medical care, and number of health care visits.

According to the Commonwealth Fund report, Hispanics and Asian Americans stand out as the least well served by the health care systems because of communication problems. Thirty-nine percent of Asian Americans have an Asian-American physician compared with 82% of whites who have a white doctor. Twenty-seven percent of Asian Americans reported one or more of the following problems: their doctor did not listen to everything they said, they did not understand their doctor fully, or they had questions but did not ask them during their visits (Collins et al., 2002). Chinese Americans (37%) felt less likely to feel welcome at their doctor's office, with the Chinese, Koreans, and Vietnamese

the least likely among minorities to be satisfied with their health care services and insurance plans (Collins et al., 2002; Hawks, 1996).

In relation to disparities resulting from clinical encounters and interactions between a doctor and a patient, Balsa and McGuire (2003) propose a unified conceptual model to show three possible mechanisms resulting in disparities: prejudice in the form of physicians being less willing to interact with members of minority groups; clinical uncertainty associated with differential interpretation of symptoms from minority patients; or distinct prior engagements and stereotypes held about health-related behaviors of minority patients. Because race is always observable, group categorizations may result in miscommunications regardless of benevolence on the part of the health care provider (in this case, physicians).

Cultural Beliefs, Values, and Attitudes as Possible Barriers

According to the Hughes (2002), Asian Americans, particularly Chinese, Vietnamese, and Filipinos, are more likely to agree that it is better to take care of one's own health and that staying healthy is a matter of luck. This may explain why 52% of Asian Americans versus 39% of white, 40% of blacks, and 34% of Hispanics reported that they did not follow their doctor's advice. The reason was that they disagreed with the advice. Furthermore, 32% of Asian Americans and 25% of Hispanics said they did not follow the doctor's advice because it went against personal beliefs, compared with 19% of whites and 13% of blacks.

Asian Americans are slightly more likely than the general population to use herbal medicine (20% versus 23%). They are twice as likely to use acupuncture (6%) and services of traditional healers (6%). Thirty-eight percent of Vietnamese and 36% of Japanese use herbal medicine, 24% of Koreans use acupuncture, and 14% of Chinese consult with traditional healers (Hughes, 2002).

Asian Americans are also less likely to report leaving it up to their doctor to make the right decisions for their health. They believe that their doctors are less likely to understand their background and values and feel that they are looked down upon by their physicians. About 45% of Asian Americans reported that family and friends were the most frequently reported source of health information. Twice as many (11%) believe they would get better care if they were not of a different race or ethnicity than the overall population (5%) (Hughes, 2002). This lack of trust and understanding is a huge barrier to seeking and adhering to health care regimens for Asian Americans/Pacific Islanders.

Native Hawaiians, regardless of how distantly persons were related, still are considered brothers and sisters. This relationship stems from their roots from the `oha, or the *taro corm,* and is defined as `ohana. The `ohana included parents, grandparents, children, ties of blood and non-related persons, and the `aumakua, or family god (Lindo, 2004). Affection and warmth are the values of the `ohana. This included those "hanai" or adopted into different families and who are treated equally as family members. A recent controversial case involved an adopted young white boy who applied to a school reserved for those with Hawaiian blood. The child was considered "Hawaiian" by his family because of his status in the Hawaiian family. Unfortunately, not everyone shared these views.

In the `ohana there is a sense of shared involvement, mutual responsibility, interdependence and helpfulness. The belief that life is interconnected relates to dependence on others for survival and open sharing of food and resources (Lindo, 2004). To this day, the Hawaiian culture is known worldwide for its "aloha" spirit of sharing, graciousness, and love.

A culture also can be understood by its proverbs and sayings. Although many proverbs are universal, two Japanese and Hawaiian proverbs illustrate some of the specific values and beliefs of each of these cultures. A Japanese proverb states, *Deru kui wa utareu* ("A protruding post is hammered down"). A Hawaiian proverb states *E noho iho i ke opu weuweu, mai ho`oki`eki`e,* or "Remain among the clumps of grass and do not elevate yourself," which has been further interpreted as "Don't show off. Don't get puffed up and big-headed," but to be *ha`aha`a* (humble), which does not mean timid, submissive, and spineless. These sayings reflect a value of inner self-confidence that gives rise to quiet strength and self-reliance and is seen as far more admirable than self-importance, arrogance, and egotism. Another Hawaiian saying, `Ike aku, `ike mai, kokua aku kokua mai; pela iho la ka nohana `ohana (Pukui, 1983), translates to "Recognize others, be recognized, help others, be helped; such is a family relationship." The explanation given for this is that many native Hawaiians live with their extended family and family is the most important part of life for them. This saying teaches why they should put family first. In the `ohana or family, you know others and they know you, you help others and know you will be helped if there is anything you need (Lindo, 2004).

These proverbs exemplify the value of humility and not elevating oneself and the deep ties with the family,

in contrast to the Western values of independence, assertiveness, self-reliance, and self-promotion. In general, values and beliefs in the Asian American/Pacific Islander culture focus on thinking of the good of the family, culture, the individual, and finally to the outer world. These are reflected in behaviors of socialization and obligations within the family first, then to the culture, the individual, and finally to others. These values are illustrated in the socialization patterns of obligations within the family with leftover time for social events with colleagues and acquaintances.

Another Hawaiian saying is, *Nana ka maka; ho`olohe ka pepeiao; pa`a ka waha,* or "Observe with the eyes; listen with the ears; shut the mouth." Thus one learns (Pukui, 1983). The Japanese also have similar sayings: "Silence surpasses speech" and "The inarticulate speak longest." (Takashima, 1981). This may explain silence and lack of questioning of health care providers on the part of Asian Americans/Pacific Islander, and may be misconstrued as acceptance and/or understanding.

Beliefs, values, and attitudes regarding the importance of family, not standing out, and difficulty with trust, respect, and communication with health care providers tend to pull this group inward to those close to them for support and care. This can be a double-edged sword because more traditional Western forms of care may be rejected to the detriment of their health. Other beliefs, such as a strong sense of self-care and personal beliefs, in Asian Americans may be reasons for noncompliance with health care.

Social Capital. Closely related to cultural values for Asian Americans/Pacific Islanders is the notion of social capital. Coleman (1990) referred to social capital as the networks of community relationships that facilitate trust and motivate purposeful action. The concept of social capital is defined by attributes such as mutual trust and reciprocity drawing on the work of Putnam (1993) and by its evidence of relationships among persons in a community, shared norms, and shared activities that advance shared norms (Mechanic, 2000). Because social capital is multifaceted, it has been operationalized with measures of social participation and interaction or trust (Bolin, Lindgren, Lindstrom, & Nystedt, 2003). Recently, interest in the effect of social capital on health and health care has been growing.

Two key elements related to Asian American/Pacific Islander culture and values are general community trust and generalized reciprocity. Ahern and Hendryx (2003) refer to reciprocity as norms of cooperative behavior by which persons are inclined to support and help each other. They describe trust in relation to the physician's or health care practitioner's ability to make accurate diagnosis and provide appropriate treatment while acting in the best interest of the patient. They found that social capital seemed to mediate how health care is perceived and is delivered in communities, or that the level of trust, engagement, and reciprocity influences the levels of trust individuals perceive in their health care providers. Bolin et al. (2003) have developed a theoretical model of the family as producer of health and social capital. However, their operational definition of social capital was having a close friend outside the family and is more similar to the social support concept than what is generally defined as social capital.

How does social capital relate to culture, ethnicity, and barriers? In Hawaii, one Chinese-Hawaiian attorney explained, "We owe our first obligation to our family and our second to our high school classmates. After that, we make choices" (Markrich, 2004, p. B1). The high school classmates refer to childhood friends and illustrate concentric circles of social capital with the family being in the center (Figure 63-1). This illustration may explain why although there is significant social capital in Asian American/Pacific Islander groups, there is low trust in physicians.

Help-Seeking Behaviors. Strong family ties discourage one from going outside the group culture to seek help from others. A brief review of the literature of Asian-American help-seeking behaviors was reported by Espirat, Inouye, Gonzales, Owen, and Feng (2004). They found that Asian Americans sought and received help in the family; sought help more from informal sources (family and friend) versus formal sources (health care professionals); resolved problems on their own; sought help from formal sources only when there was conflict within the family or when symptoms were severe; and sought help depending on differences in acculturation and availability of family networks. These studies focused on specific Asian ethnic groups and gave helpful information on preferences of these groups.

Lack of Mentoring. The literature on faculty and nurse mentoring highlights how the relationship stimulates growth in research and scholarship, promotes socialization and adjustment, increases networking, provides emotional support, and assists with the reappointment process (Jacelon, Zucker, Staccarini, & Henneman, 2003; Mundt, 2001; Snelson et al., 2002; Washington, Erickson, & Ditomassi, 2004). However, the literature contains little regarding benefits specific to cross-cultural/ethnic or ethnic/cultural matches.

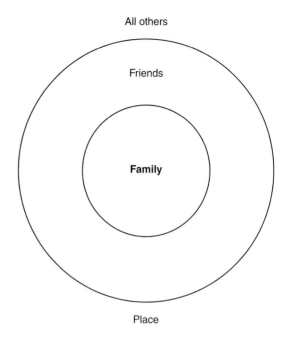

FIGURE 63-1 Social capital illustration of Asian Americans/ Pacific Islanders.

Although there is a belief that mentoring with a similar minority as a role model is more successful, there are no studies supporting this belief. A few (Griffiths & Tagliareni, 1999) conclude that the important variables are personality style and compatibility.

Do Asian Americans/Pacific Islanders mentor and accept mentoring from members of their same group? In the case of nursing, nothing has been reported in the literature. Many reasons exist for this, from the small numbers of senior-level Asian Americans/Pacific Islanders in the nation to the smaller number of nurses who are of senior capacity in academia and administrative positions. In attempting to identify a minority match for their students, Griffiths and Tagliareni (1999) found too few were available, and their project had to rely on expertise offered by majority mentors.

Is there another reason? These historically collectivistic groups should fall naturally into such relationships. However, could collectivistic groups relate specifically to family relations and not include mentoring or accepting mentoring from too far outside the circle? The literature on help-seeking behaviors suggests that help may not be readily accepted by members of the same group because of the value of independence from outsiders. Is this a need for self-reliance, a value of not being "a burden" or a natural inclination of non-help-seeking behaviors?

However, many Asian American/Pacific Islander nurses have been mentored by senior white faculty or administrators. They are encouraged, supported, and pushed by others outside their ethnic/cultural groups. Some of this may be cultural, as exemplified in the discussion of culture in the previous section. One may not stick out in one's own group but may in others.

Lack of Strategic Plans. The President's Advisory Commission on Asian Americans and Pacific Islanders (2001) found that less than half of the federal agencies had conducted a needs assessment or study to identify, quantify, or evaluate Asian Americans/Pacific Islanders' needs or had grant programs for which Asian American/Pacific Islander were a funding priority. However, recently the National Institutes of Health has developed its Strategic Research Plan and Budget to Reduce and Ultimately Eliminate Health Disparities as a first step in implementing Public Law 106-525, the Minority Health and Health Disparities Research and Education Act of 2000. The report states that "because of concerns about current definitions, we are unable to provide the Congress with valid and reliable data on minority health disparities research" (U.S. Department of Health and Human Services, 2002, p. 32). The National Institute for Nursing Research, with a long history of supporting research on minority health developed its strategic plan with research, infrastructure, and outreach goals and activities (Phillips & Grady, 2002). The entire strategic plan is available on the institute Web site (http://ninr.nih.gov/ninr/). It is noteworthy that the National Institute for Nursing Research specifically targets minority nurses interested in pursuing research careers. Furthermore, the institute has partnered with the National Coalition of Ethnic Minority Nursing Associations to develop initiatives and disseminate research opportunities. The coalition has taken a step in including all five minority organizations—the Asian American/Pacific Islanders Nurses Association, the National Alaska Native American Indian Nurses Association, the National Association of Hispanic Nurses, the National Black Nurses Association, and the Philippine Nurses Association of America—as equal partners to identify future directions for improving the health of racial and ethnic minority populations and increasing the number of minority nurse investigators.

FUTURE DIRECTIONS/RECOMMENDATIONS

Changes in the ethnic backgrounds of the population and the increased understanding of disparities shape nurses' approaches to Asian Americans/Pacific Islanders.

TABLE 63-1

Targets and Points of Intervention

Points of Intervention	Target
Hospital, clinic, public health, government, universities	Disease
Decrease barriers, increase access	Individual
Mentoring, training, coaching	Health care provider
Cohesion/social support/family support	Group
Social capital, neighborhoods, clubs, gatekeepers	Community
Culturally specific interventions, cultural brokers, interpreters	Culture/ethnic group
Information interventions (Balsa & McGuire [2003]) and support for research that causes the disparities, best match of services to needs of minorities	Policy makers

Research, practice, and education can focus on the points of intervention in Table 63-1 and are discussed further. At the disease level, the focus should be clinical intervention research to specify the epidemiology of diseases and the Asian American/Pacific Islander's unique responses to diseases and interventions. These then can be tailored specifically for the different subgroups within the larger Asian American/Pacific Islander group. At the individual level, strategies should be investigated to decrease barriers and increase access such as providing services in nearby neighborhoods at churches, markets, or other convenient and safe places; providing help with transportation; and possible matching of health care provider and Asian American/Pacific Islander. Research on the results of these interventions also should be done to determine efficacy of outcomes.

For health care professionals, the government now is providing support to increase minority nurses for those who feel more comfortable accepting help from their own. Mentoring programs and support for research careers for Asian Americans/Pacific Islanders could lead to more focused research specific to this group. Because of the importance of family, at the group level, providers should include family members in decision making for health care and learn more about the family's specific health care practices and behaviors. Including family or significant others along with the participants in research studies may increase minority participation in clinical trials and increase adherence to medical and nursing interventions.

For Native Hawaiians, a sense of place or being one with the community is at the nexus of their well-being and health. Place takes on spiritual connections with health and healing. Similar to social capital but more expansive, place is about relationships or connections to natural elements, the self, and others and belongingness (Oneha, 2000). The implications for practice are to take a broader ecological and spiritual perspective when working with Native Hawaiians. Sensitivity to inclusion and respect for history are crucial to practice and research. With Asian Americans, trust and reciprocity are important concepts for practice and research.

At the cultural level, inclusive, descriptive research on specific complementary health care practices of all the different subgroups should be conducted. The use of native healers or elders from the specific groups is consistent with health care practices of some Pacific Islander cultures and should be accepted and included in treatment plans. Esperat et al. (2004) suggest the use of cultural brokers as informal levels of support to navigate the barriers to health care. At the policy level, Balsa and McGuire (2003) suggest information-based policies may be one step in countering decisions health care providers make based on uncertainty, and rules-based actions may be more effective when stereotyping or prejudice is an issue related to treatment.

SUMMARY

Disparities in services may result from poorly matched services to needs. To make an impact on the disparities gap, more research is needed on the specific causes for these disparities, culturally specific responses to interventions, and interventions that include not only the individual but also the family, friends, and environmental sensitivity.

REFERENCES

Ahern, M. M., & Hendryx, M. S. (2003). Social capital and trust in providers. *Social Science and Medicine, 57,* 1195-1203.

Balsa, A. I., & McGuire, T. G. (2003). Prejudice, clinical uncertainty and stereotyping as sources of health disparities. *Journal of Health Economics, 22,* 89-116.

Bolin, K., Lindgren, B., Lindstrom, M., & Nystedt, P. (2003). Investments in social capital: Implications of social interactions for the production of health. *Social Science & Medicine, 56,* 2379-2390.

Coleman, J. S. (1990). *Foundations of social theory* (pp. 300-321). Cambridge, MA: Harvard University Press.

Collins, K. S., Hughes, D. L., Doty, M. M., Ives, B. L., Edwards, J. N., & Tenney, K. (2002). *Diverse communities, common concerns: Assessing health care quality for minority Americans.* New York: Commonwealth Fund.

Espirat, M. C., Inouye, J., Gonzales, E. W., Owen, D. C., & Feng, D. (2004). Health disparities among Asian Americans and Pacific Islanders. In J. J. Fitzpatrick, A. M. Villarruel, & C. P. Porter (Eds.), *Annual Review of Nursing Research* (Vol. 22, pp. 135-159). New York: Springer.

Griffiths, M., & Tagliareni, E. (1999). Challenging traditional assumptions about minority students in nursing education: Outcomes from Project IMPART. *Nursing and Health Care Perspectives, 20*(6), 290-295.

Hawks, B. L. (1996). Barriers to health improvements for Asian Americans. *Asian American and Pacific Islander Journal of Health, 4*(1-3), 50-54.

Hughes, D. L. (2002). *Quality health care for Asian Americans* (No. 525). New York: Commonwealth Fund.

Institute of Medicine. (2002). *Unequal treatment: Confronting racial and ethnic disparities in health care.* Washington, DC: National Academy Press.

Jacelon, C. S., Zucker, D. M., Staccarini, J. M., & Henneman, E. A. (2003). Peer mentoring for tenure-track faculty. *Journal of Professional Nursing, 19*(6), 335-338.

Lindo, C. K. (2004). *The Spirit of `Ohana and the Polynesian Voyagers.* Retrieved February 4, 2005, from http://www.pvs-hawaii.com/History_Culture/spirit.htm

Markrich, M. (2004, June 6). Are we losing "social capital" in Hawai`i? *The Honolulu Advertiser,* pp. B1, B4.

Mechanic, D. (2000). Rediscovering the social determinants of health. *Health Affairs, 19*(3), 269-276.

Mundt, M. H. (2001). An external mentor program: Stimulus for faculty research development. *Journal of Professional Nursing, 17*(1), 40-45.

National Center for Health Statistics. (2003). Table 31. Leading causes of death and numbers of deaths, according to sex, race, and Hispanic origin: United States, 1980 and 2001. In *Health, United States, 2004.* Retrieved April 8, 2005, from http://www.cdc.gov/nchs/data/hus/hus04.pdf

Oneha, M. (2000). *Ka Mauli O Ka `Aina A He Mauli Kanaka (The life of the land is the life of the people): An ethnographic study from a Hawaiian sense of place.* Unpublished doctoral dissertation, University of Colorado, Denver.

Phillips, J., & Grady, P. A. (2002). Reducing health disparities in the twenty-first century: Opportunities for nursing research. *Nursing Outlook, 50,* 117-120.

President's Advisory Commission on Asian Americans and Pacific Islanders. (2001). *Interim report to the president and the nation* [Executive summary]. Rockville, MD: Author.

Pukui, M. K. (1983). *`Olelo No `eau: Hawaiian words of wisdom.* Retrieved April 8, 2005, from http://www.geocities.com/TheTropics/Shores/6794/olelono1.html

Putman, R. (1993). *Making democracy work: Civic traditions in modern Italy.* Princeton, NJ: Princeton University Press.

Ricketts, T. C., & Gaul, K. (2004). Number of minority health professionals: Where do we stand? *North Carolina Medical Journal, 65*(6), 381-384.

Snelson, C. M., Martsolf, D. S., Dieckman, B. C., Anaya, E. R., Cartechine, K. A., Miller, B., et al. (2002). Caring as a theoretical perspective for a nursing faculty mentoring program. *Nurse Education Today, 22,* 654-660.

Takashima, T. (1981). *Kotowaza no izumi* (Fountain of Japanese Proverbs). Tokyo: Hokuseido Press.

U.S. Census. (2000). Washington, DC. U.S. Government Printing Office.

U.S. Census Bureau. (2001, December). *The Native Hawaiian and other Pacific Islander population: 2000.* Washington, DC: U.S. Government Printing Office.

U.S. Census Bureau. (2004, December). *We, the American Asians.* Washington, DC: U.S. Government Printing Office.

U.S. Department of Health and Human Services. (2002). *National Institutes of Health: Strategic Research Plan and Budget to Reduce and Ultimately Eliminate Health Disparities* (Vol. 1). Washington, DC: Author.

Washington, D., Erickson, J. I., & Ditomassi, M. (2004). Mentoring the minority nurse leader of tomorrow. *Nursing Administration Quarterly, 28*(3), 165-169.

Yeo, S. (2004). Language barriers and access to care. In J. Fitzpatrick, A. Villarruel, & C. Porter (Eds.), *Annual Review of Nursing Research* (pp. 59-73). New York: Springer.

Bridging Cultures

Hispanics/Latinos and Nursing

SARA TORRES ◆ HELEN CASTILLO

Hispanics/Latinos and the nursing profession will be faced with a tremendous challenge in the coming decade: to increase the representation of Hispanics/Latinos in the nursing profession at all levels.

The growing demographic multiculturalism of America is viewed in a positive light, yet it poses a challenge and a dilemma; that is, meeting the health care needs of an ethnically diverse population in an infrastructure that is philosophically and economically unprepared to do so. Statistics indicate that 87% of all nurses are non-Hispanic whites from middle- and working-class backgrounds (Health Resources and Services Administration, 2000). The underrepresentation of racial and ethnic minority nurses and other health professions has been linked to the continued disparities in health care outcomes for these populations (Smedley, Stith, & Nelson, 2002). The only way for the nursing profession to increase the number of Hispanics needed to meet existing nursing service demands is to become more culturally diverse. In this context, cultural diversity refers to the variety of ethnicities and cultures within the nursing profession that need to reflect the societal makeup of the country and nursing patients/clients. Many variables exist and clearly are not simply a matter of making a choice.

Cultural diversity, however, is *not* occurring in nursing for several reasons. Baccalaureate and graduate degree nursing programs are especially challenged to increase the number of new student admissions and to facilitate the admission process for Hispanics. This challenge includes providing flexibility and allowing course credits for registered nurses (RNs) with associate's degrees in nursing (ADNs) who wish to pursue bachelor's or master's degrees. The highest education credential of most Hispanic nurses is the ADN, with a significantly lower number of Hispanic nurses attaining bachelor's, master's, and doctoral degrees than the rest of the RN population in the United States.

Given the financial limitations of Hispanics in this country, most are educated in 2-year ADN programs and in the few remaining 3-year hospital-based diploma schools of nursing. These programs attract students primarily because they provide earning power earlier than the 4-year (bachelor of science in nursing [BSN]) degree programs and have less stringent entrance criteria requirements. Thus the majority of Hispanics continue to enroll in 2-year programs, limiting their long-term mobility in the nursing profession, unless they continue into baccalaureate education and beyond.

Hispanic nurses who attend 2- and 3-year nursing programs usually are not appointed to positions of nursing leadership and responsibility because of the lack of advanced preparation in these programs that is provided in higher education. Additionally lacking are Hispanic mentors in higher education and nursing leadership positions who can promote other Hispanics. Hispanics who do hold leadership positions are deluged with requests to participate in activities that demonstrate cultural diversity and visibility of the agency by including an academically prepared Hispanic nurse. Together, selective discrimination and family and financial responsibilities make it more difficult for Hispanics to continue their studies, often precluding them from attaining master's and doctoral degrees.

Few Hispanics have been employed at the level of director or dean in the history of nursing in the United States. The few visible Hispanics in leadership positions further limit opportunities for students to view Hispanics as role models in nursing. In a study, Villaruel and Peragallo (2004) discussed the importance of leadership development among Hispanic nurses and the barriers and supports to that development.

Role modeling is the product of a complex set of social, economic, and educational factors. High dropout rates, poor academic preparation, and inadequate facilities and equipment in underserved communities, together with the low expectations of Hispanic students by teachers, contribute to the small pool of Hispanics who ultimately achieve professional careers and serve as role models for others. More significantly, these low numbers reflect an educational system that remains ill-prepared to develop Hispanic students to achieve their fullest potential. Why are Hispanics/Latinos not entering nursing in correlation to the growing population of Hispanics? According to National Sample Survey of Registered Nurses conducted in 1996 (Health Resources and Services Administration, 2000), RNs in the United States numbered 2.6 million. Only 40,600 of these nurses were Hispanic, a meager 1.6%. Further, about 7% of Hispanic nurses hold master's or doctoral degrees compared with about 12% of black nurses and 10% of non-Hispanic white nurses. These are dismal statistics considering that the number of Hispanic communities and their populations are increasing rapidly, but the numbers of Hispanic nurses are not growing proportionately. From a nursing leadership perspective, two major questions arise. First, how aware are nursing leaders of this critical issue? Second, what steps are being taken to resolve this issue? Data from national and state levels are disturbing illustrations that validate the underrepresentation of Hispanics in nursing education and practice. These data support expressed concerns at the baccalaureate and graduate levels, from where most nursing leaders evolve.

Nursing faculty and government agencies must address the recruitment, retention, and attrition problems in nursing programs from a Hispanic/Latino perspective. The U.S. workforce is expected to be more diverse and complex, and nursing must anticipate these effects and long-term implications in order to prepare graduates accordingly. Recruitment efforts need to be improved dramatically to reflect the cultural diversity of society within the nursing profession. Although not consciously intended, health care agency recruiters often select nurses who appear similar to themselves instead of considering as the first priority their patient population preferences and their psychosocial needs. Thoughtful consideration of patients' needs must be brought to the awareness level of nursing staff members, recruiters, and administrators who are ultimately responsible for effecting change.

USE OF THE TERM HISPANIC/LATINO

The term *Hispanic/Latino* is used interchangeably with preferences seeming to be geographical; that is, divided by locale. For example, the term *Hispanic* often is used in the Midwest and the East Coast, whereas *Latino* is preferred on the West Coast. Yet Hispanics living along the 2000-mile United States-Mexico border prefer to self-report as Mexican American, Chicano, or Hispanic. To distinguish between these terms as having a historical base from which negative or positive images and connotations arise is important. Because long-standing cultural values and military conflicts such as the historic Battle of the Alamo between Mexico and the United States, Hispanic/Latino terms remain controversial and generate strong feelings and emotions. These terms are distinctive and arise partly from the period of history in which ethnocultural labels were applied. Perhaps the terms are a function of the age of the "labeled" and the stage of their acculturation. Throughout this chapter, *Hispanic* and *Latino* will be used interchangeably.

OVERVIEW OF THE HISPANIC/LATINO POPULATION IN THE UNITED STATES

The demographic profile of the Hispanic/Latino population is changing in the United States. According to the U.S. Census Bureau (2000a), the Hispanic population more than doubled from 1980 to 2000. In 1980, there were 14.6 million Hispanics in the United States. From 1980 to 1990, the population grew by 7.7 million to 22.4 million. During the 1990s, the Hispanic population increased by 13 million, reaching a population of 35.3 million persons, or 12.5% of the total population. By the year 2010, Hispanics are projected to make up 13% of the U.S. population, 17% by 2030, and 23% by 2050. In 1990, about 1 of every 10 Americans was Hispanic, and this number is expected to rise to 1 of every 5 by 2050. Since 1970, this tremendous Hispanic population increase has been attributed to several factors. Among them are a higher birth rate than the rest of the population, substantial ongoing immigration, and improvements in census-reporting procedures.

The largest group of Hispanics/Latinos in the United States are Mexican Americans (58.5%), followed by Central or South Americans (28.4%), Puerto Ricans (9.6%), and Cubans (3.5%) (Grieco & Cassidy, 2001). Although found in every state, nearly 9 of every 10 Hispanics/Latinos live in just 10 states. Of the total population of California and Texas, 32.4% and 32%, respectively, are of Hispanic origin. Combined, California and Texas are home to more than half of the nation's Hispanics. The additional 8 states of New York, New Jersey, Florida, Illinois, Arizona, New Mexico, Colorado, and Nevada round out the top 10 states with the largest Hispanic populations.

Hispanic Americans are more likely than non-Hispanics to live in metropolitan areas and central cities. Approximately 90% of Hispanics lived in metropolitan areas in 1990 compared with about 76% of non-Hispanics (U.S. Census Bureau, 1995). In 1997, about 23% of Hispanic families lived below the poverty level compared with about 12% of non-Hispanic white families (U.S. Census Bureau, 2000a). According to the U.S. Census Bureau (2000b), in 2000 nearly 47 million persons accounting for 18% of the population were 5 years of age and older and spoke a language other than English at home. Of this number, 8% did not speak English well or at all, whereas Spanish was spoken by more than 17 million persons or 8% of those 5 years of age and older. Among Spanish-speaking persons, 8.3 million could not speak English well or at all, and Spanish speakers represented 54% of all non-English speakers in the United States.

HISPANIC/LATINO WOMEN IN LEADERSHIP ROLES

The question arises, Why do so few Hispanic/Latino women aspire to leadership roles? In the Hispanic culture, few women are in leadership roles because leadership traditionally has been viewed as a competitive male attribute, especially in business and health care circles. Consider the traditional physician-nurse dyad in which the physician typically has been male and the nurse has been female. Today, these roles are changing as more women enter male-dominated health care and other disciplines such as law, engineering, and business. Conversely, more men also are entering nursing and other health care–related professions. In the past, Hispanic/Latino women were relegated to "ama de casa," which translates to "housewife." The independent, well-educated, entrepreneurial woman until recently had not been accepted readily in the traditional Hispanic family because men had been expected to provide financial and other supports for wife and family while the wife remained at home. In the past, Hispanic males were considered poor providers if they were unable to carry this role. As Hispanic women have initiated stronger leadership efforts and sought opportunities for higher education, their numbers are increasing. Far from representative of the Hispanic population, this group needs to grow significantly. Mentoring by peers and other female leaders is sorely needed, regardless of their ethnicity or culture and especially by Hispanic/Latino women. The new leadership role of the Hispanic/Latino woman is emerging and needs to be addressed fully.

PROBLEMS FACING HISPANICS/LATINOS IN NURSING

The deteriorating health status of the growing Hispanic population of the United States is disturbing. Hispanics disproportionately are affected by cardiovascular disease, obesity, hypertension, diabetes, certain cancers, alcoholism, and drug abuse, in addition to dental diseases, and human immunodeficiency virus/acquired immunodeficiency syndrome. More Hispanic nurses are needed to care for the specific health and cultural needs of Hispanic patients in a culturally competent manner that includes language comprehension in a culturally accepting environment.

Few if any data are available on the career mobility of Hispanics in nursing. The term *career mobility* implies that an individual moves from one career level to another, laterally or to a higher level. The problems of career development and mobility are applicable to the whole of nursing and not to Hispanic nurses alone. Historically, however, career advancement in nursing has been difficult and limited for Hispanics primarily because of their lack of advanced educational preparation in nursing and related disciplines such as management. However, with the promotion of the BSN, master's, and doctoral degrees in nursing, along with the major restructuring taking place in health care facilities today, an ever-increasing number of nurses are moving beyond basic ADN and BSN preparation. A study by Villaruel, Canales, and Torres (2001) contributed to the discussion by identifying bridges and barriers to educational mobility as perceived and experienced by Hispanic nurses.

The mobility of Hispanics in nursing has been limited for two basic reasons. First, although the proportion of Hispanics enrolled in nursing programs has increased during the past decade, the increase has been well below the Hispanic population parity. Second, Hispanics continue to enroll in ADN programs, limiting their future mobility and leadership opportunities in the profession. Certainly, although the many options in nursing do allow lateral career moves more easily, mobility into leadership positions clearly is restricted by a "glass ceiling" effect (Parsons & Reiss, 2004).

As mentioned before, the problem of career mobility for Hispanic nurses is intensified by cultural, social, and educational differences. In addition, because Hispanic/Latino nurses lack contact with important professional role models, their opportunities to be socialized in the dynamics of self-advancement are fewer than for their non-Hispanic counterparts. New Hispanic nurses often do not look beyond the prospect of their first position. Instead, they view their "job" as a satisfying career of helping others rather than also as a first step in the progression of a lifetime professional career. If nurse educators are to promote career mobility within the existing ranks of Hispanic nurses, they must initiate career development programs that include leadership and management skills development and provide a variety of resources to guide Hispanics through the educational process. Because many Hispanics are first-time college students in their families, their educational efforts need to begin as early as middle school and high school and continue through higher education in colleges and universities.

Hispanic nurses must prepare themselves academically and acquire the necessary experience and expertise in clinical areas of specialization. Additionally, Hispanic nurses must develop their leadership skills and other relevant formal and informal skills to increase their competitive edge and succeed in attaining leadership posts. They need to learn the unwritten rules of success and find out how they "fit" into the culture of the organization. These skills are essential to command positions of responsibility and prestige in nursing. Institutions that espouse support need to assist Hispanic/Latino nurses in their career development and mobility by providing opportunities for career planning, by addressing professional issues, by rewarding nurses for direct patient care and other contributions, and by facilitating their education. Additionally, the nurse should prepare short-term and long-term personal goals for career development that define benefit for the nurse and the employing agency.

Models of career mobility and professional advancement for Hispanic/Latino nurses also need to be developed by professional organizations such as the American Nurses Association, the National League for Nursing, and the American Association of Colleges of Nursing. Models need to promote and support the advancement of underrepresented Hispanics/Latinos at all levels of nursing practice within the scope of the mission of the agency. Needed are strategies that will develop well-prepared and effective leaders among the ranks of nursing practice at state, national, and international levels.

Role socialization is the process by which an individual comes to internalize certain knowledge, skills, behaviors, values, and attitudes that are integral to one's chosen profession. Role modeling is the method of teaching professional attitudes and behaviors by being the person students emulate; it becomes the process by which a person takes on the values and behaviors of another through identification. For Hispanics/Latinos, the dearth of visible role models is a major contributing factor to a lack of career orientation that exists among the Hispanic nursing population. Attrition from nursing because of dissatisfaction and limited career commitment have been linked to inadequate socialization into nursing for the long term. Insufficient exposure to appropriate role models and lack of collegial support and resources are also contributing factors.

What potential currently exists for career development among Hispanic/Latino nurses in the United States? Hispanics/Latinos must be educated and socialized into professional nursing; their leadership potential must be encouraged through leadership opportunities and mentoring. The supply of Hispanic/Latino nurses graduating from nursing programs continues to be disproportionately low compared with the representation of Hispanics in the general population. In 2000, only 2% of all graduates of basic RN programs (including ADN, diploma, and baccalaureate programs) were Hispanic/Latino—too few to respond to the ever-increasing need for Hispanic/Latino professionals as this population grows. Although increasing numbers of Hispanic/Latinos graduate from these programs every year, retention of students in these programs is critical to maintain the number of qualified students eligible to progress into graduate studies. Options need to be made available to Hispanic/Latino nurses. The same factors that influence career development and mobility of Hispanics, such as culture, family support, diplomacy, bilingualism, risk taking, and personal goals, also restrict their leadership opportunities if these factors are lacking.

With the known available pool of young Hispanics/Latinos in the nation, it is time to capitalize on their abilities by facilitating financial aid and providing new opportunities for higher education. Innovative measures are needed to encourage Hispanic/Latino nurses to pursue graduate education and leadership opportunities that will promote career mobility and develop them as future role models.

FUTURE DIRECTIONS

The factors that will promote successful career development and mobility among Hispanic nurses include career counseling, career development models, mentoring approaches, networking systems among peers, and role modeling. Taxis (2002) advocates active, specific recruitment of Hispanic/Latino nursing students at every level of education. Career development for Hispanic/Latino nurses should include incentives and recognition for practice, development of clinical and management ladders, and institutional support for their education and professional advancement. Additional incentives should include financial support for nursing faculty such as academic leaves of absence, paid sabbatical opportunities for further study and research, and release time to utilize new knowledge and gain clinical expertise. Institutions need to support the professional development of their members, including attendance at conferences and participation in professional organizational activities. Career development requires further support for participation in focused programs of personal development, personal financial management, and policy development. Career development also means the inclusion of Hispanic/Latino nurses in agency committees and on policy development boards.

The need to increase the number of Hispanics entering the profession of nursing remains high. Educators must provide flexibility in class schedules to allow students to succeed in their basic preparation and must provide information and incentives to encourage Hispanic/Latino nurses to pursue higher education. Accelerated tracks, including RN options for licensed vocational nurses, BSN options for nurses with ADNs, and master's options (including specialty completion programs), will increase the opportunity for more Hispanic/Latino nurses and nurses in general to achieve doctoral study. The retention of Hispanic/Latino nurses in generic nursing programs is also critical. Additionally, the voice of Hispanic/Latino nurses in the political arena needs to be heard to secure substantial grants for educational programs, stipends for students, faculty development funds, and curricular change in this time of economic cutbacks. State and federal governments need to develop databases that provide tracking information about Hispanic students to appropriate agencies.

Strategies must be developed that inform the public at every level about the comprehensive needs of Hispanic/Latino nursing students in this country. Together, educators can develop short-term and long-term strategies that open pathways of opportunities for the success of Hispanic/Latino nursing students. Participative and cooperative endeavors between the private business sector and nursing programs must be fostered for the recruitment, retention, and graduation of Hispanic/Latino nursing students, especially in higher education. Additionally, networking systems among peers continue to be a priority for the development of information databases and centralized key group efforts.

Education has always been an important indicator of success in American society. Studies indicate that Hispanics have not attained an educational level sufficient to compete aggressively in the labor market, especially at the upper end of the health care professions. Hispanics/Latinos and the nursing profession are faced with a tremendous challenge in the coming decade to increase the representation of Hispanics at all levels of nursing and to provide true opportunities for leaders whose cultural sensitivity will affect the quality of health care delivered by culturally competent responsive health care service providers. In that process, the continuing education of professional nursing staff members will be enhanced and awareness levels will be raised.

Issues relating to the supply and demand of nursing professionals in the United States continue to change dramatically as major shifts in financial and human resources continue to unfold. Nursing resources have been reallocated from hospitals to community-based facilities and to new structures such as mini-hospitals, elderly care centers, community nursing organizations, and health screening stations in malls and other centers of commerce. Additionally, the critical need is to respond to the growing underserved bilingual and culturally diverse Hispanic population—a need that has not yet been met and continues to be an elusive goal.

The dilemma of poor health care for Hispanics and underrepresentation of Hispanics in nursing is demonstrated by the following issues:

1. A disproportionate number of Hispanics are socioeconomically and educationally disadvantaged. As a result, a high attrition rate exists and continues to rise throughout the educational pipeline.
2. The present and future enrollment of Hispanic secondary education students will continue to represent a large prospective applicant pool for nursing. However, the pool is concentrated in school districts that traditionally have limited educational resources, give little attention to engendering goal-oriented students toward nursing careers, and lack culturally appropriate recruitment models for Hispanics.
3. Hispanic college enrollment is concentrated in community colleges. According to the October 1998 Current Population Survey (U.S. Census Bureau, 1999), 53% of all Hispanic college students were enrolled in community colleges versus 31% of white non-Hispanic college students and 37% of black college students. Nursing enrollment data also indicate that most Hispanics continue to enroll in ADN programs instead of baccalaureate programs (Health Resources and Services Administration, 2000).

4. Hispanic nurse professions employment data in 1996 illustrate the substantial underrepresentation and general lack of progress in increasing employment numbers for Hispanics. More than 11% of the total U.S. population is Hispanic, whereas less than 2% of the RN population is Hispanic (Health Resources and Services Administration, 2000). Hispanic nurse enrollment and program completion trends also suggest the lack of significant progress in the representation of Hispanic nurses in the health professions. This continuing disparity is widening between Hispanic enrollments in nursing and degree completion and is not anticipated to increase given the school-age Hispanic student populations reported.

5. The literature is sparse, and documented program interventions to increase opportunities for Hispanics in nursing are few. Nursing representatives have demonstrated inadequate leadership in addressing these important issues in public and private educational institutions.

Three central recommendations address these issues:

Recruitment: Increase the applicant pool of Hispanics/Latinos in higher education programs for pre-nursing and nursing students.

Retention and graduation: Retain Hispanics/Latinos in nursing education programs for pre-nursing and nursing students through graduation.

Career mobility: Promote the career mobility and leadership of Hispanic/Latino nurses in collaborative and creative opportunities funded jointly by private and community-based funding agencies.

Within the profession is a lack of understanding about cultural perspectives and needs that often leads to conflict. Workforce and workplace conflicts are often disruptive. Anger that may be present may be difficult to verbalize and is exhibited in other ways, often increasing the intensity of individual and group conflicts. Discussions about cultural differences and similarities are needed to encourage nurses to work together effectively, constructively, and productively.

Communication patterns are learned and are culturally based. With Hispanics/Latinos, verbalization may be limited as a result of fear of conflict, reprisal, deference, or feelings of intimidation and violence. Communication and language barriers in health care settings must be recognized and discussed. With the insufficient number of bilingually prepared nurses, the few who are bilingual become overburdened with requests not only to serve as "translators" for an entire institution but also to assist in other greater responsibilities. Language differences that should be viewed as assets often become barriers that serve to further isolate Hispanics/Latinos in the work environment.

A natural affinity and commonality between groups of Hispanic/Latino nurses draws them together. Within these groups they find support, collegiality, and guidance that they do not receive from society as a whole. Additionally, insufficient emphasis is placed on the significant differences among various Hispanic/Latino cultural groups. The tendency is to place all cultural groups together and label them broadly as Hispanic/Latinos without allowing for these differences, especially socioeconomic differences.

Institutional ethnocentrism exists. If nurses are to deliver culturally competent and appropriate care, the unique differences among cultures, such as health care beliefs, sick role responses, and the meaning of illness, need to be addressed openly and nonjudgmentally. The institutional racism and discrimination that may exist need to be reassessed and eliminated by working together in collaborative environments that foster positive care and nursing outcomes.

Economic, familial, and many other societal factors interfere with the advancement of many Hispanic/Latino nurses. These and other barriers also prevent them from entering the nursing profession or preclude advancement in the profession. For the majority of Hispanic nurses attaining at least an ADN or BSN, this accomplishment is momentous. Many are the first college or university graduates in their families. This accomplishment is equally important for many who have faced and overcome obstacles during the completion of their degrees. Because of these constraints, many Hispanic/Latino nurses complete degree requirements as part-time students and frequently extend the time to graduation.

Hispanics quickly are becoming the largest culturally and linguistically different group in the United States based on acculturation and socioeconomic stages. Hispanic cultural values and family experiences provide the foundation for research and for many positive, culturally based intervention models that can be integrated into efforts for increasing Hispanic student enrollment, retention, career mobility, and leadership in nursing.

The major strides expected of Hispanics were not achieved this decade, partly because systems informally have inhibited such progress with "glass ceilings." This obstacle is clearly evident in the lack of educationally prepared Hispanics in nursing and the absence of Hispanics in health care leadership positions regardless of their capabilities. However, qualified Hispanics may choose not to enter the subtle second-class status afforded them in acquired leadership roles assigned by non-Hispanics. Some critics condescendingly assume that Hispanics/Latinos achieved these positions for reasons of ethnicity alone.

Stronger links between academic and service settings must be established, such as the development of career ladders between hospitals and local colleges or universities. Hospitals and other health care agencies need to build mutually beneficial partnerships with schools and nursing programs via paid preceptorships, adjunct faculty roles, and other creative alternatives used to provide financial and other assistance to students and the academic programs. The new generation of professional nurses and educators has the tremendous responsibility of opening doors that will secure professional growth, development, and mobility for Hispanic/Latino nurses in education, practice, and research. The process of advocating for access to health care for Hispanics in the United States must continue, and the time for planning has passed. The time for strategic action is now.

REFERENCES

Grieco, E. M., & Cassidy, R. C. (2001). *Overview of race and Hispanic origin.* Retrieved August 1, 2005, from http://www.census.gov/prod/2001pubs/c2kbr01-1.pdf

Health Resources and Services Administration. (2000). *The registered nurse population: National Sample Survey of Registered Nurses—March 2000.* Retrieved August 1, 2005, from ftp://ftp.hrsa.gov/bhpr/nursing/sampsurvpre.pdf

Parsons, L. C., & Reiss, P. L. (2004). Breaking through the glass ceiling: Women in executive leadership positions. *Scientific Nursing, 21*(1), 33-34

Smedley, B. D., Stith, A. Y., & Nelson, A. R. (Eds.). (2002). *Unequal treatment: Confronting racial and ethnic disparities in health care.* Washington, DC: National Academies Press.

Taxis, J. (2002). The underrepresentation of Hispanics/Latinos in nursing education: A deafening silence. *Research and Theory for Nursing Practice, 16*(4), 249-262.

U.S. Census Bureau. (1995). *Housing in metropolitan areas: Hispanic origin households* (Bulletin 95-4). Washington, DC: U.S. Government Printing Office.

U.S. Census Bureau. (1999). School enrollment: Social and economic characteristics of students (update). In *Current population reports P20-521.* Washington, DC: U.S. Government Printing Office.

U.S. Census Bureau. (2000a). Housing in metropolitan areas: Hispanic origin households (SB/95-4). Washington, DC: U.S. Government Printing Office.

U.S. Census Bureau. (2000b). *Table 4. Languages spoken at home by persons 5 years and over, by state: 1990 census.* Retrieved August 1, 2005, from http://www.census.gov/population/socdemo/language/table4.txt

Villaruel, A. M., Canales, M., Torres, S. (2001). Bridges and barriers: Educational mobility of Hispanic nurses. *Journal of Nursing Education, 40*(6), 245-251.

Villaruel, A. M., & Peragallo, N. (2004). Leadership development of Hispanic nurses. *Nursing Administration Quarterly, 28*(3), 173-180.

Bridging Cultures

American Indians and Nursing

BETTE KELTNER ◆ DEBRA SMITH ◆ MECHEM SLIM

Health disparities in America have been acknowledged as a systematic and moral division. Issues of equity and human capital play into discussion that profiles fundamental hurdles posed in the lives of ethnic minorities in the United States. For American Indians, lower life expectancy and higher age-adjusted mortality rates exist and define many aspects associated with individual, family, and social life course (Andersen, Belcourt, & Langwell, 2005). The incidence and prevalence of diseases such as diabetes, sudden infant death syndrome, and alcoholism coexist with high rates of injury and suicide. Data show that morbidity, mortality, and the burden of disease are magnified in these communities. Although disorder-specific prevalence rates far exceed expectations, the most resonating approach to resolving disparities calls for a holistic approach to resolving these issues for American Indians and Alaska Natives (Eschiti, 2004).

American Indian culture is a complex social structure and a deeply embedded personal life experience. Some American Indian cultural symbols and stories recently have become popular among persons involved in New Age movements and certain groups seeking to incorporate images of diversity into their agendas. Yet culture is much more than art, music, and exotic foods. These facets of culture are vibrant expressions of history, values, beliefs, and resources. This history and these values, beliefs, and resources shape tradition. Culture guides behavior and decision-making and ascribes meaning to action and circumstance. Culture tells these peoples how to raise their children, treat their mothers-in-law, and spend their time and money. The culture appeals to more persons to enjoy fry bread on occasion than to run to greet the sun each and every morning. At the same time that interest in American Indian culture is increasing, concomitant racist advertising in public forums offers bounties for killing American Indians. Also at the same time are insidious forces inviting the gradual undermining of culture through culturally dissonant programs and services. Today, contemporary versions of massacre and marginalization exist. The most remarkable characteristic of American Indian culture is its resilience, thus far, to such assaults.

BUILDING BRIDGES

Addressing health disparities in ethnic minority groups involves connections that have not occurred sufficiently to date. American Indians have been isolated by poverty, inadequate services, and lack of coordination through interdisciplinary approaches to complex problems. Furthermore, communities themselves have experienced exploitation and disregard of traditions essential to health behavior and health service use. The purpose of a bridge is access, directly to connect two places separated by substantial barriers. Sometimes the two points of connection can be seen; sometimes they cannot be seen at all, or only major landscape features can be seen. Mountains, rivers, and canyons are metaphors for cultural distance. The reason that nurses need the metaphorical bridge is based on their obligation to provide health care for all people. Building bridges involves considerable time and effort. Nurses have become more involved in identifying cultural competence as a critical aspect of practice for American Indians (Holkup, Tripp-Reimer, Salois, & Weinert, 2004; McCauley, 2004; Struthers, Eschiti, & Patchell, 2004). Specific skill sets are needed to provide good care to culturally diverse people. The issue of culturally competent care is important as a quality indicator for effective nursing practice.

We who write this chapter are three American Indian (Indian) nurses who are involved in different professional roles. We represent different tribes, different professional paths, and different contributions to the profession. This diversity reflects the exciting options of our profession and exemplifies a small part of the interesting within-group cultural diversity of American Indians.

As Indian nurses we care passionately about cultural competence and our careers as a vehicle to bring the best of dominant science to enhance the spiritual continuity of our culture. Our professional training and the wisdom of our elders point to the possibility of untoward side effects that can come even in actions filled with good intentions. Side effects can be serious, even fatal. We are eager to embrace technology and its benefits so long as these do not short-circuit the soul. The "missionary mindset" (Keltner, 1994) typically is not brought to Indians by people of faith today, it is brought by people of science and the helping professions streaming onto reservations (in good weather) and urban Indian centers armed with solutions to the many problems they have assessed. The major fault line in achieving cultural competence is the inability to appreciate the different experience and perspective of other people's lives. Looking only at the visible cultural markers—even important things such as art, music, and food—is insufficient to understand how people live. A discovery that one of your relatives reports "Indian blood" somewhere in your personal lineage may spark interest in the culture but does not convey understanding of a lived experience. The chapter we present provides a *framework* rather than a *blueprint* for building bridges between Native Americans and nursing. We seek to give readers information about tools to develop blueprints, the kinds of raw material that will be needed, and where to go to get the material for building bridges. The bridges we support are those that will not desecrate the beauty of the landscape.

BACKGROUND

Overview

Approximately 2 million citizens have identified themselves as American Indian in the U.S. census. American Indians are the only ethnic group for whom self-identification is insufficient for most purposes. To receive benefits as a "real" American Indian (authenticity can be challenged), a person must be enrolled in one of the 558 federally recognized tribes. These tribes exist with sovereign nation status in a treaty relationship with the U.S. government. Therefore although many individuals claim some Indian heritage, degrees of acculturation are marked not only by life experience but also by specific pedigree. Diversity among tribes can be considerable. A pan-Indian perspective will always be limited. Tribes of the Northwest rely on fish as a staple food and fundamental to the economy. In the arid Southwest, some tribes consider fish sacred and would never eat them.

A Southeastern tribe developed a popular tourist business but constantly was plagued by tourists wanting to see tipis. Because few buffalo roamed the heavy forests and mountains, tipis were not part of this tribe's history. However, a tipi was installed for business purposes. If tourists took time to visit the museum, they would learn that the tribal ancestors lived in longhouses made from the abundant wood given to them by their Creator.

As a group category, American Indians often are forgotten or misrepresented. A very public image of Indian people is rooted in elementary school history books and Hollywood Western movies. In general American culture, specific notions about how ethnicity among American Indians should be validated persist. Carrying out the federal government assignation of ethnicity, it is common to question whether a person is "full-blood Indian," a question never asked of persons from other ethnic groups.

A current distorted image of casino wealth has become a popular topic for journalists and television personalities. Gaming has operated on some Indian reservations since the early 1980s. Only 198 of the 558 federally recognized tribes have gaming compacts. The top 20 gaming operations (less than 10% of tribes that operate gaming) account for 55% of total gaming revenue (National Indian Gaming Association, 2005). The key indicator for financial success in gaming is proximity to metropolitan areas. Most reservations were selected to be isolated with few known natural resources when they were established. Urban growth has changed this scenario for some reservations, and consequently, they have some advantages related to developing this type of recreational industry. Just as state governments use taxes to operate programs and services for their constituents, the reservations use casino profits to increase the number of programs and services for tribal members. Recent revenue generation from gaming has transformed a few tribal operations but for the most part has been insufficient to erase centuries of neglect. A public perception that wealth has infused all Indian reservations and enriched Indian people is seriously wrong. The Indian Health Service, which undergirds the primary service system, spent an average of $1914 per patient in the year 2003 (Roubideaux, 2005). One should note that basic income is highly correlated with health and social well-being and, as such, is of concern for Indian people and society at large. However, although there is naturally within-group variation, Indian cultures are fundamentally nonmaterialistic. Although economic needs profile large for

Indian leaders, a position of aggressive acquisitiveness is rare. Pursuit of wealth is different than establishing an economic base for basic needs. Poverty clearly is a major component of disparate health and a prominent issue for Indian people. Economic inequities underlie much of the health disparities.

Social Systems

The formal social structures that exist in the world shape how resources are allocated and services are delivered. These structures are symbols of values and history. Many aspects of daily life arise from social systems. One cannot understand how to work with American Indians until one knows about basic structures of social systems that have powerful effects on Indian health. Indian social structure is rooted in a sense of place and people. The actual geography and animal and plant life can have historic, spiritual, and social meaning. The solution of relocation away from Indian reservations is proposed repeatedly as one way to mediate problems of unemployment and inaccessible services. A common and not necessarily unreasonable question from a dominant culture perspective is to pose the possibility that Indians who are very poor or suffer serious hardship related to isolation move away from their homelands. Moving for advancement is an entrenched American value. Relocation has a long, unhappy history in Indian country starting with the reservation system itself.

The nineteenth century was one in which the U.S. government fought many battles with Indian people wanting to preserve their land and way of life. At the conclusion of conquests, tribes generally were sent to new places typically known to be insufficient to sustain life. Even in times of peace and posttreaty agreement, Indians could be moved away from their assigned lands if it were perceived to be of value to European immigrants. The Indian Removal Act of 1836 forced the fraudulent relocation of Indians in the Southeast by federal troops to an area called "Indian Territory" where, according to the New Echota treaty, the land could never be annexed by another state or territory. Within a generation it became the state of Oklahoma. This relocation is called the Trail of Tears because of the high mortality among Indian people who left their land and belongings at gunpoint to walk from North Carolina, Tennessee, Georgia, and Alabama to Oklahoma. Two quotations remind readers about the values of land to Indians (Eagle/Walking Turtle, 1995, p. 10):

1. "They made us many promises, more than I can remember, but they never kept but one; they promised to take our land, and they took it."

2. "The Great Spirit raised both the white man and the Indians. I think he raised the Indian first. He raised me in this land. It belongs to me. The white man was raised over the great waters, and his land is over there. Since they crossed the sea, I have given them room. There are now white people all about me. I have but a small spot of land left. The Great Spirit has told me to keep it."

In the late 1940s and early 1950s, another federal relocation called for Indian people to leave their reservations and allotment lands to move into major U.S. cities. This relocation plan was to entice Indian families into places with more job opportunities. A sense of place is associated with extended family, cultural referents, and spiritual base. Relocation of various types and plans has undermined, sometimes violently, the basic cultural strengths that unite and sustain families and tribes.

To understand the sense of communal grief and pain shared by most Indian communities today, one first must understand relocation that occurred in "boarding schools." For many years, Indian children (as young as 4 years old) routinely were removed by the federal government from their parents and homes and sent to boarding schools to be assimilated into the American culture. At the boarding schools Indian children were not allowed to speak their language or to have contact with their families, were disciplined with beatings, and too often were sexually abused. The removal of Indian children from the home tore the fabric of family life. The children did not learn appropriately how to parent the next generation and did not know their culture or traditions, and this caused a major break between the generations. In effect, families did not know each other, and within the space of a few generations, the functioning family systems almost became extinct. Indian people today conjecture that the real reason the boarding schools were established was to eliminate Indian people entirely. The effects of the boarding school system are felt today with poor parenting skills, alcohol and drug abuse, and related social ills. Consequent to varied forms of assault through relocation, evidence of historical trauma is exhibited in a variety of mental health concerns (Struthers & Lowe, 2003).

Self-determination is a nearly sacred value among American Indians for long-standing cultural reasons and for political position. Indian tribes are sovereign governments, meaning that they have an inherent right or power to govern (American Indian Resource Institute, 1993). At the time Europeans "discovered" America, Indian tribes were autonomous and sovereign by nature. Because the Europeans inconsistently treated the Indian tribes as separate governments or foreign nations, the legal status of Indian tribes was uncertain. The U.S. Supreme Court clarified the situation by establishing the sovereign status of Indian tribes in 1823 (Canby, 1988). American Indians could not vote in U.S. elections until the Indian Citizenship Act of 1924, even though Indian men fought in American wars before that time. Although tribal sovereignty has specific limits, the pledges by the federal government to provide health and education to Indians in exchange for massive amounts of land make public support for human services among Indian people unique. Government assistance is perceived to be "payment" rather than "welfare."

Tribal government structure varies somewhat from tribe to tribe but has its own sets of dynamics and exerts tremendous influence. Tribal leaders may be called chief, president, governor, or chairman. Governing bodies exercise advisory and decision-making functions for the tribe. If health professionals propose to collaborate with Indian tribes in any way, they must understand tribal government and its scope of responsibilities. This takes considerable time and effort and absolutely cannot be bypassed. Community partnerships are essential for working with American Indians (Holkup et al., 2004; Marks & Graham, 2004). Such models of care have been shown to have a ripple effect, enhancing efficacy and efficiency across a range of health care problems (Deters, Novins, & Manson, 2004).

KEY CHARACTERISTICS OF AMERICAN INDIAN CULTURE

Natural Strengths and Resilience

Indian health and human service summaries generally focus on needs and deficits related to poverty and disorders. When visiting reservations and Indian communities, many persons come away with an image of deficits: substandard roads, public services, and housing. These facts do become prominent for service providers because they are associated with need for care. However, one must understand important aspects associated with natural strengths and resilience among Indians. The cited abysmal health indicators and markers of poverty and lack of services are indeed all too real. These effects stem in large part from intentional and neglectful social initiatives designed to obliterate Indian culture and Indian people. The fact of survival among Indian people points to cultural strengths worthy of note. Furthermore, Indian culture has been undermined to great extent by "helpers"—individuals who believe that solutions for

perceived problems can be imposed from outside without regard to community values, beliefs, and practices. Resilience research is important for American Indians. Negative profiles become contextualized with honor and recognition in a burgeoning field of study that describes and quantifies elements that mark human flourishing in the face of adversity (Keltner & Walker, 2003).

Indian family and community supports can be remarkably strong and supportive. The sense of interconnectedness and reliance on family ties mediates many of the visible deficits on which visitors to Indian communities remark. As with any small and close group, tensions and rivalries can play out in different ways. However, Indians typically have strong family obligations and communal identity. Expressions of obligation and identity take a variety of forms. Identity is very much associated by family and tribe. An obligation to assist family and tribe is an important cultural value. This is sometimes perceived as "keeping each other down," but the same values are those that prompt action, such as taking relatives into one's home or writing a chapter together. For many tribes, there is no such thing as an orphan. Examples of multigenerational extended family households are common, and even more common are clusters of houses on reservations that house extensive extended family close together. The American tradition of launching young adult children far away to school or jobs is juxtaposed by Indian traditions such as burying an umbilical cord near a family dwelling so that the child will never go far from home.

A variety of circumstances may cause Indian people to move away from a place where they feel rooted. Economics do impose pressures for some Indians to relocate for jobs. A pattern that is recognized easily but is not well documented by the U.S. Census is the fact that moving "to town" for a job can be a relatively temporary experience, for months or a year at a time, after which one returns to live "at home" on the reservation or allotment land. Another major force prompting Indians to move is a need for sophisticated or specialized medical services unavailable on most reservations. This relocation is not based on choice or preference but on fundamental need.

A case study in point illustrates this situation. A father, mother, and their four children lived in a small home that is part of a family compound on an isolated section of a large remote Indian reservation. The youngest child repeatedly is misdiagnosed by the nearest Indian Health Service providers, resulting in the child becoming blind, deaf, and severely mentally retarded because of untreated meningitis. As the child turns 4 years old, nourished via a gastrostomy and with the developmental level of a newborn, the frequency and nature of specialized medical needs requires the family to move to the nearest major city, a distance of 500 miles away from home. Caregiving, which previously was shared among extended family members, now rests exclusively on the parents. Not only are the parents exhausted and overwhelmed (and frightened) by their duties, older family members are no longer available for guidance with the older children. The older brothers of the "sick child" who previously played primarily with cousins fell into violence as victims and perpetrators. The father could no longer participate in ceremonies and tribal activities. Instead he had a series of low-level jobs providing constant messages about his low value to society. The young mother suffered from lack of instrumental and emotional support in raising all of her children. She had been a confident and effective mother in her home community but had not grown up with a model or expectation of independent family units. Her attempts to sustain the important traditions and daily family routines were undermined when she was given an overwhelming script from clinics, hospitals, schools, and social service agencies about what she should be doing. The child, for whom this upheaval had occurred, received surgery and other sophisticated therapies while missing the daily touch, prayers, and sense of belonging and acceptance that the tribe would have given her. This relocation was successful in many terms but came at a price that undermined natural family strengths and family supports.

Characteristics of Resilience

The origins of resilience, a phenomenon of thriving under stress and duress, may be multifaceted but centers primarily on family life and spiritual beliefs and practices. Resilience comes partly from individual factors but primarily from collective experience. Families and communities shape experience and response to events and circumstances in ways that are important to characteristics of resilience. Although risk and resilience are calibrated on an individual basis, Indians who circumvent probable risk regularly identify family and community support and their spiritual traditions and practices as sources of strength.

Almost always, American Indians are spiritual people. Faith or "religion" is an integral part of daily life not separated by time and place. Interest has arisen recently concerning the dominant culture in traditional Native American spiritual practices, meaning particularly those ancient beliefs known to tribes when Europeans

first arrived. And although clearly a lineage has sustained these beliefs and practices, a revival of sorts also has occurred among Indians who have reclaimed these beliefs after generations of disconnect from them. Certainly, these renewed practices have strengthened many individuals, families, and communities. Spiritual beliefs, however, have a dynamic nature—a particularly critical quality as they interact with current circumstances and events. The dynamic nature is characteristic of responses to contemporary issues with enduring core values. An important note is that there is a wide diversity of ancient spiritual beliefs among tribes.

Sometimes selected practices from Native American spiritual beliefs are incorporated into multigenerational Christian traditions. Diversity of religious practices and beliefs includes the fact that many families have more than 300 years of tradition in a Christian faith and deliberately choose to continue with these beliefs. This does not itself make them less "Indian." Therefore Indians who actively use sweat lodges also may be devout Catholics. Other Indians may adhere to only one or the other system of beliefs and forms of worship. A priori assumptions regarding specific beliefs are inappropriate even though it is well known that most Indians attribute resilience to being involved in some type of daily spiritual practices.

Another key characteristic of resilience has been the Indians' ability to discern the importance of family and community. This type of collective wisdom is associated with expected behavior and may be symbolized in stories, proverbs, or community rules for etiquette. Respecting and caring for persons with disabilities and family role expectations epitomize how important it is for individuals to have an obligation for others and not only oneself. Information such as this is passed down through family generations. Nursing homes to care for the elderly have never figured prominently in Indian communities. Indians have a sense of obligation to care for the elderly at home and a role for them to function in their families and communities. Many elders have acquired the ability to pass down the most critical aspects of culture that make their people unique and strong. Wisdom is also manifest in knowing what aspects of the dominant culture can be useful or helpful or congruent with traditional values. Most Indian people use some aspects of Western health care, even if it is combined with traditional healing methods. Many people, however, use Western health care only as a last resort—a reverse picture of white Americans who sometimes turn to native practices when unsatisfied with conventional Western health care.

Resilience has not been without price. The social costs for Indian people associated with the powerful cultural assaults directed toward them have been high. Many of these cultural assaults (such as bounties, boarding schools, relocation programs, and explicit termination policies) have aimed at overt extermination. Social costs have come in the form of pervasive effects such as high rates of poverty, domestic violence, and substance abuse. In recognizing cultural strengths and sources of resilience, these qualities may be celebrated and leveraged for addressing some of the more difficult challenges now facing Indian tribes. Most importantly, interventions and services should be examined carefully to determine whether, in the purpose of assistance, aspects of strength and resilience could be undermined (Keltner & Ramey, 1993).

Health Needs

The cause of disorders leading to disease or death can be categorized as having genetic, environmental, infectious, and situational antecedents. As increased understanding for the natural history of disease and injury emerges, it becomes clear that for most disorders there are interactive effects among these etiologic agents. American Indians share common risk for many disorders with the general population. The leading causes of death for Indians residing in Indian Health Service areas were heart disease followed by malignant neoplasms. However, Indians have unusually high risk for diabetes, sudden infant death syndrome, alcohol abuse, developmental disabilities, and spinal cord injuries. Regional and tribal variations in risk exist among certain conditions (such as sudden infant death syndrome, which is 6 times higher than average for Indians in the Great Plains). The Indian Health Service (1997) service area age-adjusted death rates illustrate that overall Indians experience mortality rates substantially higher than t he general population in key conditions: alcoholism (579% greater), tuberculosis (475% greater), diabetes mellitus (231% greater), accidents (212% greater), suicide (70% greater), pneumonia and influenza (61% greater), and homicide (41% greater).

In addition to death, Indian people have higher frequency of complications and disability associated with common health problems. Besides morbidity and mortality, the burden of disease and disorder is exponentially increased because of poverty and isolation. For example, rehabilitation hospitals assist patients in learning to ride buses and use common assistive devices such as ramps. However, on reservations there is no public transportation. Indian tribes, which have sovereign nation status, do not have to adhere to the federal Americans

with Disabilities Act. Ethnic disparities in morbidity, mortality, and burden occur because of many factors, including genetic predisposition, environmental risk and infectious agent exposure, lifestyle, and inaccessible or poor-quality or inappropriate health care.

Standard health indicators of morbidity and mortality point to the extent of health needs among Indian people. Data collection for Indian people is subject to greater error than other ethnic groups because raters (health professionals) often take it upon themselves to identify a patient's ethnicity or race based on skin color or surname. Indian people may "look" Hispanic or fail to have what the rater considers to be a "real" Indian last name. A common saying is that persons are born Indian but die white because birth certificates are more likely to use self-identified data than do death certificates. Furthermore, Indians are more likely to be born close to home and transferred to mainstream medical centers for dying. Geocoding and more specific data-tracking mechanisms are elucidating how the interactive effects of ethnicity and location account for some of the variance in health disparities for American Indians (Krieger, Chen, Waterman, & Rehkopf, 2005; Probst, Moore, Glover, & Samuels, 2004; Puukka, Stehr-Green, & Becker, 2005).

In spite of known underreporting, health indicators for Indian people show a bleak picture. Rates of disease, injury, and death are disproportionately higher among minorities in the United States, and American Indians profile significantly in this differentiation. These epidemiological ethnic disparities, after decades of documentation, now are being addressed within a systematic research agenda at the National Institutes of Health (Eaglestaff, McClain, & Fernback, 2003). American Indians, as with other underserved minority groups, experience higher frequency of serious disease, injury, and death. However, also in common with other underserved minority groups is extreme suspicion associated with research participation based on history of exploitation. Specific events vary, but examples of using and abusing Indian people in a quest for mainstream knowledge is all too full of unhappy exemplars. Treatment testing for tuberculosis has a history for Indians similar to that of African Americans in the Tuskegee experiments on syphilis. Therefore an effective research agenda to reduce ethnic disparities is not impossible, but it is complex and not amenable merely to generalizing standard protocols to a new participant population.

For all tribes, a traditional belief is that treatment is treatment of the whole person. Although this is common rhetoric in health care, it should be an essential premise in the care of Indian people. Many disorders are perceived to have origins that speak to lack of balance or harmony, violating a taboo, or disarray in social relationships. Few Indian people refuse to have any type of conventional medical treatment, but most feel it is necessary or at least important to have traditional healing practices performed as well. Prayers and ceremonies engage major social supports and rely on ancient wisdom. In some tribes, prayers are never for oneself but only for others—a symbolic expression of healthy interpersonal adaptation, avoiding problems of self-absorption common in some people in the dominant culture. Traditional indigenous healing practices have breadth and depth in nature and use (Novins, Beals, Moore, Spicer, & Manson, 2004; Struthers et al., 2004). Prayer has been associated with positive health outcomes for elderly Indians (Meisenhelder & Chandler, 2000). Many traditional remedies are characterized by elements of social support, familiarity, and a more egalitarian model contrasted to a prescriptive model.

Expectations regarding health and the meaning of health are different in different societies. Good health and optimal functioning are valued in all cultures, and the richness of cultural practices to support health across many different traditions is important knowledge for nurses to have. A variety of tribal traditional beliefs provide traditional explanation and treatment for certain disorders. For example, in one tribe it is believed that epilepsy is a sign of sibling incest. This creates an overlay of special needs associated with conventional treatment of this disorder. Some health disorders, nonspecific in Western terms, require and respond to traditional treatments. Sometimes these disorders have symptoms that might be described as predominately psychosocial, perhaps a symptom such as sleeplessness commonly associated with depression. Traditional treatments can be highly successful in reducing many such symptoms. Rarely does an Indian person believe that there should be no suffering in life—there are too many visible experiences with suffering and pain. Indians have many ways to live a healthful life and have varied ways among tribes to treat a wide range of disorders. However, meaning and purpose often are ascribed to health problems that cannot be changed. The attribution of meaning and purpose assigned to a serious health disorder, whether terminal or chronic, aids individuals in coping and adaptation.

Health Behavior

Behavioral expectation can vary across cultures. Even though human development follows a fairly typical trajectory, the identification of key milestones is known to vary from culture to culture. In some Indian tribes, the age of the first word is a less important developmental marker for social-cognitive development than is the first smile or laugh, and the occasion of a naming ceremony or christening may stand out more in parental memory than does the age of first steps. Child development milestones achieved by almost all human beings have been catalogued by Western professionals with special emphasis on indicators marking independence from the family unit. These milestones are important, but not all cultures have celebrated them in the same ways. Similarly, role expectations establish some parenting practices. In a study of several different parenting practices among different ethnic groups in the San Francisco Bay area, it was found that American Indian parents expected their children to dress themselves at an earlier age and care for themselves and younger children at an earlier age (Joe & Malach, 1992). An appreciation of the meaning associated with developmental milestones is helpful for nurses.

Lifestyle, including daily habits, is well known to serve risk or protective functions for individual health. Lifestyles develop in many ways but most commonly arise from cultural practices within families. Routines from toothbrushing to activity patterns are formulated in childhood. Such practices are not immutable but sometimes are value laden. Pima Indians who were experiencing enormous health problems associated with type II diabetes improved the overall health when they reclaimed their tribal tradition of running. Many short-term interventions yield good outcomes that lack sustainability. Among the most remarkable features of the Pima Indian exercise intervention is that it was linked directly to tribal custom and responsibility for the program became embedded within the tribe rather than a service provided by external health providers (Wingood & Keltner, 1999). Effectiveness in achieving good health outcomes, particularly in the area of health promotion is facilitated by honoring rather than ignoring the culture. Issues related to sustainability, an imposing challenge, also are enhanced when culturally competent methods are used.

One of the most well-known health risk behaviors is smoking. In many tribes, smoking is linked directly to lung cancer, heart disease, low birth weight, and other known consequences of tobacco use. Smoking is a health behavior that hurts Indian people as much as it harms other people. Correlates of smoking include family influences and alcohol use (Nez Henderson, Jacobsen, & Beals, 2005). Tobacco use includes other modalities such as chewing. In some tribes more than half of adolescents and adults use tobacco in some way (Robinson, 2003). In many health arenas, tobacco is abhorred, for good reason, with many health professionals believing that tobacco should be outlawed. One should note, however, that tobacco has a different history, and sometimes different uses, among Indian people. Tobacco is a New World discovery—a crop that early Europeans learned about when first meeting Indians in America. Tobacco has long been used in different ways and continues to be associated with certain spiritual ceremonies. Tobacco is the appropriate gift for medicine people. Therefore the dominant culture's war on tobacco, which would ban it, misses the distinction between use and abuse of this substance. It can be hard to make a case to decrease smoking when specific ceremonial uses are not acknowledged.

Alcohol addiction is another health behavior sometimes associated in stereotype with Indian people. Rates of alcoholism and alcohol-related disorders are extraordinarily high in many tribes. Most reservations are "dry"–that is, they do not sell alcohol—but this does not correlate with lack of alcohol consumption. Stores and bars often are established on reservation borders with the express purpose of selling to Indians. Although many Indians are teetotalers, it is also true that most Indians have been affected by alcohol in some way, personally or with close family members. Motor vehicle injuries and domestic violence are highly correlated with intoxication. The experiences of poverty, isolation, and unemployment interact with a biological delay in alcohol metabolism among Indians and also with social drinking patterns originally introduced by hard-drinking trappers or traders intending to take advantage of Indians in an intoxicated state. The effects of these different factors make alcohol abuse an important health behavior concern for many tribes. Binge drinking is especially problematic as a habitual pattern and is associated with periods when money is available.

Increasingly, tribal leaders are implementing successful alcohol treatment and prevention programs, incorporating culture-specific principles and methods. Issues related to health behavior appear to be most amenable to change when solutions come from within the community. Certainly, sustaining good health outcomes has been a particular challenge because Indian reservations often have not had the type of formal infrastructure to continue programs that have shown promise. Sustainability is enhanced when programs are "owned" by the local community and continuity is supported from within the group.

Violence is a pervasive threat for American Indians (Manson, Beals, Klein, & Croy, 2005). Lifetime injury rates for men (62% to 67%) and women (66% to 70%) show a substantial health threat within the communities in which American Indians live. Domestic violence is a behavioral phenomenon having serious and pervasive effects on health. A public and personal profile is associated with domestic violence. The public image exists as data, media reports about individual situations, and work done by service providers involved in health and social services. The visible parts of domestic violence rate include epidemiological estimates about nature and frequency, services specific to intervention such as offender treatment, services such as emergency care that require nurses to be alert for signs of unreported abuse, law enforcement involvement, and stories revealed in newspapers and on news programs. Domestic violence commonly is associated with other health and social ills such as alcohol abuse, stress, unemployment, and family dysfunction. Indians experience these correlates in higher frequency. Domestic violence is by no means an Indian problem, but in communities with high numbers of Indian people, the public perception of domestic violence among Indians can be magnified. Domestic violence has a personal dimension as well. The most enduring effects of this experience are generally psychological and cannot be seen. Potential conflicts in this thorny area became increasingly problematic because one common solution to child abuse has been removal of Indian children from their families. In the past, Indian children have been placed primarily in institutions or in care of white families, adding to cultural assault. The Indian Child Welfare Act has kept children within their tribal communities unless there is compelling reason to do otherwise.

Health Services

Indian people are not explicitly excluded from using typical health services options, but the Indian Health Service (IHS) is part of the "agreement" of giving Indian people services in exchange for land. Indian Health Service is an organization with three aims: in partnership with American Indian and Alaska Native people, (1) the mission is to raise their physical, mental, and social health to the highest level; (2) the goal is to ensure that comprehensive, culturally acceptable personal and public health services are available and accessible to all American Indian and Alaska Native people; and (3) the foundation is to uphold the federal government obligation to promote healthy American Indian and Alaska Native people, communities, and cultures and to honor and protect the inherent sovereign rights of tribes (Nolan, 2005).

The appropriation for IHS is $3.0 billion toward a tribal needs based budget of $19.4 billion (Roubideaux, 2005).

Provision of health care for Indians was determined by the U.S. Supreme Court in the 1830s. In 1954 the responsibility for providing health care to Indian people shifted from the Bureau of Indian Affairs (which is in the Department of Interior) to the IHS as a branch of the U.S. Public Health Service. The Indian Health Service is the principal federal health care provider and health advocate for Indian people, and its goal is to raise the health status of Indians to the highest level possible. Indians often refer in shorthand to IHS or PHS (Public Health Service, the broader entity in which IHS exists) as their source of health care service. The operation of the IHS delivery system is managed through local administrative units called service units. A service unit is the basic health organization for a geographic area served by the IHS program, just as a county or city health department is the basic health organization in a state health department. The IHS is composed of 12 administrative units called area offices. Area offices consist of 150 service units, of which 84 are operated by tribes. The IHS operates 37 hospitals, 61 health centers, 4 school health centers, and 48 health stations. Approximately 1.5 million people need IHS services.

Health system changes abound in today's world, and there have been some major changes in IHS as well. Paramount among these changes has been the opportunity to decentralize health care through tribal compacting or contracting. The Indian Self-Determination and Education Assistance Act of 1974 (P.L. 93-638) has been vital in encouraging Indian tribes and people to assume active participation in the program and services conducted by the federal government for Indian people. The act states that "The prolonged federal domination of Indian service programs has served to retard rather than enhance the progress of Indian people and their communities by depriving Indians of the full opportunity to develop leadership skills crucial to the realization of self-government, and has denied to the Indian people an effective voice in planning and implementation of programs which are responsive to the true needs of Indian communities" (Prucha, 1990, p. 274).

The Indian Health Care Improvement Act of 1976 was developed to lessen or remove the gap between Indian health conditions and those of the total population. Congress provided for increased funding for health services, urban health centers, and the determination of the feasibility of Indian medical schools (Prucha, 1990). The Indian Self-Determination Act (P.L. 93-638) allowed Indian tribes to assume partial control over the provision of their health and social services. Today, the IHS is in the process of restructuring. This is the first attempt in 40 years by the IHS to restructure in order to provide better services for Indian people. The need for change was prompted by external and internal factors. External factors include the change in the general health care industry and its impact on the ability of IHS to provide quality care at a reasonable cost. The "reinvention" of government has included streamlining government from the bottom up so that downsizing of federal employees within IHS reduced approximately 1000 full-time equivalents in a system known to be seriously underfunded. The possibility of converting federal support to block grants to states jeopardizes a focal understanding of Indian health needs. Among the internal forces affecting the need for a system change include sophistication of the Indian health care consumer and increasing abilities of tribal management to assume the delivery of health care for their communities (Design for a New IHS, 1995).

The Indian Health Design Team was created in 1995 to examine the issues of Indian health care, IHS, and tribal health care provision and to recommend changes in the IHS structure. In part, the Indian Health Design Team recommendations include to restructure IHS organization above the local (tribal) level; let tribes determine their own course of action; provide support from IHS for the unique needs of the tribes; authorize, upon request, flexibility to the tribal government in managing its budget authorize alternative sources for tribal health care agencies essential business and professional support functions; and authorize the tribes to purchase and develop billing and accounts receivable systems that are equal to the private sector. Therefore Indian tribes recently have been able to compact or contract directly with the federal government for their portion of the health care money that would have been retained by the federal government at the IHS level rather than distributed to the tribes. To date, 44 tribes have entered into such a compact with the federal government. Although there is a federal obligation to provide health care for Indian people, the future for Indian health care often is called into question because federal funds for Indian health are appropriated annually and frequently are challenged and negotiated downward by members of Congress.

BUILDING BRIDGES

Communication

The fundamental resource for building a cultural bridge is communication. Cultural competence is care that respects knowledge and traditions in different cultures and uses both in pursuit of better health.

Verbal and nonverbal communication skills are key to culturally competent care. The statement that white professionals talk too much and listen too little is generally true. Much may be noted about communication styles among Indians, first and foremost being that there is considerable within-group variation as one would expect from any large group of people. Probably there are many more Indian styles of understated or subtle ways of talking that may be misinterpreted as "slow" than are found in the overall population. Indians are more likely to be comfortable with silence and even use silence as an expression of respect for what has just been said. This communication style can interfere with the current expected pace for health care services. As with any group that has experienced discrimination and marginalization, suspicion or caution often arises when one is communicating with outsiders. Such barriers cannot be circumvented in a single session. A system is needed that strives for consistency and follow-through of commitments.

Some Indian traditions identify self-promotion as bad manners. Indeed, humor—a wonderful human characteristic that Indians also have in abundance—is often self-deprecating among Indians. The particular belief that self-promotion is inappropriate runs counter to many core principles in advocacy groups, including health advocacy groups such as parents of children with disabilities. Relatively few Indians have college degrees, a tool that aids in making system and service change. Advocacy training can empower Indian families who lack formal education with knowledge and skills that combine with their own traditions of resilience to improve health and well-being for themselves and their children. Change will not come naturally for all Indians to be assertive in this way.

Communication can be impeded simply by the fact that health professionals have a culture almost to themselves. Words, concepts, and values are used that are particularly associated with health care. One example of this is the continued search for knowledge and value of new information. This is a facet almost everyone can appreciate in the abstract but can become confusing in practice. When a young mother takes her child for a well-baby visit and is advised that feeding strained foods in the first months is "bad" for her child and that her baby should be put to sleep on his back, the information can be interpreted as conflicting. Not only have older women in the family probably recommended something different, personnel in the same clinic were dispensing opposite advice just a few short years ago. The major point of conflict is when value judgments are ascribed (feeding a child strained fruit at the age of 4 weeks is "bad"). Rarely are explanations for changes given and certainly not in the amount of detail to be understood. Grandmothers not only give instrumental assistance and care in child rearing but also rarely change their minds about what is good and appropriate care. Communication, therefore, becomes a critical part of health care delivery—not just what is said, but how it is said.

When linguistic diversity is spoken about in the United States, it rarely is recognized that certain tribal languages, such as Navajo, continue to be the primary or only language for some Indian people. For others who speak English, experience with serious illness may inhibit their understanding of English or require the use of words and phrases of particular intimacy that only native words can suffice. When one works with people who speak a language different from English, one should learn as much of that language as possible. Interpreters will be needed at times. The use of interpreters is a skill in itself (Wingood & Keltner, 1999). Anyone who knows multiple languages knows that precise translations are not always possible. Another aspect of the use of interpreters is to pay attention to who is serving in this role. Young school-age children often are pressed into this duty, but it is of course inappropriate for a young child to inquire, for example, about the dates of his mother's last menstrual period. Although this may seem self-evident, such courtesies routinely are violated among many people who use interpreters. In some tribes, communication customs exist about when and how men speak to women such as mothers-in-law. Communication is important to building bridges between cultures, but it is essential to recognize the complexity and iterative nature that good communication should have.

Research and Measurement

As the discipline of nursing becomes more empirical, research tools that measure common health phenomenon take on a larger profile. As previously mentioned, meaning can be ascribed by context and experience. Concern about validity of measures with ethnic populations that have been underrepresented in research is ongoing. Serious concern exists about abbreviating the careful instrument development process used in dominant research programs through shortcuts. Shortcuts in this area are not only poor science but also can lead to faulty conclusions and perpetuation of cycles of misunderstanding and poor practice. Many examples are available of popular instrumentation that can be inappropriate for use with Indian tribes. A common question on the Family Resource Scale, for example, inquires about resources to take a "vacation" or "have time alone." In a community with long-standing high (85% to 95%) unemployment and where being with family members is more valued than time alone, the original meaning of these questions is not in concert with the context.

A common problem for American Indian people is that they are "used" by researchers who seek them out for interviews. Although this avoids the many pitfalls associated with inadequate instrumentation and state of the art for tools to be used among Indians, there are potential problems. Qualitative methodologies not uncommonly are chosen by some researchers less for reasons of interest and more because of their personal limitations in quantitative skills. This particular motivation does not bode well for meaningful findings through narrative data. Analyses must be just as rigorous using qualitative techniques. Even words in English may have particular meaning for people. In a detailed analysis of qualitative data to learn about Indian families' adaptation to children with disabilities in seven different tribes, Keltner (1994) learned that parents of children with disabilities expressed many occasions of burnout. Burnout (stress) is not atypical for families with these types of challenges, but it simply did not ring true with what had been learned in interviews with 150 families. When examining the interviews transcriptions more carefully, it was discovered that families were referring to their houses burning down rather than to emotional stress. Several potential problems of interpretation of data can occur from a researcher's perspective. American Indians have a long history of exploitation, and marking the perceived problems and deficiencies for a group of people can bring harm—particularly when validity can be reasonably challenged.

Concurrent Challenging Life Circumstances

As a health professional addresses a disorder such as diabetes or childhood asthma, the professional should consider the entire context of a patient's experience. One cannot easily disentangle interactive effects of either of these disorders in the presence of domestic violence, crowded living conditions, long distance to health care facilities that are sometimes of questionable quality, alcoholism, and diet options that have the variety of commodity or trading post sources. Something as basic as distance and travel can be misunderstood. Many Americans think of "rural" as something like Vermont or Alabama. Distances in Wyoming, Arizona, and New Mexico where we have lived are vast and empty by comparison with the rural image that many Americans hold. As service delivery models emphasize varied efficiencies, the difficult life circumstances associated among Indians overlook some of the most potent forces in determining morbidity, mortality, and burden of disease.

Partnership Models

The only paradigm for effective health care among American Indians is using some variation of an appropriate partnership model. This is important because involvement is more engaging than command, exploitation can be minimized, and essential information about history, communication styles, resources, and challenging life circumstances can be discerned more readily. Partnerships contribute to an overall goal of self-determination.

Partnership in health care initiatives, in research and practice, has become de rigueur in our vocabulary if not actual function. Improvements toward developing partnerships in which Indian leaders and health care professionals work toward common goals have been steady. Such models take a lot of time and personal effort. Partnership models are beginning to demonstrate how such an approach can lead to more effective and enduring results (Keltner & Ramey, 1993; Petersen, Trapp, Fanale, & Kaur, 2003).

AMERICAN INDIANS AND NURSING

Building bridges should be based on seeing the beginning and the destination associated with a desired connection. The Native American worldview of a circle of life and a circular way of living is common. Among the many different tribes are terms and images related to a sacred circle, sometimes called a sacred hoop. This image is considered sacred because it epitomizes family and cultural continuity. Dwellings and ceremonies from most tribes often have used circular or curved walls or borders that illustrate this perspective. The image of a circle is different from the way Americans typically envision a bridge. Bridges as Americans know them are linear and direct. Bridges in the physical sense may be seen as essentially unidirectional for different parties. People may pass with different destinations or purposes or perhaps even go back and forth but with a sense that one direction is definitely "to" and the other direction is essentially "from." A linear image is fundamentally different from a circular one. A circular worldview captures a notion of multiple iterations and retains a sense of returning to the beginning time and time again. Within a circular framework there would always be much give and take across the metaphorical bridge, illustrating the partnership paradigm for working with American Indians. The contrasting images of a circle and a straight line serve as a symbolic reminder of how different assumptions and styles of different cultures can be. From a pragmatic point of view, the pace of interactions is distinctly different in a circular lifestyle. People sometimes comment on "Indian" time, meaning a significantly slower pace. Cultural rhythms for Indians traditionally have been tied to cycles of nature such as seasons, rather than segmented by repeated minutes and hours. Much benefit can be gained through sharing knowledge and traditions. A metaphorical bridge that encompasses a circular worldview will be a preferred cultural fit with most Indian communities.

Need for Nursing

Health care needs among American Indians are not only extensive but also complex. As major health care providers, nurses are prepared to deliver care to people with a variety of needs and within contexts that also may vary substantively. In earlier times, most nurses may never have met Indians in the course of their practice. As mobility dramatically increases and outreach becomes a health care responsibility in a technological world, nurses are more likely to serve Indians. The epidemiological data document ethnic disparities in risk for disorders and deleterious outcomes among Indians. Concerns can be grouped according to mortality, morbidity, and burden. Health needs too often are complicated by challenging life circumstances and inadequate community infrastructure to address these needs. Nurses involved in primary care, public health, trauma, and rehabilitation are greatly needed to provide service to diminish the ethnic disparities that are so troublesome in society. Nursing practice and research must engage in culturally competent actions to provide effective care. Standards for cultural competence have not been well defined.

What Is Culturally Competent Nursing Care for American Indians?

Care and comfort certainly can be provided by Indian-to-Indian nursing care. Such a model has many merits because special sensitivity would increase the likelihood that personal needs would be met. Not enough Indian nurses are available to meet the need, however. Only 0.4% of nursing graduates in 2002 were American Indians (Mee, 2005). Another good way would include caregivers from a different culture who have acquired

a certain level of cultural competence. Nevertheless, it is always reassuring to see visible representation of one's own culture somewhere in the immediate health services. If an Indian person enters a hospital or clinic, seeing other Indians in professional roles communicates some reassurance that the Indian way of life matters to the institution.

The question arises from time to time whether non-Indians actually can provide culturally competent care for Indians. We believe emphatically that they can but that cultural competence is a skill with as much knowledge, sophistication, and the need for continual updating as any other skill within nursing. Cultural competence has three key components: sensitivity, specificity, and synergy. *Sensitivity* is the essential respect afforded to a culture with long-standing strengths and traditions that are positive and sustaining. Being culturally sensitive means possessing a certain humility as an outsider or "nonexpert" in domains that are valuable and beneficial to good health. *Specificity* means assuming a responsibility to learn about specific cultural traditions of a people—words of a native language, knowledge about cultural healers, and healing traditions—and an engagement or referral to those experts who can best assist persons in gaining, regaining, or maintaining optimal health. *Synergy* is a characteristic that combines traditions from two life forces and pathways to provide complementary rather than separate or competing health care supports. Cultural competence, therefore, is something that can be taught and learned.

Need for American Indian Nurses

For reasons of philosophy and pragmatism, it is essential that Indians become part of the health care delivery system. A fundamental social value exists in opening education and professional training to people who have long been underrepresented and excluded from participation. Knowledge and professional advancement can be enhanced with a diversity of background perspectives. How cultural competence can be articulated or communicated without the participation of Indian health professionals, including Indian nurses, is hard to imagine. A variety of educational preparation models for nurses are available. Several tribal colleges have nursing programs, mostly at the vocational and associate-degree level. Indian nurses are more likely than other Indian health professionals to remain in their own communities and even within the service systems that provide care for Indians. This permits nurses to have important opportunities in the design and implementation of culturally competent care. Many nurses serve on tribal councils and are becoming increasingly prominent in certain arenas as tribes assume more responsibility for their own health care programs. The opportunity to advance nursing practice is especially unique in this context.

Increasingly important is having minority persons in positions of influence in clinical decision making, setting administrative standards, in shaping health services, and most importantly, in directing health care resources. A persistent barrier to leadership is that the basic, and too often the only, educational preparation Indian nurses have attained has inherent limits. Many, many more Indian nurses have practical licensure and associate's degrees than bachelor's or advanced degrees. Among Indian nurses who have standard professional degrees, they are more often from the least selective, least prestigious baccalaureate schools. Education quality and networking opportunities vary according to these parameters of preparation. Nursing has multiple roles, and it is important that the best fit for the individual be made.

When mere overall numbers are examined, however, minorities most seriously are underrepresented within the professional field in the positions of influence. Significantly fewer key administrators and policy makers, academic leaders and full professors, senior scientists and nursing leaders are from any minority group but, most particularly, are American Indian. A need exists for direct care to be culturally competent, but just as important is that systems of inquiry, program, and service also have the capacity for cultural competence. As the overall presence of nursing dramatically declines in highly selective universities in the United States, there are even fewer opportunities for minority representation in leadership roles in schools with superior education, unparalleled professional networks, and sophistication. At the same time, the best educational institutions in the United States are recruiting many more young Indians into careers other than nursing. Although in important ways this expands opportunities for Indian youth, they are more likely not to return to their home communities than are Indians who choose nursing careers. Most definitely a need exists for bright young members of minorities to enter highly selective schools of nursing because they are being aggressively recruited for other professions. The intellectual vigor and potential scope of influence that minorities can bring to benefit the general public are magnified greatly through this educational stream.

Professional organizations are important networks for support and development. The unity for all nurses through local and national professional organizations fosters such growth. Indian nurses are dispersed widely across the United States but also have a unified organization, the National Alaska Native American Indian Nurses Association (NANAINA). In addition to support and networks, NANAINA provides a voice to advocate for cultural competence and for addressing special health care needs for Indian people. Although the organization is a relatively small and young, NANAINA is increasing its public profile and scope of involvement. An annual summit is held for members and supporters who are interested in promoting Indian health and Indian nursing. In the spirit of advancement and collaboration, NANAINA is a founding member of the National Coalition of Ethnic Minority Nurse Associations. The coalition is composed of NANAINA, the National Black Nurses Association, National Association of Hispanic Nurses, Asian American/Pacific Islanders Nurses Association, and the Philippine Nurses Association. The opportunity to leverage greater political position and support each other's organizations is an important step toward decreasing ethnic disparities in health outcomes.

The National Coalition of Ethnic Minority Nurse Associations has moved forward to provide a forum to produce minority nurse scientists with assistance of a $2.6 million grant from the National Institute of General Medical Sciences. American Indian mentors and mentees are part of this systematic program to develop research capacity in nursing. The skill, advanced education, and networking connections for American Indian nurses are vital steps in developing leaders in this field.

REFERENCES

American Indian Resource Institute. (1993). *Indian tribes as sovereign governments*. Oakland, CA: Author.

Andersen, S. R., Belcourt, G. M., & Langwell, K. M. (2005). Government, politics, and law: Building healthy tribal nations in Montana and Wyoming through collaborative research and development. *American Journal of Public Health 95*(5), 784-789.

Canby, W. C. (1988). *American Indian law in a nutshell* (2nd ed.). St. Paul, MN: West Publishing.

Design for a New HIS. (1995). *Recommendations of the Indian health design team executive summary*. Unpublished manuscript.

Deters, P. B., Novins, D. K., & Manson, S. M. (2004). Editorial [on circles of care]. *American Indian and Alaska Native Mental Health Research, 11*(2). Retrieved July 23, 2005, from http://www.uchsc.edu/ai/ncaianmhr/pdf_files/11(2).pdf.

Eagle/Walking Turtle. (1995). *Indian America* (4th ed., pp. 10-11). Sante Fe, NM: John Muir Publications.

Eaglestaff, M. L., McClain, M., & Fernbach, K. (2003). *American Indian infant mortality meeting: Community driven strategies.* Report of a meeting sponsored by the National Institute of Child Health and Human Development in Rapid City, SD, January 22-23, 2003. Washington, DC: U.S. Department of Health and Human Services.

Eschiti, V. S. (2004). Holistic approach to resolving American Indian/Alaska Native health care disparities. *Journal of Holistic Nursing, 22*(3), 201-208.

Holkup, P. A., Tripp-Reimer, T., Salois, E. M., & Weinert, C. (2004). Community-based participatory research: An approach to intervention research with a Native American community. *Advances in Nursing Science, 27*(3), 162-175.

Indian Health Service. (1997). *Trends in Indian health.* Rockville, MD: Indian Health Service, Office of Planning, Evaluation and Legislation, Division of Program Statistics.

Joe, J. R., & Malach, R. S. (1992). Families with Native American roots. In E. W. Lynch & M. J. Hanson (Eds.), *Developing cross cultural competence: A guide for working with young children and their families* (pp. 89-119). Baltimore, MD: Brookes.

Keltner, B. (1994). *American Indians and adaptation* (Grant No. R01HD31863-01). Washington, DC: National Institute of Child Health and Human Development.

Keltner, B., & Ramey, S. (1993). Family issues. *Current Opinion in Psychiatry, 5,* 638-644.

Keltner, B., & Walker, L. (2003). Resilience for those needing health care. In E. H. Grotberg (Ed.), *Resilience for today: Gaining strength from adversity* (pp. 141-160). Westport, CT: Praeger.

Krieger, N., Chen, J. T., Waterman, P. D., & Rehkopf, D. H. (2005). Painting a truer picture of US socioeconomic and racial/ethnic health inequalities: The Public Health Disparities Geocoding Project. *American Journal of Public Health 95*(2), 312-323.

Manson, S. M., Beals, J., Klein, S. A., & Croy, C. D. (2005). Social epidemiology of trauma among 2 American Indian reservation populations. *American Journal of Public Health 95*(5), 851-859.

Marks, E. L., & Graham, E. T. (2004). *Establishing a research agenda for American Indian and Alaska Native Head Start programs.* Washington, DC: Head Start Bureau, Administration on Children, Youth, and Families, U.S. Department of Health and Human Services.

McCauley, M. (2004). Going the distance for American Indians. *Nursing, 34*(12), 46-47.

Mee, C. L. (2005). The *other* nursing shortage. *Nursing, 35*(2), 6.

Meisenhelder, J. B., & Chandler, E. N. (2000). Faith, prayer, and health outcomes in elderly Native Americans. *Clinical Nursing Research 9*(2), 191-203.

National Indian Gaming Association. (2005). Retrieved July 23, 2005, from http://www.indiangaming.org

Nez Henderson, P., Jacobsen, C., & Beals, J. (2005). Correlates of cigarette smoking among selected Southwest and Northern Plains tribal groups: The AI-SUPERPFP Study. *American Journal of Public Health, 95*(5), 867-872.

Nolan, L. (2005). *Priorities of the Indian Health Service.* Paper presented at Indian Health Care in the 21st Century: A Case Study in Disparities, May 9, 2005. Retrieved July 23, 2005, from http://www.kaisernetwork.org/health_cast/hcast_index.cfm?display=detail&hc=1423

Novins, D. K., Beals, J., Moore, L. A., Spicer, P., & Manson, S. M. (2004). Use of biomedical services and traditional healing options among American Indians. *Medical Care, 42,* 670-679.

Petersen, W. O., Trapp, M. A., Fanale, M. A., & Kaur, J. S. (2003). Evaluating the WEB training program for cancer screening in Native American women. *Holistic Nursing Practice, 17*(5), 262-275.

Probst, J. C., Moore, C. G., Glover, S. H., & Samuels, M. E. (2004). Person and place: The compounding effects of race/ethnicity and rurality of health. *American Journal of Public Health 94*(10), 1695-1073.

Prucha, R. P. (1990). *Documents of United States Indian policy* (2nd ed.). Lincoln: University of Nebraska.

Puukka, E., Stehr-Green, P., & Becker, T. M. (2005). Measuring the health status gap for American Indians/Alaska Natives: Getting closer to the truth. *American Journal of Public Health, 95*(5), 838-843.

Robinson, R. (2003). *Minutes of the National AI/AN Smoking Cessation Workgroup.* Atlanta, GA: Centers for Disease Control and Prevention.

Roubideaux, Y. (2005). *Overview of Indian health issues.* Paper presented at Indian Health Care in the 21st Century: A Case Study in Disparities, May 9, 2005. Retrieved July 23, 2005, from http://www.kaisernetwork.org/health_cast/hcast_index.cfm?display=detail&hc=1423

Struthers, R., Eschiti, V. S., & Patchell, B. (2004). Tradition indigenous healing: Part I. *Complementary Therapies in Nursing & Midwifery, 10,* 141-149.

Struthers, R., & Lowe, J. (2003). Nursing in the Native American culture and historical trauma. *Issues in Mental Health Nursing, 24,* 257-272.

Wingood, G., & Keltner, B. (1999). Sociocultural factors and prevention programs affecting the health of ethnic minorities. In J. Raczynski & R. DiClemente (Eds.), *Handbook of health promotion and disease prevention* (pp. 561-579). New York: Kluwer Academic.

ETHICS, LEGAL, AND SOCIAL ISSUES

Ethical, Legal, and Social Concerns in a Changing Health Care World

PERLE SLAVIK COWEN ◆ SUE MOORHEAD

As the world of health care changes and the concerns for cost control escalate, it is increasingly difficult to keep a focus on the needs of people and the underlying legal, ethical, and social issues that surround health care decision making. Escalating health care costs clearly stress the national economy, and per capita health care expenditures for insured persons have been increasing at rates that are sharply disproportionate to overall inflation and worker earnings. Evidence of instability in insurance coverage is growing, with increasing premiums, increasing required co-payments, and limitations in health benefits. As health care insurance becomes more costly, the number of uninsured grows in a vicious circle. This creates increased health care costs as the costs of uncompensated care are passed on to the government and insured consumers in the form of higher charges. Many experts believe that increases in health care spending will continue into the distant future and are simply unsustainable.

As the debate over the future of health care continues, much of the discourse is based on an assumption that the problem is a lack of resources. Therefore the argument continues that rationing in some form is the only solution. This basic assumption requires examination. Is the problem a lack of resources, or is it rather a matter of how these resources are spent? Is it fair and just that more than 25% of health care expenditures are spent in processing the paperwork necessary to keep the providers paid and running economically viable businesses? Is it right and just that more than 45 million persons in the United States have no health care insurance and are effectively cut out of the health care system? Whose problem is it? Health care currently is rationed with the wealthy able to access elaborate and costly care while the poor are freely able to choose inadequate health care. Although this is a de facto form of rationing, full disclosure and rationing in broad daylight is advocated as an alternative. The tendency is to blame the victim rather than to accept that this is the responsibility of everyone.

In the future, ethical, social, and legal questions will be pushed to a new level with the current advances in the genetic field and the possibility of detecting genetic problems at a much earlier stage. A whole new world of options, each fraught with new legal and ethical issues, is emerging that will further complicate decision making and allocation of resources.

As you read the chapters in this section, we urge you to keep in mind some of the broader issues that have been addressed. Are the problems based on a lack of resources, or are they a reflection of a lack of ability to debate hard issues and reach a reasoned consensus that is fair and just? Much of health care decision making has been pushed out of the clinical domain, which was predominantly a case-by-case approach, and into the world of business, which makes decisions based on financial concerns. The general public usually has been left out of the decision-making process. In this section, some issues are raised that should be a matter of public debate. These issues are certainly a matter of debate within the nursing community.

In the opening chapter, Dunn-Lopez addresses the ethics of U.S. health care reform. This debate chapter presents arguments for the question "Should health care be rationed?" Two definitions of rationing are provided, the most common referring to "the denial of certain health care services to those who have enough money to buy them." The more difficult definition refers to "the persistent and systematic denial of health care services to those who cannot afford them." In setting up the debate, Dunn-Lopez includes perspectives from both definitions and points directly at two major forces driving the need for economic and ethical reform. She identifies solid indicators of an economic crisis in health care and cites four major reasons: increasing technology, aging population, increased pharmaceutical costs, and the high cost of providing hospital care to the uninsured. She says that the ethical issues concerning inequalities in health care are equally compelling and notes that the uninsured rate varies disproportionately by age, race, and income. An interesting review of historical influences builds to the failed attempts in the United States to provide universal access, and she provides an interesting pro-con debate based on philosophical underpinnings. The "equal opportunity for welfare" is presented as a bridge. Under this principal, individuals with access to insurance would continue to purchase insurance within a structure created for the uninsured to access insurance at a realistic and equitable price. Noting that under this view bad outcomes for those who choose not to participate would be tolerated. Dunn-Lopez reviews universal access health care insurance issues, noting that proposals have had a difficult time determining fair minimum packages, often encountering microallocation issues. A stark discussion of rationing decisions for vulnerable populations includes age-based rationing, rationing based on birth weight of premature infants, and rationing of intensive care unit services. Dunn-Lopez says "nurses are in a position to see the direct outcomes of those compromised by the current method of allocation." How nurses address the issues of health care rationing should be governed by a concern for justice for the powerless, vulnerable, and disenfranchised.

In the first viewpoint chapter, Markus, an attorney, addresses the intertwining of nursing and patient advocacy roles and questions whether there is a conflict of interest. She clarifies that "advocate" is a verb (to support, vindicate, or recommend publicly) and a noun (one who assists, defends, or pleads for another) and states that these legal definitions translate into three fundamental duties in the health care setting: (1) to ensure that patients are informed of their rights in a particular situation, including the right to refuse treatment; (2) to support patients in decisions they make; and (3) to protect patients, which includes reporting threats to their well-being. Markus posits that with the "development of biomedical technology and the corresponding fragmentation of medical care came a shift in nurses' primary loyalty from the physician and institution to the patient." She provides an extensive review of numerous cases and judicial findings related to legal protection for nurse patient advocates in nonstatutory and statutory claims, Nurse Practice Acts, conscience acts, whistleblower acts, and constitutional provisions, and she discusses current confusion in the courts. Markus recommends that specific language be incorporated into each state Nurse Practice Act or its regulations "based on a widely acknowledged code of ethics, such as the American Nurses Association *Code of Ethics for Nurses,* to clarify the distinction between moral and ethical decisions." This is

an interesting and well-written chapter that all nurses should read and all state nurses' associations should consider critically.

In the next chapter, Zink, Potter, and Chirlin address some of the complex issues across the life cycle that nurses face in practice settings. Although institutional ethics committees are in place in most settings, they have limitations placing nurses in a particularly difficult position. Another complication is the lack of emphasis on ethical and legal issues in the basic nursing curriculum. Some of the issues nurses faced in the practice setting that have profound ethical implications include cost-containment approaches, end-of-life decisions, pain management, "futile" care, genetic and reproductive issues, informed consent and confidentiality, and incompetent caregivers. The authors advocate nursing ethics committees, clinically based ethics education, and ethical rounds in practice settings. They note that the "push for cost containment finds us fearful for those without financial access to service and suspicious of the clinical decisions that are being made in the voice of profit for managed care organizations and increasingly in the not-for-profit sector in the name of financial viability."

Although nurses are faced with complexities related to the ethics of clinical decision making, they also may be confronted with problems such as sexual harassment in the workplace. Fielder carefully outlines the specific conditions defining sexual harassment. The chapter provides information about courses of action that might be taken. Fielder stresses the importance of institutional policies for handling sexual harassment. The author states that "male and female nurses need to understand what constitutes sexual harassment, and they must be made aware of the actions that need to be taken to protect themselves and their rights if sexual harassment occurs."

The remaining chapters in this section turn to specific ethical and social issues. Groves addresses the problem of health care for the poor and underserved. The author identifies the underserved as "the uninsured, the underinsured, the poor, and the working poor who do not receive adequate and quality health care." She believes that uninsured and underinsured persons receive less health care (usually too little and too late), less primary prevention, less care for their chronic conditions, and worse care in the hospital. Eighty-five percent of the uninsured are part of families with working members, and racial and ethnic minorities are more likely to be uninsured. This is a reflection of less education and lower-income employment that provides less health coverage. Groves states that the health care cost to society for poor and uninsured is not just the actual dollar amount of uncompensated care ($35 billion in 2001) but the decreased health capital of the underserved who have poorer health, premature mortality, and greatly increased unnecessary morbidity at an estimated cost of $65 billion to $130 billion. The author provides a solid review of previous legislation and new policies and solutions. Groves emphasizes that nurses can be a strong political force and can create change to move people out of poverty and provide real opportunities for improved health. This is an important chapter that pines to the roots of nursing.

One of the particularly troubling ethical problems confronting nurses who care for the elderly relates to the treatment of patients with Alzheimer's disease. Edwards states that 22 million individuals are expected to have Alzheimer's disease by the year 2050, and nearly half of those age 85 and older may have the disease. With a growing population of patients older than 80, this problem will increase in the years ahead. The author advocates that in decision making regarding care of patients with Alzheimer's, the first step is determining the capacity of the individual to participate in decision making and, to the degree possible, to respect the patient's choices. Advance directives are particularly useful. One of the major ethical concerns is creating unreasonable burdens for caregivers while weighing the rights of the patient against those of the caregivers. Nurses can be caught in particularly problematic decisions when the proxy for the patient may make decisions, such as that of withholding medication, that the caregiver may feel obligated to refuse to obey. Advance directives and communication with caregivers are advocated in reaching ethically viable decisions.

Kjervik specifically addresses issues related to advance directives. Noting the fundamental value in society of individualism, advance directives are a way of empowering patients. After describing the main types of advance directives, the author clarifies their ethical aspects. The value of a living will is that it is a clear way of stating what a patient wants at a specific point before a crisis. The major objections to advance directives are (1) the paternalistic view of health care providers that they know best; (2) living wills, which are made at a point when the patient is not in a crisis situation; and (3) the slippery slope between living wills and murder or genocide. Nurses play a key role in the development and implementation of advance directives.

Next, Silva and Williams breathe new life into the discussion of managed care and the violation of ethical principles. They posit that quality, quantity, and access to

health care have faltered because accelerating health care costs resulting in ethical concerns about the violation of ethical principles underlying managed, or more accurately, (mis)managed care. To understand how nurses' perceive ethical issues related to the restructuring of health care, particularly managed care, the authors conducted a qualitative study with a sample of 15 nurses enrolled in a doctoral program who had 20 or more years of nursing experience in a wide variety of settings. The participants were asked to share professional or personal stories or comments related to the restructuring of health care that they had experienced. The qualitative analysis resulted in identification of four discrete categories of violated ethical principles: respect for persons, respect for autonomy, of not harming persons, and of justice. The nurses' subjects' stories are grouped by category and are presented through a series of riveting vignettes. The authors offer suggestions for how "ethically compromised organizations and the nurses within them can empower themselves so that ethical principles are honored." This elegant chapter is at once a classic and is simply a must read for nurses and legislators.

In the final chapter in this section, Zoloth contends that "clinical ethics can be learned, via a method of decision making that clearly defines and describes a narrative. Nurses can lead the way toward the interpretation of that narrative; can ensure that the voice of the patient and the family is clearly articulated, and that the choices and the values that inform them remain central to treatment decisions." The author describes clinical ethics as resting on the core claims of bioethics and drawing on traditions in moral philosophy, theology, and the philosophy of law. She suggests that cases such as Schiavo—following Quinlan, Cruzan, Barber, and Drabeck—seem to define the parameters of the field; however, such court cases might be avoided if a consistent policy of locally based ethics review is enacted. Zoloth's detailed description of bioethics case consultation and how it works in the clinical setting is enlightening.

Nurses stand in the gap between patients and the health care system. As pressures build from all sides—the profit-making motives of big business at the expense of humane and quality patient care—the escalation of a wide array of social problems are intertwined inextricably with health. Nurses are obliged to examine the moral, ethical, and legal implications that govern their practice. Never have the challenges been greater. With challenge comes opportunity, however, the opportunity to rise to the fore in being a voice for the powerless and the disenfranchised and to speak out on behalf of patients.

Ethics of Health Care Reform

Should Health Care Be Rationed?

KAREN DUNN LOPEZ

Health care providers make decisions daily regarding the allocation of health care to individuals. Generally, providers in the United States are comfortable with the idea of not providing every available treatment alternative to every patient in every situation (American Thoracic Society, 1997; Asch & Ubel, 1997; Fletcher, Lombardo, Marshall, & Miller, 1997). However, "rationing" is a contentious issue. For the public and many providers, rationing is associated with the unpalatable idea of denying certain health care services to individuals in need (J. Wells, 1995). In addition to the negative connotations of rationing, the word has inconsistent definitions, therefore obscuring public understanding and thwarting substantive discussions of health care reform. The most common meaning of the term *rationing* in the context of health care refers to the denial of certain health care services to those who have enough money to buy them (Aaron & Schwartz, 1990; R. Wells, 2002). However, a complete discussion of rationing is impossible without acknowledging the second definition of the term that refers to the persistent and systematic denial of health care services to those who cannot afford them. Despite discomfort with the concept of rationing, the unremitting increase in health care costs signals that Americans will not have the luxury of postponing a thorough and pragmatic discussion of health care rationing much longer (Aaron & Schwartz, 1990; Fleck, 2002).

The goal of this chapter is to foster an understanding of the factors associated with the need for health care reform and the many ethical issues that are relevant to this discussion. Although many other countries have experience in health care rationing, this debate focuses on the United States, including major historical influences on the evolution of health care allocation and the projected trends for the future. The pro and con arguments for rationing in health care include perspectives from both definitions of the word *rationing*.

FORCES ASSOCIATED WITH THE NEED FOR U.S. HEALTH CARE REFORM

The need to proceed with health care reform in the United States is driven by two major forces: economic and ethical. Economically speaking, the rising cost of health care has been a major concern to the overall U.S. economy for several decades (Aaron & Schwartz, 1990). Health care is the single largest sector of government spending (Heffler et al., 2004). The continuing rise in health care cost relative to gross domestic product means that the United States is forced to decrease relative spending in other important areas of the economy (housing, education, job training, defense, police, transportation, and fire services). In addition to the increased cost to the federal government, the out-of-pocket costs to individual consumers also has increased (Strunk & Ginsburg, 2004).

Several forces are involved in driving up the cost of health care in the United States. Perhaps the most important force is the continued rate of technical innovation in health care (Aaron & Schwartz, 1990; American Thoracic Society, 1997; Fletcher et al., 1997). Research in health care often is supported through government agencies, such as the National Institutes of Health, and is costly. Successful research generates new demand for new health care services (Butler, 1999). No signs of a future decline in health care innovation are apparent, for technological possibilities seem without limit (Nyland, 2005). In addition, U.S. citizens, providers, and policy makers highly value research and technology in health care (American Thoracic Society, 1997; Fleck, 2002). Insured Americans, compared with citizens of other developed countries, have a strong preference for choosing what services they want and believe they are entitled to every health service they desire (Buchanan, 1998; Butler, 1999). A second, but less important reason for increasing health

611

BOX 66-1

Major Reasons for Increasing Health Care Costs

1. Technology
2. Aging population
3. Increased pharmaceutical costs
4. High cost of providing hospital care to uninsured

BOX 66-2

By the Numbers: Signs of Continued Economic Crisis in Health Care

1. Rising number of uninsured
   - 40 million in 2000
   - 43.6 million 2002
2. Rising health care expenditures
   - Increased 9.3% in 2002 (highest in a decade)
3. Rising health insurance premiums
   - Increased by 13.9% in 2003 (third consecutive year of double-digit increases)

From *Healthcare costs and instability of insurance: Impact on patient's experiences with care and medical bills.* (2004). Washington, DC: U.S. House of Representatives.

care costs, relates to demographic changes of the aging population. As disease and disability become more prevalent with age, so does the consumption of health care services (American Thoracic Society, 1997). A third factor driving increased health care costs is pharmaceuticals. The cost of pharmaceuticals has been increasing at a staggering rate for several years (Aaron & Schwartz, 1990; Heffler et al., 2004). Although fewer blockbuster drugs were introduced in the last few years, economic forecasters predict that drug-spending growth will continue to exceed total health care spending growth over the next several years (Heffler et al., 2004). The high cost of providing care to the uninsured is the fourth major force behind increasing health care costs. Individuals without insurance continue to seek health care but often are diagnosed later, incur more costly services, and have worse outcomes than those with insurance (Thorpe, 2004). Although hospitals try to extract payment from the uninsured, (Institute of Medicine, 2004a; Thorpe, 2004), the vast majority of uninsured cannot pay these medical bills. The cost of uncompensated care is passed on to the government, which pays up to $25 billion annually to reimburse for this care, and to insured consumers in the form of higher charges (Thorpe, 2004) (Box 66-1).

Escalating health care costs clearly place stress on the national economy but directly affect individual consumers as well (Mayes, 2004; Strunk & Ginsburg, 2004). Per capita health care expenditure for insured persons has been increasing at rates that are sharply disproportionate to overall inflation and worker earnings (Gabel et al., 2004; Strunk & Ginsburg, 2004). Evidence is increasing of instability in insurance coverage with increasing premiums, increasing required co-payments, and limitations in health benefits (*Healthcare Costs,* 2004; Mayes, 2004). As health care insurance becomes more costly, the number of uninsured grows (Emanuel, 2002; Strunk & Ginsburg, 2004), creating further opportunity for increased health care costs. Many experts believe that increases in health care spending

will continue into the distant future and are simply unsustainable (Emanuel, 2002) (Box 66-2).

Economic reasons alone provide sufficient justification for discussing new ways to contain health care costs that include the taboo subject of rationing (Fleck, 2002; Strunk & Ginsburg, 2004). However, the ethical issues concerning inequities in U.S. health care are equally compelling. Instead of having a system that provides some amount of basic health care services to all citizens, the United States has a fragmented market-based approach (Geyman, 2004). Approximately two thirds of the population obtains private health insurance via employer-sponsored health plans that provide a wide range of services. Trends indicate, however, that services increasingly are being limited (Emanuel, 1994). Services are available to elders (older than 65) and the chronically ill via the government-sponsored Medicare program. Far fewer services are offered to the very low-income individuals via the government-sponsored Medicaid program and to moderately low-income, uninsured children via the State Children's Heath Insurance Program (Emanuel, 1994). Not one state is able to provide health insurance to all persons under the poverty line (Beauchamp & Childress, 2001). This approach leaves approximately 16% of the population, or 45 million persons, uninsured (DeNavas-Walt, Proctor, Mills, & U.S. Bureau of the Census, 2004). Contrary to public misconception that the majority of the uninsured are unemployed, 65% to 80% of the uninsured are working families who work in businesses that do not offer insurance and who cannot afford the high cost of private insurance (Thorpe, 2004; Geyman, 2004). The uninsured rate varies disproportionately by age, race, and income with an uninsured rate for children in poverty of 19%

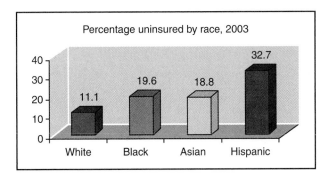

FIGURE 66-1 Percentage of uninsured persons by race, 2003. (From DeNavas-Walt, C. Proctor, B.D., & Mills, R.J. (2004). *U.S. Census Bureau current population reports. Income, poverty, and health insurance coverage in the United States: 2003.* Washington, DC: U.S. Government Printing Office.)

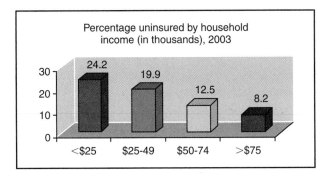

FIGURE 66-2 Percentage of uninsured persons by household income (in thousands of dollars), 2003. (From DeNavas-Walt, C. Proctor, B.D., & Mills, R.J. (2004). *U.S. Census Bureau current population reports. Income, poverty, and health insurance coverage in the United States: 2003.* Washington, DC: U.S. Government Printing Office.)

and a range from 11% for non-Hispanic whites to 33% for Hispanics (DeNavas-Walt et al., 2004). Most statistics of uninsured underestimate the problem by asking only about status. When asked if they had been without health insurance in the previous year, 52% of minorities and low-income (less than $20,000/year) persons reported being without health insurance for some months of the year (*Healthcare Costs,* 2004). These statistics also do not note the problem of underinsurance that include exclusions for preexisting diseases, waiting periods, and maximum lifetime benefits (Beauchamp & Childress, 2001) (Figures 66-1 and 66-2).

In addition to inequities in access to health care, the U.S. approach to health care leaves several other areas of inequities, including the following:

1. A disproportionate share of income is devoted to health care, with the poorest 10% paying 20% on average of their income toward health care expenses, whereas the 10% with the highest income paid 8% on average (Bodenheimer, 2003).

2. The practice of billing uninsured individuals considerably more than the negotiated insurance rate for the same services is unfair (*Healthcare Costs,* 2004; Bartlett & Steele, 2004). In addition, some hospitals charge high interest rates and place liens on the homes of patients who do not pay their bills. Among those with problems paying medical bills, 27% reported they had been unable to pay for food, heat, or rent so as to pay medical bills (*Healthcare Costs,* 2004). In addition, 51% below average income reported not filling prescriptions because of the cost (Blendon et al., 2002).

3. Unequal distribution of the insurance risk pool occurs, such that non–group insurance often has a smaller, sicker risk pool and thus charges much higher rates than those who purchase through medium or large employers (Beauchamp & Childress, 2001; Buchanan, 1998; Holahan & Pohl, 2002). This flaw in the distribution of risk also burdens the public sector as they provide insurance to the seriously chronically ill (Geyman, 2004).

4. Those with poor health, preexisting conditions, or family history of disease often are denied insurance coverage (Beauchamp & Childress, 2001).

5. The cost of employer-based insurance varies widely from state to state (Branscome, 2004).

6. Wide disparities in health outcomes exist between the poor and not poor (Institute of Medicine, 2004a; Isaacs & Schroeder, 2004; Jennings, 1994; Vladeck, 2003).

7. Health outcome disparities for racial and ethnic groups, particularly blacks, are significant even after adjusting for socioeconomic differences (Institute of Medicine, 2004b; Thrall & Friedman, 2003).

The United States spends substantially more on health care than other countries (Aaron & Schwartz, 1990; Vladeck, 2003). Despite the rising cost of health care and inequities in health care, many feel that the market-based approach to health care in the United States is superior and that the United States has the best health care in the world (Starfield, 2004). International comparisons suggest otherwise. The United States has the distinction of being the only industrialized nation without universal health care insurance. A recent study of 13 industrialized nations found the United States with the lowest percentage of low-birth-weight newborns, neonatal and infant mortality rates, and years of potential life lost. The United States was in the lowest quartile for life expectancy and age-adjusted mortality (Vladeck, 2003). In addition, dissatisfaction with the current structure of health care in the United States is growing among physicians and consumers (Emanuel, 2002). A study of five industrialized countries found the sharpest inequities in the United States. Low-income U.S. adults reported being much more likely to be dissatisfied than their low-income counterparts in Australia, Canada, New Zealand, and United Kingdom, citing worsening access and difficulty seeing specialists. In addition, 51% of U.S. respondents indicated that the United States needed to undertake fundamental changes in the way health care is delivered, and 28% advocated rebuilding health care delivery completely. The United States also had the highest proportion of the public who reported problems paying medical bills (Blendon et al., 2002).

Others who deny the need for major health care reform claim that reforms aimed at elimination of wasteful practices in health care would allow the United States to continue to provide all beneficial health care services. Although previous reforms have been useful, they have provided only one-shot savings. Various other approaches have been used in the past to cut health care cost and improve access; however, these incremental efforts have been dwarfed by exponential increases in available health care technology that drives the demand for ever-increasingly expensive health care and have not diminished the number of uninsured (Aaron & Schwartz, 1990) (Figure 66-3).

HISTORICAL INFLUENCES ON U.S. HEALTH CARE REFORM

The roles of the U.S. government and the private sector in providing access to health care have been shaped by changing economic and social conditions. This section provides an overview of some of the major influences, most of which originated in response to specific conditions rather than as incremental steps to a national agenda for health care delivery. One of the earliest health care insurance companies began in 1929 as the country began to experience the outcomes of the stock market crash that began the Great Depression. The administrator of Baylor Hospital entered into an arrangement to provide care to a group of teachers on a prepaid basis that eventually became Blue Cross Insurance (Fletcher et al., 1997). Although technically not health care, in 1935 in the midst of the depression, Franklin Roosevelt established Social Security. This provided public dollars to support unemployed and needy older Americans who could no longer be provided for via charity (Vladeck, 2003). In the 1940s, during World War II, wage controls were placed on American employers, giving rise

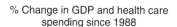
% Change in GDP and health care spending since 1988

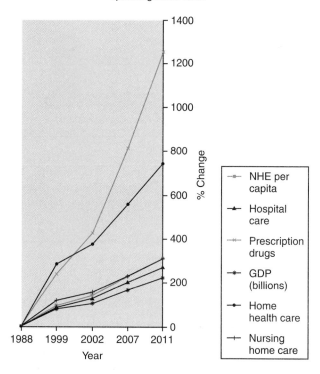

FIGURE 66-3   Percentage change in gross domestic product and health care spending since 1988. *GDP,* Gross domestic product; *NHE,* national health expenditure. (From Center for Medicare and Medicaid Services. (2005). *National health care expenditures and projection, Table 1: National health expenditures and selected economic indicators, levels and average annual percent change 1998-2011.* Retrieved January 2, 2005 from http:// new.cms.hhs. gov/NationalHealthExpendData/ downloads/nheprojections 1998-2011.pdf.)

to employer-based health insurance as employers used health insurance to compete for workers. In 1948, President Truman proposed single-payer public health insurance, but his plan was denounced by the American Medical Association and was labeled by some as a communist plot. In the 1960s the U.S. government took a major step toward increasing health care access to two of its most vulnerable population groups via Medicare, which provided public health insurance to those over age 65, and Medicaid, which provided public insurance to the poor (Fletcher et al., 1997). In the 1970s, health care costs soared because of unexpected costs of the Medicare program. In response, President Nixon sought to control costs through price controls that proved too complex to enforce. Nixon also proposed a mandate requiring employers to provide health insurance, but this initiative failed (Aaron & Schwartz, 1990). In the

1980s, Medicare shifted to a prospective payment system for hospitalized patients, whereby hospitals were reimbursed based on the patient's diagnosis (diagnosis-related groups) (Geyman, 2004). The private sector followed suit through similar prospective payment systems within managed care companies. Although these programs successfully halted the rate of Medicare expenditure growth, they are regarded widely as only having shifted costs to hospitals and employers (Fletcher et al., 1997; Geyman, 2004; Mayes, 2004). In the early 1990s, newly elected president Clinton proposed a plan for universal public health care coverage that he believed would solve problems of escalating health care costs and increases in the number of uninsured (Brock & Daniels, 1994). As was the case with President Truman's attempt to enact universal coverage, the plan failed with major stakeholders putting forth massive "information" campaigns that misled the public by labeling the proposal "socialized medicine" (Geyman, 2004). A disappointed President Clinton went on to make incremental changes in health care reform such as the State Children's Health Insurance Program, which makes insurance available to uninsured children who do not qualify for Medicaid, and the Health Insurance Portability and Accountability Act, which protects workers from loss of health insurance when they change or lose their job. Despite these incremental advances in health care access, the overall rate of uninsured has not changed (Holahan & Pohl, 2002), and as previously described, costs continue to escalate. More recently, some states moved in the opposite direction of improved access by restricting eligibility to Medicaid and the State Children's Health Insurance Program (*Healthcare Costs,* 2004). The current administration, under President George W. Bush, favors plans that are much more modest and an increased role of the private sector to help solve the economic and access problems of health care. Included in his plans are the following (Republican National Committee, 2005):

1. Tax credits (up to $1000 per individual and $3000 per family) to purchase insurance, which is far less than the cost of individual insurance plans
2. Health savings accounts, which offer a tax deductibility to individuals for health care spending but do little for poor individuals and families who do not have enough income to cover basic needs and are therefore unable to save
3. Medical malpractice reform, which is not regarded as being a major player in the escalation of health care costs
4. Small business purchasing pools

In summary, the major attempts to provide universal access in this country over the last 50 years have failed. Incremental changes, although well intentioned, have left Americans with an increasingly complex array of choices, escalating costs that many in the business industry are no longer willing to pay (Buchanan, 1998), and gross inequities in access to care and health outcomes. The economic incentives for reforming U.S. health care are virtually irrefutable, yet the methods of reform are yet to be determined. The concept of rationing necessary care is inescapable in the current context of an ever-increasing array of innovative and expensive health care services available to the individual consumer. Despite discomfort with the word *rationing,* as a matter of national policy the United States, access to routine health care services are denied to vulnerable population groups. The health care system systematically denies access to care based on the ability to access employee-based insurance or one of the government insurance programs. This method of rationing denies potentially beneficial care to approximately 16% of U.S. citizens. The ethical challenge is to determine more fair ways to allocate health care services in the United States that will fulfill the requirements for fiscal solvency (Daniels & Emanuel, 1996).

ETHICAL ISSUES IN HEALTH CARE REFORM

Ethicists agree that health care is an important focus of concern in the field because good health is needed to participate fully in society (Beauchamp & Childress, 2001; Butler, 1999; Emanuel, 1994). Furthermore, ethicists argue that structures for health care allocation are the responsibility of a just government and should not be left to chance forces (Butler, 1999). What has been missing in the U.S. debate about health care reform is the societal (versus individual) perspective. Several ethical principles will guide this debate:

◆ Beneficence: The duty to do good for patients that requires balancing of benefits against risks and costs (Beauchamp & Childress, 2001; Spencer, 1997)
◆ Nomaleficence: The duty to avoid the causation of harm (Beauchamp & Childress, 2001)
◆ Social justice: The way in which the basic structures of major social, political, and economic institutions are arranged such that everyone has a fair share (Butler, 1999)
◆ Distributive justice: "Fair equitable and appropriate distribution determined by justified norms that structure terms of social cooperation" (Butler, 1999, p. 226)

- Utilitarianism: A principle that emphasizes social efficacy and maximum benefit (Beauchamp & Childress, 2001)
- Collective social protection: A principle that focuses on the similarity between health care and other needs to which the government provides access, such as crime control, firefighting, sanitation, and pollution control (Beauchamp & Childress, 2001)
- Egalitarianism: A principle that focuses on the equal worth of persons and fair opportunity (Beauchamp & Childress, 2001)
- Autonomy: A principle of respect for the decision-making capabilities of individuals (Beauchamp & Childress, 2001)
- Libertarianism: Under this principle, "a just society protects rights of property and liberty, allowing persons to improve their circumstances and protect their own health on their own initiative" (Beauchamp & Childress, 2001)

Pro Argument

The majority of ethical principles support the idea of providing universal health care coverage within a just society (Emanuel, 2002). Principles of social justice provide general support for reforming the approach to allocation of health care so that all citizens have a fair share of access to health care. In addition, justice often requires favoring aggregation of modest benefits to many over substantial benefits to a few (Daniels & Emanuel, 1996). The principle of fair equality of opportunity permits inequality in distribution of health care as long as everyone has an opportunity to access basic health care (Emanuel, 2002). Collective social protection finds similarities between health care and other needs that the government provides for and helps one formulate the argument that if the government provides equal access to those services, it also has the obligation to provide for equal access to health care. Although the principle of beneficence catches health care providers in a conflict, for health care providers who interact chiefly with individuals, the principle of beneficence does not require unlimited care to individuals at great cost to society (Fletcher et al., 1997; J. Wells, 1995). Furthermore, even those who favor libertarian ideals must acknowledge that it is not possible to have unlimited choice in some areas (Brock & Daniels, 1994).

Con Argument

The United States has long favored the libertarian tradition in which health care is distributed through a free market ideal (Beauchamp & Childress, 2001).

This approach allows individuals to protect their health by their own initiative with minimal government intrusion. Many in American society believe that this approach is the best because it respects individual autonomy and self-determination (Fletcher et al., 1997; J. Wells, 1995). Under this view, health care systems that are characterized by a great degree of equity place unacceptable cost on individual liberty (Menzel, 2003). Distributive justice emphasizes the role of social cooperation in determining allocation. Several attempts have been made in the United States to adopt universal coverage. The fact that universal coverage has been defeated every time indicates that this endeavor may not reflect the values of American society and may not be realistically achievable in the context of social cooperation required by distributive justice.

Bridging the Ethical Gap

At its most basic level, the conflict between individual and societal needs and justice and liberty and clinically possible and economically affordable health care seems to be an endless ideological battleground (American Thoracic Society, 1997). Menzel (2003) argues for an alternative view of distributive justice called "equal opportunity for welfare" as a way to bridge this divide. Under this principle, "People should not be worse off than others through no fault or voluntary choice of their own." In the United States, those with the access to insurance would continue to purchase insurance. A structure could be created for those without access to insurance to provide access at realistic and equitable price. Bad outcomes for those who choose not to access insurance would be tolerated based on their voluntary choice not to purchase insurance. This preserves more of a role of individual choice to satisfy the libertarian view and offers a chance for equality in access. What should emerge is a third sense of rationing that provides for equal opportunities for access to health insurance while allowing individuals with financial resources choice to access services beyond the basic package, as well as tolerating individuals who choose not to access insurance (Beauchamp & Childress, 2001; Fletcher et al., 1997).

Gaps in Ethical Guidance

Although most ethical principles support universal access health care insurance as a way to distribute health care fairly, the ethical theory does not provide enough guidance to inform what the concrete content of a fair minimum basic package of health care insurance should include in times of a vast assortment of potentially beneficial services and limited resources (Buchanan,

1998; Emanuel, 1994; Jennings, 1994; Reinhardt, 1997). The concept of distributive justice concerns how to distribute resources fairly and requires that one look to "justified norms" to develop a fair allocation of health care. The problem of how to determine what the "justified norm" is could range from allocating care when normal opportunity is impaired to providing enough care to ensure individual happiness (Butler, 1999). Furthermore, norms are constantly changing. This point is especially relevant in health care because potentially beneficial treatments are introduced frequently. A sharper definition of this concept of distributive justice for health care is needed for real-life application. The principle also requires that society be engaged meaningfully in social cooperation in determining allocation. Examples of this kind of social engagement are rare in the United States, and it has proved difficult to establish what this minimum basic health care should be. One of the examples of this type of process took place in Oregon in the mid-1990s when multiple methods—including telephone surveys, educational forums, and town hall meetings—were used to engage Oregonians in determining which services to allocate to the Medicaid population (Daniels, 1994; Bodenheimer, 1997). Critics of this experiment in rationing found that many treatments, such as incapacitating hernias, were left off the treatment list and questioned how the outcomes could be in accord with social justice even when the process involved a high degree of social cooperation (Beauchamp & Childress, 2001). Utilitarian theories require one to look at social efficacy, which may lead one to the slippery slope of microallocation determined by an individual's value to society.

Ethical Dilemmas in Microallocation Rationing Decisions: Vulnerable Populations

Age-Based Rationing. How much and what care should be pursued for the elderly at a time when technical possibilities may be virtually limitless is of concern to ethicists (Nyland, 2005). Some argue that priority for health care spending should be given to the young because elders have had a chance to live their life (Butler, 1999). In general, older patients have less life expectancy and less opportunity to benefit from life-sustaining treatments (Clarke, 2001). Others assert that elders have a moral duty to die rather than continuing to pursue costly medical care near the end of their life (Hardwig, 2000). Justice and egalitarian philosophies value life at any age and require persons to be treated equally (Butler, 1999; Clarke, 2001). Others assert that if viewed in terms of an entire life span, elders will have had a fair

and equal opportunity to health care over the entire course of their lives even if they do not receive as many services when they are older (Beauchamp & Childress, 2001; Butler, 1999).

Rationing Based on Birth Weight for Premature Infants. Neonatal intensive care unit technology has made it possible for very-low-birth-weight infants to have long-term survival. This technology is costly, and the children who are born prematurely at very low birth weight grow to need many additional forms of specialized care throughout their lifetime. Some have argued that this expensive technology be rationed. A recent analysis of this issue notes that this practice would increase racial disparities in health care further because of a higher rate of very-low-birth-weight infants that are black. The authors also felt that setting a birth weight cutoff point at which care is not offered would deny care to many infants who would have long-term survival (Stolz & McCormick, 1998).

Rationing of Intensive Care Unit Services. The critically ill are another group that may be likely targets for rationing decisions because intensive care services are in increased demand and are expensive. A task force of the American Thoracic Society (1997) along with legal and bioethical consultants developed a framework for fair allocation of intensive care unit beds. The task force arrived at the following principles to allocate services:

- Sufficient medical need
- Sufficient potential for benefit
- Equal access regardless of ability to pay and personal character

Aged-based rationing was discarded because it does not take into account the risk of death in a young person who may be critically ill with a low chance of benefit (American Thoracic Society, 1997). Although the framework is not explicit, it takes significant steps in the right direction that will assist hospitals to formulate policies.

THE RESPONSE OF THE PROFESSION

In 1991, *Nursing's Agenda for Healthcare Reform* was released and endorsed by 76 nursing and health care organizations (American Nurses Association, 1991). This document is regarded as a benchmark for collaborative work in health care policy development for nursing (American Nurses Association, 1991; Betts, 1993, 1996; Lassa, 1993). Although health care reform efforts failed in the early 1990s, nursing took a proactive stance and was involved in the process of planning for reform. It may be time again for nurses to consider their role in health care reform efforts. Nurses are in a position to see the direct outcomes of those compromised by the current method of allocation of health care services. Although it will be a challenge to engage the current administration, ethical principles require that nurses continue to advocate in the public arena. At a minimum, all nurses should understand the economic issues and understand the effects that the current approach to health care allocation has on society at large.

REFERENCES

Aaron, H., & Schwartz, W. (1990). Rationing health care: the choice before us. *Science, 247*(4941), 418-422.

American Nurses Association. (1991). *Nursing's agenda for health-care reform.* Washington DC: American Nurses Publishing.

American Thoracic Society. (1997). Fair allocation of intensive care unit resources. *American Journal of Respiratory and Critical Care Medicine, 156*(4), 1282-1301.

Asch, D., & Ubel, P. (1997). Rationing by any other name. *New England Journal of Medicine, 336*(23), 1668-1671.

Bartlett, D., & Steele, J. (2004). *Critical condition: How health care in America became big business and bad medicine.* New York: Doubleday.

Beauchamp, T., & Childress, J. (2001). *Principles of biomedical ethics* (Vol. 5). New York: Oxford University Press.

Betts, V. T. (1993). Priorities in health care reform. *Imprint, 40*(4), 55-56.

Betts, V. T. (1996). Nursing's agenda for healthcare reform: Policy, politics, and power through professional leadership. *Nursing Administration Quarterly, 20*(3), 1-8.

Blendon, R., Schoen, C., DesRoches, C., Osborn, R., Scoles, K., & Zapert, K. (2002). Inequities in healthcare: A five country survey. *Health Affairs, 21*(3), 182-191.

Bodenheimer, T. (1997). The Oregon health plan: Lessons for the nation. *New England Journal of Medicine, 337*(10), 720-723.

Bodenheimer, T. (2003). The movement for universal health insurance: Finding common ground. *American Journal of Public Heath, 93*(1), 112-115.

Branscome, J. (2004). *State differences in the cost of job-related heath insurance, 2002* (Statistical Brief No. 51). Rockville, MD: Agency for Healthcare Research and Quality.

Brock, D., & Daniels, N. (1994). Ethical foundations of the Clinton administration's proposed health care system. *Journal of the American Medical Association, 271*(15), 1189-1196.

Buchanan. A. (1998). Managed care: Rationing without justice, but not unjustly. *Journal of Heath Politics, 23*(4), 617-634.

Butler, J. (1999). *The ethics of heath care rationing.* London: Cassell.

Clarke, C. (2001). Rationing scarce life-sustaining resources on the basis of age. *Journal of Advanced Nursing, 35*(5), 799-804.

Daniels, N. (1994). Four unsolved rationing problems: A challenge. *Hastings Center Report, 24*(4), 27-30.

Daniels, N., & Emanuel, E. (1996). Is justice enough? Ends and means in bioethics. *Hastings Center Report, 26*(6), 9-10.

DeNavas-Walt, C., Proctor, B. D., Mills, R. J., & U.S. Census Bureau. (2004). *Income, poverty, and health insurance coverage in the United States: 2003.* Washington, DC: U.S. Government Printing Office.

Emanuel, E. (1994). Where civic republicanism and deliberative democracy meet Ezekiel J. Emanuel. *Hastings Center Report, 24*(6), 5-13.

Emanuel, E. (2002). Health care reform: Still possible. *Hastings Center Report, 32*(2), 32-34.

Fleck, L. (2002). Rationing don't give up. *Hastings Center Report, 32*(2), 35-36.

Fletcher, J., Lombardo, P., Marshall, M., & Miller, F. (1997). *Introduction to clinical ethics* (2nd ed.). Hagerstown: University Publishing Group.

Gabel, J., Levitt, L., Pickgrein, J., Whitmore, H., Holve, E., Rowland, D., et al. (2004). Job-based health insurance in 2001: Inflation hits double digits, managed care retreats. In C. Harrington & C. Estes (Eds.), *Health policy: Crisis and reform in the U.S. health care delivery system* (pp. 318-323). Sudbury, MA: Jones and Bartlett.

Geyman, J. (2004). Myths as barriers to health care reform in the United States. In C. Harrington & C. Estes (Eds.), *Health policy: Crisis and reform in the U.S. health delivery system* (pp. 29-35). Sudbury, MA: Jones and Bartlett.

Hardwig, J. (2000). *Is there a duty to die?* New York: Routlege.

Healthcare costs and instability of insurance: Impact on patient's experiences with care and medical bills. (2004). Washington, DC: U.S. House of Representatives.

Heffler, S., Smith, S., Won, G., Clemens, M., Keehan, S., & Zezza, M. (2004). Health spending projections for 2001-2011: The latest outlook. In C. Harrington & C. Estes (Eds.), *Health policy: Crisis and reform in the U.S. health care delivery system* (pp. 250-259). Sudbury, MA: Jones and Bartlett.

Holahan, J., & Pohl, M. (2002, May/June). Changes in insurance coverage: 1994-2000 and beyond. *Health Affairs,* pp. W162-W171.

Institute of Medicine. (2004a). Care without coverage: Too little too late. In C. Harrington & C. Ester (Eds.), *Health policy: Crisis and reform in the U.S. health care delivery system* (pp. 94-95). Sudbury, MA: Jones and Bartlett.

Institute of Medicine. (2004b). Unequal treatment: Confronting racial and ethnic disparities in health care. In C. Harrington & C. Estes (Eds.), *Health policy: Crisis and reform in the U.S. healthcare delivery system* (pp. 71-78). Sudbury, MA: Jones and Bartlett.

Isaacs, S., & Schroeder, S. (2004). Class: The ignored determinant of the nation's health. *New England Journal of Medicine, 351*(11), 1137-1142.

Jennings, B. (1994). Beyond distributive justice in health reform. *Hastings Center Report, 24*(6), 5-13.

Lassa, T. (1993). Health care reform plan should benefit nurses. *Nurse Practitioner, 18*(6), 7.

Mayes, R. (2004). Causal chains and cost shifting: How Medicare's rescue inadvertently triggered the managed-care revolution. *Journal of Policy History, 16*(2), 144-174.

Menzel, P. T. (2003). How compatible are liberty and equality in structuring a health care system? *Journal of Medicine and Philosophy, 28*(3), 281-306.

Nyland, S. (2005). Do you want to live forever? *Technology Review, 108*(2), 37-45.

Reinhardt, U. (1997). Wanted: a clearly articulated social ethic for American health care. *JAMA: The Journal of the American Medical Association, 278*(17), 1446-1447.

Republican National Committee. (2005). *President's Bush's agenda to improve healthcare.* Retrieved January 7, 2005, from http://www.gop.com/GOPAgenda/AgendaPage. aspx?id=4

Spencer, E. (1997). Economics, managed care, and patient advocacy. In J. Fletcher, P. Lombardo, M. Marshall, & F. Miller (Eds.), *Introduction to clinical ethics* (pp. 239-254). Hagerstown, MD: University Publishing Group.

Starfield, B. (2004). Is U.S. health really best in the world? In C. Ester (Ed.), *Health policy: Crisis and reform in the U.S. health care delivery system* (pp. 46-51). Sudbury, MA: Jones and Bartlett.

Stolz, J., & McCormick, M. (1998). Restricting access to neonatal intensive care: Effect on mortality and economic savings. *Pediatrics, 101*(3), 344-348.

Strunk, B., & Ginsburg, P. (2004, June 9). *Tracking health care costs: Trends turn downward in 2003.* Retrieved January 7, 2005, from http://content.healthaffairs.org/cgi/content/ full/hlthaff.w4.354/DC1

Thorpe, K. (2004). Protecting the uninsured. *New England Journal of Medicine, 351*(15), 1479-1481.

Thrall, T. H., & Friedman, E. (2003). Blind to bias. *Hospitals and Health Networks, 77*(8), 36-38.

U.S. Bureau of the Census. (2003). *Current population survey.* Washington, D.C.: U.S. Bureau of the Census.

Vladeck, B. (2003). Universal health insurance in the United States: Reflections on the past, the present, and the future. *America Journal of Public Heath, 93*(10), 16-19.

Wells, J. (1995). Health care rationing: Nursing perspectives. *Journal of Advanced Nursing, 22*(4), 738-744.

Wells, R. (2002). Can rationing be fair? *Hastings Center Report, 32*(5), 4-5.

CHAPTER
67

The Nurse as Patient Advocate

Is There a Conflict of Interest?

KAREN MARKUS

Lorraine, a middle-aged widow, is wheeled into the busy emergency department of a large urban teaching hospital. She has been severely beaten and raped, sustaining multiple jaw fractures and pulmonary contusions from blows to the chest. Both wrists are fractured. Doctors insert an endotracheal tube via a tracheotomy to treat her pulmonary edema and provide an airway for reconstructive facial surgery. Although alert, she is able to communicate only by slight head movements. Before she was intubated, however, Lorraine whispered that she had gotten a good look at her assailant. Thus the detective in charge of her case is eager to get a description of the perpetrator, who is suspected of being a brutal serial rapist.

Lorraine's nurse, an emergency room veteran, suggests deflating the cuff of Lorraine's endotracheal tube and briefly occluding the opening of the tube to allow her to whisper. The attending physician vetoes the suggestion on clinical grounds and accuses the nurse of being overzealous in her advocacy on behalf of female assault victims. He believes Lorraine should not answer the detective's questions until after surgery, when her condition is more stable. The nurse, convinced that time is of the essence if the culprit is to be apprehended, obtains Lorraine's consent to her plan. She verbally informs Lorraine of the risks, assuring her that she will be there to handle anything that might go wrong. She does not inform the attending physician.

The nurse justifies her actions on the grounds that she is complying with Lorraine's wishes and contributing to the greater good, yet she is uneasily aware that she is disobeying the attending physician's order and promoting her own agenda. The nurse deflates the cuff and Lorraine manages to whisper "white guy, dark hair" to the detective before she regurgitates, aspirates, and arrests.[1]

Melodrama notwithstanding, this scene identifies types of conflict that occur daily in health care facilities nationwide: between patients and external entities, such as law enforcement agencies or even family members; between physicians and nurses; between patients' wishes and their own best interests. Many, if not most, of these conflicts implicate nurses' duty to advocate for their patients.

What does it mean to be a patient advocate, however? The word *advocate* is a verb and a noun. As a verb,

advocate means "[t]o support, vindicate, or recommend publicly." The noun form describes "one who assists, defends, or pleads for another."[2] These legal definitions translate into three fundamental duties in the health care setting: (1) to ensure that patients are informed of their rights in a particular situation, including the right to refuse treatment; (2) to support patients in decisions they make; and (3) to protect patients, which includes reporting threats to their well-being.[3]

The complexity of the medical environment requires the use of professional judgment to apply this model of advocacy on a case-by-case basis. Application of the model in actual practice may be problematic, however, because legal support for patient advocacy is unsettled. Little legal guidance is available to instruct nurses in how to carry out the patient advocate role. As the following survey of case law illustrates, standards of nursing practice are vague regarding patient advocacy. Nurse Practice Acts may provide minimum guidelines but often do not define unprofessional behavior adequately. A paucity of general laws exists regarding nurses' right to make ethical decisions. Codes of ethics are unlikely to provide legal protection for the nurse who acts as a patient advocate and often are too abstract for the courts to apply.

Thus ambiguous and inconsistent legal holdings have caused confusion about the behavior subject to sanction. For example, conduct that has been sanctioned includes granting a cancer patient's request to discuss treatment alternatives,[4] reporting illegal practices to a government agency,[5] and refusing to perform kidney dialysis for a patient with a terminal condition.[6]

Conflict stems from the fact that although nursing is an independent profession with its own body of knowledge and legal accountability,[7] the vast majority of nurses do not legally function as independent practitioners. Rather, they serve employers within the bureaucratic structure of institutions and implement the orders of physicians.[8] In the first instance, conflict may arise from countervailing pressures on hospitals. Although liability provides hospitals with an incentive to avoid negligence, hospitals are also under economic pressure to increase revenues by treating the largest number of patients with smallest possible number of nurses. Consequently, the nurse's ethical mandate may diverge from her[9] employer's goals. Second, the unique body of knowledge encompassed by nursing, as distinct from that of medicine, may contribute to conflicts. Whereas medicine focuses on pathology, nursing focuses on patients' response to health problems and the nursing needs that arise therefrom, wherein lie many quality of life issues.[10] Thus a nurse's view of her obligations may diverge from a physician's.

When patient advocacy involves a nurse's duty to support the patient in a decision contrary to the beliefs of the physician, institution, or society as to what is "right," divergent loyalties may lead to fundamental conflicts that can expose the nurse to considerable risk. The nurse who adopts a position that is adverse to that of the physician or the institution that employs her may face a difficult personal and professional dilemma.

SOURCES OF THE PATIENT ADVOCATE DUTY

The duty of advocacy stems from the impact of illness on patients' autonomy and ability to make decisions, which places nurses in a powerful position. The experiences to which individuals increasingly are subjected as institutionalized patients create a responsibility to assist them to cope with this environment. Consequently, along with the development of biomedical technology and the corresponding fragmentation of medical care came a shift in nurses' primary loyalty from the physician and institution to the patient. This attitudinal shift was recognized by the American Nurses Association in 1976, when it amended its *Code of Ethics for Nurses* to replace directives about respect for and obedience to the physician with statements affirming the duty of patient advocacy.[11]

State nursing practice laws and their corresponding administrative regulations also may impose an affirmative duty to advocate for patients. In California, for instance, registered nurses have an explicit duty to act "as the client's advocate, as circumstances require, by initiating action to improve health care or to change decisions or activities which are against the interests or wishes of the client, and by giving the client the opportunity to make informed decisions about health care before it is provided."[12]

LEGAL PROTECTION FOR PATIENT ADVOCATES

A common legal claim made by health professionals sanctioned for acts of patient advocacy is in tort for wrongful discharge. The majority of nurses, who are not covered by employment contracts, are subject to the employment-at-will doctrine, a judicially created rule that permits termination of employment by either party without cause. To prevail in this type of claim, the nurse must convince the court that her conduct fell within a public policy exception to the employment-at-will rule. For instance, a nurse may allege that her conduct was supported by important public concerns, such as patient welfare and safety, which warrant preventing her employer from discharging her in retaliation for professional decisions made in the best interests of her patient. However, judicial acceptance of a public policy defense against wrongful discharge appears to depend primarily on whether the source of the public policy that supports the nurse's conduct is statutory or nonstatutory.

Nonstatutory Claims

Courts generally have been unwilling to accord public policy status to nonstatutory sources of policy, such as professional oaths and codes of ethics. A leading case, *Pierce v. Ortho Pharmaceutical Corp.,*[13] involved a research physician who alleged that she was forced to resign in response to her refusal to work on the development of a drug she believed was hazardous to public health. She argued that continuing to work on the drug would violate her vow to do no harm as a medical doctor under the Hippocratic Oath and urged the New Jersey Supreme Court to recognize this proscription as public policy, thereby giving rise to a cause of action for wrongful discharge.

Although acknowledging the harshness of the at-will doctrine, the court nevertheless ruled that the general language of the Hippocratic Oath falls short of the standard required for judicial elevation to the level of public policy. The court stated that an employee has a cause of action for wrongful discharge only when the discharge is contrary to a "clear mandate" of public policy, which emanates from sources such as legislatures and regulatory agencies. However, the court tempered this pronouncement by stating in dicta, "In certain instances, a professional code of ethics may contain an expression of public policy." The court placed the burden of proof on the employee to identify a specific expression of public policy for the judge to evaluate on a case-by-case basis.

VIEWPOINTS

The court criticized the physician for failing to use a professional code of ethics to buttress her ethical objections to the drug experiments, recognizing that professional employees "owe a special duty to abide not only by federal and state law, but also by the recognized codes of ethics of their professions." The broad reach of this statement was limited, however, by the proviso that this duty does not permit employees to prevent their employers from pursuing their business. The court admonished professional employees to distinguish business decisions that offend their personal morals from violations of their professional code of ethics. However, the court failed to identify a method by which to make this sometimes difficult distinction.

Despite the statement by the New Jersey Supreme Court that a code of ethics can serve as a source of public policy, 5 years later, in *Warthen v. Toms River Community Memorial Hospital*,[14] a New Jersey Court of Appeals refused to recognize the American Nurses Association *Code of Ethics for Nurses* as such. In that case, a nurse specialist who was assigned to dialyze a terminally ill double amputee patient in renal failure had to terminate the procedure on two occasions because the patient suffered cardiac arrest and severe internal hemorrhaging. The nurse notified her supervisor in a timely manner of her "moral, medical, and philosophical objections" to performing a procedure that further complicated a terminal patient's condition. When the nurse subsequently refused to provide dialysis as ordered, she was terminated.

Although acknowledging the nurse's good faith effort to comply with her professional code of ethics, the court held that the *Code of Ethics for Nurses* does not provide the clear mandate of public policy required by *Pierce* because it defines "a standard of conduct beneficial only to the individual nurse and not to the public at large." The court articulated the fear that it would be virtually impossible to administer a hospital if nurses were allowed the freedom to decide whether to treat patients based on their personal beliefs.

The court closed the door further on the use of professional codes of ethics when it stated, "The source of public policy is the statutes enacted by the legislature and in the decisions of the courts; there we find what acts are considered harmful to the public." Significantly, the court assigned the role of identifying public policy to the judge, comparing it to the judge's duty to interpret statutes. Thus the court took away from the jury, which tends to be more plaintiff-oriented, the issue of whether a clear public policy mandate exists to support a nurse's ethical conduct.

Statutory Claims

Courts have been more willing to limit the at-will rule when the discharge violates a legislatively declared public policy. Nevertheless, attempts by nurses to derive public policy exceptions from existing legislative sources have yielded inconsistent results. The main legislative sources employed in defense of patient advocacy are (1) Nurse Practice Acts; (2) right of conscience acts, most of which focus on objections to participating in abortion and sterilization procedures; (3) whistle-blower statutes; and (4) constitutional provisions, especially if the employer is a public institution.[15]

Nurse Practice Acts. The first hurdle when using a Nurse Practice Act to contest a nurse's discharge is to convince the court that it contains an expression of public policy. Thus in *Francis v. Memorial General Hospital*,[16] a New Mexico court denied the wrongful discharge claim of a nurse who refused to float to a specialized unit on the grounds that it would jeopardize patient safety. The nurse argued that to do so would violate his licensing statute, but the court instead focused on the floating policy of the hospital, stating that not only did it fail to violate public policy but also that it implemented the important public policy of ensuring adequate staffing in a cost-effective manner. Clearly, the court, viewing nurses as a fungible commodity, did not appreciate the degree of specialization required for competent nursing practice.

Similarly, in *Lampe v. Presbyterian Medical Center*,[17] a Colorado court declined to elevate a Nurse Practice Act to the level of public policy. In that case, the head nurse of an intensive care unit who was ordered to reduce overtime expenditures believed she could not do so without jeopardizing patients and was fired for being "unwilling to fulfill the requirements of her job description." The nurse relied on the legislative declaration of policy in the Colorado Nurse Practice Act, which required her to act in manner consistent with the health and safety of her patients. She contended that had she obeyed her employer's order to reduce overtime, she would have violated the statute under which she was licensed. The court, however, refused to interpret the broad policy statement of the statute to impute a legislative intent to "modify the contractual relationships between hospitals and their employees in such situations." Thus the plaintiff's claim for relief was denied because of the lack of prescriptive specificity in the statute governing her professional behavior.

In contrast, *Tuma v. Board of Nursing*[18] illustrates the proscriptive inadequacy of a Nurse Practice Act.

The plaintiff, an instructor of clinical nursing, was assigned to administer chemotherapy to a terminal leukemia patient because of her special interest in the needs of dying patients. The patient pleaded with the nurse to return that evening to discuss a controversial alternative treatment. She did so, but the chemotherapy was continued and the patient died 2 weeks later after experiencing serious adverse side effects.

Although there were no allegations that she had caused harm to the patient, hospital personnel complained to the Board of Nursing that the nurse "had interfered with the physician-patient relationship." Subsequently, a hearing officer concluded that her discussion of treatment alternatives constituted unprofessional conduct in violation of the Idaho Nurse Practice Act. Although the act explicitly conformed to the policies and practices of the American Nurses Association, the nurse was not permitted to testify regarding the *Code of Ethics for Nurses*. The Board of Nursing affirmed the hearing officer's decision and suspended her license for 6 months.

On appeal, the Idaho Supreme Court found nothing in the language of the Nurse Practice Act to put the nurse on notice that her license would be suspended if she engaged in the contemplated behavior. The court decried depriving the nurse of a property right as important as a license to practice her profession in the absence of guidelines established by the Board of Nursing. Therefore, it held that the Board of Nursing had violated the nurse's constitutional due process rights by suspending her license on the grounds of unprofessional conduct without an explicit statutory definition of such conduct.

However, sufficiently detailed legislation authorizing the practice of nursing may support a public policy exception to the at-will doctrine. Thus in *Deerman v. Beverly California Corp.,*[19] a North Carolina court vindicated a nurse who was fired for responding to a family's specific inquiries about the deteriorating condition of a nursing home resident. When the family was unable to contact the patient's physician, the nurse had advised selecting another physician because the patient was not receiving appropriate care. Although the court expressed reluctance to recognize exceptions to the at-will employment doctrine absent "substantial justification grounded in compelling considerations of public policy," it found that the Nurse Practice Act did create public policy.

The court gave great weight to the comprehensiveness and specificity of the Nurse Practice Act and its administrative regulations, which enabled the court to comprehend that the practice of nursing includes "'assessing,' a patient's health, which entails a 'responsibility' to communicate, 'counsel,' and 'provid[e] accurate … guidance to clients [and] their families.'" Thus the court concluded that firing the nurse violated public policy because her comments were proffered in fulfillment of her statutory responsibilities.

Conscience Acts. Following the U.S. Supreme Court decision in *Roe v. Wade,*[20] a majority of states enacted so-called "conscience acts."[21] Some of these acts are limited to prohibiting discrimination against employees who object to participating in abortions; others extend to procedures such as sterilization and artificial insemination. The Illinois Right of Conscience Act,[22] however, has broad language that covers medical personnel who exercise their conscience with respect to "any phase of patient care." Nevertheless, in *Free v. Holy Cross Hospital,*[23] the Right of Conscience Act did not support the public policy argument of a hospital shift supervisor who was ordered to transfer a patient to another facility. When the nurse could not locate a receiving hospital, she was instructed to proceed with the transfer "even if removal required forcibly putting the patient in a wheelchair and leaving her in the park." Her attempt to intervene on behalf of the patient resulted in her immediate discharge by the vice president of the hospital.

The court rejected the nurse's wrongful discharge claim because it interpreted the Right of Conscience Act to apply to moral convictions arising from sincerely held religious beliefs, as opposed to ethical concerns relating to her duty as a registered nurse. Because the nurse did not allege that the order she refused to carry out violated her religious beliefs, the court declined to use the act to create a public policy exception to her employer's right to discharge her. Furthermore, although the court stated that the nurse's ethical concerns fell within the province of the Illinois Nursing Act, it did not address using it as an alternate legislative source of public policy.

Whistle-Blower Acts. Legal remedies for nurses who suffer retaliation for reporting unsafe practices or conditions vary from state to state. Most states have laws that address "external whistle-blowing," which involves reporting an employer or colleague to an agency outside the organization.[24] Such a statute was used by the vice president of nursing of a New York hospital to challenge her termination successfully in *Kraus v. New Rochelle Hospital Medical Center.*[25] In that case the court held that the nurse was discharged wrongfully for reporting a physician who had noted falsely on patient records that he had performed bronchoscopies and had forged patients' signatures on the accompanying informed consent forms.

Some states have extended statutory protection further to "internal whistle-blowers" who report health and safety issues within their own organization.[26] These laws often contain a presumption that any adverse treatment of an employee within a specified period of time after reporting is retaliatory, thus shifting the burden of proof to the employer. Nevertheless, in *Gonzales v. Methodist Retirement Communities,*[27] one such law failed to protect a Texas nurse practitioner, who was fired the day after she argued with the medical director of a nursing home about the disposition of a patient who was injured when he fell out of a geriatric chair. Believing that it was obvious that the fall resulted from neglect, she did not explicitly state the cause of the fall when she verbally reported it. Interpreting the language of the statute narrowly, the court held that the law did not cover her report because she omitted to alleged neglect. Thus a law intended to encourage employees to report unsafe practices or conditions did not protect a nurse who did so.

Constitutional Provisions. Nurses who can claim constitutional protection may fare better in suits involving retaliation for patient advocacy. Thus in *Jones v. Memorial Hospital System,*[28] an intensive care nurse, who was discharged for writing a magazine article about conflicts between the duty of hospital personnel to prolong life and patients' right to die with dignity, argued that the discharge violated the freedom of speech clause of the Texas Constitution because the issues she addressed were a matter of public concern. Although it upheld her claim, the court emphasized the narrowness of the public policy exception to the at-will rule, concluding that a hospital is free to discharge a nurse on any grounds that are not constitutionally protected.

More extensive protection exists for nurses employed by public hospitals, which as governmental entities are under federal constitutional constraints. For instance, in *Rookard v. Health and Hospitals Corp.,*[29] the Second Circuit federal court of appeals reinstated a director of nurses who had supervised more than 1000 employees until she was demoted to an entry-level position for reporting wasteful and illegal practices. The court held that the hospital had violated her First Amendment right of free speech regarding matters that are of public concern.

CONFUSION IN THE COURTS

Ethics must be distinguished from morals. Ethics focuses on rational methods for choosing the best course of action among conflicting alternatives, whereas morality refers to action in accordance with prescribed rules of conduct.[30] However, although cautioning health professionals against confusing moral precepts with ethical considerations, courts have failed to provide guidelines with which to accomplish this task. Thus the *Warthen* court's characterization of a nurse's refusal to perform renal dialysis as moral, rather than ethical, led it to deny the nurse's public policy claim. More important, the failure of the court to articulate standards by which to make this distinction deprived nurses of guidance for future conduct because the nurse's philosophical objection to dialysis arguably fell into the realm of a responsible ethical decision. Two years later, the *Free* court further blurred the distinction between ethical guidelines and moral beliefs when it ignored the broad language of the Illinois Right of Conscience Act by limiting its coverage, on similar facts, to moral convictions with respect to "euthanasia, sterilization or abortion."

Moreover, the *Warthen* court erroneously concluded that the plaintiff's reliance on the American Nurses Association *Code of Ethics for Nurses* was solely for her own benefit when it stated, "By refusing to perform the procedure she may have eased her own conscience, but she neither benefited the society-at-large, the patient, nor the patient's family." On the contrary, the *Code of Ethics for Nurses* is a policy document intended to promote the quality of patient care, rather than the personal interests of individual nurses.[31]

Case law demonstrates that nursing advocacy must be supported specifically by statute. Without legislative acknowledgment of nurses' need for legal protection in their role as patient advocates, compliance with this ethical and legal mandate will continue to be risky. Because of the relative openness of the courts to Nurse Practice Acts as sources of public policy, amendment of these statutes explicitly to include the duty to advocate for patients is likely to be more effective than enactment of freestanding laws, such as conscience or whistle-blower protection acts. Furthermore, revision of current laws governing the professional conduct of nurses will decrease the potential for misapplication and will provide the clear mandate of public policy required by the courts.

Therefore language that sets forth nurses' duty to advocate for patients should be incorporated into each state Nurse Practice Act or its regulations. This language should be based on a widely acknowledged code of ethics, such as the American Nurses Association *Code of Ethics for Nurses,* to clarify the distinction between moral and ethical decisions. This will enable the nursing profession and the courts to apply consistent guidelines more accurately to identify conduct that is protected by public policy.

REFERENCES

1. ER: *White Guy, Dark Hair* (NBC television broadcast, Nov. 18, 2004).
2. Black's Law Dictionary 51 (5th ed. 1979).
3. Ellen W. Bernal, *The Nurse as Patient Advocate,* Hastings Center Rep., July/Aug. 92, at 19 [hereinafter *Bernal*].
4. *Tuma v. Bd. of Nursing,* 100 Idaho 74, 593 P.2d 711 (1979).
5. *Rookard v. Health and Hosps. Corp.,* 710 F.2d 41 (2d Cir. 1983).
6. *Warthen v. Toms River Cmty. Mem'l Hosp.,* 199 N.J. Super. 18, 488 A.2d 229 (1985).
7. *See generally,* William O. Morris, *The Negligent Nurse—The Physician and the Hospital,* 33 *Baylor L. Rev.* 109 (1981); Walter T. Eccard, Note, *A Revolution in White: New Approaches in Treating Nurses as Professionals,* 30 Vand. L. Rev. 839 (1977).
8. *The Registered Nurse Population: Findings from the National Sample Survey of Registered Nurses* 19 (U.S. Dep't. of Health and Human Servs., March 2000), at ftp://ftp.hrsa.gov/bhpr/rnsurvey2000/rnsurvey00-1.pdf (last visited Dec. 22, 2004).
9. For the sake of brevity, female pronouns are used to refer to nurses because as of 2000, men constituted only 5.4% of the registered nurse population, up from 2.7% in 1980. Id. at 17.
10. "The practice of nursing … means those functions, including basic health care, that help people cope with difficulties in daily living that are associated with their actual or potential health or illness problems or the treatment thereof." Cal. Bus. & Prof. Code § 2725(b) (West 2004).
11. *Bernal, supra* note 3, at 21 (citing *Code of Ethics for Nurses with Interpretive Statements* (American Nurses Ass'n, 1976)).
12. 16 Cal. Code Regs. § 1443.5(6) (2004).
13. 84 N.J. 58, 417 A.2d 505 (1980).
14. 199 N.J. Super. 18, 488 A.2d 229 (1985).
15. Bruce G. Davis, *Defining the Employment Rights of Medical Personnel within the Parameters of Personal Conscience,* 1986 Det. C.L. L. Rev. 847, 848-49 (1986) [hereinafter *Davis*].
16. 104 N.M. 698, 726 P.2d 852 (1986).
17. 41 Colo. App. 465, 590 P.2d 513 (1978) (citing Colo. Rev. Stat. Ann. § 12-38-201).
18. 100 Idaho 74, 593 P.2d 711 (1979) (citing Idaho Code § 54-1414).
19. 135 N.C. App. 1, 518 S.E.2d 804 (1999) (quoting N.C. Gen. Stat. § 90-171.20) (alterations in original). *See also Kirk v. Mercy Hosp. Tri-County,* 851 S.W.2d 617 (Mo. Ct. App. 1993) (the nursing practice act's description of professional practice was detailed enough to create public policy, which the hospital had violated by firing the nurse who persisted in protesting substandard care that resulted in patient's death).
20. 410 U.S. 113 (1973).
21. *Davis, supra* note 15, at 849.
22. 745 Ill. Comp. Stat. Ann. 70/3 (West 2004).
23. 153 Ill. App. 3d 45, 505 N.E.2d 1188 (1987) (citing former Ill. Stat. Ch. 1111/2, ¶ 5303).
24. California Labor Code section 1102.5 (West 2004), which protects employees against retaliation for disclosing to a government or law enforcement agency conduct that violates a state or federal statute, is a typical external whistleblower statute.
25. 216 A.D.2d 360, 628 N.Y.S.2d 360 (1995) (citing New York Labor Law § 740(2)).
26. In 1999, fifteen years after it passed Labor Code section 1102.5, the California Legislature enacted Health & Safety Code section 1278.5 (West 2004) specifically to protect health care workers who file grievances or complaints with facility administrators.
27. 33 S.W.3d 882 (Tex. Ct. App. 2000) (citing Tex. Health & Safety Code Ann. § 242.133 (Vernon 1997)).
28. 677 S.W.2d 221 (Tex. Ct. App. 1984).
29. 710 F.2d 41 (2d Cir. 1983).
30. *Integrated Clinical Experience Ethics Booklet,* ch. 2 (Univ. of Neb. Med. Ctr.), at http://www.unmc.edu/psm/students/ice/ethicsbook/ethics-morals.htm (last updated Dec. 16, 2004).
31. The first and third provisions of the *Code of Ethics for Nurses* exhort nurses to provide services "unrestricted by considerations of social or economic status, personal attributes, or the nature of health problems" and "to safeguard the client and the public when health care and safety are affected by the incompetent, unethical, or illegal practice of any person." *Code of Ethics for Nurses with Interpretive Statements* (American Nurses Ass'n, Silver Spring, Md., © 2001 nursesbooks.org), at http://nursingworld.org/ethics/1985prov.htm (last visited Dec. 20, 2004) (reprinted with permission from American Nurses Ass'n).

Ethical Issues and Resources for Nurses Across the Continuum

MARGO R. ZINK ◆ JEANNE POTTER ◆ KRISTI CHIRLIN

The health care system of today provides an unending supply of bioethical challenges amid its enormous complexity and rapid change. Life can be sustained, often precariously, for long periods. However, life support frequently may be done in an intensive care environment or through artificial fluid, nutrition, or sophisticated pharmacology. Technology has been extended into the home setting, where ventilator-dependent children and adults can be maintained for indefinite periods. The explosion of genetic information has seeded an array of ethical concerns, including threats to confidentiality, misuse of information resulting in discrimination, denial of health care coverage, selective reproduction, and questioning of the value of life with genetic imperfections.

A push for cost containment finds nurses fearful for those without financial access to service and suspicious of the clinical decisions that are being made in the voice of profit for managed care organizations and increasingly in the not-for-profit sector in the name of financial viability. Concerns for cost have reduced staffing levels in some health care settings to an extent that may compromise health care workers' duty to patients. Patients entering the health care system not uncommonly fear that their rights may be violated and their expectations will not be met. Their concern often is related to informed consent, use of restraints, medication errors, pain management, or research. Health care professionals have a responsibility to identify good practice and to regulate practice to protect the client and to ensure that quality services are provided (Wood, 2001).

Nurses must maintain vigilance and competence within this complex health care system to identify and address actions or events that ethically may compromise them or the patients for whom they are responsible. Sources of assistance in the domain of ethics include professional codes or standards and formal ethics structures. Nurses must use sound nursing knowledge coupled with critical thinking skills in order objectively to assess the facts of a situation and related legal implications (Wood, 2001).

CODE FOR NURSES

Nurses' involvement in ethical issues has been well documented in the literature and through professional organizational efforts. The "Nightingale Pledge" of 1893, patterned after the Hippocratic Oath, is accepted as the first nursing code of ethics. The *Code of Ethics for Nurses with Interpretative Statements,* published by the American Nurses Association, provides a framework from which nurses in any setting can engage in ethical analysis and decision making. The *Code* originally was adopted by the American Nurses Association in 1950 and periodically has been revised. A major revision to the 1985 version of the *Code* was under way for some time. These revisions have prompted nurses to assess the value of the *Code* on practice across settings (Ketefian & Norris, 2002; Turkoski, 2000). Following are the nine final components of the *Code* (American Nurses Association, 2001):

1. The nurse, in all professional relationships, practices with compassion and respect for the inherent dignity, worth, and uniqueness of every individual, unrestricted by considerations of social or economic status, personal attributes, or the nature of health problems.
2. The nurse's primary commitment is to the patient, whether an individual, family, or community.
3. The nurse promotes, advocates for, and strives to protect the health, safety, and rights of the patient.
4. The nurse is responsible and accountable for individual nursing practice and determines the appropriate delegation of tasks consistent with the nurse's obligation to provide optimum patient care.

5. The nurse owes the same duties to self as to others, including the responsibility to preserve integrity and safety, to maintain competence, and to continue personal and professional growth.
6. The nurse participates in establishing, maintaining, and improving health care environments and conditions of employment conducive of the provision of quality health care and consistent with the values of the profession, through individual and collective action.
7. The nurse participates in the advancement of the profession through contributions to practice, education, administration, and knowledge development.
8. The nurse collaborates with health professionals, the public, and others in promoting community, national, and international efforts to meet health needs.
9. The profession of nursing, as represented by professional associations and their members, is responsible for articulating nursing values, for maintaining the integrity of the profession and its practice, and for shaping social policy.

The statements of the *Code* and the interpretation guide nursing practice and maintain high quality in nursing care. The *Code* directs nurses to practice with compassion and respect for every individual (Milton, 2003). The current revisions in the code fail to address the current dilemmas of practice.

ETHICS FORUMS

Institutional Ethics Committees

Recognition of bioethics as an important aspect of health care management spawned the development of institutional ethics committees (IECs) beginning in the early 1980s. With the broadly held purposes of education, policy development, and clinical consultation, these committees provide a forum in which to address difficult patient choices. Staff education and the establishment of clear policies for areas such as informed consent, limitation of treatment, and end-of-life issues are typical committee topics. Clinical consults are routinely available to health care team members, patients, and families to assist with ethical dilemmas. The IEC provides a more systematic and principled approach to multidisciplinary decision making that can link ethical and social values and medical technology across the health care continuum. Nurses working in long-term care and home care have been in leadership positions in the establishment of ethics committees.

Institutional ethics committees have a limited membership and do not consistently address the specific concerns of nurses. These committees are able to offer a forum for only a few nurses, leaving the majority of nursing staff in most settings without an opportunity to participate. Although nurses have been highly visible among the membership, bringing strong clinical voice and patient-focused approaches to committee activity, they have been in the minority of representation.

Dodd, Jansson, Brown-Saltzman, Shirk, and Wunch (2004) examined the extent to which nurses engage two specific ethical behaviors:

◆ Ethical activism: Nurses attempt to make hospitals more receptive to nurses' participation in ethics deliberations.
◆ Ethical assertiveness: Nurses participate informally in ethics deliberations.

In a research study of 165 nurses from several major hospitals, Dodd (2004) found that nurses' perceptions of the receptiveness of other hospital health professionals strongly influenced their participation in focused ethical meetings. These findings were found to have implications on specific content for nurses' ethics education and on expanding the extent to which nursing participates in ethical forums. Dierchx de Casterle, Meulenbergs, van de Vijver, Tanghe, and Gastmans (2002) concluded that nursing participation in ethical discussions actually could function as a catalyst for improved nursing care.

Daily nursing practice problems, nursing dilemmas related to increased high-tech care in acute and home care settings, the allocation of decreasing resources, long-term care, and reductions and reallocations of professional staff generally are not addressed in an IEC.

Nursing Ethics Committees

Nursing ethics committees usually are organized more informally than the IECs and allow nurses an opportunity to prepare for involvement in IECs. Some criticism has been that nursing ethics committees (NECs) compete with IECs, although they generally have much less decision-making power than the IEC. Although there continues to be a trend in most health care settings for a multidisciplinary ethics committee, a need remains to provide a specific avenue for nurses to seek advice on ethical issues more unique to the profession. The primary function of an NEC is the identification, exploration, and resolution of ethical issues in nursing practice. The NEC also should provide the availability of education for nurses in bioethics and nursing ethics. This committee has long been described as a foundation for the preparation of nurses for participation in interdisciplinary decision making about ethical issues. The committee also should serve as a resource group for other nurses in an institution and should be a clearinghouse for the review of nursing ethics materials. Committee members have a responsibility to be involved with review of departmental policies related to ethics and involvement with nursing ethics research.

Ethical rounds can be another framework to provide nurses and other disciplines working with specific patients the opportunity to address current ethical dilemmas involved with care. These discussions can deal with current ethical issues or projected problems in the delivery of care to a specific patient or patient population. The formation of groups composed only of nurses cultivates the knowledge and skills required to engage in ethical decision making. The NECs critique real or situational case studies, test various problem-solving techniques, and assess ethics related to nursing practice.

NURSES' EDUCATIONAL PREPARATION

Nurses continue to have inadequate preparation for effective handling of ethical issues, despite the fact that accrediting bodies for nursing education programs and health care organizations require that nursing ethics content be provided. Milton (2004) explored the distinction of ethics content at various levels of nursing education. The active participation of nursing students in the process of teaching ethics will enhance the process (Dinc & Gorgulu, 2002). Volker (2003) proposes that there actually may be a distinct nursing ethic, which examines theories, standards, and inquiry distinct to nursing practice.

First, nurses need preparation in ethical concepts, decision making, and pertinent legal standards. This knowledge is necessary to participate articulately in interdisciplinary ethics discussions. Second, many issues relating to the nurse's role as a patient advocate requires a forum in which these issues can be clarified. Appropriate nursing development of the advocacy role has emerged as a crucial element in nursing practice, especially in light of reimbursement declines and managed care.

Specific ethics content in nursing education at the undergraduate or graduate levels presently is not required by state curriculum or nationwide accreditation bodies. Gastmans (2002), however, recommends that ethical content reflect the theory of nursing, based on the following three components of a fundamental view of nursing ethics:

◆ Nursing as moral practice
◆ Intersubjective character of nursing
◆ Moral perception of nursing

Based on these fundamental views, Gastmans (2002) suggests the following consideration for ethics education for nurses:

◆ Attitude versus action-oriented ethics education
◆ Integral versus rationalistic ethics education
◆ Contextual model for ethics education

Nurses working in hospital settings are caring for patients with higher acuity, more social stressors (e.g., homelessness, violence, isolation, poverty, and illiteracy), and reduced hospital lengths of stay. These conditions provoke enormous ethical concerns in the area of beneficence. Can effective patient education occur with a short hospital stay? When is a patient ready for discharge? What are the institutional obligations to ensure patient safety after discharge? What if a patient has no financial means for needed post-hospital care if the insurance payer limits continued care?

Nurses, however, in direct clinical roles are suited especially to be involved in ethical decision making because of the sustained relationships with patients and families that these roles provide. The nurse in this role is best able to understand the patient's pain, suffering, achievements, and disappointments. The nurse may be the first to become aware of an ethical issue. Education in ethics should be provided to the nurse across the continuum during initial orientation and ongoing through continuing education offerings. This education should address specific application of ethical principles to acute and home care settings. The future of nursing management appears to be heading toward decreased numbers of graduate-prepared individuals. Without this support, it may be necessary to provide ongoing support for nurses in high-autonomy settings. This may lead to improved orientation and ongoing competence.

ISSUES IN PRACTICE

Although the *Code of Ethics for Nurses* provides a framework for critical thinking and adherence to identified core principles, it has limited use in addressing the individual daily practice issues encountered by nurses. Such issues are situational and so often are created or influenced by multiple factors, such as clinical status, patient values, family dynamics, institutional policy, organizational culture, and patient outcomes. Nurses do not always have a clear understanding about their role in ethical deliberations or even in the way ethical decisions are made. Nurses frequently feel powerless in these situations.

Maintenance of professional boundaries can be another challenge in the home setting, the patient's turf.

The home care provider who fails to establish and maintain professional boundaries often develops an emotional connection with the patient that may override clinical judgment. Milton (2002) examines the nursing phenomenon of acting faithfully in the nurse-client relationship. The obligation to act in good faith, fulfill agreements, and maintain an appropriate relationship are components of this relationship. Trust has long been considered central to this nurse-client relationship (Peter & Morgan, 2001). The absence of truth, where client rights may have been violated, is another dilemma faced by nurses, particularly cited by Turkoski (2001) in the home setting.

Cost Containment and Allocation

Policy debates have increased at local and national levels concerning universal access to care and the allocation of increasingly limited health care resources. Nurses must be knowledgeable about the numerous issues with ethical implications that can affect allocation determinations with the ultimate goal of universal access to care (Sarikonda-Woitas & Robinson, 2002). Managed care organizations are changing the infrastructure of health care delivery and are placing limitations on access to health care, which has ethical implications for the entire health care continuum. The four fundamental principles underlying the process of decision making in a managed care environment include patient self-determination, well-being, equality, and competence.

The first principle of self-determination is that patients define their values and assume responsibility for their lifestyle and health care practices. A managed care delivery scheme imposes certain lifestyle practices on patients, whether desired or not. The well-being of the patient is a second principle to consider in the decision-making process. The health profession, especially nursing in the community or home setting, has long focused on this through health promotion teaching. The issue of equality is an underlying moral principle in ethics. This principle also can be seen as a vital component in the decision-making process; arbitrary decisions about patient care essentially are eliminated in this principle. This, however, also implies that different needs of patients are treated in different ways. Other considerations of the decision-making process involve the assessment of the patient's ability and competence to be involved in this process. When managed care guidelines are dictated, how much decision-making ability will the health professional or the patient have about any desired alternatives?

Although managed care organizations pose many challenges on the ethics of health care delivery, they also minimize some previously existing unethical practices. The focus on maximum quality and cost-effectiveness places more demands on the provider than has occurred in the past, coupled with increased accountability. In the old, unstructured, noncompetitive health care environment, providers were not accountable to the patient for providing the best quality care for the best price. In this managed, integrated market, competition is strong, and so quality becomes a benchmark when alliances and mergers take place. Public reporting has increased the consumers' awareness of quality measures.

Futility

With the extreme sophistication of high-tech care, providers and patients struggle with defining the futility of care options. Nurses are central members of the health team participating in identifying the value of particular treatment options and in meeting the desired attainable goals of the patient. Choices as diverse as artificial ventilation, chemotherapy, dialysis, artificial nutrition, and hemodynamic support must be made within the context of overall prognosis for recovery and rehabilitation potential. These choices are seldom those of the patient or family alone; rather they are influenced more and more by the insurance payer. Home health providers who have gained the trust of the caregivers are often in the position of being asked to guide treatment decisions.

Now sophisticated catheters and infusion pumps for the delivery of all types of medications, including antibiotics, parental nutrition, and analgesics, are available for home use. Home ventilator systems and other high-tech equipment now can be adapted to the home setting at a significantly lower cost than institutionalized care. A feeling of intrusion and loss of privacy can accompany high-tech home care. Additional burdens are placed on caregivers, who must oversee these technologies and provide skilled care on a 24-hour daily basis. Family and friends must learn about these high-tech interventions with sometimes limited instruction before the patient's discharge. Home care nurses with a caseload of patients who all require high-tech care can experience burnout because of the intensity of the care and the extensive documentation requirements. Ethical dilemmas arise for the staff and the agency when nurses are assigned patients with high-tech care needs beyond their experience level and qualifications. In all settings, nurses are required to demonstrate their competency skills to ensure safe practice. Nurses have a responsibility to identify a procedure they do not feel qualified to perform. Technology in the home setting can create a conflict between the beneficent obligations of the home care provider and the autonomy of the patient and family.

Informed Consent and Confidentiality

The right to full disclosure of health care information has become a keen patient right that creates ethical dilemmas in practice. What is full disclosure? When has valid informed consent been given? When is truth telling secondary to other ethical principles? What is the role of the nurse in the informed consent process? Who is entitled to give information to patients? How has computerization of patient data affected the issue of informed consent?

The patient in any health care setting has the right to be informed of his or her plan of care, any charges the patient may be obligated to pay, and when discharge from services will take place. Patients also have a right to be informed of what staff will be involved in their care and these individuals' qualifications. The home care patient must be informed of how to voice a complaint through the agency or through a state hotline number.

Information management systems in today's acute care settings are highly computerized. Maintaining security of information access and distribution is a responsibility of nurses not to be taken lightly. The "need to know" standard guides caregivers when friends, family, or high-visibility patients are under care to ensure that medical information is not accessed unnecessarily. Nurses serve as guardians of the patient's medical record for others seeking access.

Home telemedicine technology poses additional ethical issues in health care. Sanner (2004) describes a statewide telehealth project used to deliver high-quality care while facing a nursing shortage, a growing aging client population, and continued financial restraints. The advent of this innovative health care delivery system brings a new array of ethical issues.

End-of-Life Decisions

Moving from cure to comfort in patient care is often difficult for patients and providers. Health care workers, by nature and training, want to cure. This strong goal at times can inhibit facing a terminal situation squarely and openly for patients. Nurses are key players in moving the health care team toward recognition of end-of-life situations and the needed comfort care and psychosocial support. Recognizing the individual patient's need for hope while addressing the gravity of a terminal status and quality-of-life issues is an art

developed with experience and is essential to effective nursing practice in any setting.

Genetic, Reproductive, and Stem Cell Issues

Genetics Issues. The Human Genome Project has definite medical, social, and legal implications, and nurses, especially those dealing with neuroscience disease, are in an integral role in this genetics age (Tazbir, 2001). Diekelmann & Diekelmann (2000) posit that the genetic age presents new issues for examining ethics and values in nursing practice.

Reproductive Issues. Clearly, the collective social fabric is divided on the moral and ethical issues entwined in reproduction. Nurses are at the forefront of many of these issues, including birth control, abortion, artificial insemination, in vitro fertilization, and use of fetal tissues. Selective abortions for multiple pregnancies and embryo implantation in postmenopausal women may raise many new questions. Is it ethical to give birth control information to minors? Should nurses participate in abortions? Should any social or sexual condition limit the availability of artificial insemination for an individual? When six fetuses are created by medical manipulation, is it ethical selectively to reduce the number to enhance the chances for survival of those remaining? Should a 60-year-old woman receive an embryo implant? The distinction of reproductive versus therapeutic cloning is an associated ethical topic. Opposition to reproductive cloning centers around three areas: (1) health risks from gene mutation, (2) emotional risks, and (3) abuse of the technology (Lachman, 2004). Therapeutic cloning, however, has received more support in the medical community because this technology is aimed at transplanting an individual's own DNA into an unfertilized egg to grow stem cells.

Stem Cell Issues. Ethical issues arise because of the origin of the stem cells. Sources of stem cells include bone marrow and cord blood. How should fetal tissues be obtained or used for medical research or treatment? Anti-abortion groups oppose use of embryo stem cells on ethical grounds (Lachman, 2004).

Palliative Care

The Robert Wood Johnson Foundation recently has funded training programs for nurses and physicians in palliative end-of-life care. The End-of-Life Nursing Education Consortium is a comprehensive educational program provided nationally to improve end-of-life care by nurses. The content of this course includes pain and symptom management, issues related to withdrawal and withholding care, and nutrition and hydration (Lachman, 2004).

Children. Pediatric palliative care takes several critical issues into consideration that include the following, according to Rushton (2004):

1. Needs change in drastic ways as children grow.
2. Life-threatening medical conditions in children tend to require more intensive care than similar situations in the adult population.
3. Greater variation occurs in the responses of children than adults.
4. As a child develops, it is difficult to predict the outcome to therapy.
5. The death of a child is considered by some to be more intense and of longer duration.
6. Someone else is making decisions for the child.

Major differences of opinion can occur between the health care professional and the family in relationship to the child's overall prognosis. If the treatment increases the child's pain and burden, then this must be weighed against merely prolonging an agonizing existence. Is the infant/child in pain? Should the focus of care shift from prolonging life to promoting comfort? The Children's Hospice International (2005) reported that fewer than 1% of children who could benefit from hospice in the United States ever receive it, even though the American Academy of Pediatrics issued a policy in 2000 supporting palliative care as an essential alternative of pediatric care. The ethical difference between withholding a life-support measure and withdrawing it once started may have a thin line according to some (Rushton, 2004). The natural parental desire to protect a child may conflict with the reality of the child's death. Rushton indicates that greater burdens are placed on the medical community and caregivers the more severe the child's medical situation. This severity supports greater justification for allowing the child to die, especially when the treatment burdens outweigh the benefits to the child.

Adult. Despite an increasing pharmacological and therapeutic arsenal, patients continue to perceive and fear pain associated with their illness. Nurses are vital in evaluating pain and advocating for effective pain management. Pain control is one of the most common problems with cancer patients. Hospitalizations can be prolonged when appropriate home pain control measures are not available. A well-designed home care pain management program can deal effectively with concerns such as potential narcotic overdose, poor intravenous access, and complications from a long-term intravenous catheterization. Aging, misconceptions, assessment, and an awareness of the nonpharmaceutical alternatives

that are available must be considered in pain program design. Misunderstandings concerning the dimensions of a patient's pain can interfere with adequate assessment and treatment of pain (Gallagher, 2001).

Pain relief does not equate to euthanasia. Relieving a patient's pain is the humane thing for any health care professional to do within the boundaries of practice. The patient, however, should have the chance to decide for himself or herself whether pain management intervention is needed. Issues of health care rationing and cost containment may be in conflict with degrees of suffering allowed. Ethical dilemmas may arise when nurses are not allowed to implement an effective pain management program because of reimbursement restraints.

SUMMARY

The *Code of Ethics for Nurses* provides practicing nurses across settings with a framework for ethical decision making. The *Code*, although it was updated finally in 2001, still does not speak to the current dilemmas of practice. Although IECs serve a vital role within the broad areas of education, policy, and consultation for the acute care nurse, they do not provide a broad resource for the educational and practice issues faced daily by nurses. Significant data show that nurses are prepared inadequately to address the burgeoning complexities of bioethics.

Traditional ethical issues facing nurses today—such as end-of-life decisions, incompetent health care workers, "futile" care, and pain management—are taking on added dimensions in the world of cost containment and managed care. Informed consent and confidentiality have taken on more complexity in light of enhanced computerization of patient data and data transmission capabilities. Advancements in technology pose continued ethical dilemmas in the fields of genetics and reproduction.

The academic environment must evaluate carefully the need for more foundational knowledge of ethics at all levels of nursing education. Nurses continue to need an organized avenue to bring forth ethical issues and discuss solutions in a nonthreatening environment. Nursing ethics committees and forums and patient ethic rounds provide the profession with avenues to voice ethical concerns and problem solve on resolutions.

REFERENCES

American Nurses Association. (2001). *Code of ethics for nurses with interpretative statements.* Washington, DC: Author.

Children's Hospice International. (2005). *About children's hospice, palliative, and end-of-life care.* Retrieved July 19, 2005, from http://www.chionline.org/resources/about.phtml

Diekelmann & Diekelmann. (2000).

Dodd, S., Jansson, B., Brown-Saltzman, K., Shirk, M., & Wunch, K. (2004). Expanding nurses' participation in ethics: An empirical examination of ethical activism and ethical assertiveness. *Nursing Ethics, 11*(1), 15-17.

Diekelmann, N., & Diekelmann, J. (2000). Learning ethics in nursing and genetics: Narrative paragogy and the grounding of values. *Journal of Pediatric Nursing 15*(4).

Dierchx de Casterle, B., Meulenbergs, T., van de Vijver, L., Tanghe, A., & Gastmans, C. (2002). Ethics meetings in support of good nursing care: Some practice-based thoughts. *Nursing Ethics, 9*(6), 12-22.

Dinc, L., & Gorgulu, R. (2002). Teaching ethics in nursing. *Nursing Ethics, 9*(3), 259-268.

Gallagher, B. (2001). Managing pain in elderly patients at home. *Nursing, 31*(8), 18.

Gastmans, C. (2002). A fundamental ethical approach to nursing: some proposals for ethics education. *Nursing Ethics, 9*(5), 494-507.

Ketefian, S., & Norris, D. (2002). The recent revision of the code of ethics for nurses with interpretative statements (American Nurses Association). *Research Theory in Nursing Practice, 16*(4), 219-221.

Lachman, V. (2004). Frontiers of biomedicine. *Advances for Nurses, 8*(8), 19-22.

Milton, C. (2002). Ethical implications for acting faithfully in the nurse-person relationship. *Nursing Science Quarterly, 15*(1), 21-24.

Milton, C. (2003). The American Nurses Association code of ethics: A reflection on the ethics of respect and human dignity with the nurse as expert. *Nursing Science Quarterly, 16*(4), 301-304.

Milton, C. (2004). Ethics content in nursing education: Pondering with the possible. *Nursing Science Quarterly, 17*(4), 308-311.

Peter, E., & Morgan, K. (2001). Explorations of a trust approach for nursing ethics. *Nursing Inquiry, 8*(1), 3-10.

Department of Education Project of National Significance Award #H325N000055 to California State University.

Rushton, C. (2004). Ethics and palliative care in pediatrics. *American Journal of Nursing, 104*(4), 54-64.

Sanner, T. (2004). Using telehealth to address the nursing shortage. *Home Healthcare Nursing, 22*(10), 695-699.

Sarikonda-Woitas, C., & Robinson, J. (2002). Ethical health care policy: Nursing's voice in allocation. *Nursing Administration Quarterly, 26*(4), 72-80.

Tazbir, J. (2001). The Human Genome Project: Ethical and legal considerations for neuroscience nurses. *Journal of Neuroscience Nursing, 33*(4), 180-183.

Turkoski, B. (2000). Home care and hospice ethics: Using the code for nurses as a guide. *Home Healthcare Nurse, 18*(5), 308-316.

Turkoski, B. (2001). Ethics in the absence of truth. *Home Healthcare Nurse, 19*(4), 218-222.

Volker, D. (2003). Is there a unique nursing ethic? *Nursing Science Quarterly, 16*(3), 207-211.

Wood, J. (2001). Ethical decision making. *Journal of Perianesthesia Nursing, 16*(1), 6-10.

Sexual Harassment

ANNE M. FIEDLER

Sexual harassment has been a problem facing health care professionals for many years. Sexual harassment is especially pervasive in nursing because of the large number of women and the physical nature of the profession. A survey of registered nurses attending the Memphis State University Nursing Program reported that 60% of the respondents said that they had been sexually harassed within the last year, and 25% of them reported that it affected their ability to work normally (Goldberg & Reagan, 1985). However, this phenomenon is not limited to the United States. In a recent study from five medical centers in Israel, 90% of the nurses participating in the study reported experiencing some type of sexual harassment, with 33% indicating that the harassment was severe (Bronner, Peretz, & Ehrenfeld, 2003).

Another survey involving sexual harassment policies in hospitals (Kinard, McLaurin, & Little, 1995) found that although 95 of the 97 hospitals included in their study had formal sexual harassment policies, 299 complaints of sexual harassment were filed in these hospitals. Even more interesting is the fact that all of the cases did not deal with traditional forms of sexual harassment, that is, men harassing women. Thirty-seven of the 299 cases (12.4%) involved male employees making charges against women.

The Equal Employment Opportunity Commission (EEOC) calculates that approximately 7% of all reported claims come from the health care industry. These complaints come from various sources such as hospitals, physicians' offices, dentists' offices, health facilities, and nursing and personal care facilities (Esters, 1996). This is important because in today's health care environment of tight cost containment, the large awards being made by the courts today in sexual harassment cases could have a major impact. For example, in a major class action suit, Mitsubishi Motors Manufacturing agreed to pay $44 million to 350 women for numerous instances of sexual abuse by co-workers and supervisors. Even more important, the indirect costs of sexual harassment from lowered employee morale, decreased productivity, and increased turnover may be even greater than those awarded by the court.

Even with all of the attention that sexual harassment has been getting in the media in the past years and also because of differing court interpretations, gender bias, and insufficient training as to what constitutes sexual harassment, employers and employees often are confused as to what constitutes sexual harassment. Often sexual harassment goes "unreported and unresolved" partially because people on both ends aren't always sure what it is (Sherer, 1995). Much behavior, although considered sexual harassment by some, is done out of ignorance of the feelings of the other person and not malice. Therefore, it is important to define sexual harassment as described by the courts and the EEOC and to understand the perceptions of men and women in nursing of traditional and nontraditional sexual harassment. The purpose of this chapter is to start with an encompassing definition of sexual harassment as interpreted by the EEOC and the courts, followed by a discussion on why even with clear definitions, different persons in the nursing profession still may hold different perceptions of what constitutes harassment. After discussing employer liability for harassment, I will look at ways to deal with the problem of sexual harassment in the workplace from the administrator's and the employee's perspective.

SEXUAL HARASSMENT DEFINED

Sexual harassment was not defined by the federal government until 1980 when the EEOC issued guidelines that declared sexual harassment to be a violation of Title VII of the Civil Rights Act of 1964 (EEOC, 2006). These guidelines define two types of sexual harassment: "quid pro quo" and "hostile environment." Quid pro quo harassment occurs when submission to or rejection of such conduct by an individual is used as the basis for employment decisions affecting that individual. In these cases, harassers use threats or rewards to back up their sexual advances.

Hostile environment involves unwelcome sexual conduct, including actions or materials in the workplace that unreasonably interfere with the individual's job performance by creating an "intimidating, hostile, or offensive working environment." The issue of whether sexual harassment violates Title VII reached the Supreme Court in 1986 in the hostile environment case, *Meritor Savings Bank v. Vinson* (1986). The guidelines interpret the condition of a hostile environment using the "reasonable person" standard, determining that "the harasser's conduct should be evaluated from the objective standpoint of a reasonable person." The victim only has to demonstrate that the behavior of the defendant was physically threatening or humiliating or that it interfered with the employee's work.

The enactment of the Civil Rights Act of 1991 (EEOC, 2005b) also has had an impact on sexual harassment cases. This law allows for punitive and compensatory damages for sexual harassment victims. More important, the current EEOC guidelines allow the courts to hold employers financially liable for the sexual misconduct of their employees.

Sexual Harassment of Men

Cases involving males being sexually harassed by females on the job are far less common than cases of males harassing females. In a survey, 4.6% of the men reported that they had been sexually harassed at work, but 61.8% failed to report their harasser (Byron, 1994). There may be three reasons for this difference between genders. The first is that women perceive that if they want sex, it is usually readily available. The second reason is based on the fact that sexual harassment is generally a power issue, and even today, far fewer women are in positions of power than men. The third reason that few men are filing cases against women is because they are embarrassed and afraid that they will be ridiculed. However, evidence indicates that this is changing. In 2003, the EEOC (EEOC, 2005a) received 13,566 charges of sexual harassment. Almost 15% of those charges were filed by males. This is up from approximately 9% in 1993.

Research has shown that in environments where men are working primarily with women, they are more likely to receive unwanted sexual attention than men that work primarily with men (Jackson & Newman, 2004). This can have serious implications for men in the nursing profession, which is dominated by women.

In those nontraditional cases in which men are being sexually harassed by women, the rights of the individual are more likely to be overlooked. Often the powers in the health care organization may not take the charges seriously. This can be costly to the organization. The courts are beginning to award some large settlements in these types of cases, such as in *Gutierrez v. Martinez and Cal Spa* (1993), in which a jury awarded $1 million to a man who was harassed by a woman. In this case, a female supervisor had a relationship with a male laborer who was promoted into management. When he announced his engagement, he was demoted and his office was torn down. A jury in California found Maria Martinez guilty of sexual harassment in this quid pro quo case.

When organizations do not take such cases seriously, they are often responsible for a large portion of the award. Gloria Aldrich (*Gutierrez v. California Acrylic Indus., Inc.,* 1993), an attorney who has represented several male victims who have won in sexual harassment cases, says that sexual harassment is based on power. She believes that as more women move into positions of power, more women will be viewed as perpetrators. As an increasing number of men join the nursing profession, nurses can expect to see more cases of men being harassed by their female supervisors.

Same-Sex Harassment

In some studies, approximately 14% of the cases reported were same-sex harassment cases (Schuyler, 1994), and since the 1998 Supreme Court ruling outlawing same-sex harassment, the number of cases filed has continued to rise (Anonymous, 2004). For example, in a recent case a major U.S. car dealer had to pay $500,000 to salesmen who were being harassed by their male managers. Some experts even believe that the reported number of these cases may err on the low side because many employees are too embarrassed to file charges or they are afraid to file because they fear that they may be labeled as a homosexual.

Before 1998, many potential same-sex cases were not filed or reported because it was often not clear at the district court level whether same-sex harassment is a violation of the law. In the 1998, Joseph Oncale sued Sundowner Offshore Services under Title VII for being sexually assaulted by his same-sex co-workers and supervisor on an oil rig in the waters off Louisiana. This case had nothing to do with sexual orientation. Oncale was a heterosexual family man. The Supreme Court decision ruled on behalf of the plaintiff, making sexual harassment illegal, whether it is same-sex or opposite-sex harassment. Although fewer women file same-sex harassment charges than men, same-sex sexual harassment among women does occur. In *Pointdujour v. Mount Sinai Hospital* (2004), a clerk registrar in the emergency room at Mount Sinai Hospital brought a Title VII (gender discrimination) action against her former employer and one of its nurse managers. Marie Carmen Pointdujour claimed that defendants retaliated against her by firing her after she complained that a female co-worker had subjected her to same-sex sexual harassment.

PERCEPTIONS OF SEXUAL HARASSMENT

Some sexual harassment activities are malicious. However, often these behaviors are due to ignorance clouding perceptions of what actually would be considered harassment even though it is stated clearly by the courts and in the EEOC guidelines. Today, because of high-profile cases such as $44 million class action suit against Mitsubishi, most persons clearly understand the concept of traditional sexual harassment, where a man sexually harasses a female. They also understand the concept of a quid pro quo case in which sexual behavior affects an employment decision. Less clear, but still perceived as harassment, is the hostile environment case involving things such as the lewd comments and the pats on the bottom. However, much of the American public is still unclear as to what constitutes sexual harassment in less traditional cases such as when a woman harasses a man or in same-sex harassment cases. Therefore supervisors or employees may not be as quick to recognize sexual harassment when it occurs in these nontraditional cases.

Understanding the basis for these differing perceptions is important so that nurses can begin to correct them. Researchers (Gutek & Cohen, 1987; Gutek & Morasch, 1982; and Kanter, 1977) have suggested that traditional sex roles are part of the way of viewing the world and that these views can spill over into the workplace and can be used to explain the differing perceptions of sexual harassment. These roles include viewing women as passive, nurturing, and dependent. They also include the viewing of females as sex objects. Others (Foulis & McCabe, 1997) have suggested actual gender differences that result from gender-typing at an early age influence attitudes toward sexual harassment. Sexually harassing behavior often is seen as appropriate and normal to some males. If this is true, men are more likely to be accepted in the role of harasser than women. This could result in a significant difference between how the nurses perceive opposite-sex harassment when a female nurse is being harassed by a man and how they perceive harassment where a male nurse is being harassed by a female.

When a person's occupation was of a traditional nature relating to gender (e.g., nurses are women, physicians are men, and hospital chief executive officers

are men), sexual harassment is perceived to a lesser extent, but sexual coercion is perceived to a greater extent (Burgess & Borgida, 1997). This can be explained using sex-role spillover based on the belief that stereotyping and social categorization actually "spill over" into the workplace (Gutek & Morasch, 1982). If the occupation or workplace is male dominated—that is, men hold the power, such as in the health care industry, which is dominated by male chief executive officers and male doctors—the chance of sex-role spillover is greater for a woman working in that environment. When a woman is working in a female-dominated occupation or environment, the attributes of their gender role become apparent. Because women dominate the hands-on patient care activities, men dominate the hospital chief executive officer positions, and more physicians are male than female, one would expect traditional gender roles to emerge in each of these situations. This results in acceptance of sexually harassing behavior. Therefore a conscious effort must be made to change these perceptions. Serious training and conditioning must be used to counteract this traditional gender conditioning.

Persons carry mental scripts defining what is and what is not sexual harassment. These scripts or viewpoints tend to be subjective (Gutek & Morasch, 1982). An important note is that these viewpoints have nothing to do with the actual laws or the EEOC guidelines that define different types of harassment. These viewpoints are different for men and women (Popovich et al., 1995; Travis & White, 2000; Richman, Rospenda, & Flaherty, 2004). Therefore if men and women in the nursing profession have different sexual harassment scripts, there may a significant difference between how men and women in nursing perceive different forms of sexual harassment. This may mean not only that the differences in gender-based perceptions need to be addressed but also that differing perceptions of non-traditional harassment need to be addressed in training sessions.

According to human resources professionals, although most supervisors have a fairly clear concept of the law, many rank-and-file employees are still unaware of everything that constitutes sexual harassment (Firestone & Harris, 1994). A recent study found that women in white-collar jobs were significantly more knowledgeable about what constituted sexual harassment than women in blue-collar jobs (Icenogle, Eagle, Ahmed, & Hanks, 2002). Employers often meticulously train supervisors regarding sexual harassment, the law, company policies, and implications. However, this message may not reach nonsupervisory personnel. This could be for several reasons. Employees may find the training repetitive and boring or may not take it seriously. Employers also may feel that teaching employers about sexual harassment may result in an increase in the number of sexual harassment complaints. Research has shown that co-workers are actually responsible for more sexual harassment than supervisors (Firestone & Harris, 1994). A nationwide survey of hospital human resource managers found that most hostile environment sexual harassment allegations and most formal charges were levied against co-workers (Kinard & Little, 2002). This finding may be because administrators and employees do not hold the same perceptions of what constitutes sexual harassment. Such disparity of perceptions has been shown to be true for the nursing profession (Fiedler & Hamby, 2000).

LIABILITY

Not only is sexual harassment damaging to victims, but also it can result in financial liability to health care organizations, even if the employer in unaware of the harassment activity. Two Supreme Court decisions in 1998 clarified employer liability for sexually harassing acts of their supervisors. In *Burlington Industries, Inc. v. Ellerth* (1998) and *Faragher v. City of Boca Raton* (1998), the Supreme Court found that employers are subject to vicarious liability for unlawful harassment by supervisors.

The standards for employer liability are different for quid pro quo cases than for hostile environment cases. In quid pro quo cases, the burden of proof is on the employer. Even if the employer did not know about the harassing behavior, the only defense is to prove that the harassment did not occur. In a hostile environment case, the employer still may be liable; however, the employer may be able to avoid liability or limit damages by establishing a defense that includes the following two elements: the employer exercised reasonable care to prevent and correct promptly any harassing behavior, and the employee unreasonably failed to take advantage of any preventive or corrective opportunities provided by the employer or to avoid harm otherwise. Because an employer is subject to vicarious liability for unlawful harassment if the harassment was committed by a supervisor with immediate (or successively higher) authority over the employee, it is important to be aware as to whether the person who engaged in unlawful harassment had supervisory authority over the person filing the complaint. According to the EEOC guidelines, an individual qualifies as an employee's "supervisor"

if the individual has authority to undertake or recommend tangible employment decisions affecting the employee or the individual has authority to direct the employee's daily work activities (EEOC, 2005)

Fiedler and Hamby (2000) also found that nurses who are sensitized to sexual harassment by previous episodes of harassment regard it as more severe behavior. This does not mean that nurses or administrators must be sensitized by actual harassment. Training techniques, such as role-playing and behavior modeling techniques, probably will be nearly as effective and less traumatic.

PREVENTION OF SEXUAL HARASSMENT

Prevention is the best tool to eliminate sexual harassment in the workplace. To avert sexual harassment in the workplace is imperative not for only ethical and motivational reasons but also for the financial reasons as discussed before. A prevention program should have three parts: a policy statement, a training component, and a reporting and enforcement procedure.

Policy Statement

First, the organization should have a strong policy statement that makes it clear that sexual harassment will not be tolerated and that defines sexual harassment so that all employees have a clear understanding of what constitutes harassment. This policy should include legal definitions of harassment and examples of behavior. Employers should communicate the policy to employees the day that they are hired and should reinforce the message periodically. The policy can be communicated through several methods, including the following:

◆ Directives from top management
◆ Oral sessions including role plays
◆ Printing of the policy in the employee handbook
◆ Posting of information on electronic and traditional bulletin boards

Today's health care environment is ethnically diverse. Whatever method is used, the information should be communicated in the language in which the employee is the most comfortable. If any significant part of the population is illiterate, the information on sexual harassment should be presented and communicated in oral form in the employees' native language.

Training

Training can be one of the most important components of a sexual harassment prevention program. A health care organization that has a policy regarding sexual harassment gains no benefit if the employees do not understand all of the nuances of what constitutes sexual harassment. Employees also must internalize the concept that any form of sexual harassment is wrong.

The training should consist of several components. The first component should define sexual harassment clearly, including clear statements describing exactly what may be considered harassing behavior from the viewpoint of the victim and the organization. The second part of the training should include scenarios that illustrate examples of this behavior. This could include short, written vignettes or films that show harassing behavior. Inclusion of a third section involving role-play exercises in which participants can practice responses to harassment. This sensitization will help to align perceptions of harassment with the legalities of this issue.

Enforcement

A policy without an enforcement component is useless. This enforcement procedure should begin with a process in which the victim of the harassment can file a complaint. Immediate and appropriate action must be taken when an employee complains.

The organization should have at least two or three alternate persons with whom a person can file a complaint. The organization should not make the mistake of having the direct supervisor as the only person to whom one can go because the supervisor might be the perpetrator.

A second important note is that the policy must be enforced equitably at all levels. In some organizations, such policies are enforced readily with the rank-and-file employees such as when technicians or nurses are the perpetrators, but the policy often is ignored when the infraction involves top administrators or physicians. Finally, health care organizations need to be aware that any person who reports sexual harassment activities is to be protected from retaliation.

FILING WITH THE EQUAL EMPLOYMENT OPPORTUNITY COMMISSION

If the health care organization cannot or will not solve the sexual harassment problem to the employee's satisfaction, a victim can file a charge at any field office of the EEOC. The addresses and telephone numbers for these offices can be found on the EEOC Web site (*www.EEOC.gov*).

The victim must be made aware of the time limitation that a sexual discrimination (harassment) charge must be filed with the EEOC within 180 days of the alleged discriminatory act *or* within 300 days if a state or local employment practice agency enforces a law prohibiting such discriminatory practices. When a claim is filed with the EEOC, the EEOC pays all legal costs of the complainant, but the employer must cover its own legal fees.

SUMMARY

With the heightened awareness of sexual harassment issues generated by cases in the news media, the EEOC (2005) has received an increase of approximately 129% in sexual harassment claims from 1992 to 2003. Most health care organizations have policies and procedures for dealing with sexually harassing behavior. This may not be enough. A national survey of hospital human resource managers found that allegations of sexual harassment in hospitals are increasing and that the largest number of these charges are being brought by nurses (Kinard & Little, 2002). This demonstrates that health care workers still are not understanding what constitutes harassment or that they understand and are behaving inappropriately anyway, leaving themselves and their employers open to potentially huge financial liabilities.

Male and female nurses need to understand what constitutes sexual harassment, and they must be made aware of the actions they need to take to protect themselves and their rights if sexual harassment occurs. More fundamentally, policies against harassment must be disseminated to all health care workers. Physicians who are often not actual employees of the organization and are therefore much less likely to participate in training sessions than the nurses, technicians, and other health care workers also must be made aware of sexual harassment policies. Finally, nonthreatening procedures must be in place so that when a problem occurs, the victim feels comfortable reporting the situation so that the problem can be resolved by the health care organization without the intervention of government agencies.

REFERENCES

Anonymous. (2004, September 28). Sexual harassment of men doubles in decade. *Personnel Today,* p. 10.

Bronner, G., Peretz, C., & Ehrenfeld, M. (2003). Sexual harassment of nurses and nursing students. *Journal of Advanced Nursing, 42*(6), 637-645.

Burgess, D., & Borgida, E. (1997). Sexual harassment: An experimental test of sex-role spillover theory. *Personality and Social Psychology Bulletin, 3*(1), 63-79.

Burlington Industries, Inc. v. Ellerth, 118 S. Ct. 2257 (1998).

Byron, C. (1994). Work ethics: Sexual harassment. *Men's Health, 9,* 86-91.

Equal Employment Opportunity Commission. (2005a). Retrieved December 29, 2005 from http://www.eeoc.gov/stats/harass.html

Equal Employment Opportunity Commission. Retrieved January 11, 2006 from eeoc.gov/abouteeoc/35th/milestones/1980.html

Equal Employment Opportunity Commission. (2005b) Retrieved December 29, 2005 from eeoc.gov/policy/cra91.html

Esters, S. D. (1996). Sex-harassment policies seen needed in hospitals. *National Underwriter, 100*(40), 9-13.

Faragher v. City of Boca Raton, 118 S. Ct. 2275 (1998).

Fiedler, A., & Hamby, E. (2000). Sexual harassment in the workplace: Nurses' perceptions. *Journal of Nursing Administration, 30*(10), 497-503.

Firestone, J. M., & Harris, R. J. (1994). Sexual harassment in the U.S. military: Environmental and individual contexts. *Armed Forces & Society, 21,* 25-43.

Foulis, D., & McCabe, M. P. (1997). Sexual harassment: Factors affecting attitudes and perceptions. *Sex Roles, 37*(9/10), 773-798.

Goldberg, G. L., & Reagan, J. T. (1985). Sexual harassment: A problem for the health care supervisor. *Health Care Supervisor, 3*(3), 55-65.

Gutek, B. A., & Cohen, A. G. (1987). Sex ratios, sex spillover, and sex at work: A comparison of men's and women's experiences. *Human Relations, 40,* 97-115.

Gutek, B. A., & Morasch, B. (1982). Sex-ratios, sex-spillover and sexual harassment of women at work. *Journal of Social Issues, 38,* 55-74.

Gutierrez v. California Acrylic Indus., Inc., No. BC055641 (Cal.Super.Ct. 1993).

Icenogle, M. L., Eagle, B. W., Ahmad, S., & Hanks, L. A. (2002). Assessing perceptions of sexual harassment behaviors in a manufacturing environment. *Journal of Business & Psychology, 16*(4), 601-616.

Jackson, R. A., & Newman, M. A. (2004). Sexual harassment in the federal workplace revisited: Influences on sexual harassment by gender. *Public Administration Review, 64*(6), 705-718.

Kanter, R. M. (1977). *Men and women of the corporation.* New York: Basic Books.

Kinard, J., & Little, B. (2002). Sexual harassment in the health-care industry: A follow-up study. *Health Care Manager, 2*(4), 46-52.

Kinard, J., McLaurin, J., & Little, B. (1995). Sexual harassment in the hospital industry: An empirical inquiry. *Health Care Management Review, 20*(1), 47-53.

Meritor Savings Bank v. Vinson, 106 S. Ct. 2399, 40 EPD 36,159 (1986).

Oncale v. Sundowner Offshore Services. Inc., 98 1.1:OR 9001, (1998).

Pointdujour v. Mt. Sinai Hospital, No. 02 Civ. 4470, 2004 U.S. Dist. LEXIS 629 (N.Y. App. Div. 2004).

Popovich, P. M., Jolton, J. A., Mastrangelo, P. M., Everton, W. J., Somers, J. M., & Gehlauf, D. N. (1995). Sexual harassment scripts: A means to understanding a phenomenon, *Sex Roles, 32,* 5/6, 315-335.

Richman, J. A., Rospenda, K. M., & Flaherty, J. A. (2004). Perceived organizational tolerance for workplace harassment and distress and drinking over time (harassment and mental health). *Women & Health, 40,* 4, 1-23.

Schuyler, N. (1994). Close encounters of a new kind. *Working Woman, 4*(19), 11-12.

Sherer, J. L. (1995). Sexually harassed. *Hospitals & Health Networks, 69*(2), 54-57.

Travis, C. B., & White, J. W. (Eds). (2000). *Sexuality, society, and feminism* (pp. 323-354). Washington, DC: American Psychological Association.

Health Care for the Poor and Underserved

SARA GROVES

OVERVIEW

The poor and underserved of the United States have never received health care equal to Americans with higher socioeconomic status. Lack of care for minorities was brought to the forefront in the 1985 landmark Heckler Report, the *Report of the US Department of Health and Human Services Secretaries Task Force on Black and Minority Health* (Heckler, 1985). In a more contemporary discussion, the five reports of the Institute of Medicine on *Insuring America's Health* (2001-2004) have spelled out the problems clearly and have provided four prototypes that could reform the health care system. Today the need to eliminate disparities among racial and ethnic minorities is one of two goals for *Healthy People 2010* (US Dept of Health and Human Services, 2000). Even a *Journal of Health Care for the Poor and Underserved* and an Association of Clinicians for the Underserved exist. What has happened in the richest country in the world that this problem of health care distribution has not yet been solved?

Health care in the United States should be an entitlement for all individuals. In 2001 the United States spent $1.4 trillion on health care, 14.1% of the U.S. gross domestic product (McCarthy, 2003). Yet health disparity still exists, resulting in part from not having adequate and universal health care for all U.S. residents. Universal health care coverage lacks broad-based political support. Those without health care are disenfranchised, not a strong political block to vote for change. Those with health care have other political priorities. Financially, one out of seven families has difficulty paying the medical bills, and in 2003, these same families were less likely to seek out medical care and purchase prescription medication. Adults without insurance are less than half as likely to get medical care for serious health problems (Institute of Medicine, 2001). Is the goal then to achieve universal high-quality health coverage for the poor and underserved? Several groups have proposed inclusive state health plans that

would provide this care, and other plans stress the positive economics of a universal single-payer system.

PREVIOUS SOLUTIONS

President Franklin D. Roosevelt, in his State of the Union address in January 1944, reviewed his "Economic Bill of Rights." One of his major thrusts was the right for all Americans to have adequate medical care. President Roosevelt already had provided the population with its first economic safety net, the Social Security Act of 1935. Senator Robert Wagner, with the support of President Roosevelt, unsuccessfully introduced a bill in February 1939 to create a national compulsory health insurance program administered by the states. President Truman, likewise, repeated the request for legislation for a compulsory national health program from 1945 to 1951 without success (Centers for Medicare and Medicaid Services, 2004a, p. 1).

Finally in 1965, following a proposal from President Johnson to pay for health care for the elderly and poor children, Congress established the Medicaid and Medicare programs under amendments to the Social Security Act. The Medicaid program was designed to pay medical bills for low-income Americans who had no other way to pay. Medicaid is a basic health insurance program for the poor and an insurance program for persons with chronic or long-term health care needs. In the last 39 years, as a federal/state matching program, Medicaid has expanded greatly (Centers for Medicare and Medicaid Services, 2004b, p. 2). Currently, the Medicaid program has 50 million beneficiaries and is projected in 2005 to exceed $300 billion; the federal government portion will be $190 billion. In addition, 45 million persons still are without any health insurance. Currently, several safety nets provide access to quality health care for the poor and underserved and include state-funded primary care clinics, Federally Qualified Health Centers, local health departments, other nonprofit clinics supported by public funds, faith-based organizations, private foundations, and local contributors. Are these the permanent solutions?

THE CURRENT PROBLEM

The underserved are the uninsured, the underinsured, the poor, and the working poor who do not receive adequate and quality health care. Uninsured and underinsured persons receive less health care, usually too little and too late. They also receive less primary prevention, less care for their chronic conditions, and worse care in the hospital. In the United States, 16.5% of patients under age 65 are uninsured. In 2001, 85% of the cost of health care for the uninsured ($34 billion to $38 billion) was paid for by the public sector, frequently at the local level, placing great strain on the overall health of the immediate community. Concentration of uninsured and poor can add to the community burden of disease (Institute of Medicine, 2003b).

Medicaid provides health insurance, guaranteeing health care for the very poor. However, the growing cost of this program threatens its continuation at the currently funded level. At the Families USA Conference in Washington in January 2005, Senators Clinton and Kerry expressed hope that the Medicaid program funding would not be cut from the current 50 million Americans who receive benefits. Senator Clinton is concerned that state Medicaid funds will be capped through block grants, placing more burdens on states that already have significant budget constraints. Kerry is concerned about the 11 million uninsured children who could be covered with Medicaid funding if the program were expanded (Kenen, 2005). Senator Obama, newly elected from Illinois, was also at the conference and expressed concern that President Bush invest in fixing the Medicaid and Medicare programs that appear more broken than the Social Security system (Rathbun, 2005).

The potential problem of limiting federal money to the states for Medicaid is reflected in Pennsylvania. In 2004 the state spent about 25% of it $51 billion state budget on health care for the poor. The number of their Medicaid recipients, a continuing reflection of poor economic recovery, is projected to increase in 2005 by 8%, with continuing double-digit health care inflation (Levy, 2004). The state does not know how it will pay for increased health care expenditure for the poor and uninsured if the federal government decreases its contributions. The National Governors Association has asked the federal government not to cut Medicaid as

a way to cut the federal deficit. This decrease in resources could undermine already fragile safety nets for the poor and underserved (Chapman, 2004).

The number of uninsured, increasing at about 1 million each year, is growing faster than the population and even in areas where there is economic prosperity (Institute of Medicine, 2001). Eighty-five percent of the uninsured are part of families with working members (Institute of Medicine, 2002). Racial and ethnic minorities are more likely to be uninsured, a reflection of less education and lower-income employment that provides less health coverage. Most families do not choose to be uninsured (Institute of Medicine, 2001). The Institute of Medicine (2002) found that the health and economics of the whole family suffered when even one member was uninsured.

The health care cost to society for poor and uninsured is not just the actual dollar amount of uncompensated care ($35 billion in 2001) but the decreased health capital of the underserved who have poorer health, premature mortality, and greatly increased unnecessary morbidity at an estimated cost of $65 billion to $130 billion (Institute of Medicine, 2003a). The Institute of Medicine (2002) concluded, based on its dollar estimates, that the benefits to society of providing universal health care coverage were greater than the social cost of the increased burden of disease to the uninsured.

THE NEW SOLUTIONS

In 2000 the United States was ranked thirty-seventh by the World Health Organization in health care. The low ranking was not reflective of how much is spent per capita, but rather on whether health care is fair and equitable (Mastel, 2000). There are several possible answers to making health care fair and equitable. The Institute of Medicine (2004) has offered four solutions for universal health care coverage:

1. Expand current public programs such as Medicaid and Medicare and provide a new tax credit to those who purchase private insurance.
2. Offer individual selections of health insurance plans from the work place, public programs (Medicare and Medicaid), or individual purchase.
3. Place responsibility on the individual to obtain his or her own insurance using tax credits with Medicare intact.
4. Enroll everyone in a single-payer system administered and funded federally with no other public programs.

Some of these policy solutions already are being pursued actively. At the same time, many of the safety nets are being enhanced to provide health care in the interim.

New Policies

One health policy promotes universal state health insurance. Health Care for All (2004) is a legislative campaign in several states, including Massachusetts, California, Maine, and Maryland. The goal of the campaign is that everyone in the state will have health insurance, giving everyone access to affordable, quality health care. Most of the plans are a coalition of health plans with governmental and private monetary support to increase federal and state coverage, employer plans (including small businesses), and individual policies. Maryland, in its health initiative, wants to make sure the plan is community based (Maryland Citizens' Health Initiative, 2004). The state has 1100 organizations that include religious, health, local community, labor and business groups. The state is working with current public and private insurance groups to guarantee universal affordable insurance plans. The strategy is built on private sector coverage with 80% of Maryland residents receiving care through preexisting plans. Other components include supporting the small group market, monetarily supplementing small businesses and individuals to purchase health insurance, and providing more affordable drug prescriptions for seniors through a statewide buying pool to supplement the current new Medicare program.

Health Care for All in California and the Missourians for Single Payer Health Care program (2004) promote comprehensive universal health care using a single-payer public insurance fund. Friedenberg (2000), a physician, supports this solution as providing a more equitable system. He suggests that the medical community take more initiative in selecting a single-payer model. He outlines a system that would moderate price, control the overproduction of medical specialists, guarantee universal coverage, and allow for choice of providers. Dr. Friedenberg recommends that the Medicaid and Medicare programs be modified to provide this universal health coverage. He sees these insurance systems as working well, with no need to create a new format. Dr. Friedenberg proposes that individuals, with additional private payment, could upgrade their care, but everyone definitely would receive quality basic care. McCormick, Himmelstein, Woolhandler, and Bor (2004) sampled 904 Massachusetts physicians and found that 64% favored single-payer

national health insurance and 70.3% did not want the insurance industry to continue playing a major role in medical care delivery. Many of the doctors commented on how well Medicare works for themselves and their patients.

One new policy, in addition to universal health coverage, is the allocation of research dollars to develop improved technology to save lives by medical advances, thereby decreasing the inequities of health outcomes among the poor and underserved. Woolf, Johnson, Fryer, Rust, and Satcher (2004) examined this as a potential solution. What they found was that better drugs, better devices, and better procedures did result in lives saved between 1991 and 2000, averting 176,633 deaths in the United States. However, this number of averted deaths could be increased to 886,202 if the age-specific mortality rate for whites and African Americans were equal. The authors clearly assert that instead of investing millions of dollars in technology, investing this money in resolving the causes of higher mortality in African Americans would save 5 times as many lives (Woolf, 2004). Robbins and Webb (2004) also verified that African American adults, living in neighborhoods with high poverty rates, had high excessive mortality. Between 1999 and 2001, 5305 excessive deaths occurred among African Americans in Philadelphia compared with the same gender and age-specific rates for non-Hispanic whites. Robbins and Webb found a strong, graded association between neighborhood poverty and mortality.

Enhanced Safety Nets

The Association of Clinicians for the Underserved currently is making efforts to improve the health of the poor and underserved by educating health practitioners in a transdisciplinary role. This enhances the efficiency of health care in a situation with limited resources (Rhee, 2004). Other communities have designed and implemented innovative approaches to deliver care to the uninsured. This approach usually occurs with strong partnerships between private and official agencies and with strong continual financial commitment to meet the identified need. The New York Academy of Medicine, with Robert Wood Johnson Foundation funding, examined 20 such programs to provide a synthesis of what communities can do to meet the needs of their uninsured (Andrulis & Gusmano, 2000). The report also provides guidelines for policy implication at the state and federal level.

Free clinics, another safety net, were first established to provide medical care in the 1960s. They are by definition a service that is private and community-based and has no charge for services. In 2004, Volunteers in America identified more than 1000 functioning free clinics in the United States (Geller, Taylor & Scott, 2004). Keis, DeGeus, Cashman, and Savageau (2004) reported on three free clinics in Massachusetts. The clients on average were poor, uninsured, and female. Many of the long-term clients (less than 25% of the total visits) had limited health insurance but used the clinic for free prescription medication. In another survey of volunteer-based (free) clinics in seven Midwestern states, the 106 clinics clearly provided a substantial safety net for the poor and uninsured with 200,000 total visits. The most common services were primary care and pharmaceutical assistance, with 75% of the clinics also providing some specialty care. For many, the focus was on the adult, given that Medicare, Medicaid, and state children insurance programs serve the young and the elderly. In these free clinics with budgets (mean) of $237,170, there were almost no paid staff (Geller, Taylor, & Scott, 2004). These authors again emphasized that free clinics are a bandage for the medical system. They provide no comprehensive care, long-term care, or hospital care. For many poor Americans the free clinic is health care of last resort.

ALTERNATIVE SOLUTION

There is another solution. Walker, Mays, and Warren (2004) suggest that nurses, as health professionals, have not been adequately cognizant of the broad assortment of health determinants that affect the racial/ethnic disparities of morbidity and mortality. Lack of medical care accounts for only 10% to 15% of premature deaths (McGinnis, Williams-Russo, Knickman, 2002). Isaacs and Schroeder (2004) noted, "ensuring adequate medical care for all will have only a limited effect on the nation's health." Others have found that the difference in health persists among different socioeconomic statuses even when health risk behaviors are controlled (Lantz et al., 1998). Lu, Samuels, and Wilson in 2004 found that health behavior and health insurance only explained 10% to 16% of the socioeconomic differences in health in the population covered by the 2000 Kentucky Behavioral Risk Factor Surveillance System. Would there be more impact on the health of the poor and underserved population if public health officials paid attention to other factors such as changing demographics, economics, environment, and globalization? Is there now too much emphasis on health insurance issues and access to quality health care and not

enough on poverty? Nurses and policy makers need to put more weight on optimizing the health of the entire population.

To correct the inequities for the poor and underserved now becomes even more complicated. The answer is not as simple as providing universal health insurance or quality technical medical care. The answer is not providing more education in the area of health promotion and disease prevention. Nurses need to influence the more distal health determinants that are part of a complex continuum of causality. Macinko, Starfield, and Shi (2003) divide distal health determinants into two broad classifications: national policies and culture. National policies include economics, international relations, and income distributions. Culture refers to a wide set of beliefs that influences the population's choice of political and legal institutions that include social participation, institutional development, lifestyle choices, and individual overall priorities. These are the determinants of macroeconomics, healthful environments, positive sociodemographics, and education. This is where nurses need to influence policy and determinants related to health. This solution would be a complete reorientation of where nurses would put resources.

Adverse socioeconomic conditions place obstacles in the way of the poor and underserved to be healthy. They need literacy to understand and communicate health needs, but they also need literacy to have adequate employment. They need secure employment to have adequate housing and health insurance for their family. They need to know they have adequate and consistent food, services, safety, and protection to provide and care for their family, reducing stress in their lives. Families can neither nurture nor place appropriate emphasis on health promotion and disease prevention until the family is secure and stable in a secure and stable community.

Consistently, research and surveillance shows an inverse relationship between race and premature death. That same inverse relationship is also true for social class. Isaacs and Schroeder (2004) note that in general, this class pattern of premature death is true in a progressive fashion from the poor to the rich. They acknowledge that smoking, poor nutrition, less activity, environmental hazards, lack of insurance, and being African American increase risk. However, they show that rates of premature cardiac death between poor and rich are significantly greater than between African Americans and white. What the defining factor of class is that creates poor health is not clear. Isaacs and

Schroeder acknowledge that stress could be one of these mechanisms.

Without concern about the lack of positive distal opportunities for the poor, the whole community can be at risk. The lack of social justice is a disgrace, but inequities in health care also can be a problem for all members of society. In areas of high unemployment and low-paying jobs, the limited tax base contributes to limited resources for public education, health, and policing. As Woodward and Kawachi (2000) suggest, this can lead to increases in infectious disease, community violence, and substance addictions that affect the entire community.

The poor and underserved should have the same health as other Americans. Obviously, they should have access to comprehensive primary health care, prescriptions, and inpatient hospital care, equal in quality that given to those with more economic resources. Nurses can provide the health care, they can advocate for their clients, and they can help set policies for universal health care coverage. However, I call for more assertive action. Nurses, as a group, can be powerful in demanding better inner-city schools and better jobs with better pay. Nurses can work to build strong communities that promote social cohesion. Nurses can be a strong political force, creating change to move people out of poverty and provide real opportunity for health.

REFERENCES

Andrulis, D., & Gusmano, M. (2000). *Community initiatives for the uninsured: How far can innovative partnerships take us?* New York: New York Academy of Medicine.

Centers for Medicare and Medicaid Services. (2004a). *History of Medicare and Medicaid.* Retrieved January 10, 2005, from http://www.cms.hhs.gov/about/history/ssachr.asp

Centers for Medicare and Medicaid Services. (2004b). *Medicaid: A brief summary.* Retrieved January 10, 2005, from http://www.cms.hhs.gov/publications/overview-medicare-medicaid/default4.asp

Chapman, J. (2004, December 31). *US: Bush administration targets medical care for the poor.* Retrieved January 22, 2005, from World Socialist Web Site: http://www.wsws.org/articles/2004/dec2004/medi-d31.shtml

Friedenberg, R. (2000). Perspective. Managed care and social justice. *Radiology, 217,* 11-13.

Geller, S., Taylor, B., & Scott, H. (2004). Free clinics helping to patch the safety net. *Journal of Health Care for the Poor and Underserved, 15,* 42-51.

Health Care for All. (2004). *Real Change for real people in Massachusetts.* Retrieved November 13, 2005, from http://www.hcfama.org

Heckler, M. M. (1985). Report of the Secretary's Task Force on Black and Minority Health. Washington, D.C.: U.S. Department of Health and Human Services.

Institute of Medicine. (2001). *Coverage matters: Insurance and health care.* Washington, DC: National Academies Press.

Institute of Medicine. (2002). *Health insurance is a family matter.* Washington, DC: National Academies Press.

Institute of Medicine. (2003a). *Hidden costs, value lost, uninsurance in America.* Washington, DC: National Academies Press.

Institute of Medicine. (2003b). *A shared destiny: Effects of uninsurance on individuals, families, and communities.* Washington, DC: National Academies Press.

Institute of Medicine. (2004). *Insuring America's health: Principles and recommendations.* Washington, DC: National Academies Press.

Isaacs, S., & Schroeder, S. (2004). Class—the ignored determinant of the nation's health. *New England Journal of Medicine, 9*(351), 1137-1142.

Keis, R., DeGeus, L., Cashman, S., & Savageau, J. (2004). Characteristics of patients at three free clinics. *Journal of Health Care for the Poor and Underserved, 14,* 603-617.

Kenen, J. (January 27, 2005). Sen. Clinton says Bush plans harm health care for poor. *Reuters Foundation.* Retrieved January 29, 2005, from http://www.alertnet.org/thenews/newsdesk/N27656956.htm

Lantz, P., House, J., Lepkowski, J., Williams, D., Mero, R., & Chen, J. (1998). Socioeconomic factors, health behavior and mortality: Results from a nationally representative prospective study of US adults. *Journal of the American Medical Association, 279*(21), 1703-1708.

Levy, M. (2004, December 19). Affording health care for the poor getting harder for Pennsylvania. *Buck County Courier Times* (Levittown, PA).

Lu, N., Samuels, M., & Wilson, R. (2004). Socioeconomic differences in health: How much do health behaviors and health insurance coverage account for? *Journal of Health Care for the Poor and Underserved, 15,* 618-630.

Macinko, J., Starfield, B., & Shi, L. (2003). The contribution of primary care systems to health outcomes within Organization for Economic Cooperation and Development countries, 1970-1998. *Health Service Research, 38*(3), 831-865.

Maryland health care for all! Coalition. Retrieved November 17, 2005 from http://healthcareforall.com/HTML1.phtml

Mastel, R. (2000, June 21). Despite big spending, U.S. ranks 37th in study of global health care. *Los Angeles Times,* p. A22.

McCarthy, M. (2003). US health-care system faces cost and insurance crises. Rising costs, growing numbers of uninsured, and quality gaps trouble world's most expensive health-care system. *Lancet, 362*(9381), 375.

McCormick, D., Himmelstein, D., Woolhandler, S., & Bor, D. (2004). Most physicians endorse single-payer national health insurance according to Harvard study. *Archives of Internal Medicine, 164,* 300-304.

McGinnis, J., Williams-Russo, P., & Knickman, J. (2002). The case for more active policy attention to health promotion. *Health Affair, 21,* 78-93.

Missourians for Single Payer Health Care. (2004). *Single payer universal health care.* Retrieved January 15, 2005, from http://mosp.missouri.org/

Rathbun, A. (2005, January 28). Obama blasts Bush on health care. *Northwest Indiana Times.* Retrieved, November 17, 2005 from http://nwitimes.com/articles/2005/01/28/news/illiana/52639b8595d1125986256B

Rhee, K. (2004). Creating a national, transdisciplinary community of clinicians who serve the underserved. *Journal of Health Care for the Poor and Underserved, 15,* 1-3.

Robbins, J., & Webb, D. (2004). Neighborhood poverty, mortality rates, and excess deaths among African Americans: Philadelphia, 1999-2001. *Journal of Health Care for the Poor and Underserved, 15,* 530-537.

U.S. Department of Health and Human Services. *Healthy People* 2010. 2nd ed. With Understanding and Improving Health and Objectives for Improving Health. 2 vols. Washington, DC: U.S. Government Printing Office, November 2000.

Walker, B., Mays, V., & Warren, R. (2004). The changing landscape for the elimination of racial/ethnic health status disparities. *Journal of Health Care for the Poor and Underserved, 15,* 506-521.

Woodward, A., & Kawachi, I. (2000). Why reduce health inequalities? Journal of Epidemiology Community Health, *54,* 923-929.

Woolf, S. (2004). Society's choice: The tradeoff between efficacy and equity and the lives at stake. *American Journal of Preventive Medicine, 27,* 49-56.

Woolf, S., Johnson, R., Fryer, G., Rust, G., & Satcher, D. (2004). The health impact of resolving racial disparities: An analysis of US mortality data. *American Journal of Public Health, 94,* 2078-2081.

Legal, Ethical, and Moral Considerations in Caring for Individuals With Alzheimer's Disease

NANCY EDWARDS

As we enter the twenty-first century, the growth of the elderly population, the cost of health care, and the advances in medical technology and science continue to have a profound impact on the health care system. This transformation in the health care system raises ethical, legal, and moral issues. The special nature of persons with Alzheimer's disease (AD) and the natural trajectory of their disease require special care on the part of the health care team to meet the ethical challenges and to establish health care goals that result in consistent, reasoned, and compassionate care.

The United States spends more than $100 billion annually to treat Alzheimer's disease, making it the third most costly disease in the United States after heart disease and cancer (Holston & Schutte, 2004). More than half of these costs are related to caregiving. Furthermore, by one estimate, barring prevention or a cure, 22 million individuals are expected to have AD by the year 2050. Scientists estimate that as many as 4.5 million Americans suffer from AD. The disease usually begins after the age of 60, and risk increases with age. Although younger persons may get AD, it is much less common. About 5% of men and women over age 74 have Alzheimer's disease, and nearly half of those age 85 and older may have the disease (Alzheimer's Disease Education & Referral Center [ADEAR], 2003a). In light of the increase in absolute numbers of elderly, dementia obviously will be a national health problem of increasing proportion.

The cost of Alzheimer's disease care is astronomical. One study found that for a 6-month period, the cost could rise to more than $30,000 per patient, depending on the severity of symptoms. In most cases, neither Medicare nor most private health insurance covers the necessary long-term care that frequently is required.

Care for a 6-month period costs approximately $20,000 for a typical high-functioning patient, compared with $35,000 for a patient with severe dementia. The unpaid caregiving provided by family and friends combined with the caregivers' lost productivity, is often more than the direct medical costs with per patient estimates as high as $47,000 per year (Small, McDonnell, Brooks, & Papadopoulos, 2002). The average lifetime cost per patient is estimated to be more than $174,000. With limited health care and financial resources, issues related to care demand and delivery must be examined.

The progressive decline in cognitive functioning and physical abilities that characterize Alzheimer's disease raises numerous issues, which vary and evolve throughout the course of the illness. Those who are afflicted with the disease, their families, and health care providers will have to face these issues. These issues must be examined in light of patient autonomy, justice, veracity, beneficence, and nonmaleficence.

DETERMINATION OF CAPACITY

One of the first issues to be considered is respecting patient choice regarding the right to know the diagnosis, participation in treatment, and informed consent. Often the diagnosis of dementia automatically leads to the assumption that individuals are incapable of making decisions for themselves. Nurses are in a key position to evaluate the decision-making capacity of persons with dementia in long-term care facilities, acute care settings, primary care clinics, and the home.

The principle of autonomy is fundamental to the U.S. legal system; that is, individuals are entitled to make their own decisions. To the extent possible, the legal and health care communities support the concept of self-determination. Loss of competency, or decision-making capacity, is an inevitable consequence of Alzheimer's disease, but nurses must remember that the diagnosis of Alzheimer's disease is not an automatic declaration that the patient has lost all decision-making capacity. A 1914 decision noted, "Every human being of adult years and sound mind has a right to determine what shall be done with his own body" (*Schloendorff v. Society of New York Hospital*). Each adult is presumed competent to make personal decisions unless the evidence demonstrates that the person is incompetent. The words *competent* and *incompetent* are legal terms and should be relegated to the legal setting; however, the reality of the health care setting compels professionals to make competency judgment each day. Some have suggested that the term *capacity* would be more appropriate when referring to the health assessment necessary to determine the ability to make health decisions (Caralis, 1994; Weiler, 1994).

Capacity is not an all-or-nothing condition but rather a continuum that incorporates wide variations between total capacity and total incapacity (Sands, Ferreira, Stewart, Brod, & Yaffe, 2003). A major issue for physicians and other clinicians in evaluating and treating patients with Alzheimer's disease is judging an individual patient's decision-making capacity to handle a number of tasks, including competence to consent to medical treatment or to manage finances. Individuals with Alzheimer's disease may be unable to make complicated, detailed decisions such as estate or financial matters, but they may well maintain the ability to make decisions regarding their health care. Marson and Harrell (2000) identified five standards necessary for competency. First is the expression of treatment choice, or being aware of what treatment is being offered. Second is the ability to make reasonable choice. Third is having the capacity to appreciate the emotional and physical consequences of the choice. The fourth standard is that the person can appreciate rational reasons for the treatment choice. The fifth standard is that the individual can understand the treatment situation and the associated risks and benefits. Therefore assessment of capacity must be considered in light of the preceding standards (Box 71-1).

Numerous tests are used to assess capacity, from simple interviews to objective measures such as the Folstein Mini-Mental State Examination (Folstein, Folstein, & McHugh, 1975). The difficulties with the objective tests presently used are that the tests do not contain capacity-specific assessment measures. One must remember that the concepts of cognition and judgment are not synonymous. Assessment of the individual for the ability to understand treatment options and consider treatment alternatives in light of all the risks and benefits is essential. If the person is able to do that, alone or with support, the person must be given the opportunity to determine the course of medical treatment.

BOX 71-1

Definitions

Autonomy: The capacity to think, decide, and act on the basis of thought and decisions freely and independently (Purtilo, 1999). The right of independence and self-determination.

Beneficence: The requirement to do good. This includes a holistic approach to the individual, including the patient's beliefs, thoughts, values, and judgments.

Health care representative: An individual appointed to make health care decisions on another's behalf if that persons becomes unable to make such decisions.

Incapacity: Being incapable of managing property or providing self-care or both. Incapacity may stem from infirmity, insanity, mental illness, alcoholism, excessive drug use, or neurological deterioration. Although these conditions may contribute to incapacity, an individual who has one or more of these problems is not necessarily incapable.

Justice: Equitable distribution of burden and benefits. It is the obligation to be fair to all individuals regardless of race, creed, religion, gender, or socioeconomic status.

Living will: A document in which one states one's wishes and desires to have or not to have life-prolonging procedures such as respirators, surgery, or feeding tubes, which may delay but would not prevent imminent death.

Nonmaleficence: The principle to do no harm intentionally or unintentionally.

Power of attorney: A document that gives another person the authority to handle one's personal matters.

Veracity: The principle to tell the truth. It requires that the health care worker be honest and not intentionally deceive or mislead the patients.

ADVANCE DIRECTIVES

The reality is that 90% of all individuals will have an extended period of illness before they die. This is especially true for the patient with Alzheimer's disease/dementia, the course of which can run for 2 to 20 years. In an era of advanced medical technology, it is more important than ever to have an advance care plan (Murphy, 2005). This allows the person to maintain autonomy when loss of capacity can be anticipated. This can be accomplished through the completion of estate wills, living wills, and durable powers of attorney for the health care. These documents allow individuals with Alzheimer's disease who maintain competency to determine what health care measures they would like to be carried out as their disease progresses.

One area of difficulty that often occurs is that the person who makes the prospective directives (decisional autonomy) most likely will not have the ability to carry out these decisions (executional autonomy). In many situations the consequences of these decisions fall on the family and caregiver. The child of the person with Alzheimer's disease now has to expend a large amount of time, energy, and money to follow through with the directives. Rhymes (1995) states that the presumption in favor of autonomy assumes that persons possess the capacity to decide, to carry out decisions, and to manage and be accountable for the consequences of their decisions. If there comes a time when they are not able to carry out and manage their decisions, the presumption of autonomy must be considered. This is especially true when the execution of those decisions creates unreasonable burdens on the caregivers or other persons who have a legitimate interest in avoiding undue stress and demands on their time and resources. Rhymes contends that "Guidelines which advocate that decisions that can be articulated should be accepted, may abrogate the rights of an entire class of others who are affected by those decisions" (p. 1437). What may occur is that when caregivers decide to meet the predetermined guidelines, it may be at the expense of others in terms of financial, emotional, and social resources. Often caregivers are required to use financial resources needed by other family members, invite outside caregivers into the home to assist in the caregiving tasks, and split limited time between family and the care recipient. If caregivers decide that they cannot meet the predetermined guideline, they often live with the guilt that accompanies such decisions. One must consider that long-term care decisions involve not only the autonomy of the person with Alzheimer's disease but also those who are expected to provide the caregiving support.

DO NO HARM

In addition, ethical and moral conflicts can appear when a person who is delegated to make health care decisions (proxy) follows a course of action that seems not to be in the patient's best interest. One must be careful to avoid the paternalistic route; that is, if the patient or proxy decides on a course of treatment that is not recommended or that threatens the patient's well-being, it must not be dismissed automatically for the Alzheimer's disease patient's "own good." For example, if the proxy decides that antibiotics will not be given in case of pneumonia, one must look at all sides of the situation and not just insist that antibiotics be given.

However, the health care provider has the duty to act as the patient's advocate if necessary. If the course of treatment decided by the proxy is not considered in the patient's "best interest," the health care provider has a moral obligation to take into account possible motives. Such motives may be caregiver burden—emotional, physical, or financial; financial gain such as inheritance, pension, or disability payments; or possibly abuse or neglect. The principle of nonmaleficence requires health care workers to do no harm. This does not imply that every time proxies disagree with health care providers that they are acting for their own gain but that each case must be investigated on its own merits with an open mind. One must consider all aspects of the case to reach an ethical decision. In most institutions, ethics committees are available as sounding boards to consider the positive and negative aspects of such decisions and to provide support and feedback to the health care provider.

DISCLOSURE OF DIAGNOSIS

Protecting patients from harm while respecting their autonomy sometimes creates difficult ethical dilemmas that health care providers must confront. The patient's right to know is now a well-established priority, with patients demanding more equality within the doctor-patient relationship and wishing to be more actively involved. Giving a diagnosis can allay patients' fear of "going mad" or "being stupid" if it is seen in the context of a biological disorder or illness rather than negative personality characteristics. In a recent study, 39% of individuals with dementia had not been told of their diagnosis, and roughly 75% of patients had not been informed about management or prognosis. Three reasons commonly are given for nondisclosure: the uncertainty of the diagnosis, the feeling of futility, and protecting the individual from undue stress. Being told the diagnosis may aid the issue of psychological adjustment, enabling patients to share their anxieties with professional and informal caregivers and thereby relieving some of their uncertainties (Pinner & Bouman, 2003). The patient has the right to know the diagnosis in enough time to be able to make the appropriate advance decisions for his or her health care. The principle of veracity requires the health care worker to be honest. It states that the truth must always be told. The family, however, may contend that withholding information is not the same as being dishonest. At that point the family must be informed that the person with the diagnosis of Alzheimer's disease has a moral and legal right to be present and to receive a specific diagnosis unless he or she waives it. If the dementia is advanced at the time the diagnosis is made, disclosure may no longer be an issue.

Regarding autonomy, as much as patients have a right to be informed of their diagnosis, they equally may wish to waive that right of autonomy. When considering whether to disclose would be in the best interest of the patient, one should ensure that there is not undue influence of another person's needs and that emotional factors such as fear or depression that are overwhelming to the patient are identified and addressed so that individual may face the situation from a position of strength (Pinner & Bouman, 2003).

If disclosure is to occur, the disclosure should occur in a setting that encourages the person and his or her support system to be present so that the information can be presented to all simultaneously and so that emotional support can be given. Pinner and Bouman (2003) outlined some suggested guidelines for diagnosis disclosure. The guidelines are the following:

1. Use a multiprofessional approach to answer questions and make recommendations.
2. Consider telling patient and caregiver together.
3. Allow each separate time to talk and ask questions.
4. Arrange follow-up meetings to continue discussions.
5. Discuss how the disease might progress.
6. Agree on a care plan.
7. Provide written educational materials.
8. Provide a list of community resources and contacts.
9. Arrange for further support.

In this type of setting, the expectations of the patient and family and their perceptions of the disease can be discussed in an open forum. The health care provider can advise the person with Alzheimer's disease and the family to discuss and agree on a plan of care that incorporates the personal values and resources of all involved.

DRIVING

Driving represents independence, competence, and control. Driving is a way to access health care, buy necessities, be productive, and stay connected to family, friends, and the community. In protecting the persons with Alzheimer's disease and the community from harm, one must consider when driving privileges should cease. The diagnosis of Alzheimer's disease in itself is not sufficient reason to revoke driving privileges. One difficulty in the decision is that there is no precise test to indicate that the person with Alzheimer's disease is no longer capable of driving. Deciding when to limit or stop driving can be a confusing issue for individuals diagnosed with dementia and their caregivers. Most information about dementia warns against driving but does not describe when or how to stop. Some caregivers must assume the responsibility for monitoring and regulating the driving of a person with dementia (The Hartford, 2000).

Consideration has been given to reporting persons with the diagnosis of Alzheimer's disease to the motor vehicle department. This mandated reporting would compromise patient confidentiality and might even deter an individual from seeking diagnosis and treatment. What is vital is that communication lines remain open between the person with Alzheimer's disease, caregivers, and health care professionals.

If restriction of driving becomes necessary, negotiation with the person with Alzheimer's disease and the family may result in the person's agreeing to limit driving, such as driving only in the daytime hours. Later, the decision can be made as to when the driving privileges should be terminated. The family must consider that when driving ceases, other arrangements should be made to ensure that transportation would be available when necessary. It is important that the person with Alzheimer's disease does not feel that he or she is a burden to others and thus unnecessarily to restrict his or her freedom.

RESTRAINTS

Ethical dilemmas related to behavior control may occur as the disease progresses. Wandering occurs in 26% of homebound persons with Alzheimer's disease and in

59% of institutionalized patients with Alzheimer's disease. In addition, many persons with Alzheimer's disease have episodes of aggression and agitation. Many methods have been tried to manage these behaviors, including chemical and physical restraints. Any restraint should be a last resort. Instead, efforts should be made to try to determine whether there is an underlying cause for the behaviors and to correct those causes. For example, sometimes individuals act out because they are in pain or they are constipated or hungry, and they cannot make their needs known. As health care providers, nurses have the responsibility to do no harm and to look for the least invasive intervention. Medications are necessary in some instances, but ethical problems arise when behavior-controlling medications are given at doses that interfere with what cognitive function remains. The person with Alzheimer's disease should be given the lowest effective dose of medications for the shortest duration possible. These medications should be given only for specific purposes, such as control of anxiety, and should be used cautiously. Medications should be used in the lowest possible doses and should be increased only when all other interventions have been exhausted.

Physical restraints are usually not necessary and in fact may be hazardous to the person. A physical restraint is considered anything that restricts or controls an individual's freedom of movement. In many instances, the person with Alzheimer's disease does not understand the purpose of the restraints, and in most instances the restrained person becomes more agitated. Often as the person is attempting to get free from the restraint, a fall occurs, resulting in an injury. For example, a person may fall trying to crawl over a side rail and, as a result, fall from a higher distance than if the rail had not been raised. The ethical dilemma that occurs is the person's right to freedom and autonomy and the health care provider's duty to prevent harm. In many instances, the health care provider is fearful of liability if the person with Alzheimer's disease falls. Physical restraints are rarely a necessity and then should be used for a brief period, and the person must be monitored carefully while being restrained.

END-OF-LIFE ISSUES

Although Alzheimer's disease is a progressive disease, death usually occurs from pneumonia, sepsis, or other infectious diseases that may result from the immobility that frequently occurs. Therefore the person with Alzheimer's disease may want to consider what life-prolonging procedures he or she would want. A living will can be made to help health care professionals determine what the patient wishes when the patient becomes incapable of making his or her wishes known. In addition, a living will helps the health care representative make decisions based on the patient's wishes. The health care representative document specifies who individuals designate to make health care decisions for them should they become unable to make decisions for themselves. Advance directives often eliminate legal battles that may occur when family members disagree. The documents allow the health care professional to support the family or health care representative to make the difficult end-of-life decisions. Goals for end-of-life care should be discussed between the person with Alzheimer's disease, the family, and the health care professionals. The parties should clarify whether the long-term goal is that of comfort and emotional well-being or that of prolonging life. A cohesive decision about the goal will make future health care decisions more clear.

One must remember that health care professionals and caregivers should not equate the right to refuse treatment with assisted suicide or euthanasia. If a person with Alzheimer's disease requests no life-prolonging procedures and this wish is not followed, the community may begin to lose trust in the health care system. If this occurs, persons erroneously may believe that they do not have control of their future health considerations and view suicide or assisted suicide as a viable alternative.

An important end-of-life issue that legislators and policy makers must address is the availability of hospice care to families of persons with Alzheimer's disease. The present difficulty is that to qualify for hospice care, the physician must certify that death is imminent and likely will occur within 6 months. Persons with Alzheimer's disease need hospice care for extended periods, and hospice workers need to be prepared for the long-term demand of the care of the person with Alzheimer's disease. Research suggests that services currently available only to patients who are hospice eligible (such as bereavement and counseling services before death for the family and pain control for the patient) would benefit the more than 6 million unpaid caregivers who provide care to individuals with dementia (ADEAR, 2003b).

GENETIC TESTING

The progress being made in the area of genetic testing to predict Alzheimer's disease makes the exploration of ethical and moral implications a necessity. Over the past several decades, researchers found that some

Alzheimer's disease cases, specifically those with early onset, ran in families. Early-onset Alzheimer's disease in persons younger than 50 years has been linked to chromosomes 1, 14, and 21 (Mayeux & Schupf, 1995) and represents less than 1% to 3% of all cases of Alzheimer's disease. Amyloid precursor protein gene mutations were linked to chromosome 21. The amyloid precursor protein gene encodes amyloid precursor protein, a large protein that contains beta amyloid protein, which is a core component of senile plaques. Plaques are a characteristic finding in the brains of individuals with Alzheimer's disease. In 1995, mutations of the presenilin I gene were identified on chromosome 14. These mutations lead to a particularly aggressive form of Alzheimer's disease with average ages of onset between 30 and 50 years of age (Sherrington et al., 1995). Following the discovery of presenilin I gene, another gene associated with early onset was identified on chromosome 1. This gene was identified in a group of families with Volga German ancestry and accounts for a small number of individuals with early-onset Alzheimer's disease (Levy-Lahad et al., 1995). For families in which these genes were identified, characteristics include disease onset before ages 60 to 65 and autosomal dominant patterns of influence. All three of these cases demonstrate an autosomal dominant pattern.

In contrast to the rare variations (mutations) identified in the genes associated with early-onset Alzheimer's disease, common variations (polymorphism) within genes have been identified that influence an individual's risk for developing more common late-onset Alzheimer's disease. An association of apolipoprotein E (APOE) with the onset of the most common familial late-onset Alzheimer's disease is only a beginning of what is to be learned. Apolipoprotein E, a protein located on the chromosome 19, is found in three variations in the population. These variations are called alleles. The alleles are named APOE $\varepsilon2$, $\varepsilon3$, or $\varepsilon4$. Each person inherits one allele from his or her mother and one from the father, resulting in one of six combinations ($\varepsilon2/\varepsilon2$, $\varepsilon2/\varepsilon3$, $\varepsilon2/\varepsilon4$, $\varepsilon3/\varepsilon3$, $\varepsilon3/\varepsilon4$, $\varepsilon4/\varepsilon4$). The APOE $\varepsilon3/\varepsilon3$ allele combination is the most common, occurring in 59% of the population. Roses (1996) found that the inheritance of two specific combinations of the 4 allele ($\varepsilon3/\varepsilon4$ or $\varepsilon4/\varepsilon4$) is associated with an increased risk for earlier age of onset of Alzheimer's disease compared with the other genotypes. The combination $\varepsilon3/\varepsilon4$ is found in 21% of the white population, whereas the combination $\varepsilon4/\varepsilon4$ is found in only 2% (Roses, 1996). The presence of the allele indicates an increased risk for Alzheimer's disease, although factors that indicate which persons with the $\varepsilon4$ allele actually may have

Alzheimer's disease develop are under investigation but are presently known. Interestingly, the presence APOE-$\varepsilon2$ has a protective function, decreasing overall risk and increasing age of onset (Bretsky, Guralnik, Launer, Albert, & Seeman, 2003). Mayeux and Schupf (1995) state that "while the apolipoprotein E genotype may be undeniable as a genetic risk factor for AD [Alzheimer's disease], it does not provide sufficient information to be an adequate predictive genetic test" (p. 1281). Currently, predictive genetic testing for the presence or the absence of the APOE4 allele is not recommended.

Several issues arise from this. First, the question must be asked whether this is a health care need or a health care desire. With the high costs of health care, the principle of justice must consider health care for all. For example, cosmetic surgery in most cases is considered a health care desire. In these cases an individual who had such desire but did not have the economic resources to fulfill those desires would have no basis for claiming unjust treatment. Therefore one must assess the new technological advances as to what benefit they will have and who will benefit.

The second issue arises from the prospect that genetic information may be entered into a computer, where it may become accessible to others. This presents the issue of privacy. If genetic testing becomes more prominent, issues of job or insurance discrimination may arise. In addition, if this information is used as a type of genetic testing, a protocol must be in place to ensure that appropriate counseling and support systems are available.

One suggested use of genetic testing is with an older individual who is suspected of having dementia. The additional information gained by the testing would be a benefit if as a result it would reduce the cost of evaluation or if the diagnosis could be confirmed. This predictive testing also could be used for the purposes of family planning issues once the testing has been refined and the meaning associated with the presence of the gene has been determined and solidified.

With the increasing incidence of Alzheimer's disease, the ethical, legal, and moral issues affect nurses as they deal daily with the patient with Alzheimer's disease, his or her family, and other caregivers. Care must be provided in a way that is compassionate not only for the patient but for the entire support system. Nurses must be forward thinking enough to help facilitate the discussion and planning of future health care needs. Nurses must consider the principles of autonomy, justice, veracity, beneficence, and nonmaleficence as they counsel, educate, and provide care for persons with Alzheimer's disease and their caregivers.

REFERENCES

Alzheimer's Disease Education & Referral Center. (2003a). *Alzheimer's disease fact sheet.* Retrieved July 14, 2005, from http://www.alzheimers.org/pubs/adfact.html

Alzheimer's Disease Education & Referral Center. (2003b). *First study of Alzheimer's caregivers and end-of -life cites both remarkable resilience, need for support.* Retrieved July 14, 2005, from http://www.alzheimers.org/nianews/nianews61.htm

Bretsky, P., Guralnik, J., Launer, L., Albert, M., & Seeman, T. (2003). The role of APOE-epsilon4 in longitudinal cognitive decline: MacArthur studies of successful aging. *Neurology, 60,* 1077-1081.

Caralis, P. (1994). Ethical and legal issues in the care of Alzheimer's patients. *Medical Clinics of North America, 78*(4), 877-893.

Folstein, M. F., Folstein, S. E., & McHugh, P. R. (1975). Mini-Mental State: A practical guide for grading the cognitive state of patients for the clinician. *Journal of Psychiatric Research, 12,* 189-198.

The Hartford. (2000). *A practical guide to Alzheimer's, dementia and driving.* Retrieved July 14, 2005, from http://www.thehartford.com/alzheimers/

Holston, E., & Schutte, D. (2004). The clinical utility of genetic information in the care of persons with Alzheimer's disease. *Medsurg Nursing, 13,* 415-419.

Levy-Lahad, E., Wasco, W., Poorkaj, P., Romano. D., Oshima, J., Pettingell, W., et al. (1995). Candidate gene for the chromosome 1 familial Alzheimer's disease locus. *Science, 269,* 973-977.

Marson, D., & Harrell, L. (2000). Executive dysfunction and loss of capacity to consent to medical treatment in patients with Alzheimer's disease. *Seminars in Clinical Neuropsychiatry, 4*(1), 41-49.

Mayeux, R., & Schupf, N. (1995). Apolipoprotein E and Alzheimer's disease: The implications of progress in molecular medicine. *American Journal of Public Health, 85*(9), 1280-1284.

Murphy, B. (2005). *Planning for future health care decisions: What you should know.* Retrieved July 14, 2005, from the Alzheimer's Association Web site: http://alz-nca.org/caretips/adv-dir.asp

Pinner, G., & Bouman, W. (2003). What should we tell people about dementia? *Advances in Psychiatric Treatment, 9,* 335-341.

Purtilo, R. (1999). *Ethical dimensions in the health profession.* Philadelphia: Saunders.

Rhymes, J. (1995). When the bill comes due for the autonomy of demented older adults, who pays? *Journal of the American Geriatric Society, 43*(12), 1437-1438.

Roses, A. (1996). Apolipoprotein E and Alzheimer's disease: A rapidly expanding field with medical and epidemiological consequences. *Annals of the New York Academy of Science, 802,* 50-57.

Sands, L., Ferreira, P., Stewart, A., Brod, M., & Yaffe, K. (2003). Does dementia caregivers' burden affect their reports of their relative's depression. *Gerontologist, 43*(S1), 272.

Schloendorff v. Society of New York Hospital, 211 N.Y.125 (1914).

Sherrington, R., Rogaeva, E., Levesque, G., Ikeda, M., Liang, Y., Chi, H., et al. (1995). Cloning of a gene bearing missense mutations in early onset familial Alzheimer's disease. *Nature, 375,* 754-760.

Small, G., McDonnell, D., Brooks, R., & Papadopoulos, G. (2002). The impact of symptom severity on the cost of Alzheimer's disease. *Journal of the American Geriatric Society, 50,* 321-327.

Weiler, K. (1994). Legal aspects of nursing documentation for the Alzheimer's patient. *Journal of Gerontological Nursing, 20*(4), 31-40.

Advance Directives

Promoting Self-Determination or Hampering Autonomy

DIANE K. KJERVIK

A commitment to individualism (autonomy) is one of the fundamental values in the United States. Individual freedom is seen as the hallmark of a democratic political system. Soldiers continue to fight and die for freedom from governmental oppression and for freedom of the individual to say and do what is desired. The Bill of Rights in the U.S. Constitution promises freedom to speak one's own mind, to associate with persons and groups with whom one wishes to associate, the right to practice one's own religion, and the right of privacy.

Concomitant with the orientation to individual freedom is a corresponding right to make decisions about where one lives, what one does with one's property, and in terms of health care, what one will allow to be done with one's body. As Justice Cardozo stated, "Every human being of adult years and sound mind has a right to determine what shall be done with his own body; and a surgeon who performs an operation without his patient's consent commits an assault, for which he is liable in damages" (*Schloendorff v. Society of New York Hospital,* 1914). Assumed in this statement of the law is the necessity of a "sound mind" and the belief that without an opposing affirmation, consent is not present. Interestingly, the health care system presumes more often than the legal system that consent is present unless refusal is noted in do not resuscitate (DNR) orders, other advance directives, and communications with providers.

The concept of informed consent has become widely accepted in health care and legal circles as the standard for entering into a patient/health care provider contract for services. Part of the reason for implementing informed consent in health care is to empower the patient by providing information about services to be given so that the patient is able to make a more meaningful choice among the options available (Kjervik & Grove, 1988). With knowledge of the options presented in a clear and consistent fashion, the patient becomes aware of his or her ability to participate actively and with authority in the decision-making process. In this way the patient becomes an active participant in the health care decision-making process, and the power imbalance created by the lack of information is redressed (Katz, 1984). A corollary of the right to consent to treatment is the right to refuse treatment (*Cruzan v. Director, Missouri Department of Health,* 1990) Advance directives in the health care context usually state what the patient does not want done and, in effect, refuses to have done. Nurses are considered by some to be among the best qualified to discuss advance directives with patients and their families (Henderson, 1997; Silverman, Fry, & Armistead, 1994). However, few studies have addressed specific roles nurses play in the discussion of advance directives other than comparisons with physicians' roles (Baggs & Schmitt, 2000). Patients trust nurses, and as studies have shown, patients consider quality at the end of life to include feeling a sense of control and avoidance of inappropriate prolongation of dying (Hanson, 2004; Cameron, 1999; Singer, Martin, & Kelner, 1999). Whether advance directives achieve the goal of promoting autonomy has been debated recently and raises the question of whether ideals match with reality. Nurses and their patients strive to achieve the goal of peaceful death despite pressures from others to prolong the patient's life, but whether advance directives facilitate the process is open to question.

TYPES OF ADVANCE DIRECTIVES

Advance directives are legal mechanisms that enable a person to make decisions about financial arrangements or health care services before the occurrence of a situation in which the person is unable to make such decisions. Advance directives enhance individualism by providing a written document signed by the person that indicates what that person wants done under certain specified circumstances. When properly legally executed, these documents serve as a valid statement of the person's wishes and cannot be invalidated without compelling reasons.

Advance directives include those relating to financial affairs such as wills, trusts, representative payeeships, powers of attorney, and joint tenancy (Weiler, 1989). These financial advance directives provide that a substitute decision maker, such a personal representative in the case of a will or a trustee in the situation of a trust, is empowered to act on behalf of the person who executed the document. The purpose of articulating these wishes in advance is so that the individual's wishes will be predominant, rather than the wishes of persons who are likely to receive direct benefit from the estate of the individual. These legal arrangements have been available for a considerable time to handle financial matters. Directives also can be given to a third party about care for oneself rather than one's property such as those relating to health care: the living will, DNR, do not hospitalize order, and the durable power of attorney for health care (Rosovsky, 2004).

The living will is a document that states that under certain circumstances, such as terminal illness, an individual prefers to have certain choices exercised on his or her behalf if unable to participate in decision making. In 1976, California became the first state to enact legislation that allowed advanced decision making for end-of-life situations (Fade, 1995). The typical direction of the living will is that life-sustaining activities such as the provision of food, fluid, and cardiopulmonary respiration are to be withheld so that the person may die a peaceful death. Without this kind of direction, a hospital or independent health care provider would feel obligated to maintain life for fear of a lawsuit alleging wrongful death. Mental health directives also are becoming more common in states, and Medicare and Medicaid patients' rights standards for hospital participation recognize the importance of these directives (Rozovsky, 2004). For instance, North Carolina enacted a statute that allows a patient to develop an advance instruction for mental health treatment (NC ST sec. 122C-72, 1998), and the New York Office of Mental Health issued a policy encouraging the use of written statements by psychiatric patients who would identify the types of treatments they prefer to receive during crises ("18 Deaths," 1994). Fifteen states have enacted psychiatric advance directives (Duke University Program on Psychiatric Advance Directives, n.d.). A psychiatric crisis can precipitate life-death consequences as with other illnesses, and many patients who have been through emergency episodes can identify what works well for them. However, some authors have questioned vigorously the ability of living

wills to effectuate a patient's choice (Fagerlin & Schneider, 2004).

The durable power of attorney for health care, sometimes referred to as a health care proxy, enables the person to name another person to be a substitute decision maker under the circumstances of impaired functioning on the part of the person executing the document (Rozovsky, 2004). If the person is impaired to the point of being unable to decide what to do, then the substitute decision maker can make the decision. Most states have enacted laws that provide for the living will and durable power of attorney for health care (Cate & Gill, 1991; *Choice in Dying*, 1992). All states but Massachusetts, Michigan, and New York have laws governing living wills (Fade, 1995), and all states have laws allowing health care powers of attorney (Last Acts, 2002). The usefulness of these advance directives in assisting clinical decision making is not yet clear, although Rozovsky (2004) points to problems that may occur if a proxy is unavailable or unwilling to assume responsibilities of the role and the possibility of ambiguity regarding the proxy's scope of authority. One team of researchers concluded that advance directives were irrelevant to decision making regarding resuscitation of seriously ill patients (Teno et al., 1994). Another study showed that family members of dying patients perceived that 10% of patients did not receive care they preferred at the end of life (Lynn et al., 1997).

An important development is the portable DNR document that patients carry with them or the provider sends with the patient to the hospital; for example, from a nursing home. Forty-one states now use out-of-hospital DNRs that are especially helpful in situations where emergency medical service personnel are called to help and must follow the physician-ordered DNR (Last Acts, 2002; State Initiatives in End-of-Life Care, 1999). Portability of advance directives is important for persons who travel from state to state, and uniformity of law among states also would enhance the effectiveness of the directives. Of course, it is vital that hospitals and other health care agencies develop protocols for handling DNR orders to avoid subsequent charges of negligence (Rozovsky, 2004).

ETHICAL ASPECTS OF ADVANCE DIRECTIVES

Although advance directives are legal mechanisms to support substitute decision making, ethical principles underlie the development of the statutes and the practice related to advance directives. The concept of autonomy, which is a fundamental ethical principle, is related

VIEWPOINTS

closely to the freedom of the individual to choose what is to be done with his or her body. Likewise, as Faden and Beauchamp (1986) have pointed out, the principles of justice and beneficence also are served by the implementation of informed consent. Katz (1984) discussed the history of silence between physicians and patients that has led to the doctrine of informed consent. Nurses and patients have not experienced the same degree of silence in relation to nursing care. This could be because nursing care involves patient participation and discussion about the implementation of nursing tasks. In addition, nurses have long espoused the importance of mutuality between nurse and patient.

Caring for patients (beneficence) is manifest in the concern for the individual's decision-making capability and the importance of empowering the individual to be part of the decision-making process. To give patients a voice in what happens with their health care is a beneficent act that is respectful of varying human values and recognizes differences among human beings regarding life and death matters. To feel compassion for the person who is facing difficult choices exemplifies the ethic of care, a new orientation to ethics that attends to feelings that hold relationships together (Beauchamp & Childress, 2001).

The principle of justice is served by giving all individuals a fair share of attention to their wishes about the prolongation of their lives. Whether a person is rich or poor, African-American or Caucasian should make no difference in the decision about whether to end one's life. Deontologically, the rules to be served by advance directives are those relating to the freedom of the individual to choose what will be done with his or her own body and the value of the individual's life and death. Teleologically, the goal to be served is that of peaceful and dignified death for all patients within the health care system.

Empowerment is also an ethical concern from the vantage point of coerciveness by a more powerful party in the decision-making process. Coercion or manipulation makes the choice of less powerful individuals meaningless. Cooperation and conflict resolution among human beings is enhanced by empowering all persons in the relationship. In the case of advance directives for health care, empowerment of the nurse and patient is an ethical matter. If the nurse has far more power than the patient in the interactions, the decisions made by the patient are suspect as lacking autonomy. Therefore the patient must be empowered to speak his or her mind with the nurse as the patient discusses the decisions to be made. Responsible assertiveness is a communication technique that can assist and empower a client to speak. As Lange and Jakubowski (1976) point out, "responsible assertion means not deliberately using personal power to manipulatively overpower weaker people in conflict situations" (p. 58). Therefore the more powerful individual has the responsibility to encourage and teach assertive behavior to a less powerful person. An advance directive can strengthen the patient's ability to speak her or his own mind by providing a visible, concrete form of the statement of preference. The nurse too, is empowered by advance directives, because information is made available to the nurse about the patient's orientation to life and death. This information assists the nurse to implement the nursing process. In one study, nurses indicated that working with patients to help them with advance directives promoted communication among patients, families, and health care providers and increased staff knowledge about advance directives (Silverman et al., 1994).

The living will is a clear way of stating what the patient values at a point in time that is outside the framework of the time of crisis; that is, when a patient is admitted to a hospital or a nursing home. Under circumstances of these critical admissions to a health care facility, the staff and family of the patient often must make decisions without benefit of prior consideration and decision by the patient. Effective December 1991, federal law mandated that hospitals and other health care facilities inform patients of their rights under state law to have living wills and durable powers of attorney for health care (*Patient Self-Determination Act,* 1990). The Joint Commission on Accreditation of Healthcare Organizations also has endorsed this requirement of health care agencies (Rozovsky, 2004). Although informing incoming patients of these rights is useful, the time of admission is not the most fruitful time for development of this thought- and emotion-provoking document. However, the federal mandate to agencies and health care workers raises their awareness of the importance of these documents to patients, families, and society, and the effect of this attitudinal change presumably is passed on to patients.

Another fundamental ethical issue underlying advance directives is the value placed by society on life. In *Cruzan v. Director, Missouri Department of Health* (1990), it became apparent that U.S. Supreme Court justices were divided on the importance that could be attached to life per se in relation to quality of life. The majority of the justices in the Cruzan case believed that life per se was worth preserving and that a state had the right to set the parameters for using advance directives. The minority opinion emphasized the quality of life and the right of an individual to determine when that quality of life had deteriorated to the point that intrusive measures were no longer justified.

Considerations of the quality of life must always address the question of who is to determine the quality of life. Living wills and durable powers of attorney for health care are premised upon the belief that the patient determines what quality of life means for her or him. Other individuals who are willing to be more paternalistic in their orientation say the quality of life is to be determined by health care providers or the government. In reality, the quality of one's life can be ascertained clearly only by oneself based on an evaluation of whatever criteria the individual decides constitutes quality. One's values are a critical element in ascertaining the quality of one's life and can be evaluated by use of a values history such as that developed by the Center for Health Law and Ethics at the University of New Mexico (Cate & Gill, 1991) or the *Five Wishes* document of the Commission on Aging with Dignity in Florida, which allows persons to indicate values and preferences for their care at the end of life (Aging with Dignity, 1999). One study showed that older persons often continue to rely on others to make decisions and so lack enthusiasm about creating advance directives even when they receive written information about them (High, 1993) The trend toward surrogate decision making laws (Fade, 1995) responds to the need some persons have to rely on others to make difficult choices. For instance, the recent case of Terri Schiavo in Florida exemplifies the struggle families have when faced with the decision of removing life-sustaining treatments and their desperate use of the legal system to help resolve these conflicts (*Schiavo ex rel Schindler v. Schiavo*, 2005).

OBJECTIONS TO ADVANCE DIRECTIVES

Several arguments are raised in opposition to advance directives. The first is the paternalistic belief that the health care provider, usually physician, knows what is best for the patient. In its modern form, this paternalistic attitude cloaks itself in a discounting of the patient's choice to stop treatment by arguing that the patient is incapable of deciding because of psychological illness, such as the newly touted demoralization syndrome in which the experience of meaninglessness leads to the wish to die (Kissane, 2004). Paternalism has been eroded considerably by consumer activism and by other health care providers who are interested in sharing power with other members of the health care team and

their patients. The designation of "patient" is even undergoing challenge and revision because of its emphasis on a one-up/one-down position between doctor and patient. As consumers become more active and interested in their own health care, they expect to be part of the decision-making process and ultimately to make their own decisions. Certainly, there are rare cases where individuals do not want to be bothered with decisions about their health care. However, these cases are less frequent as consumers become more sophisticated about health care alternatives and therefore are interested in asserting their own voice or relying on a relative who knows their preferences. One reason consumers are interested in asserting their own voice is their experience with inadequate diagnostic and treatment decisions by health care providers that have resulted in injury to patients and corresponding large medical malpractice awards. However, even though individuals may seek control at the end of life, the percentage of those who have living wills remains at around 20% (Fagerlin & Schneider, 2004), so many choose not to use this particular advance directive in spite of legislative and other efforts to encourage persons to execute living wills.

Another argument against living wills asserts that these directives do not reflect an incompetent patient's interests accurately. Because these documents are formulated when the person is competent and presumably has different interests, it is argued that later when the person becomes incompetent, the best interests are served in entirely different ways than what the patient long ago envisioned (Fagerlin & Schneider, 2004; Robertson, 1991). Following this line of reasoning, one's will and choice would have to be recorded continuously for a living will or any other form of advance directive to be considered valid. Contracts, wills, and trusts would have to be invalidated because they were developed before the time they are acted upon. Clearly, this is an absurd result that would create tremendous dysfunction in several areas of the law. However, the durable power of attorney option allows for the patient's proxy in the immediate situation to decide what, in these circumstances, the patient would want. So although the living will may not represent the patient's decision accurately, the proxy decision maker may do so.

A third argument points to research that shows patients are willing to grant their surrogates leeway in the way the living will is interpreted and do not expect strict adherence to wishes they have stated in their living wills (Sehgal et al., 1992). The response to this argument is that specification as to areas of leeway and principles to be followed can be enumerated and, indeed, should be enumerated in the living will itself. Alternatively, the proxy decision maker acting under the durable power of attorney for health care can be instructed orally by the patient as to the leeway to be given. Decisions of the surrogate thus can reflect an accurate and full discussion with the patient. McPherson and Addington-Hall (2003) point out that proxies best express the correct wishes of the patients when service provision and observable symptoms are at issue; however, correct reporting of the patient's subjective state (feelings and pain experiences) is less accurate. So careful monitoring by nurses of these subjective states will be an important contribution to the care of these patients.

A fourth argument is that living wills are not available when needed; many patients do not take them to the hospital or give their physicians copies (Fagerlin & Schneider, 2004). Again, for those who feel strongly about control over end-of-life decisions, they will make sure written documents are made available to health care staff.

Probably the most vociferous argument against living wills has been raised in legislative sessions in which opponents warn of a slippery slope between living wills and murder or genocide. This argument can be rebutted by the realization that the law examines carefully any coercion or manipulation involved in entering into a living will as with any other legal contract. Therefore only documents that are the will of the patient are to be followed. No independent judgment by health care professionals that a given patient or a given group of patients should die would control the situation in which a living will is in effect. The law would not want to reach the absurd result that no contract or other legal document could be entered into if there were any possibility of coercion or manipulation. Ethical and legal rules must be adopted based on their ability to organize human behavior. These rules cannot be controlled by the fear of numerous possibilities of human evil. As far as coercion and manipulation go, not to allow a person to determine what will be done with his or her body during a terminal illness is a form of coercion as well, one in which the outside person decides that the life of another should be preserved at all costs. This argument against living wills also overlooks the fact that some persons indicate in their living wills that they wish every possible means to be used to keep them alive (request directives). As Steinhauser et al. (2000) have found, cultural variations exist in the wish to have all treatment provided; for example, nonwhite ethnic groups

prefer all treatments. A slippery slope in the other direction could be imagined in which a patient's wish overrules resource allocation decisions, an equally absurd result. In fact, some evidence exists that living wills are not well-followed (Fagerlin & Schneider, 2004), so the concern that patients will die because of overzealous effectuation of the living will is unrealistic.

ADVANCE DIRECTIVES IN RELATION TO NURSING PRACTICE

Nursing process can be enhanced by use of advance directives. As part of the assessment of the patient's goals in relation to severity of health care status, the nurse can discuss provisions that exist in the patient's living will or durable power of attorney for health care. Members of the health care team must respond to provisions of the living will, so they need to understand the meaning of the document to the patient, and they need to understand what the law within their state requires for the document to be considered valid. In a much publicized case in Texas in 1992, the patient and his family were distraught when the health care facility did not follow the patient's living will because state law requires that two physicians certify the patient as terminally ill and only one physician had done so (Gamino, 1992). Other legal cases have been brought in Ohio and North Carolina when patients' express wishes were not followed (Martin, 1997). Close work with the attorney for the facility is necessary to make the legal mandates clear to staff and administrators.

A values history can give a picture of the patient's beliefs about organ donation, respirators and independent functioning, for instance. If the patient has no advance directive, discussion of personal values may assist the patient to make a choice to execute a living will. Knowing the patient's belief about artificial extension of life, the nurse can plan and implement care that is respectful of the patient. Care can be evaluated according to standards developed by the patient in addition to those imposed from the outside that have to do with technical choices such as which antihypertensive drug to prescribe. If the patient chooses to have no heroic measures exercised, the nurse will be present to assist with comfort measures. Interventions in the direction of this goal rather than the goal of preserving life might create moral conflict for some nurses. In the future, nurses may be called upon to take a more active role in assisting with death (Johnson & Weiler, 1990). Nursing must take an active part in the debate about aid-in-dying, because without doubt, nurses will be called upon to play a close, active role in the process (Kjervik, 1997). The American Nurses Association (1994) issued a statement about nurse-assisted suicide that makes clear that direct assistance with suicide is not an accepted standard in nursing. Interestingly, however, carrying out the patient's wishes for withdrawal of treatment as specified in a written advance directive is legally and ethically acceptable as previously argued.

Nurses are moral agents who are responsible for their own conduct. As Theis (1990) has noted, "To conceive of the nurse as one who simply follows directives without moral reflection concerning the treatment being rendered fails to recognize the moral status of the nurse as an individual with standards of personal conscience and professional ethics." The nurse cannot assist the patient to examine values without having a sense of her or his own values. Therefore part of the process of caring for the patient involves self-reflection and decision making about how one views one's own life and death. Nurses can act as role models for behaviors considered valuable for the patient to demonstrate; for example, by having their own living wills (Weber & Kjervik, 1992). Because the range of persons with advance directives is from less than 10% of the public to 28% (Crisham, 1990; Last Acts, 2002; Teno et al., 1994), nurses' role modeling is especially important.

Patients who have advance directives demonstrate health-promoting behaviors. By stating values and preferences manifestly in writing, the patient shows the strength to be an active participant in the maintenance of health rather than a passive observer and recipient of the preferences of others. In the process of preparing an advance directive, the patient imagines his or her own possible incapacitation. Through the use of this imagery, the patient is able to consider all alternatives including the opportunity to have choice over life-and-death options. The act of imagining and then creating a written statement of choice is strengthening to patients who often feel like victims in the health care setting.

Advance directives also act as preventive measures. Just as primary prevention in health care means the practice of health promoting and disease preventing behaviors, risk management in the law means preventing legal difficulties. Advance directives prevent legal problems in the future when the viewpoint of the patient may be at issue. Economically, respecting the patient's choice may reduce escalating health care costs by ruling out a number of expensive procedures. As Katz (1984) suggests, "first patient opinions" may be less costly than "second medical opinions."

The encouragement of advance directives also may provide an opportunity for nurses to apply a relational ethic of care. Parker (1990) describes this ethic as a process of sharing relational stories of caregiving. This process is based on reciprocity and interconnectedness among human beings. To talk with patients about their stories of the meaning of life and death to them assists them to make decisions about advance directives. Self-disclosure by the nurse enriches the process and contributes to mutual understanding and concern. Deliberate conversations about death and dying issues are recommended by Badzek, Leslie, and Corbo-Richert (1998). Requests for assisted suicide or euthanasia have disappeared following support by nurses and family members, pain management, and treatment of depression (Severson, 1997).

An important foundation on which the realization of an ethic of care; the principles of justice, beneficence, and autonomy; and the legal goal of self-determination are based is the relationship between the nurse and patient. Trust is imperative to this relationship and can be enhanced by the execution of advance directives. Katz (1984) poses several assumptions that are part of a trusting, mutual relationship in the context of informed consent:

1. There is no single right or wrong answer for how life, health, and illness should be lived. Numerous treatment options exist, and suffering can be alleviated in a variety of ways.
2. Health care providers and patients have vulnerabilities and conflicting motivations, interests, and expectations. Sameness of interests cannot be presumed; it must be confirmed in conversation.
3. Both parties relate to each other as equals and unequals. Professionals share professional expertise and patients their personal expertise. At the outset, neither knows what each can do for the other.
4. Human behavior contains rational and irrational elements. These elements must be accepted in health care providers and patients. Incompetence should not be presumed for either when signs of irrationality appear.

The assumptions enumerated by Katz indicate that the physician must engage in dialogue with patients about health care choices, options, and decisions. Advance directive documents can be considered an "invitation to conversations about patients' real concerns and values, goals of treatment, and a plan of care serving those goals" (Hanson, 2004, p. 204). Such a thorough conversation of a "spectrum of clinical interventions that are increasingly complicated" may be an expression of a form of translational ethics that is based upon autonomy and informed consent (Kagarise & Sheldon, 2000, p. 39). Although nurses do not demonstrate the silence referred to by Katz, the assumptions still are important for nurses to consider. Nurses should recognize the variety of "right" answers available to patients, should be aware of their own vulnerabilities and be able to discuss these with patients, should recognize their equalities and inequalities with patients, and should become comfortable with their own irrational sides. As Katz (1984) states, "trust must be earned through conversation." In the face-to-face encounter with the patient mutual understanding develops. With the understanding comes more effective decision making about health care choices.

SUMMARY

Nurses play a key role in the development and implementation of advance directives. Nursing values of mutuality, open and direct communication, caring and health promotion and prevention support the use of advance directives for health care. A shared decision-making model is a natural for nurses and patients and is helpful during the dying process (Hiltunen, Medich, Chase, Peterson, & Forrow, 1999). As Rozovsky (2004) notes, "when properly executed, living wills eliminate indecision and family disputes" (p. 772) Portability of advance directives makes them more available when needed even when one is traveling outside one's home state. Patients are challenged to be honest and forthright in expressing their wishes. The skill nurses have in developing trusting relationships with patients can be used as a model for other health care professionals who are burdened with silence or unsupportiveness in their relationships with patients. The Patient Self-Determination Act of 1990 provides the impetus for nursing involvement with patients on the topics of living wills and durable powers of attorney for health care. Now, nurses must engage patients, their families, and other health care providers in deliberate discussions about the end of life.

We help our patients speak.

We help them look deep within

For truth, conflict and decision.

Then we accept their paths

As we accept our own.

REFERENCES

Aging with Dignity. (1999). *Five wishes.* Tallahassee, FL: Commission on Aging with Dignity.

American Nurses Association. (1994). *Position statement on assisted suicide.* Washington, DC: Author.

Badzek, L. A., Leslie, N. S., & Corbo-Richert, B. (1998). End-of-life decisions: Are they honored? *Journal of Nursing Law, 5*(2), 51-63.

Baggs, J., & Schmitt, M. (2000). End-of-life decisions in adult intensive care: Current research base and directions for the future. *Nursing Outlook, 48*(4):158-164.

Beauchamp, T. L., & Childress, J. F. (2001). *Principles of biomedical ethics* (5th ed.). New York: Oxford University Press.

Cameron, M. E. (1999). Completing life and dying triumphantly. *Journal of Nursing Law, 6*(1), 27-32.

Cate, F. H., & Gill, B. A. (1991). *The Patient Self-Determination Act: Implementation issues and opportunities* (pp. 65-73). Washington, DC: Annenberg Washington Program of Northwestern University.

Choice in dying: Right-to-die case & statutory citations. (1992, March 17). New York: Choice in Dying.

Crisham, P. (1990). Living wills: Controversy and certainty. *Journal of Professional Nursing, 6*(6), 321.

Cruzan v. Director, Missouri Dept. of Health, 110 S. Ct. 2841, 111 L. Ed. 2d 224, 58. USLW 4916 (US Mo., June 25, 1990).

Duke University Program on Psychiatric Advance Directives. (n.d.). Retrieved June 28, 2005, from the Services Effectiveness Research Program, Department of Psychiatry and Behavioral Sciences, Duke University Medical Center Website: http://pad.duhs.duke.edu

18 Deaths in NY psychiatric facilities instigate changes: Ethical concerns about restraints apply equally to mental patients. (1994). *Medical Ethics Advisor, 10*(12), 162-163.

Fade, A. E. (1995). Advance directives: An overview of changing right-to-die laws. *Journal of Nursing Law, 2*(3), 27-38.

Faden, R. R., & Beauchamp, T. L. (1986). *A history and theory of informed consent.* New York: Oxford University Press.

Fagerlin, A., & Schneider, C. E. (2004). Enough: The failure of the living will. *Hastings Center Report, 34*(2), 30-42.

Gamino, D. (1992, May 15). A living will fails to ensure dignified death. *Austin American-Statesman,* pp. A-1, A-12.

Hanson, L. C. (2004). Palliative care: Innovation in care at the end of life. *North Carolina Medical Journal, 65*(4), 202-208.

Henderson, M. L. (1997). Advance directives for patients with cancer. *Cancer Practice, 5*(3), 186-188.

High, D. M. (1993). Advance directives and the elderly: A study of intervention strategies to increase use. *The Gerontologist, 33*(3), 342-349.

Hiltunen, E. F., Medich, C., Chase, S., Peterson, L., & Forrow, L. (1999). Family decision making for end-of-life treatment: The SUPPORT nurse narratives. *Journal of Clinical Ethics, 10*(2), 126-134.

Johnson, R. A., & Weiler, K. (1990). Aid-in-dying: Issues and implications for nursing. *Journal of Professional Nursing, 6*(5), 258-264.

Kagarise, M. J., & Sheldon, G. F. (2000). Translational ethics: A perspective for the new millennium. *Archives of Surgery, 135,* 39-45.

Katz, J. (1984). *The silent world of doctor and patient* (pp. xiv, 28-29, 47, 102-103, 228). New York: Macmillan.

Kissane, D. W. (2004). The contribution of demoralization to end of life decision-making. *Hastings Center Report, 34*(4), 21-31.

Kjervik, D. K. (1997). Assisted suicide: The challenge to the nursing profession. *Journal of Law, Medicine & Ethics, 24*(3), 237-242.

Kjervik, D. K., & Grove, S. (1988). A legal model of consent in unequal power relationships. *Journal of Professional Nursing, 4*(3), 192-204.

Lange, A. J., & Jakubowski, P. (1976). *Responsible assertive behavior: Cognitive behavioral procedures for trainers* (p. 58). Champaign, IL: Research Press.

Last Acts. (2002). *Means to a better end: A report on dying in America today.* Washington, DC: Author.

Lynn, J., Teno, J. M., Phillips, R. S., Wu, A.W., Desbiens, N., Harrold, J., et al. (1997). Perceptions by family members of the dying experience of older and seriously ill patients. *Annals of Internal Medicine, 126*(2), 97-106.

Martin, R. H. (1997). Advance directives: Legal implications for nurses. *Journal of Nursing Law, 4*(2), 7-15.

McPherson, C. J., & Addington-Hall, J. M. (2003). Judging the quality of care at the end of life: Can proxies provide reliable information? *Social Science & Medicine, 56*(1), 95-109.

NC ST sec. 122C-72, GS sec. 122C-72 (1998).

Parker, R. S. (1990). Nurses' stories: The search for a relational ethic of care. *Advances in Nursing Science, 13*(1), 31-40.

Patient Self-Determination Act of 1990, 42 U.S.C.A. (1395 cc (f) (1) (A) (I)(1991 Supp. pam.), PL 101-508 (4206, 104 Stat. 1388-115 (1990)).

Robertson, J. A. (1991). Second thoughts on living wills. *Hastings Center Report, 21*(6), 6-9.

Rozovsky, F. A. (2004). *Consent to treatment: A practical guide* (3rd ed., suppl. 4). New York: Aspen.

Schiavo ex rel Schindler v. Schiavo, 403 F.3d. 1233 (2005).

Schloendorff v. Society of New York Hospital, 211 N.Y. 125, 129-130, 105 N.E. 92, 93 (1914).

Sehgal, A., Galbraith, A., Chesney, M., Schoenfeld, P., Charles, G., & Lo, B. (1992). How strictly do dialysis patients want their advanced directives followed? *Journal of the American Medical Association, 267*(1), 59-63.

Severson, K. T. (1997). Dying cancer patients at the end of life. *Journal of Pain Symptom Management, 14*(2), 94-98.

Silverman, H. J., Fry, S. T., & Armistead, N. (1994). Nurses' perspectives on implementation of the Patient Self-Determination Act. *Journal of Clinical Ethics, 5*(1), 30-37.

Singer, P. A., Martin, D. K., & Kelner, M. (1999). Quality end-of-life care: Patients' perspectives. *JAMA: The Journal of the American Medical Association, 281*(2), 163-168.

State Initiatives in End-of-Life Care. (1999). Implementing end-of-life treatment preferences across clinical settings. *National Program Office for Community-State Partnerships to Improve End-of-Life Care,* Issue 3.

Steinhauser, K. E., Christakis, N. A., Clipp, E. C., McNeilly, M., McIntyre, L., & Tulsky, J. A. (2000). Factors considered important at the end of life by patients, family, physicians, and other care providers. *JAMA: The Journal of the American Medical Association, 284*(19), 2476-2482.

Teno, J. M., Lynn, J., Phillips, R. S., Murphy, D., Youngner, S. J., Bellamy, P., et al. (1994). Do advance directives affect resuscitation decisions and the use of resources for seriously ill patients? *Journal of Clinical Ethics, 5*(1), 23-30.

Theis, E. C. (1990). Life-sustaining technologies: Ordinary of extraordinary? *Focus on Critical Care, 17*(6), 445-450.

Weber, G., & Kjervik, D. K. (1992). The Patient Self-Determination Act: The nurse's proactive role. *Journal of Professional Nursing, 8*(1), 6.

Weiler, K. (1989). Financial abuse of the elderly: Recognizing and acting on it. *Journal of Gerontological Nursing, 15*(8), 10-15.

CHAPTER
73
Managed Care and the Violation of Ethical Principles

Research Vignettes *

MARY CIPRIANO SILVA ◆ KATHLEEN O. WILLIAMS

> The changes in the way health care organizations are run in response to managed care is nothing short of a complete reversal from what we knew before. It has been equivalent to reeducating an entire profession about what the essence of their job really was.
>
> **PARTICIPANT 10**

What is the then and the now that Participant 10 is addressing? The ideal then consisted of provider-patient control of health care decision making, direct provider-patient access to specialist care, a philosophy of attending to patients' needs before profit taking, and seemingly unlimited access to resources. The now, of course, refers to managed care, which is a broad term referring to a variety of activities performed by organizations that are structured systematically to control "*cost, quality, quantity,* and *access*" (Dombeck & Olsan, 2002, p. 223) to health care. Of these four characteristics, too often costs have dominated within managed care organizations (MCOs). Consequently, the viewpoint we take here is that managed care, with its focus on cost cutting, too often has sacrificed quality, quantity, and access to health care. The result has been ethical concerns about and violation of ethical principles underlying managed, or more accurately, (mis)managed care.

First, what were some of the variables and events that provided the impetus for managed care? After World War II, enormous advances in research with subsequent development of lifesaving drugs and technologies emerged. This growth was enhanced with the introduction of the Medicare and Medicaid programs in 1965. These initiatives provided access to health care to millions of Americans who previously were disenfranchised from this care, including the aged, disabled, and impoverished. These initiatives also reflected the altruism and social consciousness of Americans (Dombeck & Olsan, 2002).

The explosion in knowledge and technology and an expanded populace able to access health care also brought pressure on public and private sector payers of health care to cut costs, resulting in the establishment of MCOs. These organizations use gatekeepers, specific practice protocols, contractual agreements between payers and providers, and provider and consumer incentives, and they govern the place, provider, type, and quantity of a patient's care (Dombeck & Olsan, 2002).

The development and the power that MCOs have on everyday care have many health care professionals, including nurses, acknowledging moral distress (Erlen, 2001). Nurses are challenged daily to practice in environments that have taken on business models and processes that seek the bottom line in order to survive financially. These environments may be alien to the ethical principles that have been an inherent part of nurses' professional practice. These ethical principles include respecting persons, respecting autonomy, preventing harm, and ensuring justice (American Nurses Association [ANA], 2001; Beauchamp & Childress, 2001; Erlen, 2001; Silva, Fletcher, & Sorrell, 2004).

METHOD

To understand better how nurses' perceived ethical issues and principles related to the restructuring of

*We thank the College of Nursing and Health Science at George Mason University for the funding of this study; Sally Bulla and Mary Frances Kordick for their assistance, respectively, with data collection and analysis; and the 15 research participants who poured their hearts out and presented to us the gift of their stories.

health care, in particular, managed care, we conducted the following qualitative study. Only parts of the study methodology and data are presented.

Nurses Speak Out

Fifteen nurses enrolled in a doctoral program in a southern state participated in this study. These nurses, all with 20 or more years of nursing experience, worked in a wide variety of settings including operating rooms, nursing homes, emergency rooms, critical care units, women's health and midwifery, nursing education, nursing administration, and public health.

The study participants were interviewed, and the interviews were taped and transcribed with the participants' permission. The 15 participants were asked to share professional and/or personal stories or comments about ethical issues related to the restructuring of health care that they had experienced. The interviews lasted from 30 to 60 minutes.

Nurses' Stories and Comments

Vignettes of the nurses' stories and comments were generated through NVivo—a qualitative research computer program; however, the following four categories were identified by the researchers. Data supporting each category and ethical principle violated were selected because they were the best fit vignettes from the data.

Disrespect for Persons: Confusion and (Dis)continuity of Care. The principle of respect for persons is defined in provision one of the *Code of Ethics for Nurses with Interpretive Statements*: "A fundamental principle that underlies all nursing practice is respect for the inherent worth, dignity, and human rights of every individual" (ANA, 2001, p. 7). The following vignettes ultimately highlight violation of this principle with the study participants as providers and as recipients of care.

When I was with _____ County, it was a dreadful situation, because we had a population who had Medicaid, and then managed Medicaid came in and took our patients to another system. This is a population that is low education, primarily Spanish speaking, who had many complex needs. After one year, they did not renew the contract. The managed care group … just fell through the cracks, but then they just came trickling back to us. And talk about a lack of continuity of care. It was a nightmare.

PARTICIPANT 7

Interviewer: But the managed care population, the small managed care population that you have, ends up going to another lab?

Participant: That's right, including her Pap smear. It becomes an added problem for the patient. I do the physical piece, but she'll leave then with her baggie of lab that we've drawn or her Pap smear and she'll be responsible for dropping it off at a certain drawing station or lab. … So it's very disjointed in terms of providing holistic care to the patient, because it's a separate billing process altogether. The lab is separate from the physical finding, the physical data that we collect. Very, very sad.

PARTICIPANT 12

I am in a HMO now, and every time I need a referral, I have to go into the office and wait in a line of people to even talk to someone. Sometimes it can be ten minutes that you stand in front of a door waiting for someone to acknowledge you, that you are there. Once they acknowledge you, you get sent to another line, the referral lady line, where you wait then for the referral. Or you just get some information at that point. Yeah. Wouldn't it be convenient if they would mail that referral to you? However, they don't. You have to go back, and you have to go back a day or two later. They will let you know when it's completed, then you have to go back into the same office, go through the same procedure, and go back to the referral lady to pick up your referral. So the amount of time that is involved in that is sometimes copious. It's extreme, and it drives me absolutely crazy.

PARTICIPANT 15

I was to have surgery at a large university hospital. Had gotten the referral from my primary physician. Went to a surgical group at the university and said, "Are you sure that you have my pre-cert and that you have that taken care of?" Simply because I knew at the time managed care was new and that there needed to be a precertification for any kind of surgery or procedure. Talked to the people, and I was probably obsessive about it. Probably talked to them about three times to make sure that they had received it and had taken care of things as they should be. Well, they had. I had the procedure to the tune of about four or five thousand dollars. At the end, when the bill came, the bill said I owed four to five thousand, because they hadn't gotten the precertification. This totally infuriated me. This was the university where I worked, so I may have had more pull than the average guy, but I went down and talked with the people and had actually made notes that I had made calls. And the person that I talked to when I made these calls confirmed that. Therefore, the university itself had to eat the charges.

PARTICIPANT 15

In the preceding four vignettes, respect for persons was violated, whether it was the research participants themselves or the patients/clients for whom they cared. This violation was personified by betrayal, by lack of genuine concern, and by lack of listening. Participant 7 felt betrayed when managed Medicaid dropped the ball

VIEWPOINTS

regardless of what happened to the clients or nurses. With Participants 12 and 15, the managed care environments were ones in which provider convenience trumped genuine concern for clients. Participant 15 also was angered by a managed care surgical group that did not listen to her or follow through with her concerns about precertification.

Dombeck and Olsan (2002), in discussing MCOs, address disrespect for persons in terms of violation of personhood. They say,

> [Professionals] might, however, abandon the old loyalties and their old values, do their jobs silently, and not raise ethical objections for fear of jeopardizing their place in the institution. Thus ... their moral voice becomes less audible and their moral face becomes less present in the institution. ... There is a subtle loss of personhood. (p. 230)

This loss of personhood results in frustration, decreased loyalty, and eroded trust among nurses (Ray, Turkel, & Marino, 2002), as well as confusion and (dis)continuity of care for patients/clients (Erlen, 2002) as attested to by the three study participants. However, ultimate disrespect for nurses in MCOs results in nurses who become so dis*ill*usioned with their profession that they become ill or leave nursing (Dworkin, 2002; Ray et al., 2002).

Loss of Autonomy: Routines, Regulations, and Rules That Bind. Autonomy means self-governing or self-determining capacities and/or actions. According to Beauchamp and Childress (2001), the principle of respect for autonomy and the violation of this principle mean

> at a minimum, to acknowledge ... [a] person's right to hold views, to make choices, and to take actions based on personal values and beliefs. Such respect [for autonomy] involves respectful *action*, not merely a respectful *attitude*. ... whereas disrespect for autonomy involves attitudes and actions that ignore, insult, or demean others' rights of autonomy. (p. 63)

The following vignettes ultimately highlight violation of the ethical principle of respect for autonomy with the study participants as providers and as recipients of care.

> As a nurse-midwife I prescribe birth control pills to many of my clients for contraception as well as therapeutic benefit. And last week I found out that one of my patients, and this is not the first time I've heard this, but this is the first time it's happened to me; her managed care policy or her insurance policy was switching the pills every six months depending on

what the managed care plan was covering that particular era. And so, unbeknownst to me, who's prescribing the medication, this woman was having her pills switched every six months as a routine, just because of that particular prescriptive policy. And if you know anything about prescribing drugs, birth control pills are something you just cannot switch without having implications or side effects. And so this woman was having breakthrough bleeding and occasional headaches. This was something she routinely had to go through every six months, depending on what her prescription plan was covering that particular era. I was extremely angry, and we now have to write a letter in support of having her stay on one particular brand so that she doesn't have the side effects that I described earlier. So, it was just terrible, the fact that I was not in charge of her medication regimen. It was outside, like insurance people who were deciding what pill she was going to be on, which is taking the control away from the provider, which is not right for the woman. The patient obviously was suffering. And it's just not a good thing.

PARTICIPANT 12

> There's an interesting daily we deal with, an interesting ethical, regulatory conflict. We're a large hospice. We provide a great number of services. There are some services we provide [to the] patient at no cost. But we have to be extremely careful what we do, because we could be accused of bridging services, enticing people to hospice services or of other things that are seen as outside the realm of the regulatory process. I'm an idealist, but I see all of these things [bridging services] as good care. And I see these concerns about not bridging services as being barriers to care. And we need to work with HCFA and HRSA and all the folks downtown to move us beyond these rigid models and look at people individually and look at really providing care. I think the model we have right now is who do we have to give care to rather than who ought we to give care to or who deserves it. And that, I think, is the decision we all need to wrestle with.

PARTICIPANT 14

> You know there are providers, usually nurse reviewers, on site in hospitals every day. Some three days a week, some every day of the week, who are actually reading charts and right behind us are writing progress notes for the day, taking a look at Does this case meet medical intensity to be here? Are things happening here that could happen in the outpatient setting? They often leave documentation behind of the sort that says it would appear that we are not meeting intensity and inviting us to give them a call and give a clinical rationale for what we are doing. Others are more cut and dry—basically you've got 24 hours to finish this treatment plan and move on.

PARTICIPANT 9

> I had to admit one of my children who was 11 or 12 years old at the time into a mental health institution because he was diagnosed with anorexia. It was a very painful experience for me,

for our whole family. And the only way he was going to get well was to go and be diagnosed because, at that point, he wasn't diagnosed totally and his behavior really became erratic. And so we had some situations in our home that were not safe anymore with him because of his behavior, and I knew that he needed help. So we ended up taking him to a mental health facility. And he was admitted and was there for six days and clearly was not ready to be discharged. … And I was very concerned that maybe there was brain injury or something that was really causing this because nobody seemed to be able to give me any answers. And one day I went in to visit him, and I was informed that he was going to be discharged that day. And, as a nurse, I knew he was nowhere ready to be discharged. I fought it. I called the doctor, and I protested it and said that the insurance company could not do this. I didn't care whether they thought he needed to be discharged or not, and the whole issue was that they only provided so many days of care for his treatment. So I was requesting to have additional tests done because in my mind they needed to rule out everything. And, so, because of the intercession of the physician, he ended up calling the managed care company and negotiating with it. So, we were able to get a couple more days out of his stay. And, I remember really being fearful of our whole health system, because I remember working as a nurse previous to managed care and that would never have happened. So, it was a very frightening experience for me and really gave me a better appreciation of how our health system has changed.

PARTICIPANT 3

The preceding four vignettes show how routines, regulations, and rules that bind can profoundly affect nurses' best practices and decision-making capacities. Thus Participant 12 was robbed of her decision-making prescriptive authority by a routine that she found harmful to her clients. Participant 14 was boxed in by regulations that created barriers to good nursing care. Participant 9's nursing care was hampered by rules that govern medical intensity standards. Likewise, Participant 3, whose son also was a recipient of care, was hampered by insurance company rules that limited days of care in a mental health facility. The experience left her fearful of the health care system.

All of the preceding four research participants were experiencing the pain of loss of autonomy. This pain manifested itself in anger, caution, frustration, and fear. Ulrich, Soeken, and Miller (2003) studied the predictors of autonomy in 245 nurse practitioners who were associated with health maintenance organizations (HMOs) in Maryland. They concluded that when HMO penetration was higher, when the number of clients enrolled in HMOs was higher, and when perceived concern about ethics was higher, nurse practitioners' perceptions of

their autonomy was lower. Because perception is often more important than fact, this conclusion is important because it could influence negatively nurse practitioners' perception of their autonomy and thus decrease their decision-making power in HMOs. Instead, the ideal outcome would be increased autonomy for nurses rather than routines, regulations, and rules that bind.

Inflicting Real or Potential Harm: Money Talks, aka the Bottom Line.   The do no harm principle in nursing can be found as far back as the Nightingale *Pledge for Nurses* and as recent as the 2001 *Code of Ethics for Nurses with Interpretive Statements*. According to the code (ANA, 2001, p. 14),

> As an advocate for the patient, the nurse must be alert to and take appropriate action regarding any instances of incompetent, unethical, illegal, or impaired practice by any member of the health care team or the health care system or any action on the part of others that places the rights or best interests of the patient in jeopardy.

When the do no harm principle is violated, then the best interests of the patient or family also are violated, resulting in damages (e.g., physical, psychological, and financial), impairments, injuries, negligence, disabilities, risk of death, and even death. The following vignettes ultimately highlight the link between costs and violation or potential violation of the ethical principle of do no harm with the study participants as providers and as recipients of care.

> There was a lady in Mississippi who contracted polio when she was 12, was a quadriplegic all her life. She was ventilator dependent, living in her own home for 53 years. She turned the magical age of 65 and immediately was dropped from [HMO]. All of a sudden, [HMO] is saying we can no longer provide these home care services you've been having 24 hours, seven days a week. … So she, very wisely, called the press. And they had Dateline, 20-20, 60 Minutes, I don't know, somebody was at her house interviewing her, taking pictures of this, this horrible, bed-ridden patient, for 50 some odd years. … She also knew she needed to get her congressman involved. And low and behold, guess who came to her rescue but Senator _____, who couldn't be more powerful. So, he got on [HMO's] butt, and guess who's providing 24/7 care for this woman. Now, should she be provided that care? I mean, she is sick. It was promised to her father, kind of, but it's not in writing. So there is something to be said about that. And do you move a 65-year-old out of an environment where she's been very well cared for? Obviously, if you can live for 53 years on a vent, in bed, you've been very well taken care of. And do you disrupt that whole thing, and basically write her death sentence if you send her to a nursing home or provide lesser care?

PARTICIPANT 8

Ethical issues I would think [are] things such as when there's a sick child, sick parent, sick spouse, and they get turned down as far as some of the treatments that may in fact be beneficial for them. I think, you know, what are we looking at? We're looking at the value of the costs versus value of life. When you're looking at quality of life, ethically. When you send somebody home when they're not really ready to go, and there's nobody in the home to take care of them, you're looking at the quality, that person's life versus what it's saving as far as money. These are all ethical issues.

PARTICIPANT 15

Organizationally, we used to spend a lot of time talking about systems that would improve clinical outcomes. And the way we chose which systems to look at, we chose who the sickest patients were, or where the patients were most at risk, or what the single driver was, or what the best was for the patient. Because, in that era, everything was good for the hospital or the organization. That changed. We worked backwards. We started looking at outcomes data in terms of financial data. Identifying which were the major DRGs [diagnosis-related groups] where we lost money. It didn't matter whether they were high volume or high risk to the patient; it just was the organization lost money; hence they would attract our attention. And so all of the organization's energy went to reducing the cost in areas where the organization had the most to gain, rather than where the patient did. And that became a fundamental, philosophical shift. It was subtle; then it became pervasive. Everything, then, became cost reduction. And fitting the patient in, you squeezed him in. ... You began scripting, truly people would send you scripts telling you what you would say to employees when you began to do things like close units, even though they were high volume, because they didn't bring in enough money. ... Or you cost shifted and made your outpatient visits twice as expensive as they had been in the past, because you still had a reimbursement percentage for those procedures that were high. People knew that. People watched that. That was nothing less than a horrible manipulation.

PARTICIPANT 10

I have some cardiac problems. And, evidently, the local anesthetic that is used for dental work causes sensitivity and throws me into some cardiac abnormalities. I have a crown that I need very badly. And yet, the dentist is terrified and I'm terrified to do this in his setting. And he spent a couple of months calling insurance companies and all. I'm going to have to be done in a monitored setting, whether it's an emergency room or an outpatient or a surgical center or somewhere. Rather than giving me the local anesthetic, I'm going to have to be done with some light nitrous or with something with cardiac monitors and the whole works. ... My dentist has called other dentists, and they will just say, "Well, the insurance companies won't pay for this anesthesia." If it's medically indicated, they have to. This just doesn't make sense to me. ... As soon as the medicine goes in, I get hypotensive and really, really sick. ... I also have a secondary dental plan, but the question seems to be who would have to pay for the anesthesia, because it's my heart that indicates that I would need the anesthesia. It seems to me that should be covered by [my insurance company]. But, [my insurance company] doesn't cover crowns, so it's just this big ole complicated mess.

PARTICIPANT 14

The preceding four vignettes show how doing real or potential harm relative to costs can jeopardize the best interests of the patient or family. Thus Participant 8 was able to foresee serious consequences, even death, if the 65-year old woman with polio was denied care by her HMO. Participant 15 raised the ethical issue of denying needed care—a harm—to persons in order to save money. Participant 10 highlighted the harm or potential harm that can happen to patients and nurses when an entire organization puts money before ethics. Participant 14 is caught in the middle regarding which of two insurance companies will pay for the anesthesia needed to have dental work done. This feud between the insurers leaves Participant 14 without badly needed dental care.

Ray et al. (2002), in a qualitative study that included 32 registered nurses and 14 executives in health care settings, sought to develop theory that explained "the basic social process for balancing cost while maintaining organizational caring within the economically driven health care environment" (p. 7). The core category that emerged from their research was the loss of trust, which the authors attributed to health care organizations being driven by the bottom line to ensure their survival. As with our study participants, several nurses in this study also commented on the importance of the bottom line over adequate staffing or quality patient care. When the latter two factors are compromised, the result is the infliction of real or potential harm.

Injustice: Limited or Lack of Access to Health Care. Simply stated, the ethical principle of justice means giving persons what they are due or owed. Other words associated with justice are *fairness* and *equality*. Herein we are talking about justice as it relates to access to health care. The ANA *Code of Ethics for Nurses with Interpretive Statements* (2001) notes, "the nurse supports initiatives to address barriers to health, such as poverty, homelessness, unsafe living conditions, abuse and violence, and lack of access to health services" (p. 24). The following vignettes ultimately highlight violation of the ethical principle of justice as it relates to access to health care, with the study participants as providers and as recipients of care.

Well, we just found out last week that we can no longer see these women. That they have to go to their primary care provider to make an appointment to get their medication renewed. We can't see them anymore in the well-women clinic for their Pap smear; they have to go to their primary care provider. I think that's an ethical problem. Because we specialize in women's health, and we have specialties; all of us who work in that clinic are midwives or nurse practitioners; most are OB-GYN nurse practitioners or women's health nurse practitioners. I think I'm the only adult nurse practitioner, but I've got years and years of women's health experience. And, the primary care providers, I'm sorry, are not as good in women's health, geriatric women's health, as providers in our clinic. So, they are not getting a service, a medical service that they really could use. By being denied, they're being denied access to a particular type of care. And that's a shame.

PARTICIPANT 1

Clients had the choice of getting a [managed care] card, getting their services through that. And, we helped, we facilitated that, feeling that was the way to go. We were real excited, actually came up with a plan where we started retooling public health nurses so that they became more home based. We decreased the number of clinics as the clients went more and more into [managed care]. Got access to private physicians, along with those who had insurance. We were really excited, shifted the nurses, and wrote a grant. Got a great health families' program where nurses were working in the home for child abuse, linking families, just a wonderful program. [Managed care company] went out of business with Medicaid. Ended their relationship with Medicaid. There were no other providers; those children streamed back into our now decreased child health clinics. We had to increase the child health clinics and double the workload of the nurses because we had no additional positions. And we are still struggling with that; we are still struggling with balancing increased child health clinics and nurses' commitments to home-based visiting case management. The state is going to find another managed care provider, but that sort of problem of a managed care provider saying, "I changed my mind," and next month you have all those Medicaid clients back.

PARTICIPANT 6

As midwives we follow the midwifery philosophy of care, which includes a midwifery model of care. And that being that birth is a natural, normal progression, life change, life event. And we try not to intervene except when appropriate. And, so, as an educator, when I teach the midwifery model of care in the classroom, we teach the students to sit down with the woman and form a bond, a relationship, so that a partnership can be developed between the patient and the provider, or the midwife. Well, since managed care has come about, what I find the students reporting back to me is that in the classroom we teach it one way, the midwifery model way, where we sit down and converse and have a partnership with the patient. But when the student then goes into the clinical setting that model of care cannot always be realized. It has a lot to do with the numbers of patients that have to be seen by the provider, and, if first of all, the patient even has access to the midwife.

PARTICIPANT 12

Stepped out, put my weight on my foot, and my foot hurt. Hadn't done anything to it that I knew of. I will give you a little background; I'm a jogger. Continues to hurt at the base of the great toe. I go to my gatekeeper at [HMO] who says, "xray it," and "there's nothing wrong with it." But it was hurting, and it was swelling, and it was getting inflamed looking. So, I end up on crutches, no other xrays, none. Pain medicines. So this physician decided, even though the sed rate was not up, it must be some arthritic issue. He did not send me to a specialist, even though I requested one. Did not send me to an orthopedic doctor [although] I requested one. Refused. Time went on. I was on crutches for three months; it developed into RSD. Reflexive sympathetic dystrophy. I was off work for three months. Ended up then with an orthopedic doctor, who diagnosed it as RSD, because my gatekeeper doctor just couldn't figure it out.

PARTICIPANT 15

The preceding four vignettes show how the violation of the ethical principle of justice as it relates to access to health care can vary. With Participant 1 the use of primary care providers as the entry point into the health care system denied women access to the special expertise about women's health that midwives and women's health nurse practitioners possess. With Participant 6 a managed care provider abruptly ended its relationship with Medicaid and left a cohort of children with limited or no access to nurse providers. As with Participant 1, Participant 12 had a problem of access—in this case, student access—to the special expertise of and philosophy about midwifery. Participant 15 was denied access to a health care specialist by her HMO gatekeeper, who refused to refer her to one.

Several authors address the ethical principle of justice and its two component parts: access to health care and allocation of resources (e.g., Beauchamp & Childress, 2001; Emanuel, 2000; Volbrecht, 2002). Our focus here, based on the preceding vignettes, is limited or lack of access to health care within MCOs. Erlen (2002) presents a case study of such a situation. Nurses in a home health agency are experiencing moral distress because some of their patients' insurance companies dropped them; the insurance companies also discontinued nurses' visits because the patients already had received the allowable number. Some of the nurses tried to continue to see the patients but ran into other problems such as lack of reimbursement and liability. In addition, the nurses inquire why persons in business are making health care decisions. The patients, too, are upset and confused.

Erlen (2002) then discusses the concept of access to health care. First, she offers a definition of access credited to Emanuel (2000): "Access refers to whether people who are—or should be—entitled to health care services receive them" (p. 8). Second, she notes that, under conditions of unlimited resources, access to care is not restricted. Third, she identifies some of the conditions under which access to care may be restricted: (1) insufficient providers, (2) hours facilities are closed for care, (3) remote location of facilities, (4) lack of transportation to facilities, (5) lack of services for child care, (6) rejection of services by provider gatekeepers, and (7) rejection of referrals to specialists by provider gatekeepers. The voices of the four research participants addressing limited or lack of access to health care help to support Erlen's preceding seven conditions.

DISCUSSION

Before discussing this chapter and recommendations for nursing and health care, we noted some limitations of the study. First, the nurses included in this study were highly educated; different stories and comments may have emerged from other nurses. Second, the four categories we identified from the data were not always mutually exclusive; for example, the category "limited or lack of access to health care" often interfaced with the category of "money talks, aka the bottom line." Third, the vignettes we selected from the data might not be the ones that other nurses would have selected.

In this chapter we have taken the viewpoint that managed, or more accurately (mis)managed, care has resulted in ethical concerns about and violation of ethical principles. Through qualitative research, we supported our viewpoint by identifying and describing four categories of unethical principles (i.e., disrespect for persons; loss of autonomy; inflicting real or potential harm; and injustice) and by listening to the voices of the study participants. Now we turn our attention to discussion of this chapter when the research data are viewed as a whole rather than categorically.

Our data suggest that the establishment of an ethical climate in MCOs may be difficult. Hinderer and Hinderer (2001) offer three reasons for this difficulty:

1. Ethical considerations typically are not given a high priority in bureaucratic organizations.

2. Accountability is diffused.
3. Ethical concerns can be divisive and can be viewed as intractable.

How then does an MCO change its ethical climate from one that violates ethical principles to one that supports them? We offer the following three recommendations:

1. *Create an ethical culture.* Culture embodies shared values and beliefs that are transmitted over time to those within the culture. Given that MCOs are one type of culture and that ethical values and beliefs are one aspect of that culture, an ethical assessment of an MCO should occur first. This is a top-to-bottom assessment. Because an ethical climate begins at the top, the leaders of the organization must themselves be ethical and committed to a visible and sustainable culture of integrity. Some suggestions for accomplishing this goal include (1) incorporate ethical values into the mission statement and strategic plan; (2) give representatives from throughout the organization a voice in the writing of the ethical component of the mission statement and strategic plan; (3) place the mission statement and strategic plan in highly visible places throughout the organization and on its Web site; and (4) designate persons who have responsibility and accountability for designing and maintaining the ethics infrastructure of the organization, including how ethical violations will be handled (Doran, 2003).

2. *Understand moral distress and how to decrease it.* Moral distress represents the uncomfortable to anguished feelings that occur when persons cannot maintain their integrity because of institutional constraints. The outcomes of moral distress include "guilt, anger, frustration, powerlessness, and loss of meaning in one's work" (Volbrecht, 2002, p. 133). Although our study participants did not use the term *moral distress,* many of them experienced it as our research vignettes poignantly showed. With pressure from MCOs to cut costs, including costs related to nursing, moral distress has become common among nurses. According to Erlen (2001), the following strategies may help to address and to decrease moral distress: (1) encourage ongoing and planned dialogue among nurses through a supportive environment that allows them to discuss their concerns and feelings among themselves and with their superiors; (2) establish a support system that may be formal or informal and that includes mentors who are experienced with ethical dilemmas and moral distress; (3) provide ethics education that includes case studies and conferences, ethics grand rounds, ethics consultants, and

continuing education programs in ethics; and (4) understand policies and procedures in one's organization that address ethics, and revise them or advocate for them when needed.

3. *Use the power inherent in the ANA* Code of Ethics for Nurses. The 2001 ANA *Code of Ethics for Nurses with Interpretive Statements* empowers nurses. First, authors of the code note that "It is the profession's nonnegotiable ethical standard" (p. 5). Understanding the power and implications of this statement should help nurses decrease moral distress in ethically compromised MCOs. Nurses are not out there alone; they have, in the code, an ally and an advocate for what is the right, the good, and the ethical in their professional practice. Second, the 2001 ANA *Code of Ethics for Nurses with Interpretive Statements* also addresses the inner nurse regarding ethical self-respect, unity of character, and personal integrity. The nurse has a duty to personal and professional self to maintain her or his ethicalness. In addition, according to the code, "Nurses have a duty to remain consistent with both their personal and professional values and to accept compromise only to the degree that it remains an integrity-preserving compromise" (ANA, 2001, p. 19). Thus this code addresses an external ethical standard (the written code) and an internal ethical standard (the nurse's character). Working together, and in combination with other nurses, these standards compose ethical nurse power that helps to change ethically tainted organizations.

SUMMARY

Our viewpoint has been that managed care, with its focus on cost cutting, too often has sacrificed quality, quantity, and access to health care. The result has been violation of the ethical principles of respecting persons, respecting autonomy, preventing harm, and ensuring justice. These violations manifested themselves in the study data as confusion and (dis)continuity of care; as routines, regulations, and rules that bind; as money

talks, aka the bottom line; and as limited or lack of access to health care. We offered three suggestions for how ethically compromised organizations and the nurses within them can empower themselves so that ethical principles are honored: (1) create an ethical culture, (2) understand moral distress and how to decrease it, and (3) use the power inherent in the ANA *Code of Ethics for Nurses.*

REFERENCES

American Nurses Association. (2001). *Code of ethics for nurses with interpretive statements.* Washington, DC: Author.

Beauchamp, T.L., & Childress, J. F. (2001). *Principles of biomedical ethics* (5th ed.). New York: Oxford University Press.

Dombeck, M. T., & Olsan, T. H. (2002). Ethics and managed care. *Journal of Interprofessional Care, 16,* 221-233.

Doran, S. J. (2003). The business imperative behind a sound ethics program. *Managed Care Quarterly, 11,* 49-51.

Dworkin, R. W. (2002). Where have all the nurses gone? *Public Interest, 15,* 23-38.

Emanuel, E. J. (2000). Justice and managed care: Four principles for the just allocation of health care resources. *Hasting Center Report, 30*(3), 8-16.

Erlen, J. A. (2001). Moral distress: A pervasive problem. *Orthopaedic Nursing, 20*(2), 76-80.

Erlen, J. A. (2002). When there are limits on health care resources. *Orthopaedic Nursing, 21*(4), 69-73.

Hinderer, D. E., & Hinderer, S. R. (2001). *A multidisciplinary approach to health care ethics.* Mountain View, CA: Mayfield.

Ray, M. A., Turkel, M. C., & Marino, F. (2002). The transformative process for nursing in workforce redevelopment. *Nursing Administration Quarterly, 26*(2), 1-14.

Silva, M. C., Fletcher, J. J., & Sorrell, J. M. (2004). Ethics in community-oriented nursing practice. In M. Stanhope & J. Lancaster (Eds.), *Community and public health nursing* (6th ed., pp. 134-135). St. Louis, MO: Mosby.

Ulrich, C., Soeken, K., & Miller, N. (2003). Predictors of nurse practitioners' autonomy: Effects of organizational, ethical, and market characteristics. *Journal of the American Academy of Nurse Practitioners, 15,* 319-325.

Volbrecht, R. M. (2002). *Nursing ethics: Communities in dialogue.* Upper Saddle River, NJ: Prentice Hall.

Learning a Practice of Uncertainty

Clinical Ethics and the Nurse

LAURIE ZOLOTH

As the entire nation watched, the bitterly divided family spoke of their grief and of their loss. On every side of the issue, and from every living room and kitchen, millions became involved in the strangely public, intensely private, long dying of Teresa Schiavo (University of Miami Ethics Program, 2005). For nurses, the drama was especially poignant, for nurses knew that the case was neither unprecedented nor uniquely tragic: such are the ethical dilemmas of any critical care setting (Ackerman & Strong, 1989) and of every long-term care facility. Such is the setting for many families—conflicted in what they ought to do and divided by the intensity of the ethical choices before them in the modern health care setting. Nursing care is now so skilled and medicine and technology so well crafted that many deaths in the clinical settings in which nurses work are ones that are "considered deaths," meaning that they involve difficult choices about when to withdraw the most aggressive therapies. For the nurse, ethical dilemmas always involve the most complex use of skill, compassion, and reflection; and the dilemma that involves a withdrawal of therapy that in some cases is indicated, and in others not, enmeshes the nurse in a necessary but uncertain practice (Kuczewski & Pinkus, 1999; La Puma & Schiedermayer, 1994). The contention of this chapter is that clinical ethics can be learned, via a method of decision making that clearly defines and describes a narrative. Nurses can lead the way toward the interpretation of that narrative and can ensure that the voice of the patient and the family is articulated clearly and that the choices and the values that inform them remain central to treatment decisions.

In this chapter, the claim is made for humility and mastery. As in the Schiavo case, there will be many chances for error. Some will be avoidable through a serious use of this method, and with practice and the trust of a good ethics committee. Others will be difficult to avoid. The reality of ethics at the bedside in nursing care is that the case by case, story by story, word by word, one will develop a community of responsibility and of response-ability for ethical decision making embedded in many aspects of the clinical practice of nursing itself.

The goal of this chapter is to defend and describe a process and a method for clinical decision making when there is an ethical conflict about how to proceed. The contention of the chapter is that a well-trained nurse will be a vital part of this process, and further, that if a good process of clinical ethics is used early in the tragic course of illness and injury, the wrenching dramas such as the Schiavo case may be avoided.

ORIGINS AND DEFINITIONS

Ethics asks the question "What is the good act, and what makes it so?" "How do I know?" asks the thoughtful practitioner, "Why do we act as we do in situations of ethical conflict?" Indeed, how does the practitioner balance her or his personal reactions and values with the many others who also face the decision?

Like much of nursing, ethical decision making cannot be enacted alone, nor by one practitioner or profession. Cases emerge over time, as diagnoses change and hoped-for treatment results fail, and suddenly, as families are confronted with new tragedies for which they are utterly unprepared (Pence, 1995). As a nurse, you will have far more experience with such cases—but for all of your expertise, you will not be an expert on the values, dreams, and faith of any particular family—hence the question of "the good act" is a complex problem.

Good ethics works best when the health care team and the family and patient balance the public and the private acts of choice, in a small room in the middle of the day, in the middle of the clinical context, in the midst of complex lives, and at the heart of small, individual tragic necessities that medicine places before families. Life-and-death decision making is the largest of problems, placed within the smallest venue called public, meaning the moral crossroads where doctors, families, patients, and staff meet. What should be the character of that meeting? What does such a practice mean? What is the future of such a fragile enterprise, one that is deliberative and set in the context of uncertainty (Kushner & Thomasma, 2001)?

The practice of clinical ethics suggests that at such a crossroads, having a road map and a guide for one who is not a native to the country but who is a stranger there is a useful thing. Hence it was that when the first nationally clinical ethics drama was discussed in the literature, that of Karen Ann Quinlan, there was a tentative suggestion that perhaps clinically based committees, "prognostication committees," might be of use in addressing moral dilemmas in the clinic, instead of adversarial, awkward judicial proceedings. From that nearly tangential observation, the practice of clinical ethics consultation committees has arisen (Wear, 1998). For most nurses who serve in hospital settings, the institutional ethics committee will be the place for the discussion of issues that arise at the bedside. For some, ethics consultation teams or individual ethicists will be used. In all of these cases, the informed participation of the nurse will be essential for the discussion. Nursing ethics is devoted to the idea that every voice—no matter how fragile or disempowered—must be heard in the process and that every reasonable option must be mapped and presented for discussion and consideration.

Training in clinical ethics begins with an accounting of its history. Clinical ethics began as a manifestation and application of the larger field of bioethics, which also considers dilemmas such as stem cell research, health care policy, and clinical research on new drugs. Clinical ethics, in contrast, is the study of and the resolution of actual cases as they present in the health care setting by physicians, social workers, therapists, and nurses who were called upon to make reflections on these cases.

Central to the discussion in the first years of clinical ethics was the notion that it brought a complicated mix of methods to the task. The field was concerned with pragmatic details and hence with the theory of pragmaticism or case-based, trial-and-error analysis. Normalizing the practice, however, was at that point, and is still, a contentious matter, for it touches on three issues that are unresolved. First, what is the nature of and standards for training as a clinical ethicist?

Second, should a licensing board regulate the practice? Finally, are there a series of best practices or, more strongly, an efficacious method for a clinical practice?

For many in the field, personal experiences or professional encounters of ethical dilemmas in health care led to clinical ethics. Hence many of the first participants were nurses, drawn from intensive care units, neonatal intensive care units, end-of-life settings, and acute care pediatrics. In these environments nurses have played a signal role, drawing on their pragmatic and cause-based approaches to decision making. For most, the pressing ethical dilemmas concerned the withholding of care and withdrawing of care in the setting where technology was utilized most fully. As the withdrawal of first artificial ventilation, then chemotherapy, and finally nutrition and hydration was rationalized (Faden, Beauchamp, & King, 1986), the attention of the field also began to consider classes of patients with whom one could make distinctions around the care withdrawal cases (Forrow, Wartman, & Brock, 1988). Cases began to emerge that concerned children and infants, that concerned formerly competent patients, and patients that were conscious and treatable, yet unhappy with their quality of life and not prepared to continue. Finally, as health care costs rose steadily, and the limits of the intensive care unit were extended, nurses and doctors themselves began to raise questions about treatment limitation, starting an entirely new sort of discussion about a unilateral physician- or hospital-driven policy decision that care was "futile" and hence could be withdrawn against the families wishes.

Cases such as Schiavo—following Quinlan, Cruzan, Barber, and Drabeck (*Barber v. Superior Court*, 1983; Legal Information Institute, 1990; *Matter of Quinlan*, 1976)—seem to define the parameters of the field. Yet such court cases might be avoided if a consistent policy of locally based ethics review is enacted. At stake for each nurse is whether a fully robust, fully open model of *moral community* could be built within the institution in which the nurse serves. To be certain, good ethical deliberation needs several preconditions to work well: accurate medical facts, a dedicated group of health care providers committed to an egalitarian process, and a stable health care setting in which to operate.

THE PROCESS OF CLINICAL ETHICS: AN EMERGING DISCIPLINE

Clinical ethics is the discipline of bioethics in the clinical setting, with dilemmas that first may emerge at the bedside, although many have their origins in health care policy. Clinical ethics processes are required by regulation and licensing agreements, but how to enact them varies. The nurse should be aware that clinical ethics rests on the core claims of bioethics, drawing on traditions in moral philosophy, theology, and the philosophy of law (Beauchamp & Childress, 2001). These claims also emerge from long-standing histories of debate in medicine and in nursing that stressed principles of beneficence (seeking to do the good) and nonmaleficence (do no harm). After the tragic history of the Nazi genocide, medicine and nursing had to face a new challenge, for doctors and nurses enthusiastically had supported the practice of medicalized torture (Lifton, 1988; Muller-Hill, 1988). Much of modern bioethics is rooted in the careful consideration of how to avoid training medical personnel who would "follow orders" blindly even when such orders direct immoral actions. New science and breakthroughs in medical technology also drove the discipline of bioethics: dialysis and organ transplantation, new experiments, and new research questions raised new ideas for consideration. Scandal and tragedy also drove the debate: in the 1970s, for example, revelations about the conduct of research in the Tuskegee syphilis trials, in which a cohort of all African American men in Mississippi was studied to track the late stages of disease and in which treatment of penicillin was withheld when it was discovered (Jones, 1974). In this case, nurses acted to convince the men of the worth of the trial and did not alert anyone to the withholding of key data from the men, much less inform the patients of the full scope of their condition and its treatment. In fact, in each of the cases of serious research misconduct, physicians did not act alone: nurses knew and did little to protect their patients. This came to be understood as a clear violation of an emerging role of the nurse.

Nursing grew as a profession at the same historical period that medicine intensified. Hence the question changed from "Can we intervene to save the patient?" to "Ought we to intervene to save the patient?" at the same time that nurses began to have a greater role in interventions. Many treatments that prolonged life formerly in the hands of doctors, such as intravenous line placement, gastrointestinal tube placement, and decisions about ventilation, were ones that implicated the nursing staff.

Along with the increasing empowerment and professionalization of nursing came the movement of empowerment of patients; hence truth telling, the hospice movement, acquired immunodeficiency syndrome, and breast cancer patient activism had an impact on the relationships of power, shifting the alliance between doctors, hospitals, nurses, and patients. Against this history ethical dilemmas are played out (Faden & Beauchamp, 1998; Maholwald, 1999).

What Is the Role of the Nurse in Clinical Ethics?

What do nurses mean by ethics and clinical ethics, and what does it mean to "do" ethics consultation? Why is clinical consultation different from a long chat with a clever and thoughtful colleague?

Bioethics is the application of the philosophical discipline of ethics found in moral and analytic traditions. As such, bioethics is an application of the discourse of ethics and not a branch of medicine, nursing, or the thoughtful, humanistic, and reflective "part" of medicine and nursing. Yet nurses have long had a practice that engages many of the issues in clinical ethics and that uses many of the classic tools of the tradition.

Clinical ethics is the deliberate consideration of treatment decisions faced by patients, families, and staff in the clinical setting. Clinical ethics involves a reflective process by which facts in the case are gathered and considered, the ethical questions are raised and analyzed, and different resolutions are suggested for the next step in clinical care. These suggestions have the force of moral persuasion: they then are carried out or are not carried out by the treatment team. The nurse may participate in this process at one or several levels: as sentinel and advocate for the patient, as messenger or translator of the problem, as participant in the ethics committee or team, or as nurse-expert.

Discussion follows of some of the many possible roles that must be considered in thinking about this question of what role the nurse can play in clinical ethics.

Nurse as Advocate for the Patient. When the nurse acts as a patient advocate, the nurse must assume that he or she is acting as the one who speaks on behalf of patients, often when the patients cannot speak for themselves. The role is familiar for the nursing profession: to articulate the narrative of the patient and to argue on behalf of the patient's needs. In this capacity, the nurse is the "insider" in the debates; asked to speak for the patient, she in a sense has that patient as her "client," articulating the case for what the patient would desire (Braddock, Edward, Hasenberg, Laidley, & Levison, 1999; Brock, 1987; Lidz, Appelbaum, & Meisel, 1988). In this role, the patient or family may confide in the nurse about their unhappiness with the treatment, the moral dilemma the treatments are creating, or the simple wish to end treatments.

Nurse as "Existential Messenger." Karen Stanley (1997) has called the nurse the "existential messenger" who carries the reality of end-of-line care and end-of-life realities between the health care team and the patient. In the dilemmas of bioethics, nurses can act as messengers or translators between one world—the hospital, its needs and functions and competing justice claims from other patients—and the needs of the patient, who may speak in another language, come from another culture, or have an utterly different perspective on the story of illness. In this account the nurse plays a role as neither insider nor outsider to the conflict. The role differs from advocacy in that the nurse understands that other patients and other needs compete with this patient's needs. In this role the nurse may be the first person to suggest that an ethical conflict has arisen, in which there is a conflict between family members over deep values or decisions, or the nurse may be the intermediate figure who recognizes a dissonance between the treatment goals and the actual process of the therapies, or one who can understand that the staff is morally anguished about treatment choices.

Nurse as Participant in Clinical Ethics Services or Committees. The bedside nurse often will be called on to be part of an ethics consultation process, which is a mandated part of the accreditation process of the Joint Commission on Accreditation of Healthcare Organizations. The nurse may be a part of a small, trained team or may work as a member of a larger committee.

Nurses Who Become Ethics Consultants. Ethicists typically come as outsiders and as strangers bringing outsider perspectives to the inside culture—secret knowledge, hierarchies, ritual activities, and alliances that exist within the clinical venue. This role was accepted at the beginning of the field when theologians and philosophers entered the clinical world not as insiders with clinical expertise but as strangers with a unique perspective and skill in identifying and framing the questions (Meisel & Kuczewski, 1996). However, with specialized training and education, nurses may leave the classic role of bedside nursing to act as ethics consultants. Moreover, the preference on some level is for the ethicist to be an "insider," for the role of the nurse to be expanded, merely to include this activity without additional cross-disciplinary training in philosophy or ethics, and crucially, for the loss of what nurses considered essential—estrangement from the encounter. Keeping the sense of being "outside" the debate when one is a nurse-ethicist means making a distinction between one's role as caregiver and one's role as "navigator" in an ethics process.

When nurses are clinical ethicists, they are not "captains of the ship," for it is the role as a navigator that marks the practice of ethics consultation as distinctive. Clinical ethicists and nurses who act in that capacity must know the map of the terrain; have an acute understanding of the language, scope, and force of previous arguments in the literature; must understand the way that the culture of the clinical world is organized and expressed; and hence must avoid pitfalls.

Clinical ethics, because it derives its potency from the work of language, as opposed to the care and touch-based behaviors characteristic of nursing, is a form of communicative ethics, rooted in the idea that the moral dilemma occurs in a particular context, at a particular moment in history, and within a particular moral community. When ethics committees meet, the space created is described as architectural in the literature—a moral space—creating a climate supportive of moral discourse within a highly structured world of medicine. In part, nurses' awareness of this complex context leads to the final point: The scope of the work for the nurse who is attentive to ethics, who finds herself or himself working with an ethics committee, is to be understood as broad. "Doing" clinical ethics means making ethics an integral part of the organization of the medical institution and of raising the ethical issues in day-to-day practice, and not just at times of crisis, from clinical to organizational ethical issues.

What Clinical Ethics Is Not: Psychotherapy

Clinical ethics ought to be a task of heightening awareness of conflict, not mediating. Varieties of mediation and of therapeutic encounter do not substitute for ethics, for at its core, grave moral conflict and its encounter is not a matter that can be negotiated or a matter of contract, but a conflict about the very meaning of being. Ethics is a practice that requires the development and enhancement of a pragmatic skill over time. Clinical ethics requires application and testing in the clinical arena. One cannot master a body of knowledge without application, for at the bedside and in the consultation the theories meet the rigorous test of facticity. Ongoing practice, peer review, responsivity, and mentoring are required to develop a serious practice of excellence.

Finally, developing a practice of nursing ethics, like any other aspect of nursing practice requires colleagues and peer review, for reflective knowledge does not emanate from a single point, nor is clinical ethics a matter of one person's opinion. Clinical ethics is a matter of interruption and dissent. As ethicist Robert

Gibbs (2000) notes, ethics is modeled on the speaker who is interrupted by the question. Because the nurse is so often one who hears so many questions, the nurse's practice is by nature "interrupted" by the needs of the other, making the nurse ideally prepared to participate in clinical ethics cases.

A History of Different Models

From the first mention of ethics committee–like bodies—first made in the case of Karen Ann Quinlan and Baby Doe regulations, in which they are merely suggested—to the formal Joint Commission on the Accreditation of Healthcare Organizations guidelines, in which they are required, there has been a development in the concept of methods for clinical ethics consultation (Unicorn Media for Concern for Dying, 1984). An interesting history of ethics consultation can be drawn in which at first ethics committees were the dominant accepted model for a long time, yet after which, the use of a full committee for consultation fell out of favor in many venues and has been replaced by competing models, most notably, the use of a single expert (medical model) or the use of a subcommittee for case consultation. This chapter defends the large committee/moral community model, although other models can be used well and are found widely in practice. Nurses can lead the way in the construction of a committee at their facilities, and if so, a strong argument could be made for the sort of moral community that an ethics committee can create. What is the nature, goal, and function of an ethics committee? Let us turn to the answer.

First, the nature of most clinical ethical dilemmas is such that they are characterized by fundamental value questions about which reasonable persons can and will disagree so that no one person nor a group of three can express such complex dissent fully; hence a good ethics process will foster a lively debate on the different values at stake in every dilemma. Second, the nature of expertise in the process is the acquired skill at lifting up each moral appeal and helping to shape these into concrete and discreet clinical choices—thoughtfully to ask the questions, not to provide the answers. Unlike for a medical consultant, such a task is never performed in isolation. Finally, the nature of ethical discourse is such that it is best accomplished in a face-to-face inclusive conversation with all those involved, most importantly of course, the patient and the family. Nurses should always seek this inclusive conversation and should ensure that patients and families are the fulcrum in the framing of the conversation, for ethics consultation is a conversation with them, not about them.

Creating the Moral Community

Ethics committees can be structured best around two issues: first, of membership, and second, in underlying rationale. How should the membership of an ethics committee be established? The selection of members is not a random process but rests on the establishment of mutual regard for all of the professionals involved in the health care team, in the respect for the community in which the medical center is located, in a consideration of the dignity of leadership itself, and in the need for a ethicist who is, complexly, philosopher, educator, and navigator and who has the rhetorical authority to direct discourse. A supportive environment for genuine ethics discourse and the development of a sustainable moral community rests first in the selection of leadership and then a model of nurse-physician co-chairs who model equality and inclusiveness in the most basic structure of the committee process.

Selection of members is also a key methodological choice. A strong philosophical commitment to diversity of ideas, backgrounds, life experiences, social economic statuses, values, and moral locations is critical. A wide and broad search for members of the institution and local community to seek representation of the variety of deeply held values that are inflected on health care decisions must be a part of a strong committee's relationship to the community that it serves. This commitment raises serious issues for many committees and, here I might argue, in this commitment committees best come to understand themselves and their role. For whom is ethics consultation "done"? Why the performance of ethics in medicine? The understanding that the consultation is one in which a moral community as a whole—staff, patient, family, and the social world that is shared and is placed within the community, the nation, and the many complex relationships and moral obligations—is a core understanding. Bioethicist Jonathon Moreno (1997) argues that one "decides together" and hence "does" ethics only within a moral community and subject to the network of norms and duties that hold it firm. Hence building the community is the first task, and this central task will be at the heart of clinical ethics. In clinical ethics consultation, the entire committee is trained to understand and hear cases that come before it. Thus in the method I suggest, the community is a "responsive" one, which means the patient (if possible), the family, and the staff come together with the committee to discuss the options available to them and to ask the question *What is the right act, and what makes it so?* The product of the encounter is the process itself, a collaborative process that allows all voices to be heard and a decision to be made about the best course to take (Macklin, 1987).

CASE CONSULTATION

Clinical ethics not only is a matter of anticipating that case and building a moral community in which it can be heard fully and understood thoughtfully but also must be, if it is to be transmitted successfully as a discipline, a teachable and replicable skill. This is where the theory of consultation and the pragmatic practice of case review are tested, so the method of consultation ought to be a standard, replicable conversation, one that allows patient and staff to depend on a time frame, a process, and an order of debate (Dubler & Liebman, 2004). This argues for a clear method of clinical consultation, which must be used. The method I and my colleagues have used since 1988 is divided into three steps: the first part is the gathering of the essential narrative of the case and the context, the second part is the delineation of credible options, and the final part is the deliberation among the options and the justification of the chosen one among many—the conclusion of the narrative. The method is casuistic in that it places the particular case against others in the practice of the committee, it is principle based in that it uses the justifying language of bioethics, and it is narrative in that it uses the shape of the narrative structure of the consultation to arrive at a conclusion.

The nurse will need to master several skills as a basis for all work in bioethics: the nurse will have to learn how to identify moral dilemmas, to seek and reflect on a personal and professional sense of what is ethical behavior and what makes it so. Next, the nurse must reflect thoughtfully on the difference between the nurse's moral "location" and that of her patients and why there may well be a difference in such moral locations. Finally—and perhaps most critically—the nurse must find and consolidate the ability to speak up when the nurse perceives an ethical problem, no matter how difficult and no matter what the personal consequences. These are the components in the process of moral agency, and the nurse must be a thoughtful moral agent, or no process of case consultation can be valid.

To a great extent, the ability of the nurse to be a thoughtful moral agent is the core of all of clinical ethics. Such ability can be nurtured and can be developed. The contention here that simple moral agency and simply "speaking up" is not enough. Being a thoughtful moral agent also requires a step-by-step method of case consultation.

What Is the Purpose of a Methodology in Bioethics Case Consultation?

The use of a distinctive and carefully considered method is a promise to consider the case at hand, for the committee to reflect carefully and consistently. Each member needs to approach the case with attention to the principles of equality and equity, with a systematic and replicable method, and with the intention of learning from the experiences. The mix of participants who will hear the case may vary, but the method they will use will be consistent. The nurse who feels that he or she has a case to bring to the committee should prepare what to present before the discussion begins. Such a method is grounded in respect for the clinical experience of the staff and for the history and collective wisdom of the medical team as it faces every case. Such a method also displays respect for the independence and perspective of the patient and for the patient's family and community. The ethics conversation is a special kind of discourse aimed at the creation of protected space, a "moral space" or "moral community" in which to face difficult moral decisions that arise in the course of medical treatment.

The leader of the ethics discussion next describes how the process will proceed, essentially in three parts. In the first, the committee members will gather all the relevant information about the case. In the second, they will describe all the possible options they could pursue. In the third, the members openly will consider how to justify or defend their choice of one of the options. The following is one example of how this method works in the clinical world: The method begins with a ritual of sorts; what one argues shapes the discourse. In a paragraph read aloud, one states the primary claims (Zoloth & Rubin, in press):

> *The Formal Opening:* All cases begin with a reading of the formal opening statement. This marks the considered beginning of the discussion.
>
> *"Welcome to the ethics committee. We meet here today to discuss the case of _____. In meeting here, we welcome you all in the spirit of searching for the good and right act, and we know that we are here out of the best motives, in a spirit of good will and openness. Everyone here is entitled to speak freely without fear of ramifications. If anyone has any prejudices about this case, or any reason that they ought to be excused from our discussion, we ask them to say so at this time. Confidentiality is basic to the committee's work, and our promise of confidentiality is absolute. All opinions expressed in the room will be considered confidential and are not to be discussed in any other venue. Our primary focus is on the patient, and we will keep in mind in all of our deliberations the voice and the interests of the patient. It is not our only concern. The wisdom of the entire team is important to us. Our goal is to build*

a moral community to surround the patient and the decisions about the welfare of the person in our care. In this work the experience of each team member is of equal importance. We welcome families to join us if they choose. We understand and value the special place that families have at the core of the healing process. It is an imperative voice, and we are eager to listen closely to what the family has to say. We are not a tribunal, not a court; we are not here to judge the family or to rule on the decisions that are faced by the team. We welcome the primary caregivers who may be here for the first time, and we want to assure you that your special relationships and advocacy will be honored as well. With your help, and with your frank speech, we can, as a committee, reflect on and recommend some possible courses for action today. We may need to meet again. Ethics cases are often complex and sometimes need to be revisited. Our goal is not to provide you with an answer, but with a process by which you can come to a decision about the next step in your plans."

My claim is that clinical ethics consultation falters without clear methods for the case itself. A formally read statement creates the time and space for reflection.

The case then unfolds with the primary spokesperson, named as the one who brings the case, explaining in his or her own words why the case is an ethical dilemma and what choice is faced with such difficulty. This process contains six elements:

1. *The presumption of good will* (from Emmanuel Kant's idea that the basis for ethical action is a good will): If there are members or guests who have discernible motives that could be considered prejudicial to the case, they ought to be identified.

   Nurses, residents, or others with relatively less power in the hospital may have a hard time accepting the notion that they can speak freely in front of administrators or physicians without later ramifications. Central to the goals of the committee is that all can speak freely without such fear.

2. *Confidentiality:* Confidentiality is basic to the functioning of the committee. The principle of confidentiality is absolute. All opinions and statements must never become a matter of general hospital discussion, in any capacity, in any other venue.

3. *Patient-centered decision making:* Patients are at the center of the medical enterprise itself. Their ultimate vulnerability informs the efforts of all health care personnel. This is especially true in the hospital setting. The internal ethics committee has a clear focus on the independent voice and interests of the patient.

4. *Collegial relationships:* The wisdom of the nurse, the community members, the social worker, the administrator, and the physician who sit on the committee are of equal importance. No position in the hierarchal system by itself gives special weight to the words of any member; all are important to the main enterprise—the building of the moral community.

5. *Families are welcome:* Families are offered participation in the process of the consultation unless the conflict only exists between members of the staff. The family must not be made to feel that they are at a tribunal. They will not be judged by the committee. Kinship does not mean ownership of the patient, but kinship is critical in health care human values. Although the family's input is an imperative voice for the committee to hear, it is not an absolute voice. Often the dilemma exists precisely because the views of the family and the views of the team are divergent.

6. *The primary caregivers:* The internal ethics committee acknowledges the special place at the table of the patient's primary caregivers. The primary team members should understand that the relationship and their advocacy will be honored and that their opinions and responses will be at the core of the discussion. All primary caregivers on the staff are urged to come to the meeting and should be reminded that nothing is "unsafe" to say at the meeting itself.

A recommendation and not a decision is the goal of the meeting: the process of discourse is central, but the final decision remains within the physician-patient relationship.

The next step of the process is the actual hearing of the case (Davis, 1991). Any member of the health care team may bring a case to the committee, and the patient or family may bring a case. Sometimes the issues will present primarily as a physician-nurse conflict or as a "breakdown in communication." But often what staff may identify as communication problems are really sincere conflicts in values and ethics. The leader of this process should be trained to separate ethical conflicts from other issues that may arise and to decide with the presenter the best venue for discussion. The presenter will be asked for an initial problem statement. If the nurse is the one bringing the case, the nurse must think about how to frame the ethical problem and ask, "What is troubling about this case?" and how one's values, belief structure, and intellectual commitments underlie the issues at stake.

Hearing the case is done via a formal process as well, with each participant telling their part in the narrative: first the medical story (for good ethics can rest only on good medical facts); then the patient's own story (for the wishes of the patient are primary); then the context of the narrative: social, familiar, workplace, friends, culture, religion; and then the account of the nurse.

The medical facts section begins with a concise medical history: the diagnosis and the prognosis and the history and result of each medical intervention. The following questions should be asked: What was expected of each medical intervention? What were the short- and long-term expectations of care? What went wrong? What proceeded as expected? What has the health care team done? Is the patient dying? Is the patient stable? What is the research about the disease? What have other consults determined? What are the relevant laboratory findings? Where are we in the trajectory of illness? What are the outcome measures, if available?

When patient preferences are considered, these questions should be raised: What does the patient want? (The conscious adult patient and the older child must be asked what he or she wants.) Is the patient competent, and is the patient capable of making a statement (verbal or nonverbal) of her or his desires? (Be clear about the distinction between a patient's competence and capacity.) What does the patient say exactly? What did the patient write before this if the patient cannot speak for herself or himself? What did the patient write or say to a legal surrogate? (This may be the agent named in the Patient Self-Determination Form, a form suggested in many state laws as a requirement for inclusion in the hospital admissions process if the patient is over 18). The committee must ask, Could the patient's desire be understood from any conversation that the patient may have had with family and friends? (In many cases, a healthy young adult never writes a will or leaves instructions of this kind.) Even children technically not yet competent (under the age of 18) still may have an understanding of their situation, especially if they have been ill for a prolonged period, and will need to be a part of a process geared to obtaining assent to procedures, which is the standard in pediatric cases (American Academy of Pediatrics, n.d.).

In the section on family systems these are the questions that should be asked: We assume that the family makes the decisions in the best interest of the child, unless we are in possession of evidence pointing to the contrary. In the adult patient, we assume that families love and care for one another unless we have evidence to the contrary, and we assume that families may have access to special private knowledge about patient's wishes. We use the term *family* in the broadest sense, asking, for example, Who are the real decision makers in the family? How old are the parents in pediatric cases? What is the meaning of this illness for them?

What is the meaning of tragedy or death? Who will speak for the family? Who speaks as the translator of the medical team's needs to the family? Who will care for the patient? Who has cared for the patient? What does this person know of the patient's treatment preferences? What is the living arrangement of the family? Are there other children? Grandparents? Who visits the patient? What are the nature, frequency, and consistency of the visits? Under what constraints (social, economic) does the family operate? Has this family every experienced an event like this before? Is placement an option for this family? Other relatives who may care for the patient? Do class, race, or gender affect the family in a particular way?

These are the questions that must be asked about community involvement: Who is the community of meaning for the patient and the family? Is religion a feature of their lives? What is the nature of the involvement with the religious community? Does this faith tradition have any particular practices or regulations that we need to be aware of? Are there other communities that are relevant? (Powell, 1995) Unions? Neighborhoods? Friends at work? Political groups? Scouting? School? Illness support communities? What was the patient's life like before this illness? What communities and rituals helped this family in their daily life, before the drama of the hospital? Does this patient work? What is the work of the adults in the family? What is the ethnic and racial background of the family?

When the discussions turn to social and economic factors, these are the questions that must be asked: What is the real cost and who will pay? What are the social and economic resources of the family? What are the social and economic costs to the hospital for this care? Will a third-party payer pay for the care? What are the restraints on this arrangement? Is placement (institutional or foster) possible?

For this method, nursing and other staff input is key. What is the opinion of the team that is caring for the patient? Is this opinion mutually shared and expressed, or is there disagreement among the staff? Has the team ever had a case like this on this unit? In another institution? In their own family? Remembering that no statement will place anyone in jeopardy, let each staff member express his or her opinion of the problems in the case. Remember to include all shifts and ancillary team members, not just physician and nurses. For example, what is the role and voice of the house staff?

The section on the daily life of patients should include an hour-by-hour description of the events in a patient's day and night as witnessed by the team and parents. What is sought is not the "quality" of life but an objective account of what interventions occur and how the patient reacts to them. The committee needs to know whether the interventions are painful and/or intrusive? What is the level of pain medication that is needed and the frequency of its administration? Are there periods when the patient is comfortable, resting, and interactive?

Finally, extra issues may arise, and these may be the ones about which the nurse has information. The nurse should reflect on whether any information about the patient, the family, the team, or the hospital is morally relevant to the discussion? Are there important political or public relations issues? Are lawsuits threatened? Is the press involved? Are there transitions in the team or unit? Are there research interests at stake? Teaching interests?

In the method I suggest, the bedside nurse is key, and I urge the nurse to give a careful account of the patient's situation, hour by hour if necessary. Why is this so central? For many methods, the search is rather more abstract: the committee is urged to think about the "quality of life issue." But every nurse can testify to the vagueness of that phrase, for the quality of a life is an indeterminate thing.

List All Options for the Patient

The second part of the method is to list all the options for an outcome of the ethical dilemma. Decide at the outset whether some of these are desires that cannot be met under the actual physical circumstances. Listing the *IDEAL PICTURE* and then noting the team's distance from this and noting the team's *WORST FEAR* are important. Then narrow the information from the widest range to two or more decision options. Each decision will have consequences, some beneficial, some burdensome, on the various actors identified, not just on the patient. Note the consequences for the family, the team and even for the larger society. At this point in the process, not to attach values to the outcomes is important. Simply list what the results are likely to be if each course is taken, and the effect on the various actors. The final part of the method focuses on the evaluation of these options.

The Normative Part of the Process

Ethics asks the question "What is the right act and what makes it so?" But *each person* needs to reflect and then speak to the question, and this at first may be difficult for a nurse to do in the multidisciplinary setting of the

committee and in front of families and patients. Yet truthful telling is what is needed. The leader of the committee process must ask, "In light of this case, which option do you recommend, and how do you justify that choice?"

The appeal to *consequences* is only one ethical appeal, but it is an important one. The focus is on the utility of the outcome and the happiness of the parties involved. For this argument, one must consider each option and the positive and negative outcomes for each choice. Other appeals must be considered. Second is the appeal to *rights*. Basic rights involve obligations. What rights are basic in the case: The right to informed consent? The right not to be killed? Next, the committee must consider the appeal to *respect for persons* (sometimes called autonomy). The committee values certain action that allows for human flourishing and values individuals who have the potential for such action. The committee also must consider the appeal to the *virtues:* integrity, compassion, courage, honesty, fidelity, and role-specific duties. An appeal often difficult to reveal but of critical importance is the appeal to *cost-effectiveness and justice.* The nurse must consider: Are there critical justice concerns in this case? Other ways to justify ethical decisions include references to *casuistic reasoning* (case-based). The nurse may be influenced if she has had a case like this and must ask, What did I learn from that case that is morally relevant to this new one? Some ethicists justify by using a *"narrative"* or foundational story to explain their position. Does the telling of your story or the details of this one affect your recommendation? (Brody, 1988).

After all these remarks are heard, it is time to understand what salient legal issues must be known, yet although these issues are relevant, unless the nurse is trained in the law, the nurse does not have a role to debate these issues. After the discourse about essential values and ethics is concluded, salient legal considerations and legal precedents are discussed after the committee has reflected on the ethical aspects of the case. The point of the process is *the* process; hence the patient and family and staff are present to hear the response and suggestion of the ethics committee. The expectation is that all the best recommendations will emerge and will be followed. The case process is concluded when the record of the discussion is written for the chart, and if possible, the ethics committee will meet with the nurses who could not attend the case consultation to talk to the nurse about the issues engaged in the case.

Is the method I and my colleagues have crafted the only one? Unlike some processes in medicine, there likely will not be a one "best practice" for a method of ethical deliberation. Yet I would argue that good nursing ethics must include an attention to method, to a definable and defensible process, and to far more than merely the good talk of a wise practitioner.

In the last 3 years a robust literature on the efficacy of clinical ethics practices has emerged. Success is difficult to standardize and difficult to measure with rigor. Is the goal the "satisfaction" of staff or of patients? (And what if they disagree as they did in the original dispute?) Is it reduction of terrible adversarial relationships that ends in acrimonious legal action? Is it length of stay? Is it some measurable growth in institutional knowledge about bioethics, which might be a surrogate for institutional wisdom about bioethics? (Howe, n.d.). The nurse will need to be aware of the ongoing research on clinical ethics consultation, to be sure, but the contention of this chapter is that a well-trained nurse can help families avoid the tragic and public fate of the Schiavo family.

Beyond Case Consultation: A Broader Vision of the Clinical Ethics Role

Public accountability is required in this process. The ethics committees should be publicly available, and their existence must be communicated to the public at large. The nurse can advocate for brochures in patient care areas, stories about the committee in the in-house newsletters, and a robust education effort for nurses and ancillary staff, a robust program of bioethics rounds, for ongoing ethics educational programs, including ground rounds, in-service meetings within clinical disciplines, and interdisciplinary meetings and ethics journal clubs, with binders in every unit. Nursing ethics is more than clinical ethics consultation; it will mean an ongoing commitment to teaching about ethical dilemmas, talking to families and patients about their emerging ethical concerns, and reassuring all involved in the process that millions of individuals face these choices in medical care and that there are resources for supporting choices for treatment continuance and for its withdrawal.

Classic Resistance and Suggested Responses

Despite the details of this description and despite the widespread existence—at least in theory—of ethics committees, the practice of their existence is more vexed, and the nurse may well encounter some resistance to the idea of ethics committees and to the process of ethics deliberation. This resistance will be a feature of the field for the next several years. Such resistance includes the following: "We don't really have any ethical dilemmas," or "Almost all ethical dilemmas are really communication problems," or "Having a whole committee is unworkable," or "We can't have patients or families; it will detract our focus, it will be intimidating to them," or "There's no time for this or money for this."

Ultimately, however, one must remember that ethical dilemmas are deep and fundamental disagreements that do not yield easily to even the best communicative strategies, much less to mediation or facile compromise (Althea & Ewens, 1998; Anderlik & Pentz, 2000; Bok, 1983; Boleyn-Fitzgerald, 2001; Lynn, 1991; Stone, Patton, & Heen, 2000), and the literature shows that families welcome and are fully capable of the serious moral activity within the ethics committee process and that time spent in focused, serious, and rigorous discussion with a clear method and a disciplined process does in fact take less time than long hours of acrimony and despairing discussion or lament. Although there is much to discover with careful research on clinical ethics and although there are indeed several troubling issues that still remain about how, when, and with whom to do clinical ethics, it is now clear that early intervention in the ethical dilemmas faced by patients is a vital and robust part of good nursing practice.

FOR FURTHER REFERENCE

For nurses interested in pursuing the discussion further, the author recommends the fellowship of others (American Medical Association, 1992). Colleagues in ethics can be found in the professional association of bioethics, the American Society for Bioethics and Humanities *(www.asbh.org)*. The association grew out of an earlier society, the Society for Bioethics Consultation, which was itself an outgrowth of a meeting at the Society for Health and Human Values. The latter was a group of humanities professors within medical schools who had begun a practice of consultation on cases in medical centers and was an interdisciplinary mixture of consultative methods and practitioners, with varied training and authority. The American Society for Bioethics and Humanities is now a vivid public square for the discourse of bioethics, and the nurse who is interested in the practice of clinical ethics should feel enthusiastically welcomed into the debate. The case stories that each nurse will bring can lead the way toward a deeper, more complex, and more compassionate practice of bioethics. The voice of the nurse, and the wisdom found only in the unique encounter that is nursing, ought to be a part of every discussion of ethical choices. The contention of this chapter is that there may be no better or more important story to attend to in bioethics than the one that a nurse, trained to hear, can tell.

REFERENCES

Ackerman, T. F., & Strong, C. (1989). *A casebook of medical ethics.* New York: Oxford University Press.

Althea, A., & Ewens, A. (1998). Tensions in sharing client confidences while respecting autonomy: Implications for interprofessional practice. *Nursing Ethics, 5*(5), 441-450.

American Academy of Pediatrics. (n.d.). *Bioethics.* Retrieved August 7, 2005, from http://www.aap.org/sections/bioethics/

American Medical Association. (1992). *The ethical question: Medical education kit* [videorecording]. Chicago, IL: American Medical Television.

Anderlik, M. R., & Pentz, R. D. (2000). Genetic information, legal, genetic privacy laws. In T. J. Murray & M. J. Mehlman (Eds.), *Encyclopedia of ethical, legal and policy issues in biotechnology* (pp. 456-468). Hoboken, NJ: John Wiley & Sons.

Barber v. Superior Court, 147 Cal. App. 3d 1006, 1015 (1983).

Beauchamp, T., & Childress, J. (2001). *Principles of biomedical ethics* (5th ed.). New York: Oxford University Press.

Bok, S. (1983). The limits of confidentiality. *Hastings Center Report, 13*(1), 24-31.

Boleyn-Fitzgerald, P. (2001). An egalitarian justification of medical privacy. In J. M. Humber & R. F. Almeder (Eds). *Privacy and health care* (pp. 55-68). Totowa, NJ: Humana Press.

Braddock, C. H., Edward, K. A., Hasenberg, N. M., Laidley, T. L., & Levinson, W. (1999). Informed decision making in outpatient practice: Time to get back to basics. *JAMA: The Journal of American Medical Association, 282,* 2313-2320.

Brock, D. W. (1987). Informed consent. In D. VanDeVeer & T. Regan (Eds.), *Health care ethics* (pp. 118-116). Philadelphia: Temple University Press.

Brody, B. A. (1988). *Life and death decision-making.* New York: Oxford University Press.

Davis, D. S. (1991). Rich cases: The ethics of thick description. *Hastings Center Report, 21*(4), 12-17.

Dubler, N. N., & Liebman, C. B. (2004). *Bioethics mediation: A guide to shaping shared solutions.* New York: United Hospital Fund of New York

Faden, R. R., & Beauchamp, T. L. (1998). *A history of informed consent.* New York: Oxford University Press.

Faden, R. R., Beauchamp, T. L., & King, N. M. P. (1986). *A history and theory of informed consent.* New York: Oxford University Press.

Forrow, L., Wartman, S. A., & Brock, D. W. (1988). Science, ethics, and the making of clinical decisions. *JAMA: The Journal of American Medical Association, 259*(21), 3161-3167.

Gibbs, R. (2000). *Why ethics?* (pp. i-xiii). Princeton, NJ: Princeton University Press.

Howe, E. G. (Ed.). (n.d.). *The Journal of Clinical Ethics.* Hagerstown, MD: Norman Quist.

Jones, J. (1974). *Bad blood: The case of the Tuskegee syphilis experiments.* New York: Free Press.

Kuczewski, M. G., & Pinkus, R. L. (1999). *An ethics casebook for hospitals: Practical approaches to everyday cases.* Washington, DC: Georgetown University Press.

Kushner, T. K., & Thomasma, D. C. (Eds.). (2001). *Ward ethics: Dilemmas for medical students and doctors in training.* New York: Cambridge University Press.

La Puma, J., & Schiedermayer, D. (1994). *Ethics consultation: A practical guide.* Sudbury, MA: Jones and Bartlett.

Legal Information Institute. (1990). *Supreme Court collection.* Retrieved August 4, 2005, from http://straylight.law.cornell.edu/supct/html/88-1503.ZS.html

Lidz, C. W., Appelbaum, P. S., & Meisel, A. (1988). Two models of implementing informed consent. *Archives of Internal Medicine, 148*(6), 1385-1389.

Lifton, R. (1988). *Nazi doctors: Medical killing and the psychology of genocide.* New York: Basic Books.

Lynn, J. (1991). Why I don't have a living will. *Law, Medicine & Health Care, 19*(1-2), 101-104.

Macklin, R. (1987). *Mortal choices: Bioethics in today's world.* New York: Pantheon.

Maholwald, M. (1999). *Women and children in health care.* New York: Oxford University Press.

Matter of Quinlan (excerpts). (1976). Retrieved August 4, 2005, from http://www.csulb.edu/~jvancamp/452_r6.html

Meisel, A., & Kuczewski, M. (1996). Legal and ethical myths about informed consent. *Archives of Internal Medicine, 156,* 2521-2526.

Moreno, J. (1997). *Deciding together.* New York: Oxford University Press.

Muller-Hill, B. (1988). *Murderous science.* New York: Oxford University Press

Pence, G. (1995). The Bouvia case. In *Classic Cases in Medical Ethics* (2nd ed., pp. 41-47). New York: McGraw-Hill.

Powell, T. (1995). Religion, race and reason: The case of LJ. *Journal of Clinical Ethics, 6*(1), 77-80.

Stanley, K. (1997). *City of hope: Ethics of pain management* [Speech]. Los Angeles, CA.

Stone, D. F., Patton, B., & Heen, S. (2000). *Difficult conversations: How to discuss what matters most.* East Rutherford, NJ: Penguin.

Unicorn Media for Concern for Dying. (1984). *Dax's case* [videorecording]. New York: Filmmakers Library.

University of Miami Ethics Program. (2005). *Schiavo case resources.* Retrieved August 4, 2005, from http://www.miami.edu/ethics/schiavo_project.htm

Wear, S. (1998). *Informed consent: Patient autonomy and clinician beneficence within health care* (2nd ed.). Washington, DC: Georgetown University Press.

Zoloth, L., & Rubin, S. B. (2004). *ASBH handbook for learners of clinical ethics.*

VIOLENCE PREVENTION AND CARE: THE ROLE OF NURSING

Violence: The Expanding Role of Nursing in Prevention and Care

PERLE SLAVIK COWEN ◆ SUE MOORHEAD

In metropolitan and rural areas, in cities and small towns, Americans are concerned and perhaps fearful that violence has permeated the fabric of their communities and degraded their quality of life. This is understandable since in the last 10 years Americans have experienced violence directly or indirectly. Americans have seen numerous international acts of terrorism; a domestic terrorism attack in Oklahoma City in 1995; the horrors of the series of attacks on September 11, 2001, using American aircraft; the bioterrorism attacks using anthrax abroad and in the United States in the fall of 2001; and the wars in Afghanistan and Iraq. Natural disasters such as hurricanes and tsunamis have occurred, and communities experience daily random and senseless acts of violence toward individuals or groups and the maltreatment and murder of children, women, dependent adults, and elders through family violence. This list clearly illustrates the presence of violence around the globe.

Most persons experience these sorrows indirectly through mass media, social networks, or from other sources. However, Americans know, without ever seeing or hearing, that nurses were involved directly in treating and caring for the victims of all of these tragedies. Fulmer, Knapp, and Terranova note in their chapter that the news reports after 9/11 were filled with stories of heroic firefighters and policemen, but these stories did not focus on nurses. In fact, most reports were completely silent on the role and contributions of professional nursing. Without fanfare, nurses in these metropolitan areas mobilized instinctively and immediately to assist area hospitals and those at Ground Zero. Nurses calmly assumed leadership roles to help care for those injured.

This section does not have a debate chapter; it provides a spotlight on the many leadership and care roles of nursing in violence prevention, including child maltreatment, domestic violence, elder mistreatment, gun safety prevention, terrorism events, homeland security, wars,

bioterrorism, and combat. Few professions have the knowledge, skills, and courage to serve on these frontlines. Nurses provide comfort and protection to victims of violence and their families and organize community and national relief efforts, and as the most trusted of all professionals their presence calms public anxiety. Nursing is the antithesis of violence.

In the opening chapter, Cowen addresses the problem of child maltreatment. In 2003 an estimated 906,000 children were victims of maltreatment, with 63.2% experiencing neglect, 18.9% physical abuse, 9.9% sexual abuse, and 4.9% emotional or psychological maltreatment. Tragically, an estimated 1500 children died of abuse or neglect, with 79% of these younger than 3 years old. Cowen describes characteristics of maltreatment types and gives an overview of cultural, social, and family factors. Cowen explores biological research that has begun to provide insight into the physiological pathways underlying numerous deleterious long-term psychological effects. She discusses potential lifetime developmental and negative health effects that may require treatment throughout the life span and are of importance to practitioners of all age cohorts. Cowen posits that early identification and long-term intervention have the potential for reducing or preventing these deleterious consequences. Cowen states that "nursing's role as advocate is often the critical determinant of whether at-risk children and youth or adult survivors of child maltreatment are identified and receive the therapeutic interventions and tangible services they need."

In the following chapter, Cowen delves into issues associated with child neglect and the pivotal role of nursing in prevention. Child neglect is described as the most prevalent, most lethal, and least empirically studied form of child maltreatment, and she notes that it has been associated with a plethora of adverse physical, psychological and educational outcomes. Specific types of child neglect discussed include abandonment, educational, emotional, health care, physical, and supervision. Cowen reviews research indicating that child neglect is correlated strongly with poverty, single-parent caretakers, unemployment, and multifaceted family problems. She explores risk factors, developmental consequences of neglect, assessment tools, and nursing roles and therapeutic approaches in supporting families at risk for child neglect. The author emphasizes early identification of at-risk children and details the positive outcome findings following nursing preventive interventions, particularly home health visitation programs. She discusses research findings that indicate this program "was successful in improving parental care as reflected by fewer childhood injuries and ingestions, fewer subsequent pregnancies, greater work force participation, reduced use of public assistance and food stamps, and fewer state verified reports of child abuse and neglect between the children's fourth and fifteenth birthdays."

Taylor presents an overview of issues related to nursing care of African-American women exposed to intimate partner violence. She leads us to examine the personal-social context of African American women seeking therapy and to consider their individual perspectives and needs. She describes why "support groups as collective exchanges are culturally anchored approaches that can provide a therapeutic safe environment for African American women recovering from a variety of social, psychological, emotional, and physical traumas." Taylor says that "Cultural and ideological barriers, such as racism, classism, and sexism shape African American women's experience and recovery from relationship violence differently from white women." She discusses the need for African-American leadership and member composition in therapeutic sessions, stating that racially homogeneous groups are preferred because for many women this group environment maximizes the comfort level; provides more opportunities to disclose more fully the events in their lives; and counters social isolation that is prevalent in abusive situations and in environments that foster discrimination and racism. She closes with a series of questions intended to stimulate discussion of these points. This is a well-written chapter that addresses important racial issues in treatment of victims of violence.

Lemko and Fulmer provide a detailed overview of issues related to elder mistreatment. They point out, "Although there is strong support for legislation related to elder mistreatment, senators rarely demonstrate their dedication to this issue, and unfortunately, there has been no national legislation on elder mistreatment." Currently, only 2% of the budget for abuse prevention

is allotted to elder mistreatment (physical, psychological and sexual abuse, neglect, abandonment, exploitation or financial abuse, and self-neglect). As the baby boomer population (those born from 1946 to 1964) is getting older, the interest in aging issues is said to be increasing; however, the authors say that in the medical community, elder mistreatment has been labeled as a Pandora's box because many health care providers feel they do not have adequate time to screen older adults for elder mistreatment or the necessary training to conduct such crucial evaluations. It is estimated that 1.2 million to 2 million older adults, or approximately 6% of older adults, are mistreated annually. The authors review symptoms of elder mistreatment and characteristics of the victim and caregivers and identify nursing assessment challenges. Lemko and Fulmer lament the lack of an empirical research base for interventions in elder mistreatment and underscore the need for victim advocacy.

In a change of direction, Hazinski tackles the issues of preventive gun safety, noting that although firearm injuries in all ages have decreased in the United States since 1993, they remain a leading cause of death in adolescents and young adults. She emphasizes, "Many unintentional firearm injuries and firearm suicides can be prevented if firearms are inaccessible to unsupervised children and adolescents." Hazinski recommends that nurses become knowledgeable about evidence supporting gun safety legislation and identifies specific interventions to reduce firearm injuries and fatalities. She cautions that if a nurse is the primary practitioner caring for a patient with a history of depression, alcohol or drug abuse, or violent behavior, the nurse should discuss the risks of guns in the household and encourage the family to eliminate guns from the household. The nurse should ensure that parents are aware of the data regarding risks when a gun is in the home of an adolescent, particularly if that adolescent has a history of depression or substance abuse. This is an important chapter because it underscores a problem that often is not addressed until a tragedy has occurred.

Fulmer, Knapp, and Terranova recount the role of nursing in one of the darkest days in American history in their chapter on nursing during terrorist events. This is a riveting chapter that takes the reader through nursing concerns and activities following the terrorist attacks on the World Trade Center towers and the Pentagon. They were there, and so were several of their nursing students. They also discuss care experiences following the potential exposure of postal workers to anthrax. The authors state, "Today, curricula in health professions schools have to include content of large-scale disaster preparedness and planning." Is this so? The recent response to Hurricane Ophelia indicates that nurses remain weak in disaster preparedness, and we wonder how many professors and their students think this is being addressed adequately in their institutions. The authors provide a wealth of information to launch this discussion and identify information resources and Web sites. They state that the Department of Homeland Security has begun to fund a series of Centers of Excellence to research what must be known in terrorist times. Nurses must be involved in these centers in order to generate the research and prepare the best practice protocols for what can happen next. Fulmer, Knapp, and Terranova set a new level of expectation and baseline for the nursing profession related to terrorism sequelae and disaster care. They also raise many disconcerting and compelling issues. This chapter is well written and is at once a classic and a must-read chapter.

Appropriately, Chaffee, Lavin, and Slepski next address nursing practice in homeland security. They review the development of homeland security, noting that it was known as "civil defense" in the 1950s, that it morphed into the Federal Emergency Management Agency in 1979 after a series of natural disasters in the 1960s and 1970s, and that following the impact of 9/11 the "U.S. Congress established the U.S. Department of Homeland Security to help America prepare for, respond to, and recover from potential terrorist attacks, including those involving weapons of mass destruction." The authors state that more than 22 distinct agencies and more than 170,000 personnel were reorganized into one department with the mission to protect the American homeland. This should raise some good class debate regarding systems and organizational management issues. The authors provide a thorough discussion of the historical role of nursing in emergency preparedness and specifically detail the leadership role of nursing in homeland security through an extensive list of nurses in key leadership positions. The authors discuss nursing practice in homeland security at the individual level and organizational level, the role of nursing professional associations, and nursing practice in homeland security at the state and federal levels and provide educational resources to assist emergency preparedness. They identify several colleges of nursing that are incorporating disaster preparedness and mass casualty content into classes at the undergraduate and graduate levels. This is a highly informative and enlightening chapter and provides guidance that is sorely needed.

In the next chapter, Garfield provides a compelling discussion of the conflicting values and roles that nursing faces in global conflicts. He first presents a solid framework in evolving terminology, epidemiology, and nature of war, conflict, and violence. He cites grim statistics noting that "the fortyfold rise in the number of deaths among soldiers in the twentieth century greatly exceeded a doubling of the global midcentury population. Military deaths per million population rose eighteenfold from the nineteenth to the twentieth century. Genocide and democide-related deaths also rose in the twentieth century as the centralization of large political and economic systems and the emergence of new technologies made mass killings possible." He brings forth an objective worldwide view of violence trends, and it is disturbing. He delivers an engrossing review of the roles for nursing in a world of conflict, saying that nursing has remained largely invisible in the accounts of organizations associated with war, relief, and humanitarian assistance. He notes that "Today, among nongovernmental organizations such as Save the Children and Doctors without Borders, few know that there are as many nurses as doctors serving in crisis areas around the world." Garfield advocates for research that focuses on civilian women, who are frequently the "forgotten victims" in conflict, and better training for nurses to deal with the harsh realities of global conflict. This is an extraordinary chapter, and it delivers many important messages.

Rebmann follows with a discussion of emergency preparedness for nursing related to bioterrorism and emerging infections. According to the Centers for Disease Control and Prevention, bioterrorism has become the most imminent threat to U.S. national security. The author says that "the 2001 anthrax bioterrorism attack used only a small amount of a weaponized noninfectious agent (approximately 2 to 3 oz of anthrax) and a relatively ineffective dissemination device (letters), and resulted in only 22 cases of anthrax and 5 deaths." Rebman details the recent threat of emerging pathogens on health care and public health systems in the United States since exposure to West Nile virus, monkeypox, mad cow disease, Norwalk virus, and severe acute respiratory syndrome. She emphasizes that nurses constantly are faced with the potential of new infectious disease threats and illustrates through mathematical modeling "the need for additional planning and response capabilities to respond to potential future events." Although the medical model is essential to bioterrorism management, the author underscores that "many nursing-specific issues have been neglected, including potential implications of long-term care for survivors, the mental health impact on health care workers and their families, and therapeutic communication for grieving victims' families." Rebmann deftly provides a through review of possible barriers that have kept nurses unprepared for this threat, and it serves as a solid wake-up call.

In the final chapter, Abrams looks at the environmental, cultural, technological, clinical, and psychological demands of combat nursing with emphasis on the nation's most recent involvement in the jungles and the deserts. She provides a historical background to combat nursing and the many changes, noting that "although currently 350,000 women are serving in the U.S. military, the majority serves in non-nursing capacities. One in every seven military personnel serving in Iraq is a woman. Contrast that with Vietnam when women composed less than 3% of U.S. military personnel who served, and 80% to 90% of that total number was Navy, Air Force, or Army nurses." She converses easily about the effect of war on the environment and the effect of the environment on the nurses, including health, hygiene, and predators. She describes the need to understand the culture of the land in order to obtain needed supplies and equipment from a local market and to preserve relationships with the home government. Abrams gives an overview of clinical skills, training needs, and the lingering psychological effects of serving as a nurse in combat and points out that "those who have served in a medical capacity during a time of war experience the same emotional and psychological ramifications as those who were involved directly in combat." This chapter provides a genuine and sensitive look at the many issues faced by nurses in combat.

In this section perhaps the reader should allow some time between chapters to absorb and reflect on the content. The topics address emotional, difficult, and complex issues in nursing and in the world. Garfield notes, "Our ideas of nursing are shaped by images of nurses in war. It was war, after all, that brought Florence Nightingale into public prominence and provided her with a powerful platform for military and social reform. But therein lays the paradox. For although war may shine a light on nursing, it often can blind the observer to what nurses actually do."

Child Maltreatment

Developmental and Health Effects

PERLE SLAVIK COWEN

> Children's talent to endure stems from their ignorance of alternatives.
>
> *Maya Angelou, I Know Why the Caged Bird Sings, 1969*

Child maltreatment is a complex problem that requires a host of multidisciplinary professionals to identify, treat, and provide preventive interventions. Nurses specializing in maternal-child, pediatric, trauma, school, and mental health areas have long been aware of the immediate trauma and impaired developmental and health consequences associated with child maltreatment. Biological research has begun to provide insight into the physiological pathways underlying numerous deleterious long-term effects. Recent research also has identified a host of negative health consequences for adult survivors of child maltreatment that may require treatment throughout the life span and are of importance to practitioners of all age cohorts.

Nursing interventions in child maltreatment cover a broad spectrum of roles and approaches throughout the individual's and family's life span. Different levels of family functioning require adaptations in the nursing role, therapeutic approach, and helping activities. Primary preventive interventions are directed at the general population in order to prevent or reduce the occurrence of child maltreatment, whereas secondary preventive interventions are targeted at high-risk groups and tertiary interventions are focused on preventing further injury or harm to children who have been maltreated. Clearly, a need exists for preventive and treatment interventions that focus on the potential lifetime developmental and health effects of childhood victimization. Early identification and long-term intervention have the potential for reducing or preventing the deleterious consequences associated with the physical and emotional trauma of child maltreatment. Nursing's role as advocate is often the critical determinant of whether at-risk children and youth or adult survivors of child maltreatment are identified and receive the therapeutic interventions and tangible services they need.

TYPES AND CHARACTERISTICS OF CHILD MALTREATMENT

The 1974 Federal Child Abuse and Treatment Act (P.L. 93-247) guides child protection; was amended and reauthorized in 1978, 1984, 1988, 1996, and 2003; and has continued to expand and refine the scope of law (U.S. Department of Health and Human Services, 2004). The act defines child abuse and neglect as "any recent act [harm standard] or failure to act [endangerment standard] on the part of a parent or caretaker, which results in death, serious physical or emotional harm, sexual abuse or exploitation, or an act or failure to act which presents an imminent risk of serious harm" (p. 44). Specific types of maltreatment defined include physical abuse, neglect (physical, educational, health care, and emotional), emotional abuse, and sexual abuse. States and researchers typically may expand and specify additional neglect categories (Table 75-1). It is important for nurses to be familiar with the specific state reporting statutes and definitions within their practice areas.

Individual cases may present with multiple types of maltreatment, in varying degrees of severity, with resultant physical, psychological, and developmental harm to the child. Research has indicated that children who experience chronic maltreatment versus transitory maltreatment have significantly more emotional problems (anxiety, depression) and a tendency for more behavioral problems (aggression, social withdrawal)

TABLE 75-1

Types of Child Maltreatment*

Type	Definition
Physical abuse	Intentional physical acts by the caregiver that caused or could have caused physical injury to a child younger than 18 years of age, including punching, beating, kicking, biting, burning, unreasonable confinement, and repeated acts of punishment or assault.
Health care neglect	Failure by the caregiver to provide necessary health care or medical or mental health treatment, including required immunizations, prescribed medications, recommended surgery, or other intervention in case of serious disease or injury, although financially able to do so or when offered financial or other means to do so.
Neglect/deprivation of necessities	Failure by the caregiver to provide needed age-appropriate care although financially able to do so or when offered financial or other means to do so, including minimum shelter, food, clothing, and supervision necessary to maintain life or health; abandonment; expulsion from the home or refusal to allow a runaway to return home; and educational neglect.
Sexual abuse	Involvement of the child in sexual activity to provide sexual gratification or financial benefit to the perpetrator, including contacts for sexual purposes, molestation, statutory rape, prostitution, pornography, exposure, incest, or other sexually exploitive activities.
Psychological maltreatment	Refusals or delays in psychological care; inadequate attention to a child's needs for affection, emotional support, attention, or competence; exposure of a child to extreme domestic violence; and permitting a child's maladaptive behaviors.

*States may group or specify of maltreatment categories.

(Ethier, Lemelin, & Lacharite, 2004). Numerous research studies also have provided empirical support for a substantial overlap between domestic violence and child maltreatment (Appel & Holden, 1998; Edleson, 1999; Hartley, 2002).

Physical abuse includes the intentional use of physical force resulting in bodily harm, anguish or pain and includes acts of violence such as striking (with or without an object), hitting, beating, pushing, shaking, kicking, pinching, burning, inappropriate administration of medications, and age-inappropriate physical restraints. Some researchers contend that the resultant physical injuries are seldom intentional and are instead the parent's "heedless intention" to control the child (Wolfe, 1999). Head trauma, third-degree burns, and other serious injuries result in large numbers of children becoming severely disabled from physical abuse (Kolko, 2002). Of course, the physical injuries, scars, and disabilities represent only the visible signs of physical abuse, and as noted later, the emotional scarring may unfold throughout the life span.

Generally, child neglect is defined as the failure of the child's parents or caretakers to provide the child with the basic necessities of life when financially able to do so or when offered reasonable means to do so, including minimally adequate care in the areas of shelter, nutrition, health, supervision, education, affection, and protection. State statutes often classify specific subpopulations of neglect by the type of action that the parent or caretaker fails to take, and researchers have identified the existence of child neglect in many forms, including abandonment, educational, emotional, physical, and supervision. The most common form of child neglect involves failure to supervise the child properly, leading to physical harm or death (U.S. Department of Health and Human Services, 2000).

Although there is basic agreement as to what constitutes severe physical child neglect, other specific types and individual cases of neglect include variables that create legal and ethical dilemmas that complicate the recognition and reporting of neglect. These dilemmas include (1) legal exemptions related to parental disability, poverty, or religious practices (Dubowitz & Black, 2002; Johnson, 1993); (2) lack of professional training and guidelines for determining medical neglect of specific diseases (Johnson, 1993); and (3) dilemmas related to the excessive demands on the parents/caretakers of children who are technology-dependent or disabled (Cowen & Reed, 2002; Hogue, 1993; Sullivan & Knutson, 1998, 2000). Child neglect is not a dichotomous variable; it occurs along a continuum from mild to severe with many factors blurring the boundaries

VIEWPOINTS

between these extremes. Because many parents engage in some kind of neglectful behavior, at least occasionally, the issues of severity and chronicity are critical in assessing the future risk to the child and in designing realistic interventions. Several factors are considered in assessing the severity of neglect, including the frequency, duration, and type of neglect; age of the child; potential consequences to the child's development; and the degree of danger to the child. Fatal neglect has been associated with chronic deprivation of the basic necessities of life (Krugman & Dubowitz, 2003; Rosenberg, 1994; Wilkey, Pearn, Petrie, & Nixon, 1982) and with situational failures to supervise the activities of young children (Committee on Injury and Poison Prevention, 2001; Margolin, 1990; Mierley & Baker, 1983; Rosenberg, 1994).

Practitioners vary in their individual opinions as to what constitutes health care neglect by specialty, cultural background, and the population they are serving. In general, a solitary omission in health care is unlikely to cause harm in average children. Nonetheless, a pattern of omissions in care, such as failure to immunize, could have detrimental effects for even the healthiest children (Dubowitz, 1999b). In addition, there are times when failing to seek or comply with care for a single incidence can have a devastating effect, such as failure to have a severe head injury evaluated or in cases of meningitis (Dubowitz & Black, 2002). In cases of severe health care neglect, parents are unable, unwilling, or unmotivated to seek all forms of preventive care, and direct assistance is required to locate a provider and transport families to services (Dubowitz & Black, 1994). The parents are often unable or unwilling to meet the needs of a child with a chronic condition, and this may result in significant morbidity or mortality for health conditions such as asthma, diabetes, or cystic fibrosis (Dubowitz & Black, 2002). It has been asserted that parents should be considered responsible for health care neglect only if a layperson reasonably could be expected to appreciate the need for health care (Dubowitz et al., 2005).

Sexual abuse is any form of sexual contact with a child for which consent is not or cannot be given (by nature of age) and includes rape, sodomy, coerced nudity, exposure or voyeurism, molestation, prostitution, and sexually explicit photography. This includes sexual contact that occurs as a result of force, regardless of the age of the participants, and all sexual contact between an adult and child. State statutes specify the age an individual can consent to sexual contact, and this typically ranges between 14 and 18 years of age.

Contact between an older and younger child also can be abusive if there is a significant disparity in age, size, or development (Berliner & Elliott, 2002). All states have laws prohibiting sexual abuse of children; however, each state individually defines and labels prohibited activities, and thus criminal statutes vary among states (Meyers, 1998). State child abuse statutes may include only acts committed by caretakers and address other contacts through criminal statutes.

The characteristics of sexual abuse may vary depending on the data source (clinical or general population), type (intrafamilial versus extrafamilial), duration (limited versus ongoing), severity, frequency, and use of force and age of the child (Berliner & Elliott, 2002; Kendall-Tackett, 2003). The vast majority of offenders are male, with girls at higher risk of victimization than boys and with both sexes more at risk if they have lived without one of their natural parents, have a mother who is unavailable, or perceive their family life as unhappy (Finkelhor, Hotaling, Lewis, & Smith, 1990; Homes & Slap, 1998). The mean age for sexual abuse initiation is approximately 9 years old with a range from infancy to 17 years of age (Berliner & Elliott, 2002). Multiple episodes of sexual abuse are reported as common, with an incidence of up to 50% in nonclinical samples (Saunder, Kilpatrick, Hanson, Resnick, & Walker, 1999) and 75% in clinical samples (Ruggiero, McLeer, & Dixon, 2000). Attempted or completed oral, vaginal, or anal penetration is reported to occur in approximately 25% of nonclinical groups (Finkelhor & Dziuba-Leatherman, 1994) and in more than 50% of clinical samples (Elliott, Browne, & Kilcoyne, 1995; Ruggiero et al., 2000).

Psychological maltreatment has been conceptualized as consisting of psychological abuse and neglect that may occur alone or in association with all other forms of child maltreatment (Hart, Brassard, Binggeli, & Davidson, 2002). Professional guidelines developed through review by content experts resulted in the following broad conceptual statement: "a repeated pattern of caregiver behavior or extreme incident (s) that convey to children that they are worthless, flawed, unloved, unwanted, endangered or only of value in meeting another's needs" (American Professional Society on the Abuse of Children, 1995, p. 2). The American Professional Society on Abuse of Children also identified six categories of psychological maltreatment—spurning, terrorizing, isolating, exploiting/corrupting, denying emotional responsiveness, and mental health, medical, and educational neglect—and has further developed detailed subcategories (Hart et al., 2002).

Research findings indicate that "spurning" may be as damaging to a child's psychological development as physical abuse and that "denying emotional responsiveness" may be the most devastating of all forms of maltreatment (Erickson & Egeland, 2002).

PREVALANCE

During 2003, child protective services agencies received an estimated 2.9 million referrals of abuse or neglect (a rate of 39.1 referrals per 1000 children) concerning approximately 5.5 million children, and they accepted more than two thirds of those referrals for investigation or assessment. An estimated 906,000 children were victims of abuse or neglect, with 63.2% experiencing neglect, 18.9% physical abuse, 9.9% sexual abuse, and 4.9% emotional or psychological maltreatment. The rates of victimization by maltreatment type have fluctuated slightly from year to year with child neglect consistently the predominate type (Figure 75-1). The youngest children had the highest rate of victimization (Figure 75-2) with children younger than 1 year of age accounting for 9.8% of victims (U.S. Department of Health and Human Services, 2005).

Tragically, an estimated 1500 children died of abuse or neglect (rate of 2.00 children per 100,000) with attribution by maltreatment type as 35.6% neglect; 28.9% multiple maltreatment types; 28.4% physical abuse;

6.7% psychological, other, or unknown; and 0.4% sexual abuse (Figure 75-3). Among the children who died, 78.7% were younger than 3 years old; 10.2% were 4 to 7 years old, 5.4% were 8 to 11 years old, and 5.7% were 12 to 17 years old (Figure 75-4). Infant boys (younger than 1 year old) had the highest rate of fatalities, nearly 18 per 100,000; and infant girls had a rate of 14 deaths per 100,000 (U.S. Department of Health and Human Services, 2005). These figures represent the lowest estimate of the problem and depend on the number of states reporting (44 states, including the District of Columbia, participated in the 2003 report), the level of involvement of child protective services, and the varying levels of comprehensive investigation into child mortality cases by local authorities and classification variances among the states in reporting deaths caused by child maltreatment.

Overall, the largest percentage of perpetrators (79.9%) was parents, and statistically this category included birth parents, adoptive parents, and stepparents (U.S. Department of Health and Human Services, 2005). The maltreatment perpetrators' characteristics included 58% women (mostly mothers) and 42% men (mostly fathers) with the women's median age 31 and the men's median age 34. However, nearly 76% of all perpetrators of sexual abuse were friends or neighbors, and 30% were other relatives, with less than 3% of all parental perpetrators being associated with sexual abuse.

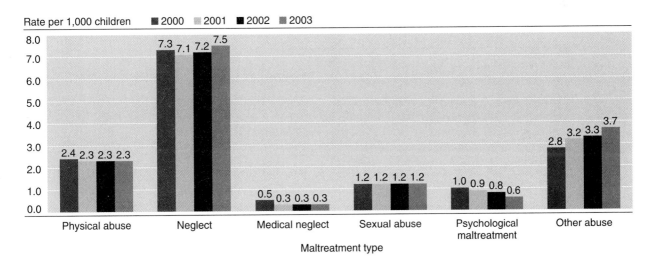

FIGURE 75-1 Victimization rates by maltreatment type, 2000-2003. (Statistics from U.S. Department of Health and Human Services, Administration on Children, Youth and Families. [2005]. *Child maltreatment 2003.* Washington, DC: U.S. Government Printing Office.)

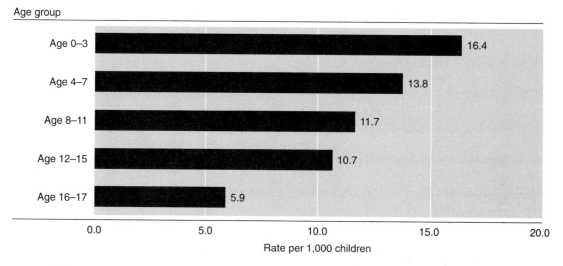

FIGURE 75-2 Victimization rates by age group, 2003. (Statistics from U.S. Department of Health and Human Services, Administration on Children, Youth and Families. [2005]. *Child maltreatment 2003.* Washington, DC: U.S. Government Printing Office.)

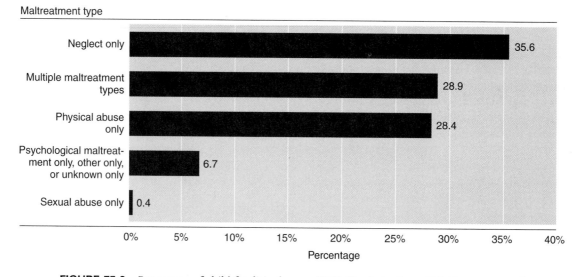

FIGURE 75-3 Percentage of child fatalities by age, 2003. (Statistics from U.S. Department of Health and Human Services, Administration on Children, Youth and Families. [2005]. *Child maltreatment 2003.* Washington, DC: U.S. Government Printing Office.)

Theoretical Perspectives

Theoretical perspectives on the causes and correlates of child maltreatment are many and varied (Cicchetti & Carlson, 1989). The inability of the single-dimensional models adequately to address the known characteristics of child maltreatment has resulted in multidimensional models including the ecological model of child maltreatment (Garbarino, 1977). This model is derived from ecological model of human development (Bronfenbrenner, 1977) and is a paradigm for examining the complex interactions among parental and child characteristics, intrafamilial and extrafamilial stressors, and the social and cultural systems that affect families. The model offers a framework for considering available supports and resources in relation to a topology of four levels that have been adapted to include individual,

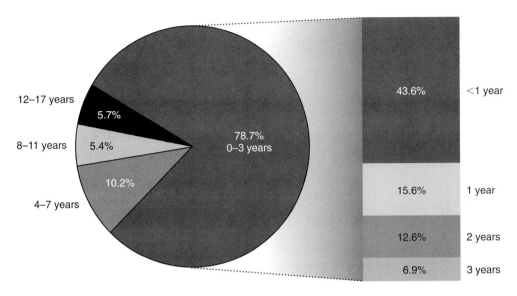

FIGURE 75-4   Fatalities by type of maltreatment, 2003. (Statistics from U.S. Department of Health and Human Services, Administration on Children, Youth and Families. [2005]. *Child maltreatment* 2003. Washington, DC: U.S. Government Printing Office.)

familial, social, and cultural (Howze & Kotch, 1984). Additionally, the model provides a framework for understanding the relationships among stress, social support systems, and child maltreatment and is adapted further to provide guidance to child maltreatment preventive intervention efforts (see Figure 75-1, p. 687).

Risk Factor Identification

The importance of early identification and intervention lies in its potential for reducing or preventing the occurrence of child maltreatment. Those variables that have been associated with child maltreatment can be classified into four separate domains: sociocultural, family, parental/caretaker, and individual characteristics of the child (Table 75-2). Stress arising from these domains may be situational, acute, or chronic. However, one should note that to date, research has not indicated that there are any factors present in all child maltreatment circumstances that are absent in all nonmaltreatment circumstances. Additionally, individual risk characteristics may be more related to specific types of maltreatment. Thus there is no litmus test for child maltreatment, only related risk factors the identification of which provides the opportunity for preventive interventions to be directed at stressful environments, interpersonal relationships, and parental psychosocial problems with securement of the child's safety and optimal growth and development as the desired outcomes.

Sociocultural Factors

Although child maltreatment is reported among all socioeconomic groups, it is reported disproportionately among poor families (National Research Council, 1993a; Sedlak & Broadhurst, 1996). Physical child abuse and child neglect have been highly correlated with poverty, whereas neglect has been found to be concentrated among the poorest of the poor who typically resided in inadequate housing (Pelton, 1985, 1994; Sedlak & Broadhurst, 1996; Wolock & Horowitz, 1984). Income level also has been associated with the severity of neglect, with higher-income families generally associated with less severe forms of neglect, presumably because they have more resources at their disposal (Crittenden, 1996). In the Third National Incidence Study (NIS III), neglect was identified 44 times more often in families with annual incomes under $15,000 compared with those earning more than $30,000 (Sedlak & Broadhurst, 1996). Low economic status is associated with a range of factors associated with poverty, such as unemployment, limited education, large numbers of children, and social isolation (Crittenden, 1999).

In 2004, 38% (70 million) of U.S. children lived in low-income families (less than 100% of federal poverty level), with 21% (11 million) of these in living in abject poverty (100% to 200% of the federal poverty level). Among children under age 6, 42% (9.6 million) lived in low-income families, with 20% (4.6 million) living

TABLE 75-2

Risk Factors Associated with Child Maltreatment

Domain	Risk Factors
Sociocultural	• Inaccessible health care because of financial and/or nonfinancial barriers (e.g., geographical)[19,43] • Lack of community resources, respite and crisis child care,[13,14] and prevention services[35] • Poverty[4,6,21,28,47,48,54] • Societal tolerance for children living in poverty[11,20,34] • Unemployment[28,54]
Family	• Chaotic family organization with high levels of conflict and low levels of verbal expression and communication[26,27] • Domestic violence[32,39] • Interaction or fit between parent and child[33,47,51] • Large number of children in family[26] • Life stressors and/or distress[16,26,42] • Low levels of coping and problem-solving skills and higher incidence of psychosocial problems and perceived stress[2,27] • Religious/folk beliefs that are injurious[52] • Single-parent head of household[7,20,42,48] • Social isolation and low level of social support[1,8,18,20,26]
Parent/caretaker	• Adolescent parent[30,49] • Anxiety[10] • History of maltreatment as child[3,9,17,40,42,48] • Immature, childlike personality related to low self-esteem, poor impulse control[26] • Lack of positive relationship with own mother[12,41] • Limited household and financial management skills[7] • Limited parenting competencies[25,44] including decreased or dysfunctional parent/child interactions[43] and stress related to the parenting role[23] • Limited social competencies[7,26] • Low level of maternal education[26,35,36] • Maternal depression[20,23,37] • Mother cohabiting with male unrelated to children[24,45] • Poor parental physical health and presence of stress-related symptoms[13,22] • Rapid repeat birth[22] • Spouse abuse[46] • Substance abuse[10,20,31,42,44]
Child	• Developmental or physical disabilities[15,50] • Children of young adolescent mothers[20,30,38] • Chronic illnesses[13,15] • Gender (females for sexual abuse,[5] males for physical abuse)[53] • Low-birth-weight or premature infants[13,15] • Prenatal neglect (inadequate prenatal care, in utero exposure to cocaine or other drugs)[10] • Temperament described as "difficult" by mother[29] • Young age[54]

Note: The following references are representative and not exhaustive: (1) Albarracin, Repetto, & Albarracin, 1997; (2) Ammerman & Patz, 1996; (3) Banyard, Williams, & Siegel, 2003; (4) Baugher & Lamison-White, 1996; (5) Berliner & Elliott, 2002; (6) Brooks-Gunn & Duncan, 1997; (7) Burke, Chandy, Dannerbeck, & Watt, 1998; (8) Campbell, 1997; (9) Carter, Joyce, Mulder, & Luty, 2001; (10) Cash & Wilke, 2003; (11) Children's Defense Fund, 1997; (12) Coohey, 1995; (13) Cowen, 1998; (14) Cowen, 2001; (15) Cowen & Reed, 2002; (16) Crittenden, 1996; (17) Crouch, Milner, & Thomsen, 2001; (18) DePanfilis, 1996; (19) Devaney, Ellwood, & Love, 1997; (20) Dubowitz, 1999b; (21) Dubowitz & Black, 2002; (22) El-Kamary et al., 2004; (23) Ethier, Lacharite, & Courture, 1995; (24) Fagan, 1997; (25) Feldman, Ducharme, & Case, 1999; (26) Gable, 1998; (27) Gaudin, Polansky, Kilpatrick, & Shilton, 1996; (28) Gillham et al., 1998; (29) Harrington, Black, Starr, & Dubowitz, 1998; (30) Jaffee, Caspi, Moffitt, Belsky, & Silva, 2001; (31) Jaudes & Ekwo, 1995; (32) Jellen, McCarroll, & Thayer, 2001; (33) Kim & Cicchetti, 2004; (34) Korbin, 1994; (35) Kotch, Browne, Dufort, & Winsor, 1999; (36) Kotch et al., 1995; (37) Lutenbacher & Hall, 1998; (38) Maynard, 1997; (39) McGuigan & Pratt, 2001; (40) Milan, Lewis, Ethier, Keshaw, & Ickovics, 2004; (41) Morton & Brown, 1998; (42) Nelson, Cross, Landsman, & Tyler, 1996; (43) Pagelow, 1997; (44) Peterson, Gable, & Saldana, 1996; (45) Rector, Fagan, & Johnson, 2004; (46) Rumm, Cummings, Krauss, Bell, & Rivara, 2000; (47) Slack, Holl, McDaniel, Yoo, & Bolger, 2004; (48) Smokowski & Wodarski, 1996; (49) Stevens-Simon & Barrett, 2001; (50) Sullivan & Knutson, 1998; (51) Toth & Cichetti, 1996; (52) Trotter, Ackerman, Rodman, Martinez, & Sorvillo, 1983; (53) U.S. Department of Health and Human Services, 2005; (54) Wang & Daro, 1998.

in poverty. Also for those under age 6, 52% have at least one parent who works full-time year-round; 30% have at least one parent who works part-time or full-time for part of the year. The largest group of low-income families of children under age 6 by race and ethnicity is white children (3.8 million, 29%) followed by Latino children (3.1 million, 65%), black children (2.1 million, 64%), and Asian children (0.2 million, 23%) (National Center for Children in Poverty, 2005).

Child maltreatment rates also have been found to be higher in poorer neighborhoods with fewer social resources than in equally deprived neighborhoods where social resources (such as respite and crisis child care) were perceived to be higher (Garbarino & Kostelny, 1992; Sedlak & Broadhurst, 1996). Although the indirect stress of poverty may lead to child neglect, there is little doubt that poverty is directly hazardous to children. Poor parents are required to be hypervigilant of the environment (deteriorated housing, fires, lead poisoning, crime), manage scarce financial resources, and provide constant supervision of children with little or no margin for error (Cutts, Pheley, & Geppert, 1998; Erickson & Egeland, 2002; Pelton, 1994). Poor children are more likely than rich or middle-class children to experience material deprivation and poor health, die during childhood, score lower on standardized tests, be retained in grade or drop out of school, have out-of-wedlock births, and experience violent crime and more often are reported as victims of child maltreatment (Brooks-Gunn & Duncan, 1997; Dubowitz et al., 2005; Duncan & Brooks-Gunn, 2000). However, unlike other forms of child maltreatment, sexual abuse does not appear to be related to socioeconomic status (Berliner & Elliott, 2002).

The relationship between poverty and child maltreatment is complex; most poor parents are not abusive, and poverty alone is not a sufficient or necessary antecedent for child maltreatment (National Research Council, 1993b). The ecological perspective argues that as the environment in which a family lives becomes more stressful, or is perceived as such, the parents may rely more and more on coercion and violence to control irritating daily events, including interactions with their children (Bronfenbrenner, 1977; Garbarino & Kostelny, 1992; Howze & Kotch, 1984; Slack, Holl, McDaniel, Yoo, & Bolger, 2004; Smokowski & Wodarski, 1996).

Child neglect particularly has been related to the inaccessibility or unaffordability of health care (Barnett, Miller-Perrin, & Perrin, 1997). Since its inception in 1997, the State Children's Health Insurance Program has provided low-income children with vital health care coverage in concert with Medicaid. However in 2000, 6.7 million children who qualified for these programs remained uninsured (Hoffman & Pohl, 2002) primarily because of parental lack of knowledge of program availability or the perceived complexity of enrollment and renewal procedures. Historically, the health care of the poor has been the providence of nursing, and the nurse-coordinated efforts to increase enrollment of poor children into this program likely will be the most successful.

Family Factors

Disruptions in all aspects of family relations, not just parent-child, are often present in the families of maltreated children, with anger and conflict pervasive in abusive families and social isolation more prevalent in neglectful families (Albarracin, Repetto, & Albarracin, 1997; Burke, Chandy, Dannerbeck, & Watt, 1998; Crittenden, 1999; Gable, 1998; Gaudin, Polansky, Kilpatrick, & Shilton, 1996). Chaotic family organization with high levels of conflict and low levels of verbal expression and communication is reported as more predominate among families of maltreated children (Gable, 1998; Gaudin et al., 1996). Family structure also has been associated with the probability of child maltreatment. Children living with a single parent are at significantly greater risk of physical abuse and neglect, most likely because of added stress, fewer resources, lower socioeconomic status, and less opportunity to share child-rearing burdens than two-parent homes (Dubowitz, 1999a; Nelson, Cross, Landsman, & Tyler, 1996; Smokowski & Wodarski, 1996; Wolfe, 1999). Children who live in father-only homes are almost twice as likely to be abused physically than those living with mothers alone (Sedlak & Broadhurst, 1996).

Maltreatment, particularly physical and educational neglect, also has been found to be more common in larger families where additional young children result in greater responsibilities, tasks, and caregiver demands (Gable, 1998; Wolfe, 1999). Additional family factors that have been linked to child maltreatment include geographical or social isolation from family and friends (Albarracin et al., 1997; Campbell, 1996; Caselles & Milner, 2000; DePanfilis, 1996; Dolz, Cerezo, & Milner, 1997; Dubowitz, 1999a; Gable, 1998; Kolko, 2002); younger parents with lower education levels and a larger number of closely spaced children (Jaffee, Caspi, Moffitt, Belsky, & Silva, 2001; National Research Council, 1993b; Stevens-Simon, Nelligan, & Kelly, 2001); life stress and distress (Crittenden, 1996; Gable, 1998; Nelson et al., 1996); violent family interactions characterized by marital discord, domestic violence, and sibling violence (Hartley, 2002; Jellen, McCarroll, & Thayer, 2001; McGuigan & Pratt, 2001); and violent, antisocial families with a history of aggressive or criminal behavior outside of the family (Abel, Becker, Cunningham-Rathner, Mittleman, & Rouleau, 1988; Lanning, 2002; Pagelow, 1989; Patterson, 1982).

Physically abusing families are characterized by negative daily interactions, anxious relationships between family members, and members who respond more negatively to aversive communication or interactions (Cicchetti & Rogosch, 2001; Crittenden, Partridge, & Claussen, 1991; Lynch & Cicchetti, 1991). Research findings indicate that hostility and aggression often underlie abusers' smiles and affectionate behavior, which may explain the process whereby children (and the adults they become) are more likely to distrust and misuse ordinary communication signals (Crittenden, 1995, 1996; Gable, 1998; Howes, Cicchetti, Toth, & Rogosch, 2000).

Neglect is usually pervasive in the lives of all family members, with parents and children often perceiving themselves to be powerless and viewing attempts at goal achievement to be futile. Evidence indicates that child neglect is more likely to be associated with single-parent households (Burke et al., 1998; Dubowitz, 1999b; Smokowski & Wodarski, 1996), chaotic family organization (Gable, 1998; Gaudin et al., 1996), lower social economic status (Slack et al., 2004), large number of children in the family (Gable, 1998), social isolation (Albarracin et al., 1997; Campbell, 1997; DePanfilis, 1996; Gable, 1998), and domestic violence (Jellen et al., 2001; McGuigan & Pratt, 2001). Researchers have reported the co-occurrence of several risk factors (single parent, substance abuse, maternal depression, and chronic mental illness) for domestic violence and child neglect and suggest domestic violence screening in families cited for child neglect (Hartley, 2002). Substance-abusing families also have been reported to exhibit unique characteristics and behaviors that heighten the risk for child neglect (Dunn et al., 2002). Vulnerable families also may include those in situational crisis related to life stressors such as death, divorce, relocation, and unemployment (Crittenden, 1996).

Family factors that have been related to child sexual abuse include an estranged family; a mother who is absent, ill, or otherwise not protective of the child; unusual sleeping or rooming conditions; the erosion of social networks; and the lack of social support for the mother (Finkelhor, 1984, 1993; Gomes-Schwartz, Horowitz, & Cardarelli, 1990; Weiss, Longhurst, & Mazure, 1999). Empirical studies have found that ongoing sexual abuse often occurs with other forms of family dysfunction. Studies have reported that families with a child who has been sexually abused (including familial and nonfamilial abuse) are less cohesive, more disorganized, more dysfunctional (Elliott & Briere, 1994; Mannarino & Cohen, 1996a, 1996b), less likely to encourage independence and moral-religious values, and less involved recreationally (Ray, Jackson, & Townsley, 1991) than families of nonabused individuals. Researchers have noted that although it appears that families in which incest has occurred do exhibit greater dysfunction, the pathology possibly is as much an outcome of the incest as the cause (Briere, 2000).

As previously noted, psychological maltreatment may occur alone or in association with all other forms of child maltreatment. Research suggests that the most common and long-lasting effects of physical abuse, sexual abuse, and neglect tend to be related to the embedded accompanying psychological experiences and that psychological maltreatment occurring alone is associated with negative effects equal to or greater than other forms of abuse (Hart et al., 2002). Thus family characteristics of all other types of child maltreatment must be considered within the context of family factors associated with psychological maltreatment. Studies have characterized the families of psychologically maltreated children as having more psychosocial problems, poor coping skills, greater levels of perceived stress (Hickox & Furnell, 1989), avoidant coping styles, total disregard for the child's emotional experience (severe parental criticism, embarrassment and humiliation of the child) (Claussen & Crittenden, 1991; Egeland, Sroufe, & Erickson, 1983; Shipman & Zeman, 2001), and negative emotional socialization of children (Krause, Mendelson, & Lynch, 2003). Researchers have postulated that vulnerable families also may include those in situational crisis related to life stressors such as death, divorce, relocation, and unemployment (Crittenden, 1996).

Parental/Caretaker Factors

Dissimilar approaches to child rearing can emerge from the interaction of two fundamental dimensions of parenting: the degree of parental "authority" and the degree of parental "sensitivity" (Maccoby & Martin, 1983). Parents who are demanding but fail to recognize their child's limitations and needs typify the pattern of physically and psychologically abusive parents, whereas parents who place few demands and provide little or no structure typify a neglectful, uninvolved style of parenting (Wolfe, 1999). Specific characteristics of parental personality have been reported extensively to increase the likelihood of abusive or neglectful behavior and are reviewed only briefly in this section (Table 75-2).

Identified parental/caregiver risks for child maltreatment include a history of depression, anxiety, and antisocial relations that are associated with subsequent disruption in social relations, social support, decreased or dysfunctional parent-child interactions, and an inability to cope with stress (Albarracin et al., 1997; DePanfilis, 1996; Dubowitz, 1999b; Éthier, Lacharité, & Couture, 1995; National Research Council, 1993b; Wolfe, 1999); excessive hostility, anger, harsh parenting, and disturbances of affect and other psychological characteristics that may be associated with a history of maltreatment during childhood (Banyard, Williams, & Siegel, 2003; Carter, Joyce, Mulder, & Luty, 2001; Crouch, Milner, & Thomsen, 2001; Milan, Lewis, Ethier, Keshaw, & Ickovics, 2004; Nelson et al., 1996; Whipple & Webster-Stratton, 1991); substance abuse, which has been implicated in rendering parents less able or less willing to interact with their children and in aggressive acts toward children (Cash & Wilke, 2003; Dubowitz, 1999b; Jaudes & Diamond, 1985; Nelson et al., 1996; Peterson, Gable, & Saldana, 1996), as well as impeding their development related to maternal ingestion during pregnancy (Cash & Wilke, 2003); and domestic violence or a history of violent or antisocial behavior (Appel & Holden, 1998; Edleson, 1999; Hartley, 2002; Jellen et al., 2001; McGuigan & Pratt, 2001).

Additional characteristics that have been associated with neglectful parents include an immature, childlike personality related to low self-esteem, poor impulse control, limited financial and household management skills, and limited social competencies (Brooks-Gunn & Duncan, 1997; Burke et al., 1998; Gable, 1998). Abusive parents have been found to demonstrate inappropriate expectations of the child; disregard for the child's needs and abilities; role reversal with expectations that the child will meet their needs; beliefs that the child intentionally annoys them; and inconsistent, rejecting, and punitive child-rearing practices (Cicchetti & Rogosch, 2001; Crittenden, 1996, 1999; Hart et al., 2002; Krause et al., 2003; Shipman & Zeman, 2001). Poor parental physical health and stress-related symptoms have been related to child physical and emotional neglect (when the parent is physically or psychologically immobilized and unable to provide care) and child physical and emotional abuse (Cowen, 1998; Crittenden, 1996; El-Kamary et al., 2004).

Aggressive and violent behavior also has been associated with the following underlying health conditions: (1) illnesses including hypoglycemia, seizure disorders, central nervous system vasculitis, hyperthyroidism, infections, cardiopulmonary insufficiency, dehydration with resulting electrolyte imbalances, severe pain, and brain lesions such as tumors, abscesses, and trauma-related conditions; (2) exposure to toxins including carbon monoxide, hydrocarbons, inorganic mercury, and boric acid; (3) ingestion, overdose, or withdrawal from psychoactive drugs including alcohol, benzodiazepines, amphetamines, phencyclidine (PCP), corticosteroids, digitalis, lidocaine, pentazocaine, narcotic analgesics, and those drugs with anticholinergic effects that can produce atropinism (atropine, scopolamine, anti-parkinsonian, neuroleptics, and tricyclic antidepressants); and (4) major mental disorders including schizophrenia and bipolar affective disorders (Barry, 1984).

Child Factors

Certain child health, intellectual, and developmental characteristics have been reported to contribute to an increased risk of child maltreatment. Some researchers contend that the "goodness of fit" between child and parent characteristics influences the child's vulnerability to maltreatment (Black, Feigelman, & Cureton, 1999; Dubowitz & Black, 1994). Others have postulated that additional or heightened care burdens placed on an already stressed or incapable family system may result in a breakdown of parental coping abilities (Cowen, 1998; Dubowitz, 1999b; Pianta, Egeland, & Erickson, 1989; Sullivan & Knutson, 2000). Professional reporting dilemmas related to the excessive care requirements of technology-dependent children on their parents/caretakers have been reported (Johnson, 1993). Nurses are familiar with parental caregiver fatigue and burnout related to caring for children with demanding chronic illnesses and the resultant "unable to contact parents" situations that may occur for a few days following a nonacute readmission for a chronic problem. In such cases, the nationwide lack of adequate respite care for children with disabilities could be noted equally as an etiological factor.

As previously noted, children 3 years of age or younger, particularly children less than 1 year of age, are the most frequently reported victims of maltreatment, with 79% of child maltreatment fatalities occurring in this age group (U.S. Department of Health and Human Services, 2005). Other vulnerable child characteristics include difficult temperament as perceived by mother

(Harrington, Black, Starr, & Dubowitz, 1998); conduct disorders (Whipple & Webster-Stratton, 1991); oppositional defiant disorders (Ford et al., 1999); factors related to increased care demands such as prematurity and low birth weight (Cowen, 1998, 2001; Herrenkohl, Herrenkohl, & Egolf, 1983); chronic disabilities and physical impairments (Cowen & Reed, 2002; National Research Council, 1993b; Sullivan & Knutson, 1998, 2000); and a large number of closely spaced children within the family (Gable, 1998).

The majority of child sexual victims are females with onset at 7 to 12 years of age as the most vulnerable age for onset (Berliner & Elliott, 2002; Finkelhor, 1993). Other characteristics of children vulnerable to sexual abuse include having a mother who is ill or disabled, living with parents whose relationship is conflicted, living with a stepfather or without one's natural parents for extended periods, living with parents who have substance abuse problems, and having few close friends (Finkelhor, 1993; Finkelhor & Baron, 1986; Finkelhor & Hotaling, 1984). Prior sexual and physical child maltreatment has been reported to make children more vulnerable to child sexual abuse (Boney-McCoy & Finkelhor, 1995). In a prospective study, all types of early child maltreatment predicted elementary school peer victimization and bullying for boys and girls (Shields & Cicchetti, 2001).

Developmental Outcomes for Children

Previous and current findings conclude that child maltreatment can have severe, deleterious effects on children's physical, cognitive, emotional, and behavioral development (Erickson & Egeland, 2002; Horowitz, Widom, McLaughlin, & White, 2001; Kendall-Tackett, 2003; Knutson, DeGarmo, & Reid, 2004; Repetti, Taylor, & Seeman, 2002). Physical and psychosocial/behavioral consequences of child maltreatment have been identified at every stage of child development. Researchers have found that child maltreatment occurring early in life is particularly detrimental to subsequent development (Hildyard & Wolfe, 2002), and significant lifetime health effects have been reported (Kendall-Tackett, 2003).

Recent biological research findings have indicated that maltreated children's exposure to extreme stress produces high levels of cortisol, and the presence of these high levels during brain development may change the brain physically for the long term (Bremner, 1999; Bremner et al., 1997). Children who have suffered chronic maltreatment have been noted to have smaller hippocampi (critical for memory) especially on the left side, smaller cortexes, and differences in limbic and brainstem functions (Frustaci & Ryan, 1999). Damage to the limbic system can result in lifelong difficulties in social relationships and with memory and learning (Perry, 2001).

Some researchers posit that the chronic stress of child maltreatment is a risk factor for acute and chronic posttraumatic stress disorder (De Bellis et al., 1999). Researchers who examined the effects of extreme deprivation on infants raised in Romanian orphanages reported that at 2 years of age, the orphanage children did not show the usual diurnal variation of cortisol levels and had significantly lower morning cortisol levels, which remained elevated relative to the lower afternoon levels compared with home-reared Romanian children in the comparison group (Carlson & Earls, 1997). In a study of 1083 emotionally disturbed 4- to 17-year-olds with no history of neglect or abuse, a history of abuse with no neglect, or a history of neglect with no abuse, the emotionally disturbed children with a history of neglect showed the lowest dopamine β-hydoxylase levels and systolic and diastolic blood pressure, which are functions mediated by the norepinephrine system (Rogeness & McClure, 1996). The researchers note that these results support animal study findings that child neglect affects the development of the norepinephrine system in a long-lasting and perhaps permanent way.

However, an important note is that each child responds differently to traumatic events; there is not one pattern of response that every child follows (Wright, Master, & Hubbard, 1997). Factors that have been identified as influencing how children will respond to traumatic events include the characteristics of the child, of the traumatic event, and of the family and social system (Perry, 2001). It has been posited that the biological response to stress depends on the interaction of several factors, including nature of the stressor (type, chronicity, severity, controllability, and predictability), prior vulnerabilities (previous stress history, genetic and social vulnerabilities), and the current family environment (Yehuda et al., 1996). The timing of maltreatment in children's lives can explain a range of symptoms in abuse survivors, with each stage of development having its own vulnerabilities and protections (Kendall-Tackett, 2003).

Long-Term Health Effects of Childhood Victimization

Numerous empirical studies consistently have demonstrated child maltreatment to be associated with a broad range of behavioral, psychological, and health problems that persist into adulthood (for review of the literature, see Kendall-Tackett [2003] and Yehuda, Spertus, and Golier, [2001]). Recent research has provided a conceptual framework for grouping the many deleterious long-term health effects of child maltreatment into five major etiological pathways (Kendall-Tackett, 2003). The following are the pathways and summaries of their characteristics (p. xiv):

Physiological pathways: Trauma changes the body; the sympathetic nervous system becomes more reactive, levels of stress hormones become permanently dysregulated, and pain thresholds are lower. Children are especially vulnerable, and such changes are likely to occur when trauma is severe.

Behavioral pathways: Adult survivors are more likely to engage in harmful behaviors, especially substance abuse and high-risk sexual activity. Kendall-Tackett notes that this category has the most empirical support.

Cognitive pathways: Adult survivors were more likely to have negative beliefs about themselves and others. Negative beliefs can undermine health and also may lead to harmful behaviors and relationships. This can explain some of the difficulties that otherwise high-functioning survivors face.

Social pathways: Adult survivors have difficulties in their adult relationships with manifestations such as revictimization, divorce, marital disruptions, and social isolation and are more likely to be poor, have a hard time in school, and to be homeless.

Emotional pathways: Depression and posttraumatic stress disorder are common sequelae of past abuse that suppress the immune system and cause myriad health problems. Instead of thinking of these as outcomes, nurses need to think of them as mechanisms that lead to poor health.

Kendall-Tackett (2003) reviews hundreds of empirical studies that examine the increased risk and higher occurrence or correlations between adult survivors of maltreatment and behavioral, psychological, and health problems. Review of these studies is beyond the scope of this chapter; however, the major negatively affected variables include (1) physiological pathways: mood and anxiety disorders and the framework for behavioral variables; (2) behavioral pathways: substance abuse, smoking, obesity and eating disorders, suicide, high-risk sexual behavior, and sleep disturbances; (3) cognitive pathways: shame, self-blame, attributional style, health perception, self-esteem and self-efficacy, mistrust and hostility, and rejection sensitivity; (4) social pathways: insecure attachments, divorce, social isolation, and dysfunctional interpersonal style, difficulties in school, learning difficulties in adults, homelessness, and revictimization; and (5) emotional pathways: depression influences on cardiovascular health, immune function, health behaviors, and increased vulnerability; posttraumatic stress disorder influences on comorbidity, reactivity, and sleep quality.

The economic and human costs of maltreatment in American society are astronomical. Billions of dollars likely are spent in treatment and social service costs and are lost in lessened productivity for a generation of maltreated children (Cicchetti & Carlson, 1989). A recent cost analysis calculated an aggregate total of $94 billion in annual costs of child maltreatment to the U.S. economy (1% of the gross domestic product) for costs related hospitalization ($3.0 billion), mental health treatment ($425 million), child welfare costs ($14.4 billion), and adult criminality ($55.4 billion) (Fromm, 2001). The human costs include a litany of death, morbidity, and psychological tragedies. The emotional damage caused by maltreatment lasts a lifetime for many of the victims.

Nursing Considerations

According to Garbarino and Sherman (1980), the unmanageability of the stress is the most crucial factor in child maltreatment, and this unmanageability is a product of a mismatch between the level of stress and the availability and potency of social support. As the largest group of health care providers and positioned on the front lines of care delivery, nurses are a powerful source of social support. To be effective advocates, nurses must be aware of the "high risk" indicators that signal potential, present, or past child maltreatment, and equally as important, they must have confidence in their assessment findings: confidence to take responsibility for translating their assessments into interventions and outcomes that may involve a host of other specialties and agencies. Their role as advocate for the child, adult, and family is often the critical determinant of whether at-risk children, survivors, and families are identified and receive the services they need.

Although some negative health variables within each domain may appear entrenched, two fundamental truisms to remember are that (1) multifaceted problems require multidisciplinary interventions (you are not in this alone) and (2) even slight remediation of stressors may change the individual's perception of those stressors (you are doing more good than you know). Nurses not only offer valuable treatment and consultation on the physiological and psychological aspects of child maltreatment but also provide direct preventive interventions and consult information on topics such as parent-child interactions, a parent's ability to care for a child, and stress management. First and foremost, nurses must consider the possibility of child maltreatment with each child, adult, or elder for whom they care and must be willing to incorporate inquiry into their assessments. A physician reported a case in which he questioned a 70-year-old woman if she had ever been sexually assaulted or abused. She responded that a brother had raped her at the age of 10; no health provider had previously tried to connect her current health problems to her past assault (Felitti, 2001).

REFERENCES

Abel, G., Becker, J., Cunningham-Rathner, J., Mittleman, M., & Rouleau, J. (1988). Multiple paraphiliac diagnosis among sex offenders. *Academy of Psychiatry and the Law, 16*(2), 153-168.

Albarracin, D., Repetto, M. J., & Albarracin, M. (1997). Social support in child abuse and neglect: Support functions, sources, and contexts. *Child Abuse & Neglect, 21*(7), 607-615.

American Professional Society on the Abuse of Children. (1995). The APSAC. *The APSAC Advisor, 8,* 1-28.

Ammerman, R. T., & Patz, R. J. (1996). Determinants of child abuse potential: Contribution of parent and child factors. *Journal of Clinical Child Psychology, 25*(3), 300-307.

Appel, A. E., & Holden, G. W. (1998). The co-occurrence of spouse and physical child abuse: A review and appraisal. *Journal of Family Psychology, 12,* 578-599.

Banyard, V. L., Williams, L. M., & Siegel, J. A. (2003). The impact of complex trauma and depression on parenting: An exploration of mediating risk and protective factors. *Child Maltreatment, 8*(4), 334-349.

Barnett, O. W., Miller-Perrin, C. L., & Perrin, R. D. (1997). *Family violence across the lifespan: An introduction.* Thousand Oaks, CA: Sage Publications.

Barry, D. (1984). Pharmacotherapy in violent behavior. In S. Saunders, A. Anderson, C. Hart, & G. Rubenstein (Eds.), *Violent individuals and families: A handbook for practitioners.* Springfield, IL: Charles Thomas.

Baugher, E., & Lamison-White, L. (1996). *Poverty in the United States, 1995* (No. Current Population Reports, P-60, No. 194). Washington, DC: U.S. Government Printing Office.

Berliner, B., & Elliott, D. M. (2002). Sexual abuse of children. In J. E. B. Myers, L. Berliner, J. Briere, C. Jenny, C. T. Hendrix, & T. A. Reid (Eds.), *The APSAC handbook on child maltreatment* (2nd ed., pp. 55-78). Thousand Oaks, CA: Sage Publications.

Black, M. M., Feigelman, S., & Cureton, P. (1999). Evaluation and treatment of children with failure to thrive: An interdisciplinary perspective. *Journal of Clinical Outcomes Management, 6*(5), 60-73.

Boney-McCoy, S., & Finkelhor, D. (1995). Psychological sequelae of violent victimization in a national youth sample. *Journal of Consulting & Clinical Psychology, 63,* 726-736.

Bremner, J. D. (1999). Does stress damage the brain? *Biological Psychiatry, 45*(7), 797-805.

Bremner, J. D., Randall, P., Vermetten, E., Staib, L., Bronen, R. A., Mazure, C., et al. (1997). Magnetic resonance imaging-based measurement of hippocampal volume in posttraumatic stress disorder related to childhood physical and sexual abuse: a preliminary report. *Biological Psychiatry, 41*(1), 23-32.

Briere, J. (2000). Incest. In A. E. Kazdin (Ed.), *Encyclopedia of psychology.* Washington, DC: American Psychological Association & Oxford University Press.

Bronfenbrenner, U. (1977). Toward an experimental ecology of human development. *American Psychologist, 32,* 513-531.

Brooks-Gunn, J., & Duncan, G. J. (1997). The effects of poverty on children. *The Future of Children: Children and Poverty, 7*(2), 55-71.

Burke, J., Chandy, J., Dannerbeck, A., & Watt, J. W. (1998). The parental environment cluster model of child neglect: An integrative conceptual model. *Child Welfare, 77*(4), 389-405.

Campbell, H. (1996). Inter-agency assessment of respite care needs of families of children with special needs in Fife. *Public Health, 110,* 151-155.

Campbell, L. (1997). Child neglect and intensive-family-preservation practice. *Families in Society, 78*(3), 280-290.

Carlson, M., & Earls, F. (1997). Psychological and neuroendocrinological sequelae of early social deprivation in institutionalized children in Romania. *Annals of the New York Academy of Sciences, 807,* 419-428.

Carter, J. D., Joyce, P. R., Mulder, R. T., & Luty, S. E. (2001). The contribution of temperament, childhood neglect, and abuse to the development of personality dysfunction: A comparison of three models. *Journal of Personality Disorders, 15*(2), 123-135.

Caselles, C. E., & Milner, J. S. (2000). Evaluation of child transgressions, disciplinary choices, and expected child compliance in a no-cry and a crying infant condition in physically abusive and comparison mothers. *Child Abuse & Neglect, 24*(4), 477-491.

Cash, S., & Wilke, D. J. (2003). An ecological model of maternal substance abuse and child neglect: Issues, analyses, and recommendations. *American Journal of Orthopsychiatry, 73*(4), 392-404.

Children's Defense Fund. (1997). *The state of America's children.* Washington, DC: Author.

Cicchetti, D., & Carlson, V. (Eds.). (1989). *Child maltreatment: Theory and research on the causes and consequences of child abuse and neglect.* New York: Cambridge University Press.

Cicchetti, D., & Rogosch, R. (2001). The impact of child maltreatment and psychopathology on neuroendocrine functioning. *Development and Psychopathology, 13,* 783-904.

Claussen, A. H., & Crittenden, P. M. (1991). Physical and psychological maltreatment: Relations among types of maltreatment. *Child Abuse & Neglect, 15*(1-2), 5-18.

Committee on Injury and Poison Prevention. (2001). Falls from heights: Windows, roofs and balconies. *Pediatrics, 107*(5), 1188-1191.

Coohey, C. (1995). Neglectful mothers, their mothers, and partners: The significance of mutual aid. *Child Abuse & Neglect, 19*(8), 885-895.

Cowen, P. S. (1998). Crisis child care: An intervention for at risk-families. *Issues in Comprehensive Pediatric Nursing, 21,* 147-158.

Cowen, P. S. (2001). Crisis child care: Implications for family interventions. *Journal of the American Psychiatric Nurses Association, 7*(6), 196-204.

Cowen, P. S., & Reed, D. (2002). Effects of respite care for children with developmental disabilities: Evaluation of an intervention for at risk families. *Public Health Nursing, 19*(4), 272-283.

Crittenden, P. M. (1995). Attachment and psychopathology. In S. Goldberg, R. Muir, & J. Kerr (Eds.), *Attachment theory: Social, developmental, and clinical perspectives.* Hillsdale, NJ: Analytic Press.

Crittenden, P. M. (1996). Research on maltreating families: Implications for intervention. In J. Briere, L. Berliner, J. Bulkley, C. Jenny, & T. Reid (Eds.), *The APSAC handbook on child maltreatment* (pp. 158-174). Thousand Oaks, CA: Sage Publications.

Crittenden, P. M. (1999). Child neglect: Causes and consequences. In H. Dubowitz (Ed.), *Neglected children.* Thousand Oaks, CA: Sage Publications.

Crittenden, P. M., Partridge, M. F., & Claussen, A. H. (1991). Family patterns of relationship in normative and dysfunctional families. *Development and Psychopathology, 3*(4), 491-512.

Crouch, J. L., Milner, J. S., & Thomsen, C. (2001). Childhood physical abuse, early social support, and risk for maltreatment: Current social support as a mediator of risk for child physical abuse. *Child Abuse & Neglect, 25*(1), 93-107.

Cutts, D. B., Pheley, A. M., & Geppert, J. S. (1998). Hunger in mid-Western inner-city young children. *Archives of Pediatrics & Adolescent Medicine, 152*(5), 589-593.

De Bellis, M. D., Keshavan, M., Clark, D. B., Casey, B. J., Giedd, J., Boring, A. M., et al. (1999). Developmental traumatology. Part II: Brain development. *Biological Psychiatry, 45*(10), 1271-1284.

DePanfilis, D. (1996). Social isolation of neglectful families: A review of social support assessment and intervention models. *Child Maltreatment, 1*(1), 37-52.

Devaney, B., Ellwood, M., & Love, J. (1997). Programs that mitigate the effects of poverty on children. *The Future of Children, 7*(2), 88-112.

Dolz, L., Cerezo, M. A., & Milner, J. S. (1997). Mother-child interactional patterns in high and low risk mothers. *Child Abuse & Neglect, 21*(12), 1149-1158.

Dubowitz, H. (1999a). The families of neglected children. In M. E. Lamb (Ed.), *Parenting and child development in "non-traditional" families* (Vol. viii, pp. 327-345). Mahwah, NJ: Erlbaum Associates.

Dubowitz, H. (Ed.). (1999b). *Neglected children: Research, practice, and policy.* Thousand Oaks, CA: Sage.

Dubowitz, H., & Black, M. (1994). Child neglect. In R. M. Reece (Ed.), *Child abuse: Medical diagnosis and management* (pp. 279-297). Malvern, PA: Lea & Febiger.

Dubowitz, H., & Black, M. (2002). Neglect of children's health. In J. E. Myers, L. Berliner, J. Briere, C. Hendrix, C. Jenny, & T. Reid (Eds.), *The APSAC handbook on child maltreatment* (2nd ed., pp. 269-292). Thousand Oaks, CA: Sage Publications.

Dubowitz, H., Newton, R. R., Litrownik, A. J., Lewis, T., Briggs, E. C., Thompson, R., et al. (2005). Examination of a conceptual model of child neglect. *Child Maltreatment, 10*(2), 173-189.

Duncan, G. J., & Brooks-Gunn, J. (2000). Family poverty, welfare reform, and child development. *Child Development, 71,* 188-196.

Dunn, M. G., Tarter, R. E., Mezzich, A. C., Vanyukov, M., Kirisci, L., & Kirillova, G. (2002). Origins and consequences of child neglect in substance abuse families. *Clinical Psychology Review, 22,* 1063-1090.

Edleson, J. L. (1999). The overlap between child maltreatment and woman battering. *Violence Against Women, 5,* 134-154.

Egeland, B., Sroufe, L. A., & Erickson, M. (1983). The developmental consequence of different patterns of maltreatment. *Child Abuse & Neglect, 7*(4), 459-469.

El-Kamary, S. S., Higman, S. M., Fuddy, L., McFarlane, E., Sia, C., & Duggan, A. K. (2004). Hawaii's healthy start home visiting program: Determinants and impact of rapid repeat birth. *Pediatrics, 114*(3), 317-326.

Elliott, D. M., & Briere, J. (1994). Forensic sexual abuse evaluations of older children: Disclosures and general population study. *Journal of Traumatic Stress, 8,* 629-647.

Elliott, M., Browne, K., & Kilcoyne, J. (1995). Child sexual abuse prevention: What offenders tell us. *Child Abuse & Neglect, 19*(5), 579-594.

Erickson, M. F., & Egeland, B. (2002). Child neglect. In J. E. Myers, L. Berliner, J. Briere, C. Hendrix, C. Jenny, & T. Reid (Eds.), *The APSAC handbook on child maltreatment* (pp. 3-20). Thousand Oaks, CA: Sage Publications.

Éthier, L. S., Lacharité, C., & Couture, G. (1995). Childhood adversity, parental stress, and depression of negligent mothers. *Child Abuse & Neglect, 19*(5), 619-632.

Ethier, L. S., Lemelin, J. P., & Lacharite, C. (2004). A longitudinal study of the effects of chronic maltreatment on children's behavioral and emotional problems. *Child Abuse & Neglect, 25*(12), 1265-1278.

Fagan, P. F. (1997). *The child abuse crisis: The disintegration of marriage, family and the American community* (No. 1115). Washington, DC: The Heritage Foundation.

Feldman, M. A., Ducharme, J. M., & Case, L. (1999). Using self-instructional pictorial manuals to teach child-care skills to mothers with intellectual disabilities. *Behavior Modification, 23*(3), 480-497.

Felitti, V. J. (2001). Reverse alchemy in childhood: Turning gold into lead. *Southern Medical Journal, 84,* 328-331.

Finkelhor, D. (1984). *Child sexual abuse: New theory and research.* New York: Free Press.

Finkelhor, D. (1993). Epidemiological factors in the clinical identification of child sexual abuse. *Child Abuse & Neglect, 17,* 67-70.

Finkelhor, D., & Baron, L. (1986). High risk children. In D. Finkelhor (Ed.), *A sourcebook on child sexual abuse.* Beverly Hills, CA: Sage.

Finkelhor, D., & Dziuba-Leatherman, J. (1994). Children as victims of violence: A national survey. *Pediatrics, 94,* 413-420.

Finkelhor, D., & Hotaling, G. T. (1984). Sexual abuse in the National Incidence Study of child abuse and neglect: An appraisal. *Child Abuse & Neglect, 8,* 23-32.

Finkelhor, D., Hotaling, G., Lewis, I. A., & Smith, C. (1990). Sexual abuse in a national survey of adult men and women: Prevalence, characteristics and risk factors. *Child Abuse & Neglect, 14,* 19-28.

Ford, J. D., Racusin, R., Daviss, W. B., Ellis, C., Thomas, J., Rogers, K., et al. (1999). Trauma exposure among children with attention deficit-hyperactivity disorder and oppositional defiant disorder. *Journal of Consulting & Clinical Psychology, 67*(5), 786-789.

Fromm, S. (2001). *Total estimated cost of child abuse and neglect in the United States: Statistical evidence.* Retrieved March 5, 2003, http://www.preventchildabuse.org/learn_more/research_docs/cost_analysis.pdf

Frustaci, K., & Ryan, N. D. (1999). Developmental traumatology. Part II: Brain development. *Biological Psychiatry, 45*(10), 1271-1284.

Gable, S. (1998). School-age and adolescent children's perceptions of family functioning in neglectful and non-neglectful families. *Child Abuse & Neglect, 22*(9), 859-867.

Garbarino, J. (1977). The human ecology of child maltreatment. *Journal of Marriage and the Family, 39,* 721-735.

Garbarino, J., & Kostelny, K. (1992). Child maltreatment as a community problem. *Child Abuse and Neglect, 16*(4), 455-464.

Garbarino, J., & Sherman, D. (1980). High-risk neighborhoods and high-risk families: The human ecology of child maltreatment. *Child Development, 51,* 188-198.

Gaudin, J. M., Jr., Polansky, N. A., Kilpatrick, A. C., & Shilton, P. (1996). Family functioning in neglectful families. *Child Abuse & Neglect, 20*(4), 363-377.

Gillham, B., Tanner, G., Cheyne, B., Freeman, I., Rooney, M., & Lambie, A. (1998). Unemployment rates, single parent density, and indices of child poverty: Their relationship to different categories of child abuse and neglect. *Child Abuse & Neglect, 22*(2), 79-90.

Gomes-Schwartz, B., Horowitz, J. M., & Cardarelli, A. P. (1990). *Child sexual abuse: The initial effects.* Newbury Park: Sage.

Harrington, D., Black, M. M., Starr, R. H., Jr., & Dubowitz, H. (1998). Child neglect: Relation to child temperament and family context. *American Journal of Orthopsychiatry, 68*(1), 108-116.

Hart, S. N., Brassard, M. R., Binggeli, N. J., & Davidson, H. A. (2002). Psychological maltreatment. In J. E. Myers, L. Berliner, J. Briere, C. Hendrix, C. Jenny, & T. Reid (Eds.), *The APSAC handbook on child maltreatment* (2nd ed.). Thousand Oaks, CA: Sage Publications.

Hartley, C. C. (2002). The co-occurrence of child maltreatment and domestic violence: Examining both neglect and child physical abuse. *Child Maltreatment, 7*(4), 349-358.

Herrenkohl, R. C., Herrenkohl, E. C., & Egolf, B. P. (1983). Circumstances surrounding the occurrence of child maltreatment. *Journal of Consulting and Clinical Psychology, 51,* 424-431.

Hickox, A., & Furnell, J. (1989). Psychosocial and background factors in emotional abuse of children. *Child Care, Health, and Development, 15*(4), 227-240.

Hildyard, K. L., & Wolfe, D. A. (2002). Child neglect: Developmental issues and outcomes. *Child Abuse & Neglect, 26,* 679-695.

Hoffman, C., & Pohl, M. B. (2002). *Health insurance coverage in America: 2000 data update.* Washington, DC: Kaiser Commission on Medicaid and the Uninsured.

Hogue, E. E. (1993). Child neglect in home care: Weighing legal and ethical issues. *Pediatric Nursing, 19*(5), 496-498.

Homes, W. C., & Slap, G. B. (1998). Sexual abuse of boys: Definitions, prevalence, correlates, sequelae, and management. *JAMA: The Journal of American Medical Association, 280,* 1855-1862.

Horowitz, A. V., Widom, C. S., McLaughlin, J., & White, H. R. (2001). The impact of childhood abuse and neglect on adult mental health: A prospective study. *Journal of Health and Social Behavior, 42,* 184-201.

Howes, P. W., Cicchetti, D., Toth, S., & Rogosch, F. A. (2000). Affective, organizational, and relational characteristics of maltreating families: A systems perspective. *Journal of Family Psychology, 14*(1), 95-110.

Howze, D. C., & Kotch, J. B. (1984). Disentangling life events, stress, and social support: Implications for primary prevention of child abuse and neglect. *Child Abuse and Neglect, 8*(4), 401-409.

Jaffee, S., Caspi, A., Moffitt, T. E., Belsky, J., & Silva, P. (2001). Why are children born to teen mothers at risk for adverse outcomes in young adulthood? Results from a 20-year longitudinal study. *Development and Psychopathology, 13*(2), 377-397.

Jaudes, P. K., & Diamond, L. J. (1985). The handicapped child and child abuse. *Child Abuse & Neglect, 9,* 341-347.

Jaudes, P. K., & Ekwo, E. (1995). Association of drug abuse and child abuse. *Child Abuse and Neglect, 19*(9), 1065-1075.

Jellen, L. K., McCarroll, J. E., & Thayer, L. E. (2001). Child emotional maltreatment: A 2-year study of U.S. Army bases. *Child Abuse & Neglect, 25*(5), 623-639.

Johnson, C. F. (1993). Physicians and medical neglect: Variables that affect reporting. *Child Abuse & Neglect, 17*, 605-612.

Kendall-Tackett, K. (2003). *Treating the lifetime health effects of childhood victimization.* Kingston, NJ: Civic Research Institute.

Kim, J., & Cichetti, D. (2004). A longitudinal study of child maltreatment, mother-child relationship quality and maladjustment: The role of self-esteem and social competence. *Journal of Abnormal Child Psychology, 32*(4), 341-354.

Knutson, J. F., DeGarmo, D. S., & Reid, J. B. (2004). Social disadvantage and neglectful parenting as precursors to the development of antisocial and aggressive child behavior: Testing a theoretical model. *Aggressive Behavior, 30*, 187-205.

Kolko, D. J. (2002). Child physical abuse. In J. E. Myers, L. Berliner, J. Briere, C. Hendrix, C. Jenny, & T. Reid (Eds.), *The APSAC handbook of child maltreatment* (2nd ed., pp. 21-54). Thousand Oaks, CA: Sage Publications.

Korbin, J. E. (1994). Sociocultural factors in child maltreatment. In G. Melton & F. Barry (Eds.), *Protecting children from abuse and neglect* (pp. 182-223). New York: Guilford Press.

Kotch, J. B., Browne, D. C., Dufort, V., & Winsor, J. (1999). Predicting child maltreatment in the first 4 years of life from characteristics assessed in the neonatal period. *Child Abuse & Neglect, 23*(4), 305-319.

Kotch, J. B., Browne, D. C., Ringwalt, C. L., Stewart, P. W., Ruina, E., Holt, K., et al. (1995). *Child Abuse & Neglect, 19*(9), 1115-1130.

Krause, E. D., Mendelson, T., & Lynch, T. R. (2003). Childhood emotional invalidation and adult psychological distress: the mediating role of emotional inhibition. *Child Abuse & Neglect, 27*, 199-213.

Krugman, S. D., & Dubowitz, H. (2003). Failure to thrive. *Family Physician, 68*(5), 879-884.

Lanning, K. V. (2002). Criminal investigation of sexual victimization of children. In J. E. Myers, L. Berliner, J. Briere, C. Hendrix, C. Jenny, & T. Reid (Eds.), *The APSAC handbook on child maltreatment* (2nd. ed., pp. 329-347). Thousand Oaks, CA: Sage Publications.

Lutenbacher, M., & Hall, L. A. (1998). The effects of maternal psychosocial factors on parenting attitudes of low-income, single mothers with young children. *Nursing Research, 47*(1), 25-34.

Lynch, M., & Cicchetti, D. (1991). Patterns of relatedness in maltreated and non-maltreated children: Connections among multiple representational models. *Development and Psychopathology, 3*(2), 207-226.

Maccoby, E., & Martin, J. (1983). Socialization in the context of the family: Parent-child interaction. In E. M. Hetherington (Ed.), *Handbook of child psychology: Socialization, personality, and social development* (4th ed., pp. 1-101). New York: Wiley.

Mannariono, A. P., & Cohen, J. A. (1996a). Abuse-related attributions and perceptions, general attributions and locus of control in sexually abused girls. *Child Maltreatment, 1*, 246-260.

Mannariono, A. P., & Cohen, J. A. (1996b). A follow-up study of factors that mediate the development psychological symptomatology in sexually abused girls. *Child Maltreatment, 11*, 246-260.

Margolin, L. (1990). Fatal child neglect. *Child Welfare, 69*(4), 309-319.

Maynard, R.A. (1997). Kids having kids: Economic and social consequences of teen pregnancy. Washington D.C.: The Urban Institute Press.

McGuigan, W. M., & Pratt, C. C. (2001). The predictive impact of domestic violence on three types of child maltreatment. *Child Abuse & Neglect, 25*(7), 869-883.

Meyers, J. E. B. (1998). *Legal issues in child abuse and neglect practice* (2nd ed.). Thousand Oaks, CA: Sage Publications.

Mierley, M. C., & Baker, S. P. (1983). Fatal house fires in an urban population. *Journal of the American Medical Association, 249*, 1466-1468.

Milan, S., Lewis, J., Ethier, K., Keshaw, T., & Ickovics, J. R. (2004). The impact of physical maltreatment history on the adolescent mother-infant relationship: Mediating and moderating effects during the transition to early parenthood. *Journal of Abnormal Child Psychology, 32*(3), 249-261.

Morton, N., & Browne, K. D. (1998). Theory and observation of attachment and its relation to child maltreatment: A review. *Child Abuse & Neglect, 22*(11), 1093-1104.

National Center for Children in Poverty. (2005). *Basic facts about low-income children: Birth to age 6.* Retrieved July 25, 2005, from http://www.nccp.org/pub_ycp05.html

National Research Council. (1993a). Consequences of child abuse and neglect. In *Understanding child abuse and neglect* (pp. 208-252). Washington, DC: National Academies Press.

National Research Council. (1993b). *Understanding child abuse and neglect.* Washington, DC: National Academies Press.

Nelson, K., Cross, T., Landsman, M. J., & Tyler, M. (1996). Native American families and child neglect. *Children & Youth Services Review, 18*(6), 505-521.

Pagelow, M. D. (1989). The incidence and prevalence of criminal abuse of other family members. In L. Ohlin & M. Tonry (Eds.), *Family violence* (Vol. 11, pp. 263-313). Chicago: University of Chicago Press.

Pagelow, M. D. (1997). Child neglect and psychological maltreatment. In K. Barnett, C. Miller-Perrin, & R. Perrin (Eds.), *Family violence across the lifespan* (pp. 107-132). Thousand Oaks, CA: Sage Publications.

Patterson, G. (1982). *Coercive family processes.* Eugene, OR: Castalia Publishing.

Pelton, L. (1985). *The social context of child abuse and neglect.* New York: Human Science Press.

Pelton, L. H. (1994). The role of material factors in child abuse and neglect. In G. Melton & F. Barry (Eds.), *Protecting children from abuse and neglect* (pp. 131-181). New York: Guilford Press.

Perry, B. D. (2001). The neuroarcheology of childhood maltreatment: The neurodevelopmental costs of adverse childhood events. In K. Franey, R. Geffner, & R. Falconer (Eds.), *The cost of child maltreatment: Who pays? We all do* (pp. 15-37). San Diego: Family Violence and Sexual Assault Institute.

Peterson, L., Gable, S., & Saldana, L. (1996). Treatment of maternal addiction to prevent child abuse and neglect. *Addictive Behaviors, 21*(6), 789-801.

Pianta, R., Egeland, B., & Erickson, M. F. (1989). The antecedents of maltreatment: Results of the mother-child interaction research project. In D. Cicchetti & V. Carlson (Eds.), *Child maltreatment: Theory and research on the causes and consequences of child abuse and neglect* (pp. 203-253). New York: Cambridge University Press.

Ray, K. C., Jackson, J. L., & Townsley, R. M. (1991). Family environments of victims of intrafamilial and extrafamilial child sexual abuse. *Journal of Family Violence, 6,* 365-374.

Rector, R. E., Fagan, P. F., & Johnson, K. A. (2004). *Marriage: Still the safest place for women and children* (No. 1732). Washington, DC: Heritage Foundation.

Repetti, R. L., Taylor, S. E., & Seeman, T. E. (2002). Risky families: Family social environments and the mental and physical health of offspring. *Psychological Bulletin, 128*(2), 330-366.

Rogeness, G., & McClure, E. (1996). Development and neurotransmitter-environmental interactions. *Development & Psychopathology, 8,* 183-199.

Rosenberg, D. (1994). Fatal neglect. *APSAC Advisor, 7*(4), 38-40.

Ruggiero, K. J., McLeer, S. V., & Dixon, J. F. (2000). Sexual abuse characteristics associated with survivor psychopathology. *Child Abuse & Neglect, 24,* 951-964.

Rumm, P. D., Cummings, P., Krauss, M. R., Bell, M. A., & Rivara, F. P. (2000). Identified spouse abuse as a risk factor for child abuse. *Child Abuse & Neglect, 24*(11), 1375-1381.

Saunder, B. E., Kilpatrick, D. G., Hanson, R. F., Resnick, H. S., & Walker, M. E. (1999). Prevalence, case characteristics, and long-term psychological correlates of child rape among women: A national survey. *Child Maltreatment, 4,* 187-200.

Sedlak, A. J., & Broadhurst, D. D. (1996). *Executive summary of the Third National Incidence Study of child abuse and neglect.* Washington, DC: U.S. Government Printing Office.

Shields, A., & Cicchetti, D. (2001). Parental maltreatment and emotion dysregulation as risk factors for bullying and victimization in middle childhood. *Journal of Clinical Child Psychology, 30,* 349-363.

Shipman, K. L., & Zeman, J. (2001). Socialization of children's emotional regulation in mother-child dyads: A developmental psychopathology perspective. *Development & Psychopathology, 13,* 317-336.

Slack, K. R., Holl, J. L., McDaniel, M., Yoo, J., & Bolger, K. (2004). Understanding the risks of child neglect: An exploration of poverty and parenting characteristics. *Child Maltreatment, 9*(4), 395-408.

Smokowski, P. R., & Wodarski, J. S. (1996). The effectiveness of child welfare services for poor, neglected children: A review of the empirical evidence. *Research on Social Work Practice, 6*(4), 504-523.

Stevens-Simon, C., & Barrett, J. (2001). A comparison of the psychological resources of adolescents at low and high risk of mistreating their children. *Journal of Pediatric Health Care, 15*(6), 299-303.

Stevens-Simon, C., Nelligan, D., & Kelly, L. (2001). Adolescents at risk for mistreating their children. Part II: A home- and clinic-based prevention program. *Child Abuse & Neglect, 6,* 753-769.

Sullivan, P. M., & Knutson, J. F. (1998). The association between child maltreatment and disabilities in a hospital-based epidemiological study. *Child Abuse & Neglect, 22*(4), 271-288.

Sullivan, P. M., & Knutson, J. F. (2000). The prevalence of disabilities and maltreatment among runaway children. *Child Abuse & Neglect, 24*(10), 1275-1288.

Toth, S. L., & Cicchetti, D. (1996). Patterns of relatedness, depressive symptomatology, and perceived competence in maltreated children. *Journal of Consulting & Clinical Psychology, 64*(1), 32-41.

Trotter, R., Ackerman, A., Rodman, D., Martinez, A., & Sorvillo, F. (1983). "Azarcon" and "Greta": Ethnomedical solutions to epidemiological mystery. *Medical Anthropology Quarterly, 14*(3), 3, 18.

U.S. Department of Health and Human Services. (2000). *Child maltreatment 1998: Reports from the states to the National Child Abuse and Neglect Data System.* Washington DC: U.S. Government Printing Office.

U.S. Department of Health and Human Services. (2004). The Child Abuse Prevention and Treatment Act: Amended by the Keeping Children and Families Safe Act of 2003. (pp. 1-77). Washington, DC: Author.

U.S. Department of Health and Human Services, Administration on Children, Youth and Families. (2005). *Child maltreatment 2003.* Washington DC: U.S. Government Printing Office.

Wang, C. T., & Daro, D. (1998). *Current trends in child abuse reporting and fatalities: Results of the 1997 annual fifty state survey* (No. 808). Chicago, IL: National Committee to Prevent Child Abuse.

Weiss, E. L., Longhurst, J. G., & Mazure, C. M. (1999). Childhood sexual abuse as a risk factor for depression in women: Psychosocial and neurobiological correlates. *American Journal of Psychiatry, 156,* 816-828.

Whipple, E. E., & Webster-Stratton, C. (1991). The role of parental stress in physically abusive families. *Child Abuse & Neglect, 15*(3), 279-291.

Wilkey, I., Pearn, J., Petrie, G., & Nixon, J. (1982). Neonaticide, infanticide, and child homicide. *Medicine, Science, & the Law, 22*(1), 31-34.

Wolfe, D. A. (1999). *Child abuse: Implications for child development and psychopathology, Volume 10.* Thousand Oaks, CA: Sage Publications.

Wolock, I., & Horowitz, B. (1984). Child maltreatment as a social problem: The neglect of neglect. *American Journal of Orthopsychiatry, 54*(4), 530-543.

Wright, M. O., Master, A. S., & Hubbard, J. J. (1997). Long-term effects of massive trauma: Developmental and psychobiological perspectives. In D. Cicchetti & S. Toth (Eds.), *Rochester symposium on developmental psychopathology: Developmental perspectives on trauma* (Vol. 8, pp. 181-225). Rochester, NY: University of Rochester Press.

Yehuda, R., Levengood, R. A., Schmeidler, J., Wilson, S., Guo, L. S., & Gerber, D. (1996). Increased pituitary activation following metyrapone administration in post traumatic stress disorder. *Psychoneuroendocrinology, 21,* 1-16.

Yehuda, R., Spertus, I. L., & Golier, J. A. (2001). Relationship between childhood traumatic experiences and PTSD in adults. In *PTSD in children and adolescents* (Vol. 20). Washington, DC: American Psychiatric Publishing.

Child Neglect Prevention

The Pivotal Role of Nursing

PERLE SLAVIK COWEN

> If our American way of life fails the child, it fails us all.
> **Pearl S. Buck, *The Child Who Never Grew***

Child neglect is the most prevalent, most lethal, and least empirically studied form of child maltreatment (U.S. Department of Health and Human Services, 2005). Child neglect has been associated with a plethora of adverse physical, psychological, and educational outcomes. Yet research on child neglect represents only a small fraction of the research on child maltreatment (De Bellis, 2005; Dubowitz, 1999b), and child neglect often is treated as a single entity under the rubric of child abuse. Child neglect, however, consists of acts of omission or failures to provide the basic care and protection that human growth requires, whereas physical abuse consists of acts of commission or inflicted injuries. Researchers have indicated that child neglect is correlated strongly with poverty, single-parent caretakers, unemployment, and multifaceted family problems (Cowen, 2001a; Myers et al., 2002; National Research Council, 1993a). Treatment for neglectful families requires multidisciplinary efforts to improve family functioning and promote a safe and supportive environment for the child. By virtue of the nature of the profession, the variety of its practice settings, and the sheer numbers of its practitioners, nursing can provide leadership in the efforts to combat this form of child maltreatment (Cowen, 1999b).

Nurses have a variety of roles in the assessment of and primary, secondary, and tertiary preventive interventions for child neglect, with child safety and optimal family functioning as the desired outcomes (Cowen, 1999a). Early identification and intervention have the potential for reducing or preventing the developmental consequences associated with the deprivations of neglect. The nurse's role as child and family advocate is often the critical determinant of whether at-risk families are identified and receive the therapeutic interventions and tangible services they need (Cowen, 1999b). In addition, nurses often have direct responsibilities for monitoring and remediating parenting patterns that have placed the child in hazardous conditions. The different levels of family functioning continually require adaptations in the nursing role, therapeutic approach, and helping activities. The purpose of this chapter is to present an overview of the problem of child neglect and the pivotal role nurses have in its prevention and treatment. This overview includes the types and characteristics of child neglect, theoretical perspectives, risk factors, and preventive considerations. In addition, areas of particular relevance to nursing practice are highlighted, such as nursing assessment, nursing interventions, and the developmental consequences of neglect for children.

BACKGROUND

During 2003, child protective service agencies received an estimated 2.9 million referrals of abuse or neglect (a rate of 39.1 referrals per 1000 children) concerning approximately 5.5 million children, and they accepted more than two thirds of those referrals for investigation or assessment (U.S. Department of Health and Human Services, 2005). An estimated 906,000 children were victims of abuse or neglect, with 63.2% experiencing neglect, 18.9% physical abuse, 9.9% sexual abuse, and 4.9% emotional or psychological maltreatment. Tragically, an estimated 1500 children died of abuse or neglect (rate of 2.00 children per 100,000), with attribution by maltreatment type as 35.6% neglect; 28.9% multiple maltreatment types; 28.4% physical abuse; 6.7% psychological, other, or unknown; and 0.4% sexual abuse.

Among the children who died, 78.7% were younger than 4 years old; 10% were 4 to 7 years old, 5% were 8 to 11 years old, and 6% were 12 to 17 years old. Infant boys (younger than 1 year old) had the highest rate of fatalities, nearly 18 per 100,000 boys of the same age; and infant girls had a rate of 14 deaths per 100,000 girls of the same age (U.S. Department of Health and Human Services, 2005). These figures represent the lowest estimate of the problem and depend on the number of states reporting (44 states, including the District of Columbia, participated in the 2003 report), the level of involvement of child protective services, and the varying levels of comprehensive investigation into child mortality cases by local authorities and classification variances among the states in reporting deaths caused by child maltreatment.

TYPES AND CHARACTERISTICS OF CHILD NEGLECT

A consensus does not exist among researchers, legislatures, and child welfare agencies as to the definition of child neglect. The 1974 Federal Child Abuse and Treatment Act (P.L. 93-247) guides child protection; was amended and reauthorized in 1978, 1984, 1988, 1996, and 2003; and has continued to expand and refine the scope of law (U.S. Department of Health and Human Services, 2004). The act defines child abuse and neglect as "any recent act or failure to act on the part of a parent or caretaker, which results in death, serious physical or emotional harm, sexual abuse or exploitation, or an act or failure to act which presents an imminent risk of serious harm" (p. 44). Specific types of maltreatment

defined include emotional abuse, neglect (physical, educational, and emotional), physical abuse, and sexual abuse. States and researchers typically may expand and specify additional neglect categories (Table 76-1). Great legal variability exists among and within state definitions because maltreatment statutes fall under three different categories: reporting laws that define who should make reports and under what conditions; dependency statutes that define which children should be made wards of the court; and criminal statutes that define a criminal act for purposes of prosecution (Erickson & Egeland, 2002). It is important for nurses to be familiar with the specific reporting statutes and definitions within their states.

Many issues are related to the definition of child neglect, perhaps underpinned by the assessment problem that neglect is the *absence* of nurturing behaviors or conditions as opposed to the presence of undesirable behaviors that can be identified in child abuse (English, Thompson, Graham, & Briggs, 2005). Some researchers have advocated for a broader, less blaming definition that views neglect from the child's perspective in that the child's basic needs are not being met and posits that not all circumstances require child protective services involvement (Dubowitz, 2003). The federal definition

TABLE 76-1

Types of Child Neglect*

Type of Neglect	Description
Abandonment	Desertion of children on a permanent or temporary basis. This can include failure to take a newborn infant home following delivery, leaving children home to fare for themselves, or failing to retrieve them from " temporary" care with a relative, child caretaker, or health care organization.
Educational neglect	Failure to comply with state requirements for school attendance, permitted chronic truancy and inattention to a child's special needs.
Emotional neglect	Refusals or delays in psychological care; inadequate attentions to a child's needs for affection, emotional support, attention, or competence; exposure of a child to extreme domestic violence; and permitting a child's maladaptive behaviors.
Health care/medical neglect	Failure to provide necessary health care, medical or mental health treatment including required immunizations, prescribed medications, recommended surgery or other intervention in case of serious disease or injury
Physical neglect	Failure to provide for a child's basic needs of shelter, nutrition, clothing, hygiene, and safety.
Supervision neglect	Failure to provide attendance, guidance, and protection to children who, lacking experience and knowledge, cannot comprehend or anticipate dangerous situations. This includes protection from environmental hazards such as poisons, electrical sockets, guns, and standing water. The parent may be in the home but impaired due to substance abuse, physical or mental illness, low intelligence, or immaturity, or may delegate their children's care to an inadequate caretaker who is obviously impaired, immature, or abusive.

* States may group or specify a variety of neglect categories.

VIEWPOINTS

also implies a certain set of accepted behaviors or care standards and designates who should be responsible for performing the behaviors or meeting the child's needs. Although parents have primary responsibility for meeting their children's needs, there is a need to acknowledge the many interacting influences that affect their ability to perform this role (Belsky, 1993; Dubowitz et al., 2005; Korbin & Spilsbury, 1999; Pelton, 1994) and perhaps to remember the African proverb "It takes a village to raise a child."

Other definitional and resultant operational issues include (1) concern regarding overwhelmed child protective services workers' prioritization of *actual* harm of a serious nature and unsubstantiation of mild and moderate *potential* harm, thereby impeding preventive efforts for at-risk children (Dubowitz & Black, 2002); (2) alarm related to the focus on short-term versus long-term harm resulting in a failure to prevent continuing care failures from contributing to significant morbidity or mortality for acute and chronic health conditions (Dubowitz & Black, 2002); and (3) failure to consider the long-term cognitive, psychological, social, emotional (Straus & Savage, 2005) and neurodevelopmental (De Bellis, 2005) detrimental effects of prolonged early neglect in ascertaining potential harm.

The child neglect categories permit specification of what parents/caretakers have failed to do; however, they do not provide insight into the severity of the neglect. Although there is basic agreement as to what constitutes severe physical child neglect, other specific types and individual cases of neglect include variables that create legal and ethical dilemmas that complicate the recognition and reporting of neglect. These dilemmas include (1) legal exemptions related to parental disability, poverty, or religious practices (Dubowitz & Black, 2002; Johnson, 1993); (2) lack of professional training and guidelines for determining medical neglect of specific diseases (Johnson, 1993); and (3) dilemmas related to the excessive demands on the parents/caretakers of children who are technology-dependent or disabled (Cowen & Reed, 2002; Hogue, 1993; Sullivan & Knutson, 1998, 2000).

In addition, there are no universal standards for child rearing. What is considered neglect in one culture may not be considered abnormal in another. For example, the norms in Western countries of allowing infants to "cry it out," children to sleep alone at night, and children to wait for meals may be considered neglect in some cultures (Schakel, 1987). Although being sensitive to variations in beliefs, health care providers should avoid the two extremes of unmoderated ethnocentrism (belief that one's cultural standards are preferable and superior) and cultural relativism (belief that every culture standard cannot be judged by another approach) (Korbin, 2002; Korbin & Spilsbury, 1999). The preferred approach is "cultural competence," which includes a repertoire of skills and knowledge that enable one to transcend cultural boundaries (Green, 1982). Cultural competence places the child's well-being first, addresses the need for a culturally informed perspective on neglect etiology, and informs culturally appropriate prevention and intervention (Korbin & Spilsbury, 1999).

Some experts suggest that several determinations should be made in culturally informed assessments based on the following questions (Korbin, 1994; National Research Council, 1993b):

1. Is the practice viewed as neglectful by cultures other than the one in question?
2. Does the practice represent an idiosyncratic departure from one's cultural practice?
3. Does the practice represent culturally induced harm to children beyond the control of parents or caretakers?

Nurses who understand the cultural-based health traditions of children's patients are able to enhance parental medical compliance and avoid mislabeling some practices as maltreatment (Davis, 2000). However, practitioners also must acknowledge that some cultural practices may cause injury or may be harmful to children, particularly if they are used exclusively to treat a condition for which more effective therapy is indicated (for example, coin rubbing for meningitis instead of antibiotics and coin rubbing). Some cultural practices have been found by health practitioners to be dangerous, such as the use of "azarcon" and "greta," indigenous medications used to cure "empacho" (an illness Hispanics define as a bolus in the stomach that must be purged) that were found to be almost pure lead (Trotter, Ackerman, Rodman, Martinez, & Sorvillo, 1983). In addition to cultural factors, standards for household cleanliness, adequate supervision, child cleanliness, and medical care may be tempered by community and economic factors (Korbin, 2002; Myers et al., 2002; Rose & Meezan, 1996).

Child neglect is not a dichotomous variable; it occurs along a continuum from mild to severe, with many factors blurring the boundaries between these extremes. Because many parents engage in some kind of neglectful behavior, at least occasionally, the issues of severity and chronicity are critical in assessing the future risk to the child and in designing realistic interventions. Several factors are considered in assessing the severity of neglect, including the frequency, duration, and type of neglect; age of the child; potential consequences to the child's development; and the degree of danger to the child. Fatal neglect has been associated with chronic deprivation of the basic necessities of life (Krugman & Dubowitz, 2003; Rosenberg, 1994; Wilkey, Pearn, Petrie, & Nixon, 1982) and with situational failures to supervise the activities of young children (Committee on Injury and Poison Prevention, 2001; Margolin, 1990; Mierley & Baker, 1983; Rosenberg, 1994).

Child neglect typically represents multidimensional caregiver problems, and neglectful families demonstrate most or all types of neglect chronically or situationally. Many children who are reported for neglect experience more than one type of neglect. Table 76-1 describes the general characteristics of different types of child neglect; however, individual cases typically include multiple types of neglect that vary in severity and frequency.

Abandonment and Supervision Neglect

Abandonment and supervision neglect actually represent different points on the continuum of failure to supervise. Abandonment occurs when parents leave their child without arranging for appropriate substitute supervision (Gaudin, 1993). Infants, particularly those impaired because of the drug addictions of their mothers, may be abandoned immediately after their birth. In these cases the infants become "boarder or resident babies" while often futile attempts are made to locate their parents. These infants become wards of the state and are placed in foster care awaiting termination of parental rights so that they can be adopted. At least 30 states have adopted a "Safe Haven for Newborns" act that allows parents, or another person who has the parent's authorization, to leave an infant up to 14 days old at a hospital or health care facility without fear of prosecution for abandonment (U.S. Department of Health and Human Services, 2000). The original intent of these statutes was to prevent the tragic death of newborns from the impulsive abandonment of them by terrified teen mothers who give birth outside of care facilities. Typically, the parent may, but need not, contact facility staff when leaving the infant and is not required to provide the family's name or medical history.

The most common form of child neglect involves failure to supervise the child properly, leading to physical harm or death (U.S. Department of Health and Human Services, 2000). In supervision neglect, children are left for hours or days at a time. Supervision is often inadequate even when the parents are present because of substance abuse, physical or mental illness, low intelligence, or immaturity. Child care also may be delegated to an inadequate caregiver who is impaired, immature, or abusive. When considering supervision neglect, one needs to consider cultural and community standards and the child's age, developmental level, and length of time the child is left alone.

Physical Neglect

Severe physical neglect is characterized by a chaotic family lifestyle with deterioration in most areas of family functioning (Dubowitz et al., 2005; Pagelow, 1997; Young, 1981). The children in severely neglectful families do not receive most of the basic necessities of life. Typically, no family routines are developed for accomplishing the activities of daily living including eating, sleeping, bathing, or household cleaning. Substandard housing is common; living areas may be littered with rotting food, garbage, and animal feces with environmental hazards present and accessible. School-age children attend school only sporadically, and their classmates or teachers often complain of foul smells related to their lack of routine hygiene.

In these families, food typically comes into the home randomly, and the children must grab it as they can. Infants in these families are often malnourished, have a history of failure to thrive, and may have intestinal disorders possibly caused by ingestion of curdled formula, although this cause may be overlooked. At its base, nutritional neglect is the failure to provide a diet of quality and nutritional balance that is developmentally appropriate (Barnett, Miller-Perrin, & Perrin, 1997). Overdilution of formula may result in insufficient calories, toddlers may be fed "junk foods" with little or no attempt to include the basic food groups, and school-aged and older children may have to fend for themselves with stale or spoiled food the only sustenance available in the home. In healthy children the first effect of malnutrition will be on the child's weight. Moderate malnutrition also affects linear growth, and severe malnutrition also affects brain growth as evidenced by microcephaly in young children (Dubowitz, 1991).

Generally, these families have many children, not because the parents want children but because they fail to plan. These families experience a high degree of cognitive impairment, social incompetencies, mental illness, and substance abuse (Burke, Chandy, Dannerbeck, & Watt, 1998; Feldman, Ducharme, & Case, 1999; Lutenbacher & Hall, 1998; Peterson, Gable, & Saldana, 1996; Pianta, Egeland, & Erickson, 1989). The families often are headed by a single mother; however, when parents do live together, their behavior tends to be similar, and they often exacerbate each other's problems (Cicchetti & Carlson, 1989; Knutson, DeGarmo, Koeppel, & Reid, 2005; Young, 1981). The parents and their older children are conscious that they are considered different from other families, and they often respond with an impotent hostility that only alienates them further (Knutson et al., 2005; Manly, Kim, Rogosch, & Cicchetti, 2001; Rogosch & Cicchetti, 2004; Williamson, Borduin, & Howe, 1991).

Moderate physical neglect is typified by lesser degrees of disorganization in family functioning and with basic functioning demonstrated in at least one area (Brooks-Gunn & Duncan, 1997; Gaudin, Polansky, Kilpatrick, & Shilton, 1996; Young, 1981). These families may have one parent working with some continuity, may have a happy relationship with an extended family member, or may be capable of some responsibility such as sending the children to school regularly or administering a medication. Meals may be erratic and of varying degrees of nutritional value. Meals are cooked, however, and an effort is made to feed the family, which marks a qualitative difference from severely neglectful families. Although the children of these families may show the results of poor nutrition, this is often a function of poverty and ignorance and not of indifference (Amling et al., 1988; Brooks-Gunn & Duncan, 1997; Pagelow, 1997; Young, 1981). Disorder and confusion may be prevalent, but most areas of parental behavior at least will demonstrate some caretaking effort. The children appear dirty, but they will not be encrusted. The parents may leave the children alone; however, it will be for hours and not days (Amling et al., 1988; Brooks-Gunn & Duncan, 1997; DePanfilis, 1996; Dubowitz, 1999b; National Research Council, 1993b; Pagelow, 1997; Young, 1981).

Health Care Neglect

The problem of health care neglect has been difficult to characterize. Practitioners vary in their individual opinions as to what constitutes medical neglect by specialty, cultural background, and the population they are serving. In general, a solitary omission in health care is unlikely to cause harm in average children. Nonetheless, a pattern of omissions in care, such as failure to immunize, could have detrimental effects for even the healthiest children (Dubowitz, 1999b). In addition, there are times when failing to seek or comply with care for a single incidence can have a devastating effect, such as failure to have a severe head injury evaluated or in cases of meningitis (Dubowitz & Black, 2002).

In cases of severe health care neglect, parents are unable, unwilling, or unmotivated to seek all forms of preventive care, and direct assistance is required to locate a provider and transport families to services (Dubowitz & Black, 1994). Parents are unable, unwilling, or inconsistent in assessing the severity of an illness or accident and thus may seek emergency care on a much delayed basis when the child's problem has advanced to a critical stage. Parents are often unable or unwilling to meet the needs of a child with a chronic condition, which may result in significant morbidity or mortality for health conditions such as asthma, diabetes, or cystic fibrosis (Dubowitz & Black, 2002). In contrast, in families with moderate neglect, children will be taken to an emergency department for acute injuries or illnesses, but the parents will ignore chronic colds, defective vision, or dental care needs. These parents are often inconsistent and inadequate in attempting to care for a child with a chronic condition (Cowen, 2001b; Dubowitz & Black, 1994).

Not all instances of health care "noncompliance" should be labeled neglect. Well-intentioned parents may at times fail to comply with health care recommendations as a result of practical problems such as poor communication, a child's refusal to take a prescribed medication, transportation problems, and inability to pay for medication and appointments. At times, the failure to seek or to delay seeking health care is simply an error in judgment. It has been asserted that parents should be considered responsible for health care neglect only if a layperson reasonably could be expected to appreciate the need for health care (Dubowitz et al., 2005).

Health care neglect and simple errors in judgment are distinct from the decision to treat children's illnesses by spiritual means. Parents of some religions believe that they are exerting their constitutionally protected religious freedom when choosing spiritual treatment. Most states agree with these parents and have provided exemptions in their child abuse and neglect statutes for spiritual treatment. Courts, however, have not recognized spiritual treatment when a child's life is in danger or the child has died (Lingle, 1996).

Educational Neglect

Educational neglect in its most severe form may include failure to comply with state requirements for school attendance or failure to provide an approved home-based school curriculum (Erickson & Egeland, 2002). This form of neglect also includes the consistently permitted truancy of the child without reason or for nonlegitimate reasons such as to care for siblings or to work (Gaudin et al., 1996). Educational neglect also involves inattention to a child's special educational needs, such as failure to follow through with special interventions or programs recommended by the school without reasonable cause (Erickson & Egeland, 1996).

Emotional Neglect

Some experts have contended that emotional neglect is the central feature of all maltreatment (Erickson & Egeland, 2002). Researchers have posited that given that neglectful parents demonstrate difficulties in meeting their children's basic needs, it would be expected that they likewise would be unresponsive to their children's emotional needs (Edwards, Shipman, & Brown, 2005). That parents who emotionally neglect their children may provide adequate physical care but not provide adequate nurturance also has been noted. In these families the parents are detached and uninvolved with their children (Schakel, 1987). Babies and toddlers may be left in their cribs for long periods, and children are seldom talked to, cuddled, or hugged. Psychological unavailability has been associated with greater developmental problems than the hostility and anger of abuse or the deprivation of physical neglect (Crittenden, 1996; Crittenden, Partridge, & Claussen, 1991) and with more cognitive impairment, anger, noncompliance, and negativistic behavior than all other types of maltreatment (Erickson & Egeland, 2002).

THEORETICAL PERSPECTIVES

Theoretical perspectives on the causes and correlates of child maltreatment are many and varied (Cicchetti & Carlson, 1989). The inability of the single-dimensional models adequately to address the known characteristics of child maltreatment, including neglect, has resulted in multidimensional models of child maltreatment. One such attempt in this direction has been proposed by Garbarino (Garbarino, 1977; Garbarino & Sherman, 1980) in his ecological model of child maltreatment, which in turn derives from Bronfenbrenner's ecological model of human development (1977) (Figure 76-1).

The Garbarino model (1977) is a paradigm for examining the complex interactions among parental and child characteristics, intrafamilial and extrafamilial stressors, and the social and cultural systems that affect families. The model offers a framework for considering available supports and resources in relation to a topology of four levels that have been adapted to include individual, familial, social, and cultural factors (Howze & Kotch, 1984). In addition, the model provides a framework for understanding the relationships among stress, social support systems, and child maltreatment. Stress arising from these domains may be situational, acute, or chronic in nature. However, one should note that to date, research has not indicated that any factors present in all child maltreatment circumstances are absent in all nonmaltreatment circumstances. Thus there is no litmus test for child maltreatment, only related risk factors, the identification of which provides the opportunity for preventive interventions to be directed at stressful environments, interpersonal relationships, and parental psychosocial problems with securement of the child's safety and optimal growth and development as the desired outcomes. A variety of sociocultural, family, parental, and child risk factors for child neglect have been reported, and Table 76-2 provides a limited overview.

SOCIOCULTURAL FACTORS

Child neglect has been correlated highly with poverty, with physical neglect found to be concentrated among the poorest of the poor, who typically reside in inadequate housing (Pelton, 1985, 1994; Sedlak & Broadhurst, 1996; Wolock & Horowitz, 1984). Income level also has been associated with the severity of neglect, with higher-income families generally associated with less severe forms of neglect, presumably because they have more resources at their disposal (Claussen & Crittenden, 1991). In the Third National Incidence Study (NIS III), neglect was identified 44 times more often in families with annual incomes under $15,000 compared with those earning more than $30,000 (Sedlak & Broadhurst, 1996). Low economic status is associated with a range of factors associated with poverty, such as unemployment, limited education, large numbers of children, and social isolation (Crittenden, 1999).

In 2004, 38% (70 million) of U.S. children lived in low-income families (less than 100% of the federal poverty level), with 21% (11 million) of these living in abject poverty (100% to 200% of the federal poverty level). Among children under age 6, 42% (9.6 million) lived in low-income families, with 20% (4.6 million) living in poverty. For those under age 6, 52% have at least one parent who works full-time year-round; 30% have at least one parent who works part-time or full-time for part of the year. The largest group of low-income families of children under age 6 by race and ethnicity is white children (3.8 million, 29%) followed by Latino children (3.1 million, 65%), black children (2.1 million, 64%) and Asian children (0.2 million, 23%) (National Center for Children in Poverty, 2005).

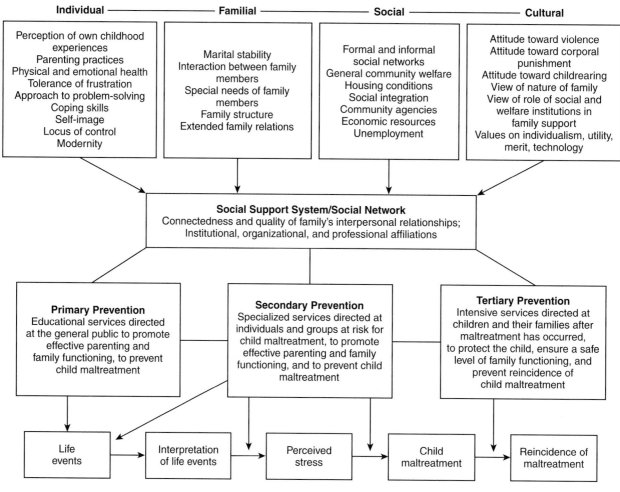

FIGURE 76-1 The ecological model of child maltreatment: implications for prevention. (Modified from Howze, D. C., & Kotch, J. B. [1984]. Disentangling life events, stress, and social support: Implications for the primary prevention of child abuse and neglect. *Child Abuse & Neglect, 8*[4], 401-409. Copyright 1984 by Elsevier Science, Ltd. Reprinted with permission.)

Child neglect rates also have been found to be higher in poorer neighborhoods with fewer social resources than in equally deprived neighborhoods where social resources (such as respite and crisis child care) were perceived to be higher (Garbarino & Kostelny, 1992; Sedlak & Broadhurst, 1996). Although the indirect stress of poverty may lead to child neglect, there is little doubt that poverty is directly hazardous to children. Poor parents are required to be hypervigilant of the environment (deteriorated housing, fires, lead poisoning, crime), manage scarce financial resources, and provide constant supervision of children with little or no margin for error (Cutts, Pheley, & Geppert, 1998; Erickson & Egeland, 2002; Pelton, 1994). Poor children are more

likely than rich or middle-class children to experience material deprivation and poor health, die during childhood, score lower on standardized tests, be retained in grade or drop out of school, have out-of wedlock births, and experience violent crime and more often are reported as victims of child maltreatment, including neglect (Brooks-Gunn & Duncan, 1997; Dubowitz et al., 2005; Duncan & Brooks-Gunn, 2000).

In addition, child neglect has been related to the inaccessibility or unaffordability of health care (Barnett et al., 1997). Since its inception in 1997, the State Children's Health Insurance Program (SCHIP), in concert with Medicaid, has provided low-income children with vital health care coverage. However, in 2000, 6.7 million children

TABLE 76-2

Risk Factors Associated With Child Neglect

Sociocultural	• Inaccessible health care due to financial and/or nonfinancial barriers (e.g., geographic)[18,42] • Lack of community resources, respite and crisis childcare,[12,13] and prevention services[34] • Poverty[4,5,20,27,45,46,50] • Societal tolerance for children living in poverty[10,19] • Unemployment[27,50]
Family	• Chaotic family organization with high levels of conflict and low levels of verbal expression and communication[25,26] • Domestic violence[31,38] • Interaction or fit between parent and child[32,45,49] • Large number of children in family[25] • Life stressors and/or distress[15,25,41] • Low levels of coping and problem-solving skills, and higher incidence of psychosocial problems and perceived stress[26] • Religious beliefs that may conflict with provision of medical care[35] • Single parent head of household[6,19,41,46] • Social isolation and low level of social support[1,7,17,19,25]
Parent/ caretaker	• Adolescent parent[29,47] • Anxiety[9] • History of maltreatment as child[3,8,16,39,41,46] • Immature, childlike personality related to low self-esteem, poor impulse control[25] • Lack of positive relationship with own mother[11,40] • Limited household and financial management skills[6] • Limited parenting competencies[23,43] including decreased or dysfunctional parent/child interactions,[42] and stress related to the parenting role[22] • Limited social competencies[6,25] • Low level of maternal education[25,33,34] • Maternal depression[19,22,36] • Parental noncompliance with medical treatment[24] • Poor parental physical health and presence of stress-related symptoms[6,12,21] • Rapid repeat birth[21] • Spouse abuse[44] • Substance abuse[9,19,30,41,43]
Child	• Developmental or physical disabilities[14,48] • Children of young adolescent mothers[19,29,37] • Chronic illnesses[12,14] • Low-birth-weight or premature infants[12,14] • Prenatal neglect (inadequate prenatal care, in utero exposure to cocaine or other drugs)[9] • Temperament described as "difficult" by mother[28] • Young age[50]

NOTE: The following references are representative and not exhaustive:
1. Albarracin, Repetto, & Albarracin, 1997; 2. Ammerman & Patz, 1996; 3. Banyard, Williams, & Siegel, 2003; 4. Baugher & Lamison-White, 1996; 5. Brooks-Gunn & Duncan, 1997; 6. Burke, et al., 1998; 7. Campbell, 1997; 8. Carter, Joyce, Mulder, & Luty, 2001; 9. Cash & Wilke, 2003; 10. Children's Defense Fund, 1997; 11. Coohey, 1995; 12. Cowen, 1998; 13. Cowen, 2001b; 14. Cowen & Reed, 2002; 15. Crittenden, 1996; 16. Crouch, Milner, & Thomsen, 2001; 17. DePanfilis, 1996; 18. Devaney, Ellwood, & Love, 1997; 19. Dubowitz, 1999b; 20. Dubowitz, et al., 2002; 21. El-Kamary, et al., 2004; 22. Éthier, Lacharite, & Couture, 1995; 23. Feldman, Ducharme, & Case, 1999; 24. Fornari, Dancyger, Schneider, Fisher, Goodman, & McCall, 2001; 25. Gable, 1998; 26. Gaudin, et al., 1999; 27. Gillham, Tanner, Cheyne, Freeman, Rooney, & Lambie, 1998; 28. Harrington, Black, Starr, & Dubowitz, 1998; 29. Jaffee, Caspi, Moffitt, Belsky, & Silva, 2001; 30. Jaudes & Ekwo, 1995; 31. Jellen, McCarroll, & Thayer, 2001; 32. Kim & Cicchetti, 2004; 33. Kotch, et al., 1995; 34. Kotch, Browne, Dufort, Winsor, & Catellier, 1999; 35. Lingle, 1996; 36. Lutenbacher & Hall, 1998; 37. Maynard, 1997; 38. McGuigan & Pratt, 2001; 39. Milan, Lewis, Ethier, Keshaw, & Ickovics, 2004; 40. Morton & Browne, 1998; 41. Nelson, Cross, Landsman, & Tyler, 1996; 42. Pagelow, 1997; 43. Peterson, Gable, & Saldana, 1996; 44. Rumm, Cummings, Krauss, Bell, & Rivara, 2000; 45. Slack, et al., 2004; 46. Smokowski & Wodarski, 1996; 47. Stevens-Simon & Barrett, 2001; 48. Sullivan & Knutson, 1998; 49. Toth & Cicchetti, 1996; 50. Wang & Daro, 1998.

who qualified for these programs remained uninsured (Hoffman & Pohl, 2002), primarily because of parental lack of knowledge of program availability or the perceived complexity of enrollment and renewal procedures. A national survey reported that 67% of low-income families with uninsured children eligible for Medicaid had tried to enroll their children; however, only 43% had been successful because of confusion about the process and difficulty producing required documents (Perry, Kannel, Valdez, & Chang, 2000). Similar SCHIP procedural barriers have been reported as impeding families from completing the renewal process, resulting in their eligible children's loss of coverage. Results from a national survey indicated that although more than 80% of all low-income, uninsured children are eligible for coverage, the parents of 62% of these children have not heard of the program in their state or do not know that enrollment in welfare is not a precondition for participation (Ross & Hill, 2003).

Many states have taken or are taking steps to simplify the application process, including allowing application for Medicaid and SCHIP on the same form; no longer counting certain family assets (value of savings accounts or vehicles) in determining eligibility for children because this asset verification cost exceeded the cost of providing the health care; no longer requiring face-to-face interviews and allowing mail submitted applications; and the use of community-based organizations to assist with enrollment, including schools, child care providers, homeless shelters, faith-based organizations, and health and human service providers (Ross & Hill, 2003). Although under federal law only Medicaid staff can determine eligibility, outreach workers can conduct the initial processing of applications, including explaining program rules and benefits, helping families fill out forms and gather documents, and submitting applications. Nurses care for low-income families in a variety of settings and are a vital link for low-income child enrollment in Medicaid and SCHIP. Thus it is important that nurses work with their state health departments and local health and community agencies to add enrollment assistance to their repertoire of interventions for these families.

Family Characteristics

Neglect is usually pervasive in the lives of all family members, with parents and children often perceiving themselves to be powerless and viewing attempts at goal achievement to be futile. Evidence indicates that child neglect is more likely to be associated with single-parent households (Burke et al., 1998; Dubowitz, 1999a;

Smokowski & Wodarski, 1996), chaotic family organization (Gable, 1998; Gaudin et al., 1996), lower social economic status (Slack, Holl, McDaniel, Yoo, & Bolger, 2004), large number of children in the family (Gable, 1998), social isolation (Albarracin, Repetto, & Albarracin, 1997; Campbell, 1997; DePanfilis, 1996; Gable, 1998), and domestic violence (Jellen, McCarroll, & Thayer, 2001; McGuigan & Pratt, 2001). Although a wide range of family functioning has been reported in neglectful families, observations of family interactions have shown neglectful families to be more chaotic, less able to resolve conflict, less cohesive, less verbally expressive, and less warm and empathetic than a matched comparison group (Gaudin et al., 1996). Researchers have reported the co-occurrence of several risk factors (single parent, substance abuse, maternal depression, and chronic mental illness) for domestic violence and child neglect and suggest domestic violence screening in families cited for child neglect (Hartley, 2002). Substance-abusing families also have been reported to exhibit unique characteristics and behaviors that heighten the risk for child neglect (Dunn et al., 2002). Vulnerable families also may include those in situational crisis related to life stressors such as death, divorce, relocation, and unemployment (Crittenden, 1996). Although previous child maltreatment research focused primarily on psychological outcomes, recent research has begun to explore the physiological impact in hopes of tailoring effective interventions (Cicchetti & Rogosch, 2001).

Parent Characteristics

Although some parents abuse and neglect their children, research has been conducted to distinguish neglectful parents from those who physically maltreat. Neglectful mothers have been found less likely to have a positive relationship with their own mothers, describing them as less warm and caring and as less able to control their anger than a matched comparison group. The partners of these neglectful mothers also were found to be less likely to live with the mother and to provide less companionship and assistance with child care than a matched comparison group did (Coohey, 1995). Additional characteristics that have been associated with neglectful parents include an immature, childlike personality related to low self-esteem, poor impulse control, substance abuse, increased incidence of maternal depression, stress-related symptoms, limited financial and household management skills, and limited social competencies (Cowen, 1998; Crittenden, 1999; Erickson & Egeland, 2002; Éthier, Lacharité, & Couture, 1995; Knutson,

DeGarmo, & Reid, 2004; Polansky, Gaudin, & Kilpatrick, 1992; Slack et al., 2004). Poor parental physical health and stress-related symptoms have been related to child physical and emotional neglect (when the parent is physically or psychologically immobilized and unable to provide care) (Brayden, Altemeier, Tucker, Dietrick, & Vietz, 1992; Cowen, 1998; El-Kamary et al., 2004).

DEVELOPMENTAL OUTCOMES FOR CHILDREN

Previous and current findings conclude that child neglect can have severe, deleterious effects on children's physical, cognitive, emotional, and behavioral development (Erickson & Egeland, 2002; Horowitz, Widom, McLaughlin, & White, 2001; Kendall-Tackett, 2003; Knutson et al., 2004; Repetti, Taylor, & Seeman, 2002). Physical and psychosocial/behavioral consequences of child neglect have been identified at every stage of child development (Table 76-3). Researchers have found that neglect occurring early in life is particularly detrimental to subsequent development (Hildyard & Wolfe, 2002) and significant lifetime health effects have been reported (Kendall-Tackett, 2003).

Recent biological research findings have indicated that maltreated children's exposure to extreme stress produces high levels of cortisol, and the presence of these high levels during brain development may change the brain physically for the long term (Bremner, 1999; Bremner et al., 1997). Children who have suffered chronic maltreatment have been noted to have smaller hippocampi (critical for memory) especially on the left side, smaller cortexes, and differences in limbic and brainstem functions (Frustaci & Ryan, 1999). Some researchers posit that the chronic stress of child maltreatment is a risk factor for acute and chronic posttraumatic stress disorder (PTSD) (De Bellis et al., 1999). Researchers who examined the effects of extreme deprivation on infants raised in Romanian orphanages reported that at 2 years of age, the orphanage children did not show the usual diurnal variation of cortisol levels and had significantly lower morning cortisol levels, which remained elevated relative to the lower afternoon levels compared with home-reared Romanian children in the comparison group (Carlson & Earls, 1997). In a study of 1083 emotionally disturbed 4 to 17 year olds with no history of neglect or abuse, a history of abuse with no neglect, or a history of neglect with no abuse, the emotionally disturbed children with a history of neglect showed the lowest dopamine β-hydoxylase levels and systolic and diastolic blood pressure, which are functions mediated by the norepinephrine system (Rogeness & McClure, 1996). The researchers note that these results support animal study findings that child neglect affects the development of the norepinephrine system in a long-lasting and perhaps permanent way.

NURSING PROCESS

Nursing roles and therapeutic approaches in supporting families at risk for child neglect have been identified based on Tapia's conceptualization (1972) of levels of family functioning (Table 76-4). This classic model underscores the need for the development of trust between the nurse and the family and the use of situational leadership to address the learning and change abilities of families at different functional levels. A specific, stepwise progression toward higher levels of functioning combined with perceived achievable goals is more effective in enhancing change than a "now and all at once" approach. The initial extensive support required in the early stages of this therapeutic nurse-client relationship tapers off as family members develop competence and confidence and internalize new values.

ASSESSMENT

Maternal-child nurses, pediatric nurses, public health nurses, community health nurses, emergency department nurses, school nurses, and primary care nurse practitioners are the most likely groups of providers to have early, direct contact with parents at risk of neglecting their children. Their role as advocate for the child and family is often the critical, pivotal determinant of whether at-risk families are identified and receive the services they need. Nurses offer valuable assessments of the physical and developmental manifestations of child neglect and provide information on topics such as parent-child interactions, a parent's ability to care for a child, and parenting stress levels. Nurses are knowledgeable of the range of developmentally appropriate behavior expected of children, and they are quick to notice behaviors that fall outside of this range. In addition, nurses have primary responsibility for monitoring and remediating parenting patterns in families in which neglect has placed the child in at-risk situations. Increasingly, overwhelmed child protective services workers are making rapid case transferals of at-risk families to public and community health nurses because they are unable to process their caseloads.

The importance of early identification and intervention lies in its potential for reducing or preventing the

TABLE 76-3

Developmental Consequences of Neglect		
	Physical Problems	**Psychosocial and Behavioral**
Infant	*Inadequate nutrition:* Failure to thrive,[8,34,49] intestinal disorders,[8] dehydration,[8,13] wasting of subcutaneous tissue,[8,25] fatigue and listlessness[8,25] *Inadequate physical development:* Delayed psychomotor and motor skills,[49] rigid posturing,[6] hyperactive reflexes,[6] hyperextension of the trunk,[6] and difficulty with the suck and swallow reflex[6] *Inadequate physical repositioning:* Flexed hips,[39] bald patches on scalp,[7,37] and flattened head[7] *Poor hygiene:* Severe diaper rash,[37,49] skin infections[37,49] *Inadequate preventive and acute health care:* Bottle mouth,[11,38] untreated ear and other infections[7,13,37,49] *Injuries/fatalities:* Choking,[7] strangulation,[7] burns and smoke inhalation related to house fires[7,9,39]	Impaired development,[23,49,50] lack of social responsiveness,[49] apathetic,[25] lack of organized attachment strategy,[22,27,28] self-stimulatory behaviors (head banging, rocking),[49] negative affect,[1] feeding problems,[6] irritability,[40] stiff body and resists being held[25]
Toddler	*Inadequate physical development:* Gross motor delays,[5] developmental milestone delays[5] *Inadequate nutrition:* Wasting of subcutaneous tissue,[8,25] failure to maintain adequate growth and development,[9,13] constant fatigue and listlessness[9,25] *Unattended physical problems:* Dental decay,[38,39,51] untreated illnesses and injuries,[7,13,14,37,49] *Injuries/fatalities:* Choking[7]; falls[7]; corrosive, hydrocarbon, and lead poisoning[7,9]; prescription or illegal drug ingestion[7,39]; drownings[9,14]; electrocution[9]; burns and smoke inhalation related to house fires[9,14,39]	Lack of organized attachment strategy[3] and continued attachment problems,[17,19] negative affect,[17] easily frustrated,[17] noncompliant,[19] delayed or retarded language development[5,49]
Preschool	*Inadequate physical development:* Motor delays,[5] microcephaly[49] *Inadequate nutrition:* Failure to maintain adequate growth and development,[9,13] constant fatigue and listlessness[9,25] *Unattended physical problems:* Dental decay,[38,39,51] language delays associated with recurrent and untreated otitis media (sometimes with partial deafness),[42,49] untreated illnesses and injuries,[7,13,14] poor hygiene,[7,39,49] unkempt appearance[7,39,49] *Injuries/fatalities:* Falls[7]; corrosive, hydrocarbon, and lead poisoning[7]; prescription or illegal drug ingestion[7,39]; drownings[9,14]; electrocution[9]; poisonings[13,39]; burns and smoke inhalation related to house fires[9,14,39]	Low self-esteem,[17] increased negative and decreased positive representations of the self and others,[52,54] confused by and less able to discriminate others' emotional displays,[44] difficulty in initiating interactions with peers,[10] poor ego control,[17] increased negative affect,[17,33] less persistent and enthusiastic, more distractible and impulsive in approach to tasks,[17,19] limited attention span,[49] decreased ability to cooperate with others[47,49]

TABLE 76-3

Developmental Consequences of Neglect—cont'd

	Physical Problems	Psychosocial and Behavioral
School age	*Inadequate physical development:* Speech disorders,[46] enuresis,[46] eating disorders[13,46] *Inadequate nutrition:* Failure to maintain adequate growth and development,[9,13] constant fatigue and listlessness,[25] obesity and morbid obesity[13] *Unattended physical problems:* Dental decay,[16,38,39] untreated illnesses and injuries,[25,37,49] poor hygiene,[37,39,49] unkempt appearance[37,39,49] *Injuries/fatalities:* Prescription, illegal drug, or alcohol ingestion[7,39]; burns and smoke inhalation related to house fires[9,14]; burns from playing with matches[14]; gun accidents[7,24]	Low self-esteem,[49] negative representation of self and others,[48] negative affect,[20] socially withdrawn,[19,35] rejection by peers,[4,19,48] internalizing[5,35] and externalizing[15,35] of problems, inattentive and uninvolved in learning,[18] poor academic achievement,[18,21,43] learning disabilities,[49] behavior problems at school,[2] aggression,[32,35] antagonism,[45] uncooperativeness,[45] antisocial behavior,[31] extended stays at or frequent absences from school,[25] poor coping skills,[49] socioemotional immaturity,[46] habit disorders (sucking, biting, rocking),[46] begging and stealing food,[25] inappropriate attention seeking,[25] assumes adult responsibilities,[25] states there is no caretaker[25]
Adolescent	*Inadequate physical development:* Problems associated with teen pregnancy[26] *Inadequate nutrition:* Failure to maintain adequate growth and development,[9,13] constant fatigue and listlessness,[9,25] obesity and morbid obesity[13] *Unattended physical problems:* Dental decay,[16,38,39] untreated illnesses and injuries,[25,37,39] poor hygiene,[37,39,49] unkempt appearance[37,39,49] *Injuries/fatalities:* Prescription, illegal drug, or alcohol ingestion[7,39]; burns and smoke inhalation related to house fires[9,14]; gun accidents[7,24]	Extra familial difficulties such as stress and involvement with deviant peers,[57] social isolation,[57] attention problems,[57] increased risk for juvenile delinquency,[36,55] prostitution,[56] running away,[2,30,40] increased risk for early initiation of sexual activity and substance abuse,[12] increased attempts at suicide,[19] increased risk of violent criminal behavior,[55] increased incidence of anxiety and depression,[29] increased risk of dissociation (predicted by neglect in infancy)[41]

NOTE: The following references are representative and not exhaustive.

1. Abramson, 1991; 2. Adams, 1997; 3. Barnett, Ganiban, & Cicchetti, 1999; 4. Bolger & Patterson, 2001; 5. Bradley, Corwyn, Burchinal, McAdoo, & Coll, 2001; 6. Chasnoff & Lowder, 1999; 7. Cowen, 1997; 8. Cowen, 1999b; 9. Cowen, 2001; 10. Darwish, Esquivel, Houtz, & Alfonso, 2001; 11. Donly & Nowak, 1994; 12. Dubowitz & Black, 1994; 13. Dubowitz & Black, 2002; 14. Dubowitz, 1999b; 15. Dubowitz, et al., 2005; 16. Edelstein, 1995; 17. Egeland, Srouffe, & Erickson,1983; 18. Erickson & Egeland, 1996; 19. Erickson & Egeland, 2002; 20. Erickson, Egeland, & Pianta, 1989; 21. Flisher, et al., 1997; 22. George, 1996; 23. Grantham-McGregor & Fernald, 2002; 24. Hazinski, in press; 25. Heindl, Krall, Salus, & Broadhurst, 1979; 26. Herrenkohl, Herrenkohl, Egolf, & Russo, 1998; 27. Hesse & Main, 2000; 28. Hildyard & Wolfe, 2002; 29. Johnson, Smailes, Cohen, Brown, & Bernstein, 2000; 30. Kaufman & Widom, 1999; 31. Knutson, DeGarmo, & Reid, 2004; 32. Knutson, DeGarmo, Koeppel, & Reid, 2005; 33. Koenig, Cicchetti, & Rogosch, 2000; 34. Krugman & Dubowitz, 2003; 35. Manly, Kim, Rogosch, & Cicchetti, 2001; 36. Maxfield & Widom, 1996; 37. Monteleone, Brewer, & Fete,1998; 38. Mouden, 1998; 39. Munkel, 1998; 40. National Research Council, 1993a; 41. Ogawa, Sroufe, Weinfield, Carlson, & Egeland, 1997; 42. Pelton, 1985; 43. Pettit, Bates, & Dodge, 1997; 44. Pollack, Cicchetti, Hornung, & Reed, 2000; 45. Rogosch & Cicchetti, 2004; 46. Schakel, 1987; 47. Shields & Cicchetti, 1998; 48. Shields, Ryan & Cicchetti, 2001; 49. Skuse,1989; 50. Strathearn, Gray, O'Callaghan, & Wood, 2001; 51. Tang, et al., 1997; 52. Toth, Cicchetti, Macfie, & Emde, 1997; 53. Toth, Cicchetti, Macfie, Maughan, & Vanmeenen, 2000; 54. Waldinger, Toth & Gerber, 2001; 55. Widom, 2001; 56. Widom & Kuhns, 1996; 57. Williamson, Borduin, & Howe, 1991.

TABLE 76-4

Nursing Roles and Therapeutic Approaches in Supporting Families at Risk for Child Neglect

Family levels*	*Infancy:* Chaotic family, barely surviving, inadequate provision of physical and emotional supports. Alienation from community, deviant behavior, distortion and confusion of roles, immaturity, child neglect, depression, failure.	*Childhood:* Intermediate family, slightly above survival level, variation in economic provisions, alienation but with more ability to trust. Child neglect not as great, defensive but slightly more willing to accept help.	*Adolescence:* Normal family but with many conflicts and problems, variation in economic levels, greater trust and ability to seek and use help. Parents more mature but still have emotional conflicts. Family has successes and achievements and is more willing to seek solutions to problems; future oriented.	*Adulthood:* Family has solutions, is stable and healthy with fewer conflicts or problems, capable providers of physical and emotional supports. Parents mature and confident, fewer difficulties in training children, able to seek help; future oriented, enjoy present.	*Maturity:* Ideal family, homeostatic balance between individual and group goals and activities. Family meets its tasks and roles well and is able to seek appropriate help when needed.
Nurse's role	*Nurturing* to provide for health and safety needs of children and family.	*Collaborating* to identify and plan to meet health needs.	*Facilitating* family follow-through on health concerns.	*Enabling* family to maintain health.	*Consulting* with families to resolve problems/crises as they arise.

child-rearing attitudes of adolescent parent and adult parent populations. Four parenting and child-rearing constructs associated with dysfunctional parenting formed the foundation from which the items were developed. They include inappropriate parental expectations of the child, lack of empathy toward children's needs, parental value of physical punishment, and parent-child role reversal (Bavolek & Keene, 1999).

The *Parenting Stress Inventory (PSI)* consists of 101 items that measure parental competence and stress. This instrument is divided into three domains. The child domain assesses the degree of stress associated with specific child characteristics separate from the stress associated solely with the parental role. The parent domain includes measures of personal stress related to depression, attachment, social isolation, spouse (partner relationships), and health. The life stress domain provides an index of the amount of stress outside of the parent-child relationship (e.g., death of a relative or loss of a job) (Abidin, 1995).

Assessment of Child Growth and Development. The *Denver II* is a screening test designed to assess a young child's development and is composed of four major categories: personal-social, fine motor-adaptive, language, and gross motor. The test is applicable for children from birth through 6 years of age. The test consists of 125 assessment items, and this instrument includes information about standardization sample differences found among ethnic groups, educational levels, and places of residence (Frankenburg, Dodds, Archer, Shapiro, & Bresnick, 1990).

The *Hawaii Early Learning Profile* is a developmentally sequenced "play-based" instrument for children ages birth to 36 months. This tool evaluates cognition, language, gross and fine motor, social, and self-help domains and was developed for lay visitors to use to familiarize parents with normal ranges of growth and development. Results of the test identify current level of skills and suggest developmentally appropriate and challenging activities for the child. The unique advantage of this tool is that it is designed for use with "special needs" or "at-risk" children and with the general population (Furuno, O'Reilly, Hosaka, Inatsuka, & Falbey, 1993).

Risk Assessment Measures. A 13-item checklist for home visitors based on known risks and developed in a retrospective study involving a matched sample of 62 known maltreating families and 124 nonmaltreating families. Interestingly, although the tool could correctly classify 86% of the cases, the best predictor of child maltreatment was the health visitor's perception of whether the parent was indifferent, intolerant, or over-anxious (Browne, 1989). The presence of parental mental illness can cause stress and adversely affect the parent-child relationship. As such, an assessment of parental mental illness provides an additional avenue to evaluate the risk for child neglect. The *Louis MACRO (Mother and Child Risk Observation)* is a tool that was developed to assess risk by interpreting the relationship between maternal mental illness and its effect on children. Two versions of this tool are designed for use with infant and toddler mother pairs, and the tool is based on three domains. The first domain relates to three aspects of "proper parenting" and includes safety, care, and emotional responsiveness. The second domain relates to the parent's opinion of child characteristics such as temperament, potential ease of care, and enjoyment. The third domain relates to maternal mental state by evaluating potential for psychosis, depression, and anxiety (Louis, Condon, Shute, & Elzinga, 1997). Methods to identify neglect, which focus on extensive home observations, include the Childhood Level of Living Scales (Polansky, Chalmers, Buttenweiser, & Williams, 1978) and the Ontario Child Neglect Index (Louds, Borkowski, & Whitman, 2004; Trocme, 1996).

NURSING CLASSIFICATION SYSTEMS

Nursing classifications—which are specific to the type of maltreatment, victim population (child versus adult), parent or caregiver risks or inabilities, and preventive level (prevention versus protection)—would offer the most guidance to practitioners and researchers. Although nursing diagnoses (NANDA International, 2005), Nursing Interventions Classification (Dochterman & Bulechek, 2004), and Nursing Outcomes Classification (Moorhead, Johnson, & Maas, 2004) demonstrate strengths in some of the preceding areas, they do not allow a seamless connection across classification systems. This requires nurses to customize or develop the nursing diagnoses, interventions, and outcomes they use in documenting the multiple aspects of child neglect.

Within nursing diagnoses, child neglect is addressed primarily through parental or caregiver risks or inabilities (e.g., risk for impaired parenting, impaired parenting, readiness for enhanced parenting, dysfunctional family processes: alcoholism, interrupted family processes, readiness for enhanced family processes, parental role conflict, risk for impaired parent/infant/child attachment, caregiver role strain, risk for caregiver role strain, ineffective coping, ineffective therapeutic regimen management, and social isolation). Victim symptoms may be addressed through a variety of physical and psychological states that result from maltreatment (e.g., imbalanced nutrition, less than body requirements; disorganized infant behavior; pain; anxiety; and fear). Nursing diagnoses are not identifiable for primary preventive concepts, however; there is a limited availability for secondary and tertiary preventive concepts (ineffective community therapeutic regimen management), although these are not specific to the concept of child neglect or to child and child-rearing populations.

The following nursing outcomes can be related to child neglect on a child/parent level parent-infant attachment; parenting: early/middle childhood physical safety; parenting: infant/toddler physical safety; parenting: adolescent physical safety; parenting performance; parenting: psychosocial safety; and parenting impaired. Others nursing outcomes indicators are available; however, they are not child specific and include child and adult victim considerations: neglect cessation; neglect recovery; abuse protection; caregiver stressors; caregiver performance: direct care; caregiver performance: indirect care; caregiver well-being; caregiver home care readiness; family coping compromised; and family coping, disabled (Moorhead et al., 2004). Although a preventive violence indicator (community risk control: violence) exists, the outcome constructs do not relate well to child neglect. The addition of community-specific poverty indicators would greatly increase their relatedness to preventive activities.

The Nursing Intervention Classification intervention "abuse protection support: child" includes identifiers for child neglect; identifies caregiver risks or inabilities; and provides a variety of primary, secondary, and tertiary preventive activities for all types of maltreatment (Dochterman & Bulechek, 2004). However, because all types of child maltreatment are incorporated under this intervention, it does provide succinct direct guidance for child neglect intervention considerations.

PREVENTIVE INTERVENTIONS

Increasing public concern about child maltreatment has resulted in the development of a diverse base of primary, secondary, and tertiary preventive interventions. Primary preventive interventions are directed at the general population to prevent or reduce child maltreatment, whereas secondary preventive interventions are targeted at high-risk groups and tertiary interventions are focused on preventing further harm to children who have been maltreated.

Examples of government-sponsored primary prevention programs that address the poverty often associated with child neglect include the Food Stamp Program, the Supplemental Food Program for Women, Infants and Children (WIC), the school nutrition programs (breakfast and lunch), Medicaid, SCHIP, Head Start, and housing assistance programs (Devaney, Ellwood, & Love, 1997). However, as previously noted, many eligible children are not enrolled in these programs. Nursing, through targeted assessment and referral, could assist in addressing this problem. Researchers have noted that at-risk families, particularly those headed by young, relatively poor mothers, are most likely to benefit from educational and supportive services (Badger, 1981; Gabinet, 1979; Olds, Henderson, Chamberlin, & Tatelbaum, 1986). In response to these findings, many secondary prevention programs have emerged. Home-based and center-based programs have demonstrated a wide range of positive client outcomes (DePanfilis, 1996; Olds, 2002; Wolfe, 1991).

A review of randomized trials of prenatal and infancy home visitation programs for socially disadvantaged women and children indicated that some home visitation programs were effective in (1) improving women's health-related behaviors during pregnancy, the birth weight and length of gestation of babies born to smokers and young adolescents, parents' interaction with their children, and children's developmental status; (2) reducing the incidence of child abuse and neglect, childhood behavioral problems, emergency department visits and hospitalizations for injury, and unintended subsequent pregnancies; and (3) increasing mothers' participation in the work force (Olds & Kitzman, 1990). The researchers noted that home visit programs with the greatest chances of success are based explicitly or implicitly on ecological models, are designed to address the ecology of the family during pregnancy and the early child-bearing years with nurse home visitors who establish a therapeutic alliance with the families, and are targeted at families with greater risk for maternal and child health problems by virtue of their poverty and lack of personal and social resources (Olds & Henderson, 1990).

A recent summary of findings from the seminal 25-year study that examined prenatal and infancy home visiting by nurses reported that the program was successful in improving parental care as reflected by fewer childhood injuries and ingestions, fewer subsequent pregnancies, greater work force participation, reduced use of public assistance and food stamps, and fewer state-verified reports of child abuse and neglect between the children's fourth and fifteenth birthdays. The researchers also found that the effect of the program on child abuse and neglect was reduced in households with higher domestic violence and recommended future program interventions that address domestic violence (Olds, 2002). Overall, the research findings on positive outcomes for home visitation programs have been mixed. The increased incidence of verified maltreatment among home visitation clients often has been explained by the increased scrutiny of the family by health and human services professionals (Gomby, Culross, & Behrman, 1999; Guterman, 2001).

Several interventions have been identified as increasing the probability of reducing child maltreatment within diverse populations, including those that do the following (Daro, 2003; Guterman, 2001):

1. Initiate services early in the parent-child relationship at birth or, if possible, when a woman becomes pregnant
2. Offer a service dosage compatible with service objectives
3. Recognize that achieving sustained change with high-risk families requires intensive, long-term efforts
4. Address participants' personal needs and their parenting responsibilities
5. Provide a specific set of developmentally appropriate services for children
6. Offer strong linkages to other local service providers

Research examining tertiary interventions (families who already have been identified as neglectful) has been less promising. One such effort titled Intensive Family Preservation is a model of crisis care aimed at maltreating families. The goal of programs that operate using this model is to prevent the unnecessary placement of children out of their home while ensuring their safety. The interventions are short-term (4 to 6 weeks) and involve a variety of therapeutic and support services designed for the needs of individual families in crisis (Bath & Haapala, 1993). Bath and Haapala found this model to be significantly less effective in dealing with neglectful families than with their physically maltreating counterparts. Other researchers reported increased recidivism rates of physical abuse, and neglect increased in at-risk families previously associated with child protective services (tertiary level) who received home health visitor interventions by public health nurses and indicated the need for different services for tertiary level (MacMillan et al., 2005).

SUMMARY

As described, child neglect represents multidimensional problems that involve the child, parent, family, community, and cultural factors. Community-wide preventive interventions that are directed at each phase of the family life cycle beginning with the prenatal period and continuing through a child's school years have been identified as the most promising child maltreatment preventive interventions (Leventhal, 1996; Myers et al., 2002; Olds, 2002). In addition, interventions need to balance the parent's problems and needs and the child's developmental needs in order to be effective.

Although some progress has been made in interventions for neglectful families, the problem of child neglect remains difficult to address. This may be due in part to the unidimensional aim of some interventions attempting to address multidimensional family problems. The programs that have succeeded in changing outcomes for high-risk children and their families differ in fundamental ways from prevailing services. Successful intervention programs see the child in the context of the family and the family in the context of its surroundings. These programs offer the following (Connell, Kubisch, Schorr, & Weiss, 1995; DePanfilis & Dubowitz, 2005):

1. Support to parents who need help with their lives before they can make use of services for their children
2. A broad spectrum of services including concrete help with basic necessities such as food, transportation, clothing, and respite child care
3. Services that are coherent and integrated, with staff crossing traditional professional and bureaucratic boundaries
4. Staff members who are fundamentally flexible and render services ungrudgingly and at a high level of intensity
5. Professionals who are perceived by clients as persons they can trust and who care about and respect them
6. Professionals who are able to redefine their roles and venture into nontraditional settings and provide services at nontraditional hours

Key components of effective nursing interventions include the nurse's ability to do the following:

- Adequately identify indicators of neglect
- Describe and document the nature of the neglect in a detailed and comprehensive manner
- Report suspected child neglect to identify proper authorities: state department of human services,

child protective services, hospital/agency social work department, police, and state child maltreatment hotline

◆ Identify necessary case management components as a key member or leader of a multidisciplinary team

◆ Promote maximum independence and self-care of the family through innovative teaching strategies

◆ Coordinate activities between acute and community settings to ensure continuity of care

◆ Provide direct care and serve as the child's advocate

◆ Provide counseling to the family to help them identify coping strategies for stressful situations

◆ Identify social support resources and assist the family in accessing needed services

◆ Determine the effectiveness of the parent's ability to meet the child's safety and care needs

◆ Coordinate efforts with child protective services to ensure the safety needs of the child are met

◆ Serve as an expert witness in cases involving legal intervention

◆ Most importantly, provide guidance in the prevention of child neglect

REFERENCES

Abidin, R. R. (1995). *Parenting stress index* (3rd ed.). Odessa, FL: Psychological Assessment Resources.

Abramson, L. (1991). Facial expressivity in failure to thrive and normal infants: Implications for their capacity to engage in the world. *Merrill-Palmer Quarterly, 37*(1), 159-182.

Adams, G. R. (1997). Runaway youth. In R. A. Hoekelman (Ed.), *Primary pediatric healthcare* (pp. 826-828). St. Louis, MO: Mosby-Yearbook.

Albarracin, D., Repetto, M. J., & Albarracin, M. (1997). Social support in child abuse and neglect: Support functions, sources, and contexts. *Child Abuse & Neglect, 21*(7), 607-615.

Amling, J. K., Illian, A. F., Miller, L., Tittle, K., Getz, S. L., Hamilton, L., et al. (1988). Child neglect: When the parents couldn't care less. *Nursing, 18*(11), 68-74.

Ammerman, R. T., & Patz, R. J. (1996). Determinants of child abuse potential: Contribution of parent and child factors. *Journal of Clinical Child Psychology, 25*(3), 300-307.

Badger, E. (1981). Effects of a parent education program on teenage mothers and their offspring. In K. G. Scott, T. Field, & E. Robertson (Eds.), *Teenage parents and their offspring.* New York: Grune & Stratton.

Banyard, V. L., Williams, L. M., & Siegel, J. A. (2003). The impact of complex trauma and depression on parenting: An exploration of mediating risk and protective factors. *Child Maltreatment, 8*(4), 334-349.

Barnett, D., Ganiban, J., & Cicchetti, D. (1999). Maltreatment, negative expressivity, and the development of type D attachments from 12 to 24 months of age. *Monographs of the Society for Research in Child Development, 64*, 97-118.

Barnett, O. W., Miller-Perrin, C. L., & Perrin, R. D. (1997). *Family violence across the lifespan: An introduction.* Thousand Oaks, CA: Sage Publications.

Bath, H. I., & Haapala, D. A. (1993). Intensive family preservation services with abused and neglected children: An examination of group differences. *Child Abuse & Neglect, 17*(2), 213-225.

Baugher, E., & Lamison-White, L. (1996). *Poverty in the United States, 1995.* Washington, DC: U.S. Government Printing Office.

Bavolek, S. J., & Keene, R. G. (1999). *Adult-adolescent parenting inventory.* Park City, UT: Family Development Resources.

Belsky, J. (1993). Etiology of child maltreatment: A developmental-ecological analysis. *Psychological Bulletin, 114*(3), 413-434.

Bolger, K. E., & Patterson, C. J. (2001). Developmental pathways from child maltreatment to peer rejection. *Child Development, 72*, 549-568.

Bradley, R. H., Corwyn, R. F., Burchinal, M., McAdoo, H. P., & Coll, C. G. (2001). The home environments of children in the United States. Part II: Relations with behavioral development through age thirteen. *Child Development, 72*(6), 1868-1886.

Brayden, R. M., Altemeier, W. A., Tucker, D. D., Dietrick, M. S., & Vietz, P. (1992). Antecedents of child neglect in the first two years of life. *Journal of Pediatrics, 120*(3), 426-429.

Bremner, J. D. (1999). Does stress damage the brain? *Biological Psychiatry, 45*(7), 797-805.

Bremner, J. D., Randall, P., Vermetten, E., Staib, L., Bronen, R. A., Mazure, C., et al. (1997). Magnetic resonance imaging-based measurement of hippocampal volume in posttraumatic stress disorder related to childhood physical and sexual abuse: A preliminary report. *Biological Psychiatry, 41*(1), 23-32.

Bronfenbrenner, U. (1977). Toward an experimental ecology of human development. *American Psychologist, 32*, 513-531.

Brooks-Gunn, J. D., & Duncan, G. J. (1997). The effects of poverty on children. In *The future of children* (Vol. 7, No. 2, pp. 55-71). Los Altos, CA: Center for the Future of Children, the David and Lucile Packard Foundation.

Browne, K. (1989). The health visitor's role in screening for child abuse. *Health Visitor, 62*, 275-277.

Burke, J., Chandy, J., Dannerbeck, A., & Watt, J. W. (1998). The parental environment cluster model of child neglect: An integrative conceptual model. *Child Welfare, 77*(4), 389-405.

Caldwell, B. M., & Bradley, R. H. (1984). *Home observation for measurement of the environment.* Little Rock, AK: University of Arkansas.

Campbell, L. (1997). Child neglect and intensive-family-preservation practice. *Families in Society, 78*(3), 280-290.

Carlson, M., & Earls, F. (1997). Psychological and neuroendocrinological sequelae of early social deprivation in institutionalized children in Romania. *Annals of the New York Academy of Sciences, 807*, 419-428.

Carter, J. D., Joyce, P. R., Mulder, R. T., & Luty, S. E. (2001). The contribution of temperament, childhood neglect, and abuse to the development of personality dysfunction: A comparison of three models. *Journal of Personality Disorders, 15*(2), 123-135.

Cash, S. J., & Wilke, D. J. (2003). An ecological model of maternal substance abuse and child neglect: Issues, analyses, and recommendations. *American Journal of Orthopsychiatry, 73*(4), 392-404.

Chasnoff, I. J., & Lowder, L. (1999). Prenatal alcohol and drug use and risk for child maltreatment. In H. Dubowitz (Ed.), *Neglected children: Research, practice, and policy* (pp. 132-155). Thousand Oaks, CA: Sage Publications.

Children's Defense Fund. (1997). *The state of America's children.* Washington, DC: Author.

Cicchetti, D., & Carlson, V. (Eds.). (1989). *Child maltreatment: Theory and research on the causes and consequences of child abuse and neglect.* New York: Cambridge University Press.

Cicchetti, D., & Rogosch, R. (2001). Diverse patterns of neuroendocrine activity. *Development and Psychopathology, 13,* 677-693.

Claussen, A. H., & Crittenden, P. M. (1991). Physical and psychological maltreatment: Relations among types of maltreatment. *Child Abuse & Neglect, 15*(1-2), 5-18.

Committee on Injury and Poison Prevention. (2001). Falls from heights: Windows, roofs and balconies. *Pediatrics, 107*(5), 1188-1191.

Connell, J. P., Kubisch, A. C., Schorr, L. B., & Weiss, C. H. (Eds.). (1995). *New approaches to evaluating community initiatives: Concepts, methods, and contexts.* Washington, DC: Aspen Institute.

Coohey, C. (1995). Neglectful mothers, their mothers, and partners: The significance of mutual aid. *Child Abuse & Neglect, 19*(8), 885-895.

Cowen, P. S. (1997). Child maltreatment: Nursing's changing role. In J. McCloskey & H. K. Grace (Eds.), *Current issues in nursing* (5th ed., pp. 731-741). St. Louis, MO: Mosby.

Cowen, P. S. (1998). Crisis child care: An intervention for at-risk families. *Issues in Comprehensive Pediatric Nursing, 21,* 147-158.

Cowen, P. S. (1999a). Abuse protection: Child. In G. M. Bulechek & J. C. McCloskey (Eds.), *Nursing interventions: Effective nursing treatments* (pp. 549-577). Philadelphia: W.B. Saunders.

Cowen, P. S. (1999b). Child neglect: Injuries of omission. *Pediatric Nursing, 25*(4), 401-405, 409-418.

Cowen, P. S. (2001a). Child neglect preventive interventions: Nursing's role. In J. M. Dochterman & H. K. Grace (Eds.), *Current issues in nursing* (6th ed., pp. 509-605). St. Louis, MO: Mosby.

Cowen, P. S. (2001b). Crisis child care: Implications for family interventions. *Journal of the American Psychiatric Nurses Association, 7*(6), 196-204.

Cowen, P. S., & Reed, D. (2002). Effects of respite care for children with developmental disabilities: Evaluation of an intervention for at risk families. *Public Health Nursing, 19*(4), 272-283.

Crittenden, P. M. (1996). Research on maltreating families: Implications for intervention. In J. Briere, L. Berliner, J. Bulkley, C. Jenny, & T. Reid (Eds.), *The APSAC handbook on child maltreatment* (pp. 158-174). Thousand Oaks, CA: Sage Publications.

Crittenden, P. M. (1999). Child neglect: Causes and consequences. In H. Dubowitz (Ed.), *Neglected children.* Thousand Oaks, CA: Sage Publications.

Crittenden, P. M., Partridge, M. F., & Claussen, A. H. (1991). Family patterns of relationship in normative and dysfunctional families. *Development and Psychopathology, 3*(4), 491-512.

Crouch, J. L., Milner, J. S., & Thomsen, C. (2001). Childhood physical abuse, early social support, and risk for maltreatment: Current social support as a mediator of risk for child physical abuse. *Child Abuse & Neglect, 25*(1), 93-107.

Cutts, D. B., Pheley, A. M., & Geppert, J. S. (1998). Hunger in mid-Western inner-city young children. *Archives of Pediatrics & Adolescent Medicine, 152*(5), 589-593.

Daro, D. (2003, Spring). Child abuse prevention: Accomplishments and challenges. *APSAC Advisor,* pp. 3-4.

Darwish, D., Esquivel, G. B., Houtz, J. C., & Alfonso, V. C. (2001). Play and social skills in maltreated and non-maltreated preschoolers during peer interactions. *Child Abuse & Neglect, 25,* 13-31.

Davis, R. E. (2000). Cultural health care of child abuse? The Southeast Asian practice of cao gio. *Journal of the American Academy of Nurse Practitioners, 12*(3), 89-95.

De Bellis, M. D. (2005). The psychobiology of neglect. *Child Maltreatment, 10*(2), 150-172.

De Bellis, M. D., Keshavan, M., Clark, D. B., Casey, B. J., Giedd, J., Boring, A. M., et al. (1999). Developmental traumatology. Part II: Characteristics of trauma and psychiatric symptoms and adverse brain development in maltreated children and adolescents with PTSD. *Biological Psychiatry, 45*(10), 1271-1284.

DePanfilis, D. (1996). Social isolation of neglectful families: A review of social support assessment and intervention models. *Child Maltreatment, 1*(1), 37-52.

DePanfilis, D., & Dubowitz, H. (2005). Family connections: A program for preventing child neglect. *Child Maltreatment, 10*(2), 108-123.

Devaney, B., Ellwood, M., & Love, J. (1997). Programs that mitigate the effects of poverty on children. In *The future of children* (Vol. 7, pp. 88-112.). Los Altos, CA: Center for the Future of Children.

Dochterman, J. M., & Bulechek, G. M. (Eds.). (2004). *Nursing interventions classification (NIC)* (4th ed.). St. Louis, MO: Mosby.

Donly, K. J., & Nowak, A. J. (1994). Maxillofacial, neck, and dental lesions of child abuse. In R. M. Reece (Ed.), *Child abuse: Medical diagnosis and management* (pp. 150-166). Philadelphia: Lea & Febiger.

Dubowitz, H. (1991). The impact of child maltreatment on health. In R. H. Starr & D. A. Wolfe (Eds.), *The effects of child abuse and neglect: Issues and research* (pp. 278-294). New York: Guilford Press.

Dubowitz, H. (1999a). The families of neglected children. In M. E. Lamb (Ed.), *Parenting and child development in "nontraditional" families* (Vol. 8, pp. 327-345). Mahwah, NJ: L. Erlbaum Associates.

Dubowitz, H. (Ed.). (1999b). *Neglected children: Research, practice, and policy.* Thousand Oaks, CA: Sage.

Dubowitz, H. (2003). Preventing child neglect: Promoting children's health, development and safety. *APSAC Advisor, 15*(2), 5-7.

Dubowitz, H., & Black, M. (1994). Child neglect. In R. M. Reece (Ed.), *Child abuse: Medical diagnosis and management* (pp. 279-297). Malvern, PA: Lea & Febiger.

Dubowitz, H., & Black, M. (2002). Neglect of children's health. In J. E. Myers, L. Berliner, J. Briere, C. Hendrix, C. Jenny, & T. Reid (Eds.), *The APSAC handbook on child maltreatment* 2nd ed. (pp. 269-292). Thousand Oaks, CA: Sage Publications.

Dubowitz, H., Newton, R. R., Litrownik, A. J., Lewis, T., Briggs, E. C., Thompson, R., et al. (2005). Examination of a conceptual model of child neglect. *Child Maltreatment, 10*(2), 173-189.

Duncan, G. J., & Brooks-Gunn, J. (2000). Family poverty, welfare reform, and child development. *Child Development, 71,* 188-196.

Dunn, M. G., Tarter, R. E., Mezzich, A. C., Vanyukov, M., Kirisci, L., & Kirillova, G. (2002). Origins and consequences of child neglect in substance abuse families. *Clinical Psychology Review, 22,* 1063-1090.

Edelstein, B. L. (1995). Disspelling the myth that 50 percent of U. S. school children have never had a cavity. *Public Health Reports, 110*(5), 522-530.

Edwards, A., Shipman, K., & Brown, A. (2005). The socialization of emotional understanding: A comparison of neglectful and nonneglectful mothers and their children. *Child Maltreatment, 10*(3), 293-304.

Egeland, B., Sroufe, L. A., & Erickson, M. (1983). The developmental consequence of different patterns of maltreatment. *Child Abuse & Neglect, 7*(4), 459-469.

El-Kamary, S. S., Higman, S. M., Fuddy, L., McFarlane, E., Sia, C., & Duggan, A. K. (2004). Hawaii's healthy start home visiting program: Determinants and impact of rapid repeat birth. *Pediatrics, 114*(3), 317-326.

English, D. J., Thompson, R., Graham, J. C., & Briggs, E. C. (2005). Toward a definition of neglect in young children. *Child Maltreatment, 10*(2), 190-206.

Erickson, M. F., & Egeland, B. (1996). Child neglect. In J. Briere, L. Berliner, J. A. Bulkley, C. Jenny, & T. Reid (Eds.), *The APSAC handbook on child maltreatment* (pp. 4-20). Thousand Oaks, CA: Sage Publications.

Erickson, M. F., & Egeland, B. (2002). Child neglect. In J. E. Myers, L. Berliner, J. Briere, C. Hendrix, C. Jenny, &

T. Reid (Eds.), *The APSAC handbook on child maltreatment* (pp. 3-20). Thousand Oaks, CA: Sage Publications.

Erickson, M. F., Egeland, B., & Pianta, R. (1989). The effects of maltreatment on the development of young children. In D. Cicchetti & V. Carlson (Eds.), *Child maltreatment: Theory and research on the causes and consequences of child abuse and neglect* (pp. 647-684). New York: Cambridge University Press.

Éthier, L. S., Lacharité, C., & Couture, G. (1995). Childhood adversity, parental stress, and depression of negligent mothers. *Child Abuse & Neglect, 19*(5), 619-632.

Feldman, M. A., Ducharme, J. M., & Case, L. (1999). Using self-instructional pictorial manuals to teach child-care skills to mothers with intellectual disabilities. *Behavior Modification, 23*(3), 480-497.

Flisher, A. J., Kramer, R. A., Grosser, R. C., Alegria, M., Bird, H. R., Bourdon, K. H., et al. (1997). Correlates of unmet need for mental health services by children and adolescents. *Psychological Medicine, 27*(5), 1145-1154.

Frankenburg, W. K., Dodds, J., Archer, P., Shapiro, H., & Bresnick, B. (1990). *Denver II technical support manual.* Denver, CO: Denver Developmental Materials.

Frustaci, K., & Ryan, N. D. (1999). Developmental traumatology. Part II: Brain development. *Biological Psychiatry, 45*(10), 1271-1284.

Furuno, S., O'Reilly, K., Hosaka, C. M., Inatsuka, T. T., & Falbey, B. Z. (1993). *Helping babies learn.* San Antonio: Therapy Skill Builders.

Gabinet, L. (1979). Prevention of child abuse and neglect in an inner-city population. Part II: The program and the results. *Child Abuse and Neglect, 3,* 809-817.

Gable, S. (1998). School-age and adolescent children's perceptions of family functioning in neglectful and non-neglectful families. *Child Abuse & Neglect, 22*(9), 859-867.

Garbarino, J. (1977). The human ecology of child maltreatment: A conceptual model for research. *Journal of Marriage and the Family, 39*(4), 721-735.

Garbarino, J., & Kostelny, K. (1992). Child maltreatment as a community problem. *Child Abuse and Neglect, 16*(4), 455-464.

Garbarino, J., & Sherman, D. (1980). High-risk neighborhoods and high-risk families: The human ecology of child maltreatment. *Child Development, 51,* 188-198.

Gaudin, J. M. (Ed.). (1993). *Child neglect: A guide for intervention. The user manual series* (pp. 1-84). Washington DC: Westover Consultants.

Gaudin, J., Jr., Polansky, N. A., Kilpatrick, A. C., & Shilton, P. (1996). Family functioning in neglectful families. *Child Abuse & Neglect, 20*(4), 363-377.

George, C. (1996). A representational perspective on child abuse and prevention: Internal working models and attachment and caregiving. *Child Abuse & Neglect, 20,* 411-424.

Gillham, B., Tanner, G., Cheyne, B., Freeman, I., Rooney, M., & Lambie, A. (1998). Unemployment rates, single parent density, and indices of child poverty: Their relationship to different categories of child abuse and neglect. *Child Abuse & Neglect, 22*(2), 79-90.

Gomby, D. S., Culross, P. L., & Behrman, R. E. (1999). Home visiting: Recent program evaluations—analysis and recommendations. *The Future of Children, 9*(1), 4-27.

Grantham-McGregor, S. M., & Fernald, L. C. (1997). Nutritional deficiencies and subsequent effects on mental and behavioral development in children. *Southeast Asian J Trop Med Public Health, 28*(2), 50-68.

Green, J. W. (1982). *Cultural awareness in the human services.* Englewood Cliffs, NJ: Prentice Hall.

Guterman, N. B. (2001). *Stopping child maltreatment before it starts: Emerging horizons in early home visitation services.* Thousand Oaks, CA: Sage Publications.

Harrington, D., Black, M. M., Starr, R. H., Jr., & Dubowitz, H. (1998). Child neglect: Relation to child temperament and family context. *American Journal of Orthopsychiatry, 68*(1), 108-116.

Hartley, C. C. (2002). The co-occurrence of child maltreatment and domestic violence: Examining both neglect and child physical abuse. *Child Maltreatment, 7*(4), 349-358.

Hazinski, M. F. (2006). *Nursing role: Preventive gun safety.* In P. S. Cowen & S. P. Moorhead (Eds.), *Current Issues in Nursing* (7th ed.). St. Louis, MO: Mosby.

Heindl, C., Krall, C., Salus, M., & Broadhurst, D. (1979). *The nurse's role in the prevention and treatment of child abuse and neglect* (No. [OHDS] 79-30202). Washington, DC: U.S. Department of Health, Education, and Welfare.

Herrenkohl, E. C., Herrenkohl, R. C., Egolf, B. P., & Russo, M. J. (1998). The relationship between early maltreatment and teenage parenthood. *Journal of Adolescence, 21*(3), 291-303.

Hesse, E., & Main, M. (2000). Disorganized infant, child, and adult attachment: Collapse in behavioral and attentional strategies. *Journal of the American Psychoanalytic Association, 48*, 1097-1127.

Hildyard, K. L., & Wolfe, D. A. (2002). Child neglect: Developmental issues and outcomes. *Child Abuse & Neglect, 26*, 679-695.

Hoffman, C., & Pohl, M. B. (2002). *Health insurance coverage in America: 2000 data update.* Washington, DC: Kaiser Commission on Medicaid and the Uninsured.

Hogue, E. E. (1993). Child neglect in home care: Weighing legal and ethical issues. *Pediatric Nursing, 19*(5), 496-498.

Horowitz, A. V., Widom, C. S., McLaughlin, J., & White, H. R. (2001). The impact of childhood abuse and neglect on adult mental health: A prospective study. *Journal of Health and Social Behavior, 42*, 184-201.

Howze, D. C., & Kotch, J. B. (1984). Disentangling life events, stress, and social support: Implications for primary prevention of child abuse and neglect. *Child Abuse and Neglect, 8*(4), 401-409.

Jaffee, S., Caspi, A., Moffitt, T. E., Belsky, J., & Silva, P. (2001). Why are children born to teen mothers at risk for adverse outcomes in young adulthood? Results from a 20-year longitudinal study. *Development and Psychopathology, 13*(2), 377-397.

Jaudes, P. K., & Ekwo, E. (1995). Association of drug abuse and child abuse. *Child Abuse and Neglect, 19*(9), 1065-1075.

Jellen, L. K., McCarroll, J. E., & Thayer, L. E. (2001). Child emotional maltreatment: A 2-year study of U.S. Army bases. *Child Abuse & Neglect, 25*(5), 623-639.

Johnson, C. F. (1993). Physicians and medical neglect: Variables that affect reporting. *Child Abuse & Neglect, 17*, 605-612.

Johnson, J. G., Smailes, E. M., Cohen, P., Brown, J., & Bernstein, D. P. (2000). Associations between four types of childhood neglect and personality disorder symptoms during adolescence and early adulthood: Findings of a community-based longitudinal study. *Journal of Personality Disorders, 14*, 171-187.

Kaufman, J. G., & Widom, C. S. (1999). Childhood victimization, running away, and delinquency. *Journal of Research in Crime and Delinquency, 36*, 347-370.

Kendall-Tackett, K. (2003). *Treating the lifetime health effects of childhood victimization.* Kingston, NJ: Civic Research Institute.

Kim, J., & Cicchetti, D. (2004). A longitudinal study of child maltreatment, mother-child relationship quality and maladjustment: The role of self-esteem and social competence. *Journal of Abnormal Child Psychology, 32*(4), 341-354.

Knutson, J. F., DeGarmo, D. S., Koeppel, G., & Reid, J. B. (2005). Care neglect, supervisory neglect, and harsh parenting in the development of children's aggression: A replication and extension. *Child Maltreatment, 10*(2), 92-107.

Knutson, J. F., DeGarmo, D. S., & Reid, J. B. (2004). Social disadvantage and neglectful parenting as precursors to the development of antisocial and aggressive child behavior: Testing a theoretical model. *Aggressive Behavior, 30*, 187-205.

Koenig, A. L., Cicchetti, D., & Rogosch, F. A. (2000). Child compliance/noncompliance and maternal contributors to internalization in maltreating and non-maltreating dyads. *Child Development, 71*, 1018-1032.

Korbin, J. E. (1994). Sociocultural factors in child maltreatment. In G. Melton & F. Barry (Eds.), *Protecting children from abuse and neglect* (pp. 182-223). New York: Guilford Press.

Korbin, J. E. (2002). Culture and child maltreatment: Cultural competence and beyond. *Child Abuse & Neglect, 26*, 637-644.

Korbin, J. E., & Spilsbury, J. C. (1999). Cultural competence and child neglect. In H. Dubowitz (Ed.), *Neglected children: Research, practice and policy* (pp. 69-88). Thousand Oaks, CA: Sage Publications.

Kotch, J. B., Browne, D. C., Dufort, V., Winsor, J., & Catellier, D. (1999). Predicting child maltreatment in the first 4 years of life from characteristics assessed in the neonatal period. *Child Abuse & Neglect, 23*(4), 305-319.

Kotch, J. B., Browne, D. C., Ringwalt, C. L., Stewart, P. W., Ruina, E., Holt, K., et al. (1995). Risk of child abuse or neglect in a cohort of low-income children. *Child Abuse & Neglect, 19*(9), 1115-1130.

Krugman, S. D., & Dubowitz, H. (2003). Failure to thrive. *Family Physician, 68*(5), 879-884.

Leventhal, J. M. (1996). Twenty years later: We do know how to prevent child abuse and neglect. *Child Abuse & Neglect, 20*(8), 647-653.

Lingle, E. A. (1996). Treating children by faith: Colliding constitutional issues. *Journal of Legal Medicine, 17*(2), 301-330.

Louds, J. J., Borkowski, J. G., & Whitman, T. L. (2004). Reliability and validity of the Mother-Child Neglect Scale. *Child Maltreatment, 9*(4), 371-381.

Louis, A., Condon, J., Shute, R., & Elzinga, R. (1997). The development of the Louis MACRO (Mother and Child Risk Observation) forms: Assessing parent-infant-child risk in the presence of maternal mental illness. *Child Abuse & Neglect, 21*(7), 589-606.

Lutenbacher, M., & Hall, L. A. (1998). The effects of maternal psychosocial factors on parenting attitudes of low-income, single mothers with young children. *Nursing Research, 47*(1), 25-34.

MacMillan, H. L., Thomas, B. H., Jamieson, E., Walsh, C. A., Boyle, M. H., Shannon, H. S., et al. (2005). Effectiveness of home visitation by public-health nurses in prevention of the recurrence of child physical abuse and neglect; a randomised controlled trial. *Lancet, 365*(9473), 1786-1793.

Manly, J. T., Kim, J. E., Rogosch, F. A., & Cicchetti, D. (2001). Dimensions of child maltreatment and children's adjustment: Contributions of developmental timing and subtype. *Development and Psychopathology, 13*, 759-782.

Margolin, L. (1990). Fatal child neglect. *Child Welfare, 69*(4), 309-319.

Maxfield, M. G., & Widom, C. S. (1996). The cycle of violence: Revisited six years later. *Archives of Pediatrics and Adolescent Medicine, 150*, 390-395.

Maynard, R. A. (Ed.). (1997). *Kids having kids. Economic costs and social consequences of teen pregnancy.* Washington, DC: Urban Institute Press.

McGuigan, W. M., & Pratt, C. C. (2001). The predictive impact of domestic violence on three types of child maltreatment. *Child Abuse & Neglect, 25*(7), 869-883.

Mierley, M. C., & Baker, S. P. (1983). Fatal house fires in an urban population. *Journal of the American Medical Association, 249*, 1466-1468.

Milan, S., Lewis, J., Ethier, K., Keshaw, T., & Ickovics, J. R. (2004). The impact of physical maltreatment history on the adolescent mother-infant relationship: Mediating and moderating effects during the transition to early parenthood. *Journal of Abnormal Child Psychology, 32*(3), 249-261.

Monteleone, J. A., Brewer, J. R., & Fete, T. J. (1998). Physical examination in sexual abuse. In J. A. Monteleone (Ed.), *Child maltreatment* (pp. 151-181). St. Louis: G.W. Medical Publishing.

Moorhead, S., Johnson, M., & Maas, M. (Eds.). (2004). *Nursing outcomes classification (NOC)* (3rd ed.). St. Louis, MO: Mosby.

Morton, N., & Browne, K. D. (1998). Theory and observation of attachment and its relation to child maltreatment: A review. *Child Abuse & Neglect, 22*(11), 1093-1104.

Mouden, L. D. (1998). Oral injuries of child abuse. In J. A. Monteleone & A. E. Brodeur (Eds.), *Child maltreatment: A clinical guide and reference* (2nd ed., pp. 59-66). St. Louis, MO: Harcourt Brace.

Munkel, W. I. (1998). Neglect and abandonment. In J. A. Monteleone & A. E. Brodeur (Eds.), *Child maltreatment: A clinical guide and reference* (2nd ed., pp. 339-356). St. Louis, MO: Harcourt Brace.

Myers, J. E., Berliner, L., Briere, J., Hendrix, C., Jenny, C., & Reid, T. (Eds.). (2002). *The APSAC handbook on child maltreamtent* (2nd ed.). Thousand Oaks, CA: Sage Publications.

Myers, J. E., & Stern, P. (2002). Expert testimony. In J. E. Myers, L. Berliner, J. Briere, C. Hendrix, C. Jenny, & T. Reid (Eds.), *The APSAC handbook on child maltreatment* (2nd ed., pp. 379-401). Thousand Oaks, CA: Sage Publications.

NANDA International. (2005). *Nursing diagnoses: Definitions & classification, 2005-2006.* Philadelphia: Author.

National Center for Children in Poverty. (2005). *Basic facts about low-income children: Birth to age 6.* Retrieved July 25, 2005, from http://www.nccp.org/pub_ycp05.html

National Research Council. (1993a). Consequences of child abuse and neglect. In *Understanding child abuse and neglect.* Washington, DC: National Academy Press.

National Research Council. (1993b). *Understanding child abuse and neglect.* Washington, DC: National Academy Press.

Nelson, K., Cross, T., Landsman, M. J., & Tyler, M. (1996). Native American families and child neglect. *Children & Youth Services Review, 18*(6), 505-521.

Ogawa, J. R., Sroufe, L. A., Weinfield, N. S., Carlson, E. A., & Egeland, B. (1997). Development and the fragmented self: Longitudinal study of dissociative symptomatology in a nonclinical sample. *Development and Psychopathology, 9*, 855-879.

Olds, D. (2002). Prenatal and infancy home visiting by nurses: From randomized trials to community replication. *Prevention Science, 3*(3), 153-172.

Olds, D. L., & Henderson, C. R. (1990). The prevention of maltreatment. In D. Cicchetti & V. Carlson (Eds.), *Child maltreatment: Theory and research on the causes and consequences of child abuse and neglect* (pp. 722-763). New York: Cambridge University Press.

Olds, D. L., Henderson, C. R., Jr., Chamberlin, R., & Tatelbaum, R. (1986). Preventing child abuse and neglect: A randomized trial of nurse home visitation. *Pediatrics, 78*(1), 65-78.

Olds, D. L., & Kitzman, H. (1990). Can home visitation improve the health of women and children at environmental risk? *Pediatrics, 86*(1), 108-116.

Pagelow, M. D. (1997). Child neglect and psychological maltreatment. In K. Barnett, C. Miller-Perrin, & R. Perrin (Eds.), *Family violence across the lifespan* (pp. 107-132). Thousand Oaks, CA: Sage Publications.

Pelton, L. (1985). *The social context of child abuse and neglect.* New York: Human Science Press.

Pelton, L. H. (1994). The role of material factors in child abuse and neglect. In G. Melton & F. Barry (Eds.), *Protecting children from abuse and neglect* (pp. 131-181). New York: Guilford Press.

Perry, M., Kannel, S., Valdez, R. B., & Chang, C. (2000). *Medicaid and children: Overcoming barriers to enrollment.* Washington, DC: Kaiser Commission on Medicaid and the Uninsured.

Peterson, L., Gable, S., & Saldana, L. (1996). Treatment of maternal addiction to prevent child abuse and neglect. *Addictive Behaviors, 21*(6), 789-801.

Pettit, G. S., Bates, J. E., & Dodge, K. A. (1997). Supportive parenting, ecological context, and children's adjustment: A seven-year longitudinal study. *Child Development, 68,* 908-923.

Pianta, R., Egeland, B., & Erickson, M. F. (1989). The antecedents of maltreatment: Results of the mother-child interaction research project. In D. Cicchetti & V. Carlson (Eds.), *Child maltreatment: Theory and research on the causes and consequences of child abuse and neglect* (pp. 203-253). New York: Cambridge University Press.

Polansky, N. A., Chalmers, M. A., Buttenweiser, E., & Williams, D. (1978). Assessing adequacy of child rearing: An urban scale. *Child Welfare, 57,* 439-449.

Polansky, N. A., Gaudin, J. M., & Kilpatrick, A. C. (1992). Family radicals. *Children and Youth Services Review, 14*(1-2), 19-26.

Pollack, S. D., Cicchetti, D., Hornung, K., & Reed, A. (2000). Recognizing emotion in faces: Developmental effects of child abuse and neglect. *Developmental Psychology, 36,* 679-688.

Repetti, R. L., Taylor, S. E., & Seeman, T. E. (2002). Risky families: Family social environments and the mental and physical health of offspring. *Psychological Bulletin, 128*(2), 330-366.

Rogeness, G., & McClure, E. (1996). Development and neurotransmitter-environmental interactions. *Development & Psychopathology, 8,* 183-199.

Rogosch, F. A., & Cicchetti, D. (2004). Child maltreatment and emergent personality organization: Perspectives from the five-factor model. *Journal of Abnormal Child Psychology, 32*(2), 123-145.

Rose, S. J., & Meezan, W. (1996). Variations in perceptions of child neglect. *Child Welfare, 75*(2), 139-160.

Rosenberg, D. (1994). Fatal neglect. *APSAC Advisor, 7*(4), 38-40.

Ross, D. C., & Hill, I. T. (2003). Enrolling eligible children and keeping them enrolled. In *The future of children* (Vol. 7, No. 2, pp. 81-97). Los Altos, CA: The Future of Children, the David and Lucile Packard Foundation.

Rumm, P. D., Cummings, P., Krauss, M. R., Bell, M. A., & Rivara, F. P. (2000). Identified spouse abuse as a risk factor for child abuse. *Child Abuse & Neglect, 24*(11), 1375-1381.

Schakel, J. A. (1987). Emotional neglect and stimulus deprivation. In M. R. Brassard, R. Germain, & S. N. Hart (Eds.), *Psychological maltreatment of children and youth* (pp. 100-109). Elmsford, NY: Pergamon Books.

Sedlak, A. J., & Broadhurst, D. D. (1996). *Executive summary of the Third National Incidence Study of child abuse and neglect.* Washington, DC: U.S. Government Printing Office.

Shields, A., & Cicchetti, D. (1998). Reactive aggression among maltreated children: The contributions of attention and emotional dysregulation. *Journal of Clinical Child Psychology, 27,* 381-395.

Shields, A., Ryan, R. M., & Cicchetti, D. (2001). Narrative representations of caregivers and emotional dysregulation as predictors of maltreated children's rejection by peers. *Developmental Psychology, 37,* 321-337.

Skuse, D. H. (1989). ABC of child abuse. Emotional abuse and delay in growth. *British Medical Journal, 299*(6691), 113-115.

Slack, K. R., Holl, J. L., McDaniel, M., Yoo, J., & Bolger, K. (2004). Understanding the risks of child neglect: An exploration of poverty and parenting characteristics. *Child Maltreatment, 9*(4), 395-408.

Smokowski, P. R., & Wodarski, J. S. (1996). The effectiveness of child welfare services for poor, neglected children: A review of the empirical evidence. *Research on Social Work Practice, 6*(4), 504-523.

Stevens-Simon, C., & Barrett, J. (2001). A comparison of the psychological resources of adolescents at low and high risk of mistreating their children. *Journal of Pediatric Health Care, 15*(6), 299-303.

Strathearn, L., Gray, P. H., O'Callaghan, M. J., & Wood, D. O. (2001). Childhood neglect and cognitive development in extremely low birth weight infants: A prospective study. *Pediatrics, 108*(1), 142-151.

Straus, M. A., & Savage, S. A. (2005). Neglectful behavior by parents in the life history of university students in 17 countries and its relation to violence against dating partners. *Child Maltreatment, 10*(2), 124-135.

Sullivan, P. M., & Knutson, J. F. (1998). The association between child maltreatment and disabilities in a hospital-based epidemiological study. *Child Abuse & Neglect, 22*(4), 271-288.

Sullivan, P. M., & Knutson, J. F. (2000). The prevalence of disabilities and maltreatment among runaway children. *Child Abuse & Neglect, 24*(10), 1275-1288.

Tang, J., Altman, D. S., Robertson, D., O'Sullivan, D. M., Douglass, J. M., & Tinanoff, N. (1997). Dental caries prevalence and treatment levels in Arizona preschool children. *Public Health Reports, 112*(4), 319-331.

Tapia, J. (1972). The nursing process in family health. *Nursing Outlook, 20*(4), 267-270.

Tertinger, D. A., Greene, B. F., & Lutzker, J. R. (1984). Home safety: Development and validation of one component of an ecobehavioral treatment program for abused and neglected children. *Journal of Applied Behavior Analysis, 17*(2), 159-174.

Toth, S. L., & Cicchetti, D. (1996). Patterns of relatedness, depressive symptomatology, and perceived competence in maltreated children. *Journal of Consulting & Clinical Psychology, 64*(1), 32-41.

Toth, S. L., Cicchetti, D., Macfie, J., & Emde, R. N. (1997). Representations of self and other in the narratives of neglected, physically abused, and sexually abused preschoolers. *Development & Psychopathology, 9*(4), 781-796.

Toth, S. L., Cicchetti, D., Macfie, J., Maughan, A., & Vanmeenen, K. (2000). Narrative representations of caregivers and self in maltreated preschoolers. *Attachment and Human Development, 2,* 271-305.

Trocme, N. (1996). Development and preliminary evaluation of the Ontario Child Neglect Index. *Child Maltreatment, 1,* 145-155.

Trotter, R., Ackerman, A., Rodman, D., Martinez, A., & Sorvillo, F. (1983). "Azarcon" and "Greta": Ethnomedical solutions to epidemiological mystery. *Medical Anthropology Quarterly, 14*(3), 3-18.

U.S. Department of Health and Human Services. (2000). *Child maltreatment 1998: Reports from the states to the national child abuse and neglect data system.* Washington DC: U.S. Government Printing Office.

U.S. Department of Health and Human Services. (2005). *Child maltreatment 2003.* Washington DC: U.S. Government Printing Office.

U.S. Department of Health and Human Services, Administration for Children and Families. (2004). *The Child Abuse Prevention and Treatment Act: As amended by the Keeping Children and Families Safe Act of 2003* (pp. 1-77). Washington, DC: Author.

Waldinger, R. J., Toth, S. L., & Gerber, A. (2001). Maltreatment and internal representations of relationships: Core relationship themes in the narratives of abused and neglected preschoolers. *Social Development, 10*(41-58).

Wang, C. T., & Daro, D. (1998). *Current trends in child abuse reporting and fatalities: Results of the 1997 annual fifty state survey* (No. 808). Chicago, IL: National Committee to Prevent Child Abuse.

Watson-Perczel, M., Lutzker, J. R., Greene, B. F., & McGimpsey, B. J. (1988). Assessment and modification of home cleanliness among families adjudicated for child neglect. *Behavior Modification, 12*(1), 57-81.

Widom, C. S. (2001). Child abuse and neglect. In S. O. White (Ed.), *Handbook of youth and justice* (pp. 31-47). New York: Plenum.

Widom, C. S., & Kuhns, J. B. (1996). Childhood victimization and subsequent risk for promiscuity, prostitution, and teenage pregnancy: A prospective study. *American Journal of Public Health, 86,* 1607-1612.

Wilkey, I., Pearn, J., Petrie, G., & Nixon, J. (1982). Neonaticide, infanticide, and child homicide. *Medicine, Science, & the Law, 22*(1), 31-34.

Williamson, J. M., Borduin, C. M., & Howe, B. A. (1991). The ecology of adolescent maltreatment: A multilevel examination of adolescent physical abuse, sexual abuse, and neglect. *Journal of Consulting & Clinical Psychology, 59*(3), 449-457.

Wolfe, D. A. (1987). *Child abuse: Implications for child development and psychopathology.* Newbury Park, CA: Sage Publications.

Wolfe, D. A. (1991). *Preventing physical and emotional abuse of children.* New York: Guilford Press.

Wolock, I., & Horowitz, B. (1984). Child maltreatment as a social problem: The neglect of neglect. *American Journal of Orthopsychiatry, 54*(4), 530-543.

Young, L. (1981). *Physical child neglect.* Chicago, IL: National Committee for Prevention of Child Abuse.

Care of African American Women Survivors of Intimate Partner Violence

JANETTE Y. TAYLOR

> Who, then, can I turn to when I hurt real bad … I find myself at therapy's doorstep. Will this counselor usher me to insanity? Because if she does not openly deal with the fact that there is a very low premium on every aspect of my existence, if she does not acknowledge the politics of Black-womanhood, now that would surely drive me nuts.
>
> *Eleanor Johnson, Reflections on Black Feminist Therapy (1983, p. 320)*

The foregoing quote from *Reflections on Black Feminist Therapy* by Eleanor Johnson (1983) informs and instructs nurses to examine the personal-social context of African American women seeking therapy and to consider their individual perspectives and responses to the needs of African American women who arrive at their doors for care. Locating Johnson's statement (1983) within the context of intimate partner violence, nurses then must ask the following: How do nurses view African American women who come to health care providers seeking counseling for a range of issues including those with histories of intimate partner violence (e.g., domestic violence)? What is the perception and reception given to women who have survived this experience? How do individual practitioners and institutions construct services to meet the needs of various women? and What are appropriate therapeutic approaches and interventions for the care of African American women who are recovering from intimate partner violence? The purpose of this brief but cogent chapter is to outline why support groups as collective exchanges are culturally anchored approaches that can provide a therapeutic safe environment for African American women recovering from a variety of social, psychological, emotional, and physical traumas.

INTIMATE PARTNER VIOLENCE AND ABUSE

Women from a variety of social and economic levels make up an estimated 2 million to 4.4 million victims each year who are involved in relationships that include intimate partner violence (Kessler, Molnar, Feurer, & Appelbaum, 2001; Plichta, 1996; Tjaden, & Thoennes, 2000). National statistics indicate that 26.3% of black women surveyed had been victims of physical violence and 4.2% had been stalked (Tjaden & Thoennes, 2000). Homicide remains the leading cause of death for African America women between the ages of 15 and 24 (National Center for Health Statistics, 1997). Because of the frequency, severity, and pervasiveness of domestic violence and sexual abuse, the National Black Women's Health Project identified the occurrence of violence and abuse as the number one health issue for black women: "The number one issue for most of our sisters is violence—battering, sexual abuse … We have to look at how violence is used, how violence and sexism go hand in hand" (Avery, 1994, p. 8). As suggested by Avery (1994) and Johnson (1983), meaningful work with African American women has to occur from perspectives that include the influence of larger social structures when addressing issues of violence. Social context matters.

Particular historical and social experiences influence the lives and health of African American women. To understand better the social context of women's lives and to formulate strategies that facilitate recovery from intimate partner violence requires a womanist/black feminist conceptual framework. Womanist/black feminist conceptual frameworks attempt to explain how women's lives are shaped by their race/ethnicity, socioeconomic class, and gender or sexuality. This helps nurses to understand the experiences of women in terms of their realities and to formulate appropriate and meaningful plans for care with victim-survivors. Womanist/black feminist frameworks provide significant insights into the lives and health of African American women (Banks-Wallace, 2000; Taylor, 1998).

SOCIAL CONTEXT AND THE DEVELOPMENT OF AN INTERVENTION FOR AFRICAN AMERICAN WOMEN

A significant component of understanding African American women and their response to domestic violence is embedded in the cultural components of their lives. Cultural and ideological barriers, such as racism, classism, and sexism, shape African American women's experience and recovery from relationship violence differently from white women (Campbell, 1993; Collins, 2000; Greene, 1994; Pinn, 1997). Widely held images of African American women contribute to the lack of outreach efforts and resources available to them. Some images lessen the ability of health care providers to identify women as victim-survivors of intimate partner violence. Hooks (1993) maintains that popular stereotypes and other negative cultural ideas give authorization to ignore the needs of African American women:

> Whenever people talk about black women's lives, the emphasis is rarely on transforming society so that we can live fully; it is almost always about applauding how well we have "survived" despite harsh circumstances or how we can survive in the future. (p. 137)

Greene (1994) continues this idea when she wrote, "African American women face a range of cultural imperatives and psychological realities that may challenge, facilitate, or undermine their development and adaptive functioning" (p. 11). Part of the continuing challenge for African American women survivors is to find resources and services. Within the health care arena the responsibility for the provision of services is located with health care providers and practitioners. Therefore practitioners must approach the development and implementation of interventions to maximize the fit between the intervention and the women's cultural background (Campbell & Gary, 1998; Cauce, Coronado, & Watson, 1998; Tripp-Reimer, 1999). One therapeutic approach that is culturally anchored is support group or solution-focused group therapy.

Group therapy is an idea being embraced by a growing number of African American women. Although there are no published statistics on the number of African American women participating in such groups, the increase in self-help book publications combined with statements from nurses, psychologists, and social workers indicate an upward trend. More women believe that they need to be replenished emotionally and spiritually and that this is accomplished best by being encircled by the strength of sisterhood.

AFROCENTRIC THERAPY: SUPPORT GROUPS AS COLLECTIVE HEALING EXPERIENCES FOR SURVIVORS

Support groups are valuable interventions for survivors of intimate partner violence because they can provide an effective healing environment. Groups as collective interventions are effective across a broad range of culturally diverse populations. In particular, group work with African American women frequently is viewed as an effective culturally anchored intervention because of a shared cultural perspective that includes groupness, sameness, and commonality as psychobehavioral modalities. Collins (2000) succinctly summarizes the development of a collective experience when she asserts, "Historically, racial segregation in housing, education, and employment fostered group commonalities that encouraged the formation of a group-based, collective standpoint" (p. 24). Group work provides a natural form of assistance since African American women are group-centered.

Group work provides an individual-collective approach that facilitates the validation and management of black women's lives (Boyd-Franklin, 1987; King & Ferguson, 1996; Pack-Brown, Whittington-Clark, & Parker, 1998). Movement between the individual-collective experiences can produce healing encounters that facilitate individual growth beyond the trauma of intimate partner violence and the daily acts of racism that often inhibit self-recovery.

In addition, groups provide an opportunity to talk about the experiences of partner violence. The subject of intimate partner violence continues to be a taboo topic in many African American communities; therefore being able to discuss abuse and violence in an accepting group of other similar women fosters a sense of connection and self-empowerment. When considering the value and function of support groups for women recovering from intimate partner violence, it is important to structure such sessions in ways that facilitate the growth and comfort of the women.

STRUCTURING COLLECTIVE EXPERIENCES FOR AFRICAN AMERICAN WOMEN

The composition of the group members is important. Often, women who seek group encounters have had individual counseling/therapy with white therapists who did not understand their sense of oppression or struggle as an African American woman. They were tired of explaining (read *justifying*) their feelings and experiences. Similarly, they were disappointed with available group sessions and the professionals leading the group, and/or the group itself was white.

Many African American women prefer working with individual or support group members that have common or shared race, ethnicity, gender, and socio-economic status. Racially homogeneous groups are preferred because for many women, this group environment (1) maximizes the comfort level; (2) provides more opportunities to disclose more fully the events in their lives (partner and cultural violence—such as racism and sexism); that is, to address issues in an environment that is closer to their social realities and to discuss topics that are central to their life experiences; and (3) counters social isolation that is prevalent in abusive situations and in environments that foster discrimination and racism.

In planning support groups or modifying existing groups, the group facilitator must consider the multiple and diverse locations of African American women. These considerations are complicated. For example, would a higher socially economic status African American woman of higher social economic status prefer a racially diverse group in the same economic status or an African American women's group with a lower social economic status? An additional consideration is the limited number of group facilitators who are culturally competent and engage in thinking through African American women's lives from a critical social theoretical perspective that understands the influence of race, class, and gender in shaping their recovery experiences. Pack-Brown et al. (1998) characterize essential qualities that culturally competent professionals must have in order to work with African American women: (1) awareness of personal biases, stereotypes, and prejudices; (2) knowledge about the clientele; and (3) ability to practice skills that are sensitive to client's life experiences.

Successful interventions with African American survivors of intimate partner violence often include group exploration of discrimination, racism, and sexism before truly productive discussions of the abuse can occur (Campbell & Gary, 1998; Heron, Twomey, Jacobs & Kaslow, 1997; Taylor, 2000). Conversations on racism may advance the therapeutic process just as discussions relative to other events block personal growth and healing. Such discussions may be initiated by the woman or the practitioner and have additional value when they occur in collective or group environments.

To broaden services to include the concerns of African American women is important. The intent is to offer options for African American women who are victim-survivors, as well as other women of color, so they do not constantly have to confront their minority status and the dynamics that thwart their journey to recovery. Additionally, the high cost of individual psychotherapy sessions exceeds many women's limited economic resources. All women need access to interventions that promote adaptive function.

Although, group identity is important, African American women also experience themselves as individuals and as members of a racial group (e.g., collective) (Kambon, 1996; McCombs, 1985, 1986; McNair, 1992; Taylor, 1998). Both social locations are crucial to African American women's self-concept and must be addressed simultaneously for recovery from abuse to occur.

SUMMARY

Increasingly, nurses and other health care providers are asked to consider the implications of the changing demographics in their communities and to accommodate a variety of cultural experiences in their practice. Health care providers cannot continue to insert African American women into predominantly white groups and then wonder, Why is she silent? Why does she have so little to say or contribute to the group? Why did she stop coming? and Why is she not beginning to resolve many (or any) of the issues that I suspect are present? Critical to African American women's healing is a thoughtfully constructed therapeutic environment. Because African American women form community through collect activities such as therapeutic support groups, groups can serve as social places where women build trusting relationships, talk about their experiences, and continue to heal and recover. Women create a healing community within a group arrangement.

This chapter opens with a quote by Eleanor Johnson (1983), who challenges therapist, advocates, practitioners, and researchers to understand the multilevel occurrences of violence in the lives of African American women. African American women encounter abuse in their intimate relationships, communities, and places of employment. Many critical questions regarding the realities of African American women need to be addressed in developing group interventions. Are there safe opportunities for women to share their stories? Are issues of social isolation addressed? Are efforts made to support familiar spiritual practices? Are there opportunities to develop healthier images of self and move toward self-determination? Are there appropriate opportunities for personal and political renewal? As you think about the conceptual framework and the complex context of African American women's lives, I encourage you to ask the additional questions:

◆ What are my images of and assumptions about African American women?

◆ What do I assume (and know) about the dynamics of domestic violence/intimate partner violence in African American communities?

◆ Where am I in relation to power and privilege with this clientele?

◆ How do I provide care and engage in therapeutic relationships with women so that they can thrive past the experience of abuse?

◆ Who should cofacilitate groups with African American women? Specifically, can non-African American (read *white*) women cofacilitate groups? If so, why? Why?

REFERENCES

Avery, B. Y. (1994). Breathing life into ourselves: The evolution of the national black women's health project. In E. C. White (Ed.), *The black women's health book: Speaking for ourselves* (2nd ed., pp. 4-10). Seattle, WA: Seal Press.

Banks-Wallace, J. (2000). Womanist ways of knowing: Theoretical considerations for research with African American women. *Advances in Nursing Science, 22*(3), 33-45.

Boyd-Franklin, N. (1987). Group therapy for black women: A therapeutic support model. *American Journal of Orthopsychiatry, 57*(3), 394-401.

Campbell, D. W. (1993). Nursing care of African American battered women: Afrocentric perspectives. In J. Campbell (Ed.), *AWHONN's clinical issues in perinatal and women's health nursing: Domestic violence* (Vol. 4, pp. 407-415). Philadelphia: J. B. Lippincott.

Campbell, D. W., & Gary, F. A. (1998). Providing effective interventions for African American battered women. In J. C. Campbell (Ed.), *Empowering survivors of abuse: Health care for battered women and their children* (pp. 229-240). Thousand Oaks, CA: Sage.

Cauce, A. M., Coronado, N., & Watson, J. (1998). Conceptual, methodological, and statistical issues in culturally competent research. In M. Hernandez & M. R. Isaacs (Eds.), *Promoting cultural competence in children's mental health services* (pp. 305-331). Baltimore, MD: Paul H. Brookes.

Collins, P. H. (2000). *Black feminist thought: Knowledge, consciousness, and the politics of empowerment* (2nd ed.). New York: Routledge.

Greene, B. (1994). African American women. In L. Comas-Diaz & B. Greene (Eds.), *Women of color: Integrating ethnic and gender identities in psychotherapy* (pp. 10-29). New York: Guilford Press.

Heron, R. L., Twomey, H. B., Jacobs, D. P., & Kaslow, N. J. (1997). Culturally competent interventions for abused and suicidal African American women. *Psychotherapy, 37*(4), 410-424.

Hooks, B. (1993). *Sisters of the yam: Black women and self recovery.* Boston, MA: South End Press.

Johnson, E. (1983). Reflections on black feminist therapy. In B. E. Smith (Ed.), *Home girls: A black feminist anthology* (pp. 320-324). New York: Kitchen Table: Women of Color Press.

Kambon, K. K. K. (1996). The Afrocentric paradigm and African American psychological liberation. In D. A. Azibo (Ed.), *African psychology in historical perspective & related commentary* (pp. 59-62). Trenton, NJ: African World Press.

Kessler, R. C., Molnar, B. E., Feurer, I. D., & Appelbaum, M. (2001). Patterns and mental health predictors of domestic violence in the United States: Results from the national comorbidity survey. *International Journal of Law and Psychiatry, 24,* 487-508.

King, T. C., & Ferguson, S. A. (1996). "I am because we are": Clinical interpretations of communal experience among African American women. *Women & Therapy, 18*(1), 33-45.

McCombs, H. G. (1985). Black self-concept: An individual/collective analysis. *International Journal of Intercultural Relations, 9,* 1-18.

McCombs, H. G. (1986). The application of an individual/collective model to the psychology of black women. *Women & Therapy, 5*(2/3), 67-80.

McNair, L. D. (1992). African American women in therapy: An Afrocentric and feminist synthesis. *Women & Therapy, 12*(1/2), 5-19.

National Center for Health Statistics. (1997). *Vital statistic mortality data, underlying causes of death, 1995-1997.* Hyattsville, MD: Centers for Disease Control and Prevention.

Pack-Brown, S. P., Whittington-Clark, L. E., & Parker, W. M. (1998). *Images of me: A guide to group work with African-American women.* Boston: Allyn & Bacon.

Pinn, V. W. (1997). The diverse faces of violence: Minority women and domestic violence. *Academic Medicine, 72*(1), S65-S71.

Plichta, S. B. (1996). Violence and abuse: Implications for women's health. In M. M. Falik & K. S. Collins (Ed.), *Women's health: The commonwealth fund survey* (pp. 237-270). Baltimore: John Hopkins University Press.

Taylor, J. Y. (1998). Womanism: A methodologic framework for African American women. *Advances in Nursing Science, 21*(1), 53-64.

Taylor, J. Y. (2000). Sisters of the yam: African American women's healing and recovery from intimate male partner violence. *Issues in Mental Health Nursing, 21,* 515-531.

Tjaden, P., & Thoennes, N. (2000). *Extent, nature, and consequences of intimate partner violence: Findings from the national violence against women survey* (ncj181867). Washington, DC: U.S. Government Printing Office.

Tripp-Reimer, T. (Ed.). (1999). *Cultural interventions for ethnic groups of color.* Thousand Oaks, CA: Sage.

SUGGESTED READINGS

Boyd-Franklin, N. (1991). Recurrent themes in the treatment of African American women in group psychotherapy. *Women & Therapy, 11*(2), 25-40.

Comas-Diaz, L. (1994). An integrative approach. In L. Comas-Diaz & B. Greene (Eds.), *Women of color: Integrating ethnic and gender identities in psychotherapy* (pp. 287-318). New York: Guilford Press.

Engel, B. (2000). *Women circling the earth: A guide to fostering community, health and empowerment.* Deerfield, FL: Health Communications.

Eugene, T. M. (1995). Swing low, sweet chariot! A womanist ethical response to sexual violence and abuse. In D. J. F. M. M. Adams (Ed.), *Violence against women and children: A Christian theological sourcebook* (pp. 185-200). New York: Continuum.

Garfield, C. A., Spring, C., & Cahill, S. (1998). *Wisdom circles: A guide to self-discovery and community building in small groups.* New York: Hyperion.

Hughes, D., & Dumont, K. (1993). Using focus groups to facilitate culturally anchored research. *American Journal of Community Psychology, 21,* 727-746.

McIntosh, P. (1995). White privilege and male privilege: A personal account of coming to see correspondences through work in women's studies. In M. L. Andersen & P. H. Collins (Ed.), *Race, class and gender: An anthology* (pp. 76-87). Belmont, CA: Wadsworth.

Metcalf, L. (1998). *Solution focused group therapy: Ideas for groups in private practice, schools, agencies, and treatment programs.* New York: Free Press.

Pierce-Baker, C. (1998). *Surviving the silence: Black women's stories of rape.* New York: W.W. Norton.

Rose, T. (2003). *Longing to tell: Black women talk about sexuality and intimacy.* New York: Farrar, Straus and Giroux.

Some, M. P. (1999). *The healing wisdom of Africa.* New York: Putnam.

Vasquez, M. J. T., & Han, A. L. (1995). Group interventions and treatment with ethnic minorities. In J. Apnote, R. Young-Rivers, & J. Wohl (Eds.), *Psychological interventions and cultural diversity* (pp. 109-127). Needham Heights, MA: Allyn & Bacon.

West, C. M. (2002). Battered, black and blue: An overview of violence in the lives of black women. In C. M. West (Ed.), *Violence in the lives of black women: Battered, black and blue.* New York: Haworth Press.

West, T. C. (1999). *Wounds of the spirit: Black women, violence and resistance ethics.* New York: New York University Press.

WEBSITES

The following national organizations may be helpful in locating group-therapy circles. Other places to find help include listings in free or community papers, community colleges, health centers, and YWCAs.

http://www.nbna.org/index1.htm
National Black Nurses Association
http://nabsw-osa.tripod.com/
National Association of Black Social Workers
http://www.abpsi.org/
Association of Black Psychologists

CHAPTER
78

Nursing Care

Victims of Violence—Elder Mistreatment

KRISTIN LEMKO ◆ TERRY FULMER

CASE STUDY

Mrs. P. is a 75-year-old woman who has been living with her son, his wife, and their four children for the past year. Mrs. P.'s husband died 18 months ago. Her son, John, is a financial analyst, and her daughter-in-law, Mary, is a clerk at the community hospital. They work full-time, and the son is often away on business. This is Mrs. P.'s second visit to the clinic in 2 weeks, complaining of shortness of breath and chest pain bilaterally. Upon examination, Mrs. P. has the following clinical data: Vital signs—Her oral temperature is 99.1° F, her pulse is 64 and regular, her respirations are 24, and her blood pressure is 118/78 while sitting. Mrs. P. is oriented to time, person, and place. A Mini-Mental State Examination shows a score of 27/30, which is excellent. She does not have any complaints of pain, but a generalized, foul odor is present, and her skin is dry and intact with ecchymotic areas on her forearms bilaterally. These areas are multicolored with bluish purple, red, and yellow areas present. The nurse suspects elder mistreatment and conducts an elder mistreatment interview and assessment. The patient confides that her daughter-in-law has been abusive to her but that it is not her daughter-in-law's fault. She states, "Mary is under a great deal of stress managing her household." Mrs. P. says that she does not want to tell her son so as not to bother him. She reports, "They are busy and have been very supportive of me."

In December 2004, nearing the end of the 108th Congress, the Elder Justice Act, proposed by the democratic Senator John Breaux (Louisiana) in February 2003, was tabled in the Finance Committee without a vote (U.S. Senate, 2004). This bill would have established an Office of Elder Justice within the Administration on Aging; an Intra-Agency Elder Steering Committee; an Elder Justice Coordinating Council; an Advisory Board on Elder Abuse, Neglect, and Exploitation; and an Elder Justice Resource Center; it also would have augmented National Institute on Aging grants. Despite the popularity of the bill and the cosponsorship of 44 senators, the bill was not a high priority for the Senate. Meanwhile, national legislators sent to their constituents an unspoken message that is politically effective but substantially empty. Who is advocating for the funding necessary to address elder mistreatment? Why was a bill with 44 Senate sponsors tabled in committee? Words but no action. As the baby boomer population (those born in 1946-1964) is getting older, the interest in aging issues is said to be increasing, and there is no question that Washington is taking notice with the National Coalition of Elder Mistreatment in 2002 and the National Research Council publication in 2003. Elder mistreatment continues to attract the attention of policy makers and legislators from virtually all political backgrounds. Although legislation related to elder mistreatment has strong support, senators rarely demonstrate their dedication to this issue, and unfortunately, there has been no national legislation on elder mistreatment. *The New York Times* reported that only 2% of the budget for abuse prevention is allotted to elder mistreatment (abuse, exploitation, neglect, abandonment, self-neglect) (Blancato, 2004). Although the issue of elder mistreatment is becoming more popular politically, progress in the field of elder mistreatment legislation and scientific funding is moving at a snail's pace.

In the public dialogue of domestic violence, elder mistreatment is considered a "late bloomer," only recently attracting national attention and gaining recognition as a critical problem. Domestic (family violence), mainly child abuse and partner abuse, drew national attention in the 1970s with the Child Abuse Prevention and Screening Act of 1974 (Bonnie & Wallace, 2003). Substantive research and interventions for child abuse and partner abuse were developed and examined in the 1980s. Mistreatment of children readily was medicalized, and screening was incorporated into the routine health assessment, and mandated child abuse education is required for licensure in many states. In 1992 the American Medical Association finally established guidelines for the screening and referral of elder mistreatment, but adequate training of health professionals has yet to be implemented systematically, and the guidelines have not been updated since publication. In the medical community, elder mistreatment has been labeled as a Pandora's box because many health care providers feel that they do not have adequate time to screen older adults for elder mistreatment or the necessary training to conduct such crucial evaluations.

News accounts of older adults who have been abandoned or abused by their families or battered in nursing homes are becoming more prevalent (National Research Council, 1992; Rather, 2000; Zeigler, 1999). By 1998 the National Research Council and the Institute of Medicine published *Violence in Families,* which addressed prevention and treatment programs for family violence. Of the 144 controlled studies on family violence that were identified in this analysis, only two elder mistreatment studies were reviewed and considered substantive to be mentioned (Bonnie & Wallace, 2003).

Several professions are involved in the detection and intervention of elder mistreatment, and nurses are key professionals for screening, assessment, and prevention of elder mistreatment (Fulmer, 2002; Fulmer, Guadagno, Bitondo Dyer, & Connolly, 2004). Isolated older adults may have infrequent connections with others. Their only interaction may be with health care professionals episodically or with daily caregivers. Nurses are in a unique position within the community to reach out to older adults because the profession has an already established rapport with community members. According to a recent Gallup poll, nurses were ranked the number one most trusted profession in America (Westbrook, 2004). Because of established rapport with the community, nurses have the opportunity to interact regularly with older adults in their practice and to offer advice about quality of life. These interactions provide the perfect milieu for routine screening for elder mistreatment. Whether in an emergency room or a half-hour intake interview, nurses should screen all older adults for elder mistreatment (Blancato, 2004). As advanced

practice nurses, modeling this behavior to staff nurses, new trainees, or new graduate nurses and emphasizing the importance for screening for elder mistreatment creates a trickle-down effect and collectively increases the awareness about this public health problem.

Nurses also should encourage interdisciplinary collaboration when working to combat elder mistreatment. A team approach to elder mistreatment has been successful in the health community (Fulmer et al., 2003). This model could be expanded further as law enforcers, attorneys, community professionals, and health professionals work together to prevent and intervene in elder mistreatment situations.

UNDERSTANDING THE PROBLEM

Estimates indicate that 1.2 million to 2 million older adults, or approximately 6% of older adults, are mistreated annually (Pillemer & Finkelhor, 1988; Bonnie & Wallace, 2003). According to the National Research Council (2003), elder mistreatment is the following:

1. Intentional actions that cause harm or create serious risk of harm (whether or not the harm was intended to a vulnerable elder by a caregiver or other person who stands in a trust relationship to the elder
2. Failure by a caregiver to satisfy the elder's basic needs or to protect the elder from harm

Five categories of elder mistreatment are (1) abuse, which encompasses physical abuse, psychological abuse, and sexual abuse; (2) neglect; (3) abandonment; (4) exploitation or financial abuse; and (5) self-neglect (Bonnie & Wallace, 2003).

As of 2003, approximately 36 million persons over the age of 65 live in the United States, making up 12% of the population. The older adult population is expected to double between 2000 to 2030, as baby boomers reach the age of 65, and then to plateau around 2050 (Figure 78-1). As the number of older adults increases, without the appropriate interventions, Americans can expect the incidence of elder mistreatment to grow proportionally (Federal Interagency Forum on Aging-Related Statistics, 2004; International Longevity Center—USA, 2004). Quantification of elder mistreatment is difficult because many cases are not reported and resources for effectively documenting suspected and substantive cases are lacking. For health professionals, especially nurses who often are confronted with elder mistreatment, it is critical to understand why an older adult may refuse help, reject an intervention, and even defend a caregiver who is abusive or mistreating them when confronted about their situation. Often, older

VIEWPOINTS

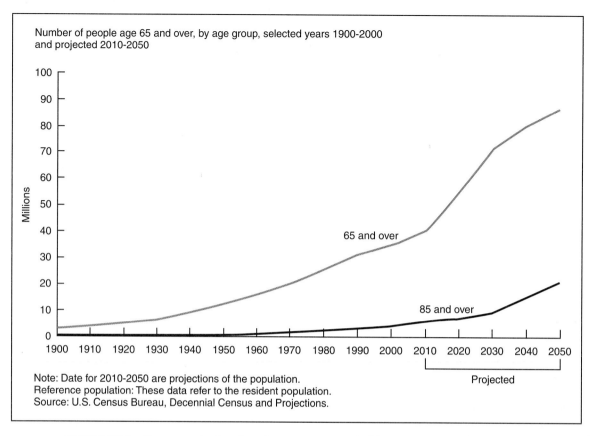

Number of people age 65 and over, by age group, selected years 1900-2000 and projected 2010-2050

Note: Date for 2010-2050 are projections of the population.
Reference population: These data refer to the resident population.
Source: U.S. Census Bureau, Decennial Census and Projections.

FIGURE 78-1   Census projection data for persons 65 and older. (From Federal Interagency Forum on Aging-Related Statistics. (2004.) *Older Americans: Key indicators of well-being.* Washington, DC: US Government Printing Office.)

adults are afraid of any change or fear the repercussions of their decision to take action (Harrell et al., 2002). Instead, they develop a tolerance for their poor treatment, consciously or unconsciously in an effort to protect themselves from further isolation or punishment from their caregiver should they report mistreatment. Many older adults feel that they are undeserving of proper treatment or that no one owes them such adequate treatment. They may not want to be considered a burden or as one who is overly demanding, they may have a sense of worthlessness and a self-view that they only cause harm or strain to their family members or caregivers.

A developing theory is that victims of elder abuse often have a history of childhood trauma, which may lead to an acceptance for low levels of care (Fulmer et al., in press). Feelings and responses of the older adult who is mistreated are often complex. Through an elevated awareness of older adults and better communication and dialogue with older adults regarding their perceptions and reactions to their situation, the advanced

practice nurse can be more effective in recognizing and managing cases of elder mistreatment.

THE CAREGIVERS

Forty percent of persons who mistreat older adults are the middle-aged adult children (National Association of Adult Protective Service Administrators, 2001). This kind of caretaker often will have a dependency on the older adult, usually financially, creating a situation of codependency. This description can conjure the image of a disrespectful or ungrateful child, even evoking the character of a criminal or a thief. However, in reality these caretakers are generally genuinely caring individuals who may be victims themselves of substance abuse, mental illness, or the stress of day-to-day life. Nurses should be vigilant to family dynamics that may indicate elder mistreatment.

Several theories attempt to explain the occurrence of elder mistreatment. Ensel and Lin (2000) address the imperative to expand the biomedical model when understanding theories of elder mistreatment to include psychological and the social component. The National Research Council (Bonnie & Wallace, 2003) further elaborates to include cultural and environmental contexts that explain the occurrence of elder mistreatment. These newer observations reflect developing theories of elder mistreatment. One such theory is the caregiver stress theory. This theory evaluates the challenges of balancing a modern lifestyle, including working and raising children, with the responsibilities of caring for an aging parent. The increased stress of an added dependent can diminish coping mechanisms that can lead to mistreatment (Glass, Laughon, & Campbell, 2004). Another leading theory is that the abuser has a psychopathology, is developmentally disabled or has a substance abuse problem (Lachs & Fulmer, 1993). The transgenerational violence theory postulates that mistreatment is a cyclical phenomenon with the perpetrator abused as a child by his or her parents and then eventually becoming an abusive adult in taking on the caregiver role. Elder mistreatment also often is associated with a web of dependency. For example, the caregiver may be emotionally and/or financially dependent on the older adult (Bonnie & Wallace, 2003). A thorough assessment of a caregiver's limitations enables a more thorough understanding of the caregiver/older adult dyad and assists in identification of appropriate interventions. For the nurse to remain nonjudgmental and to refrain from labeling perpetrators as criminals or delinquents also is important. By passing quick judgments, nurses remove themselves from a level of understanding that can be helpful in creating solutions. Abusers commonly were or are victims themselves. As health care professionals, nurses can set the example throughout the health care system of intervening without judgment.

THE VICTIMS

Like a silent illness or an asymptomatic condition, elder mistreatment can be difficult to detect among older adults. Regardless of their appearance and initial impression, older adults should always be assessed for elder mistreatment. Some shared characteristics of older adults who are mistreated pertain to sex, age, and low socioeconomic status. The most vulnerable population tends to be older adults who are female, over the age of 75, who have a low educational level, impaired functional/cognitive status, and a history of domestic violence, stressful events, and depression that may indicate

an increased risk for elder mistreatment (Dyer, Pavlik, Murphy, & Hyman, 2000; Pillemer & Finkelhor, 1989). Victims tend to be frail females (Dunlop, Rothman, Condon, Hebert, & Martinez, 2000) who live with their abusers (Lachs, Williams, O'Brien, Hurst, & Horwitz, 1997; Pillemer & Finkelhor, 1988). These women are usually dependent on their caregiver and/or are suffering from a chronic, disabling illness. These characteristics often create an increased dependency of the older adult on the caregiver. Often the caregiver will have untreated psychiatric problems or be cognitively impaired (Dyer et al., 2000; Pillemer & Finkelhor, 1989).

Even when older adults are cognizant, they may deny that they are mistreated (Lachs & Pillemer, 2004). They deny the mistreatment for several reasons. They may be fearful of retribution by the abuser, or they may fear placement in a nursing home. The potential for nursing home placement may make them anxious, or they may have come to accept their status quo and do not expect anything better. Understanding of these fears can help nurses personalize solutions.

KEY ASPECTS OF HEALTH ASSESSMENT FOR ELDER MISTREATMENT

The assessment and management of older adults who are mistreated is difficult and complex. Signs and symptoms of elder mistreatment may mimic normal signs of aging or a disease process (Lachs & Pillemer, 2004). For example, bruising may be caused by anemia or intentional abuse. Fractures may be caused by osteoporosis, a fall, or intentional trauma. In health care settings, it may be difficult to spend time interviewing a reluctant patient and/or a caregiver; consequently, the nurse misses important warning signs or evidence of elder mistreatment that can result in death.

In addition, when elder mistreatment is detected, nurses often feel they meet a brick wall in terms of creating successful solutions. Adult protective services is a community-based state agency with the purpose of intervening when mistreatment of disabled or older adults is suspected. The characteristics an older adult must possess to qualify for adult protective services varies from state to state. Often, adult protective services have burdened caseloads, and turnaround time for feedback can be excessive. Furthermore, as of this publication, no substantive evidence-based studies indicate how to intervene successfully when an older adult is mistreated. The complexities of assessment, diagnosis, and intervention can make the management of elder mistreatment a challenging and frustrating task.

PRACTICE: EVIDENCE-BASED SOLUTIONS

The empirical research base for interventions in elder mistreatment is limited, and further research is needed. Most of the recommendations include reporting and referring, yet research is needed on the effectiveness of these interventions (Bonnie & Wallace, 2003).

Victim advocacy remains a problem for older and dependent adults. Similar to child abuse and partner violence, victims often are not able to advocate for themselves or they require assistance, protection, and empowerment. Older adults fear the repercussions of speaking out, such as further social isolation or punishment. As the key players in the reduction of elder mistreatment, older adults are not admitting or accepting the existence of the problem. Their denial paralyzes policy analysis and formation, and those involved need to get involved.

Some recommendations for managing elder mistreatment include, first, always to ensure the safety of the older adult. If a patient is reluctant to accept assistance while in the hospital or the health care system, the nurse should be sure the patient knows whom to contact if an emergency situation arises. Many older adults do use the Internet and may have difficulty locating a telephone number or an appropriate agency. Second, inform patients of their rights. Because many older adults fear repercussions following elder mistreatment reporting, nurses must let them know they have the right to dictate the level of care they receive. They decide whether to press charges, and they can withdraw from treatment or an intervention plan at any time.

As nurses move forward in the development of effective intervention strategies to detect and intervene in elder mistreatment cases, it is important to maintain awareness of this grave public health problem and to share concerns, successes, and progress with colleagues. A solution to ending widespread elder mistreatment is increasing awareness and ending denial.

MRS P.: CASE SUMMARY

After a thorough health history and assessment, Mrs. P. stated to the nurse that her daughter-in-law, Mary, was overburdened because her husband was often away, that she works full time, and that Mrs. P. worried about the care of her four young grandchildren. This is an example of how caregiver stress can lead to mistreatment such as abuse and neglect. The hygiene neglect may have been unintentional, for Mary did not understand the needs or abilities of her mother-in-law, yet the physical abuse was a result of the escalating stress Mary was experiencing and maladaptive coping. The nurse notified adult protective services and recommended 3-week respite care for Mrs. P. and day care 2 times a week.

REFERENCES

American Medical Association. (1992). *Diagnostic and treatment guidelines on elder abuse and neglect.* Chicago: Author.

Blancato, R. (2004, December). Stopping abuse of the elderly. *The New York Times,* Section A, p. 32, Column 6.

Bonnie, R. J., & Wallace, R. B. (Eds.). (2003). *The National Research Council. Elder mistreatment: Abuse, neglect, and exploitation in an aging America.* Washington, DC: National Academies Press.

Dunlop, B., Rothman, M. B., Condon, K. M., Hebert, K. S., & Martinez, I. L. (2000). Elder abuse: Risk factors and use of case data to improve policy and practice. *Journal of Elder Abuse & Neglect, 12*(3/4), 95-122.

Dyer, C. B., Pavlik, V. N., Murphy, K. P., & Hyman, D. J. (2000). The high prevalence of depression and dementia in elder abuse or neglect. *Journal of the American Geriatrics Society, 48*(2), 205-208.

Ensel, W. M., & Lin, N. (2000). Age, the stress process, and physical distress: The role of distal stressors. *Journal of Aging and Health, 12*(2), 136-168.

Federal Interagency Forum on Aging-Related Statistics. (2004). *Older Americans: Key indicators of well-being.* Washington, DC: U.S. Government Printing Office.

Fulmer, T. (2002). Elder mistreatment. *Annual Review Nursing Research, 20,* 369-395.

Fulmer, T., Firpo, A., Guadagno, L., Easter, T. M., Kahan, F., & Paris, B. (2003). Themes from a grounded theory analysis of elder neglect assessment by experts. *Gerontologist, 43*(5), 745-752.

Fulmer, T., Guadagno, L., Bitondo Dyer, C., & Connolly, M. T. (2004). Progress in elder abuse screening and assessment instruments. *Journal of American Geriatrics Society, 52*(2), 297-304.

Fulmer, T., Paveza, G., Vandeweerd, C., Fairchild, S., Guadagno, L., Bolton, M., et al. (in press). Dyadic vulnerability/risk profiling for elder neglect. *Gerontologist.*

Glass, N., Laughon, K., & Campbell, J. (2004). Theories of aggression and family violence. In J. Humphreys & J. Campbell (Eds.), *Family violence and nursing practice.* Philadelphia: Lippincott Williams & Wilkins.

Harrell, R., Toronjo, C. H., McLaughlin, J., Pavlik, V. N., Hyman, D. J., & Dyer, C. B. (2002). How geriatricians identify elder abuse and neglect. *American Journal of Medical Sciences, 323*(1), 34-38.

International Longevity Center—USA. (2004). *International Longevity Center annual report: Here come the baby boomers.* New York: Author.

Lachs, M. S., & Fulmer, T. (1993). Recognizing elder abuse and neglect. *Clinical Geriatric Medicine, 9*(3), 665-681.

Lachs, M. S., & Pillemer, K. (2004). Elder abuse. *Lancet, 364*(9441), 1263-1272.

Lachs, M. S., Williams, C., O'Brien, S., Hurst, L., & Horwitz, R. I. (1997). Risk factors for reported elder abuse and neglect: A nine-year observational cohort study. *Gerontologist, 37*(4), 469-474.

National Association of Adult Protective Service Administrators. (2001). *Elder abuse awareness kit: A resource kit for protecting older people and people with disabilities.* Retrieved January 31, 2005, from http://www.elderabusecenter.org/pdf/basics/speakers.pdf

National Research Council. (2003). Older woman charges sex abuse by caregiver. (1992, June). *Seattle Post-Intelligencer,* p. 2.

Pillemer, K. A., & Finkelhor, D. (1988). The prevalence of elder abuse: A random sample survey. *Gerontologist, 28*(1), 51-57.

Pillemer, K. A., & Finkelhor, D. (1989). Causes of elder abuse: Caregiver stress versus problem relatives. *American Journal of Orthopsychiatry, 59*(2), 179-187.

Rather, D., Gonzales, V. (Anchors). (2000). "Eye on America: Nursing home abuse." *CBS Evening News* [Television broadcast]. [city]: CBS Worldwide.

U.S. Senate. (2004) *Legislation and records.* Retrieved February 1, 2005, from http://www.senate.gov

Westbrook, J. (2004, December). Americans trust nurses most, ignore news of killer caretakers. *Bloomberg News.*

Zeigler, M. (1999, March). Nurse's aid accused of abuse. *Rochester Democrat and Chronicle.*

Nursing Care

Preventive Gun Safety

MARY FRAN HAZINSKI

INTRODUCTION AND OVERVIEW

Although firearm injuries in all ages have decreased in the United States since 1993, they remain a leading cause of death in adolescents and young adults. Firearms are the leading method of suicides for all victims older than 10 years (Anderson, Minino, Fingerhut, Warner, & Heinen, 2004; Eber, Annest, Mercy, & Ryan, 2004; Vyrostek, Annest, & Ryan, 2004). Many unintentional firearm injuries and firearm suicides can be prevented if firearms are inaccessible to unsupervised children and adolescents (Eber et al., 2004).

Nurses have many opportunities to interact with community leaders, legislators, and members of the media and must be knowledgeable about evidence supporting gun safety interventions. In interactions with parents, nurses should encourage parents to store guns and ammunition safely. This chapter highlights the evidence available to support gun safety legislation and regulations and specific interventions to reduce firearm injuries and fatalities. This chapter does not address adolescent violence and gun use but focuses on gun storage and information for parents and children that is likely to reduce unintentional firearm injuries and suicides.

STATE LEGISLATION AND REGULATIONS

A variety of federal and state legislation and state and community regulations have attempted to reduce firearm injuries and fatalities (Hahn et al., 2005). These include the Brady Bill with background checks, mandatory waiting periods before firearm purchase, regulations pertaining to concealed weapons laws, child access prevention laws, and the Gun-Free Schools Act. Readers are referred to Hahn et al. (2005) for an excellent review of these laws.

The federal Brady Bill (Public Law 103-157) requires instant background checks for all firearm purchases.

However, the effectiveness of background checks is limited because records for many restriction categories (e.g., some mental health or drug addiction records) and 11.6% of all criminal records are not immediately accessible (Hahn et al., 2005).

Many states require waiting periods from 2 days (e.g., Alabama, Nebraska, South Dakota, and Wisconsin) to 6 months (New York) for purchase of a firearm. However, data are insufficient to determine the effect of waiting periods on firearm homicides and suicides. Data also are insufficient to evaluate the effects of regulations regarding establishment of registration (creation and retention of a record of firearm owners) or licensing (i.e., purchase or possession of a firearm requires a license or other authorization or certification) for the purchase of firearms (Hahn et al., 2005).

Many states have established concealed-weapons carry laws, requiring authorities to issue permits to those who wish to carry concealed weapons. Since 2000, 31 states have passed "shall issue" laws, eliminating most restrictions for carrying a concealed weapon. Evidence is insufficient to evaluate the effect of these laws on violent gun-related deaths. At this time, no law has been associated with a statistically significant reduction in firearm homicide or suicide rate (Rosengart et al., 2005), suggesting that families must take local action to reduce the risk of gun injuries.

Between 1989 and 2004, 18 states (California, Connecticut, Delaware, Florida, Hawaii, Illinois, Iowa, Maryland, Massachusetts, Minnesota, Nevada, New Hampshire, New Jersey, North Carolina, Rhode Island, Texas, Virginia, Wisconsin) passed child access prevention laws, requiring that firearm owners store firearms locked, unloaded, or both. Some states also hold firearm owners responsible when the firearms are stored improperly or when children use an improperly stored firearm to threaten or harm someone. These laws are logical because most firearms used by students in the 358 school-associated violent deaths reported from 1992 to 1999 were obtained from the perpetrator's home or from the home of a friend or relative (Centers for Disease Control and Prevention, 2003). If such firearms are inaccessible, some school-related firearm injuries or deaths might be prevented. In a 12-state study, child access prevention laws were associated with a 23% reduction (95% confidence interval [CI]: 6% to 37%) in unintentional firearm injuries among children younger than 15 years (Cummings, Grossman, Rivara, & Koepsell, 1997; Hahn et al., 2005). In a state-by-state review of firearm homicides, suicides, and unintentional injuries, state child access prevention laws also were associated with a decrease in juvenile suicide (Webster, Vernick, Zeoli, & Manganello, 2004).

The Gun-Free Schools Act (Public Law 103-382) requires that the 94% of all primary and secondary schools that receive federal funds must have a policy requiring expulsion of any student found in possession of a firearm at school. No studies have documented the effect of such policies on firearm injuries and deaths. However, in Nashville, Tennessee, the zero-tolerance policy has resulted in a eightfold to tenfold reduction of guns confiscated at schools, from an average of one or more per week before institution of the policy to four to seven confiscated during the entire school year (Bottorff, 2003).

In summary, the studies of the effect of legislation and regulations on firearm injuries and deaths have been inadequate in quality and quantity to draw any firm conclusions about their effects on firearm injuries or deaths. State child access protection laws do appear to reduce unintentional firearm injuries and firearm suicides in children, and school zero-tolerance policies for firearms appear to reduce the number of firearms brought to and confiscated at schools. Further research is needed to determine what legislation, if any, contributes to an overall reduction in the number or severity of firearm injuries.

RISKS CREATED BY HANDGUNS IN THE HOME

Several studies have documented an association between the presence of a handgun in the home and the risk of firearm injuries or death in the home. The strength of the association is stronger if the gun is stored loaded or unlocked or if there are multiple guns in the home. A debate regarding risks and benefits of guns in the home was published in *JAMA: The Journal of the American Medical Association* in 1998 (Cummings & Koepsell, 1998; Kleck, 1998).

In 1986, reports of 398 firearm-related deaths in homes in King County, Washington, were examined (Kellermann & Reay, 1986). Only 2 of the deaths were caused by intruders; the remaining 396 victims lived in or were invited visitors to the home. Only 7 (1.8%) of the 396 victims shot in the home were killed in self-defense, the remainder were victims of homicide, suicide, or unintentional injury.

Kellermann then performed a case-control study (Kellermann, Rivara, Rushforth, et al., 1993), reviewing the circumstances of homicides occurring in homes in Shelby County, Tennessee; in King County, Washington; and in Cuyahoga County, Ohio. The study matched households with homicides to similar households where homicides did not occur. Persons living in households with guns were 2.7 times (95% CI: 1.6% to 4.4%) more likely to be victims of homicide than were persons living in matched households without guns. The risk of homicide was increased further if there was previous violence or alcohol abuse in the household. The vast majority of homicide victims in this study were killed by a family member or an intimate acquaintance.

A national study (from all states except South Dakota, because it restricts use of death certificates) of violent death in the home found that guns in the home increased risk of homicide and suicide, regardless of the storage practice, type of gun, or number of firearms in the home (Dahlberg, Ikeda, & Kresnow, 2004). Males with a firearm in the home were 10.4 times more likely (95% CI: 5.8% to 18.9%) to commit suicide with a gun than males without a firearm in the home, and their risk of firearm suicide was 31.1 times higher (95% CI: 19.5% to 49.6%) than matched males without a firearm in the home. For those living in the home, the presence of a gun in the home increased the risk of a firearm homicide among those 35 years of age and older.

Studies of guns in the home and suicides in the home consistently have found an association between the availability of the guns and the likelihood of suicide. Brent (2001) reviewed this subject. In a case-control study, Kellermann, Rivara, Somes, et al. (1992) matched suicide victims who used a firearm with controls in the same community, matched for prescribed psychotropic medications, arrest record, abuse of alcohol or drugs, and education level. The researchers found that the presence of one or more guns in the home more than quadrupled (relative risk 4.8; 95% CI: 2.7% to 8.5%) the risk of suicide. In a case-control study of adolescents who committed suicide (Brent et al., 1993), the presence of any gun in the home quadrupled the likelihood of an adolescent suicide (95% CI: 1.1% to 7.5%), handguns increased the likelihood by a factor of 9.4 (95% CI: 1.7% to 53.9%), and loaded guns increased the likelihood by 32.3 times (95% CI: 2.5% to 413.4%).

A case-control study by Cummings, Koepsell, Grossman, Savarino, and Thompson (1997) verified the findings of Kellermann, Rivara, Somes, et al. (1992) and Brent et al. (1993). Cummings, Koepsell, et al. (1997) compared homicide and suicide victims in homes where a family member purchased a handgun from a licensed dealer with matched subjects of the same age, sex, and zip code of residence in the same health care plan but living in a home with no handgun purchase. Handgun purchase by someone in the family increased the relative risk of a suicide by someone in the family by a factor of 1.9 times (95% CI: 1.4% to 2.5%) and more than doubled the relative risk (95% CI: 1.3% to 3.7%) of a homicide in the family. The relative risks persisted for more than 5 years after the handgun purchase.

Although the case-control method of study may be criticized based on methods used to match subjects and controls, a large majority of the studies have found a link between presence of a gun in the home and risk of violent death in the home. If a nurse is the primary practitioner caring for a patient with a history of depression, alcohol or drug abuse, or violent behavior, or if there is such a history within the household, the nurse should discuss the risks of guns in the household and encourage the family to eliminate guns from the household. The nurse should ensure that parents are aware of the data regarding risks when a gun is in the home of an adolescent, particularly if that adolescent has a history of depression or substance abuse. These risks are substantially increased when multiple guns are present in the home and when they are stored loaded or unlocked with ammunition (see next section).

HANDGUN STORAGE PRACTICES

Based on analysis of more than 1000 published studies, it is estimated that one or more firearms are present in approximately one third of all homes in the United States. The percent of homes containing firearms is increased in the South and in rural areas. Of homes with firearms, 61% have handguns, and 60% of them have at least one automatic or semiautomatic firearm (Johnson, Coyne-Beasley, & Runyan, 2004). In reported studies, the percent of firearms in homes that are stored unlocked ranges from 49% to 53%, and the percent of firearms that are stored unlocked and loaded averages 21% to 22% (Grossman et al., 2005; Johnson et al., 2004).

A recent study compared the firearm storage practices in homes of guns used for child or adolescent suicide or unintentional shooting to the firearm storage practices of control households in the same county with guns that were not used in youth shootings (Grossman et al., 2005). The guns involved in suicides or unintentional shootings were more likely to be stored loaded, unlocked, with ammunition unlocked and in the same location than were control firearms. The four practices of storing guns unloaded, locked, with ammunition locked, and ammunition stored in a separate location were associated with a decreased likelihood of the gun being involved in a youth suicide or unintentional shooting.

In a national survey based on data reported from the 1993 National Mortality Followback Survey (this survery gathers data from next of kin regarding lifestyle practices of those who died), those who stored firearms locked or unloaded or both were much less likely to commit suicide by firearms (locked odds ratio is 0.39 [95% CI: 0.24% to 0.66%]; unloaded odds ratio is 0.30 [95% CI: 0.18% to 0.49%]) (Shenassa, Rogers, Spalding, & Roberts, 2004).

Unfortunately, even parents who do not have guns fail to appreciate the risks of guns in homes where children live or visit. In data collected from telephone interviews of adults in more than 600 houseolds with at least one child aged less than 6 years living in or visiting the home regularly, firearms were described as "present" in the household but unlocked in 33% of the homes where young children lived and in 56% of the homes where young children visited (Coyne-Beasley, Runyan, Baccaglini, Perkis, & Johnson, 2005). Another telephone survey of rural and urban households documented that overall 20% of the homes with or without children reported at least one firearm. The presence of children in the home was not associated with greater likelihood of safe storage; only 20% of gun-owning respondents who had children reported storing guns locked compared with 29% of those without children (Connor, 2005).

Parents appear to have unrealistic expectations regarding the actions of children when finding a gun. In a telephone survery, when asked what their child would do if their child found a gun, 87% of parents surveyed stated that their child would not touch a gun (Connor & Wesolowski, 2003). I have found this attitude when talking to parents after an unintentional firearm injury: parents report that they hid the gun and did not realize that the child knew where it was.

These findings suggest that gun owners do not appreciate the risks that guns pose when children are in the house. The surveys also suggest that parents need to be reminded of risks that guns pose in homes where children visit and in homes where children live. Parents would never hide Christmas presents in the same location every year, yet they often report hiding a gun in the same location for many years and are surprised to find that their child has found it.

EDUCATION OF CHILDREN REGARDING GUN RISKS

A number of educational programs have been developed to reduce risks of unintentional gun injuries during childhood. However, evidence of their ability to change behavior is limited.

The "Respect not Risk" program of firearm safety for third graders was reported as well-received with no data indicating the effect of the program on the behavior of students in simulated situations with guns (Liller et al., 2003). The Emergency Nurses Association program "Gun Safety, It's No Accident" also was reported to increase knowledge regarding gun safety, but it is not clear that this knowledge will translate to a change in behavior or a reduction in gun injuries (Howard, 2005).

The Eddie the Eagle GunSafe Program, developed by the National Rifle Association, uses cartoon videos to tell children that if they find a gun, "Stop, don't touch, leave the area, and tell an adult." Three studies compared the Eddie the Eagle program with another program of behavioral skills training that included exercises designed to teach children to role-play and model safe behavior when supervised around guns. Although both programs helped the children discuss safe behavior around guns, only after the behavioral skills training program did children demonstrate desired safety skills during role-play or in supervised scenarios where guns were present. These safety skills were demonstrated at follow-up assessments at 2- to 8-week intervals (Gatheridge et al., 2004; Himle, Miltenberger, Flessner, & Gatheridge, 2004; Himle, Miltenberger, Gatheridge, & Flessner, 2004).

COMMUNITY AND MEDIA ACTIVITIES

Trauma centers can join with community organizations and the media to promote safe gun storage. Trauma centers can identify parents of injured children who are willing to become advocates for safe gun storage. Appearance of these parents, and perhaps their injured children, on news segments describing the importance of safe gun storage can provide powerful messages to parents and children alike.

SUMMARY

This chapter highlights the evidence available to support common interventions to reduce firearm injuries in children. Nurses have the opportunity to discuss home safety with parents during well-child checkups and other encounters with families. Although some parents will deny gun ownership if directly asked, the nurse may be most effective by talking about the fact that many homes in which children live or visit have guns and parents need to be aware of safe ways for guns to be stored. Nurses should encourage the four practices of storing guns unloaded, locked, with ammunition locked, and ammunition stored in a separate location. These factors consistently have been associated with decreased likelihood of a gun being involved in a youth suicide or unintentional shooting.

REFERENCES

Anderson, R., Minino, A. M., Fingerhut, M. A., Warner, M., & Heinen, M. A. (2004). Deaths: Injuries, 2001. *National Vital Statistic Reports, 52*(21), 1-87.

Bottorff, C. (2003, January 30). Police report fewer guns found in Metro schools. *The Tennessean,* p. 3B.

Brent, D. A. (2001). Firearms and suicide. *Annuals of the New York Academy of Sciences, 932,* 225-240.

Brent, D. A., Perper, J. A., Moritz, G., Baugher, M., Schweers, J., & Roth, C. (1993). Firearms and adolescent suicide. A community case-control study. *American Journal of Diseases of Children, 147*(10), 1066-1071.

Centers for Disease Control and Prevention. (2003). Source of firearms used by students in school-associated violent deaths: United States, 1992-1999. *Morbidity & Mortality Weekly Report, 52*(9), 169-172.

Connor, S. M. (2005). The association between presence of children in the home and firearm-ownership and -storage practices. *Pediatrics, 115,* e38-e43.

Connor, S. M., & Wesolowski, K. L. (2003). They're too smart for that: Predicting what children would do in the presence of guns. *Pediatrics, 111,* e109-e114.

Coyne-Beasley, T., Runyan, C. W., Baccaglini, L., Perkis, D., & Johnson, R. M. (2005). Storage of poisonous substances and firearms in homes with young children visitors and older adults. *American Journal of Preventive Medicine, 28*(1), 109-115.

Cummings, P., Grossman, D. C., Rivara, F. P., & Koepsell, T. D. (1997). State gun safe storage laws and child mortality due to firearms. *JAMA: The Journal of American Medical Association, 278,* 1084-1086.

Cummings, P., & Koepsell, T. D. (1998). Does owning a firearm increase or decrease the risk of death? *JAMA: The Journal of American Medical Association, 280,* 471-473.

Cummings, P., Koepsell, T. D., Grossman, D. C., Savarino, J., & Thompson, R. S. (1997). The association between the purchase of a handgun and homicide or suicide. *American Journal of Public Health, 87*(6), 974-978.

Dahlberg, L. L., Ikeda, R. M., & Kresnow, M. J. (2004). Guns in the home and risk of violent death in the home: Findings from a national study. *American Journal of Epidemiology, 160*(10), 929-936.

Eber, G. B., Annest, J. L., Mercy, J. A. & Ryan, G. W. (2004). Nonfatal and fatal firearm-related injuries among children aged 14 years and younger: United States, 1993-2000. *Pediatrics, 113,* 1686-1692.

Gatheridge, B. J., Miltenberger, R. G., Huneke, D. F., Satterlund, M. J., Mattern, A. R., Johnson, B. M., et al. (2004). Comparison of two programs to teach firearm injury prevention skills to 6- and 7-year-old children. *Pediatrics, 114,* e294-e299.

Grossman, D. C., Mueller, B. A., Riedy, C., Dowd, M. D., Villaveces, A., Prodzinski, J., et al. (2005). Gun storage practices and risk of youth suicide and unintentional firearm injuries. *JAMA: The Journal of American Medical Association, 293*(6), 707-714.

Hahn, R. A., Bilukha, O., Crosby, A., Fullilove, M. T., Liberman, A., Moscicki, E., et al. (2005). Firearms laws and the reduction of violence: A systematic review. *American Journal of Preventive Medicine, 28*(2 Suppl. 1), 40-71.

Himle, M. B., Miltenberger, R. G., Flessner, C., & Gatheridge, B. (2004). Teaching safety skills to children to prevent gun play. *Journal of Applied Behavior Analysis, 37*(1), 1-9.

Himle, M. B., Miltenberger, R. G., Gatheridge, B., & Flessner, C. A. (2004). An evaluation of two procedures for training skills to prevent gun play in children. *Pediatrics, 113,* 70-77.

Howard, P. K. (2005). Evaluation of age-appropriate firearm safety interventions. *Pediatric Emergency Care, 21*(7), 473-479.

Johnson, R. M., Coyne-Beasley, T., & Runyan, C. W. (2004). Firearm ownership and storage practices, US households, 1992-2002: A systematic review. *American Journal of Preventive Medicine, 27*(2), 173-182.

Kellermann, A. L., & Reay, D. T. (1986). Protection or peril? An analysis of firearm-related deaths in the home. *New England Journal of Medicine, 314*(24), 1557-1560.

Kellermann, A. L., Rivara, F. P., Rushforth, N. B., Banton, J. B., Reay, D. T., Francisco, J. T., et al. (1993). Gun ownership as a risk factor for homicide in the home. *New England Journal of Medicine, 329,* 1084-1091.

Kellermann, A. L., Rivara, F. P., Somes, G., Reay, D. T., Francisco, J., Banton, J. G., et al. (1992). Suicide in the home in relation to gun ownership. *New England Journal of Medicine, 327,* 467-472.

Kleck, G. (1998). What are the risks and benefits of keeping a gun in the home? *JAMA: The Journal of American Medical Association, 280,* 473-475.

Liller, K. D., Perrin, K., Nearns, J., Pesce, K., Crane, N. B., & Gonzalez, R. R. (2003). Evaluation of the "respect not risk" firearm safety lesson for 3rd-graders. *Journal of School Nursing, 19*(6), 338-343.

Rosengart, M., Cummings, P., Nathens, A., Heagerty, P., Maier, R., & Rivara, F. (2005). An evaluation of state firearm regulations and homicide and suicide death rates. *Injury Prevention, 11*(2), 77-83.

Shenassa, E. D., Rogers, J. L., Spalding, K. L., Roberts, M. B. (2004). Safer storage of firearms at home and risk of suicide: A study of protective factors in a nationally representative sample. *Journal of Epidemiology & Community Health, 58*(10), 841-848.

Vyrostek, S. B., Annest, J. L., & Ryan, G. W. (2004). Surveillance for fatal and nonfatal injuries: United States, 2001. *Morbidity and Mortality Weekly Reports Surveillance Summaries, 53*(SS07), 1-57.

Webster, D. W., Vernick, J. S., Zeoli, A. M., & Manganello, J. A. (2004). Association between youth-focused firearm laws and youth suicides. *JAMA: The Journal of American Medical Association, 292,* 594-601.

Nursing Care During Terrorist Events

TERRY FULMER ◆ ROSE P. KNAPP ◆
REBECCA A. TERRANOVA ◆ IAN PORTELLI

Intentional terrorism is an unfortunate reality in today's society. After experiencing the horrors of September 11, 2001, individuals, families, agencies, and communities now are required to conduct their lives more cautiously. In the immediate days after 9/11, the news was dense with stories of heroic firefighters and police officers. Little was said of "the nurse." In fact, most reports were completely silent on the role and contributions of professional nursing. Without fanfare, nurses in the metropolitan area mobilized instinctively and immediately to assist area hospitals and those at Ground Zero after the first news of the attacks. Nurses calmly assumed leadership roles, setting up makeshift triage centers, and provided needed care to victims on the streets and in area gymnasiums, churches, community centers, and of course the hospitals. Many spent the next several days at varied sites putting aside personal fears, concerns, and families in order to meet care demands imposed by such horrifying disregard for human life. For those of us in nursing, none of this is surprising. Nurses, of course, are required to stay and work during disasters, but countless numbers of nurses volunteered to help beyond any requirements. Professional nursing has always been and will continue to be instrumental in meeting the physical and psychological needs for the health of the public.

Clara Barton, Florence Nightingale, the Visiting Nurse Service, Bellevue emergency department—each brings vivid and immediate images to mind. Nurses were not a part of the vivid imagery that followed the terrorist attacks on the World Trade Center towers or the Pentagon, but nurses were there in full force.

The multifaceted professional role of nursing encompasses caregiver, leader, educator, and emotional support system to the public nurses served. Many nurses are active participants in developing terrorism education and safety programs in their local and regional communities. The contributions of the 2.4 million nurses in America during terrorist or disaster events only now are becoming better documented and studied.

Less than 12 hours after the first plane hit the north tower of the World Trade Center, Manhattan was cut off from the rest of the world. No cars or trucks flowed along the city streets. Nearly everything was shut down: stores, theaters, restaurants, and even coffee shops normally open 24 hours a day were closed. "The city that never sleeps" shut down precipitously and slept uneasily that night. It took days for traffic into Manhattan to flow again. Fortunately, the city never lost electricity or water; but what if it had? Before September 11, 2001, few residents of Manhattan would have thought about having extra batteries, water, or ready-to-eat food for 3 days since there are numerous supermarkets, delicatessens, and coffee shops with 24-hour service. What if the delivery of food, produce, and other goods into Manhattan was halted for a week or longer? Today, curricula in health professions schools have to include content of large-scale disaster preparedness and planning.

THE INDIVIDUAL RESPONSE OF NURSES

When disasters occur, nurses respond. That is the way nurses are—ready to use their knowledge and skills to help those in the community (local or global) who are in distress. Whether the disaster is a flood, hurricane, earthquake, fire, chemical spill, train derailment, or airplane crash, nurses are there. Nurses were there on September 11 and at the recent tsunami that devastated Indonesia and its environs, and as a matter of course, they provide assistance to those affected by any tragedy. Even before that day, American nursing leadership had begun to confront the need to prepare for the newest type of disaster, one that results from intentional terrorism. Until the first bombing of the World Trade Center towers and Oklahoma City, the nursing profession had not been familiar with what would constitute post-terrorist care like nurses in other countries, such as Israel and Ireland, have long had to confront. The profession has always anticipated its role in disaster, but not intentional terrorism. Terrorism is certainly different.

Nursing skills are at the ready when persons are bleeding or have stopped breathing, but nurses heretofore have not had to prepare for unexpected intentional infliction of human suffering, when they can fully expect to get harmed in the process. In war zones such as Iraq, the expectation is that others are trying to inflict injury or death. In terrorist events, of course, there are no rules or guidelines for how to prepare and how to react, until now. The Department of Homeland Security has begun to fund a series of Centers of Excellence to research what must be known in terrorist times, and how nurses must be involved in these centers in order to generate the research and prepare best practice protocols for what can happen next.

In New York City on September 11, 2001, a core group of nurses from the city, joined by nurses from the tri-state area and all over the country, played an instrumental role in setting up and staffing makeshift triage centers in the community and at Ground Zero. Initially, some nurses mobilized to area hospitals, while many set up triage units in local gyms, churches, and public buildings. They immediately cared for those fortunate persons who escaped the Twin Towers and others who were in the immediate area of the disaster. The emergent care of these victims included flushing foreign bodies from their eyes, administering nebulizer treatments, showering rancid soot off of the victims, caring for superficial lacerations, and providing extensive emotional support to this group of persons who experienced something that most human beings would never witness in their lifetime. Several nurses went directly to Ground Zero and set up triage centers to care for the potential victims, which became the primary medical station for rescue workers over the next several months during the recovery phase of the disaster.

Several nursing students from the area universities also assisted in the care and support of the victims. They worked alongside experienced nurses, who, despite their own fears about the event, put the needs of the community first and functioned heroically in a chaotic environment. This experience most assuredly will affect all of the future practice of this unique group of nursing students who witnessed nursing at its best.

NURSING DURING TERRORISM AND FAMILIES

Nurses know how to mobilize families in times of crises. Facilitating the development of family disaster plans with family, friends, and in the community is an excellent area for nurses to become involved. Nurses can present basic preparedness information to parent-teacher associations and church groups. The necessary information can be found on the American Red Cross Web site, and nurses can anticipate an entirely new body of knowledge related to disaster preparedness over the next months and years. Nurses who help themselves and others develop a family emergency plan well in advance of a disaster can minimize the "confusion and disorientation" that naturally occur during a disaster (Durham, & Williams, 2002, p. 67) and can provide family members with a sense of control (American Psychiatric Association, 2003). For example, children can be allowed to select a favorite toy and book to put in their "Go-Bag." Developing a plan for a run-through of a disaster drill at home to see what works the best can help develop a sense of mastery and security that can decrease panic in case of an event. Information on how to develop a family emergency plan can be found on numerous Web sites and has been distributed widely in American newspapers over the past 2 years (Table 80-1). Families with school-aged children need to know how to contact school officials to find out about the specific disaster plan of the school and school procedures in advance of any need for implementation. For nurses to help families understand the importance of knowing what plans are in place at the work setting also is important. All nurses need to know procedures in advance in

TABLE 80-1

List of Internet Resources	
Web Site	**URL**
International Nursing Coalition for Mass Casualty Education	http://www.incmce.org/
American Red Cross: Get Prepared	http://www.redcross.org/services/prepare/ 0,1082,0_239_,00.html
Department of Homeland Security	http://www.dhs.gov/dhspublic/theme_home2.jsp
Centers for Disease Control and Prevention: Emergency Preparedness and Response	http://www.bt.cdc.gov/
Center for Health Information Preparedness, NYU School of Medicine	http://chip.med.nyu.edu/

order to anticipate how they will determine whether loved ones are safe or in need. French, Sole, and Fowler-Byers (2002) studied Florida nurses affected by Hurricane Floyd in 1999. Nurses who were working when the storm hit voiced concern for the safety of their families, making it difficult for them to focus on their patient care responsibilities.

NURSES IN EMERGENCY CARE SETTINGS

Emergency departments everywhere usually can expect to be flooded with not only patients but also volunteers during terrorist events. Oklahoma City and 9/11 taught that the public can and will respond and will try to participate in a meaningful role. Thousands of citizens came to hospitals around the city to volunteer after 9/11, only to find there were no roles. Next time, will nurses be prepared to assign meaningful roles that assist the public health infrastructure? This is an important new arena to orchestrate. Nurses are the majority of personnel in any hospital, and when hospitals suddenly are flooded with volunteers, we believe that nursing can help organize the public into important teams such as communications groups, facilitators for the walking wounded, and assistants to aid health care personnel. True, credentialing issues need to be worked out, but that seems trivial in light of the opportunities for using the passion and the energy of the public in terrorist times. We believe nursing schools have important roles to play in delineating these plans and that nursing faculty have an important leadership role to play. Nurses cannot be invisible or silent.

In the months that followed September 11, 2001, the emergency department in central New Jersey treated dozens of postal workers from area district post offices who handled mail that possibly was exposed to anthrax. Nurse practitioners in urgent care units of the emergency department were responsible for providing primary care to these postal workers. Initially, they were directed from the New Jersey State Health Department to obtain nasal smears for anthrax and then to treat the postal workers with ciprofloxacin (Cipro) or doxycycline. After a few days, another directive informed the nurses to obtain nasal smears only and not treat the postal workers with ciprofloxacin or doxycycline. This particular group of postal workers worked side by side with the other group and discussed the different medical approaches they received in the emergency department. Needless to say, care that was delivered during this period was confusing, and it appeared to the patients that there was uncertainty in the practice protocols.

The public will understand and tolerate a certain amount of uncertainty, but not for long. All nurses need to become educated in issues of terrorism and bioterrorism for the future. Nurses cannot be inconsistent in their treatment of potentially lethal exposures, causing undue anxiety in the public that is already anxious about exposure to toxins.

As a result of the anthrax episode, it has become imperative that regulatory agencies such as the Centers for Disease Control and Prevention and individual state departments of health develop consistent plans of care for any biochemical exposure. Nurses must avail themselves of education, training, and resources to ensure that they are knowledgeable about the most current and appropriate care protocols.

During 9/11, disaster-preparedness plans were put into effect. However, the enormity of the event coupled with the number of fatalities defined the need for a reevaluation of current disaster plans, which must include a catastrophic disaster plan for another potential terrorist attack of the magnitude of 9/11. Traditionally, disaster plans and triage are implemented to maximize the number of survivors, determine severity quickly and accurately, and prioritize care and support. Emergency department nurses are educated as triage officers who categorize and tag patients for treatment based on strict criteria ranging from critical injuries requiring immediate intervention to the deceased/near death victims whose treatment would be incompatible with life. This system is used universally in most institutions during any mass casualty incident. However, when a catastrophic event such as on September 11, 2001, occurs, other measures must be instituted, such as providing alternative sites for triage and medical care, providing emotional support to a population that witnessed and experienced the catastrophic event, and most importantly education of health care professionals and members of the community about what their roles would be if such a horrific event would repeat itself. We believe that universities can and should anticipate their roles in providing safe shelter and health assistance during terrorist events. For example, every university professor, administrator, and student should be surveyed to determine what, if any role, that person might play in a terrorist attack. Of course, no one can say with certainty if they actually will play that role in the actual situation, but cataloging the possible roles university members might play during a disaster not only assists the public health infrastructure but also provides meaningful roles and potentially can prevent the swamping of health care facilities that took place during 9/11.

TERRORISM, NURSES, AND THE COMMUNITY

After the initial shock and devastating impact of the morning events, many nurses on the evening of September 11 went to the area emergency departments to await the victims. They waited for many hours into the early morning outside the emergency departments and finally were notified that tragically no victims were found. They were asked to be available to help the next day if needed. The nurses were not needed in the emergency departments the next day because of the large number of fatalities. Taking preparedness to the community level can begin within the neighborhood. As members of one of the most trusted professions in the United States, nurses are in the position to disseminate accurate preparedness information to those who live closest to them. Nurses are also in a position to identify persons at risk (the frail elderly and adults or children with special needs) and to assist them to develop an emergency plan. Who are the retired health care practitioners in the neighborhood? They are a valuable resource that can be enlisted in a disaster response and recovery. Churches, synagogues, mosques, senior citizen centers, parent-teacher associations, and community boards are forums in which nurses could provide disaster-preparedness education to the community. Nurses have always brought energy and creativity to whatever they do. Preparing themselves, their families, and their communities for a bioterrorism attack is a viable area for nurses to take the lead.

Municipalities must support this education by providing supplemental funds for such programs. In August 2004, the Agency for Healthcare Research and Quality released a position statement stating that during a widespread terrorist attack that area hospitals would be overwhelmed by patients and that alternate care sites such as stadiums, schools, and recreation centers would be required to handle the overflow of victims. This plan also would necessitate community education so that the lay public who work in these facilities would be able to assist nurses and other health care providers in delivery of appropriate and timely care to any victims of a terrorist attack. Adequate funding to high-risk municipalities for preparedness and response-related activities is essential but remains a problem. New York City, for example, is twenty-ninth out of 54 municipalities in funding per capita in 2004 for bioterrorism according to data from the Health Resources and Services Administration and Centers for Disease Control (Sweeney, 2004). One can conclude that for municipalities to educate its nurses, health care providers, and community, increased funding must be made available to provide these much-needed bioterrorism programs.

THE PSYCHOLOGICAL RESPONSE TO TERRORISM

On September 11, 2001, Americans lost their sense of national security. All Americans were affected in some way by the events of 9/11. Several studies looked at the effects of 9/11 from the mental health and general health perspectives at the local, national, and global levels (Galea et al., 2002; Herman, Felton, & Susser, 2002; Ho, Paultre, & Mosca, 2002; Silver, Holman, McIntosh, Poulin, & Gil-Rivas, 2002; Vlahov, et al., 2002). Although preliminary findings indicate substantial anxiety related to future acts of terrorism and lifestyle changes resulting from increased levels of stress that potentially could lead to increased risk of cardiac events, Silver et al. (2002) noted that "active coping in the immediate aftermath of the attacks was the only strategy that appeared to be protective against on-going distress" (p. 1243). They describe active coping as planning or seeking support. Silver et al. also point out that "potentially disturbing levels of trauma-related symptoms can be present even in individuals who are not directly exposed to a trauma, particularly when the trauma is a massive national tragedy such as the September 11 attacks." The prevalence of symptoms in a "substantial proportion of individuals may...represent a normal response to an abnormal event" (p. 1243). According to the National Center for Post-Traumatic Stress Disorder (2003), one of the most common observations seen after all disasters is *resilience*. An individual is considered resilient if after having faced adversity, he or she has a "sense of mastery or effective coping" (Kulig, 2000, p. 378). Critical attributes identified by Kulig include "rebounding and carrying on, having a sense of self and determination, and being prosocial" (p. 378). Resilience also can be described as positive growth in the face of adversity. Communities can be resilient as well. Kulig defines community resilience as "the ability of a community to not only respond to adversity but in doing so, reach a higher level of functioning (p. 375). Being prepared for a disaster, whether naturally occurring or an act of terrorism, can be empowering for the individual and the community. Preparedness can be an act of healing. Falk (2001, p. 4) describes public health nurses conceptualization of empowerment "as an active, internal process of growth that was rooted in one's own cultural/religious/personal belief systems, reached toward actualizing one's full potential, and occurred within the context of a nurturing nurse-client relationship." According to the American Psychiatric Association (2003), participating in volunteer activities can be empowering and can help individuals develop resilience.

PREPARING FOR TERRORISM: WHAT NURSES CAN DO

Nurses focus on safety as the most basic of physiological needs. For nurses effectively to reassure and inform the community and foster a safe environment, they must be competent and knowledgeable to function during a mass casualty disaster in which significant numbers of lives are lost and the usual community resources are ineffective to manage the response. With increased awareness of this need, several resources are currently available for nursing education on common biological and chemical warfare and terrorism.

Americans now live in a state of heightened security, checking to see whether the threat level is at yellow, orange, or red and not knowing whether the next event will be biological, chemical, or nuclear. What is clear is that the increasing certainty of future terrorist acts against the United States requires that nurses be ready to continue to serve at the forefront of disaster preparedness, response, and recovery whatever their area of practice. Every nurse has the responsibility to be aware of these threats and to become educated to intervene appropriately in the event of a mass casualty incident.

In March 2001 the International Nursing Coalition for Mass Casualty Education met to create a resource focused on educating "nurses to provide emergency care during bioterrorism-related mass casualty events" (American Association of Colleges of Nursing, 2001). Courses have been established for nurses. The University of Texas at Austin School of Nursing has developed a Mass Casualty Disaster Nursing Course. This course includes the active participation by the students in disaster planning and teaching community disaster education classes, and the students become resources for their workplace to meet Joint Commission on Accreditation of Healthcare Organizations requirements for emergency planning in their individual institutions. Another resource is the U.S. Army Medical Research Institute of Chemical Defense, which offers classroom and satellite broadcasts on biological and chemical warfare and terrorism. The course focuses on pathophysiology and on diagnosis and treatment of casualties of chemical and biological weapons. The course includes emergency treatment, triage, decontamination, and evacuation of casualties. Another example is the Vanderbilt University School of Nursing program that has developed DVDs and online courses that are available to help teach appropriate curricula for the future. Courses such as these should be standard curriculum in undergraduate and graduate nursing programs, and health care institutions also should require mandatory training for current and future nursing staff.

Disasters occur every day. Nurses always serve their communities in times of disaster through employment or volunteer activities with the American Red Cross as members of the Disaster Health Service or Disaster Response Teams. The American Red Cross provides excellent training on all aspects of disasters (logistics, mass care, sheltering, and damage assessment) that is useful for nurses.

The federal government has established the Medical Reserve Corp. for all health care providers who will be called upon to participate in mass immunization programs in the event of a biological disaster. Disaster Medical Assistance Teams operate under the auspices of the National Medical Disaster System, a branch of the Department of Homeland Security. Regional Disaster Medical Assistance Teams are located in many parts of the country and are activated for national disasters. Teams were sent to New York following 9/11. The National Medical Disaster System Web site is http://www.ndms.dhhs.gov/.

SUMMARY

No one could have imagined the devastation that was inflicted intentionally on 9/11. Americans will never get over the fact that fellow human beings planned and carried out actions that murdered innocent victims. Americans can take comfort in the way the nursing profession responded and the way the community responded to the needs of others. Our purpose is to help set a new level of expectation and baseline for the profession related to terrorism sequelae and disaster care. As demonstrated by the nursing care after 9/11, nurses united and mobilized as a profession, despite their own fears and anxieties, into unchartered territory to ensure the well-being of others by becoming advocates for the community. It would be unrealistic to think that this horrific event could not be repeated. As nurses plan their vision for the future, nurses and nursing students must be educated properly in terrorism and bioterrorism to ensure that they can be even more effective in another catastrophic event.

REFERENCES

Agency for Healthcare Research and Quality. (2004). New tool helps state and local officials locate alternate health care sites during a potential bioterrorism emergency. Press Release, July 27, 2004. Retrieved August 23, 2004 from http://www.ahrq.gov/news/press/pr2004/altsitespr.htm

American Association of Colleges of Nursing. (2001). *American Association of Colleges of Nursing leads efforts to further the education of nurses to combat bioterrorism.* Retrieved October 20, 2004, from http://www.aacn.nche.edu/Media/NewsReleases/bioterrorism.htm

American Psychiatric Association. (2003). *Coping with anxiety during high risk terrorist alerts: Advise from the American Psychiatric Association.* Retrieved October 13, 2004, from http://www.psych.org/news_room/press_releases/coping withanxietyduringhighalerts021203.pdf

Durham, B., & Williams, J. (2002). Civilian preparedness: Disaster planning for everyone. *Topics in Emergency Medicine, 24*(3), 66-70.

Falk, R. (2001). Empowerment as a process of evolving consciousness: A model of empowered caring. *Advances in Nursing Science, 24*(1), 1-16.

French, E. D., Sole, M. L., Fowler-Byers, J. (2002). A comparison of nurses' needs/concerns and hospital disaster plans following Florida's Hurricane Floyd. *Journal of Emergency Nursing, 28*(2), 111-117.

Galea, S., Ahern, J., Resnick, H., Kilpatrick, D., Bucavalas, M., Gold, J., et al. (2002). Psychological sequela of the September 11 terrorist attacks in New York City. *New England Journal of Medicine, 346*(13), 982-987.

Herman, D., Felton, C., & Susser, E. (2002). Mental health needs in New York State following the September 11th attacks. *Journal of Urban Health: Bulletin of the New York Academy of Medicine, 79*(3), 322-331.

Ho, J., Paultre, F., & Mosca, L. (2002). Lifestyle changes in New Yorkers after September 11, 2001 (Data from the Post-Disaster Heart Attack Prevention Program). *American Journal of Cardiology, 90,* 680-682.

Kulig, J. (2000). Community resiliency: The potential for community health nursing theory development. *Public Health Nursing, 17*(5), 374-384.

National Center for Post-Traumatic Stress Disorder. (2003, September). *Effects of traumatic stress in a disaster situation.* Retrieved October 12, 2004, from http://www.ncptsd.va.gov/facts/disasters/fs_effects_disaster.html

Silver, R. C., Holman, E. A., McIntosch, D. N., Poulin, M., & Gil-Rivas, V. (2002). Nationwide longitudinal study of psychological response to September 11. *JAMA: The Journal of the American Medical Association, 288*(10), 1235-1239.

Sweeney, J. (2004). Talking Points. Handout from Homeland Security/Bioterrorism Meeting. August, 2004. Albany, NY.

Vlahov, D., Galea, S., Resnick, H., Ahern, J., Boscarino, J., Bucavalas, M., Gold, J., & Kilpatrick, D. (2002). Increased use of cigarettes, alcohol, and marijuana among Manhattan, New York, residents after the September 11th terrorist attacks. *American Journal of Epidemiology, 155*(11), 988-996.

SUGGESTED READINGS

American Nurses Association. (2004a). *ANA activities: Bioterrorism and Disaster Response.* Retrieved October 20, 2004, from http://www.nursingworld.org/news/disaster/

American Nurses Association. (2004b). *National nurses response team: Volunteer opportunities for registered nurses.* Retrieved October 20, 2004, from http://www.nursingworld.org/news/disaster/response.htm

American Psychiatric Association. (2001a). *Coping with a national tragedy.* Retrieved October 14, 2004, from http://www.psych.org/news_room/media_advisories/copingdisaster92001.cfm

American Psychiatric Association. (2001b). *Stress management for health care providers.* Retrieved October 14, 2004, from http://www.psych.org/disasterpsych/links/stressmgmthealth.cfm

American Psychiatric Association. (2001c). *When disaster strikes.* Retrieved October 14, 2004, from http://healthyminds.org/whendisasterstrikes.cfm

American Psychological Association. (2004). *Resilience in a time of war.* Retrieved October 12, 2004, from http://www.apahelpcenter.org/dl/resilience_in_a_time_of_war.pdf

Bleich, A., Gelkopf, M., & Solomon, Z. (2003). Exposure to terrorism, stress-related mental health symptoms, and coping behaviors among a nationally representative sample in Israel. *JAMA: The Journal of the American Medical Association, 290*(5), 612-620.

Centers for Disease Control and Prevention. (2002). Community needs assessment of lower Manhattan residents following the World Trade Center attacks—Manhattan, New York City, 2001. *Mobidity and Mortality Weekly Report, 51,* 10-13.

Chaffee, M., Conway-Welch, C., & Sabatier, K. (2001, July-August). *Nursing leaders plan to educate nurses about response to mass casualty events.* Retrieved October 20, 2004, from http://www.nursingworld.org/tan/01julaug/casualty.htm

Cox, E., & Briggs, S. (2004). Disaster nursing: New frontiers for critical care. *Critical Care Nurse, 224*(3), 16-22.

Dickerson, S. S., Jezewski, M. A., Nelson-Tuttle, C., Shipkey, N., Wilk, N., & Crandall, B. (2002). Nursing at Ground Zero: Experiences during and after September 11, World Trade Center attack. *Journal of the New York State Nurses Association, 33*(1), 26-32.

Eastwood, G. L. (2003). Academic health centers and the war on terrorism. *Journal of Public Health Management Practice, 9*(5), 433-436.

Ellis-Stoll, C., & Popkess-Vawter, S. (1998). A concept analysis on the process of empowerment. *Advances in Nursing Science, 21*(3), 62-68.

Gaffke, B. (2002). The nursing profession and disaster preparedness. *Chart, 99*(5), 9.

Herman, J. (1998). Recovery from psychological trauma. *Psychiatry and Clinical Neurosciences, 52*(S5), S145.

Ihlenfeld, J. T. (2003). A primer on triage and mass casualty events. *Dimensions of Critical Care Nursing, 22*(5), 204-207.

Johnston-Roberts, K. (1999). Patient empowerment in the United States: A critical commentary. *Health Expectations, 2,* 82-92.

Kiesz, K. (2002). Response to bioterrorism/emergency preparedness. *Washington Nurse, 32*(4), 44-45.

Kuokkanen, L., & Leino-Kilpi, H. (2000). Power and empowerment in nursing: Three theoretical approaches. *Journal of Advanced Nursing, 31*(1), 235.

Lambert, C. E., Jr., & Lambert, V. A. (1999). Psychological hardiness: State of the science. *Holistic Nursing Practice, 13*(3), 11-19.

Langan, J. C., & James, D. C. (2005). *Prepared nurses for disaster management.* Upper Saddle River: Pearson Prentice-Hall.

Low, J. A. (1999). The concept of hardiness: Persistent problems, persistent appeal. *Holistic Nursing Practice, 13*(3), 20-24.

Magai, C., Consedine, N. S., King, A. R., & Gillespie, M. (2003). Physical hardiness and styles of socioemotional functioning in later life. *Journal of Gerontology, 58B*(5), 269-279.

National Center for Post-Traumatic Stress Disorder. (2003). *Self-care and self-help following disasters.* Retrieved October 12, 2004, from http://www.ncptsd.va.gov/facts/disasters/fs_self_care_disaster.html

Nyatanga, L., & Dann, K. L. (2002). Empowerment in nursing: The role of philosophical and psychological factors. *Nursing Philosophy, 3,* 234-239.

Persily, C. A., & Hildebrandt, E. (2003). The theory of community empowerment. In M. J. Smith & P. R. Liehr (Eds.), *Middle range theory for nursing.* New York: Springer.

Pollack, S. E. (1999). Health-related hardiness with different ethnic populations. *Holistic Nursing Practice, 13*(3), 1-10.

Ryles, S. M. (1999). A concept analysis of empowerment: Its relationship to mental health nursing. *Journal of Advanced Nursing, 29*(3), 600-607.

Urbano, M. T. (2002). *American Nurse.: Nursing coalition for mass casualty education steps up initiatives.* Retrieved October 20, 2004 from http://www.nursingworld.org/tan/janfeb02/masscas.htm

Urbano, M. T. (2003). What can nurses do to prepare for terrorist acts? *ISNA Bulletin, 29*(1), 1, 3-4.

Vasquez-Brooks, M. (2003). Health-related hardiness and chronic illness: A synthesis of current research. *Nursing Forum, 38*(3), 11-20.

Veenema, T. G. (2003). *Disaster nursing and emergency preparedness for chemical, biological and radiological terrorism and other hazards.* New York: Springer.

Weiner, B., Irwin, M., Trangenstein, T., & Gordon, J. (2004). *Emergency preparedness curriculum in US nursing schools.* Retrieved October 13, 2004, from International Nursing Coalition for Mass Casualty Education Web site: http://www.incmce.org/surveypage.html

CHAPTER

81

Nursing Practice in Homeland Security

MARY W. CHAFFEE ◆ ROBERTA P. LAVIN ◆ LYNN A. SLEPSKI*

INTRODUCTION TO HOMELAND SECURITY

Before 2001 few individuals had heard of "homeland security." Since then, homeland security has emerged as a critical national issue. Homeland security has exploded as a growth industry in many sectors, including intelligence, physical security, and health care. To explore nursing practice in homeland security, it is important to define homeland security and to understand the role of the health care system in homeland security.

Homeland security has existed in the United States for a long time, but it was not always referred to by that name. In the 1950s, homeland security was "civil defense." For baby boomers, that should bring to mind the "duck and cover" song and fallout shelter drills. A series of natural disasters in the 1960s and 1970s led to the establishment of a federal agency (the Federal Emergency Management Agency) in 1979 to take the lead on coordinating the response to major disasters.

IMPACT OF 9/11

Most citizens of the United States had a sense of security before the terror attacks of September 11, 2001. The nation was surrounded by two oceans and two friendly neighbors. We had survived the Cold War without a single missile being lobbed. Terror attacks occurred regularly in distant places such as Israel and Ireland, but they were far away and usually did not involve Americans. Then the writing on the wall

became clearer. Attacks occurred on U.S. military personnel in a housing unit, the Khobar Towers, in Saudi Arabia. Two U.S. embassies were bombed in Africa. In 1993 the World Trade Center was bombed, and that faded quickly from memory. While the United States was debating whether O.J. was guilty and was learning the Macarena, hatred for the American way of life was brewing in the Mideast. The American sense of safety and complacency evaporated when four airliners were hijacked by Islamic terrorists and were used as high-yield explosives.

WHAT IS HOMELAND SECURITY?

Following the terror attacks on the United States, the term *homeland security* spilled into American discussions. But what exactly is it? In broad terms, homeland security is all activities undertaken to do the following:

◆ Prevent harm to American citizens and property
◆ Defend the nation against attack
◆ Prepare to respond to events that cause damage and casualties
◆ Recover from any attack, disaster, or event that causes large numbers of casualties

Homeland Security or Homeland Defense?

The federal government defined homeland security initially as "A concerted national effort to prevent terrorist attacks within the U.S., reduce America's vulnerability to terrorism, and minimize the damage and recover from attacks that do occur" (Office of Homeland Security, 2002). The term *homeland defense* is broader than *homeland security;* it includes all traditional military activities. The Department of Defense defines *homeland defense* as "the protection of U.S. sovereignty, territory, domestic population and critical defense infrastructure against external threats and aggression" (Tomisek, 2002). Because many military

*The views expressed in this chapter are those of the authors and do not necessarily reflect the official policy or position of the Department of the Navy, the Department of Defense, the Department of Homeland Security, the Department of Health and Human Services, the Uniformed Services University of the Health Sciences, or the U.S. government. No funding support was received from these entities.

homeland security activities are coordinated with civilian emergency preparedness and because a strong health care system (military, federal, and civilian) is essential to national security, the term *homeland security* is an umbrella covering many activities.

Homeland security activities are a linked system of diverse entities that work together to protect U.S. citizens. The system includes emergency management, emergency medical services, disaster preparedness, public health, infection control and surveillance, and many others. Woven together, these activities form a tapestry that protects the nation.

ROLE OF THE HEALTH SYSTEM IN NATIONAL SECURITY

The reader may be thinking now, "Isn't homeland security the responsibility of the military services and intelligence agencies?" Yes, intelligence agencies have a specific role in gathering intelligence about threats. The Department of Defense uses military power to protect and defend the nation. However, many other critical threads exist in the homeland security tapestry, and the health care system is a vital one.

A Very Dark Winter

A revelation occurred in the United States in 2001. It became clear that the U.S. health care system, including the health care workforce, was an integral part of national security. Here is an example. An exercise named Dark Winter was conducted to determine how an outbreak of smallpox would affect the United States. As the exercise unfolded, a few cases of smallpox spread to 25 states in 13 days, overwhelming hospitals, local government resources, and the economy and ultimately threatening the stability of the federal government (ANSER Institute for Homeland Security, 2002). This exercise demonstrated how a health care crisis will have powerful and far-reaching impact. Because of exercises such as Dark Winter and actual events, a strong, well-prepared, and resilient health care system was recognized as being critical to national security.

WHAT IS THE ROLE OF NURSING IN HOMELAND SECURITY?

Nursing Practice in Homeland Security: A Historical Perspective

Nurses have understood the importance of civic responsibility since the time of Florence Nightingale's efforts during the Crimean War. Indeed by her definition, "a nurse means any person in charge of the personal health of another" (Nightingale, 1969, p. 139). During a time of crisis, nurses commonly provide care to their neighbors, their community, and their nation, but nurses need to do more than just provide direct patient care. Being in charge of the personal health of a person includes working at the community or at the national level to ensure that appropriate policy and planning is in place to provide an effective, systematic approach to care during a disaster.

Nurses have played a significant role in civil defense since World War II. The importance and scope of that role has intensified over time with the changing international political situation, especially with the growing need for preparation for disaster or an act of terrorism. Many of the responsibilities nurses took on during the 1950s and 1960s are needed today. Additionally, a greater need exists for nurses to take an active role in community leadership focused on preparation for disaster response.

In the 1950s, nurses were trained to respond to nuclear attack. Eight hours of training was considered a significant investment by health care agencies, but nurses who were trained then were able to go into communities and answer the questions of their neighbors about not only nursing care issues but also other important issues such as emergency supplies that each family should have (Mills, 1951). The nurse was a vital community link in peacetime preparation and a factor in relieving the burden on hospitals during a war. Indeed, the qualities of a nurse that make her or him vital to civil defense today are best said in the words of the National Organization for Public Health Nursing (1951): "communities … may need special emergency control measures requiring public health nursing service, skill, and organizational ability" (p. 70). Then as now, one of the greatest contributions of nursing to emergency preparedness is the ability to organize. Nurses are taking leadership roles in planning for mass casualties, strengthening the workforce, and identifying the research agenda.

Nursing Roles in Homeland Security

Nurses participate in homeland security activities in a variety of ways at many levels; some are obvious, others are less so. Every nursing activity that contributes to emergency preparedness and effective response supports homeland security (Table 81-1). The following are some examples of how nurses have become involved in homeland security:

◆ A doctorally prepared nurse leads bioterrorism research efforts at the Agency for Health Care Quality and Research in Rockville, Maryland.

TABLE 81-1

Examples of Nursing Activities in Homeland Security

	Homeland Security Goals		
	Prepare for Emergency Response	**Prevent Harm**	**Respond to Emergencies**
Examples of nursing activities	Know own response role.	Keep immunizations up to date and participate in immunization programs.	Obtain training to respond effectively in emergencies.
	Have family preparedness plans in place to permit emergency response.	Learn to recognize threatening infectious diseases.	Maintain clinical skills for emergency response.
	Volunteer for a community or national response team.	Use self-protection measures.	Exercise regularly to fine-tune plans

♦ A Navy nurse serves on the Chemical Biological Incident Response Force of the U.S. Marine Corps, based in Indian Head, Maryland.

♦ Nurses around the United States volunteer to serve on national disaster medical response teams that are activated to respond to major disasters.

♦ Three Navy nurses serve as the emergency management officers of hospitals.

♦ The first director of the Department of Health and Human Services Secretary's Operations Center was a nurse.

♦ A nurse in Washington, D.C., volunteers with the American Red Cross as an instructor in the Masters of Disaster education program for children and adolescents.

♦ A nurse serves as the editor of the journal *Disaster Management & Response*.

♦ An emergency nurse serves as a homeland security policy analyst in Washington, D.C.

♦ A nurse has served as the director of emergency preparedness activities in the New York region of the Veterans Administration health care system.

NURSING PRACTICE IN HOMELAND SECURITY AT THE INDIVIDUAL LEVEL

The role of the nurse in disaster preparedness starts with the same responsibilities as with every other citizen. Every nurse should do the following:

♦ Keep first aid and basic life support credentials updated.

♦ Have a disaster kit.

♦ Know how to shelter-in-place.

♦ Have a family disaster plan.

♦ Prepare one's own family to care for themselves or be cared for without the nurse in the family present.

♦ Identify what the nurse's role will be during an emergency and discuss that plan with family members.

For the professional nurse, preparedness requires basic competencies. Dr. Kristine Gebbie developed core competencies for the public health workforce that has value for nurses. The core competencies include the ability to do the following (Center for Health Policy, 2001):

1. Describe the public health role in emergency response in a range of emergencies that might arise.

2. Describe the chain of command in emergency response.

3. Identify and locate the agency emergency response plan (or the pertinent portion of the plan).

4. Describe the nurse's functional role(s) in emergency response or demonstrate the role(s) in regular drills.

5. Demonstrate correct use of all communication equipment used for emergency communication (e.g., telephone, fax, and radio).

6. Describe communication role(s) in emergency response: within agency, media, general public, and personal (family, neighbors).

7. Identify limits to one's own knowledge/skill/authority, and identify key systems resources for referring matters that exceed those limits.

8. Apply creative problem solving and flexible thinking to unusual challenges within the nurse's functional responsibilities and evaluate effectiveness of all actions taken.

9. Recognize deviation from the norm that might indicate an emergency and describe appropriate action (e.g., communicate clearly within the chain of command).

NURSING PRACTICE IN HOMELAND SECURITY AT THE ORGANIZATIONAL LEVEL

Nurses who work in hospitals, clinics, schools, public health departments, and other organizations have important roles in homeland security. Regardless of the workplace, every nurse should do the following:

◆ Know the emergency response or disaster preparedness plan of the organization.
◆ Know the nurse's role in responding to disaster.
◆ Take advantage of all training opportunities to improve effectiveness of response in a disaster.
◆ Actively participate in all disaster response drills and encourage others to take them seriously.
◆ Know what the organizational plan is to increase patient care capacity in a disaster (i.e., how do you put an extra 50 trauma patients on a full 24-bed surgical ward?).
◆ In hospitals and clinics, nurses should be familiar with the Joint Commission on Accreditation of Healthcare Organization standards for emergency management.

During every major disaster, nurses have decided whether to report to work, volunteer, evacuate, or stay home to care for their families. Consider the hurricanes that hit Florida in 2004. Some nurses were fired for failure to report to duty during the storms. Planning in advance, knowing the policy of the organization where employed, and discussing the plan with a supervisor must occur before an incident.

NURSING PROFESSIONAL ASSOCIATIONS AND HOMELAND SECURITY

Many professional nursing associations have launched efforts to prepare their members to participate in emergency preparedness and response activities. The American Nurses Association and the U.S. Public Health Service launched a partnership to establish "National Nurses Response Teams." These teams are being prepared to conduct mass chemoprophylaxis (large-scale administration of medication) and mass immunization. These activities may be needed in the event of natural disease epidemic or a bioterror attack. Few communities have an adequate number of nurses to provide medication or vaccines to thousands or millions of citizens.

The International Association of Forensic Nurses (2001) passed a resolution calling for worldwide support of nursing education that includes mass disaster preparedness. The International Council of Nurses (2001) issued a position statement describing the need to increase the ability of the nursing profession "to provide adequate health services before and after a disaster occurs by their participation in prevention, mitigation, preparedness and relief operations."

NURSING PRACTICE IN HOMELAND SECURITY AT THE STATE AND FEDERAL LEVELS

Many states now have volunteer registries of nurses who are willing and prepared to respond during a disaster. One of these is the Medical Reserve Corps. Corps volunteers serve the needs of their local communities in activities such as screenings and immunizations. At the national level, nurses may join the National Nurse Response Team or a Disaster Medical Assistance Team (DMAT). These teams train together to respond to disaster on a local and national level. National Nurse Response Team and DMAT nurses are paid a salary, travel expenses, and per diem by the federal government and are covered by federal regulations while provided care during a period of activation, so licensure restrictions are not a problem. Riley (2003) describes the purpose, structure of service, process of becoming a DMAT member, and her own experience in serving on a DMAT team mobilized to New York City on September 11, 2001. Volunteer opportunities exist with the American Red Cross. The American Red Cross is one of the largest disaster relief agencies with more than 40,000 nurse volunteers.

U.S. Department of Homeland Security

The U.S. Congress established the U.S. Department of Homeland Security to help America prepare for, respond to, and recover from potential terrorist attacks, including those involving weapons of mass destruction. More than 22 distinct agencies and more than 170,000 personnel were reorganized into one department with the mission to protect the American homeland.

Homeland security is a shared responsibility, requiring coordination of federal, state, local, and private sector strategies. To that end, the Department of Homeland Security has embarked on a number of initiatives aimed at improving emergency response. Two major initiatives nurses should be aware of are the National Response Plan and the National Incident Management System.

The National Response Plan provides a single, comprehensive, all-hazards approach resulting in a coordinated and effective response, regardless of the cause, size, or nature of the event (Department of Homeland Security, 2004b). The National Response Plan can be implemented partially or fully based on a threat, in anticipation of a significant event, or in response to an Incident of National Significance, defined as a high-impact event that requires a coordinated and effective response by federal, state, local, and tribal private sector and nongovernmental partners in order to save lives, minimize damage, and provide for long-term community recovery. The plan incorporates best practices and procedures from incident management disciplines—homeland security, emergency management, law enforcement, firefighting, public works, public health, responder and recovery worker health and safety, emergency medical services, and the private sector—and integrates them into a unified structure. The plan forms the basis of how the federal government coordinates with state, local, and tribal governments and the private sector during incidents. The National Response Plan establishes protocols to help protect the nation from terrorist attacks and other natural and manufactured hazards; save lives; protect public health, safety, property, and the environment; and reduce adverse psychological consequences and disruptions to the American way of life.

In 2003, President George W. Bush issued a directive ordering the development of the National Incident Management System (White House, 2003). The system provides a consistent nationwide template to enable all government, private sector, and nongovernmental organizations to work together. The system establishes standards that reach across all levels of government and all emergency response agencies (Department of Homeland Security, 2003).

Nurses work in a variety of leadership roles within Department of Homeland Security. In the Federal Emergency Management Agency, nurses conduct credentialing, manage disaster teams and programs, and function as emergency coordinators. In the U.S. Coast Guard, nurses provide health care and direct programs such as quality assurance and health promotion. Department of Homeland Security nurses conduct training and exercises and function as subject matter experts in a variety of terrorism areas. Many contribute to developing national policy and serve on national-level groups such as the Interagency Incident Management Group. The group is a federal headquarters-level, multiagency coordination body that facilitates

federal domestic incident management for Incidents of National Significance. The Interagency Incident Management Group provides coordination for federal operations and resources, establishes reporting requirements, and conducts ongoing communications with its partners to maintain situational awareness, analyze threats, assess national implications of threat, conduct operational response activities, and coordinate actual or potential incidents (Box 81-1).

U.S. Department of Health and Human Services

The U.S. Department of Health and Human Services is responsible for coordinating public health and medical response in major disasters. The Department is responsible for "coordinated Federal assistance to supplement State, local, and tribal resources in response to public health and medical care needs (to include veterinary and/or animal health issues when appropriate) for

---

BOX 81-1

Captain Lynn Slepski's Journey to Homeland Security

Captain Lynn Slepski, U.S. Public Health Service, serves as the Principal Science and Technology Advisor to the Integration Staff and the Science and Technology Operations Integration Director in the U.S. Department of Homeland Security. Captain Slepski has worked in numerous nursing specialties, including critical care, emergency, and preventive medicine and is a certified clinical nurse specialist in community health and a health promotion director. Since 1995, much of her nursing practice has centered on emergency response and emergency operations at the national level, where she has functioned as a Response Coordinator for the Commissioned Corps Readiness Force in the U.S. Department of Health and Human Services Office of Emergency Preparedness and as a counterterrorism expert in the Food and Drug Administration. She is a deployable member of the Public Health Service and the PHS-1 Disaster Medical Assistance Team and has led numerous deployments, including the response to the first anthrax attack on Capitol Hill. Captain Slepski points to her combat experience while an intensive care unit nurse manager during OPERATION DESERT SHIELD/DESERT STORM, extensive training, and multiple deployments with the Public Health Service Commissioned Corps Readiness Force as factors preparing her for her current role.

potential or actual Incidents of National Significance and/or during a developing potential health and medical situation" (Department of Homeland Security, 2004a). These activities are defined in Emergency Support Function 8, a part of the U.S. National Response Plan. Emergency Support Function 8 has five functional areas: assessment, surveillance, medical personnel, medical equipment and supplies, and coordination of federal health and medical assistance (Box 81-2).

The U.S. Public Health Service plays a significant role in homeland security by providing surge capacity for the nation's response to mass casualty incidents. Public Health Service commissioned corps officers can be deployed rapidly to areas of greatest need. The nurse category, the largest category of Public Health Service officers workforce, is the most frequently requested asset. They usually respond in coordination with existing local resources to the site of the incident and work closely with nurses from the American Red Cross.

The Department of Health and Human Services is also responsible for the health care and public health sector critical infrastructure protection coordination. This responsibility includes working closely with medical material, occupational health, and health care professionals. Two of the organizations with which

the department has worked are the International Nursing Coalition for Mass Casualty Education and the Association of State and Territorial Directors of Nursing. Through these efforts, nurses are working on methods to coordinate nursing communication better during crises and to improve sharing of critical homeland security information.

U.S. Department of Defense

The U.S. Department of Defense is one of three partners in the National Disaster Medical System. The system is the national health care safety net in the event of a major disaster with casualties that overwhelm a specific location. In the event of a major catastrophe in the United States, the Department of Defense, the U.S. Veterans Administration health care system, and the Department of Health and Human Services work together to provide hospital beds and health care for victims of disaster. Nurses in the Department of Defense are trained for deployment to the combat theater, and many nurses receive additional trauma training. All health care providers in the Department of Defense now are required to complete training in response to chemical, biological, radiological, nuclear, and explosives events. In the event Department of Defense personnel are called upon to support other U.S. agencies in responding to a disaster in the United States, Department of Defense nurses will be valuable in supplementing civilian resources (Box 81-3).

Department of Defense nurses have responded to many emergencies and are a part of many national emergency preparedness efforts. The U.S. Navy deployed its 1000-bed hospital ship, USNSCOMFORT, to New York City following the terror attacks of 2001. Navy nurses served aboard ship, providing care and respite to disaster responders. Responders from all the military services cared for victims of the attack on the Pentagon. Department of Defense personnel stand by to provide emergency response during events of national importance in the Washington, D.C., area. Military nurses travel with the President and Vice President to ensure immediate emergency care is available at all times—a vital step in providing for the continuity of government. Department of Defense personnel, with other federal personnel, mounted an extensive response to the anthrax contamination of Capitol Hill in 2001.

The Air Force Medical Services have several self-contained emergency care systems including the Expeditionary Medical Support and the Air Force Theatre Hospital. The Expeditionary Medical Support was deployed to Houston, Texas, following massive

---

BOX 81-2

Captain Roberta Lavin's Journey to Homeland Security

Captain Roberta Lavin is a U.S. Public Health Service nurse officer who serves as the Chief Policy Officer for the Assistant Secretary for Public Health Emergency Preparedness in the Office of the Secretary, Department of Health and Human Services. She was detailed to the Department of Health and Human Services Secretary's Operations Center after the anthrax attack of 2001 and became the first director before the establishment of the Office of Public Health Emergency Preparedness, where she currently serves. Captain Lavin is a certified family nurse practitioner who maintains an active practice. She has had a diverse career including work in mental health, correctional health, and immigration health. While at the Division of Immigration Health Services, she became involved in disaster response while serving as the coordinator of the Emergency Medical Response Team. She attributes her assignment in homeland security to her organizational ability and critical thinking.

BOX 81-3

Captain Mary Chaffee's Journey Into Homeland Security

Captain Mary Chaffee is a Navy Nurse who has served on active duty and in the reserve component for 21 years. She is an emergency nurse with a background in health policy, nursing administration, critical care, and informatics. Following the terror attacks of September 11, 2001, she was assigned to serve in the Emergency Operations Center of the Federal Emergency Management Agency and then served as the director of the Navy Medicine Office of Homeland Security. She believes she was selected to lead the initial homeland security efforts of the U.S. Navy Medical Department because she had a sustained record as an effective leader, innovator, and problem solver. Captain Chaffee is a member of the board of directors of the International Nursing Coalition on Mass Casualty Education and serves on the editorial board of the journal *Disaster Management & Response.* She guided the development of a hospital-preparedness program that was recognized as a runner-up in the 2004 Harvard University/John F. Kennedy School of Government "Innovations in American Government" award program in homeland security.

flooding that paralyzed all hospitals in the city in June 2001 (Skelton, Droege, & Carlisle, 2003). Army nurses serve in a variety of roles supporting homeland security, including on Special Medical Augmentation Response Teams. These teams are trained and equipped to respond to trauma, chemical, and biological events and burns, and to provide care for psychiatric and other needs (Barajas, Stewart, & Combs, 2003).

EDUCATIONAL PREPARATION IN HOMELAND SECURITY AND EMERGENCY PREPAREDNESS

Mandatory Continuing Education

Many nurses have found that they need to learn more about emergency preparedness and response, and many programs are available for this (Table 81-2). Only two states, Texas and Nevada, require continuing education in emergency preparedness for nurses. Texas, for example, every two years in the registered nurse licensure cycle requires two hours of continuing education relating to preparing for, reporting medical events resulting from, and responding to the consequences of an incident of bioterrorism (Texas Legislature, 2003).

How to Assess Quality in Education Programs

Until the establishment of national-level role competencies and training standards, anyone can proclaim themselves to be an "expert" in homeland security. How does one judge quality and select carefully? Consider the source. Is the provider a reputable firm, associated with a university or a federal entity? What are the qualifications of the faculty? Is continuing education credit offered by an appropriate governing body? Until credentialing standards are enacted, awareness-level courses in disaster preparedness and terrorism from the National Response Plan and the National Incident Management system are good choices.

Educational Competencies

Several professional groups are working to establish core competencies for nurses. These groups include the American Red Cross (2003), the Association of Teachers of Preventive Medicine (2003), and the International Nursing Coalition for Mass Casualty Education (2003). The International Nursing Coalition for Mass Casualty Education is composed of representatives from major schools of nursing and organizations such as the American Nurses Association; the American Academy of Nursing; the American Association of Colleges of Nursing; the National League for Nursing; the National Council for State Boards of Nursing; the nursing education accreditation commissions (National League for Nursing Accrediting Commission and Commission on Collegiate Nursing Education); the U.S. Air Force, Navy, and Army Nurse Corps; the U.S. Public Health Service; and major nursing specialty organizations. The International Nursing Coalition for Mass Casualty Education is developing a comprehensive plan for educating nurses and has developed core competencies for mass casualty response. Web-based training and classroom programs are in preparation.

Academic Settings

Several schools of nursing, such as at Duquesne University, John Hopkins University, St. Louis University, the University of Massachusetts at Lowell, the University of Tennessee, the University of Texas at Austin, and the Uniformed Services University of the Health Sciences, are incorporating disaster preparedness and mass casualty content into classes at the undergraduate and graduate levels.

For nurses who prefer self-designed education, many books and journals are available, and a wide variety of resources reside on the Internet (Table 81-3).

TABLE 81-2

Training Opportunities in Homeland Security and Emergency Preparedness

Sponsor	Title/Description	Web Address
Web-Based Training		
American Journal of Nursing	Five continuing education modules on topics such as agents of terrorism, smallpox, and radiological incidents	http://www.nursingcenter.com/prodev/ce_list.asp?flag=cat&id=405978
American Red Cross and Sigma Theta Tau International*	Disaster Preparedness and Response for Nurses	http://www.nursingknowledge.org/Portal/Main.aspx?pageid=36&SKU=1050
California Distance Learning Health Network[†]	48 distance learning webcasts on a variety of bioterrorism/risk management topics	http://cdlhn.com/clickhere.cfm?type=n&id=113&title=Skills%20Training%20Institute
Centers for Disease Control and Prevention[†]	Multiple archived programs such as smallpox vaccine handling and storage, plague, and mass antibiotic dispensing	http://www.bt.cdc.gov/
Domestic Preparedness Campus[†]	WMD/Terrorism Awareness for Emergency Responders WMD Incident Management/Unified Command Concept	http://www.teexwmdcampus.com/main.cfm
Emergency Management Institute[†]	Variety of relevant topics to include the National Response Plan (IS 800), National Incident Management System (IS 700), and Incident Command (IS 100), as well as disaster preparedness and response	http://training.fema.gov/EMIWeb/IS/crslist.asp
Nursing Spectrum[‡]	Biological Weapons and Emergency Preparedness Parts I and II (286B and 287B), SARS (323). Texas-specific continuing education requirement Biological Weapons & Emergency Preparedness for Nursing Licensure in Texas ($20)	http://www2.nursingspectrum.com/ce/self-study_modules/
Public Health Training Network[†]	Variety of courses	http://www.phppo.cdc.gov/phtn/default.asp
University of Albany School of Public Health[‡]	Terrorism, Preparedness and Public Health: An Introduction Six modules: all types of hazards	http://www.ualbanycphp.org/learning/registration/detail_Terrorism.cfm
U.S. Army Medical Research and Material Command and Veterans Administration[†]	Six modules dealing with smallpox, nerve agents, vaccines, chemical threat agents, and history	http://www.biomedtraining.org/webcast.htm

*Nongovernmental.
[†]Governmental.
[‡]Private.

Continued

TABLE 81-2—cont'd

Training Opportunities in Homeland Security and Emergency Preparedness		
Sponsor	**Title/Description**	**Link to Access**
	Homeland Security and Emergency Preparedness Courses	
American Red Cross*	Disaster Health Services: An Overview (ARC 3076-1)	Contact your local American Red Cross chapter.
	Homeland Security and Emergency Preparedness Courses	
	Introduction to Disaster Services (ARC 3066)	To find your chapter, search this link: http://www.redcross.org/ index.html
	Disaster Health Services Simulation (ARC 3076-2)	
George Washington University‡	Response to Emergencies and Disasters Institute (READI). Courses at the awareness, performance, and management levels	http://readi.gwu.edu/
Noble Training Center, Anniston, Ala. (Department of Homeland Security)	Healthcare Leadership Course	http://www.training.fema.gov/ EMIWeb/EMICourses/ FY%202006%20EMI%20RS% 20Schedule.doc
Quinnipiac University‡	Disaster and Mass Casualty Management Overview of responses to and management of natural and manufactured disasters	http://www.quinnipiac.edu/ x1789.xml?ID=3713
University of Texas at Austin‡	Disaster Nursing Discusses the roles of nurses in mass casualty disasters	http://www.utexas.edu/nursing/ html/disaster/utexas.html
	Certificate Courses	
Saint Louis University School of Nursing‡	Disaster Preparedness for Nurses Core and elective modules	http://www.slu.edu/colleges/NR/cne_ disaster_prep_home.html
	Advanced Homeland Security Training Opportunities for Nurses	
American Red Cross*	Clara Barton Center for Domestic Preparedness	Contact your local American Red Cross chapter
University of Pittsburg School of Nursing‡	Acute Care Nurse Practitioner Program Trauma and Emergency Preparedness Clinical Emphasis	http://www.pitt.edu/~acnp/tep.html
University of Rochester School of Nursing	Leadership in Health Care Systems— Disaster Response and Emergency Preparedness track	http://www.urmc.rochester.edu/ son/AcademicPrograms/ disaster_management.cfm
University of Ulster, Northern Ireland	Postgraduate diploma/master of science degree in disaster relief nursing	http://prospectus.ulster.ac.uk/ course/?id=1134

TABLE 81-3

Internet Resources for Nurses on Homeland Security and Emergency Preparedness

Sponsor	Topical Area	Link
American Red Cross*	Family disaster plans and disaster check list	http://www.redcross.org/services/disaster/0,1082,0_601_,00.html
American Red Cross*	Disaster FAQs	http://www.redcross.org/faq/0,1095,0_378_,00.html
Association of State and Territorial Directors of Nursing	Disaster resources for nurses	http://www.astdn.org/publications.htm
Center for Disease Control and Prevention[†]	Emergency Preparedness and Response	http://www.bt.cdc.gov/
Department of Homeland Security[†]	Threat information; how to develop an emergency plan	http://www.ready.gov/index.html
Emergency Nurses Association[‡]	Weapons of mass destruction resource list	http://www.ena.org/EmergencyPrepared/WMD/Resources.PDF
Florida Department of Health	Statewide Public Health Nursing Disaster Resource Guide	http://www.doh.state.fl.us/PHNursing/disasterguide.html
International Coalition for Mass Casualty Education[†,‡]	Basic nursing competencies for response to mass casualty situations	http://www.incmce.org/
SAMHSA Disaster Technical Assistance Center	Disaster health resources	http://www.mentalhealth.org/dtac/default.asp
U.S. Army Medical Research Institute of Infectious Diseases Blue Book[†]	Agent identification and treatment	http://www.usamriid.army.mil/education/bluebook.htm

*Nongovernmental.
[†]Governmental.
[‡]Private.

RESEARCH

Some research has been conducted related to the role and competency of nursing in disaster response and homeland security, but there is a great need to expand the knowledge base in this area. Some recent research efforts include the following:

◆ Shih, Liao, Chan, and Gau (2002) examined the impact of a major earthquake on Taiwanese nurses as rescuers.
◆ Robison (2002) explored Army nurses' knowledge of triage in a mass casualty event.
◆ Nufer and Wilson-Ramirez (2004) compared patients' needs following two hurricanes.
◆ Riba and Reches (2002) described how Israeli nurses cope with multicasualty terror attacks.
◆ French, Sole, and Byers (2002) compared nurses' needs and concerns after Hurricane Floyd.
◆ Mitani, Kuboyama, and Shirakawa (2003) examined factors affecting nurse participation in response to sudden-onset disasters.

◆ Wisniewski, Dennik-Champion, and Peltier (2004) assessed nurses' education needs in emergency preparedness.

The Agency for Healthcare Research and Quality and the National Institutes of Nursing Research sponsor research by nurses, but nursing research focused on disaster response is seriously lacking. This is not the result of governmental lack of focus but rather the apparent low priority nurses put on this research despite the climate that would suggest an urgent need. Supported by the Department of Health and Human Services, the International Nursing Coalition for Mass Casualty Education developed a research agenda for nursing related to mass casualty education. The agenda includes new uses of technology, approaches to assessment, and methods of learning.

In addition to qualitative and quantitative research, there is value in nurses documenting their experience in disaster situations and publishing these "lessons learned." Examples include Cullen's chronicle (2003) of her experience in responding to the Rhode Island nightclub fire and Jurkovich's description (2003) of nursing efforts after the attack on the Pentagon.

A complete research agenda should be developed for the profession to address unanswered questions. What approach best uses nurses during a disaster when there are too few nurses to meet the demand? Historically, what civil defense policies were effective? What types of skills are needed during the different types of disaster, and what is the best use of nurses? What is the minimum amount of training and current clinical experience needed to respond to a disaster? Which credentialing model would best ensure competent care during a disaster? What factors affect the ability of nurses to report to duty during a disaster and what action could increase the percentage of nurses reporting? Is it more effective to train more nurses or to train the community in self-care during a disaster so that every citizen is a first responder?

As the largest component of the U.S. health care workforce, nurses have a significant role to play in homeland security. Because of the constant risk of natural disaster, transportation or industrial disaster, and the new threats of terror attack, it is vital for nurses to recognize the importance of their contributions in emergency preparedness and disaster response. From senior levels of government to individual preparedness at home, nurses can make a great difference in how well prepared the United States is to respond to the next disaster.

REFERENCES

American Red Cross. (2003). *Introduction to disaster services.* Washington, DC: Author.

ANSER Institute for Homeland Security. (2002). *Dark winter.* Retrieved January 29, 2005, from http://www.homelandsecurity.org/darkwinter/index.cfm

Association of Teachers of Preventive Medicine. (2003). *Emergency response clinician competencies in initial assessment and management.* New York: Center for Health Policy, Columbia University School of Nursing.

Barajas, K., Stewart, W. A., & Combs, E. W. (2003). The Army chemical/biological SMART (SMART-CB) team: The nurse's role. *Critical Care Nursing Clinics of North America, 15*(2), 143-148.

Center for Health Policy. (2001). *Core public health worker competencies for emergency preparedness and response.* Retrieved January 28, 2005, from http://www.mailman.hs.columbia.edu/CPHP/cdc/COMPETENCIES.pdf

Cullen, A. (2003). The Rhode Island "Station Nightclub" fire: Professional revelations of an emergency nurse. *Journal of Emergency Nursing, 29*(4), 352-355.

Department of Homeland Security. (2003). *Guidance for federal interagency operations under existing emergency response plans in accord with initial national response plans.* [Unpublished document].

Department of Homeland Security. (2004, February 25). *National response plan.* Washington, DC: Author.

French, E. D., Sole, M. L., & Byers, J. F. (2002). A comparison of nurses' needs/concerns and hospital disaster plans following Florida's Hurricane Floyd. *Journal of Emergency Nursing, 28*(2), 111-117.

International Association of Forensic Nurses. (2001). *Resolution 1: Terror on September 11, 2001.* Retrieved January 12, 2005, from http://www.forensicnurse.org/news/resolut1.htm

International Council of Nurses. (2001). *Nurses and disaster preparedness.* Retrieved February 8, 2005, from http://www.icn.ch/psdisasterprep01.htm

International Nursing Coalition for Mass Casualty Education. (2003). *Educational competencies for registered nurses responding to mass casualty incidents.* Nashville, TN: Author.

Jurkovich, T. (2003). September 11th: The Pentagon disaster—Response and lessons learned. *Critical Care Nursing Clinics of North America, 15*(2), 143-148.

Mills, M. A. (1951). Civil defense: Detroit nurses prepare. *Public Health Nursing, 43*(8), 454-455.

Mitani, S., Kuboyama, K., & Shirakawa, T. (2003). Nursing in sudden-onset disasters: Factors and information that affect participation. *Prehospital and Disaster Medicine, 18*(4), 359-366.

National Organization for Public Health Nursing. (1951). Public health nursing in the national security program. *Public Health Nursing, 43,* 69-72.

Nightingale, F. (1969). *Notes on nursing.* New York: Dover Publications.

Nufer, K. E., & Wilson-Ramirez, G. (2004). A comparison of patient needs following two hurricanes. *Prehospital and Disaster Medicine, 19*(2), 146-149.

Office of Homeland Security. (2002). *National strategy for homeland security.* Retrieved January 29, 2005, from http://www.whitehouse.gov/homeland/book/nat_strat_hls.pdf

Riba, S., & Reches, H. (2002). When terror is routine: How Israeli nurses cope with multi-casualty terror. *Online Journal of Issues in Nursing, 7*(3). Retrieved February 2, 2005, from www.nursingworld.org/ojin/topic19/tpc19_5.htm

Riley, J. M. (2003). Providing nursing care with federal disaster-relief teams. *Disaster Management & Response, 1*(3), 76-79.

Robison, J. L. (2002). Army nurses' knowledge base for determining triage categories in a mass casualty. *Military Medicine, 167*(10), 812-816.

Shih, F. J., Liao, Y. C., Chan, S. M., & Gau, M. L. (2002). The impact of the 9-21 earthquake experience of Taiwanese nurses as rescuers. *Social Science & Medicine, 55*(4), 659-672.

Skelton, P. A., Droege, L., & Carlisle, M. T. (2003). EMEDs and SPEARR teams: United States Air Force ready responders. *Critical Care Nursing Clinics of North America, 15*(2), 143-148.

Texas Legislature. (2003). Nursing Practice Act, § 301.305. Bioterrorism response component in continuing education. Retrieved December 19, 2004, from http://www.capitol.state.tx.us/statutes/oc.toc.htm

Tomisek, S. J. (2002). Homeland security: The new role for defense. *Strategic Forum, 189*(2). Retrieved February 1, 2005, from http://www.ndu.edu/inss/strforum/SF189/sf189.htm

White House. (2003, February 28). *Homeland security presidential directive/HSPD-5*. Retrieved December 19, 2004, from http://www.whitehouse.gov/news/releases/2003/02/20030228-9.html

Wisniewski, R., Dennik-Champion, G., & Peltier, J. W. (2004). Emergency preparedness competencies: Assessing nurses educational needs. *Journal of Nursing Administration, 34*(10), 475-480.

SUGGESTED READINGS

McGlown, K. J. (Ed.). *Terrorism and disaster management: Preparing healthcare leaders for the new reality*. Chicago: Health Administration Press.

Shepherd, S., Copenhaver, J. B., Fanney, R. M., Campbell, R., Dwyer, A., & Duda, J. (2004). *Jane's citizen's safety guide*. Surrey, United Kingdom: Jane's Publishing Group.

Veenema, T. G. (Ed.). (2003). *Disaster nursing and emergency preparedness for chemical, biological, and radiological terrorism and other hazards*. New York: Springer.

Nursing in Wars

RICHARD GARFIELD ◆ ANNE MARIE RAFFERTY

Crises reveal the fault lines in society, but they also bring out sources of solidarity and provide an opportunity to review the resilience, resources, and capacity to respond. What implications do conflicts around the world hold for nursing?

Nurses have long been involved in issues of war and peace. War has helped to define nursing in the modern era and sometimes has been a vehicle for the advancement of the status and skill of nursing. But the two values of patriotism and humanism often have come into conflict. Are nurses supposed to "cheer our boys on" or denounce military tactics that place civilians in harm's way? Before discussing these role issues, we will provide grounding in the evolving terminology, epidemiology, and nature of war, conflict, and violence.

Collective violence may be defined as the use of force by groups to achieve political, economic, or social objectives (Zwi, Garfield, & Loretti, 2002). The classic expression of this violence has been wars and related violent political conflicts occurring within or between states (Figure 82-1).

The character of conflicts changed significantly since the end of the cold war. More and more, conflicts are characterized as follows:

◆ They entail an element of "identity politics"—the claim to power based on a particular national, clan, religious, or linguistic identity.

◆ They attempt to control the population by eliminating those with a different identity through forced resettlement, mass killings, and intimidation.

◆ They link what appear to be local, decentralized conflicts with a "globalized war economy," interacting with persons, processes, and aspirations present at the global level.

GLOBAL BURDEN OF CONFLICT

The World Health Organization estimates that about 588,000 persons died in wars in 1998 (Krug, Dahlberg, Mercy, Zwi, & Lozano, 2002). That made war the fourth most common type of injury death in that year, after unintended injuries, suicides, and homicides. Deaths from war varied from less than 1 per 100,000 population in high-income countries, to 12 per 100,000 in low- to middle-income countries. The rate varied by region from near zero in China, India, and the Americas, to 33 per 100,000 in the eastern Mediterranean and 51 per 100,000 in Africa. Across the globe, war ranked as the thirteenth most common cause of death for newborns to 1 year olds, fifth for 5 to 14 year olds, and fifth for 15 to 44 year olds in 1998.

An estimated 5% of all deaths during the twentieth century were due to the immediate or secondary impact of such collective violence. This was higher than in the seventeenth to nineteenth centuries, in which 2% of deaths are estimated to have resulted from collective violence. The fortyfold rise in the number of deaths among soldiers in the twentieth century greatly exceeded a doubling of the midcentury population of the world. Military deaths per million population rose eighteen-fold from the nineteenth to the twentieth century (Table 82-1 and Figure 82-2). Genocide and democide-related deaths also rose in the twentieth century as the centralization of large political and economic systems and the emergence of new technologies made mass killings possible.

The number of direct deaths in war peaked in 1994. Probably an average of about 300,000 persons have died because of the direct effects of wars in recent years. Indirect deaths, however, are claiming a growing proportion of all conflict-related deaths. Laying of siege, destroying essential goods and services, poisoning water supplies, or enslavement of a losing enemy often accompanied warfare in premodern times. Whereas in European war since the establishment of nation-states in the seventeenth century, soldiers of one nation engaged in direct battle almost exclusively with soldiers of a rival nation, anticolonial wars, often based on guerilla warfare, have blurred the distinction between the military and civilians. This distinction has

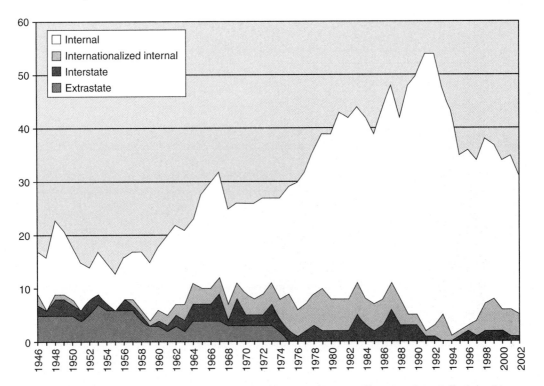

FIGURE 82-1 Conflicts by boundary type, 1946-2002. (From Wallensteen, P., & Sollenberg, M. [1999]. Armed conflict 1989-1998. *Journal of Peace Research, 36*[5], 593-606.)

TABLE 82-1

Estimated Average Annual Military Deaths in Wars, Worldwide, by Century

Century	Average Annual Military Deaths	World Midcentury Population in Millions	Average Annual Military Deaths per Million Population
Seventeenth	9,500	500	19.0
Eighteenth	15,000	800	18.8
Nineteenth	13,000	1,200	10.8
Twentieth	458,000	2,500	183.2

Data from Garfield, R. M., & Nuegut, A. I. (1991). Epidemiologic analysis of warfare: A historical review. *JAMA: The Journal of the American Medical Association, 266*(5), 688-692.

eroded further with the breakdown of national states since the end of the cold war. In many internal conflicts, often pitting the state against a section of the civilian population, torture, disappearances, and other forms of repression have been practiced in pursuit of political and ideological objectives.

The move from international to internal wars has had important implications for nursing. More and more, troops are irregular, representing a political faction or social group rather than a national army with accountability structure. Their targets also are more frequently civilians, who may be irregular troops or simply the "other" social group (Table 82-2). Targeting civilians or the infrastructure upon which their daily lives depend, has become more common, and leverage points to redress this have been lost.

A lack of a common definition of terrorism haunts international affairs; one's terrorist is another's freedom fighter. Among all definitions, *terrorism* is defined as an act of violence used by clandestine individuals.

VIEWPOINTS

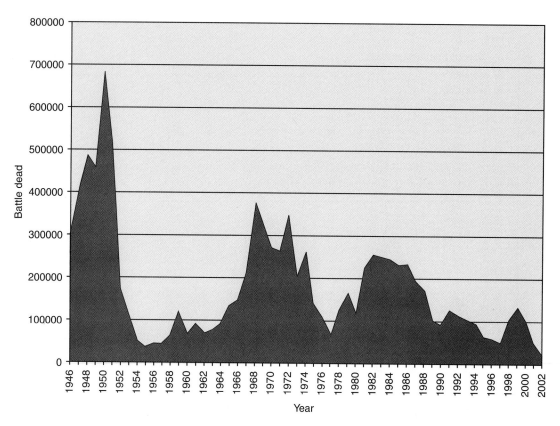

FIGURE 82-2 Battle deaths by year, 1946-2002. (From Wallensteen, P., & Sollenberg, M. [1999]. Armed conflict 1989-1998. *Journal of Peace Research, 36*[5], 593-606.)

TABLE 82-2

Battle Deaths Versus All Conflict-Related Deaths, Selected Conflicts				
Country	**Years**	**Battle Deaths**	**War-Related Deaths**	**Implied Ratio**
Angola	1974-2002	160,475	1.5 million; 50% after 1992	8.3
Democratic Republic of Congo	1998-2001	145,000	2.5 million (including 350,000 violent)	16.2
Ethiopia	1976-1991	16,000	1984-1985: 1 million to 2 million	62
Liberia	1989-2001	24,099	150,000-200,000	5.2
Mozambique	1976-1992	174,599	500,000 to 1 million	1.9
Nigeria (Biafra Rebellion)	1967-1970	75,000	500,000 to 2 million	5.7
Sierra Leone	1991-2000	12,997	1991-1995: 30,000	1.3
Somalia	1981-1996	67,250	1988 to mid-1990s: 250,000 to 350,000	2.7
Sudan	1983-2002	55,500	2 million	35
Sudan (Anya Nya rebellion)	1963-1973	20,000	250,000-750,000	11.5

The purpose is not to target that individual as such but to disrupt "life as usual" among the resident population of which they are part. Terrorism sometimes is referred to as the peacetime equivalent of a war crime because the targets of terrorist acts are most often neither combatants nor political leaders of the opposition.

During the cold war, most conflicts, especially conflicts causing the most deaths, occurred in wars between countries. Internal conflict was suppressed as part of superpower rivalry. The international forces that stimulated international conflicts and suppressed internal conflicts declined in the 1990s. The potential for international conflict has not disappeared, but the military, political, and informational gap between possible foes has widened. This set the stage for greater inequalities among those in conflict. Thus international conflict is fought on one side by ultramodern weapons launched from a distance. On the other side, small, easy-to-prepare weapons may be delivered on the body of a perpetrator, killing that individual along with the targets.

The end of the cold war unleashed the use of increasingly available small arms (Lumpe, 2000) in local conflicts. Under the Geneva Conventions of 1949, the rules of war require the application of principles of proportionality and distinction in the choice of targets. Proportionality involves an assessment of ways to minimize likely civilian casualties when a military objective involves targeting that is not exclusively military. Distinction focuses on avoiding civilian targets wherever possible. Attempts to regulate the brutality of conflicts have not kept pace with the evolving forms of conflict (Robertson, 1999). Most importantly, international humanitarian law and the Geneva Conventions are focused on states waging war and thus fail to deal adequately with conflicts within states or among multinational coalitions against a single state.

Each of these threats of conflict: depersonalized high-tech weaponry, fighting among informal, nonstate actors, and the use of indiscriminant weapons in terror attacks, increase the chance of injury or death among large groups of the population. Along with an increasing number of natural disasters and economic disruptions around the world, the number and severity of humanitarian crises and the populations affected by them have risen. Globalization also has contributed to economic disruption since the end of the cold war. For the first time in the modern era, some states are experiencing sustained economic declines. Of the 10 countries with the highest under-5 mortality rates in the world, 7 have experienced recent civil conflict (Black, Morris, & Bryce, 2003).

The majority of new wars and economic declines are in Africa, but every continent is affected by them except for North America, which after the September 11, 2001, attacks can no longer be comforted in the belief of being immune from conflict. Indeed, the disruptions caused by those terrorist attacks, the arbitrary nature of civilian victims, and the lasting impact on vulnerable groups—including women and children, family members, those with heightened anxiety, and those who lost employment—is part of a worldwide trend toward increasing impact of conflict on every day life (Human Security Centre, in press).

THE ROLES FOR NURSING IN A WORLD IN CONFLICT

Our ideas of nursing are shaped by images of nurses in war. It was war, after all, that brought Florence Nightingale into public prominence and provided her with a powerful platform for military and social reform. But therein lies the paradox. For although war may shine a light on nursing, it often can blind the observer to what nurses actually do. Nursing remains largely invisible in the historical and contemporary accounts of organizations associated with war, relief, and humanitarian assistance. It was a decade after the end of the Vietnam War until U.S. nurses' sacrifices there were honored (Freedman & Rhoads, 1987). Today, among nongovernmental organizations such as Save the Children and Doctors without Borders, few know that there are as many nurses as doctors serving in crisis areas around the world.

The history of nursing in conflict can be considered the history of the displaced person. Often nursing has no natural home or refuge within such environs. That is not to say that the record is void, only that it tends, with notable exceptions, toward a celebration of individual humanistic leaders such as Jane Delano and Clara Barton.

Locating nurses as part of a wider civic movement reduces history to heritage. Moreover, focusing on the individual can eclipse the political, the institutional, and the environmental context. In fact, war has in some ways served nursing. Nurses often have been able to improve the professional image and legal privileges from the state and to expand their role and influence in the public sphere during war.

The involvement of nursing in war is a double-edged sword, one that ultimately threatens the heart of humanitarianism. Nursing often is identified with national, patriotic interests of each warring power. Its other character is humanist and a nonnationalistic ethic of social reform and is represented by nursing leaders Lavinia Dock of the American Nurses Association and Ethel Fenwick of the International Council of Nurses. Both threads were represented by Nightingale, who on the one hand worked to improve the fighting capacity of the British army, while on the other hand she opposed the formation of the International Committee of the Red Cross because she feared it would relieve individual governments of the responsibility to protect noncombatants (Garfield, 2005). Ironically, national Red Cross associations may have done more to advance the role of nursing in the public's eyes than professional nursing organizations. Throughout the history of nursing involvement in conflict are contradictions and tensions in nurses' own understanding of a nurse's role:

- Ethically in favor of care for all, but demonstrating patriotism for one's own country and its interests
- Trying to promote humanism in the care of all while strengthening the fighting capacity of one's army
- Struggling to strengthen professionalism in nursing while acting docile under the command of doctors and political leaders

THE STRENGTHS OF NURSING

The profession of nursing is well placed to contribute to the global arena of humanitarian policy and research. Nurses bring a wealth of experience and a strong historical grounding in situations of conflict and crisis. To fulfill their potential, nursing must include, but go beyond, a clinical response to the individual patient.

First, nurses need to recognize and acknowledge their strengths and resources, and then they can build upon them to further research and policy that can work to better treat, mitigate, and prevent such crises. The strength of nursing lies in nurses' accessibility and ability to engage in advocacy in the public interest. In and outside areas of conflict in most countries there are more nurses than any other kind of health care professional. Nurses are accessible because they work everywhere and in proximity with those in need. In times of stability and times of conflict, nurses are prepared to provide care. From nurses' close relations with individuals, families, and communities, they become aware of the strengths and needs of their clients. This privileged glimpse into others' realities allows nurses to assess and respond holistically. After the September 11, 2001, attack on the World Trade Center, for example, nurses led community-based activities to reestablish community psychological health, provided assistance to harmed

individuals in recovery, and dealt with many other alterations in daily function that did not generate a physician encounter or hospital visit.

The practice of nursing includes an enormous range of skills, settings, and preparation. Because of this diversity, nurses work in many roles and in multidisciplinary teams. Common to the many types and roles of nurses is a wide recognition of the humanistic core of nursing values and practice. Nurses, even more than physicians, are trusted to have the best interests of the public in mind, to be honest, open, neutral, and disinterested agents in mending the social fabric. This trust and legitimacy are resources in rallying to a public policy agenda.

Nurses can build on these traits and contribute to an effective agenda for humanitarian research and policy. Nurses can serve as the eyes and ears of those in need and without effective voice and representation. Nurses who are practicing in such environments can work to identify the gaps, whereas nurses in other areas can advocate for change, can influence policy, and can research these gaps. For example, interventions in crisis situations focus mainly on needs and have not taken full consideration of local capacities. Colleges of nursing and professional organizations across nations, cultures, and borders can partner to assess and research these individual and community capacities to design appropriate programs and mitigate further crises.

A RESEARCH AGENDA

The effects of conflict reach beyond the wounded and dead. Many secondary and indirect effects occur, and many others may be affected. This is especially apparent in terrorism, where the social impact may be great on millions of persons, though the number of deaths is few. Family competence, psychological recovery, and reestablishing of normalcy in the community are areas in need of research from a nursing perspective. Indeed, the psychological impact and response to conflict is a unifying need among the full range of injuries, provoked or natural, individual or collective.

Much of this research should focus on women, who frequently are the forgotten victims in conflict. As the "family health worker," women frequently are involved in defining and responding to the recovery needs of the entire family. They must be enlisted to promote health, including their own, in time of crisis. In humanitarian crises in developing countries, only recently have physical abuse of women, problems of unaccompanied children, and child soldiers begun to receive attention.

Nurses are often on the frontlines dealing with women and families in both environments, and they need better training to do so. This training and practice needs to include care for their own potential needs as well.

Funds in the United States now are being directed to readiness, training for emergency response, improved communications, and upgrading of biological detection capacity. Important as these foci are, they fail to pull in the full range of nursing capacities. With a humanist perspective and a presence in key environments, nurses can do more. For example, early detection of many biological threats may occur among young persons in schools. Nurses have a long way to go to incorporate school nurses fully into systems for early detection and public health promotion. Nurses frequently are involved in assisting survivors to grieve and recover; far more preparation needs to go into developing their skill base to do this well. Nurses need to specify which of these skills is generic to all nursing and which should be developed at the specialty level.

To do population-oriented work, nurses need further integration into mass emergency response systems. They need training and practice to apply their logistical and organizational skills and their clinical skills. Communications strategies for nurses to serve in mass casualty events need to be developed. Nurses further need evaluation tools and templates to learn from and improve their systems. Each new mass casualty experience is an opportunity for systems development and improvement.

Many of those working in health care in developing countries who are from developed countries are nurses. Nurses need workforce studies to identify where they are and what roles they play. Where does service in humanitarian crisis fit into nurses' career paths? What skill levels are needed? How and when can nurses be better prepared to serve in these roles? What kinds of training work best, for nurses from developed countries and for those serving in humanitarian crises in their home countries.

Too often, nurses' approaches to ethical issues are based on individual motivation, without examination of the wider issues or systems to which the individual response contributes. Too often, nurses take on the attitudes and assumptions of other responders, such as the police or military. Like other areas of health care practice, examination of the evidence for practice in this area is needed. This examination will contribute significantly to the international agenda for humanitarian practice, policy, and research.

REFERENCES

Black, R., Morris, S., & Bryce, J. (2003). Where and why are 10 million children dying every year? *Lancet, 361*(9376), 2226-2234.

Freedman, D., & Rhoads, J. (Eds.) (1987). *Nurses in Vietnam: The forgotten veterans.* Austin: Texas Monthly Press.

Garfield, R. (2005). Nightingale in Iraq. *American Journal of Nursing, 105*(2), 69-72.

Human Security Centre. (Ed.) (in press). *Human security report 2004.* New York: Oxford University Press.

Krug, E., Dahlberg, L. L., Mercy, J. A., Zwi, A. B., & Lozano, R. (Eds.). (2002). *World report on violence and health.* Geneva, Switzerland: World Health Organization.

Lumpe, L. (Ed.). (2000). *Running guns: The global black market in small arms.* London: Zed Books.

Robertson, G. (1999). *Crimes against humanity: The struggle for global justice.* London: Penguin Press.

Wallensteen, P., & Sollenberg, M. (1999). Armed conflict 1989-1998. *Journal of Peace Research, 36*(5), 593-606.

Zwi, A., Garfield, R. M., & Loretti, A. (2002). Collective violence. In E. G. Krug, L. L. Dahlberg, J. A. Mercy, A. B. Zwi, & R. Lozano (Eds.), *World report on violence and health* (pp. 213-239). Geneva, Switzerland: World Health Organization.

Bioterrorism and Emerging Infections

Emergency Preparedness for Nurses

TERRI REBMANN

Biological terrorism is an old concept that only recently has reemerged in the literature as a current threat. In fact, according to the Centers for Disease Control and Prevention (2000), bioterrorism has become the most imminent threat to American national security. In the fall of 2001 the threat of bioterrorism became reality when a terrorist sent anthrax-laden letters to members of the media and government officials.

The past decade also has seen an increase in the number of outbreaks caused by new or reemerging organisms. These emerging pathogens are particularly challenging for health care because so little is known about the clinical description and epidemiology of each disease, such as the route of infection transmission or possible treatment options. When these pathogens surface, health care providers are forced to make medical decisions without the luxury of years of research or epidemiological data about how to treat and isolate infected patients safely. In the past decade, the United States has encountered West Nile virus, monkeypox, mad cow disease, Norwalk virus, and severe acute respiratory syndrome (SARS). In addition, the United States constantly is faced with the potential of new infectious disease threats, such as avian influenza. The threat of emerging pathogens has had a major impact on health care and public health systems in the United States and has illustrated the need for additional planning and response capabilities to respond to potential future events.

Bioterrorism and emerging infections pose a major threat to the health and safety of U.S. citizens. In today's society that allows easy and frequent travel, diseases have the potential of spreading rapidly. Germs live and travel with people; thus anywhere that people live or can travel, diseases can exist and go. Public health

professionals have long recognized that crowded or highly populated environments contribute to the spread of infectious diseases (Evans & Brachman, 1989). Previous outbreaks have shown that germs also travel with people. The 2003 outbreak of SARS illustrated the speed with which diseases can spread around the world. The SARS outbreak is believed to have begun in the Metropole Hotel in Hong Kong by a single visitor. This initial or primary SARS case is postulated to have infected at least 12 others staying at the hotel and to have exposed countless others (Centers for Disease Control and Prevention [CDC], 2003b). These secondary cases then returned home, carrying and spreading SARS to six other countries. From only a single initial case, SARS spread around the world in less than 48 hours (Figure 83-1). Within months, SARS became a global infectious disease emergency. Because infectious diseases share the same principles of transmission, a bioterrorism attack using an infectious agent, such as variola (the virus that causes smallpox) or *Yersinia pestis* (the bacteria that causes pneumonic plague when inhaled), has the same potential. Whether the event is natural (an outbreak of an emerging infectious disease) or manufactured (a bioterrorism attack) does not matter. Outbreaks of infectious diseases pose a serious threat to the health of citizens around the world.

Quantifying the potential implications of a bioterrorism attack or outbreak of an emerging infectious disease is difficult because the outcome depends on many variables, including the size of the release, the nature of the agent used, weather and other environmental conditions, and how quickly the affected community recognizes and responds to the event. The 2001 anthrax bioterrorism attack used only a small amount of a weaponized noninfectious agent (approximately 2 to 3 oz of anthrax) and a relatively ineffective

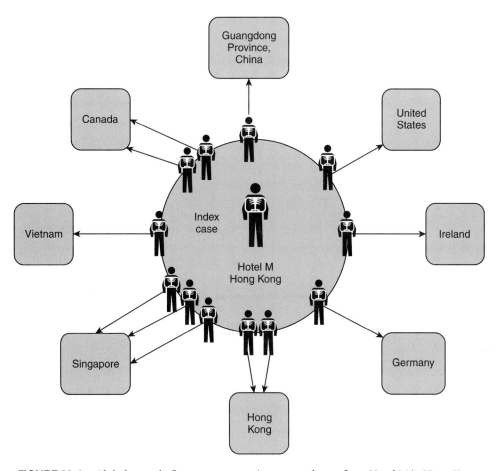

FIGURE 83-1 Global spread of severe acute respiratory syndrome from Hotel M in Hong Kong, 2003. This figure illustrates the chain of infection transmission from the Index Case to 12 other guests at Hotel M in Hong Kong. This incident is believed to have been the start of the global outbreak of severe acute respiratory syndrome. (Adapted from Centers for Disease Control and Prevention. (2003). Update: Outbreak of severe acute respiratory syndrome—Worldwide, 2003. *Morbidity and Mortality Weekly Report, 52*(12), 241-248 [Figure 1].)

dissemination device (letters), and resulted in only 22 cases of anthrax and 5 deaths (U.S. General Accounting Office, 2003). A total cost to the United States has yet to be determined, but the financial impact was devastating to many states, despite the small size of the event. If more agents had been used, a contagious organism had been chosen, or the powder had been aerosolized, there likely would have been much more associated morbidity, mortality, and cost.

In 1997 a group of researchers calculated the potential economic impact of a bioterrorism attack using mathematical modeling. This research project modeled the aerosol release of three agents (causing brucellosis, anthrax, and tularemia) and found that costs from such an attack could range from $477.7 million per 100,000

persons exposed (for a release of the brucellosis agent) to $26.2 billion per 100,000 persons exposed (when the anthrax agent is disseminated) (Kaufmann, Meltzer, & Schmid, 1997). Another model on which to base estimates of the potential costs associated with a bioterrorism attack involves the actual outbreak of SARS in Canada. In a 2003 report, the SARS outbreak that lasted less than a year in Canada was estimated to have resulted in a net cost to the national economy between $1.5 billion and $2.1 billion (Health Canada, 2003b). One feasibly may assume that an outbreak of an infectious disease resulting from a biological weapons attack in the United States would result in similar economic devastation.

The effectiveness of a bioterrorism response depends on the speed with which health care professionals recognize and respond to such an attack, which in turn depends upon their level of preparedness. The speed with which health care professionals need to respond depends on many factors, including the incubation period of the causative agent, the availability of an effective prophylactic therapy or vaccine, and the amount of agent released. For example, antibiotic distribution sites must be established rapidly (in less than 72 hours) for agents with a short incubation period, such as for anthrax and tularemia (Kaufmann et al., 1997). Following the release of agents for which antibiotics are ineffective prophylaxes, such as for smallpox, vaccination clinics must be instituted rapidly to decrease the risk of infection transmission (CDC, 2002). Failure of rapid implementation can result in higher morbidity, mortality, and costs.

A mathematical modeling study calculating the cost of early versus late intervention following a bioterrorism attack using tularemia found that there would be a net loss of $10.7 million to $115.1 million if a postexposure prophylaxis program were not begun until 6 days after exposure. When this same model examined anthrax, a net loss of $13.4 million to $283.1 million was estimated if postexposure prophylaxis were not started until 4 to 6 days after the initial exposure. Obviously, a rapid response is preferred because it would result in better outcomes in terms of physical (lower morbidity and mortality) and financial (associated costs) measures (Kaufmann et al., 1997). A rapid response requires not only effective facility and community disaster plans but also a prepared workforce that is able to respond appropriately and rapidly. Without prepared individuals, an effective response cannot be mounted.

Based on projections of the potential consequences of a bioterrorism attack and the actual reality of the immense impact of the small-scale incident using anthrax in 2001, the need for bioterrorism preparedness has become a national priority. This has been well established in the scientific literature of a variety of professions (American Academy of Pediatrics, 2000; Bernardo, 2001; Burkle, 2002; CDC, 2000; Gerberding, Hughes, & Koplan, 2002; Gwerder, Beaton, & Daniell, 2001). Despite this, many facets of health care and public health still are not engaging in bioterrorism preparedness activities. The anthrax incident of 2001 illustrated just how truly unprepared America is as a nation to respond adequately to a bioterrorism attack of any size (Altman & Kolata, 2002).

Although the possibility of a large-scale bioterrorism attack is low, the potential consequences if Americans are not prepared are staggering. The large number of victims quickly would exceed the existing capacity of the health care system, and the financial impact could reach the billions of dollars (Burkle, 2002; Kaufmann et al., 1997). In addition, the risk of an outbreak from a new or reemerging infection is feasible. The United States has encountered five such outbreaks in the past few years alone.

The good news is that the response to bioterrorism or an outbreak of an emerging infectious disease is similar. An epidemiological investigation, institution of appropriate infection control protective measures, and large-scale medication or vaccination distribution are imperative to an effective outcome from either event. Since the response to bioterrorism and emerging infections is similar, becoming prepared for one enhances readiness for the other.

Composing the largest group of health care providers, nursing is poised to be at the forefront in managing an infectious disease outbreak, regardless of whether the outbreak is naturally occurring or manufactured. If such an event occurred, nurses in all settings and specialties would be needed to help manage the emergency situation. In the acute care setting, nurses would be required to help triage and treat the large influx of patients likely to arrive. This includes not only nurses working in emergency departments but also nurses from all areas of the hospital. The initial influx of patients quickly could overwhelm the ability of emergency department personnel to handle the situation. Alternative care sites may be arranged, and these will require staffing by nurses.

Many hospitals in the United States currently are planning how to juggle a potential large influx of patients. Disaster plans often include provisions for temporarily halting some procedures and services, such as nonemergency surgeries, and pulling staff from those areas to help triage and treat the incoming patients. Nurses who usually work in operating rooms, outpatient treatment centers, and other nonemergency settings may be relocated from their daily duties to fill in during the crisis. This shifting of staff likely will burden nurses in non–acute care settings as well. As the crisis subsides and hospitals revert from emergency procedures back to day-to-day operations, long-term nursing care still will be required for the patients infected during the outbreak. This will put an added stress on non–acute care nurses, such as those working in outpatient settings, clinics, and home health care. Nurses in all areas and specialties will be affected by a bioterrorism attack or outbreak of an emerging infectious disease in their community.

As such, the nursing profession must embrace fully its responsibility in bioterrorism preparedness. Despite the fact that nurses will play a crucial role in recognizing and responding to a bioterrorism attack or outbreak of an emerging infectious disease, nursing as a profession has been slow to respond to the need for emergency preparedness. Bioterrorism articles began appearing in nursing journals around 1998, although they had been published by medicine and other health care disciplines since the early 1990s. In addition, many more bioterrorism-related articles were published in medical journals than in nursing journals (Figures 83-2 and 83-3).

Nursing must evaluate what factors have affected its slow acceptance of the need for emergency preparedness. The profession's hesitation to embrace fully this new area of study likely has affected the individual nurse's decision to engage in bioterrorism and emergency preparedness initiatives. However, other influencing factors that likely affect nurses' decisions to become better prepared for bioterrorism or an outbreak of an emerging infectious disease.

Research indicates that the majority of infection control and public health professionals (many of whom are nurses) report that a lack of training opportunities is their primary barrier to receiving bioterrorism education,

although the vast majority also report that they have received some education on this topic (Shadel, Chen, et al., 2004; Shadel, Rebmann, Clements, Chen, & Evans, 2003). Despite having received some bioterrorism education, most nurses report that they do not feel adequately prepared to respond to an attack (Rose & Larrimore, 2002). In addition, preliminary research and anecdotal information from bioterrorism planners indicates that most nurses are not participating in drills that involve exercising the bioterrorism disaster plan of their facility (Henning et al., 2004; D. Mayes, personal communication, June 8, 2004). As has been noted, the implementation of a disaster response plan through real or simulated events is the only true way to measure the level of preparedness, yet most nurses do not engage in these drills (Weil, 2003). In addition, many nurses do not engage in education or disaster plan exercise preparedness activities. What factors influence nurses' decisions to engage in bioterrorism simulation exercises and receive the education they need to feel adequately prepared?

One factor that may affect nurses' decisions to become prepared for bioterrorism or emerging infections is the misdirected education that thus far has been provided to nurses. In the nation's rush to become better prepared to respond to a bioterrorism attack,

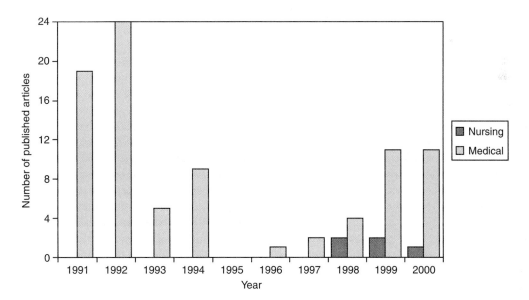

FIGURE 83-2 Number of bioterrorism articles published in nursing and medical journals, 1991-2000. There is some overlap between the two categories when the journal is written for a nursing and a physician audience. Two examples of such journals include the *American Journal of Public Health* and *Infection Control and Hospital Epidemiology*. The articles from these journals are included in the numbers for nursing and medical categories.

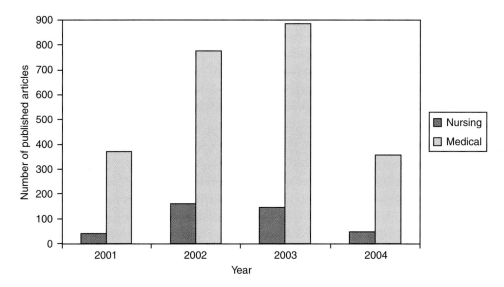

FIGURE 83-3   Number of bioterrorism articles published in nursing and medical journals, 2001-2004. There is some overlap between the two categories when the journal is written for a nursing and a physician audience. Two examples of such journals include the *American Journal of Public Health* and *Infection Control and Hospital Epidemiology*. The articles from these journals are included in the numbers for nursing and medical categories.

a paradigm for bioterrorism preparedness had to be developed rapidly. In response, an efficient, standardized approach was adopted that used a medical model as its foundation. Most articles lump bioterrorism preparedness for nurses with all other health care providers. Early bioterrorism preparedness education used the medical model and taught all professions how to identify, diagnose, and treat victims of bioterrorism. However, these are tasks of primary care providers, such as physicians and nurse practitioners; they do not apply to the vast majority of nursing specialties. Although this efficient approach has served better to prepare many health care and public health professionals in a relatively short period of time, it may have done so at the expense of the nursing profession.

The medical model is essential to bioterrorism management and should be incorporated into bioterrorism preparedness theories for all health care professions, including nursing. However, using only the medical model approach discounts the unique input and contribution of other human sciences and may lead to the neglect of critical components of bioterrorism management. Many nursing-specific issues have been neglected, including potential implications of long-term care for survivors, the mental health impact on health care workers and their families, and therapeutic communication for grieving victims' families. Nurses must

investigate and address the profession-specific barriers to bioterrorism preparedness to ensure the best response to a future bioterrorism attack. Bioterrorism preparedness educational needs that are specific to the profession of nursing, such as those described by Steed, Howe, Pruitt, and Sherrill (2004), must be defined clearly.

In addition, many articles describe bioterrorism preparedness for nurses in relation to hospital or community preparedness (American Academy of Pediatrics, 2000; CDC, 2000; Gwerder et al., 2001; Morse, 2002; O'Connell, Menuey, & Foster, 2002; Peralta, 2000; Salazar & Kelman, 2002; Shadel, Clements, Arndt, Rebmann, & Evans, 2001). Although this applies to a small subset of the discipline, it does not apply to the vast majority of nurses. Hospital and community bioterrorism preparedness are broad tasks that are the responsibility of only a few individuals rather than the responsibility of the profession of nursing as a whole.

For example, a large hospital in an urban setting most likely will have an emergency planning committee composed of individuals from numerous departments. This committee requires at least one nursing member to ensure that nursing needs are addressed in the response plan of the facility. In some hospitals, an infection control or environmental health nurse may even be the leader or coordinator of this committee. However, not all nurses employed at this facility will be members of the emergency planning committee, nor should they be.

Hospital or health care facility bioterrorism preparedness requires multidepartmental and multiagency coordination and cooperation. Not every nurse has the responsibility to assume this role. However, the majority of bioterrorism preparedness literature in nursing journals seems to imply that taking on this larger role is the responsibility of every nurse in becoming better prepared to respond to bioterrorism (American Academy of Pediatrics, 2000; CDC, 2000; Gwerder et al., 2001; Morse, 2002; O'Connell et al., 2002; Peralta, 2000; Salazar & Kelman, 2002; Shadel, Clements, et al., 2001). This task can be overwhelming to nurses who already are overworked, underpaid, and undervalued.

Another reason that nurses may have been slow to accept the need for emergency preparedness is the misdirected focus of early bioterrorism education efforts. When the threat of bioterrorism first reemerged in the 1990s, education was targeted at the traditional first responders: police and fire and emergency service personnel (Jones, 2002). As more groups joined in preparedness efforts, it became clear that health care and public health would be the "first responders" to a bioterrorism attack (CDC, 2000; Gwerder et al., 2001). Following the 1998 Presidential Decision Directive 62, federal agencies were mandated to coordinate planning efforts with health care and public health rather than only with traditional first-responder groups (CDC, 2000; Malone, 1999).

These events resulted in a shifting of priority for bioterrorism education from traditional first responders to health care and public health (bioterrorism "first responders"). However, even when health care became the focus of these new bioterrorism preparedness initiatives, nursing was neglected. Physicians were the first group to be prioritized for bioterrorism education. Physicians probably were targeted first because many experts postulate that primary care providers most likely will be the first to identify a bioterrorism attack in the community (American Academy of Pediatrics, 2000; Gerberding et al., 2002; Meyer & Morse, 2002; Patt & Feigin, 2002). This implies, however, that nurses are not considered primary care providers or that their bioterrorism preparedness is less important than physicians'.

The fact that nurse practitioners function as primary care providers has not been addressed in the literature; physicians still are considered frontline in health care bioterrorism preparedness by most planning agencies

(American Academy of Pediatrics, 2000; Gerberding et al., 2002; Meyer & Morse, 2002; Patt & Feigin, 2002). No articles specifically address the role of nurse practitioners in bioterrorism preparedness, and only a few articles use the broad term *primary care provider* or *clinician* that would encompass nurse practitioners (Bernardo, 2001; CDC, 2000; Schultz, Mothershead, & Field, 2002).

Other subsets of nursing also were excluded from the designation *primary care provider* or *frontline workers* for bioterrorism preparedness. This was demonstrated during Phase I of the smallpox vaccination that took place in winter and spring of 2003. The primary groups targeted in Phase I were hospital emergency department and public health department employees (CDC, 2002; Wharton, Chorba, Vogt, Morse, & Buehler, 2003). Although this group includes emergency department nurses, it still excludes other nursing primary care providers such as those in occupational health departments, schools, and physician's offices. Although experts have long asserted that a bioterrorism attack is most likely to be identified by a primary care provider who encounters a patient who has suspicious symptomatology, nursing has not been included in these categories of primary care provider or frontline worker.

In addition to the late inclusion in targeted bioterrorism education, another disadvantage to not being considered primary care providers or frontline workers in the bioterrorism preparedness battle is that nursing has been excluded from the majority of funding opportunities. As mentioned previously, the original funding was aimed at traditional first responders. As the political climate evolved and health care and public health became the primary focus for bioterrorism education, funding shifted to public health and hospital preparedness (Fee & Brown, 2001; Sidel, Cohen, & Gould, 2001). Of the funding allotted for primary care provider education, little or none targeted the profession of nursing. This lack of financial support may be another influencing factor for the early reluctance of nurses to join bioterrorism preparedness efforts.

Another potential influencing factor on nurses' decisions to become better prepared for bioterrorism and emerging infections is a lack of personal perceived risk. Two articles presenting the findings from a national needs assessment and risk perception survey (Shadel, Chen, et al., 2004; Shadel, Rebmann, et al., 2003) found that although the majority of infection control and public health professionals (many of which are nurses) reported that they believed that a bioterrorism attack was likely to happen somewhere in the United States within the next 5 years, few reported that they believed it was likely to occur in their community. This research suggests that although nurses have an increased risk perception of bioterrorism, they do not perceive it as a legitimate threat to their own community. Whether these health care professionals recognize the potential global threat of a bioterrorism attack using an infectious disease, regardless of where the attack is originated, is not known. It appears as though they perceive other communities to be at risk but do not realize the potential impact on their own community if infected individuals visit their area or if community members are exposed to infectious disease when traveling.

Adult learning theory seems to support this hypothesis about the positive relationship between risk perception and engaging in preparedness efforts. This theory has asserted, "adults will commit to learning when the goals and objectives are considered realistic and important to them. Application in the 'real world' is important and relevant to the adult learner's personal and professional needs" (Speck, 1996, p. 1). In other words, adults do not learn topics that they do not perceive to be personally relevant. Because research has indicated that nurses do not believe that bioterrorism is likely to affect their community, one can deduce from adult learning theory that this means that these nurses will not voluntarily seek out education on bioterrorism preparedness or participate in bioterrorism simulation exercises (Helget & Smith, 2002; Rose & Larrimore, 2002; Shadel, Clements, et al., 2001).

Other potential influencing factors include a lack of motivation, time, or administrative support. Do nurses believe emergency preparedness is important but relegate it as a lower priority than more tangible, pressing issues, such as preparing for a Joint Commission on Accreditation of Healthcare Organizations (JCAHO) survey? Perhaps nurses consider bioterrorism preparedness essential but lack the time or financial and administrative support to participate in such endeavors. These are potential factors that may affect nursing bioterrorism preparedness negatively, but they have never been studied.

On the opposite end of the spectrum are the potential influencing factors that may result in nurses' decisions to engage in bioterrorism preparedness initiatives rather than to avoid them. One such example is the political pressures applied by regulatory agencies. Many health care facilities have been threatened with the "stick" of being cited for deficiencies by regulatory agencies, such as JCAHO, if compliance is not met (American Hospital Association, 2000). Bioterrorism preparedness

in the form of revised JCAHO standards has occurred in response to social and political pressures to prepare U.S. health care facilities to respond effectively to a bioterrorism attack. From a nursing administrator perspective, adherence to these new standards may be a potential threat, or stick, if compliance is not met.

Although some specialties of nursing, such as administrators, may view regulatory mandates as a stick, others consider it an incentive, or "carrot." Some departments, such as infection control, may benefit from the addition of bioterrorism standards. This assumes, of course, that hospital administrators financially support the development of these bioterrorism preparedness strategies in order to meet the new JCAHO standards. This could result in additional funding for infection control and other nursing departments. Whether a carrot or a stick, regulatory mandate of preparedness efforts should result in better bioterrorism preparedness for nurses.

Unfortunately, all of the aforementioned potential influencing factors that may affect a nurse's decision to become better prepared for bioterrorism or emerging infections are simply educated guesses. Little or empirical data exist on which to base these assumptions. The reasons nurses choose not to engage in bioterrorism preparedness activities must be discovered so that they can be addressed. It is unfortunate that these questions are not being studied, because answering these questions is critical to determine why subsets of nurses are not pursuing preparedness initiatives.

Despite these potential influencing factors, or perhaps because of them, nursing as a profession has embraced the need for bioterrorism preparedness slowly. In the process, nursing professional organizations, conferences, and journals have begun addressing bioterrorism and emerging infections preparedness issues. Although the profession of nursing as a whole has taken on the challenge of bioterrorism preparedness, many individual nurses still are not participating in a full range of bioterrorism preparedness initiatives.

The problem with this is that nurses do not function in a vacuum. The preparedness of a facility or community depends on its employees' and members' level of preparedness. Emergency preparedness for bioterrorism, emerging infections, or other disasters is a cooperative initiative. All health professions will be required to work together if they hope to mount an effective response to a bioterrorism attack or outbreak of an emerging infectious disease. Furthermore, health care and public health will be required to work collaboratively with outside agencies, such as local, state, and federal law enforcement, fire protection, emergency medical services, and a host of other responding agencies.

Nurses will play an integral role in the response to a bioterrorism attack or outbreak of an emerging infection. Nurses must take responsibility for becoming better prepared. This is important not only to protect the safety of patients, patients' families, visitors, and staff but also to protect nurses' families and themselves.

The SARS outbreak emphasized the need for nurses to become prepared for major outbreaks of infectious diseases. Severe acute respiratory syndrome spread rapidly through households and health care settings, most notably hospitals (CDC, 2003a; Grow & Rubinson, 2003). In Canada, 40% of SARS infections occurred in health care workers, and nurses were one of the most frequently affected groups (Health Canada, 2003a). Experts postulate that nurses' SARS infections were related to two factors: (1) nurses' frequent and prolonged contact with infected patients and (2) the lack of or improper implementation of infection control procedures (Farquharson & Baguley, 2003; Health Canada, 2003a). To some extent, nurses cannot control the amount of time they spend with infectious patients, but they can protect their families and themselves by becoming familiar with proper infection control procedures and strictly adhering to such.

More stringent adherence to basic infection control practices is a necessity for all nurses, during day-to-day duties and following an outbreak of an infectious disease. Research has indicated that most health care providers, including nurses, are lax when it comes to following proper infection control. Proper hand hygiene is the single best infection control practice for controlling the spread of infectious diseases in any health care setting, yet many nurses do not do it sufficiently or often enough. Hand hygiene studies report bacterial counts ranging from 40,000 to 4.6 million on health care worker's hands, indicating that current hand-washing practices are not adequate (Boyce & Pittet, 2002).

Poor hand washing is but one example of poor compliance with basic infection control procedures that prevents the spread of disease. Another practice, respiratory hygiene, is especially important for preventing the spread of diseases in the health care setting and protecting oneself from illness. Respiratory etiquette consists of a series of infection control measures that are implemented as soon as a potentially infectious patient is encountered. Examples of respiratory etiquette interventions include covering one's nose and mouth when sneezing or coughing, the wearing of masks, and hand hygiene after contact with such a patient.

Appropriate hand hygiene and respiratory etiquette are but two components of proper infection control. Other important infection control procedures include rapid recognition of potentially infectious patients and immediate placement in appropriate isolation. Infection control and prevention strategies are critical components of preparedness for bioterrorism and emerging infections. Strict adherence to infection control will protect nurses from infectious diseases and decrease the spread of illness in all health care settings.

Every nurse must accept the personal responsibility of becoming better prepared to recognize and respond to a bioterrorism attack or outbreak of an emerging infectious disease. A better response to such an attack will result in better outcomes, including decreased morbidity, mortality, and associated costs. Bioterrorism preparedness is the responsibility of all nurses, and nurses must embrace this area of study as they have all other components of nursing science. This not only will enhance hospital and community preparedness but also will contribute to the protection of nurses' family and themselves.

REFERENCES

Altman, L., & Kolata, G. (2002, January 8). Anthrax missteps offer guide to fight next bioterror battle. *The New York Times*, p. 1.

American Academy of Pediatrics. (2000). Chemical-biological terrorism impact on children: A subject review. *Pediatrics, 105*, 662-670.

American Hospital Association. (2000). *Hospital preparedness for mass casualties*. Retrieved March 2, 2004, from http://www.mipt.org/pdf/aha082000062001.pdf/search=american%20hospital%20associatio

Bernardo, L. M. (2001). Pediatric implications in bioterrorism. Part 1: Physiologic and psychosocial differences. *International Journal of Trauma Nursing, 7*, 14-16.

Boyce, J. M., & Pittet, D. (2002). Guideline for hand hygiene in health-care settings. *American Journal of Infection Control, 30*(8), S1-S46.

Burkle, F. M., Jr. (2002). Mass casualty management of a large-scale bioterrorist event: An epidemiological approach that shapes triage decisions. *Emergency Medicine Clinics of North America, 20*(2), 409-436.

Centers for Disease Control and Prevention. (2000). Biological and chemical terrorism: Strategic plan for preparedness and response: Recommendations of the CDC Strategic Planning Workgroup. *Morbidity and Mortality Weekly Report, 49*, 1-14.

Centers for Disease Control and Prevention. (2002). *Supplemental guidance for planning and implementing the*

National Smallpox Vaccination Program. Retrieved December 10, 2004, from http://www.bt.cdc.gov/agent/smallpox/vaccination/pdf/supplemental-guidance-nsvp.pdf

Centers for Disease Control and Prevention. (2003a). Cluster of severe acute respiratory syndrome cases among protected health-care workers—Toronto, Canada, April 2003. *Morbidity and Mortality Weekly Report, 52,* 433-436.

Centers for Disease Control and Prevention (2003b). Update: Outbreak of severe acute respiratory syndrome—Worldwide, 2003. *Morbidity and Mortality Weekly Report, 52*(12), 241-248.

Evans, A. S., & Brachman, P. S. (1989). *Bacterial infections of humans: Epidemiology and control.* New York City: Plenum Medical Book Company.

Farquharson, C., & Baguley, K. (2003). Responding to the severe acute respiratory syndrome (SARS) outbreak: Lessons learned in a Toronto emergency department. *Journal of Emergency Nursing, 29,* 222-228.

Fee, E., & Brown, T. M. (2001). Preemptive biopreparedness: Can we learn anything from history? *American Journal of Public Health, 91,* 721-725.

Gerberding, J. L., Hughes, J. M., & Koplan, J. P. (2002). Bioterrorism preparedness and response: Clinicians and public health agencies as essential partners. *Journal of the American Medical Association, 287,* 898-900.

Grow, R. W., & Rubinson, L. (2003). The challenge of hospital infection control during a response to bioterrorist attacks. *Biosecurity and Bioterrorism: Biodefense Strategy, Practice, and Science, 1,* 215-220.

Gwerder, L. J., Beaton, R., & Daniell, W. (2001). Implications for the occupational and environmental health nurse. *American Association of Occupational Health Nurses Journal, 49,* 512-518.

Health Canada. (2003a). Anatomy of an outbreak. In *Learning from SARS renewal of public health in Canada* (pp. 23-42). Retrieved March 7, 2004, from http://www.phac-aspc.gc.ca/publicat/sars-sras/naylor/2_e.html

Health Canada. (2003b). Building capacity and coordination: National infectious disease surveillance, outbreak management, and emergency response. In *Learning from SARS renewal of public health in Canada* (pp. 91-112). Retrieved March 7, 2004, from http://www.phac-aspc.gc.ca/publicat/sars-sras/naylor/5_e.html

Helget, V., & Smith, P. W. (2002). Bioterrorism preparedness: A survey of Nebraska health care institutions. *American Journal of Infection Control, 30,* 46-48.

Henning, K. J., Brennan, P. J., Hoegg, C., O'Rourke, E., Dyer, B. D., & Grace, T. L. (2004). Health system preparedness for bioterrorism: Bringing the tabletop to the hospital. *Infection Control & Hospital Epidemiology, 25*(2), 146-155.

Jones, T. (2002). Bioterrorism preparedness: What progress has Congress made since September, 2001? *Policy, Procedures and Nursing Practice, 3,* 217-219.

Kaufmann, A. F., Meltzer, M. I., & Schmid, G. P. (1997). The economic impact of a bioterrorist attack: Are prevention and postattack intervention programs justifiable? *Emerging Infectious Diseases, 3,* 83-94.

Malone, B. L. (1999). Nursing's response to the use of weapons of mass destruction. *1999 ANA House of Delegates.* Retrieved July 9, 2003, from http://www.nursingworld.org/about/summary/sum99/weapons.htm

Meyer, R. F., & Morse, S. A. (2002). Bioterrorism preparedness for the public health and medical communities. *Mayo Clinic Proceedings, 77,* 619-621.

Morse, A. (2002). Bioterrorism preparedness for local health departments. *Journal of Community Health Nursing, 19,* 203-211.

O'Connell, K. P., Menuey, B. C., & Foster, D. (2002). Issues in preparedness for biological terrorism: A perspective for critical care nursing. *AACN Clinical Issues, 13,* 452-469.

Patt, H. A., & Feigin, R. D. (2002). Diagnosis and management of suspected cases of bioterrorism: A pediatric perspective. *Pediatrics, 109,* 685-692.

Peralta, L. A. (2000). Bioterrorism: An overview. *Seminars in Perioperative Nursing, 9,* 3-10.

Rose, M. A., & Larrimore, K. L. (2002). Knowledge and awareness concerning chemical and biological terrorism: Continuing education implications. *Journal of Continuing Education, 33,* 253-258.

Salazar, M. K., & Kelman, B. (2002). Planning for biological disasters: Occupational health nurses as "first responders." *American Association of Occupational Health Nurses Journal, 50,* 174-181.

Schultz, C. H., Mothershead, J. L., & Field, M. (2002). Bioterrorism preparedness I: The emergency department and hospital. *Emergency Medical Clinics of North America, 20,* 437-455.

Shadel, B. N., Chen, J. J., Newkirk, R., Lawrence, S., Clements, B. W., & Evans, R. G. (2004). Bioterrorism risk perceptions and educational needs of public health professionals before and after September 11th, 2001: A national needs assessment survey. *Journal of Public Health Management Practice, 10*(4), 282-289.

Shadel, B. N., Clements, B., Arndt, B., Rebmann, T., & Evans, R. G. (2001). What we need to know about bioterrorism preparedness: Results from focus groups conducted at APIC 2000. *American Journal of Infection Control, 29,* 347-351.

Shadel, B. N., Rebmann, T., Clements, B., Chen, J. J., & Evans, R. G. (2003). Infection control practitioners' perceptions and educational needs regarding bioterrorism: Results from a national needs assessment survey. *American Journal of Infection Control, 31,* 129-134.

Sidel, V. W., Cohen, H. W., & Gould, R. M. (2001). Good intentions and the road to bioterrorism preparedness. *American Journal of Public Health, 91,* 716-717.

Speck, M. (1996). Adult learning theory *ERS Spectrum,* 33-41. Retrieved July 25, 2003, from http://www.ncrel.org/sdrs/areas/issues/methods/technlgy/te10lk12.htm

U.S. General Accounting Office. (2003). *Bioterrorism: Public health response to anthrax incidents of 2001* (GAO-04-152). Washington, DC: Author.

Weil, K. M. (2003). Lockdown: A bioterrorism drill provides valuable information. *American Journal of Nursing, 103*(4), 64CC-64GG.

Wharton, M., Chorba, T. L., Vogt, R. L., Morse, D. L., & Buehler, J. W. (2003). Case definitions for public health surveillance. *Morbidity & Mortality Weekly Report, 39,* 1-43.

Nursing Care

Combat—Jungles to Deserts

CATHERINE H. ABRAMS

Each nation presents distinct challenges to the nursing profession when practice is moved from the controlled atmospheres of hospitals, clinics, and the home to the battlefield. However, several factors remain constant even when the arena in which nursing is practiced is changed. In addition, nurses must adjust their personal and professional lives to deal with the magnitude of care being delivered in a distinctly different and stressful way. This chapter discusses the environmental, cultural, technological, clinical, and psychological demands of combat nursing with emphasis on the most recent involvement of the United States in the jungles and the desert.

BACKGROUND

The scope and impact of nursing involvement in combat advanced with the coming of the industrial and technological ages. "Women have served in many roles throughout American history" (Wertheimer, 2005) but were not given an official role until the formation of the Army Nurse Corps in 1901 and the Navy Nurse Corps in 1908. Evidence of the changing face of nursing involvement is that although 350,000 women currently are serving in the U.S. military, the majority serve in nonnursing capacities. One in every seven military personnel serving in Iraq is a woman. Contrast that with Vietnam when women composed less than 3% of U.S. military personnel who served, and 80% to 90% of that total number was Navy, Air Force, or Army nurses.

In the March 2005 *Journal of Advanced Nursing*, Elizabeth A. Scannell-Desch, PhD, RN, suggests that much can be learned from the experiences of those who have served to prepare those who will. She emphasizes the need for nurses to be proactive in preparing themselves for this role and that the organizations sending them use programs that are intensive and realistic to assist with that preparation.

ENVIRONMENTAL DEMANDS

Not a great deal has been written about how the daily tactics and operations of war affect the environment and therefore those who live in it. One study done in 2004, *The Environmental Impacts of the Gulf War, 1991,* does explore the impact of the burning of the oil wells in Kuwait and the change in climate in many Arab nations (Linden, Jernelov, & Egerup, 2004). The use of Agent Orange to deforest Vietnam has been studied and documented within military service organizations (Veterans Health Administration, 2005). Depending on where troops were stationed during their time "in country" or the direction of the wind on any given day, there was always a chance for exposure. This exposure was something that would not manifest itself for many years to come and sometimes with devastating consequences. The impact of war on the environment is just one piece of the stress on nurses during combat.

Additionally, when traveling to a foreign country, one must prepare oneself for the weather and take time to acclimate to the new environment. Many times when nurses arrived in country, they were given 24 hours to sleep and then were expected to report for duty. Once the tour began, the expectation was that one worked as many hours as were needed to serve the wounded. This gave little time for the body to adjust in Vietnam to the pollution in the air, the extreme heat, the continuous monsoons, or even the cold.

Other environmental concerns come back to personal health. Traditionally, nurses have proved to be adaptable to whatever situation in which they are placed. They always focus on the purpose they have for being in the country and try hard to understand the impact of the environment on their ability to perform effectively. In most foreign countries, it takes time to adapt to the local water and food. Things such as taking purified water for granted and assuming that the food one eats would be prepared properly suddenly requires mental adjustments and a new awareness and vigilance. Many nurses experienced gastrointestinal upsets before learning what and where to eat or drink.

Finally, serving in a jungle or desert exposes individuals to diseases that have long been under control in the United States or other industrialized nations. This requires vaccinations and extreme attention to symptoms that could arise. In Vietnam, for diseases such as malaria to become an issue was not uncommon. Preventative mechanisms and medications were provided, but still this could not keep everyone 100% safe.

Certain predators also changed their habits based on the changing conditions during war. Examples would be the increased sighting of tigers in Vietnam and the fact that sharks entered the rivers of Iraq to feed. Both occurrences would be unusual expectations or outcomes of a major conflict. This again presents adjustments for the nurses who serve. Truly, this just added another dimension to being in a strange place, working under tiring conditions, and not knowing for sure where one could go or what one might encounter. The stress could be difficult for many.

In Iraq, Dr. Doug Rokke, former director of the Army depleted uranium project, said, "Today's troops have been fighting on land polluted with chemical, biological and radioactive weapon residue from the first Gulf War and its aftermath" (Rosenfeld, 2003). The symptoms of this exposure did manifest fairly soon and often at times with horrible consequences. In 1997, efforts were made to secure predeployment and postdeployment physicals, including blood specimens, for all soldiers. This was not done, and instead the troops were asked to fill out a questionnaire.

CULTURAL DEMANDS

Every nurse who has served in a foreign country is taught before arrival that initially one must learn to understand the culture of the land where one will be practicing. This is important not only because at times one will have to obtain needed supplies and equipment from a local market but also because one will have to preserve relationships with the government of the home country. All branches of the military prepare nurses to function in a combat situation through training and simulations of field conditions at bases in the United States. These simulations offer interaction with the culture as it has come to be known through others who served previously. In some cases, "nationals" (individuals identified by the military to be capable of interpreting language and culture) are brought to the states to participate and increase the reality and value of this work.

The culture of a country also dictates how one will act when moving about in the local economy. Understanding the cultural aspects and customs allows one to be safe and not to instigate interactions that cause more harm than anticipated. One aspect of life in the Middle East is that women do not walk outside without their faces and heads covered. Therefore military women and nurses also must ensure that they do the same. It has been reported that when the nurses would go to town unveiled, the Arab men would pinch them, not because they were trying to be fresh, but because they disapproved of women who were not veiled. Another Middle Eastern concept that is difficult for some is "women should be seen and not heard." After all of the assertiveness training for nurses during the 1970s and 1980s, it was a difficult adjustment not to respond or to follow rather than direct.

Nurses in Vietnam dealt with a custom that if one person went to the hospital, the entire family went to the hospital. It was not uncommon to approach the bed of a patient and find it difficult to determine just who required care. Instead, the whole family would be on the bed with other members possibly sleeping beneath the bed. This group would stay the entire course of care because most had traveled a great distance and did not wish to return home until the patient was well enough to go with them.

The language barrier made providing participatory care difficult. Interpreters were helpful to have when they were available. However, depending on a family member to interpret for one was dangerous. One's communication may be relayed completely the opposite of what was intended, and it was difficult to verify for accuracy. This then led to misinterpretations and unanticipated outcomes.

According to Dr. Elizabeth A. Scannell-Desch (2005), many nurses believed that peacetime military personnel exist so that they can "transfer that learning to the wartime environment." If that is the case, then training about the culture of the home country and how to act and respond is important and must be provided.

TECHNOLOGICAL DEMANDS

Technology has added new dimensions to combat nursing just as it has to the current nursing practice occurring stateside. Many technological ideas could have come from the improvisation of nurses in combat as they struggled to provide the best care for the sick and wounded. Technology also has helped nurses to keep in touch with their families and friends at home. This has helped ease some of the separation anxieties that are common.

In previous war zones, one often had to be independent of technology because it just did not exist. Adjusting practice from a hospital in the United States to a field hospital or evacuation hospital often meant that the nurse would have to improvise. Rather than having suction machines for nasogastric tubes, it might have been necessary to use bottles, establish a vacuum, and ensure that gravity would assist with the drainage. This type of nursing often took one back to the basics of training and forced the nurse to remember all pertinent anatomy, physiology, and sometimes microbiology. The development of sound, critical thinking skills helped even the most experienced nurse to function under the pressures of caring for combat casualties.

One improvisation I remember from service in Vietnam is using a Waterpik (Waterpik Technologies, Newport Beach, California) to clean wounds. We discovered shortly after my arrival in country that we were not able to clean injuries that were incurred in the rice paddies or on the dirt trails well enough to ensure that they would heal properly. One of our surgeons suggested using a pump with some sort of pressure to truly get all of the debris out of the injured body part before beginning a procedure. Once we had tried that, we then decided to add a broad-spectrum antibiotic to the chamber from which we were pumping to assist with healing. Seeing that this would aid the healing process, several of us then called home and asked all of our families to send us Waterpiks because we knew that we could sterilize the chamber and improvise with sterile tubing. We were actually able to follow several of our patients as they were transferred to other bases to receive further care before going home. The follow-up validated that our improvisation had improved the care and aided in the healing process, thus eliminating the need for multiple surgeries.

CLINICAL DEMANDS

Every nurse brings a set of clinical skills to any position where hired to serve. This is no different for nurses who serve in a combat situation. The clinical skills needed are no different from those of the emergency room nurse or the operating room nurse practicing in a noncombat situation. The hospitals or aide stations of the field are set up in a similar fashion to any other institution.

War only brings the need for quick triage and superior patient flow because of the severity of the injuries.

Whether in a jungle or desert, the most important thing for any nurse is to be self-assured and able to use the skills and talents with which they have prepared themselves for this role. One also must know one's limitations while being open to learning new skills and developing new abilities. Nurses in any battlefield situation are presented with terrible things. Coping with that reality and acknowledging it before it happens will make the task easier in many ways.

Those who had the most difficulty were those who had just completed nursing school, and this was the first duty assignment they had. Many had taken advantage of the specialty training the military offered and were able to build their professional skills with that focus. The training, such as operating room nurse training, also had components specific to combat situations and therefore aided in the preparation of nurses to serve. No matter what role one played, having solid clinical abilities allowed a higher level of functioning in this arena.

PSYCHOLOGICAL DEMANDS

Often overlooked is that those who have served in a medical capacity during a time of war experience the same emotional and psychological ramifications as those who were involved directly in combat. Coupled with this is that until recently, many returning from war were greeted with a hostile response from the general public, thus forcing any feelings they may have had to be locked inside rather than being shared.

The fact that many of the nurses were so close to the age of their patients during Vietnam and the Middle East wars made caring for those with such life-changing injuries even more difficult. Many found themselves in the role of supporter and nurturer in addition to being a nurse. Nurses would cope with these feelings in various ways from spending off-duty time with the soldiers to volunteering to work with the civilians of the country where they were serving. This allowed the nurses to find meaning in what they were doing while continuing to be faced with the negative feedback coming from the United States (National Center for Post-Traumatic Stress Disorder & Walter Reed Army Medical Center, 2004).

Showing an emotional or psychological response to the accumulation of events and the terrible wounds with which nurses were presented was interpreted as a lack of competence or lacking the emotional strength "military" nurses must possess to be successful. For many, not having the ability to express these feelings or sharing experiences with others led to continued problems when they returned home. "This is manifested by such common things as anxiety and depression; sleep disturbances and difficulties with trust in close relationships" (Leon, 2004). Leon reported in a study conducted in 1993 to assess the prepsychological and postpsychological functioning of Vietnam-era nurses that the current status of these nurses was "in the normal range." What that really means is that some still struggle with the day-to-day functions and with moving beyond the effects of dealing with the experiences they faced. Some have coped with little support. A correlation is suggested between a person's psychological functioning before participating in care delivery during war and the manner in which they dealt with these experiences.

Those who were able to develop positive coping skills were able to express their feelings while in the situation, use humor to soften emotions, or to find meaning in situations. These veterans had less difficulty returning to the life they had before service. Those who used negative coping skills such as blaming themselves for being there, for being what they were or doing what they did, withdrawing from all social contacts, and carrying around thoughts of fear for their own safety still may be trying to find that "normal" state for themselves.

Gloria R. Leon sites several studies on Vietnam and Israeli combat soldiers that have shown "how vital social support is in coping with combat situations" (Leon, 2004). The amount of exposure to traumatic wounds seen each day for hours on end also made a difference in one's ability to move positively through the experience. Even though most nurses were not in the middle of the actual fighting, they did deal with the end results. Many were sustained because they were able to recognize that their presence and their ability to provide care and comfort gave meaning to what they were witnessing. Those who used humor to cope were sometimes met with social disapproval and the feeling that they were somehow cold and callous. The advent of the television show *M*A*S*H* eased some of this because the reality of what nurses and doctors were living through while in combat was understood better.

Separation from family and friends, with the knowledge that one would not be coming home for at least 1 year, also presented challenges (Busuttil & Busuttil, 2001). The feeling of missing out on special occasions or events could lead to feelings of inadequacy or that one was "letting your family down." Those who were able to form a new wartime "family" dealt with the entire experience more successfully than those who chose isolation and introspection. These issues remained the same during the Gulf War but some of the hostilities experienced by Vietnam participants are not being felt by the military today because of more public support. This may change as the war in Iraq lingers and has the potential to become another drawn out process similar to Vietnam.

Nursing care delivery occurs in many settings, each with its own special set of challenges and rewards. Nurses who serve in combat environments are faced with dealing with circumstances and experiences that are not replicated in noncombat medical settings anywhere else in the rest of the world. They not only must consider how to adapt and deal with the environment but also must be attuned to the cultural aspects of the country where they are sent. They must mold their clinical skills to fit different expectations than is the normal during peacetime. In addition, the traumatic nature of the outcomes of war adds another facet with which to deal. These experiences have the potential to change the life pattern and alter an individual's coping skills forever. Much of the negative effects of nursing during combat can be mitigated by intense training before the nurses are placed in the hostile environment, thus giving them an opportunity to develop the needed skills on the personal and professional level before they are needed.

REFERENCES

Busuttil, W., & Busuttil, A. M. C. (2001). Psychological effects on families subjected to enforced and prolonged separations generated under life threatening situations [Special psychological trauma edition]. *Sexual and Relationship Therapy, 16*(3), 207-228.

Leon, G. R. (1993, March). Memories of war: How Vietnam-era nurses are coping today. *USA Today, 121,* 30-31.

Linden, O., Jernelov, A., & Egerup, J. (2004). *The environmental impacts of the Gulf War, 1991* (pp. vii-9). Laxenberg, Austria: International Institute for Applied Systems Analysis.

National Center for Post-Traumatic Stress Disorder & Walter Reed Army Medical Center. (2004). *Iraq War clinician guide* (2nd ed., pp. 19-32). Washington, DC: Department of Veterans Affairs.

Rosenfeld, S. (2003, April 8) *Gulf War Syndrome, the sequel: People are sick over there already.* Retrieved July 27, 2005, from http://www.tompaine.com/feature.cfm/ID/7570%20

Scannell-Desch, E. A. (2005). Lessons learned and advice from Vietnam War nurses: A qualitative study. *Journal of Advanced Nursing, 49*(6), 600.

Veterans Health Administration. (2005). *VHA office of public health and environmental hazards.* Retrieved May 15, 2005, from http://www.va.gov/oaa/pocketcard/vietnam.asp

Wertheimer, L. (2005). *Wounded in war: The women serving in Iraq.* Retrieved May 30, 2005, from http://www.npr.org/templates/story/story.php?storyId=4534450

INTERNATIONAL NURSING

Nursing

A Global View

PERLE SLAVIK COWEN ◆ SUE MOORHEAD

Nursing as a profession increasingly is confronted with the global nature of health care issues. The headlines of the news reporting famine, human immunodeficiency virus/acquired immunodeficiency syndrome (HIV/AIDS), global warming, and violence in many countries are impossible to escape. Issues facing the nursing profession are also inescapable: nursing shortages, changes in educational programs, and the aging of nurses themselves are common themes. Since the third edition of *Current Issues in Nursing* published in 1990, this book has focused on international chapters about nursing and health care in other countries. In the last edition, published in 2001, the chapters on international nursing were grouped together in the final section of the book. This edition continues that tradition and has added a new chapter on the Gambia. As the globalization of health care grows, a review of nursing and health care issues around the world seems a fitting way to end the book. Unlike the other sections of this book, there is no debate chapter to lead off this section. The chapters themselves allow for discussion and comparison and provide a platform for debate about whether health care should be nationalized or privatized or whether health care should be paid for by the government or by consumers themselves. We thank the authors who were willing to update their chapters to provide a continued overview of nursing and health care in these countries. Space limitations continue to allow us to include only a small number of countries, selected for diversity.

The chapter on Southern Africa by Seloilloe and Tlou focuses on the health care issues of fourteen African countries that make up the Southern African Development Community. These are Angola, Botswana, Democratic Republic of Congo, Lesotho, Malawi, Mauritius, Mozambique, Namibia, Seychelles, South Africa, Swaziland, Tanzania, Zambia, and Zimbabwe. Nurses in these countries provide the initial point of entry to the health care system. The major constraints

to health care for individuals and families are conflict and war, poverty, lack of autonomy for women, especially related to use of contraceptives, and the HIV/AIDS epidemic. Southern Africa remains the worst-affected subregion in the world for HIV/AIDS. Many pregnant women (more than 30%) are HIV-positive and have great chances of passing on the infection to their children. This disease is wiping out the gains made in life expectancy during the past decades in some of the countries, with some of these countries having life expectancies of only 40 years. These authors report that about 50% of hospital beds in the medical and pediatric wards in urban and rural areas are occupied by persons with HIV-related illnesses. Additional adverse effects of the disease are an increase in infections, unavailability of hospital beds, and increases in suicide rates. Nurses in Africa are extending their traditional roles to respond to the needs of the communities, and nursing education has integrated the concepts of primary care, public health, and community health. Seloilloe and Tlou conclude their chapter by outlining present and future challenges for nursing in the Southern African Development Community. These include shortages of nursing personnel, limited nursing research opportunities, risk of HIV/AIDS, and the need to mainstream a woman's perspective in health care. They state that a strong national nurses association is needed, as is proper legislation relating to nursing and nurse-midwifery. This is a fact-filled chapter that demonstrates well the enormous challenges facing nurses in this part of the world.

The next chapter moves us closer to the United States and provides a description of the health care system of our neighbor to the north, Canada. Ross-Kerr describes the Canadian health care system, which is neither free enterprise medicine nor socialized medicine and includes universal coverage for all persons, comprehensiveness of medically necessary services, accessibility of health services to all segments of the population, portability of coverage from one province to another, and public administration of the program at the provincial level. Ross-Kerr traces the development of health care in Canada from the 1800s to the present. Recently, the Supreme Court of Canada upheld the right of individuals to hold private insurance to receive timely care for health problems where access to care was problematic. This chapter provides an overview of the tax-supported system that has evolved over 45 years. Today, the limits to the system are recognized, as is the fact that some reform is needed. Approximately 75% of health expenditures are paid for by Medicare. The Canadian system has been built primarily around medical service in hospitals, with 63% of nurses practicing in acute care facilities. Emphasis, however, on maintaining patients in community-based settings is growing, stressing prevention, and health promotion and workforce trends show that the number of nurses working in tertiary care has declined over the last decade. An escalating nursing shortage is predicted over the next decade, influenced by the aging nurse workforce. Nursing graduates continue to migrate to the United States and other countries, where salaries, benefits, and the working environments are better. The Canadian education system for nurses is much like but lags behind that in the United States, with a total of eight doctoral programs now available. This chapter provides an excellent overview of the differences and similarities of the health care systems of the United States.

In the third chapter, Clark gives an overview of the past and present changes in health care and nursing in Great Britain. Her chapter demonstrates two great influences on health care and nursing in Great Britain: the past and the political party. According to Clark, many of the organizational anomalies and traditions that shape the present day system are relics of the past. The National Health System, formed in 1948, nationalized many existing services with several core values: universality, comprehensiveness, and no cost at the point of use. Currently, the British health care system is financed 95% by taxes and 5% by co-payments from patients. The government is the only third-party payer in the system. Expenditures have doubled during the past 8 years to approximately 8.4% of the gross domestic product, and this is predicted to rise to 9.2% by 2007-2008. Even with this rise, however, the cost is still barely half of the expenditure in the United States. Changes in the reigning political party bring sweeping reforms in health care. The health care systems of the four countries of the United Kingdom gradually have diverged, although the core principles of a comprehensive health care system, funded by general taxation, provided to all citizens based on clinical need, and free of charge at the point of use remain sacrosanct. Most health care is provided through the National Health System, but there is a private hospital sector and a private nursing home sector. Britain is probably the only country in the world in which at the point of initial qualification a nurse is a specialist rather than a generalist. Most nurses work for the National Health Service, but a growing number work in the private sector. Nursing education is undergoing many changes, with slow movement toward baccalaureate education. Interestingly, no nurse practice acts define the work of nurses in Great Britain, but regulation of health care providers is currently under review. This chapter is filled with many interesting facts and provides a good overview of the changes and challenges faced by the nursing profession in Great Britain, a country where history is a major influence. As Clark states, "these are turbulent times for nursing in Great Britain."

In Japan, the only Asian country in this world tour, the aging of the population, a movement toward community-based nursing, and the increasing number of nurses with baccalaureate and graduate degrees are improving the status of nursing. Takahashi and Brandi begin their chapter with an overview of the health care environment and the Japanese health care system. Some major challenges Japan has had to confront include a rapidly aging population and low birthrate; a stagnant economy; new infectious diseases such as sudden acute respiratory syndrome; and natural disasters (earthquakes, typhoons, and volcanic eruptions), all of which have been influencing health care and nursing significantly. Japanese citizens lead the world in life expectancy. The four leading causes of death in 2003 were malignant neoplasms, heart diseases, cerebrovascular diseases, and pneumonia. The overall health status of the Japanese is believed to be the best in the world. Health policy in Japan has been successful regarding standards of access, cost, and fairness. The Japanese health care system is dealing with two major challenges: cost containment and responding to the public demand for quality. Public and community health centers are integral parts of the health care system. The extended family system has shifted to a smaller nuclear family, and more elderly are living independently. There are three types of nurses, each with separate licensure. The nursing educational system is complex, and there is a major push for baccalaureate and higher degree education for nurses. In 2004, there were 25 doctoral programs in nursing; however, most graduate programs had a shortage of qualified faculty. Takahashi and Brandi provide an excellent overview of nursing practice and education in Japan, and this chapter provides an interesting comparison with other chapters in this section.

Latin America is the next stop on this tour of nursing around the globe. This chapter by de Villalobos provides an overview of another rapidly changing health care system. The vast expanse of the American continent known as Latin America extends from Mexico to Tierra del Fuego (Argentina) and is home to a host of ethnic, ecological, and economic contrasts, health being no exception. For example, consider the stark contrast in the wealth and development of southern Brazil compared with that of Haiti, believed to have the lowest standard of living in the world. Since the 1980s, Latin America has been immersed in crises involving politics, disasters, and violence. Every country in Latin America has made or is planning to make sweeping changes. Some progress has been made, including a decline in maternal and neonatal morbidity statistics, a reduction in childhood disease, and an increase in family planning. However, these changes in the right direction have not eliminated problems associated with the appearance of degenerative illnesses, chronic diseases, aging, and those conditions caused by violence of every type, drug addiction, and the physical and emotional consequences of natural disasters. Nursing in Latin America varies by country, but in all countries the challenges for the nursing profession are great, and sweeping changes are the norm. Nurses who are in short supply are being replaced by assistants. De Villalobos gives an overview of the differences in the various nursing education programs. Education is the most advanced in Brazil and Columbia, with Brazil having the largest number of undergraduate and graduate programs. A great need exists for more continuing education programs throughout all the countries. The author ends her chapter citing three challenges for the immediate future: to generate continuing practice for the services nurses offer; to have this continuity between education and practice reflected in education for nurses overall; and to establish new rules for those who deliver service. Each of these challenges involves change. The author provides an excellent summary of the many challenges faced by nurses and the nursing profession in Latin America.

In the next chapter in this section, we turn our thoughts to a different part of the globe. Smith describes in fascinating detail the current political and economic situation in Russia and, within this context, health care and the role of nursing. Russia, the largest country in the world, continues to experience a negative growth rate and a declining population. Inflation, poverty,

crime, and rising rates of communicable diseases are destroying the hope of the people. Even with some economic growth, 25% of the population of Russia continues to live below the poverty level. Salaries for health care workers, especially nurses, are dreadful. Tax evasion is a major problem, so there is no money for government reform. As many as 15 families living in public housing may share kitchen and toilet facilities. Street children are becoming an increasingly difficult Russian social problem. The estimated number of street children in Moscow is from 30,000 to 50,000, with the majority under the age of 13. Smith details these and many other problems, including the oppression of Russian women. Most Russians view nursing as a low-prestige job. Despite the general oppression of women in Russian society and of nursing as a women's profession, nursing is making some advances. Nursing organizations are beginning to develop, and nursing educational programs are being strengthened. Master's programs have been developed in the past decade, and continuing education, hospital-wide programs have been initiated. East-West collaboration is being promoted. Smith provides a gripping description of nursing and the health care system in Russia today.

The final chapter in this section of international nursing focuses on the Gambia. The Gambia, one of the smallest countries in Africa, supports a rapidly growing population. Located in West Africa where it is bordered by the Atlantic Ocean to the west and Senegal to the north, east, and south, the country historically has been instrumental in fostering the development of the slave trade because of its seaports. The Gambia has numerous ethnic groups, and each group has its own language, but the official language is English. The Gambians are mostly a conservative Muslim people, so health problems such as alcoholism or HIV infection are low compared with South Africa. The country has a severe shortage of nurses and physicians. The rainy season increases the need for health care because it results in epidemic malaria, and the precipitation also results in muddy roads, and travel for care is difficult at best. The four major components of the health care delivery system in the Gambia are central referral hospitals, the village health service, the basic health center, and the divisional health team. A number of pressing health issues in the Gambia are related to cultural beliefs and infectious disease such as trachoma, malaria, helminthic infections, dysenteries, and meningococcal disease, whereas other problems relate to reproductive health and include polygamy, female circumcision, and birth control. State registered nurses work in hospitals, health centers, and dispensaries and complete 3 years of post–high school education. The bachelor of science degree in nursing only recently has been introduced in the Gambia. The demographics of nursing are different from the United States, primarily as they relate to gender. Men are likely to enter nursing as a profession, and there is no stigma of nursing being primarily a women's profession in the Gambia. Nurses are making a major impact on public policy, particularly as it relates to hygiene education and reproductive health. Although the shortages, economic struggles, and tremendous challenges to the health of Gambians are numerous, the people of the Gambia receive free health care, and nurses are the backbone of the Gambian health care system, even though they are in short supply. This chapter provides an interesting contrast to the first chapter

in this section on South Africa and assists the reader in determining the similarities and differences in these two regions of Africa.

As these chapters suggest, the role of nurses is important in health care around the world. In spite of the differences in the health care systems and the conditions under which nurses work, nurses worldwide share common concerns about patient welfare and struggle to advance the profession and the views of nursing to make a positive impact on patient care. Political action continues to be an important part of making these changes. We salute the nurses in so many countries who are helping to make a difference. Global communication makes it possible to learn about the issues in health care in other countries and support the tremendous efforts of nurses worldwide.

CHAPTER
85

Nursing in Southern Africa

An Overview of Health Care, Nursing Education, and Practice

ESTHER SALANG SELOILWE ◆ SHEILA DINOTSHE TLOU

This chapter provides an overview of nursing education and practice in Southern Africa. The chapter analyzes the opportunities, current and future challenges, and issues facing nursing education and practice in Southern Africa. Because Africa is a vast continent with diverse cultures and nursing programs, this chapter cannot possibly cover them all. This chapter confines itself to analyzing health care, nursing education, and nursing practice within the Southern Africa Development Community (SADC).

The SADC is a group of 14 countries in Southern Africa that agreed to collaborate on matters concerning the development of their region. The countries are Angola, Botswana, Democratic Republic of Congo, Lesotho, Malawi, Mauritius, Mozambique, Namibia, Seychelles, South Africa, Swaziland, Tanzania, Zambia, and Zimbabwe. Each country is responsible for the improvement of a particular sector to benefit the whole region; for example, a country may be charged with the responsibility for health of the region and therefore be expected to initiate research and interventions that will improve the health status of all the citizens of the SADC.

HEALTH CARE IN THE SOUTHERN AFRICA DEVELOPMENT COMMUNITY

To appreciate the important role of nursing in the SADC, one needs to understand the health care system of each country, each of which is at a different stage of development and sophistication. All SADC countries, or their colonial rulers, were signatories to the Alma-Ata Declaration of 1978, which committed members to attaining socially acceptable and productive primary health care strategies (WHO-UNICEF, 1978).

Primary health care includes the provision of preventive, curative, and rehabilitative care to individuals and families at an affordable price. This care should be accessible to all age groups, from birth to death. The bulk of this care in these countries is provided by nurses who serve as the first point of contact into the health care delivery systems.

MAJOR CONSTRAINTS TO HEALTH CARE DELIVERY

Some key constraints to health care delivery in this area are conflict and war, poverty, aspects of gender and health, and the human immunodeficiency virus/acquired immunodeficiency syndrome (HIV/AIDS) epidemic.

Conflict and War

Conflict and war situations in some countries in the SADC such as Angola, the Democratic Republic of Congo, and Namibia have diverted funds from national health and social service programs to national defense. As a result, these countries have been plunged into debt, and foreign reserve levels have not enhanced investment. Developed countries with economic and business investments that would help create jobs and boost national economics have lost confidence in countries in the region and consider them more of a liability than an asset. This not only has affected the cash flow and food security at the household level but also has shifted family health-seeking behaviors and practices to food gathering and income-generation activities (Ngcongco, 1995, p. 3). The impact of conflict on the national health care system has been so enormous that formal health care is almost nonexistent in these countries.

Poverty

Poverty is another major health challenge for Southern African countries, and for some it is exacerbated by intercountry strife. All the SADC countries are still at the level of development at which the disease patterns are determined predominantly by poverty, poor nutrition, low levels of education, and conditions inconsistent with health such as poor sanitation and pollution. Even where health services are relatively free, poor families experience real problems when their dependent is referred to a major hospital in another village or town. Surveys among elderly village women in Botswana (Shaibu, 2001; Tlou, 1994), for example, revealed that lack of money was a major deterrent to seeking health care. Although the elderly are not expected to pay consultation and drug fees, they have expenditures connected with unavailability of drugs at the health facility because the drugs have to be bought from a private pharmacy. Referrals for treatment to other health care facilities pose a dilemma such as lack of transportation, which is compounded by the need for food and lodging at the referral center. These expenditures for some persons, especially older women, have meant delaying treatment or not undergoing needed treatment at all.

Gender and Health Aspect

The gender and health aspect involves especially reproductive health. In most SADC societies, women do not have the right to decide on when to have children, on the number of children they want, or on whether to have children at all. Motherhood is seen as destiny, a social responsibility, and a rite of passage into the world of womanhood. The following contribute to women's relatively poor health status: lack of autonomy, discrimination in law enforcement such as the criminalization of abortion, inadequate allocation of health resources, and failure by governments to implement remedial measures sanctioned by international agreements (Mogobe, 2000).

Health and development indicators of the SADC region, such as contraceptive prevalence rate or the percentage of women ages 15 to 49 who currently are using a modern method of contraception, is high. The term *modern* refers to the methods often offered by family planning programs and includes male and female sterilization, intrauterine devices, the pill, injectable hormonal contraceptives, male and female condoms, and female barrier methods such as diaphragms, cervical caps, jellies, creams, and spermicidal foams (Central Medical Statistics, 2001).

In ideal conditions, all women would have access to quality, reliable, and affordable methods of contraception, but in no SADC country are the conditions ideal. Family planning services usually are not woman-friendly and are "demographic targets" to be used by politicians and administrators for seeking rewards for services and targets accomplished. For example, in most countries the number of children that women desire to have is less than the total fertility rate (i.e., the total number of children that a girl will bear if her childbearing follows the current fertility patterns and she lives through her entire childbearing years). Observation indicates that for some countries the total fertility rate approximates the number of children that men desire, indicating that they control and decide on women's fertility.

Several studies have indicated the difficulty these women face in negotiating sexual relationships and that men have the most control over these issues (Fidzani, Ntseane, & Seloilwe, 2000; Molebatsi & Mogobe, 2000). Indeed, in most SADC countries, a woman cannot be sterilized (have a tubal ligation) without the written consent of her husband, but the husband does not need his wife's consent to have a vasectomy. Although no law exists in some countries to demand this, it has been a practice that has been institutionalized and observed. This power and control is so firmly established that even when the woman is not married, her future husband's rights to her fertility are protected, and she is advised simply to use another form of contraception because she might marry and the future husband may desire children (Tlou, 1997).

On the whole, demographic trends indicate improved provision of services for women in all the SADC countries compared with 10 years ago. For example, Mauritius has one of the highest levels of contraceptive use in sub-Saharan Africa, estimated at 75% of all women. Accessibility, availability, and affordability of contraceptives are good, and all health care facilities provide family planning services (Central Medical Statistics, 2000, 2001). Also, in most SADC countries the fertility rates (births per woman) have declined considerably (United Nations, 1995). The decline in fertility rate may be attributed to higher educational achievement by women. All these have contributed to the declining family size and better child spacing. The region still experiences high maternal morbidity and mortality. In some countries, for example, the maternal mortality may be as high as 200 per 1000 births. This calls for a need to train a large number of midwives to address these issues. In some areas in the countries of the SADC

VIEWPOINTS

a doctor has never set foot and health care is provided by nurses. Therefore nurses need to be empowered to deliver the care that is appropriate to the needs of the communities served.

Adolescent fertility is on the increase in some SADC countries, where about 23% of the births are to girls under 18 years of age whose bodies are not yet well developed for childbearing. Adequate care for teenage mothers before and after birth is still lacking, especially in the areas of information dissemination, education, and counseling concerning reproductive health. However, in some countries such as Botswana, youth-friendly health services have been started to address youth problems. The impact is minimal, however, because teenage pregnancy is still common (Seboni, Seloilwe, & Msimanga, 2002).

What is needed in the SADC are nurses and health care workers who are trained to reach teenagers, boys and girls, to educate them on responsible sexual behavior and the postponement of childbearing until they are physically, psychologically, and financially ready to raise a child. At the moment, the attitudes of some health care personnel toward teenagers who need contraceptive services are so discouraging that most teenagers shy away from health facilities and end up having unwanted pregnancies, or worse still, sexually transmitted diseases (Seboni et al., 2002).

HIV/AIDS Epidemic

Southern Africa remains the worst affected subregion in the world for HIV/AIDS. Antenatal data indicate that prevalence surpasses 25%, having risen sharply around the 1990s. The HIV/AIDS epidemic has had a major impact on the quality of life of citizens in the SADC. Southern Africa has some of the countries most affected by HIV/AIDS, and its negative impact on development has been felt as more and more persons infected by HIV several years ago have developed AIDS, become critically ill, and died. South Africa remains the host for about 5.3 million to 6.2 million persons living with HIV, and 50% of them are women. Unfortunately, there is no sign yet of a decline in the epidemic. Very high HIV prevalence, which exceeds 30% among pregnant women, still is being recorded in four other countries in the region, all with small populations: Botswana, Lesotho, Namibia, and Swaziland. Data comparisons have shown no decline in the epidemic because more and more persons are being infected. Infections with HIV have appeared to be stabilizing at lower levels in Malawi, Zambia, and Zimbabwe. With the exception of Angola that was torn by civil war for nearly two

generations, civilians were restricted to move around, transport links were severed, and some parts of the country were totally cut off from the outside world. Available data indicate that HIV prevalence is still low. This could suggest that these conditions could have slowed the spread of the epidemic. Overall data indicate that Southern Africa to be firmly in the grip of the AIDS epidemic (AIDS Epidemic Update, 2005). Many people in this region succumb to the HIV-related illnesses and die. Life expectancy has declined alarmingly to 40 years in some of these African countries: Botswana, Lesotho, Malawi, Mozambique, Swaziland, Zambia, and Zimbabwe.

Many pregnant women are HIV-positive and are at high risk of passing on the infection to their children in utero, during birth, or through breast-feeding. In Botswana and other SADC countries, for example, between 25% and 50% of pregnant women in various localities are HIV-positive (Sentinel Survey, 2001). Increases in opportunistic infections, especially pneumonia, meningitis, and tuberculosis have raised demands for expensive drugs for these illnesses. Financial resources are being diverted from other health services that are equally important but are not deemed urgent.

About 50% of hospital beds in the medical and pediatric wards in urban and rural areas are occupied by persons with HIV-related illnesses. This situation is likely to continue even with home-based care programs and antiretroviral therapy because of relapses and repeated admissions of patients. Increases in suicide rates have been noticed as more infected and affected persons struggle to cope with the disabling effects of the scourge. The mental health care system and social support system are finding it difficult to face up to the challenges of the HIV/AIDS epidemic.

Loss of trained personnel, including health personnel has been eminent. The impact of the HIV/AIDS epidemic on the development of human resources for the SADC is being felt as more persons are dying. The epidemic inevitably has put a lot of strain on the health care workforce, in particular nurses, with resultant high attrition rates of this cadre. Future effects of the virus on the economy will be enormous and definitely will retard or threaten most of the socioeconomic gains that have been achieved so far.

Studies in Botswana and admission data into higher education (University of Botswana, 2004) have shown no impact of HIV/AIDS on the recruitment and retention of nurses (Tlou, 1998). More younger men and women are entering the nursing profession every year, and some have to be turned away because there are too few training facilities. For instance, in 2004 there were only 80 places for second-year nursing students at the University of Botswana, and a large number of students were seeking admission into the nursing program. This led to the exceeding of the quotas by 45 students (University of Botswana, 2004).

NURSING EDUCATION AND NURSING PRACTICE

The health care systems of the SADC are organized at different levels of increasing sophistication, starting from the most basic (the mobile health stop and health post) to a major referral hospital. In all these facilities, nurses are in the forefront of the health care delivery system. Health consultations, nutrition care, health education, maternal health, patient education, and immunization of infants and children against communicable diseases have been functions and responsibilities of nurses and have been subsumed under the discipline and practice of nursing. Additionally, all the health programs that have been initiated as a way to respond to the HIV/AIDS epidemic are led mostly by nurses, such as the Prevention of Mother to Child Transmission, Voluntary Counseling and Testing, Isoniazid Preventive Therapy, rapid testing, and lately, antiretroviral therapies. Nursing, therefore, has earned for itself a unique place in the national health care system in the Southern African region.

Nursing Practice

Nursing practice is seen as a broad-based service that should meet the health care needs of individuals, families, and communities in various settings such as hospitals, schools, community centers, homes, and workplaces. The latter include mines, factories, farms, and construction sites. Even in these settings, however, nursing roles vary greatly from country to country. As Moores (1998) puts it,

> In one country a nurse may be effectively a medical assistant, in another, the only health care professional who provides a comprehensive health care service to a community. Nurses and midwives may work in hospital, in smaller first line health care centres, in towns and villages, or more remote locations, bringing care directly to individuals who need it. Some may be able to use the latest medicines, equipment and specialist skills, while others may have only the most primitive of facilities and supplies. In countries where there is a shortage of doctors, people would often have no access to preventative, curative, palliative or continuing care if it were not for the skills and expertise of nurses. (p. 2)

Indeed, nurses are extending their traditional roles to respond to the needs of their communities; for example, in Botswana, community health nurses assist communities in running income-generation projects such as sewing for youth and horticultural programs for women. In addition, workshops for traditional healers and primary school teachers also are conducted.

Nursing Education

Health care delivery is highly labor intensive and requires highly competent practitioners. According to Awases, Gbary, Nyoni, and Chatora (2004), the quality, efficiency, and equity of health services depend on the availability of skilled and competent health professionals where and when they are needed and who are trained appropriately to deliver the required services at a high standard. Nursing education in the SADC has responded to the changing needs of patients and communities by integrating concepts of primary health care, public health practice, and community health care in basic, postbasic, undergraduate, and graduate programs. Nursing practice has continued to redefine and expand its scope and parameters to meet the requirements and dictates of these primary health care–oriented national health care systems.

Conceptual frameworks for nursing and midwifery programs were broadened to include concepts and content of primary health care. Postbasic and graduate programs have been developed for nurse clinicians, family nurse practitioners, advanced midwifery and maternal and child health and family planning practitioners, and community health and community mental health practitioners to prepare nurses for providing quality nursing care and health care to individuals, families, and community groups with a variety of nursing and health care problems and needs. Because of the need for nursing leadership and management in the provision of patient care, clinical and nursing research programs also have been developed and implemented at the basic, postbasic, and graduate levels (Bachelor of Science in Nursing Curriculum, 2001).

Formal education for nurses in the SADC countries is similar to the model presented for Botswana in Figure 85-1. Most nurses are trained at the diploma level for 3 years and then may undergo 1 year of concentrated study in one of the postbasic programs to enable them to practice as registered nurses. Nurses also have the opportunity to study for a baccalaureate degree in nursing as registered nurse completers for another 2 to 3 years. This route, however, is too long and costly because it takes almost 6 to 8 years for a nurse to attain

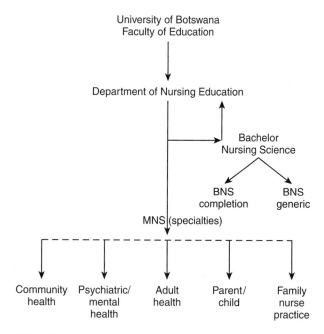

FIGURE 85-1 University of Botswana nurse education model.

a basic degree. Ways to shorten this length of training need to be explored.

Generic baccalaureate programs in nursing science admit high school graduates for a 4-year training program, after which they have the opportunity to specialize in any field of nursing at a master's degree level. Currently, the number of baccalaureate- and master's degree–prepared nurses in all the SADC countries is few, but their impact is being felt as they provide leadership in all areas of nursing care and nursing research. However, there is a much needed critical mass of nurses with higher degrees and nursing scholarship in this region in order to bring about the required change for the improvement of good quality care for the communities. Since 2000, the output for basic and graduate degrees at the University of Botswana stood at 173 graduates, and the numbers are expected to increase.

Significant developments in nursing education have been observable in the region as countries now begin to have nursing programs affiliated with universities. Over the past few years there has been a movement to start degree programs in universities. For instance, in Lesotho, Swaziland, Malawi, Zambia, and Zimbabwe, nursing programs have been started in the universities.

This movement is geared to improve the level of education for nurses and subsequently will improve the quality of care for the people. However, the shift was not a smooth one in most countries. The society at large was baffled at this trend because nursing has always been regarded as an apprentice type of vocation. Little is being realized of the changing needs of the society, which have become complex and sophisticated, requiring persons who are able to use critical thinking skills to make decisions. In some countries, such as Botswana, South Africa, and Zimbabwe, nursing education in institutions of higher learning is well anchored. The trend is expected to prevail in other Southern African countries as well.

NURSING SCHOLARSHIP IN SOUTHERN AFRICA

The unique context of the African continent is sometimes interesting with daunting challenges. Nurses with higher degrees in SADC are few, and in some countries baccalaureate programs have not been started yet. To optimize the level of scholarship in the region requires collaboration and partnerships in the development of nursing knowledge and science. Several mechanisms were used to promote this collaboration. For instance, the World Health Organization Collaborating Centers in the region, which are located at the University of Botswana, the University of South Africa, and the University of KwaZulu Natal, came together and formed an Africa Honor Society for Nurses with a main goal of promoting nursing scholarship in Africa. The honor society was inaugurated in 2001 in Pretoria, South Africa, where the foundation members were inducted (Uys, Seboni, Seloilwe, & Klopper, 2003).

In addition, a scientific meeting was held that enabled nurses to share research information. The second and third scientific conferences were held in Dares Salam, Tanzania (2003), and Gaborone, Botswana (2004), respectively. During the conference in Botswana, the honor society was admitted as a chapter at large of the Sigma Theta Tau International. This chapter is known as the Tau Lambda. The next conference will be held in Ghana in 2005. This honor society is expected to grow in strength to include all scholars in Africa who then would advance the development of nursing knowledge and science in this part of the world. Hopefully, this will decrease dependency on the Western literature that has been the case over the years.

PRESENT AND FUTURE CHALLENGES FOR NURSING IN THE SOUTHERN AFRICA DEVELOPMENT COMMUNITY

Challenging educational patterns, economic development, technological advances, and sociopolitical trends have resulted in the trend for better-educated nurses in SADC countries, but nurses still face some challenges in the delivery of health care. Among these are shortages of nursing personnel compounded by high attrition rates, lengthy periods of training, limited nursing research opportunities, HIV/AIDS, and implementation of recommendations related to women in health care.

Shortages of Nursing Personnel

In most SADC countries, nursing is a popular profession for men and women, but the number of facilities requiring nurses is growing at a faster pace than the number of trained nurses to staff them. Every graduating class is absorbed into the health care system months before commencement exercises, but nursing shortages still persist. Some of the shortages are also due to poor working conditions and inadequate information and support systems for nurses, resulting in nurses looking for "greener pastures" in neighboring countries or overseas. This brain drain has had a negative impact on the health care systems of the sending country and the receiving country, where the recruited nurses may not be familiar with the language and culture of the people they are supposed to serve. Factors often cited for migration include few opportunities for career advancement and development, economic factors, declining health services that leave practitioners in a state of helplessness and despair, and political issues that threaten the existence of these professionals (Awases et al., 2004). A possible intervention is for SADC countries to collaborate with each other in expanding the training of professional nurses and to improve working conditions of nurses to alleviate the problems of nursing staff shortages and turnover.

Long Periods of Training

Periods of training for nurses in the SADC countries are still long, spanning 6 to 8 years if one started off at a diploma level. This is wasteful in terms of resources because training centers are developing the same individual. This piecemeal kind of training also has led to nurses being dissatisfied with the way the staff development programs are implemented. Countries of the SACD need to develop curriculum that recognizes prior learning and experience. In South Africa for instance, prior learning and experience are recognized and embraced in the entire educational system. In Botswana, developments in this direction are still rudimentary. Diploma and degree programs need to be articulated and dovetailed to allow nurses in training to exit and reenter programs at whatever level they may desire; for example, at diploma, undergraduate, and graduate levels. This will be desirable because the programs of nursing education will take into consideration the different needs of the individuals. In Botswana, discussions are under way to address these curricular issues.

NURSING RESEARCH IN THE SOUTHERN AFRICA DEVELOPMENT COMMUNITY

Nursing research in the SADC is still in its infancy, but there are initiatives to encourage research, especially at university schools of nursing. Nurses prepared at higher levels, however, need to come down from the ivory tower of academic research and simplify the process so that the real implementers of care (clinical nurses) can do and use research to gain reliable information on which to base their decisions and practice. Collaborative research should be encouraged to provide expertise to those without it. More importantly, teaming up with clinicians and academicians would be more beneficial. Funding for nursing research is a major problem and is not even a priority in any of the SADC countries. Ministries of health in SADC also need to develop a research agenda and establish national research councils to guide and direct research at national levels.

HIV/AIDS

Nurses in all the SADC states have provided leadership in HIV/AIDS prevention and control and in caring for persons living with AIDS and for their families. Although there is no real research on the phenomenon, HIV/AIDS seems to be having little impact on the recruitment and retention of nursing personnel. Indeed, young persons are joining the profession in increasing numbers. Nurses as human beings, however, are at risk of HIV infection from their own sexual behavior and their behavior at the workplace. Most of the nurses are women, and they have the same biological and sociocultural vulnerability to HIV/AIDS as do women in this society. They therefore may feel powerless to protect themselves and experience anxiety and fear of contagion, which interferes with their ability to care for persons living with AIDS.

The International Council of Nurses has appealed to governments to take appropriate measures to reduce the negative impact of HIV/AIDS on nursing and midwifery personnel. The International Council of Nurses has released position statements on AIDS (1996) and on reducing HIV/AIDS risk to nursing personnel (1998). National nurses' associations in the SADC have provided information to their members on HIV/AIDS prevention and care of persons living with AIDS. Dissemination of information on universal precautions to minimize the risk of HIV transmission in the health care setting is essential. The nurses' associations in some countries—for example, Botswana—also stress the importance of responsible sexual behavior and run workshops to teach nurses skills on condom use and negotiating safer sex with partners. The SADC countries established a nurses' HIV/AIDS network called SADC AIDS Network of Nurses and Midwives in 2001. Through this forum, the HIV/AIDS fact sheets for nurses were developed and disseminated to every nurse to familiarize the nurses with the epidemic and the appropriate interventions in which they need to engage.

IMPLEMENTING RECOMMENDATIONS RELATED TO WOMEN IN HEALTH CARE

In the follow-up to the Fourth World Conference on Population and Development (1994), countries in the SADC have started to implement the recommendations related to women and health and have endorsed them in their health policies. Major constraints imposed by civil unrest and reforms in the economic sector in most countries, however, make it difficult to design comprehensive national health plans that are gender sensitive. Nurses are still not proactive in this matter and need to be in the forefront in introducing equity for women in all aspects of health.

For health care delivery, applying a fully comprehensive gender perspective would require that all health statistics be segregated and that a comprehensive women's health profile be constructed. The International Council of Nursing (1995) has issued guidelines to the national nurses' associations for countries to use in developing such a profile that includes lifestyle, environment, health care services, health service use, sexuality, and policy development. The guidelines include (1) eliminating negative cultural practices such as female genital mutilation, (2) supporting programs to reduce violence against women, and (3) promoting women's access to comprehensive health

services and health education for girls and elderly women.

OPPORTUNITIES FOR NURSES IN THE SOUTHERN AFRICA DEVELOPMENT COMMUNITY

The most important opportunities for SADC nurses are that each country has a Nurses and Midwives Act that provides for the regulation of the practice of nursing and midwifery, for the training and registering of nurses and midwives, and for the establishment of a nursing and midwifery council. The World Health Organization Collaborating Centers have undertaken some initiatives in collaborative research endeavors. These initiatives include a nursing council, a statutory institution that (1) issues registration, (2) represents the state, (3) lays down minimum requirements for the education of nurses to ensure safe practice, (4) protects the public from professional malpractice by laying down minimum requirements for practice, and (5) ensuring that only those practitioners who meet such requirements are licensed to practice.

Nursing councils are concerned with issues of accountability and the quality of nursing care. National nurses' association ensure that nursing education, nursing research, and nursing practice respond to the dictates of primary health care and that nurses assume leadership roles in health care delivery. Activities of national nurses' associations allow for (1) definition and nature of nursing practice; (2) development of education necessary for practice; (3) development, promotion, and maintenance of high standards of practice; (4) professional growth and development of individual practitioners; (5) maintenance of the honor and status of the nursing profession; and (6) improvement of the social and economic welfare of the profession.

Through bodies such as the East, Central, and Southern African College of Nursing, uniform standards of nursing education, legislation, and nursing practice are being formulated as part of having a common or similar nursing curriculum in all the countries. Reviews of current curricula or programs for nurse training are being undertaken in a number of countries, providing the opportunity for ensuring that developments in health care are reflected in the curricula and that nurses and midwives are prepared for these developments in health care roles. In Botswana, for example, basic nurse training includes management and leadership courses; the university offers master's degree courses in nursing administration; and in-service education for nurse leaders in administration is offered on an ongoing basis. Some of the students are from SADC countries, and some are from as far away as Kenya and Uganda.

SUMMARY

This chapter has outlined the important roles that nurses and nurse-midwives play in the provision of health care in the SADC. It also has outlined present and future challenges for health care and for the nursing profession and the opportunities that in the long run will enable nurses of the SADC to achieve their common objective: enhancing the health and well-being of their communities. A strong national nurses' association and proper legislation are essential to the growth and development of the nursing profession in any one country.

REFERENCES

AIDS Epidemic Update. (2005). Special report on AIDS prevention. Retrieved January 3, 2005 from http://www.unaids.org/epi2005/index.html

Awases, M., Gbary, A., Nyoni, J., & Chatora, R. (2004). *Migration of health professionals in the six countries: A synthesis report.* Congo, Africa: World Health Organization, Regional Office for Africa.

Bachelor of Science in Nursing Curriculum. (2001). Gaborone: Department of Nursing Education, University of Botswana.

Central Medical Statistics. (2000). Gaborone, Botswana: Ministry of Finance and Development Planning.

Central Medical Statistics. (2001). Gaborone, Botswana: Ministry of Finance and Development Planning.

Central Medical Statistics. (2002). Gaborone, Botswana: Ministry of Finance and Development Planning.

Fidzani, H., Ntseane, D., & Seloilwe, E. S. (2000). *Situation and response analysis of HIV/AIDS in North East District.* New York: United Nations Development Programme.

International Council of Nursing. (1995). *Women and health: Nurses lead the way.* Geneva: Author.

International Council of Nursing. (1996). *Acquired immunodeficiency syndrome.* Geneva: Author.

International Council of Nursing. (1998). *Call for action to reduce HIV/AIDS risks to nursing personnel.* Geneva: Author.

Mogobe, K. D. (2000). *A report on the utilization of reproductive services in Botswana.* New York: United Nations Population Fund.

Molebatsi, C. D., & Mogobe K. D. (2000). *Situation and response analysis of HIV/AIDS in Ngamiland district.* New York: United Nations Development Programme.

Moores, Y. (1998). *Health sector reforms: The nursing and midwifery contribution.* Paper presented at the Commonwealth Health Ministers Meeting, Barbados, November 15-19.

Ngcongco, V. (1995). *Nursing practice in the African region.* Geneva: WHO Expert Committee on Nursing Practice, World Health Organization.

Seboni, N. M., Seloilwe, E. S., & Msimanga, S. (2002). *Report on the evaluation of youth friendly services & Family Health Division, Ministry of Health.* Gaborone, Botswana Government Printer.

Sentinel Survey. (2001). Gaborone, Botswana: NACA Ministry of Health, Gaborone Printing Press.

Shaibu, S. (2001). Caregiving on the edge: Family caregiving of the elderly in Botswana. *Mosenodi, 2,* 11-17.

Tlou, S. D. (1994). The elderly and their use of the health care system. In F. Bruun, Y. Combes, & M. Mugabe (Eds.), *The situation of the elderly in Botswana* (pp. 93-99). Gaborone, Botswana: National Institute of Research.

Tlou, S. D. (1997). Indicators of health. In Botswana Society (Eds.), *Poverty and plenty: The Botswana experience* (pp. 303-315). Gaborone, Botswana: Macmillan.

Tlou, S. D. (1998). *Caring for the carers: The impact of HIV/AIDS on nursing personnel in Botswana.* Unpublished research report, University of Botswana.

United Nations. (1995). *The world's women 1995.* New York: Author.

University of Botswana. (2004). *Admission data sets.* Gaborone, Botswana: Author.

Uys, L., Seboni, N., Seloilwe, E., & Klopper, H. C. (2003). The establishment of a new chapter at large in Africa: Involving multiple schools in different African countries. *Perspectives in Nursing* (second quarter), 12-13.

WHO-UNICEF. (1978). *Alma-Ata Declaration: Primary health care.* Geneva: Author.

CHAPTER

86

Nursing in Canada

An Overview of Health Care, Nursing Education, and Practice

JANET C. ROSS-KERR

Although Canadians traditionally have supported universal health insurance coverage as a right of citizenship, public concern is growing concerning access problems, lengthy wait times, insufficient staff, and inadequate funding of the system. Public opinion polls have reflected these concerns in that 56% of the public has reported falling confidence in the system (Schafer, 2002; Milne, 2001). Although the Canadian health care system often is construed as "socialized medicine," in truth it is described more correctly as a private overlay on a public system. For example, physician services and prescription drugs fall largely within the private sector, whereas hospital and public health services are in the public domain. Even though the problems just noted have escalated in recent years, Canadians have been generally unsympathetic to the possibility of a return to private arrangements for health care that were common before federal legislation for hospital care more than 40 years ago (Axworthy & Spiegel, 2002).

Despite the relatively high level of public support for Medicare, a number of provinces have made continuing challenges to the provisions of the Canada Health Act. One such challenge has been to allow private clinics to operate under contract from health authorities. These private clinics have come under fire from citizens concerned about Medicare charging patients extra fees for expensive upgrades on items such as cataract implants, for generally higher operating costs than are found in the public system, and for the potential for creation of a two-tiered health care system. Public criticism also has focused on physicians working in private clinics who are allowed reimbursement for their services through publicly funded Medicare, a federal program that is administered jointly by the federal and provincial governments. The argument supporting the view

that private health care should not be allowed to operate alongside the public service is that the private system is likely to attract better physicians and other health care professionals and also wealthy patients, leaving the public system with substandard services, long wait times, and highly underfunded.

Although the high cost of federal health care expenditures has led to a rethinking and reconsideration of funding arrangements by successive federal governments, the federal Liberal government currently in power has maintained its fundamental commitment to the principles of Medicare. In Alberta, the provincial government attempted unsuccessfully to pass legislation allowing the private clinics to keep patients overnight following procedures such as joint replacement. Opponents of such legislation were concerned that passage of such a bill under Alberta law could jeopardize Medicare, as it is known in Canada. Under the terms of the North American Free Trade Agreement with the United States and Mexico, if one province were allowed to offer private health care, others eventually would have to make it available as well under the terms of the agreement. Although a decade ago, the National Forum on Health (1995) chaired by the prime minister championed the publicly financed system of Medicare over a private health care system, the federal government has not come up with concrete proposals to ensure that renegade provinces are not allowed to jeopardize Medicare in their own provinces or in others.

The Commission on the Future of Health Care in Canada, established in 2001 to study the problems in the health care system and recommend changes, was chaired by Roy Romanow. Strongly upholding a publicly funded system of universal health insurance, the final report of the commission recommended significantly increasing federal funding for health care and integrating priority home care services within the Canada Health Act, improved prescription drug coverage, improved wait list management, removal of obstacles to primary care reform, and increasing the supply of advanced diagnostic services and health care providers (Romanow, 2002). Although some proposals in the report have been implemented, the federal government is studying the major ones that involve significant increases in funding.

A historic decision by the Supreme Court of Canada on June 6, 2005, supported the right of individuals to hold private insurance in order to receive timely care for health problems where access to health services was problematic (Canadian Broadcasting System, 2005). In a 4-3 decision, the panel of seven justices said banning private insurance for a list of services ranging from magnetic resonance imaging tests to cataract surgery was unconstitutional under the Quebec Charter of Rights, given that the public system has failed to guarantee patients access to those services in a timely way. Although this decision may be construed as a small foray into the jurisdiction of the Canada Health Act of 1982, it nevertheless sounded a "wake-up call" to government and public health officials from coast to coast in terms of the need to develop ways and means of providing needed health services in a timely manner.

PHILOSOPHICAL BASIS OF THE CANADIAN SYSTEM OF UNIVERSAL HEALTH CARE

The rationale for the evolution of the federal health legislation program can be found in five basic principles of health care from which the standards for the legislation are derived. The first principle, *universality,* refers to the fact that under any provincial plan, 100% of insured residents must be entitled to insured services provided by the plan on uniform terms and conditions. Therefore coverage must be offered to the population as a whole rather than to select population groups. The principle of *comprehensiveness* ensured that the provincial health insurance plan must insure all insured services provided by hospitals, physicians, or dental surgeons, and similar or additional services given by other health care practitioners in provinces where legislation permits. Although extra billing and user fees were allowed before 1984 and facility fees by private clinics up to 1994, differential charges may no longer be applied on a private basis for services covered by the plan. *Accessibility* is perhaps the most difficult principle to satisfy, particularly with a sparse population scattered over a vast amount of territory. However, reasonable access to services is seen as essential even in view of the need to constrain costs.

Portability or coverage for residents of one province when they require services just after a move or during a visit to another province must be ensured in plans. *Public administration,* nonprofit operation by an organization fiscally responsible to the provincial government, also is required. In the various acts passed by the federal government relative to health insurance since 1957, progressive refinement of the standards applicable to provincial health plans based on these principles has been evident.

The incorporation of a system of health care in legislation ensures that certain defining characteristics will emerge from the philosophy and principles upon which it is based. Because the system itself is entrenched in law, if change is desired, full legislative review is required. This might be an advantage or a disadvantage depending on the issue of concern and the nature of any change deemed necessary. Approximately 75% of health care expenditures in Canada come under Medicare, and about 25% fall outside it in services not reimbursed by the plan. At the outset, the Canadian health care system evolved in a manner not unlike systems in other Western countries. The fact that the provincial plans insure hospital care and physician services means that the hospital and the physician are paramount in the system. Not surprisingly, the number of hospital beds increased at a rate much higher than the rate of population increase until legislation appeared to end the 50/50 federal/ provincial cost sharing. Outpatient care, home care, and community health services were areas not eligible for federal cost sharing at the outset. The exclusion of these forms of care from federal financing encouraged the physician-centered, in-hospital care that has been a dominant feature of the system that evolved over 40 years (Ross-Kerr, 2002). The high cost of these methods of providing care has led to a search for more effective and efficient lower-cost alternatives. The consumer movement also has heightened awareness of the need for consumers to be active participants in matters pertaining to their health. The Alma Ata agreement of 1978 by the World Health Organization member countries for health care for all by the year 2000 has carried with it an implicit challenge to encourage genuine community involvement in planning for health in ways that have not been recognized or explored previously in health care delivery systems. The challenge for health care in Canada is to tailor the legislative arrangements for health care to encourage community-based measures facilitating health maintenance, health promotion, and prevention of disease and to balance these with measures to restore health. Deber, Hastings, and

VIEWPOINTS

Thompson (1991) presaged the debate that currently is raging over the importance of reviewing and restructuring the Canadian health care system:

> Many believe that it will not be possible to sustain the current system without major modifications. Task forces and commissions in most provinces are looking at ways to shift the heavy focus on physician and institutional care to "community based" alternatives and non-physician providers. (pp. 73-74)

ESTABLISHMENT OF THE CANADIAN HEALTH INSURANCE SYSTEM

In a society in which life is deeply valued, the health of persons becomes an issue of fundamental importance. Responsibility for health was granted to the provinces in the British North America Act that established the Canadian Confederation in 1867. Health care was reserved as a federal prerogative for marine and quarantine hospitals and for aboriginal peoples. The Constitution Act of 1982, which superseded the original legislation, confirmed and continued this division of powers. Social democratic traditions along with Canada's growth and development as a colonial empire perhaps contributed more than other factors to the perception of the need to ensure the availability of health care for the population. In the aftermath of social upheavals created by the Depression and two world wars, many factors converged to create a receptive climate for consideration of public financing of individual health care expenditures. Federal/provincial agreements emerged from public debate and discussion and culminated in the implementation of a system of national health insurance to cover health care costs for all Canadians.

Although the Canadian program of insurance for hospital services at the federal level was not enacted until 1957, the stage was set for the federal legislation in previous supportive developments in the provinces. The province of Saskatchewan was clearly in the forefront of provincial developments, and after World War I, it passed legislation enabling municipalities to raise taxes to support the employment of physicians (the municipal doctor plans), the establishment of hospitals, and the development of hospitalization plans. The window of opportunity created by the firm support of the Canadian Medical Association for publicly financed health insurance in 1934 was lost through government inaction, and the Canadian Medical Association later withdrew its support in favor of private plans initiated by physicians in several provinces. Saskatchewan decided

to "go it alone" when it became the first jurisdiction in North America to enact legislation establishing a prepaid plan of hospital insurance in 1947. Although the federal government fell short of the objective of establishing a prepaid hospital insurance plan, in the first legislation dealing with health care, the federal government in 1948 passed the National Health Grants Act. Included in the act were funds for hospital construction, professional training, public health, and other provincial services, areas seen as providing the basis for the later establishment of national health insurance.

When the Hospital Insurance and Diagnostic Services Act was passed in 1957, it provided for comprehensive in-hospital patient care services with universal coverage for residents of participating provinces. Because health care fell within provincial jurisdiction, the government of each province had the right to decide whether to develop a plan to insure hospital services conforming to the federal guidelines outlined in the legislation. However, because the plan involved 50/50 cost sharing with the provinces, any province deciding to opt out of the arrangement would forgo tax dollars the federal government otherwise would contribute to health care in that province and in opting out effectively would subsidize the plans of other provinces. Initially, five provinces agreed to participate when the act came into force in 1958, and by 1961, all provinces were full participants in the program. Excepted from the national hospital insurance program were tuberculosis and mental hospitals and certain other institutions.

In adding prepayment for medical services to the hospitalization plan in 1962, the province of Saskatchewan again became the first jurisdiction to implement such legislation. The province did so over the loud protestations of Saskatchewan physicians who went on strike for 23 days beginning July 1, 1962, the date the legislation was implemented. In the face of vehement opposition from physicians, the Saskatchewan government was forced to make concessions to the medical profession in the form of allowing opting out of the plan and extra billing. Implementation of the federal agenda to add medical services to its program of prepaid health insurance undoubtedly was hastened and facilitated by the lessons learned from the Saskatchewan experience. The federal Medical Care Act thus was passed in 1966, and the controversial nature of the legislation may explain the participation of only two provinces at the time the legislation came into force on July 1, 1968, as well as the 5-year period required for all provinces to enter into an arrangement with the federal government for the prepayment of medical services. The plan allowed for coverage of physicians' services in and out of hospital but did not prevent the provinces from allowing physicians to opt out of the plan, bill patients directly, or impose surcharges on the established fee for a particular service.

In the early part of the 1970s, the escalation of expenditures and the growing size of the federal deficit caused concern over the open-ended nature of some health expenditures, in particular those for physicians' services. In 1977 the system of federal/provincial cost sharing was amended with the passage of the Fiscal Arrangements and Established Programs Financing Act. This ended the open-ended 50/50 cost sharing and introduced block funding that involved transfer of some tax points to the provinces and reduced the federal contribution to health care to 25% with additional federal contributions based on increases in the gross domestic product. In the years following the passage of this legislation, concern mounted over the increased use of co-payments termed *user fees* for institutional services and extra billing practices among physicians in provinces where this was allowed. The Liberal federal government responded to these perceived erosions of Medicare by disallowing extra billing and user fees in the Canada Health Act of 1984. Although physicians mounted a strong and vocal campaign to prevent the prohibition of extra billing, it was to no avail. A similarly perceived erosion of Medicare in the charging of facility fees by private clinics established in some province a decade later was disallowed by the federal government in 1994, and those provinces contravening the federal legislation were penalized by lowering of their federal transfer payments. The high level of concern about the structure of the health care system and the issues surrounding the provision of quality care have prompted the prime minister to establish two high-level commissions in the past decade to study health care. The National Forum on Health (1995) produced a five-volume report composed of 42 studies on particular issues of concern. Less than 6 years later in 2001, the Commission on the Future of Health Care in Canada was established under the direction of Roy Romanow to study the health care system and to recommend sweeping changes to address issues of concern to the populace (Romanow, 2002).

NURSING PRACTICE IN CANADA

As the largest group of health care professionals, nurses form the backbone of the health care system in Canada. In 2003 the nursing workforce was composed of 258,393 registered nurses, 63,138 licensed practical nurses, and 5,107 registered psychiatric nurses. In Canada, 62.5% of the registered nurse workforce practices in the hospital sector, 12.6% in community health/home care, 10.5% in continuing care facilities, 2.7% in educational institutions, 2.1% in physicians' offices, and 10.8% in other settings. In addition, 46.5% of licensed practical nurses practice in hospital settings, and 36.9% practice in continuing care (Canadian Institute for Health Information, 2004a, 2004b, 2004c). Workforce trends indicate that the proportion of nurses working in tertiary care has dropped considerably in the past decade, whereas nurses in the community health/home care sector have increased because of the health reform initiatives by which a portion of hospital-based care was moved into the community as new approaches to recovery were implemented.

Another significant trend is the aging of the nursing workforce, with the average age of a registered nurse rising to 44.5 in 2003 (Canadian Institute of Health Information, 2004b). This is undoubtedly the result of a number of factors including the downsizing of the nursing workforce in the elimination of nursing positions through cutbacks in government funding for hospitals in the health reform movement that began in the 1990s. The Canadian Nurses Association predicts an escalating shortage of nurses over the next decade, with high projected levels of registered nurse retirements combined with other factors such as graduates who leave the country because of the cutbacks in the 1990s (Ryten, 1997). According to a Canadian Council on Social Development (2000) study, nearly 1 in 10 nursing graduates migrated to the United States between 1995 and 1997. Recently, Cleverley, Baumann, Blythe, Grinspun, and Tompkins (2004) suggested that new nursing graduates continue to leave the country in search of work in the United States and elsewhere. A study by the Registered Nurses Association of Ontario (2001) found that the reason nurses in Ontario left Canada for the United States was a lack of job opportunities.

For those returning from the United States, the principal reason was availability of full-time work (Registered Nurses Association of Ontario, 2001). In 2003, 51.4% of the nursing workforce was engaged in full-time employment, whereas 42.6% worked in part-time or casual positions. Although some nurses may choose part-time or casual work to allow them to cope with their family responsibilities, many others would like to have full-time work. These nurses are unable to secure full-time positions because they are not available; many full-time positions were converted to part-time and casual positions.

Other factors are also likely to contribute to the problem, such as low salaries, inadequate benefits, and a need to enhance the quality of the working environment. The Nursing Effectiveness, Utilization and Outcomes Research Unit a joint initiative of McMaster University and the University of Toronto, has pointed to some other factors influencing the reduction in the number of those recruited to and graduating from nursing; namely, the negative light in which nursing is portrayed by the media, opportunities for women in traditionally male fields, and the fact that nursing is not portrayed as a viable career choice in elementary and high schools.

Specialization in nursing has grown exponentially with the increase in knowledge and technology in health care and the demand for nurses with advanced preparation in particular specialty areas. Specialties have tended to parallel medical specialization, and examples such as occupational health nursing, neuroscience nursing, and oncology nursing are among the 17 areas that have gained recognition under the Nursing Specialty program of the Canadian Nurses Association (2005). The Nursing Specialty program has specified requirements for sustained and current practice in the specialty, as well as basic preparation in nursing and a specialty examination the nurse must pass to receive certification in a particular specialty. This examination is set by the Canadian Nurses Association Testing Service in consultation with the specialty group. Baccalaureate and master's level education is not required for achieving certification in a designated nursing specialty under the Canadian Nurses Association program. However, nursing specialization also has occurred at the master's and doctoral levels with the emergence of the advanced practice nursing role. The health reform movement has led to a rationalization of the roles of all health care professionals, and it is clear that advanced practice nurses can deliver high-quality care at a fraction of the cost of physicians. Although specialty roles for advanced practice nurses are well-developed in the United States, these roles are just developing in Canada, where health care financing arrangements may not have been as open to this development until recently. Provincial health legislation has been amended in many jurisdictions over the past few years to provide a legal framework within which advanced practice nurses may function.

Nurses have been on record as supporting health care reform for decades. Clearly, the health care system as it has developed in Canada under a system of national health insurance has been costly. However, the health care system costs in Canada are far less than in the United States. Since the full implementation of Medicare in Canada, health care spending as a percentage of the gross domestic product consistently has been several percentage points higher. As an example, in 2003 Canada's health spending was 9.9% of GDP while that of the United States was 15% (Organization for Economic Cooperation and Development, 2005). Although many countries have established national health care systems that are publicly funded, the Canadian system relies on public and private funding. Excess capacity in some sectors including acute care, remuneration for certain categories of health care professionals on a costly fee-for-service basis, and overdevelopment of some services with little attention to whether these were needed have characterized the system. In addition, financial incentives to the provinces to develop systems based on hospital- and physician-centered care have added considerably to the overall cost of the system. Because of these incentives, the total cost of the system has been higher than would have been the case if certain other policy directions had been taken.

The political will to address structural changes in the health care system that require difficult decisions about problems, providers, services, and settings does not come easily, for political will is driven by the ability to garner votes from the electorate. Thus the shape of reform may be such that a publicly funded health care system may be less attractive to the politicians than one with more privately funded services than previously. Politicians historically have found it much easier to support the high-cost elements of the system such as physicians' services because physicians constitute a powerful pressure group in society. Thus politicians have been reluctant to address the aspects of the system that most need reform to ensure viability of the publicly funded system of health care. Among these aspects are the need to shift the acute care focus of the system to a focus that is based in community health care centers; streamlining the method of payment for health care to exclude fee-for-service and include remunerating health care professionals on a salary or contract; identifying how many professionals are needed in the system and limiting the number practicing in the system to the number required; limiting the facilities where the work of the health care system is carried on to those that are required; and closing those facilities that are not needed. Rationalization of the system could lead to the establishment of community health care centers where a range of services could be offered by health care professionals. Many health care professionals including nurses historically have been underused in the system in relation to their educational background and experience and reasonably could be expected to provide different levels of service than in the past. Introducing change in some of these areas potentially could facilitate collaboration and coordination of care and reduce costs through efficiencies achieved through common use of facilities and interdisciplinary teamwork. The need to address these matters in order to preserve a publicly funded and effective health care system is critical.

Health care reform as envisioned by nurses would see the primary focus of health care moving to the community in primary health care centers from its traditional base in tertiary care hospitals. True reform of the system requires hard decisions about care and the best ways of providing it to the people by qualified professionals. If the hands of the health care authorities are tied by a lack of jurisdiction over all services required for care, those services will continue to be fragmented and expensive. Whether the political influence of powerful groups in health care is sufficient to prevent the kind of health care reform that is needed remains to be seen.

To date, nurses have not been engaged in substantial numbers for the delivery of primary health care, but it is entirely possible that this will occur in the future with the development of community health care centers. Changes in the way in which nursing is practiced likely will continue as society becomes more aware of the benefits of health promotion and the need to develop healthier lifestyles to prevent disease. Alternatives to hospitalization for tertiary and long-term or continuing care, in the form of home care and ambulatory care, appear attractive at the personal and societal levels. One must recognize, however, that all levels of hospitalization will continue to be required to meet the needs of the people. In the rhetoric about downsizing the tertiary care hospital and moving services to the community, one must recognize that high-quality tertiary care services are critical to a well-functioning system. Nurses have been preparing for their new roles in community and long-term care settings and have the knowledge and the communication and interaction skills to assist consumers in meeting health goals. They are thus well poised and positioned to serve society in a health care system that is centered in the community and based on the primary health care model.

NURSING EDUCATION

The history and traditions of nursing education in Canada are long and impressive. A system of diploma nursing education developed following the establishment of the Mack Training School in association with the St. Catharine's General and Marine Hospital in 1874. The first university courses in nursing in Canada were offered at the University of Alberta in 1918; these first courses were in public health nursing. Subsequently, the University of British Columbia offered the first degree program in nursing in the country in 1919 under the direction of Ethel Johns. The system of diploma nursing education in hospitals and later community colleges has undergone further changes with the drive to establish the baccalaureate degree in nursing as the entry level for the profession. The increased availability of baccalaureate programs in nursing are widely believed to provide a stronger basis for the practice of nursing. Collaborative baccalaureate degree programs offered jointly between the community colleges and the universities have been developed in most provinces, and students now entering initial programs in nursing are able to study for a baccalaureate degree in nursing whether they enroll initially in a nursing program at a community college or at a university in areas where these programs are available. Baccalaureate nursing programs have been available to diploma-prepared nurses dating from the time of the early degree programs in nursing. More recently, distance programs have allowed registered nurses in more remote centers to study for their degrees even though they do not live in a major university center. The development of a context-based learning program or problem-based learning as it is termed in some centers is an innovative response to providing high-quality baccalaureate nursing education that encourages critical thinking and problem solving in nursing graduates.

Graduate programs at the master's level have been available in Canada since the establishment of the first master's degree program in nursing at the University of Western Ontario in 1959. Since then, master's degree programs have developed in every region of the country so that today they are widely available to students. The first fully funded doctoral program in nursing was established at the University of Alberta on January 1, 1991, and there are now eight PhD in nursing programs across the country (Wood, Giovannetti, & Ross-Kerr, 2004). The initiation of doctoral education has been an important milestone for the profession because preparing nurses to contribute to the discovery of nursing knowledge through theory and research will lead to improved care.

Nursing has made great progress in developing programs and ensuring that standards are high. It would appear that the long and difficult campaigns by the provincial professional associations and the Canadian Nurses Association have not been in vain, for basic nursing education has moved from the jurisdiction of hospitals to the general educational system. In evaluating the history of nursing education in the province, a progression in thinking about schools of nursing and about the system of nursing education is apparent. Nevertheless, certain principles have continued to characterize the approaches that the profession and those engaged in the educational system have taken to improve standards and monitor the quality of education in programs. The importance of engaging well-qualified instructors, selecting appropriate content, retaining a strong clinical focus, and maintaining appropriate admission standards have been concerns. The concern for standards of education and practice has been fundamental in view of the responsibility for providing safe and competent care to clients. However, dynamic leadership will be required to continue to provide direction to new generations of skilled practitioners and to ensure that their talents are used to the fullest extent for the benefit of the public.

With the development of the discipline and the expansion of the knowledge base, the appropriateness of the environment in which learning takes place is at issue. The fact that nursing is one of the last sex-segregated professions has led to attention to the potential for differential treatment, with improvement in the status of women as they gradually gain fundamental rights and privileges previously accorded only to men. Systematic undervaluing of the contributions of the profession continues to be common and is evident in the published histories of many health care institutions in which nurses usually have played significant roles in the implementation and management of care. Although it is difficult to say what will happen in the future in nursing and nursing education, nurses likely will continue to perform a highly valued service in the health care system, and they will be respected for their knowledge, skill, and contributions to the health of the people.

FUTURE DIRECTIONS

The tax-supported system of health care that has evolved in Canada over some 40 years, although not flawless, nevertheless is valued by consumers who react negatively to any suggestion that the system is imperiled. Such suggestions are the order of the day and simply part of business as usual in a not-for-profit system operated in the public sphere where interest groups and institutions alike have the opportunity to argue for funds and programs they see as being beneficial. Today, the limits to the nature and amount of care that can be provided

and the limits to growth are recognized. To ensure the continuation of the system, measures must be taken to ensure that universal availability and access to needed services are balanced by the provision of reasonably comprehensive services in a publicly funded, nonprofit, and affordable system.

The system must respond to perceptions of a need for change in the nature and context of health care. Canada has had a hospital- and physician-centered system of health care entrenched in its universal health care legislation for almost 50 years. The social determinants of health such as income, education, and the environment are important elements in the health of a nation. Universal health insurance has provided some assistance to vulnerable population groups, but other measures to address some of these problems are needed. Health increasingly is seen more broadly than simply the absence of illness, and in the presence of new approaches to the meaning of health, the nature and context of health care must change as well.

The needs of professional groups must be balanced by the needs of society. In the evolving health care system in Canada, there is a need for the health professions to work collaboratively in the best interest of the consumer. The system developed in Canada has provided high-quality medical and hospital care and has contributed significantly to improvements in the health of the people. However, despite new and impressive technological adjuncts to care, rational judgments must be made concerning the nature and context of health and health care. Social and cultural determinants of health require much study and attention to produce improved health outcomes. The political framework within which the issues relative to health care insurance plans are debated and determined will be conditioned by the economic and social realities of effecting fundamental change in the system. Decisions to move to a community-based model emphasizing prevention of disease, promotion of health, and partnerships between professionals and consumers will be difficult ones but are those that ultimately will hold the greatest potential for influencing health care positively. Issues surrounding hospital governance, education of health care professionals, the integration of boards of health care agencies on a regional basis, and restructuring of the systems for providing care and for remunerating health care professionals in a reasonable and rational way must be considered in a collaborative manner to allow the health care system in Canada to meet the challenges that are ahead in this century and beyond.

REFERENCES

Axworthy, L., & Spiegel, J. (2002). Retaining Canada's health care system as a global public good. *Canadian Medical Association Journal, 167*(4), 365-366.

Canadian Broadcasting System. (2005). *Top court strikes down Quebec private health-care ban.* Retrieved June 20, 2005, from http://www.cbc.ca/story/canada/national/2005/06/09/n ewscoc-health050609.html

Canadian Council on Social Development. (2000). *The labour market integration of new nursing graduates in Canada (1986-1998).* Ottawa, Ontario: Author.

Canadian Institute for Health Information. (2004a). *Workforce trends of licensed practical nurses in Canada, 2003.* Ottawa, Ontario: Author.

Canadian Institute for Health Information. (2004b). *Workforce trends of registered nurses in Canada, 2003.* Ottawa, Ontario: Author.

Canadian Institute for Health Information. (2004c). *Workforce trends of registered psychiatric nurses in Canada, 2003.* Ottawa, Ontario: Author.

Canadian Nurses Association. (2005). *Obtaining CNA certification: Certification for nursing specialties.* Retrieved June 24, 2005, from http://www.cna-nurses.ca/CNA/nursing/certification/ specialties/default_e.aspx

Cleverley, K., Baumann, A., Blythe, J., Grinspun, D., & Tompkins, C. (2004). *Educated and underemployed: The paradox for nursing graduands: Interim report.* Hamilton, Ontario, Canada: Nursing Health Services Research Unit, McMaster University.

Deber, R. B., Hastings, J. E. F., & Thompson, G. G. (1991). Health care in Canada: Current trends and issues. *Journal of Public Health Policy, 12*(1), 72-82.

Milne, C. (2001). *Are we being served?* Retrieved March 8, 2005, from www.pollara.ca/new/Library/surveys/healthcare Nov2001MC.htm

National Forum on Health. (1995). *The public and private financing of Canada's health system: A discussion paper.* Ottawa, Ontario: Government of Canada.

Registered Nurses Association of Ontario. (2001). *Earning their return: When & why. Ontario RNs left Canada and what will bring them back?* Toronto, Ontario, Canada: Author.

Romanow, R. (2002). *Building on values: The future of health care in Canada: Report of the commission on the future of health care in Canada.* Ottawa, Ontario: Government of Canada.

Ross Kerr, J. (2002). The organization and financing of health care. In J. Ross Kerr & M. Wood (Eds.), *Canadian nursing: Issues and perspectives* (4th ed., pp. 255-279). Toronto, Ontario, Canada: Elsevier.

Ryten, E. (1997). *A statistical picture of the past, present and future of registered nurses in Canada.* Ottawa, Ontario: Canadian Nurses Association.

Schafer, A. (2002). *The great Canadian health care debate: Values under fire.* Retrieved April 27, 2005, from http://www. umanitoba.ca/centres/ethics/articles/article8.html

Wood, M. J., Giovannetti, P., & Ross-Kerr, J. C. (2004). *The Canadian PhD in nursing: A discussion paper.* Edmonton, Alberta, Canada: Marilynn Wood and Associates.

Nursing in Britain

An Overview of Health Care, Nursing Education, and Practice

JUNE CLARK

HEALTH CARE IN BRITAIN

Most persons date the beginning of the British health care system to the introduction of the National Health Service (NHS) in 1948, but formal forms of health care have existed in Britain for several hundred years. The oldest hospital in Britain (which is still in use and still uses some of the original buildings) is St Bartholomew's Hospital in London (known as "Barts"), which was established in 1123. "Madhouses" similarly had existed for centuries, although they were not formalized as mental hospitals until late in the nineteenth century, and the training of mental health nurses did not begin until 1891. Community health services for the poor had been provided by the public authorities since the time of the first Queen Elizabeth. The major development of the formal health care system in Britain, however, took place in the nineteenth century when Britain was at the peak of its imperial power, when the industrial revolution changed Britain from an agricultural society to an industrial society in which the growth of cities created health problems that politicians no longer could ignore, when scientific medicine was beginning, and medicine and later nursing were becoming organized as professions. Every nurse has heard about Florence Nightingale and her work on hospitals and nursing education, but Florence Nightingale was very much a product of her time, and there were many other pioneers developing services that were to become, a century later, part of the "new" National Health Service.

Many of the organizational features and the cultural traditions that shape the present day health care services of Britain are the living relics of this history. For example, one of the most important features of the present British health care system that is derived from history is the arrangement by which direct access to specialist (hospital) services is not permitted (except for accident and emergency services) but depends on a referral by the primary care physician (general practitioner). This arrangement originally was negotiated during the nineteenth century by the physicians themselves as a means of protecting the respective financial interests of those who worked in hospitals and those who worked in what became primary care. Although people in other countries may interpret this as a limitation on the consumer's individual choice, it is undoubtedly a major factor in the relatively low cost of the National Health Service.

By the time of the inception of the NHS in 1948, therefore, there already existed in Britain an extensive and complex pattern of health services, although it was fragmented, patchy in its coverage, and financially unsustainable. What the National Health Service Act of 1946 did was to take the existing services and rationalize and nationalize them. That is, all services were to be made available to all citizens free of charge at the point of use, provided through public authorities (of various kinds), and financed through direct government funding derived from taxation. Over the past 60 years some of these principles have been modified in various ways (e.g., some services now require co-payment), but what has persisted are the following core values:

♦ Universality (services available to everyone as a citizen's right)

♦ Comprehensiveness (all types of services: hospital and community based, preventive and curative, from "cradle to grave")

♦ Free at the point of use (access to services based on need regardless of ability to pay)

These values remain dear to the hearts of the British people (as many governments that have tried to make changes have discovered to their cost) and are still clearly visible in the structures and processes of the NHS today.

The achievement of the 1946 act was the culmination of a great political battle in which many compromises had to be made. In particular, the service could not run without the cooperation of the medical profession, yet at that time the medical profession was opposed to several aspects of the plan. For example, medical professionals adamantly were opposed to control by local government (which they interpreted as political interference with their clinical freedom), and they were worried by the threat to their personal income derived from private practice. The compromises agreed upon with the medical profession in 1946 and for which sections of the medical profession have fought ever since, explain many of the organizational and financial features of the NHS today. For example, the resistance to working for local government explains the existence of health authorities (members of which are not elected but are appointed for their individual expertise or to represent various community interests), variously named in the years since 1946. Similarly, the right of senior hospital doctors (called "consultants") to undertake private practice alongside their salaried work in NHS hospitals explains the coexistence and pattern of private sector health care in Britain; and the fierce battle by primary care physicians (general practitioners) to work as independent contractors rather than as salaried employees explains the present organization of primary care services.

Financing of Health Care

The National Health Service is funded primarily (approximately 95%) from taxation, including a small proportion from the national insurance scheme that is compulsory for all employers and employees; approximately 5% is derived from co-payments, mainly for drugs and dental and ophthalmic services. In the NHS the only third-party payer is the government.

The assumption made in 1946 that once the "backlog" of disease had been dealt with, the costs of the NHS would become less, turned out to be a major mistake; as in all Western countries, the costs of health care have risen inexorably, and in Britain, as in most countries, cost constraint is a major preoccupation.

Until recently, expenditure on health care was low in the United Kingdom compared with other European countries, but the current "New Labor" government was elected on a commitment to increase health care spending to at least the European average. As a result, expenditure on the NHS has doubled during the past 8 years to approximately 8.4% of the gross domestic product and is due to rise to 9.2% by 2007-2008. Even with this increase, however, the expenditure is still barely half that in the United States

The health care budget is managed by the Department of Health in England and the devolved governments in Scotland, Wales, and Northern Ireland (see the following sections). After "top-slicing" for various centrally provided services, the money is devolved on a weighted per capita basis to geographically defined health authorities who spend it on providing health care services for their populations. Before 1990 the health authorities used the money directly to run the hospitals and community-based agencies; since 1990 (see the following discussion), health authorities have used the money to commission services through contracts with provider agencies called NHS Trusts. Primary care is provided, also free of charge, by general practitioners whose contracts now are managed by the same commissioning authorities. A new contract for general practitioners, negotiated in 2004, provides for a variety of item-of-service and incentive payments and reimbursement of the costs of support services (including the employment of practice nurses).

Structure and Organization of the National Health Service

The structure and organization of the NHS has changed dramatically in the past decade, but traces of the original framework still exist. For its first 30 years, the NHS was organized in three branches that reflected the structures that existed previously: hospital services were run by Regional Hospital Boards (RHBs); public health, the school health service, and community nursing services continued to be run by local government; and the general practitioners operated independently with contracts administered by Executive Councils. The three distinct organizational cultures still exist in present day services. Throughout the 1960s, there were many initiatives to bring the three branches together, and in 1974 the hospital and community services were brought together under newly created area health authorities; however, the general practitioners fought successfully to remain outside as independent contractors, a situation that still persists.

In 1979 the election of a new right-wing conservative government under the leadership of Margaret Thatcher began a series of changes in the health care system (and many other aspects of British society) that were ideological and organizational and were more radical than anything that had happened since the end of the Second World War. The 1980s saw a sequence of changes

VIEWPOINTS

that were introduced as "efficiency improvements" but that in their effects constituted radical cultural and organizational changes. The most significant change for nursing was the introduction in 1983, on the recommendation of Sir Roy Griffiths, of the concept of general management to replace the system of functional management by the traditional triumvirate of doctor, nurse, and administrator. Many senior nurses retired or lost their jobs, provoking a loss of leadership from which the nursing profession only recently has begun to recover. At the same time, the views that care in the community was cheaper and better than hospital care led to major reductions in the number of hospital beds, especially in psychiatric hospitals and hospitals providing long-term care. Health care began to become redefined as acute medical care. Many of the support services that previously had been provided "in-house" were contracted out to commercial agencies. The long-term care of frail elderly persons gradually was transferred to private sector nursing homes, which expanded dramatically in number, causing a reconfiguration of the nursing workforce that previously had been employed almost exclusively in the NHS.

The 1990 Reforms

The changes were confirmed in new legislation in 1990. The core component of the 1990 NHS reforms was the introduction of an internal market through changes in the roles of the health authorities and the hospitals and community agencies that provide health care, to create a "purchaser/provider split." Instead of using their money to run facilities themselves, the health authorities were to use it to purchase services for their resident population from the provider agencies that now were reconstituted as self-governing not-for-profit organizations called NHS Trusts. Some of the money was made available to general practitioners who chose to become "fundholders" to purchase certain services directly for their patients from trusts and other agencies. The idea was that trusts would compete with one another (and with the private sector agencies) for contracts with health authorities and fundholders, and the government believed that this competition would drive down costs and improve quality.

These changes produced a great change in the organizational culture of the NHS. On the one hand, the system undoubtedly became more cost-conscious at all levels and therefore probably more efficient. Quality assurance and outcome measurement became much more important. On the other hand, clinicians of all disciplines complained that commercial pressures interfered

with clinical freedom. Services that were regarded as uneconomical were cut, or responsibility was transferred to other sectors. Commercial competitiveness prevented the sharing of good practice. Most seriously, the negotiation by some general practitioner fundholders of contracts that gave preferential terms for their patients, produced for the first time in the history of the NHS a two-tier service that violated the basic principle of access based on need alone.

In the 1997 general election, in which the NHS was a major election issue, the Conservative government was heavily defeated, and power moved to the "New Labor" government led by Tony Blair, among whose election commitments was "restoration" of the NHS.

The New National Health Service: Modern, Dependable

Within a few months of the election the proposals of the new government were published in a white paper titled *The New NHS—Modern Dependable* (Department of Health, 1997). In line with the commitment of the new government to political devolution, however, parallel papers that differed in detail although not in their central policy were published for Wales, Scotland, and Northern Ireland. The proposals were implemented by new legislation including parallel legislation covering Scotland and Wales.

The main changes were as follows:

◆ The competitive internal market was abolished, but the split between health authorities as purchasers (renamed "commissioners") and trusts as providers was retained.

◆ A new performance framework was introduced, based on "clinical governance" in which chief executives of trusts became personally accountable for the quality of services as well as for financial management. New organizations were established to set standards and monitor quality.

◆ Fundholding was abolished, but new local primary care organizations were created, taking over from the Health Authorities (which subsequently were abolished) the responsibility for commissioning hospital services and (in England) providing community and primary care services for their local population.

◆ A duty was placed on Health Authorities, Trusts, and primary care organizations to collaborate and work in partnership with local authorities within jointly agreed health improvement programs.

◆ New ways of delivering services were established, including a national telephone help line staffed by nurses, called NHS Direct.

◆ A program of "modernisation" was introduced based on development of "new ways of working" (including shifts in traditional professional boundaries) and the use of information technology.

Each of the four countries of the United Kingdom subsequently published an "NHS Plan" that set out its policies in greater detail, with plans for implementation.

Effects of Political Devolution

In the previous edition of this book, it was possible to describe "the British National Health Service" as a centrally organized service that worked in the same way in all parts of the United Kingdom. That is no longer true. Because England is so much bigger than the other three countries, and because the Westminster Parliament is still dominant, it often is assumed that what happens in England is true for the whole of the United Kingdom. However, because responsibility for the provision of health care was devolved to the new governments established in Scotland and in Wales (because of the continuing political turbulence, Northern Ireland has moved in and out of devolution), the health care systems of the four countries of the United Kingdom gradually have diverged, although the core principles of a comprehensive health care system, funded by general taxation, provided to all citizens based on clinical need, and free of charge at the point of use remain sacrosanct. The organizational structures through which services are delivered are different in the four countries, and within the broad policy framework that is still set by the Westminster government, the relative emphasis given to various aspects of health care policy also differs—each country reflecting its own particular health problems and political ideologies.

Greer (2004) describes the differences in the following way:

◆ England has developed the concept of the *market*. It emphasizes competition, diversity, and consumer choice as the means of improving quality and has drawn heavily on American models such as the Kaiser Permanente health maintenance organization model. England makes much greater use of private sector providers, arguing that so long as the service remains free to patients at the point of use, it does not matter who provides it. Recent priorities in England have been the reduction of waiting times for elective surgery and diversifying of facilities for primary care.

◆ Wales, which is still recovering from the legacy of high morbidity and social deprivation left by its industrial past, emphasizes *localism* and in particular,

integration with local government (which is responsible for social services and environmental matters) to focus more on the determinants of health, with measures such as subsiding meals for school children and use of sports and exercise facilities for children and elderly persons. Proud of its heritage as the birthplace of the NHS, Wales demonstrates a strong political commitment to its "founding principles," for example by abolishing the co-payments required in England for drugs and eye tests.

◆ Scotland is building on a strong tradition of *professionalism,* building its policies and its organizational structures around the professional structure of medicine in contrast to the English emphasis on *managerialism*. Scotland shares with Wales a left-of-center political philosophy that is the result of its history. For example, Scotland has repudiated the concept of the market by abolishing trusts and reverting to direct provision of services by health boards.

BRITISH HEALTH CARE SYSTEM IN THE YEAR 2005

The British health care system in the year 2005 is therefore a service in transition, but one that continues to reflect some of the organizational structures of the past and is based on strong cultural values that were established in the immediate postwar period when the NHS was established. Most health care is provided through the NHS, but there is a private hospital sector (supported mainly by private insurance) that provides mainly non-emergency surgical services and a large private nursing home sector that provides long-term care for frail elderly persons. The NHS is still a national service, centrally funded from direct taxation, but in Scotland and Wales, responsibility for managing health (and education) services is devolved to the Scottish Parliament and the National Assembly for Wales; in Northern Ireland, the continuing political instability has delayed devolution.

Hospital services are similar to those in any developed country, but one of the particular strengths of the British system is its long tradition of community-based nursing services, which, like hospital services, are provided free at the point of contact to all who need them. In the British system the term *community-based services* is preferred to *ambulatory care*. District nurses provide nursing care in their own homes to persons suffering from chronic illness and following discharge from hospital; health visitors provide preventive health care and support to all families with young children;

and preventive health services are provided to children at school through the school health service. Mental health services and services for those with learning disabilities (mental handicaps) are nowadays mainly community based and are run in close collaboration with the social services of local authorities, as are community-based services for elderly persons. Long-term care for elderly persons nowadays is provided mainly in private sector care homes (often paid for by public funds). Occupational health is not included in the NHS but is provided independently by some large employers.

Primary care services are provided by family physicians called general practitioners, based in doctors' offices that usually are called "surgeries." General practitioners work in close association with community nurses who are employed by NHS Trusts and also may employ their own nurses who usually work only in the surgery. Every citizen has the right to "register" with a general practitioner of his or her choice. About 96% of the citizens do so, but there are difficulties for some mobile or homeless persons. The general practitioner contracts to provide medical services to all the persons on his or her list whenever needed. A new contract, negotiated between the government and the general practitioners in 2004, allows general practitioners to opt out of "out of hours" responsibilities, in which case the local primary care organization is responsible for providing arrangements, usually using the same doctors, but on separate contracts. Usually members of a family register with the same general practitioner and may remain registered with the same general practitioner from birth until death or until they move to another locality; this enables considerable continuity of care, which is one of the strengths of the system. The general practitioner is usually the point of first contact for persons needing health care and acts as "gatekeeper" to other services to which he or she refers patients as necessary. This position, however, currently is being challenged by new services, especially in England, such as "walk-in centres" and NHS Direct.

NHS Direct (slightly different names are used in Wales and Scotland) is a telephone help line that provides information, triage, and health advice to callers 24 hours a day, 7 days a week, and 365 days a year. Although telephone help lines have existed for many years, NHS Direct differs in that it is a national service, part of the NHS, and covers all aspects of health care. NHS Direct is primarily a nursing service (i.e., the advisers are nurses), and about half of all calls result in nursing advice alone without referral to other agencies. As a result of the 2004 General Practitioner Contract, NHS Direct increasingly is becoming the coordinating mechanism for all "out-of-hours services." NHS Direct advisers may refer patients to a hospital accident and emergency service (including calling an ambulance), but they may not refer a patient directly to a hospital specialist; that responsibility remains with the general practitioner.

Although from the patient's point of view, the services are broadly similar across the United Kingdom, the way in which they are structured and organized differs across the four countries.

England

A Secretary of State for Health appointed by the Prime Minister is directly accountable to Parliament for the running of the NHS in England. The Secretary of State is supported by the Department of Health (*www.dh.gov.uk*), which negotiates levels of funding with the Treasury, allocates resources to the health authorities, and sets national standards. At national level, numerous semiautonomous organizations have been established to be responsible for various aspects of quality assurance, regulation, and specific initiatives within the "modernisation" program. Some of these cover the whole of the United Kingdom, some only England.

At local level, geographically defined health authorities receive money from the central government to commission health services. Apart from a few Special Health Authorities that commission or provide specialist services for the country as a whole, England is divided into 28 Strategic Health Authorities (SHAs), each covering an average population of 1.8 million; their main function is the performance management of the local commissioning organizations and the NHS Trusts. In England the main commissioning organizations are the Primary Care Trusts (PCTs), each serving a population of, on average, 170,000 persons. The Primary Care Trusts, which are now responsible for approximately 75% of NHS expenditure in England, are responsible for commissioning secondary care (i.e., hospital) services and for providing primary and community health services for their resident population. Some critics suggest that PCTs are too small to undertake these functions properly, and some have merged to form larger organizations. Further changes are likely.

In England the three other main kinds of NHS Trusts that are the main providers of services to geographically defined populations are acute trusts, which are centered on a main hospital (sometimes a group of hospitals) to provide medical and surgical care; mental health trusts, which provide mental health services (hospital and community); and ambulance trusts. A few provide a combination of services or solely specialist services, such as eye or dental hospitals. Recently, as part of the commitment of the current government to local control, diversity, and patient choice, new organizations such as Care Trusts (which combine health and social care), Children's Trusts (which combine health and social services for children), and Foundation Trusts (which are given greater freedom from central control than ordinary NHS Trusts) are being created.

Wales

With a population of just under 3 million persons, Wales could be regarded as the equivalent of less than 2 of the 28 strategic health authorities in England. The devolved political powers of Wales are less than those of Scotland (i.e., it does not have full legislative powers), but they include responsibility for education and health. The National Assembly for Wales, which is elected directly by the people of Wales, receives funding in the form of a block grant from the Westminster-based Treasury, but within this budget the allocation of funds is their direct responsibility. The Minister for Health and Social Services (in Wales the two functions are combined) is accountable to the Assembly for the running of NHS Wales, supported by an executive arm known at the Welsh Assembly Government. Instead of the strategic health authorities of England, Wales has three Welsh Assembly Government regional offices covering North Wales, Mid and West Wales, and South East Wales, respectively.

Wales does not have Primary Care Trusts; most services are commissioned by 22 Local Health Boards (LHBs) that are coterminous with the local authorities that are responsible for other health-related functions such as social services and environmental health. A few specialist services are centrally commissioned. Unlike the English PCTs, the LHBs do not provide community nursing services directly. With the exception of tertiary cancer services and ambulance services, which are provided on an all-Wales basis, all services are provided by geographically defined "integrated" NHS Trusts.

Scotland

Scotland has greater devolved powers than Wales; the Scottish Parliament has full legislative power for all devolved areas, including health. Like the other countries, the Parliament has an executive arm, known as the Scottish Executive. The Minister for Health and Community Care and the Executive's Health Department have complete responsibility for health policy and for the running of NHS Scotland, with the exception of a small number of reserved areas (which include professional regulation and the control and safety of medicines).

In Scotland, health services are provided directly through 15 unified NHS boards with strategic planning, performance management, and governance responsibility for the whole of their local health systems. Since 2004, trusts have been abolished. At local level, community health partnerships have considerable influence on the deployment of the resources of the board and play a pivotal role in delivering health improvement to their local communities.

Northern Ireland

In Northern Ireland, health and social services are integrated under the umbrella of the Health and Personal Social Services Department. Under devolution, the Northern Ireland Assembly and its executive arm, the Northern Ireland Executive, had responsibilities similar to those in Wales. However, since these institutions were suspended in 2002, responsibility for health and social services has returned to the Northern Ireland Office of the Westminster parliament.

Health and social services are commissioned by four Health and Social Services Boards and are provided by 19 Health and Social Services Trusts, which are accountable directly to the Health and Personal Social Services Department. Some Trusts provide acute care services, some provide community health and social services, and some provide both.

NURSING PRACTICE

Nursing practice in any country is shaped by the health care system, by nurses' educational preparation, by the system for professional regulation, by the organizational framework in which nurses work, and by the shape of the health care workforce (e.g., the number of qualified nurses relative to the number of physicians and other health care personnel). Most nurses in Britain work within the NHS, although the recent expansion in private sector nursing homes for elderly persons means that about a third now work in the private sector. Nurses work in hospitals (mainly), community-based clinics, person's homes, schools, workplaces, and many other settings so that what constitutes "nursing practice" varies greatly.

Specialization: The Nursing "Professions"

As in many highly developed health care systems, nursing has become highly specialized—in Britain to the extent that nursing is described in legislation as consisting of three distinct professions: nursing, midwifery, and health visiting. Health visitors are always and midwives are usually also registered nurses (although direct entry to midwifery through separate educational preparation is growing). Even within "nursing" there are four different "branches" at the basic level (adult nursing, children's nursing, psychiatric nursing, and learning disabilities nursing). Britain is probably the only country in the world in which at the point of initial qualification a nurse is a specialist rather than a generalist. At the post-basic level is a wide range of other specialties and subspecialties in hospital and community practice. In addition, many specialties operate in hospital and community, sometimes specifically working across the interface to provide continuity of care to patients; for example, stoma nurses, continence nurses, and palliative care (hospice) nurses.

In Britain, no nursing practice acts define the work of nurses. The competencies required for registration as a nurse are specified by the Nurses and Midwives Council (NMC), which is the organization that regulates nursing in the United Kingdom (see the following discussion). Beyond this, what nurses were allowed to do was largely a matter of custom and practice until 1992 when the United Kingdom Central Council for Nursing, Midwifery and Health Visiting (UKCC; the predecessor of the NMC) published a seminal document titled *The Scope of Professional Practice* (UKCC, 1992). This document stressed that every nurse is personally accountable for his or her practice and that it is the nurse's professional judgment that determines what to do. In essence, this means that the only limit on the nurse's practice is his or her own competence and the policies of his or her employer. Since 1992, this principle has facilitated the development of advanced practice and many new nursing roles.

Regulation of Nursing

In the United Kingdom, nursing has been regulated since 1919, but since that time the regulatory organizations have been reformed and renamed several times. In the wake of several high-profile failures of the system of self-regulation (mainly in medicine), the regulation of medicine and nursing is currently under review.

Legislation also is being introduced to achieve the registration of support workers (assistive personnel) and professions such as social work that previously have not been subject to regulation. The organization currently responsible for the regulation of nursing, midwifery, and health visiting throughout the United Kingdom (professional regulation is not devolved to the four countries) is called the Nurses and Midwives Council. The NMC was established in 2001, replacing the United Kingdom Central Council for Nursing, Midwifery and Health Visiting. The NMC maintains the register of nurses, specifies the standard and content of the basic nursing education that is required for entry to the register, and maintains the disciplinary process under which professional misconduct may lead to the removal of a nurse's name from the register. Being "on the Register" constitutes the nurse's "license to practice." To continue to practice, nurses are required to renew their registration every 3 years, and this requires evidence of continuing education to ensure continuing competence. As part of its disciplinary function the NMC also issues guidance documents such as the Code of Professional Conduct.

Levels of Practice

In spite of the high degree of post-basic specialization, little consideration has been given until recently to differentiate *levels* of practice. For many years discussion centered on the "extended role of the nurse" (which was taken to mean the transfer of certain tasks from doctors to nurses) as opposed to the "expanded role of the nurse" (which was taken to mean a greater depth of nursing decision making). The most recent driver for change has been the need to reduce the working hours of junior hospital doctors to meet new European legislation. However, the professional lead has been taken by those nurses who have developed the role of nurse practitioner in primary health care. Currently, no system is in place in Britain for the certification or regulation of advanced practice, and the indiscriminate use of titles such as nurse practitioner and clinical nurse specialist has increased the confusion. The NMC currently is considering proposals to regulate advanced practice as part of its normal regulatory machinery. One indicator of advanced practice that has been achieved—after some 15 years of strenuous political lobbying by organizations such as the Royal College of Nursing—is prescriptive rights (known in Britain as "nurse prescribing"). Special training is required, and the formulary from which nurses may prescribe initially was very limited but gradually is being expanded.

A recent government initiative is the development of new posts for "consultant nurses," which are presented as equivalent to the role of hospital consultants (i.e., the most senior hospital doctors) although at much lower salaries. About 1500 consultant nurses are now in the United Kingdom across a wide range of specialties. Specific criteria for the role include a 50% commitment to clinical practice alongside education, research, and leadership roles.

NURSING EDUCATION

Basic Nursing Education

Britain is famous for the first school of nursing established at St Thomas's Hospital, London, by Florence Nightingale in 1858. However, as Monica Baly (1986, 1995) has shown, the reality is different from the myth, and the strength of the Nightingale tradition, based on the concepts of obedience, discipline, and vocational training by apprenticeship, has not helped more recent attempts in Britain to achieve a proper professional education for nurses. Over a period of more than 50 years from the 1930s onward, many attempts were made to reform nursing education, but as Miss Nightingale herself once wrote, "Reports are not self-executive." Moreover, nurses themselves still strongly disagree about the kind of education that is appropriate, some favoring the Nightingale model of vocational training, others the university model developed in the early days by Mrs. Bedford Fenwick.

Until the early 1990s, nurse training in Britain consisted of a 3-year hospital-based program in one of four separate specialties (general hospital nursing, children's nursing, mental nursing, and mental handicap nursing). A 2-year program was available for licensed practical nurses, known in Britain as enrolled nurses. In addition, from the 1960s onward, there were a few programs at the baccalaureate level run by universities. The nursing workforce therefore currently includes nurses prepared by a variety of routes. Since 1979, European Union requirements for mutual recognition of qualifications across Europe specify the length of basic nursing education program as 3 years or 4600 hours and also the balance between theory and practice.

In 1988, however, the government accepted in principle the recommendations of a UKCC report titled *Project 2000: A New Preparation for Practice* (1986), and programs based on these recommendations were introduced across the whole of the United Kingdom from 1990 onward. Project 2000 was a major change in

nursing education in Britain. It recommended the following:

♦ That there should be only one level of registered nurse and that training for the second level (the enrolled nurse, equivalent to the licensed practical nurse in the United States) should be discontinued
♦ That students should no longer be considered as hospital employees, but during their period of training should be supernumerary to the labor force
♦ That hospital-based schools of nursing should develop links with institutions of further and higher education
♦ That the basic program should consist of a 2-year Common Foundation Program (CFP) followed by a "Branch" program in adult nursing, children's nursing, mental health nursing, mental handicap nursing, or midwifery and should lead to a diploma in higher education

These recommendations themselves represented a series of compromises designed to resolve continuing conflicts within the profession (for example, between those who wanted a university-level generalist preparation and those who wanted to continue the traditional model), and further compromises were made during the period of negotiation with the government.

The period of implementation was fraught with difficulties. Midwives would not agree to be defined as a branch of nursing and succeeded in establishing separate programs leading to registration as a midwife (RM). To achieve higher levels for the new student bursaries that replaced salaries, the principle of "student status" was compromised by a requirement that for 1000 of the 2300 hours of required clinical practice the student would be part of the "rostered" nursing workforce. The Common Foundation Program was reduced to 18 months. Implementation coincided with cost constraint and the rapid changes in the NHS that followed the 1990 reforms, so the provision of support during clinical placements has often been less than adequate. The internal market that was applied to NHS service provision also was applied to nursing education; the purchasers/commissioners are consortia of employers who contract with the universities to train a defined number of students in each of the four branches.

Fitness for Practice

Under pressure to remedy some of the perceived deficits of Project 2000, the UKCC established another Commission for Nursing and Midwifery Education. Its report, *Fitness for Practice* (UKCC, 1999), was published in September 1999. Many of the recommendations supported the original aims of Project 2000, stressing in particular the need for greater support for students in the clinical areas and better collaboration between clinical areas and the academic departments. The report suggested that some of the contentious issues such as the funding of students and the four specialist branches should be examined further. One recommendation, however, constituted a major change in the Project 2000 program: the Common Foundation Program that Project 2000 recommended should last 2 years and that was reduced during the implementation negotiations to 18 months, was reduced further to 1 year.

Making a Difference

The proposals of the Commission were to some extent preempted, however, by proposals contained in the strategy for nursing, *Making a Difference* (Department of Health, 1999), which the government published in July 1999. Driven by the acute shortage of nurses, especially in London (which was attributed to the "over academic" nature of Project 2000 programs but which actually was caused by the major reduction in the number of training places commissioned following the 1990 NHS reforms), the government committed itself to making nursing education "more responsive to the needs of the NHS" by widening the entry gate to include more candidates without formal educational qualifications, enabling students to "step off and on" at the end of the first year of training, and increasing the practical component during the first year. Anxious about its ability to meet the workforce requirements of the NHS, the Department of Health gradually has increased its control of basic nursing education. Funding remains with the NHS and not with the Department for Education, which funds all other higher education, so integration with the university sector is incomplete; this difference is exacerbated by the level of the program (lower than the baccalaureate level, which is the usual level of a university education) and by the inability of nursing programs to conform to the normal academic year. Most significantly, traditional attitudes to students persist; many service managers and many nurses who qualified under the "old" system continue to expect high levels of practical skill early in the program and complain that the Project 2000 nurses are "too academic."

The publication of *Making a Difference,* however, coincided with political devolution and therefore applied only to England; the Welsh strategy *Realizing the Potential* (National Assembly for Wales, 1999) and the subsequent strategy for nursing education *Creating the Potential* (National Assembly for Wales, 2001) retained the commitment to expanding nursing education at the baccalaureate level with the aim of achieving all-graduate entry as soon as feasible. Since September 2004, all basic nursing education in Wales is at baccalaureate level.

At the time of writing (June 2005) all programs of basic nursing education in the United Kingdom conform to the Project 2000 model as modified by *Fitness to Practice* (UKCC, 1999):

◆ A 3-year program consists of a 1-year common foundation program, followed by a "branch programme" in one of four specialties (adult nursing, children's nursing, mental health nursing, or learning disabilities nursing).

◆ Students are supernumerary during most of their program but must complete 1000 "rostered hours" during their third year; unlike other students, they do not have to pay fees, and they are supported financially by a bursary paid by the NHS.

◆ Schools of nursing now are organizationally established within the universities, although many remain physically located in their original hospital premises.

◆ Clinical practice education is undertaken in the hospital and community settings of the NHS Trusts, where students are taught and supervised by the clinical staff and not by the university-based faculty.

◆ The program leads to professional qualification as a registered nurse, plus a diploma in higher education or a bachelor of science degree.

In spite of the difficulties, in many areas great progress has been made. Project 2000 nurses are demonstrating a more thoughtful approach to practice and improved decision-making skills. Even in England, the number of degree-level programs has expanded, and the number of nurses who qualify by this route gradually is increasing. Enrolled nurse training has been discontinued, and most enrolled nurses have "converted" to first-level registration. Nurse teachers who were themselves prepared and practiced as teachers in the "old" environment have worked hard to respond to the challenges of teaching in the university environment. More teachers are achieving master's and doctoral qualifications.

Postbasic and Advanced Nursing Education

Postbasic education has been much less contentious, although not without problems. Evidence of continuing professional development is required for renewal of registration. Programs leading to a specialist practice qualification are required to last a year and to be at the level of a first degree. Master's-level programs are developing rapidly, although there are relatively few clinical master's programs. The number of nurses achieving doctorates also is increasing rapidly. However, tensions between the NHS and the universities continue about who can best provide postbasic education and who should set standards and ensure the quality of the programs.

CHALLENGES FOR THE TWENTY-FIRST CENTURY: CURRENT ISSUES

These are turbulent times for nursing in Britain. Little consensus exists even within the profession about whether nursing should continue to develop as a full profession or whether health care needs require a more pragmatic, employer-led vocational approach. The tension shows in the continuing debates about how students should be prepared, how they should be supported financially, and who should control the level and content of this preparation. As in other developed countries, recruitment and retention of a nursing workforce adequate to meet service needs is high on the agenda, and there are debates about the ethics of recruiting nurses from other countries to meet these needs. A recently negotiated pay structure that will cover all NHS staff (Department of Health, 2003) currently is being implemented. New nursing roles are developing rapidly to meet new needs. The NHS itself constantly is changing shape in response to new government targets and initiatives. Nursing has many challenges, risks, and opportunities.

REFERENCES

Department of Health. (2005). *Agenda for change: NHS terms and conditions of service handbook.* Retrieved January 5, 2005 from http:www.dh.gov.uk/assetRoot/04/09/59/50/04095950.pdf

Baly, M. E. (1986). *Florence Nightingale and the nursing legacy.* London: Routledge.

Baly, M. E. (1995). *Nursing and social change* (3rd ed.). London: Heinemann Medical Books.

Department of Health. (1997). *The new NHS—Modern dependable.* London: The Stationery Office.

Department of Health. (1999). *Making a difference.* London: The Stationery Office.

Greer. (2004). *Four way bet: How devolution has led to four different models for the NHS.* London. The Constitution Unit, University College London.

National Assembly for Wales. (1999). *Realising the potential.* Cardiff, Wales: The Stationery Office.

National Assembly for Wales. (2001). *Creating the potential.* Cardiff, Wales: The Stationery Office.

United Kingdom Central Council for Nursing, Midwifery and Health Visiting. (1986). *Project 2000: A new preparation for practice.* London: Author.

United Kingdom Central Council for Nursing, Midwifery and Health Visiting. (1992). *The scope of professional practice.* London: Author.

United Kingdom Central Council for Nursing, Midwifery and Health Visiting. (1999). *Fitness for practice: The UKCC Commission for Nursing and Midwifery Education.* London: Author.

Nursing in Japan

Meeting the Health Care Challenges
of the Twenty-First Century

TERUKO TAKAHASHI ◆ CHERYL L. BRANDI

Japan, a country historically steeped in tradition, has been changing at an accelerated rate since the turn of the century. Some major challenges Japan has had to confront include a rapidly aging population and low birthrate, a stagnant economy, new infectious diseases such as sudden acute respiratory syndrome, and natural disasters (earthquakes, typhoons, and volcanic eruptions)—all of which have been influencing health care and nursing significantly.

HEALTH CARE ENVIRONMENT

Demographic and Social Trends

Dramatic shifts have been occurring in the population distribution of Japan. In October 2003 the total population of Japan was 127,619,000, with an age structure (including males and females) as follows: birth to 14 years, 14.0%; 15 to 64 years, 66.9%; and 65 years and over, 19.0%. However, in 1970, persons over 65 years composed only 7.1% of the total population (Kousei toukei kyoukai, 2004). In fact, the growth in the aging population in the United States is only one third that of Japan (Japan Institute for Social and Economic Affairs, 2002a). As the overall population steadily ages, the birthrate continues to spiral downward. The estimated total fertility rate in 2003 was 1.29 children born per woman (Kousei toukei kyoukai, 2004). The Ministry of Health, Labor and Welfare figures for 2003 showed the lowest number of births since 1899, when record keeping began (Curtin, 2003a). Demographers predict the population will peak in 2007 and then continuously decline, and those aged 65 and older will continue to increase so that by the year 2015, 25% of the population of Japan will be aged (Japan Institute for Social and Economic Affairs, 2002a).

Compounding the aging problem, Japan continues to lead the world in life expectancy. Children born in 2003 can expect to live to 78.36 years old if male and to 85.33 years old if female. The four leading causes of death in 2003 were malignant neoplasms, heart diseases, cerebrovascular diseases, and pneumonia (Kousei toukei kyoukai, 2004), diseases usually associated with aging.

New social patterns also are emerging in Japan. Until the late 1980s, the family unit was the foundation of social stability and order in Japanese society, with roles of each family member well defined by gender, age, and relationship to the patriarchal head of the family. Women were expected to marry, have children, and care for aging parents and/or parents-in-law. However, a quiet resistance has occurred among younger persons. With expanded occupational choices, fewer Japanese women are marrying; the average age at time of first marriage is increasing annually; and the divorce rate has been increasing, especially among couples married more than 20 years (Imamura, 2003). Overall, marriage still remains popular, but women are choosing to have fewer children and at a later age. In 2002 the average age of first-time motherhood was 28.3 years (Kousei toukei kyoukai, 2004). All of these changes affect the traditional notion of care of the aged by the eldest son and wife and have shifted a certain amount of responsibility to the elderly themselves to maintain their health and not be a burden to others (Imamura, 2003).

Social trends in Japan also have been influenced by a poor employment market for youth (Curtin, 2003b), especially during a time of a long business recession and a decline in economic growth (Japan Institute for Social and Economic Affairs, 2002b). Unemployment rates for young adults have been and are expected to continue increasing, resulting in more young persons living at home and relying on parents for longer periods of time compared with the past, later marriages (causing lower birthrates), and changing attitudes about working full time (Curtin, 2003b).

Japanese Health Care System

The overall health status of the Japanese people is thought to be the best in the world (Imai, 2002), and from an international perspective, health care policy in Japan has been successful regarding standards of access, cost, and fairness (Ikegami & Campbell, 2004). The system, which is highly regulated by the government, offers free choice of providers and equal access for all persons at a reasonably low cost (Imai, 2002). Since the establishment of a system of social security and health insurance in 1961, all citizens of Japan have been covered under a compulsory universal health insurance program. Depending on age and employment status, citizens enroll through their employers or local societies. Since 1973, medical insurance systems have covered all medical costs for patients over 70 (Kousei toukei kyoukai, 2004).

Reimbursement for all medical services occurs according to a set fee schedule, which is determined by the government and is revised every 2 years. Outpatient care is reimbursed mostly according to a fee-for-service basis, and inpatient care payments are derived from a combination of per diem and fee for service (Imai, 2002). Additionally, patients pay a small co-payment at the point of service, the amount determined by the type of insurance (Yoshikawa, Bhattacharya, & Vogt, 1996).

Public health and community health centers are integral parts of the health care delivery system in Japan, and public health nurses (hokenshi) play essential roles in both. Public health centers serve as administrative headquarters for disease prevention, health promotion, and environmental sanitation and are managed by the Japanese Ministry of Health, Labor and Welfare. In 2004, there were 571 public health centers throughout Japan. Community health centers, which numbered 2543 in 2003, are managed by cities and towns. Their main purpose is to provide direct and personalized services for health promotion. Because of legislation passed in 1994, the number of community health centers is increasing while the number of public health centers is decreasing (Kousei toukei kyoukai, 2004).

Current Trends in Health Care

The health system of Japan is dealing with two major challenges. The first involves finding ways to contain costs in an environment of a rapidly aging population and a low growth of revenues (Imai, 2002). One great concern is about the burden of an aging population on a declining workforce and the sustainability of the current pension and health care insurance systems (Japan Institute for Social and Economic Affairs, 2002c; *Universal Healthcare Insurance,* 2002). The second challenge involves responding to a public that has become more demanding regarding quality of care (Imai, 2002).

Regarding the first challenge, Japan has been reforming health care financing in a number of ways. For the first time in history, Japan experienced an actual decline in medical spending in 2002 (Ikegami & Campbell, 2004). Perhaps the most noteworthy reform began in 2000, when a new insurance that covers old-age nursing care *(kaigo hoken)* was introduced and mandated. Under this plan, any person aged 40 to 64 is covered for any age-related disease, and all persons over 65 are covered, regardless of disease. All citizens over age 40 are required to enroll in the plan and to pay premiums. The insurance covers all medical costs and home care services as directed by a care manager (Japan Visiting Nursing Foundation, 1999).

The goals of *kaigo hoken,* which is managed by municipalities, are to lessen the burden on families who are caring for frail elderly and to reduce hospital length of stay. In 2003 the average length of stay for all types of hospitals (general and psychiatric) was 36.4 days (*Kousei roudou-syou,* n.d.), reflecting a phenomenon known as "social hospitalization," in which acute care beds are used for elderly long-term care (Imai, 2002).

The Japanese government also has initiated other cost-containing measures. A new inclusive payment system, diagnosis and procedure combinations (DPCs), for acute inpatient care was introduced in 2003 at 80 main university hospitals and two national centers. The diagnosis and procedure combinations system differs from the U.S. diagnosis-related groups (DRGs) system in that fees are set per diem. Additionally, average drug prices have been cut, and various co-payment rates have increased (Ikegami & Campbell, 2004).

The second challenge, improving quality, is also driving health system change. In the traditional fee-for-service system, reimbursement has been identical for all providers regardless of quality of service, and Japanese physicians may have paid less attention to quality for the sake of quantity to sustain their incomes (Imai, 2002). For years, patients have complained about long waiting times, too-brief consultation times, and lack of information (Ikegami & Campbell, 2004; Imai, 2002). Additionally, systems for medical recording, monitoring, and reporting have been poor (Ikegami & Campbell, 2004), and there have been few quality monitoring systems

VIEWPOINTS

in hospitals (Yamagishi, Kanda, & Takemura, 2003). In 2002 the Ministry of Health, Labor, and Welfare proposed delivery system reforms that emphasize accountability and movement toward a more consumer-oriented system. To date, reforms have included a reorganization of physician education (Ikegami & Campbell, 2004).

Japan also has addressed the issue of quality through the establishment of the Japan Council for Quality Health Care in 1995. The council is a not-for-profit, independent, multidisciplinary organization that began nationwide hospital accreditation surveys in 1997. As of May 2004, 1260 hospitals were accredited, and this information is available through the Internet (Kousei toukei kyoukai, 2004).

In consideration of cost and quality, hospice has been one service that has been slow to develop, despite the fact that the idea of hospice was introduced in Japan back in 1977. The delay has been attributed to a strong cultural tradition of collaboration between family and physician in not telling a patient that he or she has cancer. In 1999, there were only 63 palliative care institutions with 1140 beds throughout Japan (Kashiwagi, 1996). However, as of October 2004, palliative care institutions numbered 138 with a total of 2608 beds, and physicians and family basically tell the patients their diagnosis ("Zenkoku kanwa kea," 2004).

NURSING PRACTICE

Definition and Role Functions: Kangoshi, Hokenshi, and Zyosanshi

The understanding of "nurse" in Japan is different compared with some other countries. Three separate occupational titles describe health care workers with basic nursing preparation: *kangoshi, hokenshi,* and *zyosanshi.* In Japan the differences are clear, and members of each category maintain a distinct identity. *Kangoshi* is translated as "nurse" in English, *hokenshi* as "public health nurse," and *zyosanshi* as "nurse-midwife." Beginning March 1, 2002, the practice of using gender-specific versions of these words to distinguish between males and females in each occupational category was abolished, but men still are prohibited from becoming *zyosanshi* ("Re-amendment to the Nurse Law," 2002). A current proposal is to consider all occupational groups as "nurses" under the umbrella name of *kangosya* (Nihon Kango Kyoukai, 2003).

A separate licensing examination is given for each type of practitioner, but each one first must hold a license as a *kangoshi.* Licensing examinations are held once a year, and licenses are granted for life. *Kangoshi* may choose to remain *kangoshi* or become *hokenshi* (public health nurses) or *zyosanshi* (nurse-midwives). Only *kangoshi* with baccalaureate degrees may take licensing examinations for *hokenshi and zyun-kangoshi* without further specialized education.

Practice settings and role functions vary among the three types of health workers. In 2002, there were 1,097,326 *kangoshi* (including *zyun-kangoshi,* or assistant nurses), approximately 90% of whom worked in hospitals or clinics. A shift in work setting from hospital to outpatient clinics and visiting nursing stations has occurred for this group. The focus of *hokenshi* is health education. In 2002, there were 38,366 *hokenshi,* with approximately 80% working in community centers or public health centers. *Zyosanshi* care for prenatal, perinatal, and postpartum patients. They independently manage uncomplicated deliveries and newborn care. In 2002, there were 24,340 *zyosanshi,* with 75.2% working in hospitals or clinics and 7.0% in private birthing centers (Kousei toukei kyoukai, 2004).

Nurse-Physician Relations

Autonomy and nurse-physician relations seem to be bigger issues for *kangoshi* compared with *hokenshi* and *zyosanshi.* The top administrator in a hospital must be a physician ("Medical Law," 2004), although a number of nurse executives have become vice presidents of nursing in recent years. Hospital physicians are perceived by *kangoshi* as powerful (Brandi & Naito, in press), and compared with the United States, physicians in Japan are more available in the hospital (Primono, 2000), and hospital nurses are more likely to rely on the physicians for direction (Lambert, Lambert, & Ito, 2004). Dating back to the Meiji era (1868 to 1912), informal groups of physicians *(ikyoku),* led by a senior professor in medical universities, have been especially controlling, leading to conditions of factionalism and autocracy, which a number of hospitals are attempting to change (Kan, 2004). With recent governmental reforms regarding physician education (Ikegami & Campbell, 2004) and as the educational level of *kangoshi* increases, hopefully the power struggles between nurses and physicians will diminish.

Role of Nursing Organizations

The Japanese Nursing Association (JNA) and Japan Nursing Federation are the two most powerful organizations in Japan for addressing the occupational and political concerns of *kangoshi, hokenshi,* and *zyosanshi.* Approximately 560,000 nurses (including *kangoshi, hokenshi, zyosanshi,* and *zyun-kangoshi* categories) belong to the JNA, which is about half the number of all employed nurses. Three of the major JNA initiatives approved at the 2004 annual JNA convention include promotion of home care and visiting nursing, promotion of medical and nursing safety and risk management, and health promotion. The JNA also continues working to stop the assistant nurse *(zyun-kangoshi)* training programs ("Tsuuzyo soukai houkoku," 2004). A *zyun-kangoshi* is similar to a licensed practical nurse or licensed vocational nurse in the United States, and the greatest opposition to JNA efforts comes from the Japan Medical Association, a powerful political group in Japan regarding medicine and welfare.

The Japanese Nursing Federation focuses on issues involving health care policy and government reform. In 2004, Chieko Nohno, a nurse-midwife and Japanese Nursing Federation member, was the first nurse to be appointed to the Japanese Cabinet as a minister of law. Nurses in Japan are proud of this achievement because her position is considered to be one of the most influential Cabinet positions.

NURSING EDUCATION

Formal Nursing Education

The history of modern nursing education in Japan began in 1885, with the establishment of the first school of nursing by Kanehiro Takagi, who studied at St. Thomas Hospital in the United Kingdom. In the late 1880s, Linda Richards, the first graduate of an American nursing school, taught at the Kyoto *Kanbyofu* School. The first nurse licensing examination was given

in 1900. In 1950 the first junior college nursing program was instituted, followed by the first baccalaureate program in 1952. The first assistant nurse program *(zyun-kangoshi)* began in 1951 in response to a critical nursing shortage (Hirao, 2003).

Presently, one has seven pathways to become a *kangoshi,* but most commonly high school graduates enter a baccalaureate, junior college, or diploma nursing program. The Ministry of Health, Welfare, and Labor regulates all three programs to ensure that students are uniformly prepared to take the national annual registered nurse *(kangoshi)* licensing examination. The Ministry of Education, Culture, Sports, Science and Technology also governs all junior college, baccalaureate, and graduate programs. The curriculum, academic credentials of all faculty members, facilities, and so forth must be reviewed and approved by this Ministry before opening and at certain intervals thereafter.

Diploma (registered nurse) programs continue to outnumber baccalaureate and associate's degree programs, but the recent and remarkable increase in baccalaureate and graduate programs for *kangoshi, hokenshi,* and *zyosanshi* is evident, as shown in Table 88-1, which was compiled from the data of multiple sources. Additionally, diploma-to-master's programs have been gaining in popularity. Even more rapid growth of graduate programs continues to be restricted by a severe shortage of qualified faculty.

Continuing Education

The JNA and the Ministry of Health, Welfare, and Labor have created many new continuing education opportunities. Programs include certified nurse specialist,

TABLE 88-1

Growth of Nursing Programs in Japan

	1975	1985	1995	2003	2004
Baccalaureate program (4 years)	10	10	40	106	121
Junior college program (3 years)	23	40	66	56	45
Diploma program (3 years)	296	382	485	500	500
Master's program (2 years)*	—	2	7	63	71
Doctoral program (3 years)[†]	—	—	6	20	25

Sources: Hirao, M. (2003). Nihon ni okeru kango kyouiku no rekishi-teki hensen [History of nursing education in Japan]. In M. Koyama (Ed.), *Kango Kyouiku no Genri to Rekishi [Principles and history of nursing education]* (pp. 68-86). Tokyo: Igaku-syoin; *Kango Kankei Toukei Shiryou-syuu [Statistical data on nursing service in Japan].* (1996). Tokyo: Kango Kyoukai Syuppankai; *Kango Kankei Toukei Shiryou-syuu [Statistical data on nursing service in Japan].* (2003). Tokyo: Kango Kyoukai Syuppankai; Sugimori, M. (1999). *Kango Kyouiku-gaku [Science of nursing education].* Tokyo: Igaku-syoin; *Syusyoku shinro zyouhou: E-naasu sentaa, gakkou zyohou [E-nurse center school information].* (n.d.). Retrieved January 20, 2005, from http://www.nurse.or.jp/sinro/index.html

*1979, Master's program established.
[†]1988, Doctoral program established.

certified expert nurse, and certified nurse administrator. Certified nurse specialist certification requires a master's degree, 5 years of clinical experience, and passing an examination. Certified nurse specialist certification is available for cancer, women's health, child health, gerontology, psychiatric and mental health, and community health nursing. Certified expert nurse certification requires 5 years of experience, completion of a 6-month training program, and passing an examination. Certified expert nurse programs exist for 17 fields, including emergency, critical care, wound/ostomy/continence, hospice care, infection control, and diabetes nursing. Certified nurse administrator certification involves a combination of experience and examinations and can be achieved at three possible levels (Japanese Nursing Association, 2002).

CURRENT TRENDS IN NURSING

In this section, whenever the word *nurse* is used, it represents *kangoshi, hokenshi,* and *zyosanshi.*

Community-Based Nursing

Recent demographic and social changes along with the introduction of long-term care insurance in 2000 certainly have been pushing Japanese nursing into community and home settings. However, the home care system in Japan already was being pioneered by visiting nurses beginning in the later half of the 1970s. In 1992, medical law dictated that a patient's home could be considered a legitimate care site, and a system of visiting nurse service stations was founded. Furthermore, for the first time in Japan, beginning in 1993, a nurse rather than a physician could be the top administrator of a health care organization (Murashima, Nagata, Magilvy, Fukui, & Kayama, 2003).

The new home care delivery systems also have resulted in some new health care occupations such as care manager. Care managers are nurses *(kangoshi)* or public health nurses *(hokenshi)* or individuals such as physicians or pharmacists with extensive experience in elderly patient care (Murashima et al., 2003; Yamazaki, 1999). A care manager assesses, plans, coordinates, and monitors cost-effective care for eligible patients after consultation with patients and families and is certified through completion of a special training program and passing an examination (Yamazaki, 1999).

Another new role is that of home care worker, a type of nurse's aide or home helper, which has been increasing in popularity since 1990 as the aging population increases. However, the emergence of this new role has forced nurses to clarify their professional nursing role in relation to paraprofessional roles, a factor of particular importance regarding future decisions about financing and reimbursement of care. One concern of home visiting nurses is providing terminal and bereavement care. Hospice facilities and agencies providing home hospice services are too few, but the demand for death at home is increasing. The medical fee for home visits for palliative care slowly has been increasing but is still insufficient (Murashima et al., 2003).

Ethics in Nursing

In the last few years, medical and nursing ethics programs have been developing rapidly. The public is becoming more attuned to issues of medical accountability and responsibility, resulting in much greater media attention to medical accidents and malpractice issues. In 2003 the JNA expanded the Code of Ethics for Nurses, originally enacted in 1988, from 10 to 15 points. The new additions emphasize a trusting relationship between persons, respect for self-decisions, and self-promotion of mental and physical health by nurses (Nihon Kango Kyoukai, 2003).

Research ethics also has been developing rapidly, especially institutional ethics review boards in universities. The Ethical Guidelines for Nursing Research was enacted by JNA in July 2004. The overall purposes of these guidelines are to protect participants in nursing research and to guide research committees in each institution (Nihon Kango Kyoukai, 2004).

Ethics also has been the focus of a number of nursing cross-cultural studies. These studies were motivated by researchers' concerns about importing Western ethical ideas and concepts to Japan, with its different sets of values and traditions (Konishi & Davis, 2001; Wros, Doutrich, & Izumi, 2004).

Research, Scholarship, and Education

With the rapid growth of postgraduate nursing education, nursing research and scholarship are advancing rapidly. Among the numerous nursing societies, the premier professional organization in Japan, dedicated to the international advancement of nursing science and dissemination of nursing knowledge, is the Japan Academy of Nursing Science. One of the most noteworthy recent accomplishments of the academy was the establishment in 2004 of the *Japan Journal of Nursing Science,* the first English-language academic journal to be published by a Japanese nursing academy (Murashima, 2004). Until recently, the barrier of language has limited the sharing of Japanese nursing research outside Japan and had limited opportunities for non-Japanese scholars wishing to publish in Japan.

Another new development has been the establishment of Center of Excellence programs, which are sponsored by the Japanese government. Beginning in 2002, nursing schools with doctoral programs could apply for funding that would promote scholarly endeavors within their institutions (Yamamoto, 2004). As of 2004, some current Center of Excellence programs include ones that are focused on disaster nursing (Yamamoto, 2004), person-centered care and health promotion (Komatsu, 2004), and nursing care that is culturally appropriate for Japanese society (Ishigaki, 2004).

Nursing education also is changing rapidly. With increasing emphasis on risk management and patient safety, the government strongly is encouraging all baccalaureate programs to adopt a more goal-directed and competency-based curriculum as described in a detailed report published in March 2004 (*Kango-gaku kyouiku*, 2004).

THE FUTURE OF NURSING IN JAPAN

With the dramatic demographic and social changes occurring in Japan and the accelerated advancement of nursing education, the picture of nursing in Japan probably will be different 10 years from now, and several predictions are offered. First, with the movement of nursing practice into the community, nurses overall will become far more autonomous in professional practice and assume a partnership role with other health professions. Second, the continued trend toward advanced formal education will result in a younger group of more highly qualified educators and scholars, capable of building the kind of nursing knowledge relevant for Japanese society and culture, as opposed to expanding knowledge borrowed from other disciplines and from Western society. These two trends will enable Japanese nursing to make even greater contributions to the global community of nurses. The future looks bright for nursing in Japan, with unlimited opportunities for continued growth and development.

REFERENCES

Brandi, C. L., & Naito, A. (In press). Hospital nurse administrators in Japan: A feminist dimensional analysis. *International Nursing Review.*

Curtin, J. S. (2003a). Family trends in 2002: Part three—Population data shows declining birthrates, fewer marriages and more divorces. *Social Trends, 41.* Retrieved December 8, 2004, from http://www.glocom.org/special_topics/social_trends/20030611_trends_s41/index.html

Curtin, J. S. (2003b). Youth trends in Japan: Part three—Increasing unemployment and poor work opportunities. *Social Trends, 40.* Retrieved December 8, 2004, from http://www.glocom.org/special_topics/social_trends/20030604_trends_s40/index.html

Hirao, M. (2003). Nihon ni okeru kango kyouiku no rekishi-teki hensen [History of nursing education in Japan]. In M. Koyama (Ed.), *Kango Kyouiku no Genri to Rekishi [Principles and history of nursing education]* (pp. 68-86). Tokyo: Igaku-syoin.

Ikegami, N., & Campbell, J. C. (2004). Japan's health care system: Containing costs and attempting reform. *Health Affairs, 23*(3), 26-36.

Imai, Y. (2002). *Health care reform in Japan. Economics department working papers No. 321.* Retrieved November 25, 2004, from Organisation for Economic Co-operation and Development Web site: http://www.olis.oecd.org/olis/2002doc.nsf/linkto/eco-wkp(2002)7

Imamura, A. (2003). The Japanese family faces the twenty-first century challenges. *Education About Asia, 8*(2), 30-33.

Ishigaki, K. (2004). Center for the creation and dissemination of a new Japanese nursing science incorporating culturally appropriate care: Establishment and development of nursing science and arts based on clinical knowledge. *Japan Journal of Nursing Science, 1*(1), 69-73.

Japan Institute for Social and Economic Affairs. (2002a). *Japan's aging society: Overview.* Retrieved December 8, 2004, from http://www.kkc-usa.org/index.cfm/1524

Japan Institute for Social and Economic Affairs. (2002b). *Japan's labor market.* Retrieved December 8, 2004, from http://www.kkc-usa.org/index.cfm/1528

Japan Institute for Social and Economic Affairs. (2002c). *Japan's pension system: Facing a bulge in retirees.* Retrieved December 8, 2005, http://www.kkc-usa.org/index.cfm/2262

Japan Visiting Nursing Foundation. (1999). *Seturitu 5-syuunen Kinen Kouenkai [Memorial lecture meeting for 5-year anniversary].* Tokyo: Japan Visiting Nursing Foundation.

Japanese Nursing Association. (2002). *JNA activities.* Retrieved January 19, 2005, http://www.nurse.or.jp/jna/english/jna/jnaact.html

Kan, S. (2004, October 9). Cure for factionalism: University hospitals try to kick their "ikyoku" addiction. *The Daily Yomiuri,* p. 12.

Kango-gaku kyouiku no arikata ni kansuru kentoukai houkoku [Report of the Committee for Baccalaureate Nursing Programs]. (2004). *Kango Jissen Nouryoku Ikusei ni muketa Daigaku Sotsugyou-ji no Toutatsu Mokuhyou [Goals for baccalaureate programs toward developing clinical competencies].* Tokyo: Ministry of Education, Culture, Sports, Science and Technology.

Kashiwagi, T. (1996). *Aisuru Hito no Shi wo Mitoru Toki [Caring for the loving person].* Tokyo: PHP Institution.

Komatsu, H. (2004). People-centered initiatives in health care and health promotion. *Japan Journal of Nursing Science, 1*(1), 65-68.

Konishi, E., & Davis, A. J. (2001). The right-to-die and the duty-to-die: Perceptions of nurses in the West and in Japan. *International Nursing Review, 48*(1), 17-28.

Kousei roudou-syou toukei-hyou deta-base shisutemu: Byouin houkoku [MHLW Statistical Database: Hospital reports]. (n.d.). Retrieved January 19, 2005, http://www.mhlw.go.jp/toukei/saikin/hw/iryosd/03/kekka04.html

Kousei toukei kyoukai [Health and Welfare Statistic Association]. (2004). *Kousei no Shihyou [Journal of Health and Welfare Statistics], 51*(9).

Lambert, V., Lambert, C. E., & Ito, M. (2004). Workplace stressors, ways of coping and demographic characteristics as predictors of physical and mental health of Japanese hospital nurses. *International Journal of Nursing Studies, 41*(1), 85-97.

Medical law. (2004). In T. Kadowaki, K. Shimizu, & H. Moriyama. (Eds.), *Kango Horei Yoran [Nursing law bulletin],* pp. 468-472. Tokyo: Nihon Kango Kyokai Shuppankai.

Murashima, S. (2004). Greeting statement. *Japan Journal of Nursing Science, 1*(1), 1.

Murashima, S., Nagata, S., Magilvy, J. K., Fukui, S., & Kayama, M. (2003). Home care nursing in Japan: A challenge for providing good care at home. *Public Health Nursing, 19*(2), 94-103.

Nihon Kango Kyoukai [Japanese Nursing Association]. (2003). Kango rinri kouryo [Code of ethics for nurses], *Kango, 55*(11), 69-72.

Nihon Kango Kyoukai [Japanese Nursing Association]. (2004). *Kango Kenkyuu ni Okeru Rinri Shishin [Ethical guides for nursing research].* Tokyo: Kango Kyoukai Syuppankai.

Primono, J. (2000). Nursing around the world: Japan-preparing for the century of the elderly. *Online Journal of Issues in Nursing, 5*(2). Retrieved July 23, 2004, from http://www.Nursingworld.org/ojin/topic12/tpc12_l.htm

Re-amendment to the nurse law: Changes to Japanese terms for nursing professionals. (2002). *Japan National Association News 32,* 2.

Syusyoku shinro Tsuuzyo soukai houkoku [Annual conference report]. (2004). *Kango, 56*(9), 39-47.

Universal healthcare insurance: Facing an increase in medical costs for the aged. (2002). Retrieved December 8, 2004, http://www.kkc-usa.org/index.cfm/2258

Wros, P. L., Doutrich, D., & Izumi, S. (2004). Ethical concerns: Comparisons of values from two cultures. *Nursing and Health Sciences, 6*(2), 131-140.

Yamagishi, M., Kanda K., & Takemura, Y. (2003). Methods developed to elucidate nursing related adverse events in Japan. *Journal of Nursing Management, 11*(3), 168-176.

Yamamoto, A. (2004). Disaster nursing in a ubiquitous society. *Japan Journal of Nursing Science, 1*(1), 57-63.

Yamazaki, M. (1999). Kaigo hoken seido no hossoku ni mukete [Toward starting a new insurance system]. In Japanese Nursing Association (Ed.), *Kango Hakusyo* (pp. 38-46). Tokyo: Kango Kyoukai Syuppankai.

Yoshikawa, A., Bhattacharya, J., & Vogt, W. B. (1996). *Health economics of Japan. Patients, doctors and hospitals under a universal health insurance system.* Tokyo: University of Tokyo Press.

Zenkoku kanwa kea byoutou syonin shisetu ichiran [Lists of approved palliative units]. (2004). *Tauminaru Kea [Terminal Care], 14,* 503-505.

Nursing in Latin America

CHAPTER

89

An Overview of Health Care, Nursing Education, and Practice

MARIA MERCEDES DURAN DE VILLALOBOS

No aspect of Latin America lends itself to generalization. The vast expanse of the American continent known as Latin America extends from Mexico to Tierra del Fuego (Argentina) and is home to a host of ethnic, ecological, and economic contrasts, health being no exception. This extreme diversity dates from before the discovery of the New World and continues to this day, with regional emphasis, and even exists among countries, despite an attempt to homogenize their culture based on little more than certain common roots and problems, which according to the experts are also common. Yet nothing could be further from reality. For example, what bigger contrast is there in Latin America than the wealth and development of southern Brazil compared with that of Haiti, which has one of the lowest standards of living in the world.

Having said as much, I should point out that the following observations on health care and nursing education and practice in Latin America are general assessments within the scope of this diversity. They should be analyzed critically and are applicable to a greater or lesser degree, depending on the circumstance. I have tried to portray the situation as it exists and what is anticipated for the future, for current conditions and decisions are basic to what could happen in the years ahead, even though this is difficult to predict.

GENERAL ASPECTS OF THE ECONOMY AND HEALTH

Since the 1980s, Latin America has been immersed in the worst political and economic crisis of its history: one that has affected every country to some extent (*Boletín del Banco Mundial*, 1999). The reasons for the crisis are many, but it has been aggravated during the last 10 years by several specific factors, such as the indiscriminate application of neoliberal policies, globalization of the economy and trade, and other policy decisions that have deepened the already serious social inequalities found within the region and have intensified the extent of human poverty (Bustelo, 1992). According to reports by the United Nations Children's Fund (2006), there has been no substantial change in these conditions to date. In addition to these problems, natural disasters and violence have devastated some parts of the continent. For example, the four countries hit by Hurricane Mitch in 1998 (Nicaragua, Honduras, El Salvador, and Guatemala) were said to be set back 50 years in terms of their economic development and suffered more than $2.3 billion in losses (*Boletín del Banco Mundial*, 1999; Bustelo, 1992).

As would be expected, the crisis has had a profound impact on health. In a generic sense, every country has made sweeping changes in its health care system or will do so in the future. During the twenty-first century, the Central and South American countries that had not instituted reforms already were encouraged to do so, as was the case in the Dominican Republic, Honduras, and Panama. The idea is to cut expenses and place responsibility for health care in the hands of the market and people themselves. Nothing is wrong with this, and these changes are sure to bring tremendous long-term benefits. For the moment, however, these changes have caused a great deal of concern among health care workers and consumers alike. Countries that consider themselves examples of reform, such as Colombia, only now—12 years later—are beginning to resolve the problems caused by haste and poorly prepared human resources in implementing reforms. These difficulties have affected not only institutions but also the population. Ultimately, the people suffer the consequences of political decisions.

The last 30 years have witnessed important developments in health care throughout Latin America. Progress toward controlling infant morbidity and mortality is obvious, without the need to mention figures, and although statistics on maternal and neonatal morbidity remain high, they have declined by almost 40%. Figures on the control of transmittable childhood diseases and on family planning are also promising. However, these changes in the right direction have yet to eliminate the problems associated with the appearance of degenerative illnesses, chronic diseases, and aging and those problems caused by violence of every type, drug addiction, and the physical and emotional consequences of natural disasters. These disasters have produced health problems that were thought to be controlled. In addition, natural disasters created a series of complex phenomena such as those derived from human migration and displacement, with the all too familiar social consequences (Pan American Health Organization [PAHO], 1994). The Latin American countries also face the urgency of coping with funding problems and developing infrastructure and human resources in keeping with the demands of the time. Although now the subject of major debate, these issues have not been addressed decisively enough, especially by health professionals (Manfredi, 1999a).

WHAT HAS HAPPENED TO NURSING?

Nursing in Latin America has developed in a context shaped by differences and similarities. Each country must be regarded differently, and by the same token, nursing cannot be viewed as a homogeneous whole. Situations vary from country to country and basically merit individual analysis. Yet one can generalize about the progress and development achieved in the nursing profession as a result of policies and strategies that have given it strength and have proved sound and flexible, according to the particular characteristics of the countries. The lessons they provide are replicable and effective. Latin American nursing has received valuable contributions within the framework of regional policies, PAHO and World Health Organization (WHO), United Nations Children's Fund, and the Dutch government; international support from the W.K. Kellogg Foundation and Ford Foundation; and institutional support from nursing institutions such as the Canadian Nursing Association and the International Council of Nurses, to name a few (Kisil & Chaves, 1994; Manfredi, 1999b). This does not mean, however, that the plight of the profession has been resolved. In fact, nursing faces a difficult and contradictory situation like none in its history, but one that is tremendously stimulating (PAHO & WHO, 1999).

The challenge to nursing is difficult because this is a time of sweeping change. Economic and health legislation has been modified, altering economic conditions in the health care sector as well. This change in health care legislation has undermined the traditional stability of the job market for health care professionals, especially nurses. Despite the growing demand for health care and a shortage of nursing professionals, the profession is plagued by unemployment (unfortunately, there are no precise figures per country). This was something that was virtually unknown in the past. The new economic reality in the health care sector took the nursing profession by surprise. The profession was unprepared to modify certain aspects of nursing practice quickly and aggressively. Nevertheless, the situation is encouraging. Nursing has a unique opportunity to play an active role in these changes and to evolve toward a new type of practice that responds to the growing needs of a population that is involved in health care decisions and is more conscious of the need for quality health care. This new type of practice is far more independent and active than what was traditional in health care systems of the past (Villalobos, 1999a, 1999b).

Accordingly, nursing is being shaped by several predominant trends. The first is the strong tendency of the market to influence decisions on the modus operandi of health care systems. This eliminates the stability of programs and personnel and fosters competition to satisfy market needs. The second trend concerns the growing challenge posed by the balance between the individual health care needs of consumers, in uncontrolled contexts (as opposed to traditional centralism and individual decisions in the private sector), and the need for cost-effective but quality intervention to improve the people's health through the use of resources organized in a sophisticated way. The third tendency is the promise of better health and the use of resources for health care at less cost. This is essentially an illusion, because the possibility of having systems like this in operation does not exist at present, and there is discontent on both sides: among health care personnel and administrators who provide service and among consumers. A fourth tendency, derived from the other three, is an uncertainty about direction and a breakdown in a number of basic parameters that guided the system in the past (Villalobos, 1999a).

In short, market forces pattern the future of nursing practice in Latin America by changes in practice and by the redefinition of health care institutions. These are significant transformations and pose important challenges to a profession that has not been sufficiently strong in the past and has taken a rather immature approach to what this uncertain future holds in store. Nurses must ask themselves What will happen to nursing? and How will deal nursing with the challenges that lie ahead? The next question is, Will Latin American nursing stay tied to tradition and struggle to maintain the status quo, or will it be capable of adapting to the need for creative and effective mobilization in response to the new needs? The answer is impossible to know, but nurses can analyze their behavior today. In doing so, nurses see that, in spite of the limitations, nursing has been a vital survivor in the field of health. Were it not for this definitive force in solving health care problems, Latin America would be in an even more precarious situation. In other words, nursing has an important heritage and a wealth of experience and can produce strategies to bolster its strength in the years ahead and to continue its role in health care maintenance.

LABOR FORCE AND PRACTICE

Enfermería en la Región de las Américas: Organización y Gestión de Sistemas de Salud [Nursing in the Americas Region: Organization and Management of Health Systems], published by PAHO and WHO (1999), offers a general overview of profiles, distribution, and legislation concerning the nursing labor force. According to the introduction to that document, "Nurses comprise 80% of the health labor force in most countries of the Americas. This means nursing is important to the development of health services and systems in every country. However, in most countries, there is a serious and persistent shortage of nursing professionals and these limited resources are distributed inadequately. The challenge for countries in the region is to make better use of their limited resources to provide safe care, until a medium and long-term improvement in quality can be achieved with a nursing labor force that is better prepared."

Demographic changes, the availability of resources, and models for health care service delivery are basic to identifying the demand for nursing personnel and the supply of nurses that could be generated to care for the population. The demand probably will grow in most Latin American countries. However, estimates indicate that the demand will not be covered. Part of the difficulty in maintaining coverage is due to the shortage in nursing personnel, especially professionals (PAHO & WHO, 1999). In this context the general tendency among countries is to regard auxiliary nursing personnel as a solution to the "shortage." Guaranteeing quality care, however, implies maintaining a balance between the

various categories of nursing. This balance can be achieved only with optimum ratios of nurses at the primary level, support personnel, and nursing assistants and auxiliary personnel (Bucham, 1993). The skill mix (nurse/auxiliary ratio or combination of personnel categories) has declined steadily during the last 10 years. The skill mix, however, does vary within a relatively broad range (from 209.7 in Cuba to 0.11 in Brazil). Moreover, because of the differences that separate countries in the Americas, a definite picture of the whole is difficult to achieve. Although the total labor force has grown as a result of an absolute and relative increase in professional and nonprofessional personnel, this growth is not enough to resolve the critical situation most countries face in terms of coverage per 10,000 inhabitants. Twelve countries have fewer than 20 nurses per 10,000 inhabitants, 7 have between 20 and 40, and no country except Cuba has more than 40 nurses for every 10,000 inhabitants (PAHO & WHO, 1999).

The ratio of physicians to nurses and the condition of health care facilities also provide an indication of the problem. The health care labor force is totally distorted, with most health care workers situated at either end of the skill and education line. The ratio of health care personnel with more years of education (physicians) is the same as those with the least amount of schooling (nurse's aides and similar personnel). Between these two extremes, the number of nursing professionals with specialized skill and knowledge appears "strangled." This relatively low number makes it difficult to ensure generalized coverage and to provide the quality demanded of health care services (some countries have 8 to 10 physicians for every nurse, and most have between 3 and 5 physicians per nurse) (PAHO & WHO, 1999). This is an indication that health care models are maintaining orthodox forms of health care, which may be the case for some time. These models emphasize curing disease through medical treatment of choice with little attention to health care management strategies.

In general, the region has no models for nursing practice. Perhaps the most valued one is the model developed in intensive care units. However, this form of nursing care, aimed at correction, was derived from the type of medical care prevailing at health care institutions. For example, the current tendency to cut costs by deinstitutionalizing care has not been aggressive enough in generating forms of nursing practice that respond to the needs of patients and the families who care for them. By the same token, and only in certain countries, innovative nursing proposals and actions have begun to emerge to satisfy the demand for care at the primary and secondary levels in a way that not only meets the demands and needs of the public but also is acceptable to insurance companies, because they decide what services are offered to the public. This also obliges the more trained members of the labor force to concentrate in the major cities, leaving large pockets of the population in suburban and rural areas and urban poverty belts without coverage of quality. These people are served by auxiliary personnel who in turn duplicate traditional care because, without appropriate nursing supervision, it is difficult to propose innovations that could improve health care conditions and people's lives.

EDUCATION

The increase in the number of nurses and auxiliary personnel is a clear indication of the increase in training. In places where this is not the case, the numbers of auxiliary personnel at least have been maintained. Again, the differences in education are broad, and there is little or no standardization in the names of programs. Bachelor's degrees or the equivalent are awarded at the university level (a 4- to 5-year program, depending on the school), and the regional tendency is to teach nursing at the university. A number of technical or technological programs (2 to 3 years) exist, and many are

attached to health ministries and schools for nurse's aides. These programs train personnel of this type in 12 or 18 months, besides offering complementary studies for aides, promoters, and attendants (the name given in Brazil to personnel who do not have a formal certificate). Most of these schools are sponsored by health ministries or the private sector (Sena, 2000). The risk now posed by nursing education at the professional, technical, and vocational level concerns the indiscriminate supply of programs that continue to turn out personnel who often fall short of the minimum qualifications for professional practice. This occurs in spite of the government controls that exist.

Generally speaking, the education subsystem trains nursing personnel to respond to the traditional needs of health care systems, and although the names of the programs are different, most have traditional curricula, even those established in recent years, including the ones mentioned before (Villalobos, 1999c). Table 89-1 provides a summary of the various programs available in the region.

The development of postgraduate education has been mixed, as illustrated in Table 89-2. Like basic education, postgraduate programs are structured in a traditional way, are taught at universities, and vary widely (Wright & Garzón, 1995). Postgraduate programs are oriented

TABLE 89-1

Types of Programs to Train Nursing Personnel in Latin America

Type of Program and Location	Duration	Degree
Additional or complementary training for aides, attendants, and promoters; health ministries and the private sector; full secondary education required for admission	8 to 12 months	Certified
Nursing assistant; health ministries and the private sector; full secondary education required for admission	12 to 18 months	Certified
Secondary education with an emphasis on health (diversified secondary schooling; Venezuela, Nicaragua, Cuba, Brazil)	Last 2 to 3 years of secondary education	Technical secondary diploma
Technicians or nurses with a degree; private or public universities or technological institutes	2 to 3 years	A technical degree or diploma in nursing
General nurses or technologists; public or private universities	3 years	A nursing or general degree
Bachelor's degree in nursing and advanced studies; public or private universities	4 to 5 years	A bachelor's degree in nursing or a professional nursing degree

Data from Pan American Health Organization & World Health Organization. (1999). *La enfermería en la región de las Américas* (Series 16, pp. 14, 15). Geneva: Authors; Sena, R. R. de. (2000). *La educación de enfermería en América Latina*. Santa Fe de Bogotá, Colombia: Gráficas Ducal.

TABLE 89-2

Postgraduate Nursing Programs in Latin America and the Caribbean

Countries	Specialization	Master's Programs	Doctoral Programs
Argentina*	0	1	1
Brazil*	102	27	11
Chile*	3	1	1
Colombia*	16	7	1
Ecuador	3	2	0
Jamaica	1	1	0
Mexico*	5	5	2
Panama	6	2	0
Peru	0	1	0
Venezuela	1	3	1
Total region	137	50	17

Data from Wright, M. da G., & Garzón, N. (1995). *Study of specialization and master's degree programs in nursing in Latin America*. Presentado en Bogotá, Colombia, en Conferencia de Postgrado en Enfermeria.
*Data for these countries have been updated with information from Nursing Schools Associations, 2005.

more toward specialization than a master's or doctoral degree. This may imply some risk for the future, considering the need for a disciplinary buildup and innovative proposals to encourage professional development. Brazil, Chile (after 2000), Colombia, and Mexico (since 1998 to 2000) are the countries where postgraduate studies in nursing at the master's and doctoral level are most developed. This could lead to serious differences, not only in post-basic professional training but also in the amount and quality of research being done in Latin America.

An interesting phenomenon revealed by the Wright and Garzón study (1995) concerns the large number of postgraduate degrees held by nurses in Latin America (up to three specializations and one master's degree for the same person), most of which are only incidental to nursing. This suggests adequate postgraduate preparation but weak education in the disciplinary component of nursing (theoretical and practical). The result is a limited emphasis on aspects particular to professional practicum and to research, both of which are essential if nursing is to develop with the priorities required to guarantee the short-term changes that are needed, especially in terms of demonstrating the importance of nursing in health care, which has to be based on scientific evidence.

Continuing education is the Achilles heel of nursing education in the region. To give a fair estimate of continuing education is impossible because there are no programs at the service level or in schools or universities that respond to the continuing education needs of health care personnel. Programs for continuing education are casuist, short-term, and sporadic. This is a serious problem, given the speed at which changes in service occur, the adoption of new technology, and the current demand for personnel (Villalobos, 1999c).

Fortunately, Latin American nursing has not been discouraged by this complex and confusing panorama. On the contrary, for more than 3 decades, Latin America has tried to find ways to solve persistent problems through regional and country proposals, with the help of organizations such as PAHO and WHO and the W.K. Kellogg Foundation, which have played a fundamental role in the development of continuing programs for improvement and innovation, and with the advice of numerous international organizations, such as the International Council of Nurses and nursing associations (the Canadian Nurses Association, the Danish Nurses Association, the one in Spain) working through alliances among countries to strengthen the professional and academic associations, and the Latin American federations (Chompre & Villalobos, 1995).

PROPOSALS FOR A PROMISING FUTURE

A number of plans, innovative projects, and programs that demonstrate the capacity of nursing to promote changes in service and education have been advanced in the wake of the 1986 Caracas Conference, the conclusions of which played an important role in producing strategies for regional development (Federation Panamericana de Facultades de Medicina, 1985). These actions have strengthened nursing by encouraging its power to negotiate at the political and executive levels and by creating successful experiences, many of which have proved effective enough to be adopted as models for care. The case of the Santander province in Colombia, educational development in Minas Gerais in Brazil, and the case of Patagonia in Argentina are examples (Chompre & Villalobos, 1995; W.K. Kellogg Foundation, 1998, 1999), as are many more in countries and local sites that are not documented, but their endeavors have proved to be of interest for health care systems.

Yet these strategies must go even further. Nursing in Latin America faces three challenges in the immediate future. The first is to generate continuing practice for the services nurses offer. This implies differentiating functions to make sure the skill mix guarantees quality coverage. Otherwise, who can guarantee that care achieves the desired result? Examples of this possibility are many. They can be found in the evaluations of UNI-Kellogg projects (a new initiative for educating human resources in health) (W.K. Kellogg Foundation, 1996, 1997, 1998), in the community-based projects sponsored by PAHO and WHO, and in experimental initiatives that have become sustainable in a number of countries. These innovative projects have done much to overcome many of the problems associated with resources and are proof that creativity and political will can produce changes in the right direction (Chompre & Villalobos, 1995; W.K. Kellogg Foundation, 1998, 1999).

The second challenge is to have this continuity reflected in education for nurses overall, for an independent analysis for each type of personnel is virtually impossible. This integration must insist on a link between teaching and service because the changing nature of nursing practice and the opportunities that lie ahead will originate a different structure. Integration will facilitate the transition from school to the workplace. Associated work must do more than ensure the skill and mobility of resources (Villalobos, 1999b). It must steer nursing research toward new avenues of investigation into care, the results of which can be used more effectively in the new continuing practice, with an eye toward lowering the cost of care and improving outcomes. Promotion of creative changes in nursing education is no easy task. Latin America has innovative experiences in the educational field, and these can be coordinated appropriately and strategies can be created to cope with the continuing crisis in these countries (Sena, 2000). Today's organizational resources—such as the associations of schools and faculties in each country, the federations, the Latin American Nursing Network, and many others—are available and are important to this effort.

The final challenge is just as intrepid as the first two. New rules are required for those who deliver service. This is not a call to eliminate the associations and interest groups that have emerged over time but a call to analyze the traditional modus operandi. From now on there will be periods of flexibility, creativity, and experimentation. Much of what made sense in the past will no longer seem important or necessary. What will predominate are measures to ensure continuity: job security, participation in decision making, opportunities for training and advancement, development of new skills required to stay in the right place, and recognition of the need to change certain roles on the job, according to age.

Change, which is so complex, hints at two situations: (1) quality care must be guaranteed, and (2) the process of change must be appropriated by nurses themselves. The health care institutions should not decide how nursing care could be improved in terms of cost-benefit. As an important part of human resources in the health care sector (80% of the total), nurses must maintain a strong position and have sufficient capacity for self-criticism and flexibility to produce the desired results. These proposals for coping with the situation as it exists today do not imply blind acceptance of what is happening in the health care sector. However, they do suggest that changes are taking place and must be dealt with. Obviously, if the new rationalization of nursing practice in Latin America is to be relevant, it must be linked to the organizational forms and systems that emerge from health services.

SUMMARY

This broad overview of Latin American nursing raises questions that will have to be answered carefully. The conditions for progress are in place. Educational and service components have been strengthened steadily and systematically in virtually every country, and the change in health care systems facilitates opportunity. So, why not respond to today's challenges in a more consistent and decisive way? Latin America is a vast region where every effort is needed to complement its development. Nursing can and will do the job, but there can be no waiting on decisions and strategies for action. Change is quick in coming, and the opportunity could be lost.

REFERENCES

Boletín del Banco Mundial. (1999). Oxford: Oxford University Press for the World Bank.

Bucham, J. (1993). *World nursing "shortages" and human resource planning.* A study group on nursing beyond the year 2000. Geneva, Switzerland: World Health Organization.

Bustelo, S. E. (1992). *La producción del estado de malestar: Ajuste y política social en América Latina. Salud Internacional, Un debate norte-sur.* Washington, DC: Pan American Health Organization, Human Resource Development Series No. 95.

Chompre, R. R., & Villalobos, M. M. de. (1995). A cooperative effort: Nursing leadership development and the W.K. Kellogg Foundation. *Nursing and Health Care Perspectives, 16,* 192-203.

Federation Panamericana de Facultades de Medicina. (1985). *La enfermería en Latinamerica: Estrategias para su desarrollo.* Caracas, Venezuela: Fondo Editorial FEPAFEM & W.K. Kellogg Foundation.

Kisil, M., & Chaves, M. (1994). *Una nueva iniciativa para la educación de los profesionales de la salud.* Sao Paulo, Brazil: Ediciones Loyola.

Manfredi, M. (1999a). *El recurso humano de enfermeria: Retos en la práctica y educación para el siglo XXI.* Santo Domingo, Dominican Republic: I Institute for Human Resource Development, Central American Nursing Group.

Manfredi, M. (1999b). *Los grandes retos de enfermería al aproximarse el siglo XXI.* Managua, Nicaragua: II Institute for Human Resource Development, Central American Nursing Group.

Pan American Health Organization. (1994). *Las condiciones de salud en las Américas* , Volume 1 & 2 (Scientific Publication No. 549), Washington D.C.: Author.

Pan American Health Organization & World Health Organization. (1999). *La enfermería en la región de las Américas* (Series 16, pp. 14, 15). Geneva: Authors.

Sena, R. R. de. (Ed.). (2000). *La educación de enfermería en América Latina.* Santa Fe de Bogota, Colombia: Gráficas Ducal.

United Nations Children's Fund. (2006). *Excluded and invisible: Executive summary.* Retrieved January 5, 2005 from http//www.unicwf.org/publications/files/SOWC_2006_English_Summary.pdf

Villalobos, M. M. de. (1999a). *Contexto socioeconómoco y el cuidado de enfermería.* Managua, Nicaragua: II Institute for Human Resource Development, Central American Nursing Group.

Villalobos, M. M. de. (1999b). *Educación de los recursos humanos de enfermería.* IV Institute for Human Resources and Leadership Development in Latin America. Como doro Rivadavia, Argentina: Universidad de Patagonia, San Juan Bosco.

Villalobos, M. M. de. (1999c). *Estrategias para la educación de enfermería en América Latina. Simposium report: Impacto de la política social en la educación y la práctica de enfermería.* Santa Fe de Bogota, Colombia: Universidad de la Sabana.

W.K. Kellogg Foundation. (1996, 1997, & 1998). Cluster evaluation reports on the UNI program (a new initiative to educate human resources for health).

W.K. Kellogg Foundation. (1998 & 1999). Cluster evaluation reports on the Leadership Development Program to trajo nursing resources in Latin America. Confidential documents.

Wright, M. da G., & Garzón, N. (1995). *Study of specialization and master's degree programs in nursing in Latin America.* Presentado en Bogotá, Colombia, en Conferencia de Postgrado en Enfermeria.

Nursing in Russia

An Overview of Health Care,
Nursing Education, and Practice

LINDA S. SMITH

UPHEAVAL IN RUSSIA

Russia is the largest country in the world; its 6,592,812 square miles make it about 1.86 times the size of the United States, yet Russia laments a declining population of only 143,525,702 people. Thus Russia is one of the most sparsely populated nations on earth. Gender differences are dramatic. Though literacy rates are close to 100% for both genders, life expectancy is just 59 years for men and 72 years for women, with an average life expectancy (both genders) of 65 (down from 69.3 in 1990). The median age for males is 34.7 years and for females is 40.7 (Central Intelligence Agency [CIA], 2004; World Health Organization [WHO], 2005). Presently, Russia is in a negative population growth rate, with a 3% population decline since 1990 (9.7 births per 1000 but 16.32 deaths per 1000). This death rate is especially alarming compared with a death rate of 11.2 per 1000 in 1990 (WHO, 2005). With a productivity level (gross domestic product) that fell 38.5% between 1992 and 1997 (U.S. Department of State, 1997), the current positive average gross domestic product growth rate of 6.5% since 1998 is promising. Even with some economic growth, 25% of the population of Russia continues to live below the poverty level (CIA, 2004).

The Independent Republic of the Russian Federation (a federation government system) became a reality on August 24, 1991, with an official, newly approved constitution on December 12, 1993 (CIA, 2004). However, as Russia struggles now to enact social reforms and a market-driven economy, inflation, poverty, crime, and a disintegrating infrastructure may be destroying hope for the Russian people (Center for Strategic and International Studies, 1999). The manufacturing base of Russia is decayed and needs major updating or replacement in order for the country to see real economic growth. Additionally, with a poor business climate that discourages foreign and domestic investment, a weak banking system, global corruption, a court system that bows to government whim, and widespread public distrust in institutions, including health care, Russians lament the stability of the old Soviet system, even as the number living below the poverty line grows to 40 million (CIA, 2004).

Many problems exist. When Mikhail Gorbachev, former president of the Soviet Union, returned from forced exile after the aborted coup in August 1991, he returned to a changed nation. Soviet Union republics declared their independence, and the communist party disintegrated (Ryan, 1992). Unfortunately, deeply ingrained social strongholds continued, such as the lack of acknowledgment for the contributions of health care professionals. Salaries for health care workers, including nurses, were then and continue to be dreadful (Curtis, Petukhova, & Taket, 1995; Osborn, 2004; Tichtchenko, 2003). Health care was a centrally ordered, government-controlled paternalistic system (Curtis et al., 1995; Tichtchenko, 2003) in which patients did not pay directly for care and health care professionals became state employees. This status permitted little autonomy or authority and has led the way to gross underfunding and a kind of gray (beyond the law) commercialization and corruption of health care services. Patients may pay bribes for services and out-of-pocket money for medications, equipment, treatment, and even food (Heilig, 1999; Osborn, 2004; Tichtchenko, 2003).

In 2002 the number of hospital beds per 100,000 persons was 1,071, and the number of hospitals per 100,000 Russians was 6.7, a 12-year decrease from 1,305 and 8.6, respectively (WHO, 2005). The number of physicians and nurses per 100,000 persons in 2004 was 417 and 786, respectively, compared with 548 and 772 in the United States (WHO, 2004). Health care concerns received a lower priority than other industrial and military endeavors. In 1990 the percent of gross domestic product (total) for health expenditures was 2.26 (WHO, 2005). This low rate led to chronic under-funding, rationing, and even in major Russian cities, a health care quality below Western standards (U.S. Department of State, 1997). Because the purpose of all health care was to increase worker productivity, the elderly and disabled became vulnerable. Long waits and medical supply shortages impaired access. To circumvent these problems, informal methods of bribing and tipping developed, as did separate elitist facilities. Primary health care principles weakened, and individual patient needs could be ignored.

Politics

With an estimated 2004 inflation rate of 13.7% (CIA, 2004), prices for almost all goods and services have increased, police are considered corrupt, and safety at night, especially for women, is a major concern. Even so, few Russians wish to turn back Glasnost reforms and return to a totalitarian regime. Unfortunately, since 1993, quiet legislation has rolled back some of the most important and hard-won human and civil rights changes in Russia. Though official government positions on human rights demonstrate some progress since 1993, the institutionalization of safeguards for these rights has lagged (U.S. Department of State, 1997). For example, in January 2000, Russian police threatened to take disrespecting journalists who report on corrupt officials to remote psychiatric institutions (Cockburn, 2000), and 24-hour surveillance for foreigners by the Federal Security Bureau, the successor to the infamous KGB, is common and even overtly boasted ("Trust, but Verify," 2000). Furthermore, though the Russian government proclaims a respect for religious freedom and the separation of church and state has been in place since 1054, Yeltsin signed a bill into law in 1997 officially to recognize the Russian Orthodox Church and to restrict activities of other religious groups (Holmes, 1997). Minority faiths may be out of favor with local authorities, and therefore overt demonstrations of prejudice and societal discrimination (i.e., anti-Semitic hate crimes) have not been prosecuted (U.S. Department of State, 1997).

In a 1998 opinion survey of 1500 Russians, fully half reported an existence so bad that they could not think of how they would live. Today, Russians' savings, hope, and trust may wane (Dahlburg, 1998). Yeltsin and now Putin, the acting president since Yeltsin's surprise resignation on December 31, 1999 (and president since May 7, 2000, and reelected president by a 71% majority in March 2004 [CIA, 2004]), have vowed to "curb all plans for seizing power" (Babakian, 1998). However, when taking office, Putin promised to reinstate a strong central government. Speculations exist that Putin, an ex-KGB officer (the Soviet equivalent to the CIA/FBI) and as of January 2000 the most popular Russian politician, will crackdown even further on hard-won, yet tenuous, civil liberties.

Though Putin has vowed in writing not to return to a Soviet state (Wines, 2000), like his predecessor Yeltsin, Putin continues to be a powerful and visible proponent of the military campaign in Chechnya. Thus the Russian military continues to demolish Grozny (the Chechen capital) apartment houses and by so doing causes multiple casualties because of highly motivated, armed Chechen rebel forces (Gordon, 2000). The military campaign in Chechnya has resurfaced some of the most criticized features of the past Soviet military and political habits (Public Broadcasting Service, 2000). Other dramatic demonstrations of terrorist activities related to the Chechen war include the tragic 3-day hostage-taking crisis in 2004 in the North Ossetian town of Beslan, where more than 335 persons, the majority of whom were children, were killed and 700 persons were injured, mostly by gunshot wounds and burns. During the siege, Putin refused to negotiate with Chechen rebel representatives, despite pressures to do so. Following the disaster, Putin vowed to conduct his own private internal investigation ("Russians Rally," 2004) into the military siege. But the Russian military, as with other government factions, has seen dramatic cuts. In 2002, Russia reduced its military by more than 15% and plans to continue to reduce the number of military personnel over the next 3 years, gradually decreasing mandatory service from 2 years to 1 and moving into a 70% volunteer force by 2010 (CIA, 2004; "Russia Says," 2002).

The foreign debt of Russia is around 28% of the gross domestic product, down from 90% during the 1998 financial crisis, with a public debt of 34%. The ruble exchange rate in 2003 was 30.7 per U.S. dollar compared with 24.6 in 1999 (CIA, 2004). Older Russians, raised on Soviet ideals now destroyed, may find their savings and pensions worthless. Three thousand homeless persons in Moscow died on the streets in 1998 (Johnstone, 1999). Street children are becoming an increasingly difficult Russian social problem. The estimated number of street children in Moscow is from 30,000 to 50,000, with the majority under the age of 13. This problem relates to the economic crisis. Many families in which parents are unable to feed their children may force their children to live on their own at early ages (United Nations Development Programme, 2002). These growing numbers of homeless children, greater than immediately following World War II, live in underground sewage systems and subways and often survive by begging and prostitution (Heilig, 1999). An additional indicator of social decline has been the dramatic increase in Russian homicide and suicide rates. Suicide deaths per 100,000 grew from 25.9 in 1990 to 36.4 in 2002; homicide deaths grew from 14.1 to 29.7 during the same period (WHO, 2005).

Infrastructure

Tax evasion is a problem in Russia, and without reliable revenue the Russian government is unable to pay for needed social services such as health care for its people. In 1997 the Russian government collected only 10.8% of its gross domestic product in taxes but spent 18.3% (Aron, 1998). Yet since 1993, Russians have been mandated to pay income taxes on April 1 of each year. Under communism, taxes automatically were deducted from each paycheck. To help remedy this problem, in 2001 the Russian government initiated a flat 13% tax on income. Though this tax requires 12 pages of forms, personal income tax revenues increased by 47% (Tavernise, 2002). Unfortunately, small and medium business growth may be thwarted because of an almost unbearable array of taxes. For example, there is a social tax of up to 35.6% (equivalent to the U.S. social security tax), a 5% sales tax, a 20% value-added tax, and a 5% advertising tax combined with property, road, net profits, and various other taxes and registration fees. To keep taxes down, many employers keep separate books, one set for the tax collector and another set disclosing actual paid salaries (Engleman, 2002b). Therefore "income" is not easily taxable.

Life in Russia can be difficult and dangerous. On January 7, 2000, the U.S. State Department warned Americans not to live or travel in the Caucasus region of Russia. Throughout this region, local criminal gangs routinely kidnap and even murder foreigners for ransom. Furthermore, unexplained acts of terrorism to government buildings, hotels, tourist sites, and public transportation sites caused the U.S. State Department to recommend travel only in groups and only with organized, reputable tour agencies. Thus throughout Russia, crimes against foreigners are a major problem. Pickpocketing, assaults, and robberies are frequent, regardless of time or place. Furthermore, "skinhead" groups and local militias may harass and attack persons of African and Asian descent. Russian roads are poor and absent of roadside assistance (U.S. State Department, 2000). Russian communications, especially in rural areas, are often outdated, inadequate, and of low density, and a large, mostly unfilled demand for mainline services continues (CIA, 2004). Connections can be uncertain or full of static. Moreover, Watkins and Rees (1999) noticed the dreadful condition of public housing. Urban-dwelling Russians live in high-rise apartment blocks, a legacy of the Soviet era with as many as 15 families sharing kitchen and toilet facilities.

For the elderly, economic inflation often means they must sell their most prized possessions, or beg, in order to live. Russian elders are also vulnerable to crime and fraud. Thus crime doubled between 1990 and 1994, yet laws remained outdated and courts overcrowded, ill prepared, and ill funded. In 1999, to complicate crime problems further, the Moscow police chief admitted that 95% of his force was on the take (Zuckerman, 1999b). This rising violence and organized crime, including major drug trafficking (CIA, 2004), has led to growing pessimism over democratic reforms. It seems likely that Russians, overwhelmed with hopelessness, may follow any politician who can guarantee law, order, and stability, regardless of the loss of civil rights.

Pollution

In Russia, congenital anomalies per 100,000 live births have increased from 1722 in 1990 to 2939 in 2002 (WHO, 2005). Because congenital anomalies and miscarriages are more common in polluted areas, most consider these changes related to rising pollution levels, in addition to poverty and unhealthful lifestyles (Knox, 2002; Winik, 2001). Furthermore, more cars are on the roads than ever before, and even in small towns, where cars rarely were seen just 7 years ago, walking across streets is life-challenging (Steinkraus, 2000).

Russian industries, unable or unwilling to install quality water and air treatment devices, continue to pollute the environment. Based on old Soviet ideology, industry intends to survive at any cost. Untreated waste is commonplace. Pesticides contaminate more than 30% of the food eaten. The prevalence of respiratory system diseases is 1.5 times higher for children living close to industrial plants and 1.5 to 2.5 times higher for children living near chemical, petrochemical, or metallurgy plants (Revich, 1999). Obviously, the ecological situation in Russia is growing worse. Currently, more than 70 million Russians drink water and breathe air exceeding permissible pollution standards by 5 to 10 times, and more than 75% of the national water supply may be contaminated. The reason is a federal budget for pollution control that is considered too little and too late (Kunin, 1997; Zuckerman, 1999b). Russian women downwind from industrial plants are encouraged not to breast-feed because of high levels of dioxin in breast milk. Thus Russian people have endured ever-higher rates of respiratory disease, mental retardation, and congenital deformities.

Increasing Morbidity and Mortality

Russian youth have suffered. Nearly 40% of Russian children may be chronically ill, and without safety matches or flame-retardant clothing, burns are common among children. Domestic violence and suicide also are rising dramatically (Zuckerman, 1999b), with a reported incidence of domestic violence between 4 and 5 times greater than in the United States (Dymchenko & Callister, 2002). Compared with the United States, the largest mortality for Russian children ages 5 to 9 was for accidents and drowning. Drowning for children ages 5 to 9 was greater than 10 times the U.S. rate. Thus mortality rates for Russian children between 1 and 14 years are comparable to the death rate for all causes of death in the United States (Centers for Disease Control and Prevention [CDC], 2002). Psychological disorders also have increased, with the number of diagnosed persons with alcohol-induced psychosis per 100,000 up to 53.5 in 2002 from 9.68 in 1990 (WHO, 2005). Alcohol further is implicated in the large number of deaths by fire, motor vehicle collisions, and work-related accidents (Green, Holloway, & Fleming, 2001). Half of this increased mortality is related to cardiovascular disorders, which reflect unfavorable social habits of smoking, alcohol intake, obesity, poor diet, and the inadequate identification and treatment of this disease category (Ashlund, 2001; Burger, 2000; Lally, 2000). Interestingly, a good portion of cardiovascular deaths, especially for young men, is related to acute alcoholism and binge drinking (Lally, 2000; Watkins & Rees, 1999).

Ever-increasing pollution, crime, inflation, unemployment, and the underfunded Russian health care system have led to increasing morbidity and mortality rates. Women are having sex earlier, but fewer women are bearing children, and Russia is losing about half a million persons per year; two of three pregnancies end in abortion ("Russian Fertility Problems," 2000).

THE DISORDERED HEALTH CARE SYSTEM OF RUSSIA

In Russia the per person per year health care expense in U.S. dollars is $115.00, compared with $4887 in the United States and $2163 U.S. dollars in Canada (WHO, 2005). According to Gaufberg (2004), though Russian society has had a dramatic shift since the fall of the Soviet empire in 1991, the health care system remains much the same and health care resources may even be more scarce. Most of the Russian citizens, he wrote, believe their health care system shows progressive deterioration. These comments concur with those made by Heilig (1999).

As mountain factories encase downwind cities in soot and the Chernobyl nuclear accident continues to take its toll, for children from birth to 17 years old, diseases such as diphtheria (rare in the United States), hepatitis, tuberculosis, syphilis, gonorrhea (CDC, 1999, 2002), and acquired immunodeficiency syndrome (AIDS) are rising or are remaining alarmingly high. Childhood diseases are increasing related to malnutrition (especially in the first year of life as evidenced by rickets, stunted growth, and obesity) and the fear parents have had regarding immunizations, though currently the immunization rates in Russia are comparable to those in the United States. Unfortunately, a tremendous growth in syphilis occurred in 1997, with 376,000 new cases, and the rate of syphilis infection for youth ages 15 to 17 is 30 times greater than the U.S. rate (CDC, 2002).

Tuberculosis mirrors social life, economic conditions, and health care policy. The number of new tuberculosis cases in 2002 has grown to 128,873, more than 2.5 times greater than 1990 rates (WHO, 2005). Tuberculosis spreads rapidly among the 1.2 million prisoners in Russia because of overcrowding, food shortages, poor health care, interrupted treatment, and poorly ventilated facilities. The incidence of tuberculosis among prisoners is 40 to 50 times greater than in civilian populations; and 30% of these infected prisoners have virulent drug-resistant strains. Tuberculosis is a main cause of death among prisoners (Engleman, 2002a; Yale University School of Nursing, 2004) and among alcohol and drug abusers, the homeless, and Russian mountain dwellers. To complicate this problem, tuberculosis drugs and diagnostic supplies are difficult to access for regional hospitals and clinics, and thus Russians with tuberculosis may be poorly diagnosed and ineffectively treated and monitored as cuts to public health care reduce access (Engleman, 2002b; Zuckerman, 1999b). Besides tuberculosis, present and former prisoners are also infected with human immunodeficiency virus (HIV)/AIDS. The number of AIDS (pronounced "speed" in Russian) cases in Russia increased 650% in 1 year (Kunin, 1997) because of intravenous drug use, an escalation in prostitution, contaminated blood supplies, sexual promiscuity, and contaminated needles. Unfortunately, even in health care facilities, reuse of disposable needles continues to be a common practice. Between 1998 and 1999, cases of HIV infection more than tripled as 14,980 new cases were recorded ("Russian Official Criticizes," 2000). Showing this continued and dramatic increase were 860,000 Russian adults with AIDS/HIV in 2003, and of these, 290,000 were female (UNAIDS, 2004).

The greatest increase in HIV/AIDS has been among intravenous drug users; since 1990 the rate has increased twenty-fold; half of all HIV/AIDS cases in Russia have occurred among intravenous drug users (Gore-Felton et al., 2003). Furthermore, substance abuse is a real concern for Russian youth who abuse chemicals such as alcohol, homemade drugs, opiates, and cannabis. The number of drug addicts rose by 50% among the total Russian population and 100% among teens. Inadequate financing of health care services and facilities has resulted in severe equipment and pharmaceutical shortages; and medications continue to be a main import for Russia (CIA, 2004). The inability of Russia to produce pharmaceuticals and medical devices is of major concern. Yet when medicines are available, they are believed to be ineffective, weak, or contaminated.

Another concern is the illness/treatment focus rather than a primary prevention focus (Maksimova, 1998). Most of the Russian health care budget is spent on secondary care, with only 2.2% allocated for the purpose of prevention of health problems. Therefore aftercare is rare for children and adults discharged from acute care institutions. As evidence of this, some hospital stays are at least 21 days long (Watkins & Rees, 1999). Interestingly, according to Douglas and Mannino (1997), hospitalized patients were compliant and tolerant of a near total lack of privacy: 4-, 8-, 12-, and even 24-bed wards are common. Clinics and hospitals have limited funds available for food, medicines, equipment, or utilities (Public Health Research Institute, 1997), and many medical institutions have been closed because of policy decisions and lack of funding. Though between 1990 and 2002, the number of hospitals in Russia dropped by 25% (WHO, 2005), a bill drafted by Vladimir Putin's government is seeking to shift the health care emphasis away from illness care and the Soviet-era patient quotas toward quality care. To do this, government officials propose to cut the number of health care workers (physicians and nurses included) by 300,000 over the next several years, and the number of hospital beds by 33%. The motive is to focus more heavily on prevention and community care and less heavily on specialization, hospital admissions, and long lengths of stay (Osborn, 2004). Currently, the average length of stay for all Russian hospitals is 14.7 days,

down from 16.6 in 1990 (WHO, 2005). Proposals are to reduce this time even further, and more physicians are being encouraged to become general practitioners (Osborn, 2004).

The Duma, the lower parliament of Russia, has promised to place health and education as top priorities, but will salaries for nurses and physicians improve? Certainly, the Duma will need to move quickly. Specialists, scientists, artists, educators, and highly skilled personnel including physicians and nurses are leaving Russia and/or their professions, taking with them the contributions they could make to Russian life. Though wages are a huge problem, numbers of professional health care workers are not. In 2004, for every 100,000 persons, the Russian Federation boasted 417 physicians, 32 dentists, 786 nurses, 47 midwives, and 7 pharmacists. In the United States, this compares with 548 physicians, 58 dentists, 772 nurses, and 68 pharmacists (U.S. midwife data not listed) (WHO, 2005).

OPPRESSED RUSSIAN WOMEN

Gender discrimination is a powerful Russian force. Under Soviet rule, most employees in nonindustry categories were women, and thus women received lower wages. This difference expanded even further after the collapse of communism as inflation rose (Ryan, 1992). Though a majority of physicians and teachers are women and Russian women are well educated, these women may lack authority and responsibility. Women can be denied opportunities and continue to be relegated to menial labor (Boe, 1993), especially in the home. Thus unemployment is highest among women and young persons (U.S. Department of State, 1997).

Life is hard for Russian women. This is especially true for women working for state enterprises (such as nurses, teachers, and doctors) where salaries have not increased proportionately to prices. Russian women compose 47% of the country's working-age population; 90% of women between 35 and 49 are working or are seeking work, but women, most often employed in routine jobs, may be overlooked when employers hire for management positions. Thus salaries for women are estimated to be half to two thirds of those earned by men, a gap that has increased steadily since the fall of the Soviet Union. This contrasts with the fact that more Russian women are university educated (63% versus 50%) (Sandul, 2002). The legal age for marriage has dropped from 18 to 14, creating conditions for increased teen pregnancy with and without marriage. Many of those teen pregnancies end in abortion because of lack of money to support a child; for example, a baby carriage. If combined salaries are 300,000 rubles per month, but a baby carriage costs 1,000,000 rubles, the carriage is an impossible commodity (Heilig, 1999). Thus chances are that a woman will have one or more abortions before her first full-term pregnancy ("Russian Fertility Problems," 2000). Abortion rates for Russian women are the highest in the world (Knox, 2002).

Russian men generally loathe participating in child care and housework such as cooking or cleaning. This near total responsibility for women for home and family is compounded because Western conveniences such as garbage disposals, dishwashers, and microwave ovens may be unaffordable. Two thirds of the jobless in Russia are female, and far more women than men have fallen into poverty. A further insult occurs when many Russian families break apart as Russian men look for younger, more attractive sexual partners. The Russian woman must pick up the pieces of a broken family (Weir, 2001).

As Russian women seek men who will stay employed, avoid alcoholism, and assist with child care, they may turn to foreign marriage brokers, prostitution, and pornography in hopes of finding love and stability. Penthouse, Playboy, and Internet sources all purport the virtues of "beautiful" Russian women. Using a mega search engine, one need only type "Russian and women" to locate hundreds, even thousands of Internet pornography and marriage brokering sites that feature Russian brides. Many sites include biographies and photographs. Unfortunately, foreign men want beautiful subservient wives and may be surprised by the independence of Russian women caused by years of defending themselves and surviving in the midst of hostile conditions. Russian women have been called "drill sergeants" by men seeking fragile femininity.

Violence against Russian women has increased dramatically. Appropriately, this secret violence has been called the "undeclared war" and represents a deep contempt by Russian men for females. As evidence, women who leave their husbands may lose their legal status and their property rights. Women often are expected to give sexual favors to employers and landlords. Partly because women do not press charges against abusing partners (they fear severe retaliation), Russian police have been loathe to exhibit empathy or even file reports when witnessing violence against women in the form of rape or domestic battles. During the Soviet rule, authorities could be consulted when battering occurred. Women could report abuses to their employer, their local party, or their trade union representatives. Now, they say there is no one to listen. Clearly, Russian women face a more stressful living environment with possible desperate financial constraints, violence, underemployment, disease, malnutrition, abortion complications, and alcohol abuses (Bennett, 1997; Knox, 2002).

Russian women also have pregnancy, labor, and delivery concerns that Russian men never face. Abortion as a right became popular when the Soviet state needed women in the work force. Now, few women have the time, money, social support, or living space to have more than one child. Abortions are permitted on request of economic or social motives. Poor Russian women may not have access to contraceptives (only 34% use them and of these, only 6% use oral contraceptives), and condoms are unpopular with Russian men, can be difficult to obtain, and are considered of poor quality. (Of the contraceptives used by married women, about half use the intrauterine device [Dymchenko & Callister, 2002]). Thus the average Russian woman has 3 to 7 abortions, contributing to the 1,782,266 abortions in 2002 and to the about 4 million abortions in 1990 (WHO, 2005).

Though the official number of abortions in Russia has declined 45% from 1990 to 2002, the rate of abortions per 1000 live births remains high at 1275.8. Russian maternal deaths per 100,000 number 33.57 (WHO, 2005). More than 20% of all pregnant Russian women are diagnosed with anemia at the time of their delivery (CDC, 2002), increasing premature birth risk. Labor and delivery occurs in birth houses or maternity units within district hospitals. Attendance at births is by institution-based midwives and in cases of high-risk, physicians are consulted (Dymchenko & Callister, 2002). The percent of cesarean births to live births is 6.6%, far less than in the United States but showing an increase from 1990 data when the rate was 0.06%. Maternal deaths are due to sepsis, toxemia, hemorrhage, abortion (25%), and ectopic pregnancy, and with 90% of Russian women in the workforce, workplace conditions can become health risks for mother and baby.

OPPRESSED RUSSIAN NURSES

Most Russians view nursing as a low-prestige job. Even the noun *nurse* (as a separate profession) does not exist. Instead, Russian nurses are called medical sisters, similar to the title given a domestic servant (Douglas & Mannino, 1997). As health care providers, Russian nurses depend on physicians for patient teaching and problem solving, often unable to exercise critical thinking and make independent decisions regarding clinical care. Physicians give orders and nurses carry them out (Alaniz, 2001; Watkins & Rees, 1999). Hard physical labor and 24-hour shift work are familiar burdens to Russian nurses, and nurses may have a patient load of between 20 and 25 patients (Steinkraus, 2003). In some hospitals, nurses work double shifts and second and third jobs and take increased patient loads or add extra housekeeping duties just to bring wages high enough to survive. When they do get paid, the salaries are among the poorest in Russia. Nursing is a female-based (about 5% male), physician-dominated (Perfiljeva, 1997), task-oriented profession. Physicians believe strongly that they, not nurses, are best able to assess patients and plan care. Thus nurses often carry out roles of respiratory (setting up and maintaining all respiratory equipment), dietary, laboratory, janitorial, and clerical personnel. The good news, however, is that nurses can receive additional salary based on years of experience, intensity of work, and level of education. The base pay for nurses with 0 to 3 years experience (no nurse category) is 1,220 rubles/month or about $41.00. Base pay will increase by 15% to 18% when the nurse has between 3 and 5 years of experience and demonstrates competence (Category II nurse). Base salary also can increase by 15% to 18% with at least 5 years of experience, recommendations, and the passing of a competence examination (Category I nurse). In the highest category (Category highest) a nurse can earn a 30% increase in base pay to 1,640 rubles/month ($54.66) after at least 8 years of experience, passing a cumulative examination (from Category I and II levels), and manager recommendations. Nurses doing extra cleaning and sterilizing during their normal shift work also can earn 15% to 25% above base pay. Low salaries and hard work have motivated nurses to seek employment with private health care facilities or to leave the profession altogether. At least one hospital in St. Petersburg reported a 30% unfilled nurse vacancy rate (Difazio, Lang, & Boykova, 2004).

CHANGES FOR RUSSIAN NURSING

Nursing Education

Before the Russian Revolution of 1917, nursing practice blended the physical, social, psychological, and spiritual aspects of human life and death. However, after the rise of communism, nursing education moved to procedure-oriented technical schools (referred to as medical schools) with little attention paid to the social sciences and humanities (Edwards, 1994; Picard & Perfiljeva, 1995). The job of nursing "still remains dependent on and subordinate to medicine. Most doctors believe this is right and proper" (Perfiljeva, 1997, p. 8). Nursing and nursing education existed under the bureaucratic, federally regulated medical model (Ivanov & Paganpegara, 2003).

Russian nursing education generally has taken place in 2-year programs, and candidates who pass an entrance examination may apply after 10 or 12 years of secondary education. Physicians traditionally serve as administrators and faculty in nursing schools. Level one nursing education includes 3 years of education, after which the graduate becomes a "medical nurse." The average age of the level-one nurse is about 18 years. Level-two nursing education includes an additional $1\frac{1}{2}$ years of full-time medical schoolwork, after which graduates earn a certificate as a nurse or an educator. Level-three nursing education includes $4\frac{1}{2}$ years of university education, after which the graduate receives certification as a nurse manager or chief nurse and is eligible to assume these types of positions (Difazio et al., 2004). Feldsher education also takes place in technically based medical schools. Feldshers have been compared with the U.S. physician's assistant. They learn advanced techniques such as suturing and birthing and may apply these techniques without physician presence. Feldshers ride in ambulances and work in a variety of settings such as polyclinics and emergency departments. Feldshers and midwives are relied upon more heavily in rural areas (CDC, 1999).

Despite the problem that Russian physicians do not believe nurses need additional schooling (V. Sarkisova, personal communication, June 2000), progress has been made in the area of Russian nursing education. A new curriculum was formulated and circulated to all basic nursing education institutions. "Following the recommendations of the first World Health Organization Conference on Nursing, this curricula is focused not only on hospital nursing, but also on community nursing" (Perfiljeva, 1997, p. 9). This community focus translated into reality when a U.S.-based $20 million health care reform project was implemented. One of its health care reform goals (subscribed to by the Russian Ministry of Health) was to enhance medical and nursing school curricula in such a way that quality, family-focused, preventative, population-based, and community-based health care would be promoted and enhanced (Maksimova, 1998; Milburn, 1997; Perfiljeva, 1997). In 1996, intensive work was under way in Russia to create standards for all the branches of nursing education, and in that same year, requirements for continuing education courses every 5 years were started. One example of a current curricular change is a required course in bioethics that has been added in nursing education programs (Tichtchenko, 2003), and a program to prepare nurse managers better (4600 hours) started in 1994, with the goal of 25 programs nationwide by the year 2000 (Ivanov & Paganpegara, 2003). In a letter to the editor in 1998,

Perfiljeva and Picard wrote of the 7-year effort to move nursing forward through the creation of master's in nursing programs. They reported that at the time of their writing, 14 universities in Russia had such programs. Support for these nursing education changes has come from educational facilities and nursing organizations located in the Scandinavian countries, United Kingdom, and North America. Thus one important advantage for Russian nursing schools has been the regular exchanges of faculty, students, and nursing administrators between Russia, the United States, and other countries (Y. Filan, personal communication, June 2000; Mikheeva, 1997; V. Sarkisova, personal communication, June 2000) such as the one from the Yale University School of Nursing (2004).

As with nursing, educating Russian physicians is the responsibility of the Russian government, for all medical schools follow established Ministry of Health curriculum. Medical education is 6 years long with an additional year of internship and 3 years of mandatory service. Russian physicians are highly specialized, and only 25% of Russian physicians specialize in general practice or internal medicine (CDC, 1999).

Before 1991, Russian nurses had little hope of advancement other than becoming a physician or feldsher, because nursing education was considered a lesser version of medicine (Wallen & Cammuso, 1997). Therefore for decades, nursing journals were authored, edited, developed, and directed by physicians. During a meeting in 1991 with representatives from the only Russian nursing journal *Meditsinskaya Sestra,* I and other delegates faced an editorial board and administration composed entirely of physicians. We discussed the complete lack of manuscripts authored by nurses and were told that "nurses cannot write." We discussed the lack of nursing representation on their board and were told, "Nurses cannot be leaders. Physicians are the ones who must lead and inform nurses." Without government funding, this journal disappeared shortly after our meetings.

As with nursing journal authors and editors, nurse educators were almost always physicians; supervisors of patients and nurses were physicians, and government standards for nurses were and continue to be established by physicians. Now this physician dominance may be changing. In 1991 the Ministry of Health in Russia developed the first college of nursing designed to promote baccalaureate nursing education with a 3-year curriculum following Western models. By 1997, there were 48 nursing colleges and an additional 10 programs planning to offer graduate nursing education (Douglas & Mannino, 1997). Beginning in 1991, the Moscow

Medical Academy, through the vision of Dr. Galina Perfiljeva, initiated a master's program in nursing. This prestigious educational facility also collaborated with Nursing College No. 1 to offer a bachelor's degree in nursing program. The master's program emphasized nursing theory, leadership, research, and education (Picard & Perfiljeva, 1995). Hence formal postgraduate nursing education has been an 8-year effort designed to "advance nursing through development of master's programs in nursing, which now include 14 universities throughout the country. The first, at the I. M. Sechenov Moscow Medical Academy (MMA) has so far graduated three classes [as of 1998] of students who are now faculty and leaders in major health care facilities" (Perfiljeva & Picard, 1998, p. 108). Certainly, the hopes of a national nursing system developed and implemented by nurses rather than physicians rests with these graduates who have been taught to write, speak, and teach about the values of the nursing profession (Picard & Perfiljeva, 1995). Though the Moscow Medical Academy became the first graduate school of nursing in the Russian Federation, as of 2004 there were four. D. Olsen from Yale School of Nursing collaborated with the Moscow Medical Academy to explore research opportunities, teach academy advanced practice nursing students, share teaching strategies with the academy graduate nursing faculty, and establish collaborative partnerships between the Yale University School of Nursing and Moscow Medical Academy ("Building an International Partnership," 2004).

As nursing education and patient advocacy improved, the need to develop continuing education programs for new and currently practicing nurses became more evident. Postgraduation, ongoing specialty training for nurses includes periodic continuing education for 1 to 4 months, after which a certificate is awarded and, depending on the specialty, additional salary. Work analyses have demonstrated the efficacy of such ongoing continuing education for nurses, which enhances professional skills via a continuous educational patient care focus (Mikheeva, 1997). Importantly, hospital-wide continuing education programs have been developed through American partnerships since 1993 (Kirgetova, 1997).

Even with additional continuing education, the nursing process was not emphasized clinically until recently and is only periodically taught in nursing education programs. Valentina Sarkisova, president of the newly formed Russian Nurses Association (RNA), explained in her December 26, 1999, correspondence that "we hope to gradually introduce the nursing process into all hospitals as we hope this technique will improve the quality of nursing care in all hospitals and give nurses increased status and prestige."

Nursing Practice

It has been said that Russian nurses must carry the health care burdens with their bare hands. Despite almost overwhelming oppression by physicians and an unyielding system, Russian nurses continue to struggle for authority and dignity within their practice. They are trying now to improve the quality of the care they provide, but there is little time and little equipment. Through their professional organization, Russian nurses continue to appeal to the Russian Ministry of Health asking for enough equipment (such as gloves, disposables, and goggles) to remain safe from blood-borne pathogens and to care adequately for their patients. Physical assessments may not be performed by nurses because these skills are considered the domain of medicine, not nursing (Ivanov & Paganpegara, 2003). Team nursing, with each nurse taking on a specific role such as medication administration or wound care, is the norm (Difazio et al., 2004). Russian nurses believe that the quality of patient care and communication has improved since the influences of the nurse exchanges. They have seen the benefits of American nurses spending time assessing, listening to, and teaching patients, and they hunger to use these skills, if given the time and resources.

In addition to independent practice, Russian nurses dream of improved working conditions in hospitals—especially the problems of high nurse/patient ratios. They look for ways to finance medical equipment and pharmaceuticals in order to avoid shortages and maldistributions. Last, they wish to impose employment standards for hospitals so that only dedicated, qualified, hard-working nurses receive positions. As in the United States, Russian nurses love their profession and care deeply for their patients (Barron, 1994). Russian health care facilities may have shortages of everything from soap, sutures, gloves, pharmaceuticals, anesthesia, diagnostic equipment, and nearly all other imaginable amenities that U.S. nurses take for granted. These items include things such as a sink and running water to wash hands and clean instruments. V. Sarkisova proclaims in nearly all communications her honest appraisal of the hard work and many burdens of nurses in Russia.

Changes that promise to improve the quality of working life for Russian nurses are occurring, however. In at least one Russian facility, and as a response to nurses' concerns, pilot programs are being established to examine 4-, 6-, 8-, and 12-hour shifts (versus 24-hour shifts). Concepts of quality control and quality improvement

also are being implemented and evaluated along with nurse job and patient satisfaction surveys. At another geriatric center, better systems for nursing documentation, nursing assessments, and nursing diagnoses proudly are implemented (Difazio et al., 2004).

Nursing Research

The master's in nursing program at the Moscow Medical Academy includes nursing research as a studied and supported endeavor, but funding is precarious. As proof, faculty at this federally funded academy received no salary for 4 months because of budget problems (Picard & Perfiljeva, 1995). Therefore publishers of U.S. nursing research journals have been encouraged to donate subscriptions to the academy. Practice-based nursing research endeavors have surfaced in the area of home health care where Russian nurses have been taught by Western colleagues to measure health outcomes and thus to validate their profession (Bjornsson, Dalgard, Fonn, & Kjeldsen, 1998). Dr. Perfiljeva (1997) explained the implementation of joint research endeavors among Russian and U.S. nurse colleagues. Additionally, specially trained Russian nurses now are participating actively in scientific research efforts through the assistance of the American International Health Alliance (Mikheeva, 1997). Thanks to these and other efforts such as nursing publications and information dissemination, evidence-based nursing is becoming a greater reality.

Nursing Organizations

Before 1992, professional nursing organizations were already in place in Russia. For example, the Moscow City Nurses Association, members of which I met during two visits to Russia, was officially registered in 1992. Nationally, in 1990, nurses from each Soviet Republic met and discussed education and practice standards (Perfiljeva & Picard, 1998). Early that year each Soviet republic sent nurses to a Ministry of Health–sponsored meeting. They met because of the perceived need to standardize nursing education and practice throughout the Soviet Union (Picard & Perfiljeva, 1995). (These goals were expressed to me during my meeting at the Soviet Ministry of Health, July 4, 1989.) The breakup of the Soviet Union slowed but never stopped these standardization efforts. In 1993, as evidence of a continued effort to improve nursing care, I met RNA President Sarkisova, along with regional representatives from more than 36 Russian districts. (Representative regions are loosely connected subgroups of this national organization.) Members of these nursing groups are the leaders of nursing in Russia: education, practice, research, and administration. During these meetings, these leaders were willing to come together to explain their problems and their concerns for the purpose of improved nursing care. My Russian colleagues asked wonderfully challenging questions regarding nursing practice models, theories, and decision-making tools. Clearly, knowledge and information that has been shared with Russian nurses from the United States have been used significantly. They told me, "We are all very interested in the medical and nursing practices in the U.S.A." In 1998, the RNA boasted 7000 members who must pay individual membership fees through a 10% allocation of their regional nurses' association fees or as individual members with a fee of 1% of their salary (Bjornsson et al., 1998). In 2000, I again was invited to speak and connect with members of the RNA during their June conference in St. Petersburg. How exciting it was to listen to nurse leader-speakers proclaim a collective professional identity and the importance of professional unity.

Several endeavors can be credited with assisting Russian nurses to organize. These include World Vision International, which provided its first of three grants in 1992 and assisted in the growth of the RNA (Milburn, 1997). World Vision International monies were channeled through the Agency of International Contacts in Moscow, and in 1996 the organization prolonged the grant for an additional 6 months. Valentina Sarkisova, RNA president, proclaimed, "thanks to the financial support, we have made many improvements for nurses" (personal communication, 1996). Importantly, besides computers, telefax, and copier, Sarkisova was able to initiate a new nursing journal produced and written by Russian nurses for Russian nurses. In volume 1, issue 1 of *Nurses Work,* I wrote of my initial 1987 contacts with Chairman Gorbachev and the Ministry of Health and of my great honor and privilege in meeting and working with beloved Russian colleagues. Thanks to an outpouring of interest from Russian nurses, during two Russian nursing conferences, a moral Code of Russian Nurses was formulated and published.

In addition to World Vision International assistance, RNA President Sarkisova has sought advice and thereby has prepared necessary documents for RNA inclusion into the International Council of Nurses. Certainly, President Sarkisova has taken her leadership position seriously. She herself is an inducted member of Sigma Theta Tau International and hopes to bring Sigma Theta Tau International chapters to Russia. In November and December of 1999, President Sarkisova presented two seminars with Swedish nursing colleagues, gave a presentation to the Russian Ministry of Health (December 27)

regarding the problems of nursing, and participated in a weeklong health program in Louisville, Kentucky. On December 26, 1999, Ms. Sarkisova asserted that "the most important thing is that nurses need to understand that they need to unite. Sure, we have professional associations on the state and regional levels, but we still have a long way to go to reach a totally national Russian nursing organization." Sarkisova spent time in 1997 attending the Swedish Congress in Stockholm. The topic was nursing and computer science, another indication that Russian nurses continue to be interested in learning needed technology to advance their profession. Consequently, in late 1999, President Sarkisova recognized the Swedish Association of Health Workers for their generous offering of materials and assistance.

I have had several opportunities to speak before the Moscow Nurses Association in Moscow, Russia, and the new beginnings and continued growth of the RNA. During these occasions, I was struck with the strength and fortitude of this visionary group. Love for our beloved profession of nursing remains as the binding force for us all. Watching these nurses struggle with almost overwhelming obstacles—yet making progress politically and professionally—was inspirational. In closing impromptu remarks, I explained honestly that, "We are nurses. We are the ones who heal the hurts of the world. We have seen and experienced great suffering, yet we survive. As sisters we'll join you as you've joined us—in one united profession. I honor and respect your courage. I love you all."

EAST-WEST COLLABORATION
What Western Nurses Will Learn

Many Western nurses lack the knowledge their Russian colleagues have regarding holistic, homeopathic health care, including herbal medicines and leach therapy. In a nation suffering pharmaceutical shortages, Russian nurses understand the art and science of massage therapy, contactless massage, acupuncture, magnetic therapy, and acupressure. With advanced training, they perform these techniques to promote patient relaxation and noninvasive pain relief. Furthermore, in the absence of mechanical tools and diagnostic workups, Russian nurses have become expert clinicians and creative improvisers. They truly have learned to treat with their hands. For decades, Russian nurses have practiced contactless massage, hands-on massage, and the application of hot wax treatments to promote analgesia and circulation. Bjornsson et al. (1998) wrote of the practice of "blood therapy" in which venous blood is drawn and then reinjected into muscle to bolster immune systems. I also witnessed the teaching of leach therapy to student nurses. During episodes of angina, nurses were taught to place six to eight leaches in a semilunar fashion around the left chest wall. The saliva of the leach (effects can last up to 6 hours) provides a nearly perfect combination of anticoagulation, analgesia, and vasodilation.

What Western Nurses Will Teach

The Russian health care system gives patients a passive, subordinate position in the health care culture. This dependency, though gradually changing, presents problems regarding patient rights and responsibilities (Curtis et al., 1995; Tichtchenko, 2003). Additionally, palliative care concepts for the treatment of terminally ill patients are new and mostly doubted philosophies (Alaniz, 2001; Wallen & Cammuso, 1997). One reason for this reluctance is the concern medical professionals have for honesty with dying patients. Nurses are taught that under no circumstance should the patient be told of an incurable disease (Salmon, 1999). For this reason, Russian nurses were alarmed during discussion sessions that stressed openness with dying patients. An example of this reluctance is the slow evolution of hospice care. In 1997, just 10 hospice centers existed in all of Russia, and the only Russian hospice team making home visits started in 1994. The chief physician at this center confessed that his physician colleagues needed education regarding hospice care, philosophy, and benefits (Wallen & Cammuso, 1997). Needed instruction in bioethics also was identified by Yale University School of Nursing (2004) Associate Professor Douglas Olsen as he prepared for a fall 2004 teaching assignment at the Moscow Medical Academy.

Western nurses share with Russian colleagues research-based nursing care that is sensitive to the patient's physical and psychological distress. Head nurses learn to use informatics systems for data entry and retrieval (Kirgetova, 1997), and knowledge and skills regarding occupational therapy and nursing management are implemented. A nursing management program and manual was developed jointly between the faculty of nursing of the University of Western Ontario and Volfograd Medical College (Canadian International Development Agency, 1999).

Additional areas of sharing will occur regarding the implementation skills, strategies, and opportunities for patient and community health education. Teaching/learning in the area of bioethics is lacking (only one journal devotes itself to the discussion of legal and moral health care issues) (Tichtchenko, 2003). Bloor, McHugh, Pearson, and Wain (2004) found that a training course in the management of aggression between United Kingdom and Russian health care professionals was enormously successful. Nursing informatics information will allow greater communication and dialogue between and among internationally based nurses. For example, with the help of new and exciting technology, telemedicine consultation and education can take place in clinical, surgical, community, and classroom settings.

The Aid to Russia Controversy

Multitudes of Russian financial and health care problems can cause Westerners to believe that giving aid to Russia is like pouring money into a huge black hole. Doubts remain over the efficacy of such endeavors. A report by the U.S. Senate Foreign Relations Committee concluded that the average Russian is "unaware of or affected by international assistance or the reforms that it is supposed to foster" ("U.S. Aid Trickles," 1994, p. 1A). Many believe that no amount of foreign aid will help until Russia can put inflation, increasing financial deficits, and skyrocketing crime in check. The frightening side of Russian economic turmoil is the tendency for high-level, underpaid Russian scientists to leave the country for more lucrative locations or to supplement meager salaries by selling sensitive knowledge and materials. This Russian brain drain is a major threat to world peace efforts and has become a complex problem, given the estimated 30,000 nuclear weapons in the possession of desperate Russians residing in more than 39 separate Russian districts ("Rescuing Russia," 1999; Zuckerman, 1999a). Nuclear, chemical, and biological weapons easily could enter black markets. Thus a stable Russia is in the interest of U.S. foreign policy.

Health and health care are enmeshed with all other social concerns in Russia, and foreign intervention is essential. For example, during the Russian school siege in Beslan in 2004, the biggest problem faced by health care services was a lack of equipment such as medication and surgical supplies (Triggle, 2004). Immediately, the Russian Red Cross appealed to the international community, and within days a Norwegian air shipment arrived containing enough medical supplies to treat 1000 patients for 10 days along with three donated ambulances, diagnostic equipment, and burn bandages (BBC, 2004). U.S. involvement has been just as important. In July 2004, then–U.S. Department of Health and Human Services Secretary Tommy Thompson announced that the Global Fund to fight AIDS, tuberculosis, and malaria would be awarded to Russia over a 2-year period in the amount of $34.2 million. While in Moscow, Thompson urged the Russian government and health care officials to demonstrate strong public leadership to stop the spread of these deadly diseases (U.S. Department of Health and Human Services, 2004). In a letter Thompson wrote in *Rossiyskaya Gazeta,* he stated his hope that the two nations could strengthen their alliance against the global enemy of disease (U.S. Embassy, Moscow, Russia, 2004).

These aid benefits would be tangible and far reaching. For example, one of the more productive joint projects has been through the U.S.-Russia Joint Commission on Economic and Technological Cooperation. From 1994 to 2004, this commission helped Russian health officials control the spread of infectious diseases (tuberculosis, HIV, and sexually transmitted diseases), improve access to quality health care (primary and preventive medicine), and promote maternal and child health, including programs for nutrition, alcohol, diabetes, and the environment (U.S.-Russia Joint Commission on Economic and Technological Cooperation, 1999). An additional program, organized through the American Red Cross (Booth, 2002) was the $1 million grant from the U.S State Department to be used to improve the efficiency and effectiveness of Russian Red Cross branches in the northern Caucasus region and to support the Russian visiting nurses program. Before this U.S.-based grant, these visiting nurses had almost no equipment. They needed thermometers, gloves, linens, syringes, disinfectant, and money. Unfortunately, not all Russians (especially ultranationalists) welcome Western help, even for health programs (Ronalds, 1998).

CULTURALLY COMPETENT NURSE-TO-NURSE EFFORTS

Assistance to Russian nurses by American colleagues is and will continue to be accomplished through the efforts of many nursing groups such as the American International Health Alliance, Project Hope, WHO, American Red Cross, and U.S.-Russian Nurse Exchange Consortium of Racine, Wisconsin. The consortium, with members in multiple U.S. states and Russia, has hosted U.S.-Russian exchanges of health care professionals since 1989.

Russian health professionals propose that education scholarships, person-to-person exchanges, and quality health care research be supported financially (Komarov, 1994; V. Sarkisova, personal communication, 2000). Russian nursing education can be supported through the LEMON Project (Learning Education Materials on Nursing), a curricular package of nursing materials developed by European nurses and sponsored by WHO (Perfiljeva & Picard, 1998). With the help of foreign money, nursing materials are translated, packaged, printed, and distributed (Picard & Perfiljeva, 1995).

Another exciting nurse-to-nurse biannual exchange between Western and Russian nurses is the Russian- and U.S.-sponsored nursing tour and cross-cultural conference titled "Building Bridges for Collaboration between U.S. and Russian Nurses." During these conferences, Russian and Western nurses have been asked to share ideas for possible professional collaborative projects (Difazio et al., 2004). As these ideas become reality, additional exchange and growth opportunities will surface, and I feel fortunate to have played a small part in the planning and implementation for them. The Russian tours have involved paper presentations, focused discussion groups, and site visits to health care and educational facilities. The next scheduled conference is in 2005.

Nurse-to-nurse efforts need to focus on teaching the teachers and leaders so that they may teach others. This is easy. Russian nurses are hungry to learn from Western peers. From personal experience, I have found my Russian colleagues to be well educated, quick to grasp concepts, enormously dedicated to their profession, and creative in their attempts to implement new knowledge and technology (Barron, 1994, p. 59; V. Sarkisova, personal communication, December 26, 1999). Milburn (1997) wrote that "our role in Russia was that of catalysts to facilitate the reform movement and its partnerships, ambassadors of our country in a country that until recently viewed the U.S. as a dreaded enemy, role models of market economic principles in an environment that is just learning the meaning of competition, teachers of nurses … on management principles needed to sustain reform, liaisons with the government health care leaders to promote changes at the local and national levels and advocates for Russia's health care consumers who today face challenges of a broken-down health care system and society" (p. 6a). Dr. Yevgeny Filan, nursing school director in Moscow wrote in June 1998, "Our colleagues from the USA have given us and our faculty a powerful impulse for creativity and we are really anticipating the continuation of this cooperation." In 2000, Dr. Filan told me of his desire to develop continuing and lasting faculty and student exchanges between and among Russian and U.S. health care education institutions.

THE FUTURE OF RUSSIA

New freedoms will help Russian nurses and other health care professionals identify and track health care issues and indexes without forced data embellishment. Computer systems are in place that will restore the true health care picture in Russia. Reform programs, started under Yeltsin and Gorbachev, will continue to move forward under President Putin's regime. Especially important will be the Russian government's budget prioritization in the area of health care and education of health care professionals. Fortunately, what Perfiljeva (1997) wrote about the need to enhance nursing care quality has been well supported throughout Russia, and slow but significant transitions have taken place. Key to these changes will be the emerging, visionary role of the professional nurse, organized nursing and professional nursing education. Nurses, once docile and subservient, have found new political and professional savvy as they confront old worn traditions of medical authority. They are showing officials that nursing decision making and independent practice can and will move Russian health care forward. "Join us now as we struggle for our identity," Russian nurses say. "We are strong and we will survive these difficult times; we are one with you as nurses. Our profession is our hope and our voice."

DEDICATION

It is with the greatest admiration that I dedicate this chapter to my nursing friends and colleagues in Russia. On a daily basis, they show all of us the ideals for which our beloved profession stands. Let us share of ourselves toward one goal and purpose—international health, love, and peace.

REFERENCES

Alaniz, J. (2001). Crossing cultures: Russian nurses navigate the unfamiliar US health care system, finding career advantages and obstacles. *Nursing & Allied Health Week, 6*(18), 20-21.

Aron, L. (1998, Summer). *AEI Russian Outlook.* Retrieved March 16, 1999 from American Enterprise Institute for Public Policy Research database: http://www.aei.org.ro/ro9464.htm

Ashlund, A. (2001). *Think again: Russia. Foreign Policy: The Magazine of Global Politics, Economics, and Ideas.* Retrieved June 9, 2002, from http://www.foreignpolicy.com/issue_julyaug_2002/Tajulyaug.html

Babakian, G. (1998, July 14). Fraying economy feeds rumors of a coup in Russia. *USA Today,* p. 7A.

Barron, S. (1994). A nursing experience in Russia. *Neonatal Network, 13*(2), 59.

BBC. (2004, September 7). *Medical aid flows to siege town.* Retrieved September 7, 2004, from http://newsvote/bbc.co.up/mpapps/pagetools/print/news.bbc.co.uk/1/hi/world/europe/36342

Bennett, V. (1997, December 6). Violence against women in Russia grows worse. *LA Times.* Retrieved January 23, 2000 from dimensional.com database: http://dim.com/~randl/russ.htm

Bjornsson, K., Dalgard, P., Fonn, M., & Kjeldsen, S. B. (1998). Nursing and health in Russia. *International Nursing Review, 45*(3), 89-93.

Bloor, R., McHugh, A., Pearson, D., & Wain, I. (2004). A training course for psychiatric nurses in Russia. *Nursing Standard, 18*(39), 39-41.

Boe, B. (1993). Boe knows Russia. *The Carthaginian, 72*(4), 6.

Booth, M. (2002, October 9). *American Red Cross nurse urges help for Russia's vulnerable populations.* Retrieved August 28, 2004, from the American Red Cross Web site: http://www.redcross.org/news/in/health/021009nurses.html

Building an international partnership: Russia. (2004, July 9). New Haven, CT: Yale University School of Nursing. Retrieved June 5, 2005 from http://nursing.yale.edu/world/programs/russia.html

Burger, E. J. (2000, January 2). An unhealthy Russia (letter). *Washington Post.* Retrieved January 3, 2000, from http://www.cdi.org/russia/johnson/4005.html##15

Canadian International Development Agency. (1999). *Canada-Russia Health and Social Development Project.* Retrieved August 18, 1999, from the Queen's University Web site: http://www.quensu.ca/crhsd/can-rus.htm

Centers for Disease Control and Prevention. (1999). *Vital and health statistics: Maternal and child health statistics: Russian Federation and United States, selected years 1985-1995* (DHHS Pub. No. [PHS] 991486). Hyattsville, MD: Author.

Centers for Disease Control and Prevention. (2002). *Maternal and child health compared in U.S. and Russia.* Retrieved July 12, 2002, from http://www.cdc.gov/nchs/releases/99facts/russian.htm

Center for Strategic and International Studies. (1999, February 18). *Net assessment of the Russian economy.* Retrieved March 16, 1999, from the Center for Strategic and International Studies database: http://www.csis.org/ruseura/rus_econ.html

Central Intelligence Agency. (2004). *The world factbook: Russia—Economy.* Retrieved January 16, 2005, from http://www.cia.gov/cia/publications/factbook/geos/rs.html#econ

Cockburn, P. (2000, January 21). Russians threaten to incarcerate 'dissident'. *The Independent* (United Kingdom). Retrieved January 21, 2000 from Johnson's Russia List: davidjohnson@erols.com

Curtis, S., Petukhova, N., & Taket, A. (1995). Health care reforms in Russia: The example of St. Petersburg. *Social Science and Medicine, 40*(6), 755-765.

Dahlburg, J-T. (1998, November 8). As Russian economy crumbles, many despair of better life. *Arkansas Democrat-Gazette,* p. 18A.

Difazio, R., Lang, D., & Boykova, M. (2004). Nursing in Russia: A "travelogue." *Journal of Pediatric Nursing, 19*(2), 150-156.

Douglas, J., & Mannino, J. F. (1997). Postconference tour highlights challenges facing Russian nurses. *Journal of Transcultural Nursing, 9*(1), 40-41.

Dymchenko, L. D., & Callister, L. C. (2002). Challenges and opportunities: The health of women and newborns in the

Russian Federation. *Journal of Perinatal & Neonatal Nursing, 16*(3), 11-21.

Edwards, D. J. (1994). Transcultural nursing: A view of the Russian health care system. *Orthopaedic Nursing, 13*(2), 47-51.

Engleman, E. (2002a, March 22). *Experts warn Russia's fight against TB is far from over.* Retrieved January 5, 2995, from Johnson's Russia List Web site: http://www.cdi.org/russia/johnson/6153-7.cfm

Engleman, E. (2002b, April 14). Russians getting sued to paying flat income tax. *The Journal Times* (Racine, WI), p. 9A.

Gaufberg, S. V. (2004, March 11). *Emergency medicine in Russia.* Retrieved August 28, 2004, from eMedicine.com Web site: http://www.emedicine.com/emerg/topic725.htm

Gordon, M. R. (2000, January 23). Putin sacks commander in Grozny. *The Sunday Oregonian,* p. A9.

Gore-Felton, C., Somlai, A. M., Benotsch, E. G., Kelly, J. A., Ostrovski, D., & Kozlov, A. (2003). The influence of gender on factors associated with HIV transmission risk among young Russian injection drug users. *American Journal of Drug and Alcohol Abuse, 29*(4), 881-894.

Green, A. J., Holloway, D. G., & Fleming, P. M. (2001). An education programme for professionals who specialize in substance misuse in St. Petersburg, Russia: Part 1. *Nurse Education Today, 21,* 656-662.

Heilig, S. (1999). A modern public health crisis: A physician speaks about healthcare in post-Glasnost Russia. *Cambridge Quarterly of Healthcare Ethics, 8,* 257-258.

Holmes, C. W. (1997, September 27). Yeltsin OKs restricting some faiths. *Atlanta Journal/Constitution,* p. B3.

Ivanov, L. L., & Paganpegara, G. (2003). Public health nursing education in Russia. *Journal of Nursing Education, 42*(7), 292-295.

Johnstone, A. (1999). Homelessness: Cold feat in Moscow. *Nursing Times, 95*(7), 30-31.

Kirgetova, G. (1997). *Improving nursing training through partnerships.* Retrieved August 20, 1999, from the American International Health Alliance database: http://www.aiha.com/english/pubs/nursbook/p26.htm

Knox, K. (2002, March 23). *Russia: Unhealthy mothers in Russia get babies off to a poor start.* Retrieved June 9, 2002, from Johnson's Russia List Web site: http://www.cdi.org/russia/johnson/6153-6.cfm

Komarov, Y. M. (1994). Quality assurance in health care: Lessons for others. *International Journal for Quality in Health Care, 6*(1), 27-30.

Kunin, V. (1997, March 5). *Russian medicine on verge of crisis.* Retrieved August 20, 1999, from the Public Health Research Institute database: http://www.russia.phri.org/b3597.htm

Lally, K. (2000, January 10). Death offers no relief for woes of Russians. *Baltimore-The Sun,* pp. 1A, 10A.

Maksimova, L. (1998, January). *Major medical projects in Russia.* Retrieved May 29, 1999, from the Business Information Service for the Newly Independent States database: http://iepnt1.itaiep.doc.gov/bisnis/isa/9801medi.htm

Mikheeva, T. (1997). *Continuous training of nursing staff as an integral part of improving the quality of medical care.* Retrieved August 20, 1999, from the American International Health Alliance database: http://www.aiha.com/english/pubs/nursbook/p27.htm

Milburn, L. T. (1997). Health reform in Russia: Challenges and success. *Prairie Rose, 66*(2), 5a-7a.

Osborn, A. (2004). Half of Russia's doctors face sack in health-care reforms. *British Medical Journal, 328*(7448), 1092.

Perfiljeva, G. (1997). Progress in Russia: Working together for change. *Reflections, 23*(2), 8-9.

Perfiljeva, G., & Picard, C. (1998). Clarification about nursing in Russia. *Image: Journal of Nursing Scholarship, 30*(2), 107-108.

Picard, C., & Perfiljeva, G. (1995). Nursing education in Russia: Visions and realities. *N&HC: Perspectives on Community, 16*(3), 126-130.

Public Broadcast Service. (2000). *Return of the czar.* Retrieved May 10, 2000, from http://www.pbs.org/wgbh/pages/frontline/shows/yeltsin/

Public Health Research Institute. (1997, June 7). *Russia is dying doctors warn.* Retrieved August 20, 1999, from Public Health Research Institute database: http://www.russia.phri.org/b6797.htm

Rescuing Russia. (1999, November 21). *Parade Magazine,* p. 20.

Revich, B. A. (1999). *Environmental epidemiology in Russia: Some results and prospects.* Centre of Demography and Human Ecology Institute of Forecasting. Retrieved August 20, 1999, from friends-partners database: http://www.friends-partners.org/oldfriends/welling/revich.htm

Ronalds, F. (1998, February 10). *The health crisis in Russia.* Retrieved August 20, 1999 from the Public Health Research Institute database: http//www.russia.phri.org/b21098.htm

Russia says cutbacks in military. (2002, January 4). Retrieved June 9, 2002, from Johnson's Russia List Web site: http://www.cdi.org/russia/johnson/6005-2.cfm

Russian fertility problems in women cause of alarm. (2000, August). *Herald and News* (Klamath Falls, OR), p. D1.

Russian official criticizes government over HIV. (2000, January 29). Retrieved January 30, 2000, from Johnson's Russia List Web site: http://www.cdi.org/russia/johnson/4079.html#3

Russians rally against terror after bloodbath. (2004, September 7). Retrieved September 7, 2004, from MSNBC.com Web site: http://msnbc.msn.com/id/5881958/print/1/displaymode/1098/

Ryan, M. (1992). Russian report: Perspectives on strikes by health care staff. *BMJ, 305*(6848), 298-299.

Salmon, I. (1999). To Russia with cling film. *Nursing Times, 95*(18), 35.

Sandul, I. (2002, March 22-28). Trying to break through the glass ceiling. *The Russia Journal.* Retrieved June 9, 2002, from Johnson's Russia List Web site: http://www.cdi.org/russia/johnson/6152-15.cfm

Steinkraus, D. (2000, August 15). Russian visits for a government lesson. *The Journal Times* (Racine, WI), pp. 1C, 3C.

Steinkraus, D. (2003, November 7). Putting soul into health. *The Journal Times* (Racine, WI), pp. 1B, 3B.

Tavernise, S. (2002, March 23). Russia imposes flat tax on income, and its coffers swell. *New York Times.* Retrieved June 9, 2002, from Johnson's Russia List Web site: http://www.cdi.org/russia/johnson/6152-14.cfm

Tichtchenko, P. (2003). Changing roles in Russian healthcare. *Cambridge Quarterly of Healthcare Ethics, 12,* 265-267.

Triggle, N. (2004, September 6). *The strain on Russia's health service.* Retrieved September 7, 2004, from the BBC News Web site: http://newsvote.bbc.co.uk/mpapps/pagetools/print/news.bbc.co.uk/1/hi/health/3631286.stm

Trust, but verify. (2000, August 28). *US News & World Report, 129*(8), p. 10.

UNAIDS. (2004). Russian Federation: HIVAIDS estimates. *UNAIDS/WHO Epidemiological fact sheet—2004 update.* Retrieved January 6, 2005 from http//www.who.int/GlobalAtlas/predefineReports/EFS2004/EFS_PDFs/EFS2004_RU.pdf

United Nations Development Programme. (2002, January-February). *International Labor Organization publicizes working street children.* Retrieved August 28, 2004, from http://195.68.179.50/eng/newsletter/01_202/page2.html

U.S. Aid trickles down to ordinary Russians. (1994, March 28). *The Journal Times* (Racine, WI), p. 1A, 7A.

U.S. Department of Health and Human Services. (2004, July 1). *Secretary Thompson announces global fund grant to Russia.* Retrieved September 7, 2004, from Global Health.gov Web site: http://www.globalhealth.gov/TGT_Russia_070104.shtml

U.S. Department of State. (1997, June). *Background notes: Russia, June 1997.* Retrieved March 16, 1999, from http://www.state.gov/www/background_notes/russia_0697_bgn.html

U.S. Embassy, Moscow, Russia. (2004, July 1). United against a common enemy: US Secretary of Health and Human Services Tommy G. Thompson. *Rossiyskaya Gazeta.* Retrieved September 7, 2004, from http://moscow.usembassy.gov/embassy/print_oped.phd?record_id=12

U.S.-Russia Joint Commission on Economic and Technological Cooperation. (1999, March 23). *Joint report of the 8th Health Committee Meeting.* Washington, DC: Author. Retrieved August 20, 1999, from the U.S. Department of Health and Human Services database: http://odphp.osophs.dhhs.gov/russia/jr8eng.htm

U.S. State Department. (2000, January 7). *Russia: Consular information sheet.* Retrieved January 30, 2000, from state.gov database: http://travel.state.gov/russia.html

Wallen, A. J., & Cammuso, B. S. (1997). Health care in the new Russia: A western perspective. *Nursing Forum, 32*(3), 27-32.

Watkins, D., & Rees, C. (1999). Healthcare crisis in Russia: A public health issue. *Nursing Standard, 13*(22), 33-35.

Weir, F. (2001, March 8). Women's day in Russia: Showers of flowers. *Christian Science Monitor.* Retrieved January 23, 2005, from http://csmonitor.com/cgi-bin/durable/2001/03/08/fp7s1-csm.shtml

Wines, M. (2000, January 2). Putin's acts hint at agenda addressing graft, economy. *The Sunday Oregonian,* p. A19.

Winik, L. W. (2001, January 28). Intelligence report: Russia in crisis. *Parade Magazine,* p. 6.

World Health Organization. (2004). *The global atlas of the health workforce.* Retrieved January 16, 2005, from http://www.who.int/globalatlas/default.asp

World Health Organization Regional Office for Europe. (2005). *Country profile: Russia.* Retrieved January 14, 2005, from http://hfadb.who.dk/hfa/hfaoverw2

Yale University School of Nursing. (2004, July 9). *YSN in the world: Russian Federation.* Retrieved August 28, 2004, from www.nursing.yale.edu/world/regions/europeRussia/russia.html

Zuckerman, M. B. (1999a, February 8). Coming to Russia's rescue. *US News & World Report, 126*(5), 68.

Zuckerman, M. B. (1999b, February 8). Proud Russia on its knees. *US News & World Report, 126*(5), 30-36.

Nursing in the Gambia

An Overview of Health Care, Nursing Education, and Practice

KENNITH CULP

The Gambia is one of the smallest countries in Africa with only 4361 square miles and no point wider than 30 miles; however, it supports a rapidly growing population. Located in West Africa where it is bordered by the Atlantic Ocean to the west and Senegal to the north, east, and south, the country historically has been instrumental in fostering the development of the slave trade because of its sea ports (Gregg & Trillo, 2003). In fact, some of this history was popularized in the Alex Haley book and television series *Roots*, which was set in the Gambia. Although historians have questioned some of Haley's facts about the slave trade in Africa (Fullen, 2002), the Gambian government has embraced the popularity of this phenomenon and rejoices at the opportunity to serve as a cultural center for those seeking to understand better the rich heritage of the African people. Banjul is the capital city of this mostly Muslim country of 1.5 million persons. Little is written about health care and nursing in the Gambia. The country is small, and most of the statistics and descriptions are based on informal reports and bulletins, newspaper accounts, state documents, and the experiences of the author (Culp, Bobb, & Marquez, 2003).

CULTURE, HISTORY, AND POLITICS

The Gambia has numerous ethnic groups, and each group has its own language, but the official language is English. The single largest tribal group in Gambia is the Mandinka, an agricultural people with hereditary nobility (Schaffer, 2003). The Wolofs are prominent in the capital city of Banjul, as are the Akus, descendants of freed slaves who rank among the bureaucratic elite. The Jola people are organized around the cultivation of rice, and the Fulas around the herding of cattle.

The Gambians are mostly a conservative Muslim people, so health problems such as alcoholism or the human immunodeficiency virus infection are low compared with South Africa. Census records are few, but in general about 85% of Gambians are Muslim, 13% are Christian, and the remaining 2% have animist beliefs (Levtzion & Fisher, 1987).

DEVELOPING DEMOCRACY

The Gambia gained independence from the United Kingdom in 1965, and the People's Progressive Party dominated Gambian politics for nearly 30 years. The People's Progressive Party was never seriously challenged by any opposition party. It was difficult for the people to criticize the government openly, and opposition parties often were fragmented. The current political system has distinct features of a "strong" presidential regime; however, a separation of powers does exist. For example, 45 of the 48 seats in the National Assembly (i.e., the Gambian Parliament), belong to the president's political party.

The major threats to democracy are social and economic issues. Foremost is "Third World" debt (Hertz, 2004), poverty, and illiteracy (Dent & Peters, 1999; Millet & Toussaint, 2003; Roodman, Peterson, & Worldwatch Institute, 2001). Many social programs such as education and health care have external influences from the World Bank and the International Monetary Fund because interest payments consume nearly half of all tax revenue, leaving little for education and health care (Millet & Toussaint, 2003; Roodman et al., 2001).

HEALTH CARE DELIVERY SYSTEM

Whenever the Gambian health care delivery system is described, one must remember that there is a severe

TABLE 91-1

Health Status: National Indicators in the Gambia				
Indicator	1973	1983	1993	Latest Estimates
Population	493,499	687,817	1,038,145	1,546,848 (2004)
Life expectancy (years)	33	42	53	55 (2004)
Male	32	40	52	53 (2004)
Female	35	44	54	57 (2004)
Infant mortality rate (per 1000 live births)	217	167	85	73 (2004)
Under 5 mortality rate (per 1000)	320	260	137	135 (2001)
Maternal mortality rate (per 100,000)	N/A	N/A	1050	730 (2001)
Fertility rate (births per woman of childbearing age)	6.1	6.4	6.1	5.6 (2004)
Fully immunized under 2 years	<27%	55%	80%	71% (2001)
Crude birth rate (per 1000 population)	49	51	46	40 (2004)
Crude death rate (per 1000 population)	30	21	19	12 (2004)

Source: Department of State for Health and Social Welfare, the Gambia.
N/A, Not available.

shortage of nurses and physicians. The term *delivery* must be taken literally because of the poor transportation infrastructure in the Gambia. A rainy season increases the need for health care because it results in epidemic malaria, and the precipitation also results in muddy roads, which are impassible. Mortality is high during the rainy season (June to November), and the young die from infectious disease. The mean survival in years is much lower in the Gambia compared with Western countries where chronic disease is the leading cause of death (Table 91-1).

The term *health care delivery* means one has something to deliver. Nurses are the backbone of the system, and the Gambia also relies heavily on lay workers in health care. Although nurses are most likely to be Gambian, the physicians are not, for in 1999, Cuba offered to help the Gambia, and today a large number of Cuban physicians are in the country. Sierra Leonean or Nigerian doctors are also in the Gambia. Of course, with the Cuban physicians come communication problems in English, but the nurses have learned to operate with minimum supervision under well-developed clinical protocols. Relief nurses from the international community are few in the Gambia; it is one country that is "poached" of its nurses to other countries as nurses, and many young persons are lured to higher-salaried nursing positions and better working conditions in Western countries. This is unfortunate and is discussed later in this chapter.

The four major components of the health care delivery system in the Gambia are (1) central referral hospitals, (2) the village health service, (3) the basic health center, and (4) the divisional health team.

Referral Hospitals

Three main referral hospitals in the Gambia handle the most complex medical problems and are analogous to tertiary care centers in the United States. However, these hospitals lack the technical expertise and advanced diagnostic equipment seen in industrial nations. Referral hospitals are located strategically in the Gambia (Figure 91-1) with the Royal Victoria Hospital as the largest hospital. Each hospital has a principal nursing officer, and he or she oversees a staff of state registered nurses (SRN), state enrolled nurses, midwives, and nurse attendants. Working conditions in these hospitals are challenging to the nurses, and often the government requires them to rotate to different regions of the country every few years. Few intravenous pumps, electronic monitoring devices, or latex gloves are on the wards. The environment is clean, and critical medications are usually available. When staff shortages exist, the nurses are required to work longer hours. Disposable equipment is nonexistent; anything that can be autoclaved or cleaned is reused. These hospitals are the best places for care at public expense in the Gambia.

Village Health Service

Primary health care in rural villages is based on village health workers and traditional birth attendants who are supervised by community health nurses. A village development committee selects the village health worker and traditional birth attendants. These workers are given 6 to 8 weeks of formal training in a centralized course with a standardized curriculum from the Department of State for Health. Village health workers treat minor illnesses

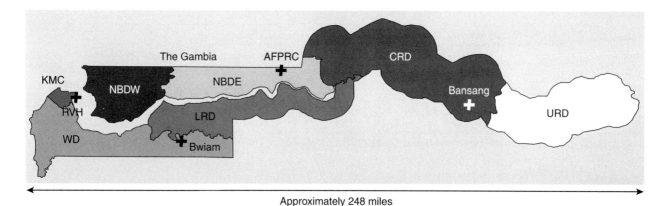

FIGURE 91-1   Hospital locations in the Gambia. *+,* Hospital; *AFPRC, Armed Forces Provisional Ruling Council; CRD,* Central River Division; *KMC,* Kanifing Municipal Council; *LRD,* Lower River Division; *NBDE,* North Bank Division East; *NBDW,* North Bank Division West; *RVH,* Royal Victoria Hospital; *URD,* Upper River Division; *WD,* Western Division.

and injuries. Traditional birth attendants function as trained birth attendants, as antenatal and postnatal advisors, and family planning distributors. Contraception is not widely accepted by rural people, and the traditional birth attendants fail in this area miserably. The community health nurse oversees circuits of 4 to 10 villages and generally transverses the countryside on motorbikes that are suited for the road conditions in rural areas, for seldom does one see a "paved" road.

Basic Health Centers

Functioning in parallel with the village health service are the basic health facilities. Basic health centers include (1) major health centers, (2) minor health centers, and (3) dispensaries. Major health centers admit small numbers of patients (10 to 20) for inpatient care, although I have directly observed many more patients in the countryside. State registered nurses (equivalent to a 3-year registered nurse in the United States) and state enrolled nurses (equivalent to the 2-year associate's degree nurse in the United States) are assigned to the inpatient wards and clinics. Nurse midwives (specialty SRNs with additional 9 to 18 months of midwifery training) are on staff to run the labor and delivery ward.

Divisional Health Teams

Divisional health teams oversee the functioning of the basic health centers and village health services in each region. These regions are mapped in Figure 91-1 and include the Western Division, Lower River Division, North Bank West and North Bank East, Central River Division, and Upper River Division. The divisional health team is multidisciplinary and is responsible for the

budgeting, material supply, monitoring, and supervision of all government health services in its administrative area. Facilities and services provided by nongovernmental organizations are also under the authority of the divisional health team because each nongovernmental organization has signed a memorandum of understanding with the government agreeing to this condition. At my last count, at least 14 nongovernmental organization–run clinical facilities were in the country. An annual planning meeting is held by the divisional health team at the end of each year to set divisional priorities and to plan programs, workshops, and other activities for the following year. Every year, planning is a struggle because the need for health care services outpaces available resources.

Other Health Care Resources

The Medical Research Council is also a major source of health care for the Gambian people. The council is analogous to a research hospital in the United States, and the author found these facilities to be fairly modern and well-staffed. The Medical Research Council is one of the major institutions left over from the British influence in the Gambia and serves a vital function in researching malaria and providing free care for the poor (Aitman et al., 2000; Bojang et al., 2001; Pinder et al., 2004). The success of the Medical Research Council has won the attention of the Bill & Melinda Gates Foundation, of Microsoft Corporation fame, which is helping to finance health projects in the Gambia. For affluent citizens, there are also private health clinics and small hospitals that provide clinical services more consistent with Western health care (e.g., disposable needles, diagnostic laboratory tests, and personalized health care services).

TABLE 91-2

Hospital Admissions and Mortality for Children Under 5 Years of Age in the Gambia, 2002

	Malaria	Pneumonia	Malnutrition	Anemia	Sepsis	Prematurity or Low Birth Weight	Trauma and Burns
Admissions (%)	57.2	17.2	3.3	6.1	4.8	1.0	1.7
Deaths (%)	36.9	10.0	6.2	12.0	9.0	5.5	2.1

Source: Department of State for Health and Social Welfare, the Gambia.

TABLE 91-3

Hospital Admissions and Mortality for Pregnancy-Related Complications in the Gambia, 2002

	Malaria	Anemia	Hemorrhage	Preeclampsia and Eclampsia	Sepsis	Pelvic Inflammatory Disease	Ectopic Pregnancy	Other
Admissions (%)	40.1	9.4	11.7	11.8	6.7	6.2	0.9	13.2
Deaths (%)	37.2	9.3	23.3	4.7	7.0	2.3	4.7	11.6

Source: Department of State for Health and Social Welfare, the Gambia.

HEALTH ISSUES

A number of pressing health issues in the Gambia are related to cultural beliefs and infectious disease. These include trachoma, malaria, helminthic infections, dysenteries, and meningococcal disease (O'Dempsey et al., 1996; Wenger, 1997). Other problems relate to reproductive health and include polygamy, female circumcision, and birth control (Luck, Jarju, Nell, & George, 2000). As mentioned before, the rates of human immunodeficiency virus infection are low, about 1% of the adult population (Schim van der Loeff et al., 2003).

Trachoma

Trachoma accounts for 10% to 15% of blindness worldwide (Kalayoglu, 2002) and is completely preventable. This illness is caused by ocular infection with *Chlamydia trachomatis*. While in the Gambia, I have observed many older adults with blindness caused by this disease. Initiatives exist to treat this disease early (Bowman, Faal, et al., 2002; Bowman, Jatta, et al., 2000; Burton et al., 2003), and nurses specially trained in eye procedures are key to this program. Besides early treatment, prevention of trachoma is based on the World Health Organization (1998) mission to eliminate trachoma by the year 2020. The World Health Organization program is based on "The SAFE" strategy: *s*urgery for in-turned eyelashes, *a*ntibiotics for active disease, *f*ace and hand washing (or promotion of facial cleanliness), and *e*nvironmental improvement to reduce transmission. For example,

Gambians are learning that trachoma is lower in children with clean faces than in those with ocular or nasal discharge or flies on the face (Schachter & Dawson, 2002).

Malaria

Malaria accounts for more than half of all hospital admissions in children 5 years and under and is responsible for more than one third of all deaths in this age group (Table 91-2). Pregnant women are also at risk, and infection results in a substantial number of hospital admissions (Table 91-3). Women with malaria are challenged with the task of delivering oxygen to the fetus; thus miscarriages and low birth weight are common (Duffy, 2003; Newman et al., 2003).

In the United States, nurses hardly ever think about malaria, but the situation is different in the Gambia. Malarial parasites are transmitted from one person to another by the female anopheline mosquito (Christophides, 2005; Hay, Guerra, Tatem, Atkinson, & Snow, 2005). Preventive measures include draining wet areas and spraying with pesticides, but anopheline resistance to insecticides does exist (MacAlister, 2001).

Malaria is diagnosed by the clinical symptoms, and the older practice of microscopic examination of red blood cells is still commonplace even though there are quicker and far less complex screening tests. These tests are based on a few drops of blood and could be used by field workers instead of laboratory personnel as is done currently (Bates, Bekoe, & Asamoa-Adu, 2004).

These "quick tests" for malaria especially would be ideal in remote areas (Bojang et al., 2001) and save lives by prioritizing patients in need of emergency transportation to the hospital.

Malaria and Children

The limited availability of antimalarial drugs outside major towns contributes to the high mortality from the disease in pregnant women, infants, and toddlers (Lesi & Meremikwu, 2004). Seasonal patterns of infection sometimes leave remote villages without effective antimalarial drugs, especially in late August. One misconception of rural people is that paracetamol will cure malaria, but it does not. Paracetamol has been in use as an analgesic for more than 30 years in the Gambia and is accepted as an effective treatment for the relief of pain and fever, but it does not decrease the parasite count. Hence the most common course of many parents is to try to provide home care for a child with malaria. This results in delayed treatment. One study found that the most common practice in the Gambia for treating a child with malaria was using paracetamol and/or tepid sponging to reduce fever (Clarke, Rowley, Bogh, Walraven, & Lindsay, 2003).

REPRODUCTIVE HEALTH

The Gambia has had a consistently high population growth rate of 4.2% for the last 3 decades. Reasons include high female fertility (5.6 nationwide) and, owing to polygamy, an even higher male fertility (approximately 12 children per father in the North Bank Division); a general reduction in infant mortality rates; and increasing in-migration from conflict-ridden areas (Ratcliffe, Hill, Harrington, & Walraven, 2002). The ability to control immigration into the Gambia is severely limited because border patrols are rare. In any case, overpopulation has resulted in crowded public schools. One account recently found in the newspaper was that 60,000 Gambian children, aged 7 to 15 years, simply have dropped out of school because of the large size of the classrooms (Ceesay, 2005).

Approximately one third of women participate in polygamous marriages (Hayase & Liaw, 1997), but the practice is as difficult to "count" because marriage licenses and legal papers are not completed routinely. No clear single reason exists why polygamy persists. Polygamy is related most strongly to culture and the social status of men, but some wives with many children and household chores may ask their husband to consider adding a wife to the family to ease the burden. Gambians generally perceive marriage as an alliance between two kinship groups and only secondarily a union of individuals (Umelo, 2004). Men are allowed four wives at any one time, but women frequently leave these family units, and divorce is common. Both of these statistics are difficult to document, but over the course of a lifetime, it is not uncommon for some men to have been married more than four times (Ratcliffe et al., 2002).

The low use of modern contraceptives is rooted in traditional behavior and communication structures, religious constraints, and low educational and literacy levels, particularly among women. Those who opposed birth control stated that they believed, "God provides for all his creatures, so there is no need to limit births," or that "Muhammed asked his followers to have many children." Others fear that birth control would lead to promiscuity and prostitution. The Gambia Family Planning Association, partnered with the Federal Republic of Germany has made great strides in disseminating accurate information about contraception to Gambian women.

Female Genital Mutilation

Another issue related to reproductive health in the Gambia is the practice of female genital mutilation as a type of circumcision (James & Robertson, 2004). This deeply embedded rite dates to ancient times. The estimated percentage of all women in the Gambia who have undergone some form of female genital mutilation ranges from 60% to 90%, but statistics are unsubstantiated. Female genital mutilation generally is carried out between the ages of 4 to 7 years, but in some cases the girl may be well into her teen years (Morison et al., 2001). A campaign to abolish female genital mutilation is active in the Gambia; however, the stance of the government on this practice is not always clear. The Gambia Committee against Traditional Practices is taking the lead role in sensitizing the public about the harmful effects of traditional practices such as female genital mutilation. The committee has directed its campaign to eradicate this practice to women, community leaders, youth, and children. The committee has carried out programs on the harmful effects of the practice for traditional birth attendants in a number of villages.

NURSING EDUCATION

State registered nurses work in hospitals, health centers, and dispensaries and have completed 3 years of post-high school education. The bachelor of science in nursing (BSN) degree only recently has been introduced in the Gambia and produces only 5 to 10 graduates per year, but this is more analogous to the RN-BSN completion program in the United States because candidates for the BSN must complete the basic SRN program before applying. Both of these programs are located in the capital city, Banjul. The SRN/midwife (SRN/M) curriculum was developed to increase the availability of maternal-child services. For the SRN/M, nurses complete 1 additional year of education to get the nurse midwifery credential, which is the state certified midwives certificate. The SRN/M nurse does not manage serious maternity cases; if there are any complications in the delivery, the person is referred to a nurse clinician with more advanced training or to an SRN/M "at risk" midwife who has completed an additional 9 months of training after the SRN/M credential.

The other levels of nursing are from a 2-year program with the resulting title of state enrolled nurse and the enrolled nurse (a 1-year program similar to the licensed practical nurse in the United States). Some state enrolled nurses focus on community health nursing. Specialty programs for the 2- and 3-year nursing graduates include ophthalmic nursing (1 year of training) and mental health nursing (less structured and offered at several hospitals). Specialized nursing is greatly needed in the Gambia. Those who complete the ophthalmic training can become a senior ophthalmic medical assistant and can manage a hospital eye unit; this level of provider can diagnose and treat ophthalmic problems and perform basic eye surgery as previously noted.

Number of Graduates

The yearly number of graduates from the SRN program is 31 to 36 students; for the SRN/M, 10 to 15 students; for the state enrolled nurse, 40 students; and for the community health nurse, about 30 students. The Gambia Nurses and Midwives Council, the regulatory body in nursing, participates in the development of all curricula in schools of nursing and participates in the final examination papers upon graduation. The license has no term limit when a student graduates and no renewal fees or continuing education requirements.

NURSING PRACTICE

The demographics of nursing in the Gambia are different from the United States, primarily as it relates to gender. Men are likely to enter nursing as a profession, and there is no stigma of nursing being primarily a women's profession in the Gambia. Much autonomy exists in nursing practice, and the nurses are assertive in advocating for the poor. Because of a severe shortage of physicians, they have less of a tendency to interfere with nursing practice.

A license to practice nursing is granted from the Gambia Nurses and Midwives Council under the Gambian Nurses and Midwives Act. The council is a professional board composed of 13 nurses and regulates nurses following graduation from a state-approved school of nursing. The Gambia Nurses and Midwives Council is also responsible for discipline, but rarely do "cases" of malpractice or clinical incompetence go to council. The need for nurses is great, and disciplinary problems usually are handled within the institution. State registered nurses perform some of the same roles as doctors, specifically prescribing medication, suturing lacerations, and performing minor surgical procedures. This practice is out of necessity and is guided by clinical protocols developed by the Department of State for Health. Some of these skills are taught in the SRN program. Traditional lay midwives are not registered with the Gambia Nurses and Midwives Council.

NURSES RECRUITED TO WESTERN COUNTRIES

Nurses from the Gambia do migrate to seek better wages and working conditions. No formal studies have been done on why nurses leave the Gambia, nor are there any programs designed to keep nurses in the country. Working conditions and finances are primary reasons for leaving the country. Major complaints among Gambian nurses relate to the number of hours they are required to work to fill critical shortages and the policy of moving between health facilities every 2 to 3 years. Low salaries and the inability of nurses to obtain a home loan or purchase an automobile are also key factors. Developed countries such as the United States, Europe, and the United Kingdom actively send nurse recruiters to the Gambia. The practice is unfortunate because the Gambian people need nurses, as can be seen from Table 91-4. The rural districts are the most difficult places to practice nursing, and most nurses employed by the government are required to relocate there during their careers.

Some have written about the ethics of nurse recruiting by Western countries and call it "nurse poaching" (Singh, Nkala, Amuah, Mehta, & Ahmad, 2003). Gambia nurses are excellent targets of "nurse poachers" because they speak English. Migration is predicted to continue until Western countries address the underlying causes of nurse shortages (Kline, 2003). No formal statistics are kept in the Gambia related to the nursing attrition problem, but attrition is estimated at 8% to 15%. Despite guidelines

TABLE 91-4

Number of Health Professionals by Division in the Gambia, 2001

Division or District	Physicians	All Nurses	Midwives	Physicians/ 1000 Population	All Nurses/ 1000 Population	Midwives/1000 Population
Western Division	85	326	142	0.11	0.41	0.18
North Bank West	9	45	17	0.09	0.46	0.17
North Bank East	29	84	19	0.27	0.79	0.18
Lower River Division	14	46	17	0.19	0.62	0.23
Central River Division	49	91	34	0.26	0.49	0.18
Upper River Division	20	64	14	0.10	0.31	0.07
Total for The Gambia	206	656	243	0.14	0.44	0.16

Source: Department of State for Health and Social Welfare, the Gambia.

and promises by developed countries that the practice should cease, the "nurse poaching" continues.

NURSING AND PUBLIC HEALTH ISSUES

Nurses in the Gambia are making a major impact on public policy, particularly as it relates to hygiene education and reproductive health. Many of the nurses in the country focus on prevention in the areas of diarrheal diseases, helminth infection, sanitation, and hand washing with soap (Hoare, Hoare, Rhodes, Erinoso, & Weaver, 1999). Enormous rural-urban differences in maternal mortality exist at least in part because of increased rates of infectious disease and poor access to maternity care in rural areas (Waters, Postic, Durocher, Donker, & Brenner, 1999). A rural woman is more likely to be followed by a traditional birth attendant and not an SRN/M when it is time for her child to be born.

Personal hygiene and poor water supplies are the main factors behind the spread of diseases such as dysentery and trachoma. Central to this is how water is accessed and carried. Clean containers were difficult to obtain until a plastic industrial operation was able to manufacture tubs and buckets at low cost. Before this development, some rural people would recover plastic containers with toxic residues left over from agrochemical applications. The environmental health of many Gambian farmers is improving; for example, moving cattle and other animals away from village compounds to decrease flies and distance people from animal waste is an excellent beginning. The environment in some urban areas is different; refuse is piling up in residential areas as overcrowding occurs. Occasionally, children are seen wading through refuse looking for something of value. Because there is no municipal collection of garbage, these activities lead to most diarrheal pathogens and infectious disease.

POVERTY AND WORKER HEALTH

Politics and economic conditions have led to poverty, and people will take whatever jobs they can get. Agriculture is the main income for many Gambians, and in the age of globalization, their main crop is groundnuts or "peanuts" as they commonly are called in the United States. Worldwide, peanut prices have fallen in recent years, and this has added to the public debt in the Gambia. Farmers in the United States normally would get a government subsidy when crop prices fall, but in the Gambia the result is more drastic (Weaver & Beckerleg, 1993).

When crop prices are poor, men and women in these rural communities must seek employment in a factory or a tourist hotel or work for the government to compensate for the loss of agricultural income. Gambians do not like to beg, and as a people are always willing to work. The International Monetary Fund and World Bank policies have meant that nations like the Gambia are loaned money on condition that they repay the loan when they succeed in the global marketplace. When this does not happen, the only option is to cut social expenditures (such as for health care and education) to repay the loans.

I focused on improving worker health and occupational safety by bringing together stakeholders in the Gambian economy (Culp, Marquez, Bobb, & Jagne, 2005). Working conditions are poor because unemployment is high, and people will work in undesirable and unsafe places so that they can provide for their families. To see how poverty, employment, and worker environment are interrelated is fascinating. For example, worker deaths in a soap factory resulted after the workers were burned from a boiler that overflowed with hot caustic soda. In the United States, an industrial accident such as this would have resulted in lawsuits and payment of workers' compensation to the victims and their families. Most likely the factory would be closed from all of the financial liability involved. This did not happen in the Gambia. In fact, if this factory would have closed, soap would need to be imported. Many more people would die from infectious disease because imported soap would cost too much for a poor farmer in a small village.

SUMMARY

The Gambia is one of the smallest countries in Africa, but it is also a nation that prides itself as being able to rise above all the problems it faces. Although there are numerous shortages, economic struggles, and tremendous challenges to the health of Gambians, health care is free. If health care were not free, disease and death rates would be much higher. Nurses are the backbone of the Gambian health care system, even though they are in short supply.

REFERENCES

Aitman, T. J., Cooper, L. D., Norsworthy, P. J., Wahid, F. N., Gray, J. K., Curtis, B. R., et al. (2000). Malaria susceptibility and CD36 mutation. *Nature, 405*(6790), 1015-1016.

Bates, I., Bekoe, V., & Asamoa-Adu, A. (2004). Improving the accuracy of malaria-related laboratory tests in Ghana. *Malaria Journal, 3*(1), 38.

Bojang, K. A., Milligan, P. J., Pinder, M., Vigneron, L., Alloueche, A., Kester, K. E., et al. (2001). Efficacy of RTS, S/AS02 malaria vaccine against *Plasmodium falciparum* infection in semi-immune adult men in the Gambia: A randomised trial. *Lancet, 358*(9297), 1927-1934.

Bowman, R. J., Faal, H., Myatt, M., Adegbola, R., Foster, A., Johnson, G. J., et al. (2002). Longitudinal study of trachomatous trichiasis in the Gambia. *British Journal of Ophthalmolgy, 86*(3), 339-343.

Bowman, R. J., Jatta, B., Faal, H., Bailey, R., Foster, A., & Johnson, G. J. (2000). Long-term follow-up of lid surgery for trichiasis in the Gambia: Surgical success and patient perceptions. *Eye, 14*(Pt. 6), 864-868.

Burton, M. J., Holland, M. J., Faal, N., Aryee, E. A., Alexander, N. D., Bah, M., et al. (2003). Which members of a community need antibiotics to control trachoma? Conjunctival *Chlamydia trachomatis* infection load in Gambian villages. *Investigative Ophthalmology and Visual Science, 44*(10), 4215-4222.

Ceesay, Y. (2005, February 9). Over 50,000 Gambian children out of school. *Gambia The Daily Observer,* p. 1.

Christophides, G. K. (2005). Transgenic mosquitoes and malaria transmission. *Cell Microbiology, 7*(3), 325-333.

Clarke, S. E., Rowley, J., Bogh, C., Walraven, G. E., & Lindsay, S. W. (2003). Home treatment of 'malaria' in children in rural Gambia is uncommon. *Tropical Medicine International Health, 8*(10), 884-894.

Culp, K., Bobb, M., & Marquez, S. P. (2003). Occupational safety and health in the Gambia. Developing concern for worker health. *American Occupational Health Nursing Journal, 51*(2), 84-88.

Culp, K., Marquez, S. P., Bobb, M., & Jagne, J. (2005). An inaugural conference on occupational health in the Gambia: Exploring the world through international occupational health programs. *American Occupational Health Nursing Journal, 53*(2), 65-71.

Dent, M. J., & Peters, B. (1999). *The crisis of poverty and debt in the Third World.* Brookfield, VT: Ashgate.

Duffy, P. E. (2003). Maternal immunization and malaria in pregnancy. *Vaccine, 21*(24), 3358-3361.

Fullen, M. K. (2002). *Great black writers: Biographies.* Greensboro, NC: Open Hand.

Gregg, E., & Trillo, R. (2003). *The Gambia* (p. v). New York: Rough Guides.

Hay, S. I., Guerra, C. A., Tatem, A. J., Atkinson, P. M., & Snow, R. W. (2005). Urbanization, malaria transmission and disease burden in Africa. *Natural Review of Microbiology, 3*(1), 81-90.

Hayase, Y., & Liaw, K. L. (1997). Factors on polygamy in sub-Saharan Africa: Findings based on the demographic and health surveys. *Developing Economies, 35*(3), 293-327.

Hertz, N. (2004). *The debt threat: How debt is destroying the Third World.* New York: Harper Business.

Hoare, K., Hoare, S., Rhodes, D., Erinoso, H. O., & Weaver, L. T. (1999). Effective health education in rural Gambia. *Journal of Tropical Pediatrics, 45*(4), 208-214.

James, S. M., & Robertson, C. C. (2004). Sorting out misunderstandings: Genital cutting and transnational sisterhood. *Archives of Sexual Behavior, 33*(1), 2-3.

Kalayoglu, M. V. (2002). Ocular chlamydial infections: Pathogenesis and emerging treatment strategies. *Current Drug Targets Infectious Disorders, 2*(1), 85-91.

Lesi, A., & Meremikwu, M. (2004). High first dose quinine regimen for treating severe malaria. *Cochrane Database System Review,* (3), CD003341.

Levtzion, N., & Fisher, H. J. (1987). *Rural and urban Islam in West Africa.* Boulder, CO: L. Rienner.

Luck, M., Jarju, E., Nell, M. D., & George, M. O. (2000). Mobilizing demand for contraception in rural Gambia. *Studies in Family Planning, 31*(4), 325-335.

MacAlister, V. A. (2001). *The mosquito war.* New York: Forge.

Millet, D., & Toussaint, E. (2003). *The debt scam: IMF, World Bank, and Third World debt.* Mumbai: VAK Publication.

Morison, L., Scherf, C., Ekpo, G., Paine, K., West, B., Coleman, R., et al. (2001). The long-term reproductive health consequences of female genital cutting in rural Gambia: A community-based survey. *Tropical Medicine & International Health, 6*(8), 643-653.

Newman, R. D., Hailemariam, A., Jimma, D., Degifie, A., Kebede, D., Rietveld, A. E., et al. (2003). Burden of malaria during pregnancy in areas of stable and unstable transmission in Ethiopia during a nonepidemic year. *Journal of Infectious Disease, 187*(11), 1765-1772.

O'Dempsey, T. J., McArdle, T., Ceesay, S. J., Secka, O., Demba, E., Banya, W. A., et al. (1996). Meningococcal antibody titers in infants of women immunized with meningococcal polysaccharide vaccine during pregnancy. *Archives of Disease in Childhood, 74*(1), F43-F46.

Pinder, M., Reece, W. H., Plebanski, M., Akinwunmi, P., Flanagan, K. L., Lee, E. A., et al. (2004). Cellular immunity induced by the recombinant *Plasmodium falciparum* malaria vaccine, RTS,S/AS02, in semi-immune adults in the Gambia. *Clinical Experimental Immunology, 135*(2), 286-293.

Ratcliffe, A. A., Hill, A. G., Harrington, D. P., & Walraven, G. (2002). Reporting of fertility events by men and women in rural Gambia. *Demography, 39*(3), 573-586.

Roodman, D. M., Peterson, J. A., & Worldwatch Institute. (2001). *Still waiting for the jubilee: Pragmatic solutions for the Third World debt crisis.* Washington, DC: Worldwatch Institute.

Schachter, J., & Dawson, C. R. (2002). Elimination of blinding trachoma. *Current Opinion in Infectious Disease, 15*(5), 491-495.

Schaffer, M. (2003). *Djinns, stars, and warriors: Mandinka legends from Pakao, Senegal.* Leiden, the Netherlands: Brill.

Schim van der Loeff, M. F., Sarge-Njie, R., Ceesay, S., Awasana, A. A., Jaye, P., Sam, O., et al. (2003). Regional differences in HIV trends in the Gambia: Results from sentinel surveillance among pregnant women. *AIDS, 17*(12), 1841-1846.

Umelo, V. (2004, March 5). How fashionable is polygamy today? *Gambia The Daily Observer,* p. 3.

Waters, K. M., Postic, M., Durocher, S., Donker, H., & Brenner, B. (1999). Feedback: Men in nursing. *Journal of Advanced Nursing, 29*(2), 523.

Weaver, L. T., & Beckerleg, S. (1993). Is health a sustainable state? A village study in the Gambia. *Lancet, 341*(8856), 1327-1330.

Wenger, J. (1997). *Haemophilus influenzae* type b (HIB) vaccine introduced in the Gambia. *African Health, 20*(1), 13-15.

World Health Organization. (1998). WHO's mission for vision. *African Health, 20*(5), 38.

Index

Page numbers followed by b indicate boxes; f, figures; t, tables.

Reader Evaluation and Feedback

We would very much like to hear feedback from our readers. Please take a few minutes to let us know what you think of the 7th edition of *Current Issues in Nursing*. Your response will help us keep the future editions of this book relevant to our readers and guide future debate topics and content areas.

1. On a scale of 1 to 5 (1= not effective, 5 = very effective) how would you rate the 7th edition for the following characteristics?

	Not helpful	Somewhat helpful	Moderately helpful	Substantially helpful	Extremely helpful
Content	1	2	3	4	5
Format	1	2	3	4	5
Usefulness	1	2	3	4	5
Thought provoking	1	2	3	4	5

2. What additional topics would you suggest? Or what topics do want to see expanded in a different direction? Include potential authors for your additions.

3. What did you like best about the book?

4. What content areas would you delete?

Please make sure we can read your response since your comments are important to us.
Thank you for your suggestions. Please mail or fax this form to:

Mail: Fax: 319-335-9990
Perle Slavik Cowen
College of Nursing, Office 472
The University of Iowa
Iowa City, IA 52242